AF334084

Common Problems in Acute Care Surgery

Laura J. Moore • Krista L. Turner • S. Rob Todd

Editors

Common Problems in Acute Care Surgery

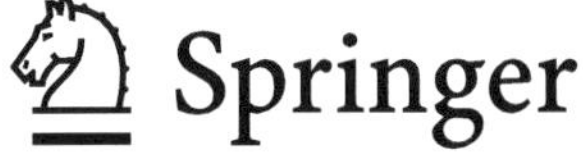 Springer

Editors
Laura J. Moore, MD, FACS
Department of Surgery
The University of Texas Health Science Center
Houston, TX, USA

Krista L. Turner, MD, FACS
Department of Surgery
Weill Cornell Medical College
The Methodist Hospital
Houston, TX, USA

S. Rob Todd, MD, FACS
Division of Trauma, Emergency Surgery
    and Surgical Critical Care
Department of Surgery
New York University Langone Medical Center
New York, NY, USA

ISBN 978-1-4614-6122-7   ISBN 978-1-4614-6123-4 (eBook)
DOI 10.1007/978-1-4614-6123-4
Springer New York Heidelberg Dordrecht London

Library of Congress Control Number: 2013931977

Foreword

Three decades ago as a surgery resident at the University of Colorado, I enthusiastically pursued trauma surgery as a tantalizing career option. I had inspirational mentors, did a variety of lifesaving operations, and had abundant translational research opportunities. I personally participated in the birth of surgical critical care. I was not alone in my enthusiasm. Across the USA, waves of talented and dedicated surgical residents throughout the 1980s choose this career pathway and prospered in this evolving field. However, for variety of reasons in the 1990s, we experienced some serious "bumps in the road" related to professional happiness.

First, we had created exclusive regional trauma centers designed to take care of all trauma patients. Smaller hospitals and community surgeons were told that this is not their problem and, given the unsavory nature of trauma care, they readily agreed. As a result, trauma center volume increased and, with declining violence in America, the focus of our clinical practice shifted away from high-adrenaline penetrating trauma operations to complex ICU care of multisystem blunt trauma patients.

Second, as we advanced through the 1990s we learned how not to operate on blunt trauma and, contrary to our heritage, we progressively became nonoperative surgeons. We had become the "baby sitters" for the other surgical specialists.

Third, as our clinical volume became overwhelming, we largely abandoned our core mission of translational research. Unfortunately, this provides a tremendous source of personal satisfaction and is a necessary pathway to academic productivity and advancement. Trauma surgery became recognized to be a high-risk burnout profession and consequently not an unattractive career option for trainees of that era.

In the early 2000s through the leadership of the American Association for the Surgery of Trauma and the Committee of Trauma of the American College of Surgeons, we began the process of redefining our specialty into acute care surgery (ACS). Our domains of clinical practice now include trauma, burns, surgical critical care, and emergency general surgery. As we progress into the 2010s this appears to be an effective model. It ensures access to safe and evidence-based emergency care, which our patients and hospitals sorely need. Additionally, there appears to be a strong interest amongst a subset of our trainees for what we do. With increasing surgical specialization, there is reluctance by most surgeons to participate in emergency surgery call. As part of our trauma call we have assumed this responsibility. As a result we now do a wide variety of emergency operations and obviously help many patients.

The 80-h work week has also "dumbed down" most surgeons in regards to surgical critical care, making our role of taking care of critically ill surgical patients crucially important. Finally, while some are critical of the ACS shift work mentality, it offers the young surgeons the opportunity to work hard but also have time off to pursue other life interests.

This book was edited by three of my previous trainees/partners who are very committed to ACS. They recognize that compared to trauma, burns, and critical care, our expertise and ownership of emergency general surgery is less secure. The purpose of this book is to define this broad field and to establish evidence-based guidelines (EBGs) related to its practice. The book is organized into three parts: (1) general principles, (2) specific disease states, and (3) ethic/legal issues and systems development. Part 2 is the "beef." It contains 26 chapters that address problems commonly encountered by acute care surgeons. Each chapter ends with a management algorithm. An algorithm is an excellent method to implement and improve EBGs. To create an algorithm, the key questions that drive decision making related to a process of care are indentified and then put in a decision tree order that best fits the process of care. The decision making is based on the best available data, and if the data is incomplete, expert opinion prevails. Importantly, this process identifies what we "do know" as well as the "gray zones," which offer future opportunity for performance improvement (PI). To be implemented into daily practice in a specific hospital, the algorithms frequently need to be modified based on local resources and biases. However, the modified algorithm can then be consistently implemented; it is possible to identify "what works" and "what does not work." In an iterative PI process, the algorithm can then be progressively refined to optimize outcomes. Trauma surgeons have traditionally embraced algorithms and so I expect these will be of great interest.

The target audience for this book includes all trainees, physician extenders, and practicing surgeons who participate in the care of patients requiring emergency surgical care.

Finally, I would like to acknowledge and thank the distinguished authors who participated in writing this book. It is an important milestone in the ever-evolving field of trauma surgery and now acute care surgery.

Gainesville, FL, USA   Frederick A. Moore M.D., F.A.C.S., M.C.C.M.

Preface

Acute care surgery is a rapidly evolving specialty that encompasses emergency general surgery, care of the injured patient, and surgical critical care. There is a growing demand for access to emergency surgical services. Unfortunately, this increased demand for emergency surgeons has been accompanied by a declining number of surgeons willing to take emergency general surgery calls. The field of acute care surgery has developed in response to this need for reliable access to emergency surgical care.

The care of the emergency surgical patient presents a complex set of challenges for surgeons. Not only must the surgeon possess the skills needed to perform an emergent operation, but also they must often do so in the setting of a physiologically deranged patient. In order to deliver optimal care, the acute care surgeon must have expertise in both surgery and critical care. They must be familiar with the current diagnostic modalities, resuscitation strategies, operative techniques, and management principles required to deliver rapid, evidence-based care for these challenging patients.

Common Problems in Acute Care Surgery addresses the common surgical emergencies encountered by acute care surgeons. The purpose of this text is to provide both trainees and practicing surgeons a comprehensive, evidence-based review of the most common clinical problems encountered by acute care surgeons. The book is organized into three main parts: The first part is focused on general principles of acute care surgery including initial evaluation and resuscitation, perioperative management of the hemodynamically unstable patient, and common critical care issues encountered in the management of these patients. The second part is focused on specific disease states that are commonly encountered by acute care surgeons. Each chapter in this part addresses a specific clinical problem by describing the epidemiology, clinical presentation, diagnosis, management (including pertinent operative techniques), potential complications, and follow-up. Each of the chapters in this second part also includes an algorithm for management of the disease state being discussed. The third and final part focuses on ethics and legal issues frequently encountered in acute care surgery.

Each of the authors in this text was selected for their expertise in the field of acute care surgery. We are grateful to the many surgeons who devoted countless hours in the preparation of this text. The end result is a practical resource to assist acute care surgeons in delivering compassionate, evidence-based care to the emergency surgical patient.

Houston, TX, USA   Laura J. Moore, M.D., F.A.C.S.

Contents

Contributors

Hassan Aijazi, M.B.B.S. Department of Anesthesiology, University of Texas at Houston Medical School, Houston, TX, USA

Rondel P. Albarado, M.D. Division of Acute Care Surgery, The University of Texas Medical School at Houston, Houston, TX, USA

Adnan Alseidi, M.D., EdM Department of Surgery, Virginia Mason Medical Center, Seattle, WA, USA

Tanner Baker, M.D. Department of General Surgery, University of Texas Health Science Center, Houston, TX, USA

Zsolt J. Balogh, M.D., Ph.D., F.R.A.C.S., FA.OrthA, F.A.C.S. Division of Surgery, Department of Traumatology, John Hunter Hospital and University of Newcastle, Newcastle, NSW, Australia

Philip S. Barie, M.D., M.B.A. Department of Surgery, NewYork-Presbyterian Hospital-Weill Cornell Medical College, New York, NY, USA

Shanda H. Blackmon, M.D., M.P.H., F.A.C.S. Section of Thoracic Surgery, Department of Surgery, Weill Cornell Medical College, Houston, TX, USA

Nicholas M. Brown, M.D. Department of Surgery, University of Texas Health Science Center, Houston, TX, USA

Sara Bubenik, M.D. Division of General Surgery, Department of Surgery, Oregon Health and Science University, Portland, OR, USA

Brittany Busse, M.D. Department of Surgery, University of California Davis Medical Center, Sacramento, CA, USA

Bennet Butler, B.S. Department of Surgery, Northwestern University Feinberg School of Medicine, Chicago, IL, USA

Edie Chan, M.D. Department of Surgery, Rush University Medical Center, Chicago, IL, USA

Christine S. Cocanour, M.D., F.A.C.S., F.C.C.M. Department of Surgery, University of California Davis Medical School, Sacramento, CA, USA

Steven M. Cohen, D.O. Department of Surgery, New York University Medical Center, New York, NY, USA

Bryan A. Cotton, M.D., M.P.H. Department of Surgery, The Center for Translational Injury Research, The University of Texas Health Science Center, Houston, TX, USA

Michelle L. Cowan, M.D. Department of Surgery, University of Chicago Medical Center, Chicago, IL, USA

Marie Crandall, M.D., M.P.H. Department of Surgery, Northwestern University Feinberg School of Medicine, Chicago, IL, USA

Andrej Cretnik, M.D., Ph.D. Trauma Department, University Clinical Center Maribor, Maribor, Slovenia

Svetang Desai, M.D. Division of Gastroenterology, Duke University Medical Center, Durham, NC, USA

Clifford W. Deveney, M.D. Division of General Surgery, Department of Surgery, Oregon Health and Science University, Portland, OR, USA

Linda A. Dultz, M.D., M.P.H. Division of Trauma, Emergency Surgery, and Surgical Critical Care, Department of Surgery, New York University Langone Medical Center, New York, NY, USA

James K. Dzandu, Ph.D. Trauma/Acute Care and Critical Care Services, John C. Lincoln Health Network, Phoenix, AZ, USA

Soumitra R. Eachempati, M.D. Department of Surgery, New York-Presbyterian Hospital-Weill Cornell Medical College, New York, NY, USA

James A. Edney, M.D., F.A.C.S. Department of Surgical Oncology, University of Nebraska Medical Center, Omaha, NE, USA

Bridget N. Fahy, M.D., F.A.C.S. Department of Surgery, The Methodist Hospital, Weill Cornell Medical College, Houston, TX, USA

Nicole Fox, M.D., M.P.H. Department of Trauma, Cooper Medical School of Rowan University, Cooper University Hospital, Camden, NJ, USA

Stephanie Gordy, M.D., F.A.C.S. Department of Trauma, Acute Care Surgery and Surgical Critical Care, Oregon Health and Science University, Portland, OR, USA

Lynn Gries, M.D. Department of Surgery, Division of Trauma, Critical Care and Acute Care Surgery, Arizona Health Science Center, University of Arizona Medical Center, Tucson, AZ, USA

Ashley Hardy, M.D. Department of Surgery, Northwestern University Feinberg School of Medicine, Chicago, IL, USA

John A. Harvin, M.D. Department of Surgery, University of Texas Health Science Center at Houston, Houston, TX, USA

Heitham T. Hassoun, M.D. Departments of Surgery and Cardiovascular Surgery, The Methodist Hospital Physician Organization, Houston, TX, USA

Tricia Hauschild, M.D. Department of Surgery, University of Utah School of Medicine, Salt Lake City, UT, USA

W. Scott Helton, M.D. Department of Surgery, Liver, Pancreas and Bile Duct Surgical Center of Excellence, Virginia Mason Medical Center, Seattle, WA, USA

Vanessa P. Ho, M.D., M.P.H. Department of Surgery, New York-Presbyterian Hospital-Weill Cornell Medical Center, New York, NY, USA

John B. Holcomb, M.D., F.A.C.S. Department of Surgery, Hermann Memorial Hospital, Houston, TX, USA

Alexzandra Hollingworth, M.D. Trauma/Acute Care and Critical Care Services, John C. Lincoln Health Network, Phoenix, AZ, USA

Randeep S. Jawa, M.D. Department of Surgery, University of Nebraska Medical Center, Omaha, NE, USA

Lillian S. Kao, M.D., M.S. Department of Surgery, University of Texas Health Science Center, Houston, TX, USA

Michael Klebuc, M.D. Department of Plastic and Reconstructive Surgery, The Methodist Hospital, Weill Medical College, Cornell University, Houston, TX, USA

Thomas M. Komar, M.D. Department of Surgery, Stroger Hospital of Cook County, Chicago, IL, USA

Roman Kosir, M.D. Trauma Department, University Clinical Center Maribor, Maribor, Slovenia

Rosemary Kozar, M.D., Ph.D Department of Surgery, The University of Texas Medical School at Houston, Houston, TX, USA

Laura A. Kreiner, M.D. Department of Surgery, The University of Texas Health Science Center, Houston, TX, USA

Anand Lodha, M.D. Department of Surgery, Methodist Hospital of Dallas, Dallas, TX, USA

Quan P. Ly, M.D., F.A.C.S. Department of Surgery, University of Nebraska Medical Center, Omaha, NE, USA

Mandy R. Maness, M.D. Department of General Surgery, Vidant Medical Center, Greenville, NC, USA

Alicia J. Mangram, M.D., F.A.C.S. Trauma/Acute Care and Critical Care Services, John C. Lincoln Health Network, Phoenix, AZ, USA

Gary T. Marshall, M.D. Department of Surgery, University of Pittsburgh Medical Center, Presbyterian University Hospital, Pittsburgh, PA, USA

Robert G. Martindale, M.D., Ph.D. Division of General Surgery, Department of Surgery, Oregon Health and Science University, Portland, OR, USA

James J. McCarthy, M.D. Medical Director of Emergency Medical Services, Texas Medical Center, Memorial Herman Hospital, University of Texas Medical School, Houston, TX, USA

David W. Mercer, M.D. Department of Surgery, University of Nebraska Medical Center, Omaha, NE, USA

Marc Mesleh, M.D. Department of General Surgery, Rush University Medical Center, Chicago, IL, USA

Frederick A. Moore, M.D., F.A.C.S. Department of Acute Care Surgery, Shands at the University of Florida, Gainesville, FL, USA

Laura J. Moore, M.D., F.A.C.S. Department of Surgery, The University of Texas Health Science Center, Houston, TX, USA

Andrew H. Nguyen, M.D. Department of Surgery, David Geffen School of Medicine at UCLA 757 Westwood Plaza, Los Angeles, CA, USA

Jacquelyn K. O'Herrin, M.D., F.A.C.S. Department of Surgery, University of Oklahoma, Oklahoma City, OK, USA

H. Leon Pachter, Department of Surgery, New York University Medical Center, NY, USA

John R. Pender IV M.D., F.A.C.S. Departments of General and Laparoscopic Surgery, Bariatric Surgery, Brody School of Medicine, Vidant Medical Center, Greenville, NC, USA

Peter Rhee, M.D., M.P.H., F.A.C.S., F.C.C.M., D.M.C.C. Department of Surgery, Division of Trauma, Critical Care and Acute Care Surgery, University of Arizona Medical Center, Tucson, AZ, USA

Harry M. Richter III M.D., F.A.C.S. Division of General Surgery, Department of Surgery, Stroger Hospital of Cook County, Chicago, IL, USA

Heena P. Santry, M.D. Trauma and Surgical Critical Care, Department of Surgery, Umass Memorial Medical Center, Worcester, MA, USA

Paul J. Schenarts, M.D., F.A.C.S. Department of Surgery, College of Medicine, University of Nebraska, Omaha, NE, USA

Martin A. Schreiber, M.D., F.A.C.S. Professor of Surgery, Chief of Trauma Surgery, Oregon Health and Science University, USA

Diane A. Schwartz, M.D. Department of Surgery , John Hopkins School of Medicine, Baltimore, MD, USA

Michelle Shen, M.D. Department of Surgery, University of Texas Health Science Center, Houston, TX, USA

Vasiliy Sim, M.D. Department of Surgery, Brookdale University Hospital and Medical Center, Brooklyn, NY, USA

Bruce J. Simon, M.D. Trauma and Surgical Critical Care, Department of Surgery, Umass Memorial Medical Center, Worcester, MA, USA

Marc Singer, M.D., F.A.C.S., F.A.S.C.R.S. Section of Colon and Rectal Surgery, NorthShore University Health System, University of Illinois at Chicago, Evanston, IL, USA

Sherry L. Sixta, M.D. Department of Surgery, Cooper University Hospital, Camden, NJ, USA

Spencer Skelton, M.D. Department of General Surgery, The Methodist Hospital, Houston, TX, USA

Ryan K. Smith, B.A. Department of Surgery, Virginia Mason Medical Center, Seattle, WA, USA

Jeffrey P. Spike, Ph.D. McGovern Center for Humanities and Ethics, University of Texas Health Science Center, Houston, TX, USA

Agathe Streiff, B.S. Department of Surgery and The Center for Translational Injury Research, The University of Texas Health Science Center, Houston, TX, USA

Joseph F. Sucher, M.D., F.A.C.S. Department of Surgery, The Methodist Hospital, Weill Cornell Medical College, Houston, TX, USA

S. Rob Todd, M.D., F.A.C.S. Division of Trauma, Emergency Surgery, and Surgical Critical Care, Department of Surgery, New York University Langone Medical Center, New York, NY, USA

Michael S. Truitt, M.D., F.A.C.S. Methodist Hospital of Dallas, Dallas, TX, USA

Krista L. Turner, M.D., F.A.C.S. Department of Surgery, The Methodist Hospital, Weill Cornell Medical College, Houston, TX, USA

Daniel Vargo, M.D., F.A.C.S. Department of Surgery, University of Utah School of Medicine, Salt Lake City, UT, USA

Laura E. White, M.D. Department of Surgery, The Methodist DeBakey Heart and Vascular Center, The Methodist Hospital, Houston, TX, USA

Abigail Wiebusch, M.D. Department of Surgery, Virginia Mason Medical Center, Seattle, WA, USA

Erik B. Wilson, M.D. Department of Surgery, University of Texas Health Science Center, Houston, TX, USA

James Wiseman, M.D. Department of General Surgery, The Methodist Hospital, Weill Cornell Medical College, Houston, TX, USA

Chang-I Wu, M.D. Columbia University Mailman School of Public Health, New York, NY, USA

Osamu Yoshino, M.D., Ph.D. Division of Surgery, Department of Traumatology, John Hunter Hospital and University of Newcastle, Newcastle, NSW, Australia

Part I

General Principles

The Careful Art of Resuscitation

Diane A. Schwartz and John B. Holcomb

Resuscitation during ongoing hemorrhagic shock attempts to restore physiologic balance by achieving rapid surgical control of hemorrhage, providing fluid and blood products, and titrating to laboratory and clinical parameters. Phases of resuscitation occur in the pre-hospital environment, emergency room, operating room, and intensive care unit (ICU) where multiple health care providers and physicians influence patient outcome by their attentiveness and diligence to this careful art.

The patient's clinical picture is dynamic, in constant flux requiring continuous attention to the details of the resuscitation. While profound hemorrhagic shock is easily recognized, it is difficult to gain control of bleeding with meaningful outcome once cardiopulmonary collapse has occurred. Subtle signs of impending hemorrhagic shock often go unnoticed or unrecognized, although they are present and often reversible at the onset of the traumatic event. Since blood and blood product are generally not available in the field, emergency medical service (EMS) and other health care personnel are relied upon to identify and treat signs of blood loss. They use direct pressure and mechanical devices, such as tourniquets, gauze, or hemostatic agents to stop visible bleeding. Internal bleeding, however, must be controlled surgically or by embolization once the patient reaches the hospital setting. Coagulopathy must be corrected and temperature optimized. It is often not until entering the emergency department that patients receive their first unit of blood or blood product, and it generally is not until reaching the operating room or interventional radiology suite that effective control of bleeding is achieved.

Hemorrhagic shock often correlates to a source of surgical bleeding. Coagulopathy, acidosis, and hypothermia wreak havoc on metabolic processes and physiologic responses during the perioperative period. In the operating theater, surgeons frequently focus on operative management, while decisions regarding transfusion, colloid, and crystalloid administration are made by the anesthesiologist. During damage control operations, bleeding is quickly controlled in preparation for further resuscitation in the ICU. Once in the ICU, serial laboratory values, continued resuscitation, and correction of the acidosis, hypothermia, and coagulopathy continue until the patient shows signs of stabilization, returns emergently to the operating room or interventional suite, or succumbs to death. This chapter outlines the general principles of resuscitation and its various aspects, historical and future perspectives, and non-trauma resuscitation guidelines.

Hemorrhagic and Hypovolemic Shock and Initial Stabilization Maneuvers

In 1946 hemorrhagic shock was induced in animal models and a stratification system emerged: simple hypotension, which was noted to always be reversible if identified and treated; impending shock, which was reversible if treated aggressively; and irreversible shock state, where hypotension, sustained by high-volume blood loss, correlated to notable metabolic derangement [1]. The authors concluded that hemorrhagic shock did not occur at a specific volume loss or blood pressure, but was rather a fluid state that required early recognition by the treating physician and immediate intervention during the reversible period.

Today hemorrhagic shock remains elusive in its definition. It encompasses the full spectrum of a complex clinical picture and accompanying findings consistent with metabolic acidosis and impending cardiopulmonary collapse secondary to blood loss, poor tissue perfusion, tissue injury, and ineffective oxygen extraction (Table 1.1, Fig. 1.1).

Hemorrhage is commonly categorized by volume and percent blood loss with specific findings at defined losses [2]. Interestingly these categories are largely based on opinion rather than objective clinical data. Clinical parameters are not markedly different from baseline in phases one and two of shock,

D.A. Schwartz, M.D. • J.B. Holcomb, M.D., F.A.C.S. (✉)
Department of Surgery, Hermann Memorial Hospital,
5410 Fannin Street, Suite 1100, Houston, TX 77030, USA
e-mail: john.holcomb@uth.tmc.edu

L.J. Moore et al. (eds.), *Common Problems in Acute Care Surgery*,
DOI 10.1007/978-1-4614-6123-4_1, © Springer Science+Business Media New York 2013

Table 1.1 Classes of hemorrhagic shock

	I	II	III	IV
Blood loss (ml)	Up to 750	750–1,500	1,500–2,000	>2,000
Blood loss (% blood volume)	Up to 15	15–30	30–40	>40
Pulse rate (per minute)	<100	100–120	120–140	>140
Blood pressure	Normal	Normal	Decreased	Decreased
Pulse pressure (mmHg)	Normal or increased	Decreased	Decreased	Decreased
Respiratory rate (per minute)	14–20	20–30	30–40	>35
Urine output (ml/h)	>30	20–30	5–15	Negligible
Central nervous system/mental status	Slightly anxious	Mildly anxious	Anxious, confused	Confused, lethargic

Reprinted with permission from American College of Surgeons. ATLS manual 7th Edition, 2004

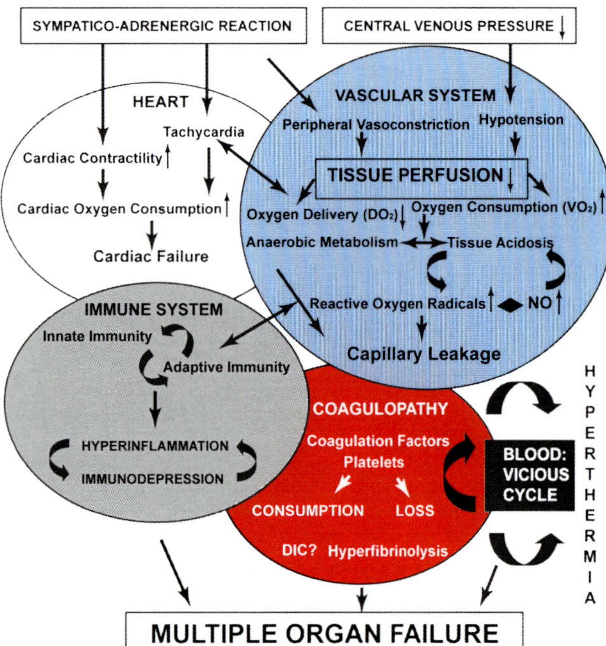

Fig. 1.1 Pathophysiology of hemorrhagic shock. Reprinted from Angele MK, Schneider CP, Chaudry IH. Bench to bedside review: latest results in hemorrhagic shock. Crit Care. 2008;12(4):218. Epub 2008 Jul 10. with permission of BioMed Central

Table 1.2 Current indications and contraindications for EDT

Indications
  Salvageable post-injury cardiac arrest:
    Patients sustaining witnessed penetrating trauma with <15 min of pre-hospital CPR
    Patients sustaining witnessed blunt trauma with <5 min of pre-hospital CPR
Persistent severe post-injury hypotension (SBP ≤60 mmHg) due to:
  Cardiac tamponade
  Hemorrhage—intrathoracic, intra-abdominal, extremity, cervical
  Air embolism

Contraindications
  Penetrating trauma: CPR >15 min and no signs of life (pupillary response, respiratory effort, or motor activity)
  Blunt trauma: CPR >5 min and no signs of life or asystole

Reprinted with permission from Mears G, Glickman SW, Moore F, Cairns CB. Data based integration of critical illness and injury patient care from EMS to emergency department to intensive care unit. Curr Opin Crit Care. 2009 Aug;15(4):284–9

patients in hemorrhagic shock need definitive control of the bleeding before there will be any chance of salvage.

Crystalloid

Choice of crystalloid as a resuscitation fluid in the face of known hemorrhagic shock remains one of the most highly debated topics in the trauma literature at this time. It seems intuitive that if a person is hemorrhaging, correction of that shock will be contingent on the repletion of blood, and that his or her coagulopathy will respond to transfusion of plasma and platelets. However, replacement of volume by crystalloid represents classical teaching and guidelines for correction of the initial phase of hemorrhagic shock [6]. Advanced Trauma Life Support (ATLS) [2] discusses placing two large-bore IVs and bolusing 2 liter of crystalloid for any patient assumed to be in hemorrhagic shock or any patient with significant blood loss. However, recent data suggest that as little as 1.5 l of fluid has negative clinical implications and numerous sources are refuting the benefit of large-volume crystalloid resuscitation in hemorrhagic shock [7].

contributing to the difficulty in recognizing shock in its early stages. In providing care to the critically injured patient, it is of utmost importance to have the ability to diagnose impending or early hemorrhagic shock. It is rather easy to diagnose severe hemorrhagic shock; however, the affected patients have already undergone cardiovascular collapse and are near death. The astute clinician will prefer to intervene earlier, when the diagnosis is more obscure. Once recognized, directed treatment of imminent shock or ongoing hemorrhage begins.

During field resuscitation, patients receive treatments necessary to control bleeding. Several centers tout an integrated database or registry to incorporate pre-hospital data to analyze outcomes (Table 1.2) [3–5]. Such pre-hospital interventions to consider in the management of hemorrhage are infusions of crystalloid and placement of tourniquets. Ultimately all

While many clinicians consider lactated Ringer's and normal saline interchangeable, they are not. Multiple studies in the swine model compare the use of various crystalloid solutions, focusing on lactated Ringer's solution and normal saline. The swine model demonstrates that if shock is induced and maintained for 30 min, followed by resuscitation with either normal saline or lactated Ringer's solution, the animals resuscitated with Ringer's lactate have better improvement in markers of shock, pH, and extracellular lung water [8]. In this study neutrophil activation contributes to cellular damage. Other studies support the neutrophil activation phenomenon; dextran is the biggest activator, followed by normal saline and then lactated Ringer's [9]. Colloid, plasma, and blood have also been implicated as morbid contributors to effects on neutrophil activation, mainly in the pulmonary system [10–12].

Lactated Ringer's, as a resuscitation fluid, yields less acidosis and less coagulopathy than seen with similar volumes of normal saline [13]. Normal saline causes a well-recognized metabolic hyperchloremic acidosis; patients resuscitated with lactated Ringer's do not achieve such levels of acidosis. Furthermore, normal saline-resuscitated patients demonstrate more blood loss than those resuscitated with lactated Ringer's [8, 14]. This has been demonstrated also in the vascular literature. In a study of aortic repairs it was shown that there was more perioperative bleeding and acidosis when normal saline was used as opposed to lactated Ringer's [15]. There was no statistically significant difference in outcome however. Even despite the better physiologic results with lactated Ringer's resuscitation as compared to normal saline, lactated Ringer's still would not be the first choice for resuscitation in a patient with hemorrhagic shock as excessive bleeding is not well controlled with replacement of volume by crystalloid [16].

While several centers still practice crystalloid-based resuscitation, many trauma centers are moving toward the practice implemented during the ongoing war in Iraq and Afghanistan where the standard of care is to transfuse blood and blood products immediately and limit the crystalloid volume during the initial resuscitation [17, 18]. Excessive crystalloid has been implicated in increased mortality and morbidity rates when used in large volume in the trauma patient [19–21].

Permissive hypotension purposefully maintains mean arterial pressure as low as possible to ensure adequate organ perfusion. If the minimum mean arterial pressure is not exceeded with over-resuscitation, the delicate new clot formation should not be disrupted prior to operative intervention [22, 23]. These authors show that by purposefully maintaining mean arterial pressure no greater than 50 mmHg, the patients in these groups are not afflicted with coagulopathy to the same degree as controls that are resuscitated to a mean arterial pressure of greater than 65 mmHg. Earlier data from animal models show no difference in ultimate outcome when hypotension is maintained; end organ perfusion and prevention of metabolic perturbations

that can occur when tissue oxygenation is inadequate are the goals of permissive hypotension [24]. That is to say that when metabolic acidosis is controlled and the mean arterial pressure is minimized on purpose, patients do not show any long-term adverse effects compared to patients whose resuscitation targets a higher mean arterial pressure. It is unclear how long patients can remain hypotensive without deleterious effects. The original descriptions of this concept date to World Wars 1 and 2. The original civilian studies on this topic show less intraoperative bleeding and overall fluid requirement and hence less postoperative morbidity when this strategy is applied [25]. Survival is improved by limiting crystalloid infusion. Furthermore overaggressive resuscitation to a physiologically normal blood pressure may contribute to ineffective hemostasis, termed "popping the clot," shown in an animal study where raising the blood pressure caused re-bleeding and increased mortality [26]. This cycle of repeated resuscitation and bleeding is ultimately detrimental to clot stability and to overall survival [27].

The use of tourniquets in the field has turned some of the most life-threatening injuries into ones where life and limb can be salvaged. The resurgent use of tourniquets has been overwhelmingly supported in the recent military data from the Iraq and Afghanistan experience, where it is shown that there are virtually no adverse effects of the tourniquet itself [28]. Even in inexperienced hands, tourniquets have been shown to prevent life-threatening exsanguination and should be applied in any situation in which extremity hemorrhage exists and prior to the onset of exsanguination [28, 29]. Mangled extremities are not more likely to require amputation when a tourniquet is applied. There are several commercial devices available and their purpose is to exert enough circumferential pressure to prevent blood from flowing into the extremity in question [30]. Contrary to older teaching, use of a tourniquet does not cause increased amputation rates [31].

Hospital Arrival

Once in the emergency department, indices of vital signs and laboratory values may assist the surgeon in separating the critically ill trauma patient from one who appears "stable." Lactate, serum bicarbonate, base deficit, hemoglobin, or tissue oxygenation are some of the most crucial lab values in determining metabolic acidosis, which occurs with poor tissue oxygen extraction and indicates shock at the cellular level [32–38]. Lactate, in the pre-hospital setting, may be more predictive of prognosis than are vital signs, which can be fairly stable until hemodynamic collapse ensues [39]. Lactate increases in under-perfused tissues and can be an early predictor of impending shock, and helps differentiate the stable patient from the one in a compensated shock state.

Base deficit is a reflection of metabolic acidosis secondary to unmeasured anions, which is typically assumed to be lactate in the trauma patient [40]. Base deficit, lactate, anion gap, and bicarbonate levels all correspond to metabolic acidosis and have all been shown to predict morbidity and mortality [41–44]. However, bicarbonate is only a single marker of acid–base status, whereas anion gap, base deficit, and lactate all have some dependence on electrolytes, pH, and buffer capacity of blood [45]. There does not seem to exist great consensus in the literature regarding which is the best predictor of mortality [46].

Up to a third of patients in the ICU show discordance between their base deficit and lactate, and in these situations it has been shown that lactate is more predictive of overall outcome, when it differs significantly from base deficit [47]. Authors from this source imply that base deficit on its own does not have the predictive capacity for mortality that lactate has. On the other hand, while lactate is the most helpful in the initial phase of resuscitation, it is not as accurate in determining the ongoing causes of metabolic acidosis in critical situations outside of trauma where lactate may not elevate, such as respiratory alkalosis and diabetic ketoacidosis.

Serum bicarbonate will correlate with base deficit only when the pH is constant, which has clinical implications in the patient whose standard chemistry is drawn from a venous line at a different time than the arterial blood gas is collected [48]. The fluctuating pH may affect the accuracy of either measurement when compared to the other. There may be a significant difference in base deficit when comparing arterial to venous samples. Venous samples may be more sensitive to changes in pH, pCO_2, and pO_2 resulting in earlier changes in base deficit [49].

Acidosis, coagulopathy, and hypothermia portend the downward spiral into fulminant hemorrhagic shock. The key to understanding hemorrhagic shock is to understand the interactions of the lethal triad and the human body's capacity to self-correct versus what must be medically and surgically repaired. Acidosis is a product of poor tissue perfusion and death at the cellular level [50]. Lactic acidosis is a finding associated with cellular anoxia. Free radical release during tissue hypoxia also contributes to overall organ dysfunction and further perpetuates the cascade [51]. The coagulopathy is secondary to dilution, platelet dysfunction, cellular damage, decreased hepatic synthesis of factors, and shunting of proteins away from creating coagulation factors and toward production of acute-phase reactants [51–55]. Hypothermia occurs secondary to decreased metabolism. It is also associated with infusion of cold or chilled blood products and crystalloid, and hypothermia itself contributes to continued perpetuation of coagulopathy [56]. Furthermore it is the mismatch between oxygen delivery and consumption with resultant organ dysfunction that defines the shock state [57]. All three elements of the lethal triad contribute and potentiate the death spiral after substantial bleeding. Interruption of this process is paramount to survival.

Evaluation of Volume Status

Distinguishing compensated shock from impending complete cardiovascular collapse can be difficult. Understanding physiology and volume status on a global scale seems straightforward—it is the clinical application of these principles to the individual patient that creates a conundrum for identifying the degree of shock. Given the application of focused assessment with sonography in trauma (FAST) exam, there has been some interest in examination of the inferior vena cava (IVC) volume during the initial assessment. This is a noninvasive, accurate, and rapid way to assess the patient's overall volume status and is easy to repeat. The technique has been described as placing the patient in the supine position and angling the probe toward the right shoulder from a subcostal view. The IVC can be measured at the entrance of the hepatic veins. Measuring in expiration appears to yield the most accurate measurement. Several small studies demonstrate that measurements of IVC diameter are incredibly fast, noninvasive, accurate measures to determine if shock is present [58–61]. Of note there can be error in measuring the IVC diameter; when accounting for volume variability, the anterior–posterior measurement has been found to be less precise than measurements taken on the oblique axis [61]. In this manuscript the minor axis was defined as the shorter axis when the IVC was viewed as an ellipse shape in horizontal orientation. Trauma patients were included in the study if they were noted to be hypovolemic on the initial ultrasound (minor axis measurement less than 15 mm, consistently measured one cm below the renal vessels) and if they received a computed tomography (CT) scan of their abdomen to further confirm results within 1 h of their diagnosis of hypovolemia. Expected expansion after fluid resuscitation was approximately 7 mm in the minor axis. It remains to be seen if this technique can be widely applied and reliably instituted as a means to identify patients who are volume depleted or dependent.

The Role of CPR During Resuscitation

One of the great follies occurring during the treatment of hemorrhagic shock is to perform advanced cardiac life support (ACLS) or cardiopulmonary resuscitation (CPR) with the notion that there will be any chance of survival. ACLS/CPR does not appear in the resuscitation algorithm of ATLS simply because it has no purpose there; it has no role in the definitive treatment of hemorrhagic shock [2]. Until the

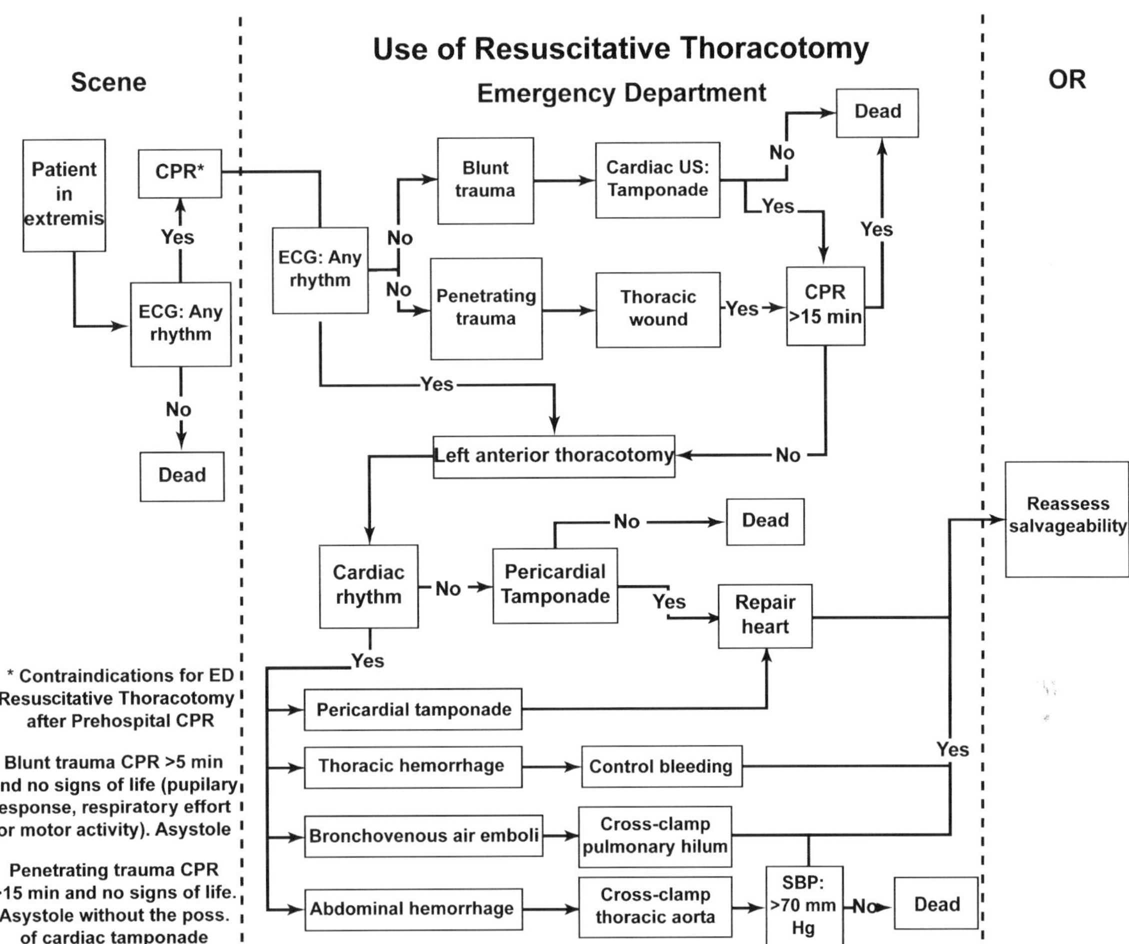

Fig. 1.2 Algorithm showing when a resuscitative thoracotomy should and should not be performed. Reprinted with permission from Mears G, Glickman SW, Moore F, Cairns CB. Data based integration of critical illness and injury patient care from EMS to emergency department to intensive care unit. Curr Opin Crit Care. 2009 Aug;15(4):284–9

source of the hemorrhage is controlled and intravascular volume restored after hypovolemic arrest, there is no other effective treatment option.

In the pediatric literature, several studies have looked at long-term survival data on children who received ACLS in the field prior to arrival at the treating facility [62]. The majority of non-survivors in this study of blunt trauma mechanisms all had either a head injury or a spinal cord injury, and the causes of death in all cases were secondary to devastating neurologic demise or neurogenic shock with cardiopulmonary collapse. Only two deaths had identifiable sources of hemorrhage, which were unable to be adequately controlled. Of the two who survived out of the total 25 who received CPR either in the field or in the emergency department, both had detectable vital signs during transport, lost vitals in the emergency department, and had protracted periods of CPR. Neither survivor had a head injury. The final conclusions from this data set were that children who received field CPR had poor prognosis and that traumatic hemorrhage, brain injury, and spinal cord injury were likely not treatable in any

manner by way of CPR. These results are consistent with previous data showing abysmal outcomes for survivability in children receiving post-traumatic CPR [63, 64].

Emergency Room Thoracotomy

Although residents often consider it a rite of passage to perform the emergency room thoracotomy (ERT) [65], the mature surgeon realizes that the ERT has its place in very few clinical circumstances (Fig. 1.2). With only a 2% overall survival rate in blunt trauma, and a 35% survival rate for patients with a single penetrating, quickly controllable injury and no or brief loss of vitals, a selective approach to deciding which patient qualifies for such an invasive maneuver is mandatory.

In 1993 a small study of 23 retrospectively reviewed cases from UC Davis-Sacramento's children's hospital showed that the parameters for ERT and survival rate paralleled those of the adult population with mortality of greater than 96%

and more than 85% based on blunt or penetrating mechanism [66]. A more selective approach to the pediatric population is now standard of care.

Once the decision has been made to commit to the ERT, several key maneuvers remain instrumental. The chest should be opened swiftly and efficiently. The skin, subcutaneous tissue, and muscle should be quickly divided at the level of the fourth intercostal space and the superior edge of the rib exposed and then followed to gain appropriate level access to the thoracic cavity. The rib space is held open using a retractor and the inferior pulmonary ligament is divided sharply with scissors up to the inferior pulmonary vein. The lung is then retracted superiorly and anteriorly with the left hand while the right hand traces the posterior ribs to the aorta. The pleural tissue about the aorta is divided sharply or bluntly dissected with a finger and the aortic cross clamp is placed. Care is taken not to injure any intercostal arteries. During this time any blood in the chest is evacuated swiftly. The pericardium can be opened anterior to the phrenic nerve with a plan of how cardiac injury will be controlled during consequent transport to the operating room. The patient should then, upon return of vital signs, be transported to the operating room where definitive surgical management can occur.

Massive Transfusion

Since no factors, other than severe head injury, have ever been identified to correlate with non-survivability, massive transfusion protocols should not be held for an assumption of impending mortality [67]. According to this article, no lab value, no injury severity score (ISS), no demographic data, and no vital sign, singly or grouped, determine a mortality score. A second manuscript from the same group of authors discusses a potential model for predicting mortality at 30 days; however, still there are cautions against using such a model to withhold much-needed blood products during resuscitation [68]. Factors most predictive of 24-h mortality are pH, base deficit, and amount of blood transfused within the initial 6 h. Factors at 30 days that are of significance include age and ISS on admission.

At Memorial Hermann Hospital in Houston, Texas, the massive transfusion protocol is activated for any patient who is suspected to require substantial transfusion, based on any one of the following: heart rate on arrival of more than 120 beats per minute, systolic blood pressure on arrival of less than 90, a positive FAST exam, penetrating or blunt trauma mechanism, or having a requirement for un-crossmatched blood in the emergency room on arrival. These recommendations come from retrospective data comparing predictive scores for massive transfusion. Using these parameters a score of two or greater was found to be 75% sensitive and 86%

specific, correlating relatively well without statistical significance to other published scoring systems [69]. The goal of this guideline is to make a continuous supply of six units of packed red blood cells (PRBC), six units of plasma (FFP), and one dose of a six-pack of platelets readily available. After 12 units of PRBC it is advised to check a fibrinogen level and if less than 100 mg/dl to administer ten units of cryoprecipitate. Serial labs are also drawn during the massive transfusion and include lactate, arterial blood gas, rapid thromboelastogram (TEG), coagulation panel, and complete blood count (CBC) with differential and platelet count. It should be noted that a TEG is available within minutes (five for a rapid TEG), whereas the coagulation panel and CBC take more than 45 min to process [70]. Additionally all code three trauma activations, which are the highest acuity patients at Memorial Hermann Hospital, are typed and crossed on arrival so that type-specific blood may be given when available.

Although directed transfusion with specific ratio has never been definitively proven to have advantage [71, 72], a 1:1:1 ratio of FFP:platelets:PRBC is maintained for trauma patients at Memorial Hermann Hospital. Data supporting the 1:1:1 FFP:platelet:PRBC ratio initially came from military literature dating from 2007, which shows an improvement in mortality for patients receiving such ratios [73]. This was later extrapolated in several studies to the civilian population and further propagated in several trauma centers as a new standard of care [74]. A review article from 2010 looked at nine additional observational studies that were published after the 2007 article [75]. While these authors agree that a 1:1:1 ratio seems to be well supported by the retrospective data thus far, they quickly focus attention to the lack of randomized controlled trials on the subject and to the inherent difficulty of maintaining a perfect ratio during a true massive resuscitation. Interestingly, there are no large randomized studies supporting the conventional method of transfusion. Additionally, they identify the prospect of using lab-guided and goal-directed transfusion recommendations, which have not at this point been prospectively studied.

A goal-directed transfusion protocol is a seemingly attractive approach for trauma resuscitation. Originally, massive transfusion protocols were designed to rapidly and reliably provide products to patients who had clinical evidence of substantial hemorrhage. Products and blood were given without a specific ratio until patients either expired or improved clinically. After introduction of the 1:1:1 ratio, which targets the coagulopathy that accompanies massive transfusion, surgeons began to question if transfusion should be automatic or rather if it should be guided by objective data and lab values. One of several manuscripts on goal-directed resuscitation [76] expresses the idea that resuscitation may be more functional and cost effective if lab values, such as TEG, are used to guide decision making during the resuscitation. This concept relies on laboratory reports being ordered, drawn, sent

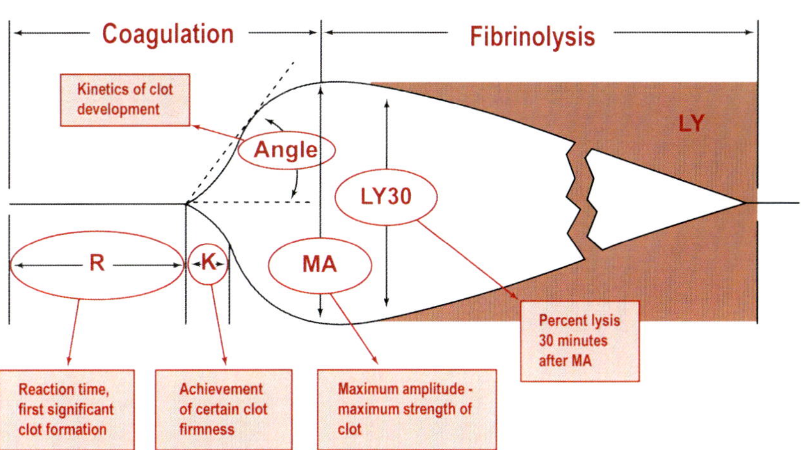

Fig. 1.3 Analytical software graphical representation of a TEG tracing. R: initial time; K: time it takes to reach clot strength; MA: maximal amplitude; LY: lysis. Reprinted with permission from Mark H. Ereth, MD. Uncontrolled bleeding after thoracic aortic aneurysm repair: a case report and interactive discussion. http://www.bloodcmecenter.org

to, and returned from the laboratory in a clinically relevant time frame. Current published data call into question the rapidity with which laboratory values can be utilized in the rapidly bleeding patient. Which reproducible ratio (if any) that a goal-directed resuscitation returns will be interesting to see. There is, at this time however, no consensus on either the 1:1:1 ratio or the use of goal-directed transfusion for resuscitation. These outstanding questions await level 1 data.

Thromboelastogram

The trauma service at the University of Texas at Houston has been using r-TEG consistently in all higher level activations for more than 18 months. The TEG is used to guide decisions on non-massively hemorrhaging patients or patients at risk of hemorrhage. TEG is a plotted graph of the effectiveness of clot formation and breakdown, and is considered more accurate to identify causes of coagulopathy in the trauma patient than is a coagulation panel [77, 78]. A recent Cochrane Review failed to show any mortality difference in patients who are resuscitated using TEG guidance versus those who follow a standardized massive transfusion protocol; however, the authors note that only five of the included nine studies evaluated mortality data as an endpoint [79]. They also note that TEG can potentially reduce the amount of transfusions if interpreted and applied during hemorrhagic shock, but that the data on this point is not definitive [79].

The TEG curves can provide information about all aspects of the clotting system, possibly even the interactions with the endothelium, which is currently an ongoing area of research [80]. The initial part of the TEG, which comprises the R time, or the activated clotting time (ACT), illustrates the amount of time to begin forming a clot (Fig. 1.3). The K time shows how long it takes to reach clot strength and quantitates the clot kinetics [81], whereas the alpha angle and the maximal amplitude (MA) show the rate of clot formation and the absolute clot strength indicating a relationship between fibrinogen and platelets, respectively. A low angle reflects a low fibrinogen concentration; a low MA means that the platelet count or function is reduced and the patient would benefit from platelet transfusion or desmopressin (DDAVP). The LY30 indicates the stability of the clot and the degree of fibrinolysis. The G value shows clot strength or firmness [82].

Normal ACT, R time, and K time indicate that clotting factors are intact and functional. Delays in any of these mean that the patient would most benefit from the administration of FFP or factor; additionally it can reflect a patient on heparin or other medication that impairs clotting. The angle and MA reflect platelet function and an increase in either suggests hypercoagulable state, whereas a decrease in either means that the platelets may not be aggregating properly. In patients with an elevated MA there is argument for administration of a daily aspirin or placement of an IVC filter (publication pending) [83]. It has been shown that an MA greater than 68 correlates with an increase in coagulability, predisposing patients to thromboembolism [84]. LY30 greater than 3% has significant consequences of increased mortality and should be treated with amicar or tranexamic acid [85–88].

Damage control resuscitation is a term coined in the military [89, 90]. It is a reproducible strategy with reproducible results and it is automatic and continuous until a physician decides that the shock state has resolved and that hemostasis has been achieved. It describes a resuscitation that uses replacement blood product, rather than crystalloid, for hemorrhagic shock. By limiting the crystalloid infused in the initial resuscitation, patients appear to have less complications and morbidity [91, 92]. There are fewer reports of compartment syndromes, a higher number of abdomens that can be closed after a damage control laparotomy, less acidosis, and less electrolyte disturbances.

Many centers now utilize a strategy of blood product resuscitation and limitation of crystalloid allocation [93]. For example Cotton and colleagues investigated the success of the trauma laparotomy when damage-control resuscitation in a 1:1:1 ratio and limited crystalloid were implemented [94]. This strategy of damage control resuscitation was found to be useful in the field. Patients in the damage control resuscitation group received approximately 10 l less of crystalloid in the first 24 h, had better short- and long-term survival, and showed signs of being less acidodic, less coagulopathic, and less hypothermic on arrival to the ICU than patients who received a traditional resuscitation. The study was a retrospective cohort that examined two similar groups of patients, finding improved morbidity and mortality rates in the group receiving better ratios and colloid. Secondary analyses showed statistically significant differences in multi-organ failure, acute lung and kidney injury, and their effects.

The length of time it takes to get access to FFP plays a role in the success of a massive transfusion protocol [92]. Several studies have examined time factors in receiving product as a way to analyze the effectiveness of a massive transfusion protocol [95–97]. At Memorial Hermann Hospital in Houston the trauma team improved availability of the initial unit of FFP by simply changing the physical location of the thawed FFP from the blood bank to the emergency department (unpublished data). This data shows an improvement in infusion time interval from 56 min to less than 5 min, which is associated with improved outcomes.

Hypertonic Saline

Crystalloid evaluation would not be complete without consideration of hypertonic saline. Hypertonic saline use is pervasive throughout the literature. Prior to the recent explosion of blood product-based resuscitation, crystalloid resuscitation was the standard of care. Hypertonic saline shows some improvement in blood pressure and arguable survival difference for patients who receive it in the pre-hospital setting [98]. There are other studies showing decreased pre-hospital fluid requirements in patients who receive hypertonic during transport [99]. Immunomodulatory effects are enhanced with single administration of 250 ml of hypertonic saline in the initial phase of resuscitation of hemorrhagic shock [100], and this could have additional effects on patients with later discovered head injury [101]. A large study of hypertonic saline showed statistical difference in outcome in pediatric head-injured patients when compared with isotonic fluid administration [102]. Hypertonic saline decreases interstitial pressure and consequently decreases bowel edema, which may be a potential benefit of using it on the patient whose abdomen is still open, as will be discussed later [103, 104]. Animal studies in the 1990s showed that there was no protective effect or difference in outcome for the patient in hemorrhagic shock with a head injury [105]. Since that time several studies examining hypertonic saline as a resuscitative fluid have been terminated secondary to futility and concerns for patient safety [106, 107]. It is still debatable that hypertonic has a physiologic or survival advantage when compared to other crystalloid formulations when used as a primary resuscitation fluid [108].

Complications of Resuscitation

Data from the days when trauma patients were resuscitated with multiple liters of saline prior to receiving their first blood product shows complications more related to the overwhelming volume of crystalloid infused than to the blood and product resuscitation [109–111]. These types of complications include compartment syndromes, high number of abdomens that cannot be closed, and grossly edematous bowel, all secondary to large volume resuscitation [112]. Complications of transfusion-related acute lung injury (TRALI) and transfusion-associated circulatory overload (TACO) are not seen frequently now because the base resuscitative fluid is colloid at lower volume not large volumes of crystalloid [113–115]. Ileus, heart failure, and difficulty with wound healing have all additionally been attributed to over-resuscitation with crystalloid.

All trauma patients who receive a massive resuscitation are at risk of abdominal compartment syndrome. One study claims that there will be an epidemic if crystalloid resuscitations are continued with such fervor and that patients are threatened by secondary compartment syndrome that occurs solely as the result of excessive crystalloid resuscitation during hemorrhagic shock [116]. Abdominal hypertension is defined as any pressure greater than 12 mmHg without evidence of multi-organ failure. Abdominal compartment syndrome is defined as any one of the following: pressure greater than 20 mmHg; progressive, identifiable organ dysfunction; and improvement following decompression. The trauma population is susceptible, even those who lack abdominal injuries and develop elevated pressures simply due to the amount of fluid they receive [112]. In Houston during the late 1990s the resuscitations during the first 24 h for a group of 128 patients requiring decompression for organ dysfunction averaged the following volumes: (26 ± 2 units PRBC, 38 ± 3 L crystalloid). Seven of these cases required urgent non-abdominal operations, where they likely received several additional units of crystalloid or colloid [117].

It is recommended to check bladder pressures and peak inspiratory pressures routinely and aggressively in patients where massive transfusion has taken place [118]. This practice of serially checking bladder pressures, based on observational data, seems to help in the early identification of abdominal hypertension, perhaps staving off the evolution to abdominal compartment syndrome [119]. Decompression can be done with placement of a temporary dressing and later planned closure with evidence of better results and earlier closure [120, 121].

Table 1.3 Different monitoring systems available in the intensive care unit

LiDCO	PiCCO	FloTrac	PAC/thermodilution
SV, SVV, CO	SV, SVV, CO	SV, SVV, CO	SV, CO, SVO2
Calibrate Q 8 h	Calibrate Q 8 h or when HD changes	Self-calibrates	Recalibration required
Arterial line; CVC or PIV	CENTRAL Arterial Line; CVC	CENTRAL Arterial Line; CVC	Uses its own catheter
Cannot be used: First-trimester pregnancy, weight less 40 kg	Independent of vent or damping of A-line	Dependent on strong wave form; arrhythmia affect reads	No contraindication
			Best used in the patient where there are two shock states, such as cardiogenic and septic

Keeping the abdomen open after a damage control laparotomy also has its disadvantages. It has been shown that ileus and bowel edema prevent advancement of feeds and definitive closure, and that these phenomena are likely related to an ongoing inflammatory response that occurs as a result of the sustained acute resuscitative phase [122–124]. It is additionally unclear whether ileus is a cause or an effect of bowel edema and vice versa [125, 126]. Three percent hypertonic saline running at 30 ml/h during the time that the abdomen is open decreases bowel edema [103]. The mechanism is thought to be due to hydrostatic gut edema induced by overaggressive resuscitation with crystalloid. The hypertonic saline gives a smaller volume of more concentrated solution, and pulls extra edematous fluid from the bowel wall. Success has been shown in the rat and subsequently in the human model.

Monitoring Systems in the Intensive Care Unit

Once the trauma patient arrives in the surgical ICU there are a number of different monitoring systems available, such as the Swan Ganz, the Vigileo, LiDCo, and PICCo, to trend cardiac output, ScVO2, stroke volume variation (SVV), and other measures of hemodynamic parameters (Table 1.3). The Swan Ganz catheter, introduced in 1970, was the first right heart catheterization device that could be placed at the bedside without the use of real-time imaging. Measurements are taken by thermodilution and continuous monitoring. The Swan Ganz catheter, also known as a pulmonary artery catheter (PAC), was used for many years under the assumption that "knowledge of the numbers" improved patient outcome. The other monitoring devices use the arterial wave form to extrapolate data.

Pulmonary Artery Catheterization

The following data references overwhelmingly show that there is no indication for the routine use of the PAC in any specific patient population (Fig. 1.4). The Connors paper from Case Western concludes that there is an overall lack of benefit to using PAC [127]. The second landmark article from 1996 is from Cooper, looking at data from 36 studies where PAC was used [128]. Citing several of them in particu-

lar he notes that there is no difference to most endpoints in any of the articles used. Specifically there is no significant difference found for mortality, ICU length of stay, hospital length of stay, or total hospital costs.

The Cochrane Review shows that of the 12 studies included to evaluate the validity of PAC use, only one has adequate power to substantiate the results. It has been found that there is no difference in mortality, complication rate, morbidity, cost, or length of stay with or without a PAC [129]. The key finding is that the PAC has been used extensively without the evidence of its merit. Studies included here are all randomized, but not all blinded; 4,687 total patients are included. The use of a PAC does not demonstrate survival advantage in any group. In 2010 noncardiac, high-risk surgical patients potentially benefit when selectively chosen for PAC if it is used to better optimize oxygen delivery and consumption for volume or inotropic support. From the Evaluation Study of Congestive Heart Failure and Pulmonary Artery Catheter Effectiveness (ESCAPE) database numerous studies from 2009 to 2011 have been published stratifying patients in different manners to revisit the issue of the PAC, heart failure management in general, and other various related issues [130–132]. There continues to be inconsistent data on the utility of the PAC in the general surgery population and fairly unclear and nonuniversal indications in the cardiac and heart failure populations.

Additionally there are other devices that are non- or minimally invasive that can assist the physician in assessing these parameters [133]. Examples include bedside echocardiography, arterial catheters, central venous pressure (CVP) monitoring, SVV, and arterial blood gas. Current indications for the use of the PAC include combined shock states, such as cardiogenic and septic, discordant ventricular heart failure, and in working up the differential of pulmonary hypertension.

General Surgery Operative Resuscitations

Consideration should be given to the application of transfusion protocols to the massively bleeding non-trauma patient and to the general surgery patient who requires fluid in the operating room, but who is not bleeding. There is extensive

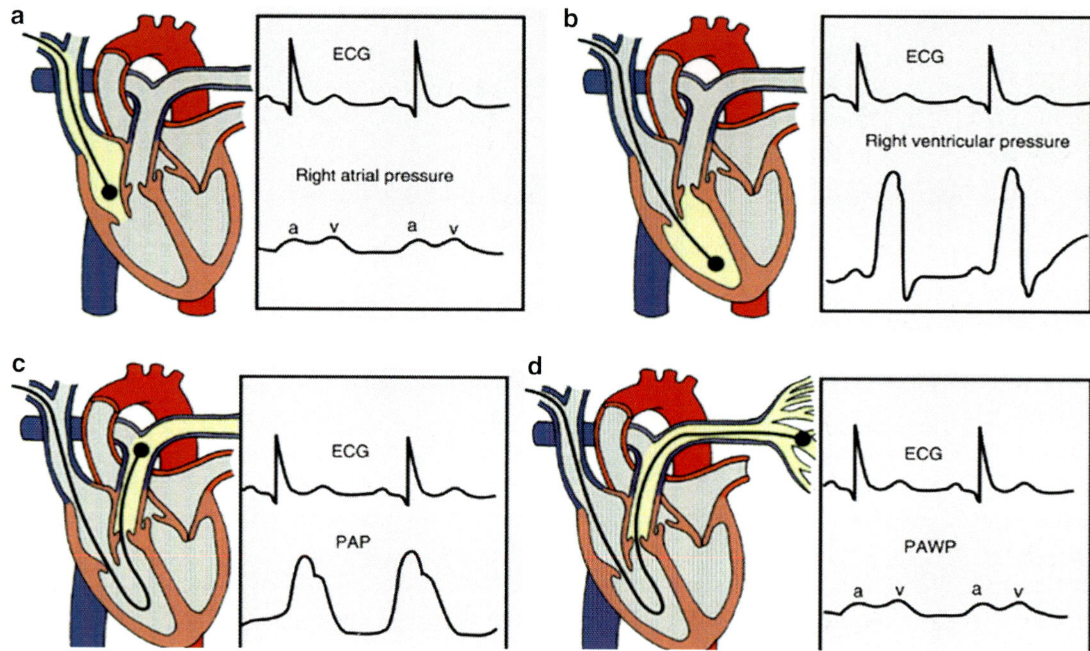

Fig. 1.4 Pulmonary artery catheter (PAC) insertion. During insertion, the waveforms change as the PAC enters the heart. (**a**) When the PAC enters the right atrium, a waveform with two upright *peaks* appears. The a waves represent the right ventricular end-diastolic pressure. The v waves represent the right atrial filling. (**b**) The catheter enters the right ventricle. Sharp systolic upstrokes and lower diastolic dips appear in the waveform. (**c**) A pulmonary artery pressure (PAP) waveform appears. The dicrotic notch in the PAP upstroke indicates pulmonic valve closure. (**d**) When the PAC "floats" into a distal branch of the pulmonary artery, the balloon becomes wedged in vessels that are too narrow for it to pass. A pulmonary artery wedge pressure (PAWP) waveform appears, with the a wave representing left ventricular end-diastolic pressure and the v wave representing ventricular filling. ECG—electrocardiogram. Reprinted with permission from Instructor's Resource CD-ROM in: Fontaine DK, Hudak CM, Gallo BM, Morton PG (eds). Critical care nursing: a holistic approach, 8th edition, copyright 2004 Lippincott Williams & Wilkins

data that aggressive intraoperative resuscitation maneuvers negatively affect fresh bowel anastomoses, contribute to edema, and inevitably increase ileus time [134]. In this study the administration of 10.5 l of IV fluid or blood product within the first 72 h corresponds to a fivefold increase in anastomotic breakdown rate. It is equally well known that non-resuscitative fluid volumes can hurt bowel anastomoses in elective general surgery cases [135]. Perioperative fluid restriction appears to be one way, other than good technique, in which surgeons can control the integrity of the anastomosis [136–138].

The Obstetric Patient

In the obstetric data, and likely similarly in other surgical subspecialties not involving trauma, resuscitation for hemorrhagic shock includes all the interventions described previously and additional specialty-specific interventions (i.e., hysterectomy). Thromboelastography is promoted in the literature, as is low-volume crystalloid, with better goal-directed, smaller volume, resuscitation [139].

Adding colloid, specifically albumin, to the resuscitation formula decreases the amount of crystalloid needed to maintain target urine output [140]. There are no reported compartment syndrome complications in this group, but albumin use in the general population for resuscitation is still not universally implemented.

The Burn Patient

The burn data is extensive, as expected. Any burn over 20% requires a balanced fluid management strategy. Several formulas exist to guide fluid resuscitation in burn patients, with all having a common goal of replacing the losses associated with the injury based on the size of the burn and maintaining urine output. All of the parameters that are used for trauma resuscitations, including base deficit, lactate, bicarbonate, and urine output 0.5–1 ml/kg/h should be used in the burn population, since these values are not exclusive to the trauma subset and are reasonably applied and extrapolated to the burn patient. All of these formulas can contribute to over-resuscitation, causing a term called "fluid creep" [141]. Boluses are not encouraged; the burn victim responds best to periodic adjustment in rate [142].

When considering the percentage of burn and calculating the predicted losses to be replaced, it is important to consider inhalation injury which adds surface area-insensitive loss. Unlike trauma, colloid is not recommended for the initial resuscitation of the burn patient; albumin should not be used in the initial resuscitation because it leaks into the interstitium and causes additional fluid loss from the vasculature [143, 144]. Of course any extra fluid volume during resuscitation manifests as edema and can result in any complication associated with over-resuscitation, including compartment syndromes [145].

Conclusion

Resuscitation is an art and requires attention to detail at all stages including pre-hospital, hospital, operating room, and ICU. The salient points from this chapter are to focus resuscitation on providing deficient products, using TEG to guide resuscitation for the non-massive transfusion patient, and monitor resuscitation with specific goals and endpoints. Interested readers are encouraged to focus on several of the resources below to enhance their knowledge and perfect their resuscitation abilities.

References

1. Wiggers HC, Ingraham RC. Hemorrhagic shock: definition and criteria for its diagnosis. J Clin Invest. 1946;25(1):30–6.
2. American College of Surgeons. ATLS manual 7th Edition, 2004.
3. Newgard CD, Zive D, Malveau S, Leopold R, Worrall W, Sahni R. Developing a statewide emergency medical services database linked to hospital outcomes: a feasibility study. Prehosp Emerg Care. 2011;15(3):303–19.
4. McGillicuddy DC, O'Connell FJ, Shapiro NI, Calder SA, Mottley LJ, Roberts JC, Sanchez LD. Emergency department abnormal vital sign "triggers" program improves time to therapy. Acad Emerg Med. 2011;18(5):483–7. 2011 Apr 26.
5. Mears G, Glickman SW, Moore F, Cairns CB. Data based integration of critical illness and injury patient care from EMS to emergency department to intensive care unit. Curr Opin Crit Care. 2009;15(4):284–9.
6. Spinella PC, Holcomb JB. Resuscitation and transfusion principles for traumatic hemorrhagic shock. Blood Rev. 2009;23:231–40.
7. Stern SA. Low-volume fluid resuscitation for presumed hemorrhagic shock: helpful or harmful? Curr Opin Crit Care. 2001;7(6):422–30.
8. Phillips CR, Vinecore K, Hagg DS, Sawai RS, Differding JA, Watters JM, Schreiber MA. Resuscitation of haemorrhagic shock with normal saline vs. lactated Ringer's: effects on oxygenation, extravascular lung water and haemodynamics. Crit Care. 2009;13(2):R30. Epub 2009 Mar 4.
9. Scultetus A, Alam HB, Stanton K, et al. Dextran and Hespan resuscitation causes neutrophil activation in swine after hemorrhagic shock. Shock. 2000;13(Suppl):52.
10. Rana R, Fernández-Pérez ER, Khan SA, Rana S, Winters JL, Lesnick TG, Moore SB, Gajic O. Transfusion-related acute lung injury and pulmonary edema in critically ill patients: a retrospective study. Transfusion. 2006;46(9):1478–83.
11. Eder AF, Herron R, Strupp A, Dy B, Notari EP, Chambers LA, Dodd RY, Benjamin RJ. Transfusion-related acute lung injury surveillance (2003–2005) and the potential impact of the selective use of plasma from male donors in the American Red Cross. Transfusion. 2007;47(4):599–607.
12. Plurad D, Belzberg H, Schulman I, Green D, Salim A, Inaba K, Rhee P, Demetriades D. Leukoreduction is associated with a decreased incidence of late onset acute respiratory distress syndrome after injury. Am Surg. 2008;74(2):117–23.
13. Todd SR, Malinoski D, Muller PJ, Schreiber MA. Lactated Ringer's is superior to normal saline in the resuscitation of uncontrolled hemorrhagic shock. J Trauma. 2007;62(3):636–9.
14. Kiraly LN, Differding JA, Enomoto TM, Sawai RS, Muller PJ, Diggs B, Tieu BH, Englehart MS, Underwood S, Wiesberg TT, Schreiber MA. Resuscitation with normal saline (NS) vs. lactated ringers (LR) modulates hypercoagulability and leads to increased blood loss in an uncontrolled hemorrhagic shock swine model. J Trauma. 2006;61(1):57–64. discussion 64–5.
15. Waters JH, Gottlieb A, Schoenwald P, Popovich MJ, Sprung J, Nelson DR. Normal saline versus lactated Ringer's solution for intraoperative fluid management in patients undergoing abdominal aortic aneurysm repair: an outcome study. Anesth Analg. 2001;93(4):817–22.
16. Bickell WH, Bruttig SP, Millnamow GA, O'Benar J, Wade CE. The detrimental effects of intravenous crystalloid after aortotomy in swine. Surgery. 1991;110(3):529–36.
17. Dubick MA, Atkins JL. Small-volume fluid resuscitation for the far-forward combat environment: current concepts. J Trauma. 2003;54(5 Suppl):S43–S5.
18. Dubick MA. Current concepts in fluid resuscitation for prehospital care of combat casualties. US Army Med Dep J. 2011:18–24.
19. Balogh Z, McKinley BA, Holcomb JB, et al. Both primary and secondary abdominal compartment syndrome can be predicted early and are harbingers of multiple organ failure. J Trauma. 2003;54(5):848–59.
20. Kowalenko T, Stern S, Dronen S, et al. Improved outcome with hypotensive resuscitation of uncontrolled hemorrhagic shock in a swine model. J Trauma. 1992;33:349–53.
21. Joshi GP. Intraoperative fluid restriction improves outcome after major elective gastrointestinal surgery. Anesth Analg. 2005;101:601–5.
22. Cotton BA, Reddy N, Hatch QM, LeFebvre E, Wade CE, Kozar RA, Gill BS, Albarado R, McNutt MK, Holcomb JB. Damage control resuscitation is associated with a reduction in resuscitation volumes and improvement in survival in 390 damage control laparotomy patients. Ann Surg. 2011;254(4):598–605.
23. Morrison CA, Carrick MM, Norman MA, Scott BG, Welsh FJ, Tsai P, Liscum KR, Wall Jr MJ, Mattox KL. Hypotensive resuscitation strategy reduces transfusion requirements and severe postoperative coagulopathy in trauma patients with hemorrhagic shock: preliminary results of a randomized controlled trial. J Trauma. 2011;70(3):652–63.
24. Skarda DE, Mulier KE, George ME, Bellman GJ. Eight hours of hypotensive versus normotensive resuscitation in a porcine model of controlled hemorrhagic shock. Acad Emerg Med. 2008;15(9):845–52.
25. Bickell WH, Wall Jr MJ, Pepe PE, Martin RR, Ginger VF, Allen MK, Mattox KL. Immediate versus delayed fluid resuscitation for hypotensive patients with penetrating torso injuries. N Engl J Med. 1994;331(17):1105–9.
26. Sondeen JL, Coppes VG, Holcomb JB. Blood pressure at which rebleeding occurs after resuscitation in swine with aortic injury. J Trauma. 2003;54(5 Suppl):S110–S7.
27. D'Alleyrand JC, Dutton RP, Pollak AN. Extrapolation of battlefield resuscitative care to the civilian setting. J Surg Orthop Adv. 2010;19(1):62–9.

28. Beekley AC, Sebesta JA, Blackbourne LH, Herbert GS, Kauvar DS, Baer DG, Walters TJ, Mullenix PS, Holcomb JB, 31st Combat Support Hospital Research Group. Prehospital tourniquet use in Operation Iraqi Freedom: effect on hemorrhage control and outcomes. J Trauma. 2008;64(2 Suppl):S28–37. discussion S37.

29. Kragh JF, O'Neill ML, Beebe DF, Fox CJ, Beekley AC, Cain JS, Parsons DL, Mabry RL, Blackbourne LH. Survey of the indications for use of emergency tourniquets. J Spec Oper Med. 2011;11(1):30–8.

30. Taylor DM, Vater GM, Parker PJ. An evaluation of two tourniquet systems for the control of prehospital lower limb hemorrhage. J Trauma. 2011;71(3):591–5.

31. Peck MA, Clouse WD, Cox MW, Bowser AN, Eliason JL, Jenkins DH, Smith DL, Rasmussen TE. The complete management of extremity vascular injury in a local population: a wartime report from the 332nd Expeditionary Medical Group/Air Force Theater Hospital, Balad Air Base, Iraq. J Vasc Surg. 2007;45(6):1197–204. discussion 1204–5.

32. Dunham CM, Siegel JH, Weireter L, Fabian M, Goodarzi S, Guadalupi P, Gettings L, Linberg SE, Vary TC. Oxygen debt and metabolic acidemia as quantitative predictors of mortality and the severity of the ischemic insult in hemorrhagic shock. Crit Care Med. 1991;19(2):231–43.

33. Siegel JH, Fabian M, Smith JA, Kingston EP, Steele KA, Wells MR, Kaplan LJ. Oxygen debt criteria quantify the effectiveness of early partial resuscitation after hypovolemic hemorrhagic shock. J Trauma. 2003;54:862–80.

34. Siegel JH, Rivkind AI, Dala S, Goodarzi S. Early physiologic predictors of injury severity and death in blunt multiple trauma. Arch Surg. 1990;125:498–508.

35. Rixen D, Raum M, Holzgraefe B, Sauerland S, Nagelschmidt M, Neugebauer EA, Shock and Trauma Study Group. A pig hemorrhagic shock model: oxygen debt and metabolic acidemia as indicators of severity. Shock. 2001;16:239–44.

36. Bakker J, Coffernils M, Leon M, Gris P, Vincent JL. Blood lactate levels are superior to oxygen-derived variables in predicting outcome in septic shock. Chest. 1991;99:956–62.

37. Convertino VA, Ryan KL, Rickards CA, Salinas J, McManus JG, Cooke WH, Holcomb JB. Physiological and medical monitoring for en route care of combat casualties. J Trauma. 2008;64(4 Suppl):S342–S53.

38. Vary TC, Siegel JH, Rivkind A. Clinical and therapeutic significance of metabolic patterns of lactic acidosis. Perspect Crit Care. 1988;1:85–132.

39. Jansen TC, van Bommel J, Mulder PG, Rommes JH, Schieveld SJ, Bakker J. The prognostic value of blood lactate levels relative to that of vital signs in the pre-hospital setting: a pilot study. Crit Care. 2008;12(6):R160. Epub 2008 Dec 17.

40. Balasubramanyan N, Havens PL, Hoffman GM. Unmeasured anions identified by the Fencl-Stewart method predict mortality better than base excess, anion gap, and lactate in patients in the pediatric intensive care unit. Crit Care Med. 1999;27:1577–81.

41. Smith I, Kumar P, Molloy S, et al. Base excess and lactate as prognostic indicators for patients admitted to intensive care. Intensive Care Med. 2001;27:74–83.

42. Husain FA, Martin MJ, Mullenix PS, et al. Serum lactate and base deficit as predictors of mortality and morbidity. Am J Surg. 2003;185:485–91.

43. Kincaid EH, Miller PR, Meredith JW, et al. Elevated arterial base deficit in trauma patients: a marker of impaired oxygen utilization. J Am Coll Surg. 1998;187:384–92.

44. Rutherford EJ, Morris JA, Reed GW, et al. Base deficit stratifies mortality and determines therapy. J Trauma. 1992;33:417–23.

45. Fidkowski C, Helstrom J. Diagnosing metabolic acidosis in the critically ill: bridging the anion gap, Stewart, and base excess methods. Can J Anaesth. 2009;56(3):247–56. Epub 2009 Feb 13.

46. Rocktaeschel J, Morimatsu H, Uchino S, Bellomo R. Unmeasured anions in critically ill patients: can they predict mortality? Crit Care Med. 2003;31(8):2131–6.

47. Martin MJ, FitzSullivan E, Salim A, Brown CV, Demetriades D, Long W. Discordance between lactate and base deficit in the surgical intensive care unit: which one do you trust? Am J Surg. 2006;191(5):625–30.

48. Lujan E, Howard R. Venous bicarbonate correlates linearly with arterial base deficit only if pH is constant. Arch Surg. 2006;141(1):105. author reply 105.

49. Schmelzer TM, Perron AD, Thomason MH, Sing RF. A comparison of central venous and arterial base deficit as a predictor of survival in acute trauma. Am J Emerg Med. 2008;26(2):119–23.

50. Rossaint R, Cerny V, Coats TJ, Duranteau J, Fernandez-Mondejar E, Gordini G, Stahel PF, Hunt BJ, Neugebauer E, Spahn DR. Key issues in advanced bleeding care in trauma. Shock. 2006;26:322–31.

51. Hierholzer C, Billiar TR. Molecular mechanisms in the early phase of hemorrhagic shock. Langenbecks Arch Surg. 2001;386:302–8.

52. Hess JR, Brohi K, Dutton RP, Hauser CJ, Holcomb JB, Kluger Y, Mackway-Jones K, Parr MJ, Rizoli SB, Yukioka T, Hoyt DB, Bouillon B. The coagulopathy of trauma: a review of mechanisms. J Trauma. 2008;65(4):748–54.

53. Moore FA, McKinley BA, Moore EE, Nathens AB, West M, Shapiro MB, Bankey P, Freeman B, Harbrecht BG, Johnson JL, Minei JP, Maier RV. Inflammation and the host response to injury, a large-scale collaborative project: patient-oriented research core: standard operating procedures for clinical care. III. Guidelines for shock resuscitation. J Trauma. 2006;61:82–9.

54. Ayala A, Wang P, Ba ZF, Perrin MM, Ertel W, Chaudry IH. Differential alterations in plasma IL-6 and TNF levels following trauma and hemorrhage. Am J Physiol. 1991;260:R167–R71.

55. Erber WN, Perry DJ. Plasma and plasma products in the treatment of massive haemorrhage. Best Pract Res Clin Haematol. 2006;19:97–112.

56. Krause KR, Howells GA, Buhs CL, Hernandez DA, Bair H, Schuster M, Bendick PJ. Hypothermia-induced coagulopathy during hemorrhagic shock. Am Surg. 2000;66(4):348–54.

57. Peitzman AB, Billiar TR, Harbrecht BG, Kelly E, Udekwu AO, Simmons RL. Hemorrhagic shock. Curr Probl Surg. 1995;32:925–1002.

58. Lyon M, Blaivas M, Brannam L. Sonographic measurement of the inferior vena cava as a marker of blood loss. Am J Emerg Med. 2005;23(1):45–50.

59. Yanagawa Y, Sakamoto T, Okada Y. Hypovolemic shock evaluated by sonographic measurement of the inferior vena cava during resuscitation in trauma patients. J Trauma. 2007;63(6):1245–8. discussion 1248.

60. Stawicki SP, Braslow BM, Panebianco NL, Kirkpatrick JN, Gracias VH, Hayden GE, Dean AJ. Intensivist use of hand carried ultrasonography to measure IVC collapsibility in estimating intravascular volume status: correlations with CVP. J Am Coll Surg. 2009;209(1):55–61. Epub 2009 May 1.

61. Murphy EH, Arko FR, Trimmer CK, Phangureh VS, Fogarty TJ, Zarins CK. Volume associated dynamic geometry and spatial orientation of the inferior vena cava. J Vasc Surg. 2009;50(4):835–42. discussion 842–3. Epub 2009 Aug 6.

62. Calkins CM, Bensard DD, Partrick DA, Karrer FM. A critical analysis of outcome for children sustaining cardiac arrest after blunt trauma. J Pediatr Surg. 2002;37(2):180–4. Source Denver, Colorado.

63. Hazinski MF, Chahine AA, Holcomb 3rd GW, et al. Outcome of cardiovascular collapse in pediatric blunt trauma. Ann Emerg Med. 1994;23:1229–35.

64. Fisher B, Worthen M. Cardiac arrest induced by blunt trauma in children. Pediatr Emerg Care. 1999;15:274–6.

65. Cothren CC, Moore EE. Emergency department thoracotomy for the critically injured patient: objectives, indications, and outcomes. World J Emerg Surg. 2006;1:4. doi:10.1186/1749-7922-1-4. Published online 2006 March 24.

66. Sheikh AA, Culbertson CB. Emergency department thoracotomy in children: rationale for selective application. J Trauma. 1993;34(3):323–8.

67. Barbosa RR, Rowell SE, Diggs BS, Schreiber MA, Trauma Outcomes Group, et al. Profoundly abnormal initial physiologic and biochemical data cannot be used to determine futility in massively transfused trauma patients. J Trauma. 2011;71(2 Suppl 3):S364–S9.

68. Barbosa RR, Rowell SE, Sambasivan CN, Diggs BS, Spinella PC, Schreiber MA, Trauma Outcomes Group, et al. A predictive model for mortality in massively transfused trauma patients. J Trauma. 2011;71(2 Suppl 3):S370–S4.

69. Nunez TC, Voskresensky IV, Dossett LA, Shinall R, Dutton WD, Cotton BA. Early prediction of massive transfusion in trauma: simple as ABC (assessment of blood consumption)? J Trauma. 2009;66(2):346–52.

70. Cotton BA, Faz G, Hatch QM, Radwan ZA, Podbielski J, Wade C, Kozar RA, Holcomb JB. Rapid thrombelastography delivers real-time results that predict transfusion within 1 hour of admission. J Trauma. 2011;71(2):407–14. discussion 414–7.

71. Murthi SB, Stansbury LG, Dutton RP, Edelman BB, Scalea TM, Hess JR. Transfusion medicine in trauma patients: an update. Expert Rev Hematol. 2011;4(5):527–37.

72. Hannon T. Trauma blood management: avoiding the collateral damage of trauma resuscitation protocols. Hematology Am Soc Hematol Educ Program. 2010;2010:463–4.

73. Borgman MA, Spinella PC, Perkins JG, et al. The ratio of blood products transfused affects mortality in patients receiving massive transfusions at a combat support hospital. J Trauma. 2007;63:805–13.

74. Holcomb JB, Wade CE, Michalek JE, et al. Increased plasma and platelet to red blood cell ratios improves outcome in 466 massively transfused civilian trauma patients. Ann Surg. 2008;248:447–58.

75. Stansbury LG, Dutton RP, Stein DM, Bochicchio GV, Scalea TM, Hess JR. Controversy in trauma resuscitation: do ratios of plasma to red blood cells matter? Transfus Med Rev. 2009;23(4):255–65.

76. Kashuk JL, Moore EE, Sawyer M, Le T, Johnson J, Biffl WL, Cothren CC, Barnett C, Stahel P, Sillman CC, Sauaia A, Banerjee A. Postinjury coagulopathy management: goal directed resuscitation via POC thrombelastography. Ann Surg. 2010;251(4):604–14.

77. Johansson PI, Stissing T, Bochsen L, et al. Thrombelastography (TEG) in trauma. Scand J Trauma Resusc Emerg Med. 2009;17:45.

78. Plotkin AJ, Wade CE, Jenkins DH, et al. A reduction in clot formation rate and strength assessed by thrombelastography is indicative of transfusion requirements in patients with penetrating injuries. J Trauma. 2008;64:64–8.

79. Afshari A, Wikkelsø A, Brok J, Møller AM, Wetterslev J. Thrombelastography (TEG) or thromboelastometry (ROTEM) to monitor haemotherapy versus usual care in patients with massive transfusion. Cochrane Database Syst Rev. 2011;16(3):CD007871.

80. Johansson PI, Ostrowski SR. Acute coagulopathy of trauma: balancing progressive catecholamine induced endothelial activation and damage by fluid phase anticoagulation. Med Hypotheses. 2010;75(6):564–7. Epub 2010 Aug 13.

81. Reikvam H, Steien E, Hauge B, Liseth K, Gjerde Hagen K, Størkson R, Hervig T. Thrombelastography. Transfus Apher Sci. 2009;40:119–23.

82. Stammers AH, Bruda NL, Gonano C, Hartmann T. Point-of-care coagulation monitoring: applications of the thromboelastography. Anaesthesia. 1998;53 Suppl 2:58–9.

83. Cotton B, Minei K, Radwan ZA, Matijevic N, Pivalizza E, Podbielski J, et al. Admission rapid thrombeolastography (r-TEG) predicts development of pulmonary embolism in trauma patients. J Trauma Acute Care Surg. 2012;72(6):1470–5.

84. McCrath DJ, Cerboni E, Frumento RJ, et al. Thromboelastography maximum amplitude predicts postoperative thrombotic complications including myocardial infarction. Anesth Analg. 2005;100:1576–83.

85. CRASH-2 collaborators, Roberts I, Shakur H, Afolabi A, Brohi K, Coats T, Dewan Y, et al. The importance of early treatment with tranexamic acid in bleeding trauma patients: an exploratory analysis of the CRASH-2 randomised controlled trial. Lancet. 2011;377(9771):1096–101.

86. Henry DA, Carless PA, Moxey AJ, et al. Antifibrinolytic use for minimizing perioperative allogenic blood transfusion. Cochrane Database Syst Rev. 2011;(3):CD001886.

87. Morrison JJ, Dubose JJ, Rasmussen TE, Midwinter MJ. Military application of tranexamic acid in trauma emergency resuscitation (MATTERs) study. Arch Surg. 2012;147(2):113–9.

88. CRASH-2 trial collaborators, Shakur H, Roberts I, Bautista R, Caballero J, Coats T, Dewan Y, et al. Effects of tranexamic acid on death, vascular occlusive events, and blood transfusion in trauma patients with significant hemorrhage (CRASH-2): a randomized, placebo controlled trial. Lancet. 2010;376(9734):23–32.

89. Hess JR, Holcomb JB, Hoyt DB. Damage control resuscitation: the need for specific blood products to treat the coagulopathy of trauma. Transfusion. 2006;46:685–6.

90. Holcomb JB. Damage control resuscitation. J Trauma. 2007;62:S36–S7.

91. Duchesne JC, Kimonis K, Marr AB, Rennie KV, Wahl G, Wells JE, et al. Damage control resuscitation in combination with damage control laparotomy: a survival advantage. J Trauma. 2010;69(1):46–52.

92. Duchesne JC, Barbeau JM, Islam TM, Wahl G, Greiffenstein P, McSwain Jr NE. Damage control resuscitation: from emergency department to the operating room. Am Surg. 2011;77(2):201–6.

93. Duchesne JC, Hunt JP, Wahl G, Marr AB, Wang YZ, Weintraub SE, Wright MJ, McSwain Jr NE. Review of current blood transfusions strategies in a mature level I trauma center: were we wrong for the last 60 years? J Trauma. 2008;65(2):272–6. discussion 276–8.

94. Cotton BA, Reddy N, Hatch QM, Lefebvre E, Wade CE, Kozar RA, et al. Damage control resuscitation is associated with a reduction in resuscitation volumes and improvement in survival in 390 damage control laparotomy patients. Ann Surg. 2011;254(4):598–605.

95. Ho AM, Karmakar MK, Dion PW. Are we giving enough coagulation factors during major trauma resuscitation? Am J Surg. 2005;190:479–84.

96. Dente CJ, Shaz BH, Nicholas JM, et al. Improvements in early mortality and coagulopathy are sustained better in patients with blunt trauma after institution of a massive transfusion protocol in a civilian Level I trauma center. J Trauma. 2009;66:1616–24.

97. Zink KA, Sambasivan CN, Holcomb JB, et al. A high ratio of plasma and platelets to packed red blood cells in the first 6 hours of massive transfusion improves outcomes in a large multi center study. Am J Surg. 2009;197:565–70. discussion 570.

98. Vassar MJ, Fischer RP, O'Brien PE, Bachulis BL, Chambers JA, Hoyt DB, Holcroft JW, The Multicenter Group for the Study of Hypertonic Saline in Trauma Patients. A multicenter trial for resuscitation of injured patients with 7.5% sodium chloride. The effect of added dextran 70. Arch Surg. 1993;128(9):1003–11. discussion 1011–3.

99. Vassar MJ, Perry CA, Gannaway WL, Holcroft JW. 7.5% sodium chloride/dextran for resuscitation of trauma patients undergoing helicopter transport. Arch Surg. 1991;126(9):1065–72.

100. Rizoli SB, Rhind SG, Shek PN, Inaba K, Filips D, Tien H, Brenneman F, Rotstein O. The immunomodulatory effects of hypertonic saline resuscitation in patients sustaining traumatic hemorrhagic shock: a randomized, controlled, double-blinded trial. Ann Surg. 2006;243(1):47–57.

101. Rhind SG, Crnko NT, Baker AJ, Morrison LJ, Shek PN, Scarpelini S, Rizoli SB. Prehospital resuscitation with hypertonic saline-dextran modulates inflammatory, coagulation and endothelial activation marker profiles in severe traumatic brain injured patients. J Neuroinflammation. 2010;7:5.

102. Simma B, Burger R, Falk M, Sacher P, Fanconi S. A prospective, randomized, and controlled study of fluid management in children with severe head injury: lactated Ringer's solution versus hypertonic saline. Crit Care Med. 1998;26(7):1265–70.

103. Radhakrishnan RS, Xue H, Moore-Olufemi SD, Weisbrodt NW, Moore FA, Allen SJ, Laine GA, Cox Jr CS. Hypertonic saline resuscitation prevents hydrostatically induced intestinal edema and ileus. Crit Care Med. 2006;34(6):1713–8.

104. Cox Jr CS, Radhakrishnan R, Villarrubia L, Xue H, Uray K, Gill BS, Stewart RH, Laine GA. Hypertonic saline modulation of intestinal tissue stress and fluid balance. Shock. 2008;29(5):598–602.

105. Sheikh AA, Matsuoka T, Wisner DH. Cerebral effects of resuscitation with hypertonic saline and a new low-sodium hypertonic fluid in hemorrhagic shock and head injury. Crit Care Med. 1996;24(7):1226–32.

106. Bulger EM, Jurkovich GJ, Nathens AB, Copass MK, Hanson S, Cooper C, et al. Hypertonic resuscitation of hypovolemic shock after blunt trauma: a randomized controlled trial. Arch Surg. 2008;143(2):139–48. discussion 149.

107. Bulger EM, May S, Kerby JD, Emerson S, Stiell IG, Schreiber MA, et al.; ROC investigators. Out-of-hospital hypertonic resuscitation after traumatic hypovolemic shock: a randomized, placebo controlled trial. Ann Surg. 2011;253(3):431–41.

108. Riha GM, Kunio NR, Van PY, Hamilton GJ, Anderson R, Differding JA, Schreiber MA. Hextend and 7.5% hypertonic saline with dextran are equivalent to lactated ringer's in a swine model of initial resuscitation of uncontrolled hemorrhagic shock. J Trauma. 2011;71(6):1755–60.

109. Coimbra R, Porcides R, Loomis W, Melbostad H, Lall R, Deree J, Wolf P, Hoyt DB. HSPTX protects against hemorrhagic shock resuscitation-induced tissue injury: an attractive alternative to Ringer's lactate. J Trauma. 2006;60(1):41–51.

110. Hatoum OA, Bashenko Y, Hirsh M, Krausz MM. Continuous fluid resuscitation for treatment of uncontrolled hemorrhagic shock following massive splenic injury in rats. Shock. 2002;18(6):574–9.

111. Solomonov E, Hirsh M, Yahiya A, Krausz MM. The effect of vigorous fluid resuscitation in uncontrolled hemorrhagic shock after massive splenic injury. Crit Care Med. 2000;28(3):749–54.

112. Balogh Z, McKinley BA, Cocanour CS, Kozar RA, Valdivia A, Sailors RM, Moore FA. Supranormal trauma resuscitation causes more cases of abdominal compartment syndrome. Arch Surg. 2003;138(6):637–42. discussion 642–3.

113. Popovsky MA. Pulmonary consequences of transfusion: TRALI and TACO. Transfus Apher Sci. 2006;34(3):243–4. Epub 2006 Jul 26.

114. Gajic O, Gropper MA, Hubmayr RD. Pulmonary edema after transfusion: how to differentiate transfusion-associated circulatory overload from transfusion-related acute lung injury. Crit Care Med. 2006;34(5 Suppl):S109–S13.

115. Haupt MT, Teerapong P, Green D, Schaeffer Jr RC, Carlson RW. Increased pulmonary edema with crystalloid compared to colloid resuscitation of shock associated with increased vascular permeability. Circ Shock. 1984;12(3):213–24.

116. Balogh Z, Moore FA, Moore EE, Biffl WL. Secondary abdominal compartment syndrome: a potential threat for all trauma clinicians. Injury. 2007;38(3):272–9. Epub 2006 Nov 15.

117. Balogh Z, McKinley BA, Cocanour CS, Kozar RA, Holcomb JB, Ware DN, Moore FA. Secondary abdominal compartment syndrome is an elusive early complication of traumatic shock resuscitation. Am J Surg. 2002;184(6):538–43. discussion 543–4.

118. Maxwell RA, Fabian TC, Croce MA, Davis KA. Secondary abdominal compartment syndrome: an underappreciated manifestation of severe hemorrhagic shock. J Trauma. 1999;47(6):995–9.

119. Sugrue M, Buhkari Y. Intra-abdominal pressure and abdominal compartment syndrome in acute general surgery. World J Surg. 2009;33(6):1123–7.

120. Hatch QM, Osterhout LM, Ashraf A, Podbielski J, Kozar RA, Wade CE, Holcomb JB, Cotton BA. Current use of damage-control laparotomy, closure rates, and predictors of early fascial closure at the first take-back. J Trauma. 2011;70(6):1429–36.

121. van Boele Hensbroek P, Wind J, Dijkgraaf MG, Busch OR, Carel Goslings J. Temporary closure of the open abdomen: a systematic review on delayed primary fascial closure in patients with an open abdomen. World J Surg. 2009;33(2):199–207.

122. Bueno L, Ferre JP, Ruckebusch Y. Effects of anesthesia and surgical procedures on intestinal myoelectric activity in rats. Dig Dis. 1978;23:690–5.

123. Livingston EH, Passaro Jr EP. Postoperative ileus. Dig Dis Sci. 1990;35:121–32.

124. Bauer AJ, Schwarz NT, Moore BA, Türler A, Kalff JC. Ileus in critical illness: mechanisms and management. Curr Opin Crit Care. 2002;8(2):152–7.

125. Balogh Z, McKinley BA, Cox Jr CS, et al. Abdominal compartment syndrome: the cause or effect of postinjury multiple organ failure. Shock. 2003;20:483.

126. Drake RE, Teague RA, Gabel JC. Lymphatic drainage reduces intestinal edema and fluid loss. Lymphology. 1998;31:68.

127. Connors Jr AF, Speroff T, Dawson NV, Thomas C, Harrell Jr FE, Wagner D, et al. The effectiveness of right heart catheterization in the initial care of critically ill patients. SUPPORT Investigators. JAMA. 1996;276(11):889–97.

128. Cooper AB, Doig GS, Sibbald WJ. Pulmonary artery catheters in the critically ill. An overview using the methodology of evidence based medicine. Crit Care Clin. 1996;12(4):777–94. Review.

129. Harvey S, Young D, Brampton W, Cooper AB, Doig G, Sibbald W, Rowan K. Pulmonary artery catheters for adult patients in intensive care. Cochrane Database Syst Rev. 2006;19(3):CD003408. Review.

130. O'Connor CM, Hasselblad V, Mehta RH, Tasissa G, Califf RM, Fiuzat M, et al. Triage after hospitalization with advanced heart failure: the ESCAPE (Evaluation Study of Congestive Heart Failure and Pulmonary Artery Catheterization Effectiveness) risk model and discharge score. J Am Coll Cardiol. 2010;55(9):872–8.

131. Chatterjee K. The Swan-Ganz catheters: past, present, and future: a viewpoint. Circulation. 2009;119(1):147–52.

132. Khush KK, Tasissa G, Butler J, McGlothlin D, De Marco T, ESCAPE Investigators. Effect of pulmonary hypertension on clinical outcomes in advanced heart failure: analysis of the evaluation study of congestive heart failure and pulmonary artery catheterization effectiveness database. Am Heart J. 2009;157(6):1026–34. Epub 2009 Apr 23.

133. Hadian M, Kim HK, Severyn DA, Pinsky MR. Cross-comparison of cardiac output trending accuracy of LiDCO, PiCCO, FloTrac and pulmonary artery catheters. Crit Care. 2010;14(6):R212. Epub 2010 Nov 23.

134. Schnüriger B, Inaba K, Wu T, Eberle BM, Belzberg H, Demetriades D. Crystalloids after primary colon resection and anastomosis at initial trauma laparotomy: excessive volumes are associated with anastomotic leakage. J Trauma. 2011;70(3):603–10.

135. Brandstrup B, Tonnesen H, Beier-Holgersen R, et al. Effects of intravenous fluid restriction on postoperative complications: comparison of two perioperative fluid regimens: a randomized assessor-blinded multicenter trial. Ann Surg. 2003;238:641–8.

136. MacKay G, Fearon K, McConnachie A, Serpell MG, Molloy RG, O'Dwyer PJ. Randomized clinical trial of the effect of postoperative intravenous fluid restriction on recovery after elective colorectal surgery. Br J Surg. 2006;93:1469–74.

137. Nisanevich V, Felsenstein I, Almogy G, Weissman C, Einav S, Matot I. Effect of intraoperative fluid management on outcome after intraabdominal surgery. Anesthesiology. 2005;103:25–32.

138. Rahbari NN, Zimmermann JB, Schmidt T, Koch M, Weigand MA, Weitz J. Meta-analysis of standard, restrictive and supplemental fluid administration in colorectal surgery. Br J Surg. 2009;96:331–41.

139. Pacheco LD, Saade GR, Gei AF, Hankins GD. Cutting-edge advances in the medical management of obstetrical hemorrhage. Am J Obstet Gynecol. 2011;205(6):526–32.

140. Lawrence A, Faraklas I, Watkins H, Allen A, Cochran A, Morris S, Saffle J. Colloid administration normalizes resuscitation ratio and ameliorates "fluid creep". J Burn Care Res. 2010;31(1):40–7.

141. Saffle JI. The phenomenon of "fluid creep" in acute burn resuscitation. J Burn Care Res. 2007;28:382–95.

142. Chung KK, Wolf SE, Cancio LC, et al. Resuscitation of severely burned military casualties: fluid begets more fluid. J Trauma. 2009;67:231–7.

143. Pruitt BA. Protection from excessive resuscitation: "pushing the pendulum back". J Trauma. 2000;49:567–8.

144. Baxter CR. Problems and complications of burn shock resuscitation. Surg Clin North Am. 1978;58:1313–22.

145. Cartotto R, Zhou A. Fluid creep: the pendulum hasn't swung back yet. J Burn Care Res. 2010;31:551–8.

Ashley Hardy, Bennet Butler, and Marie Crandall

Introduction and Epidemiology

Abdominal pain is one of the most common reasons for visits to the emergency room. Although for the majority of patients, symptoms are benign and self-limited, a subset will be diagnosed with an "acute abdomen," as a result of serious intra-abdominal pathology necessitating emergency intervention [1].

An expeditious workup is necessary when evaluating patients presenting with acute abdominal pain to determine the most likely cause of their symptoms and determine whether or not emergent operative intervention is necessary. The most appropriate therapy should then be initiated with the patient's clinical status optimized. The workup should first include a thorough but efficient acquisition of the patient's history and physical examination followed by the judicious use of laboratory and radiologic studies. The evaluation of patients with acute abdominal pain can pose a diagnostic challenge for physicians as patients may present with atypical symptoms that interfere with the usual pattern recognition that often guides decision making. These atypical presentations may help account for the over 25% of abdominal pain cases labeled as "nonspecific" or "undifferentiated" [1].

Additionally, physicians must take into account the patient's age and gender, as conditions associated with the acute abdomen may vary accordingly. Specifically, gastroenteritis, acute appendicitis, and abdominal trauma are common causes of the acute abdomen in children and young adults [2], whereas biliary disease, intestinal obstruction, diverticulitis, and appendicitis are among the most common causes in middle-aged adults and the elderly [3]. Furthermore,

pelvic pathology accounts for approximately 12% of acute abdominal pain presentations and should therefore be considered when evaluating female patients [1].

Finally, there are a variety of nonsurgical causes of abdominal pain that are cardiovascular, metabolic, and toxic in origin that should be considered when evaluating these patients.

Clinical Presentation

A thorough, yet expeditiously obtained, history and physical exam are paramount to developing the differential diagnosis for patients presenting with an acute abdomen. Various laboratory and imaging studies may subsequently be used as adjuncts to help guide decision making.

History

When obtaining a patient history, the physician should avoid questions that are leading and should focus on details of the pain. This includes information on the onset, character, duration, and location of pain as well as the presence of radiation of pain.

Regarding onset, pain that develops suddenly may be suggestive of a perforated viscus or ruptured abdominal aortic aneurysm (AAA). Pain that gradually worsens over time may be the result of conditions characterized by the progressive development of infection and inflammation such as acute appendicitis and cholecystitis.

With regard to character, pain described as "burning" may implicate the pain of a perforated peptic ulcer while a "ripping" or "tearing" sensation typically represents the pain of an aortic dissection. Pain that is intermittent or colicky should be distinguished from pain that is continuous in nature. Colicky pain is typically associated with obstructive processes of the intestinal, hepatobiliary, or genitourinary tract, while pain that is continuous is usually the result of underlying

A. Hardy, M.D. • B. Butler, B.S. • M. Crandall, M.D., M.P.H. (✉)
Department of Surgery, Northwestern University Feinberg School of Medicine, 676 N. St. Clair, Suite 650, Chicago, IL 60611, USA
e-mail: mcrandall@northwestern.edu

L.J. Moore et al. (eds.), *Common Problems in Acute Care Surgery*,
DOI 10.1007/978-1-4614-6123-4_2, © Springer Science+Business Media New York 2013

ischemia or peritoneal inflammation. The latter may occur primarily or following an initial episode of colicky pain when an obstructive process is complicated by the development of ischemia. Examples of this include cases of biliary colic that progresses to acute cholecystitis or an incarcerated loop of intestine that becomes strangulated and ischemic.

The location of pain is important to consider as various pathologic conditions tend to occur in specific regions or quadrants of the abdomen (Fig. 2.1a, b). Therefore, if the physician is knowledgeable of the disease processes that cause pain in these areas, they may be able to significantly narrow down their differential. This holds true for those with the understanding that certain conditions may result in pain that radiates or is referred to an area beyond the site of disease due to shared innervation. Classic examples of this include biliary pain that is referred to the right subscapular region, the pain of acute pancreatitis that radiates to the back, and genitourinary pain that radiates from the flank down to the groin. Finally, it is important to note any chronological variation in the pain as this may provide helpful clues to the diagnosis. One of the best examples of this is in the case of acute appendicitis, in which pain is initially perceived in the periumbilical region before localizing to the right lower quadrant (RLQ). This phenomenon reflects the transition from visceral to parietal pain as appendiceal inflammation progresses to involve and irritate the peritoneal lining.

The majority of patients presenting with acute abdominal pain have associating symptoms (e.g., nausea, vomiting, diarrhea, constipation, hematochezia) that are often helpful in making a diagnosis. Chronology of nausea is important to consider as vomiting that occurs after the onset of abdominal pain is more likely to be surgical in nature as a result of medullary vomiting centers that are stimulated by pain impulses traveling via secondary visceral afferent fibers. Additionally, constipation or obstipation may point towards an intestinal obstruction, while diarrhea (especially if bloody) is associated with gastroenteritis, inflammatory bowel disease, and intestinal ischemia.

Aggravating or alleviating factors may also provide diagnostic clues. Depending on the underlying etiology, patients may maintain certain positions to help alleviate their pain. For example, patients with peritonitis may find some relief when lying still with their knees bent, while patients suffering from a bout of acute pancreatitis prefer to sit upright and lean forward. The effect of food is also important to consider as eating may alleviate the pain of a peptic ulcer while worsening the pain of an intestinal obstruction, acute cholecystitis, or acute pancreatitis [4, 5].

The patient's past medical and surgical histories may also help to narrow down the differential. A remote history of abdominal surgery may indicate that intestinal obstruction secondary to adhesive disease is the source of a patient's complaints. Furthermore, it is important to consider the impact that coexistent medical conditions, such as diabetes, chronic obstructive pulmonary disease, and atherosclerosis, may have on patient outcomes. The fact that elderly patients are more likely to have significant comorbidities places them at increased risk for end organ damage incited by gastrointestinal emergencies [6].

Physicians should also take into account the effects of medication use. Anticoagulants may predispose to the development of rectus sheath hematomas and precipitate the gastrointestinal bleeding that is a component of the patient's underlying illness or complicating the patient's postoperative or posttreatment course. Chronic use of nonsteroidal anti-inflammatory drugs (NSAIDs) may also promote bleeding episodes along with the development of peptic ulcer disease (PUD) and its complications.

A detailed social history should also be obtained to determine if there is any significant history of tobacco, alcohol, or illicit drug use, as such behaviors can be a source of the patient's symptoms as well as complicate the patient's hospital course. Notably, a history of cocaine abuse may point towards a diagnosis of mesenteric ischemia as the underlying reason for the patient's symptoms.

The social history should consist of a detailed gynecologic history, including the date of the last menses, the presence of any vaginal bleeding or discharge, and any history of unprotected sexual activity or intercourse with multiple partners. Such information could indicate pregnancy complications, salpingitis or pelvic inflammatory disease, and other gynecologic conditions as the cause of the patient's acute abdominal complaints. Physicians should also take note of any history of recent travel to implicate infectious enterocolitis. Any exposure to environmental toxins should be determined, as lead and iron poisoning are two well-known, extra-abdominal sources of acute abdominal pain [4, 5].

Finally, the patient's family history may ascertain whether a patient's symptoms are hereditary in origin, as seen in the case of inherited hypercoagulable states, which can cause acute mesenteric ischemia secondary to mesenteric venous thrombosis.

Physical Exam

Examination of the patient presenting with acute abdominal pain should initially begin with overall appearance of the patient and vital signs. Patients who appear diaphorectic, pale, and anxious often suffer from a condition of vascular origin, including dissecting AAA, mesenteric ischemia, or atypical angina. The patient who is lying particularly still on the exam table often has peritonitis from perforated viscus or pancreatitis. Vital signs should always be interpreted knowing the status of the patient's pain, or the influence of any home medications (beta blockers masking tachycardia, for

a

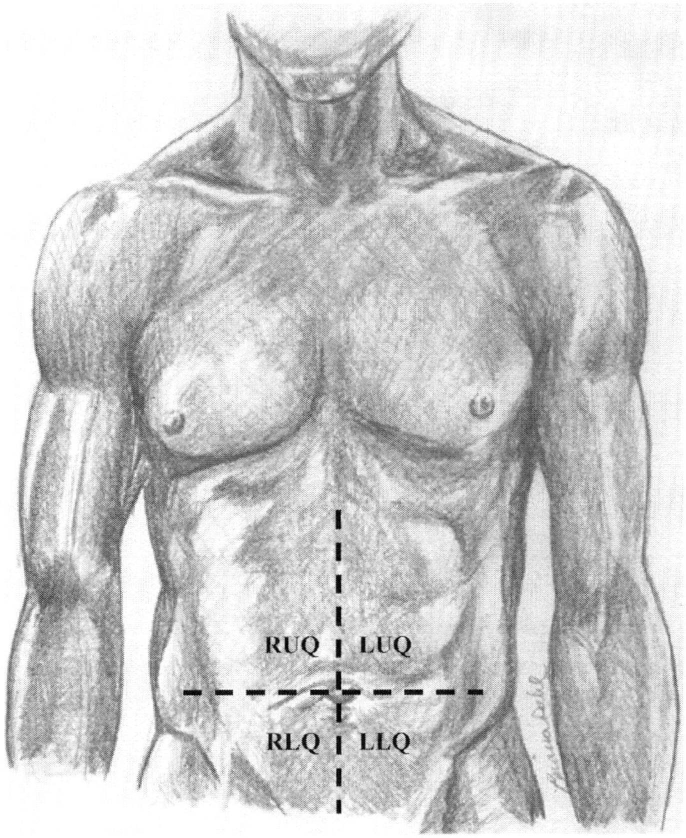

RUQ | LUQ

RLQ | LLQ

Right Upper Quadrant (RUQ)
Cholecystitis
Biliary Colic
Cholangitis
Hepatitis
Hepatic Abscess
Pancreatitis
Peptic Ulcer
Appendicitis (pregnancy)
Intestinal Obstruction
Inflammatory Bowel Disease
Pneumonia

Left Upper Quadrant (LUQ)
Gastritis
Peptic Ulcer
Pancreatitis
Splenomegaly
Splenic Rupture
Intestinal Obstruction
Inflammatory Bowel Disease
Diverticulitis (Splenic Flexure)
Pneumonia
Myocardial ischemia
Pericarditis

Right Lower Quadrant (RLQ)
Appendicitis
Inflammatory Bowel Disease
Diverticulitis (Cecal, Meckel's)
Mesenteric Adenitis
Intestinal Obstruction
Hernia
Ectoptic Pregnancy
Salpingitis
Ovarian Torsion
Ruptured Ovarian Cyst
Mittelschmerz
Nephrolithiasis
Pyelonephritis

Left Lower Quadrant (LLQ)
Diverticulitis
Appendicitis
Intestinal Obstruction
Inflammatory Bowel Disease
Ischemic Colitis
Hernia
Ectopic Pregnancy
Salpingitis
Ovarian Torsion
Ruptured Ovarian Cyst
Mittelschmerz
Nephrolithiasis
Pyelonephritis

Fig. 2.1 (**a**) Common causes of the acute abdomen based on quadrant. (**b**) Common causes of the acute abdomen based on region. Illustrations courtesy of Briana Dahl

b

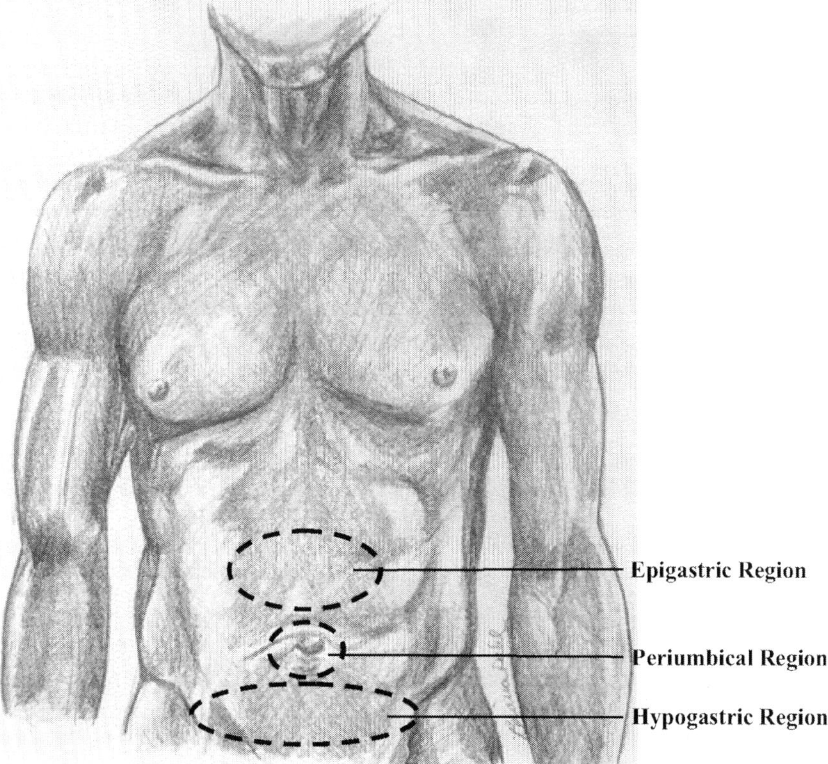

<table>
<tr><td>

EPIGASTRIC REGION
Gastritis
Peptic Ulcer
Pancreatitis
Cholecystitis
Mesenteric Thrombosis/Ischemia
Intestinal Obstruction
Myocardial Ischemia
Pericarditis

</td><td>

PERIUMBILICAL REGION
Appendicitis (Early)
Enterocolitis
Mesenteric Thrombosis/Ischemia
Intestinal Obstruction
Inflammatory Bowel Disease
Ruptured Abdominal Aortic
Aneurysm
Hernia

</td><td>

HYPOGASTRIC REGION
Appendicitis
Enterocolitis
Diverticulitis
Intestinal Obstruction
Inflammatory Bowel Disease
Hernia
Ectopic Pregnancy
Salpingtitis
Ovarian Torsion
Ruptured Ovarian Cyst
Cystitis

</td></tr>
</table>

Fig. 2.1 (continued)

example). Severity of systemic illness can be graded based on the degree of tachypnea, tachycardia, febrile or hypothermic response, and relative hypotension. Further examination of the lungs and heart could reveal signs representing primary cardiac disease or new-onset arrhythmias, which could lead to mesenteric embolic disease. The remainder of a complete physical examination should proceed expeditiously so that attention can be focused on the abdomen.

Examination of the abdomen should comprise four sequential components: inspection, auscultation, percussion, and palpation. The exam should include all areas of the abdomen, flanks, and groins.

Inspection

Inspection is the initial step of the abdominal examination and consists first of a general assessment of the patient's overall state followed by focus on the abdomen. Patients with peritonitis tend to lie still with their knees flexed as doing so provides some alleviation of their pain. Upon closer inspection of the abdomen, one should note the presence of prior surgical scars, abdominal distension or visible peristalsis, any obvious masses suggestive of an incarcerated hernia or tumor, or erythema or ecchymoses secondary to traumatic injury or hemorrhagic complications of acute pancreatitis. Caput medusa may indicate liver disease.

Auscultation of the abdomen should be performed next and involves listening for the presence or the absence of bowel sounds, for the characteristics of those sounds, and for the presence of bruits. Although this step may be the least valuable overall, as bowel sounds may be completely normal in patients with severe intra-abdominal pathology, it may nonetheless provide some information that assists the physician in making a diagnosis. For example, the absence of bowel sounds may point towards a paralytic ileus, while ones that are high pitched in nature or rushed may indicate the presence of a mechanical bowel obstruction. Finally, bruits that are detected on the abdominal exam suggest the presence of turbulent flow, which is often the case for arterial stenoses.

Percussion

Next, percussion is utilized to assess for any dull masses, pneumoperitoneum, peritonitis, and ascites. A largely tympanic abdomen may indicate the presence of underlying loops of gas-filled bowel typical of intestinal obstructions or a paralytic ileus. If findings of tympany extend to include the right upper quadrant (RUQ) however, it may be suggestive of free intraperitoneal air. Lastly, percussion can be used to detect ascites by the presence of shifting dullness or by the generation of a fluid wave. Percussion may be all that is necessary to elicit pain in the patient who has peritonitis, for whom further palpation should be deferred.

Palpation

Palpation is the final, critical step as it enables the physician to better define the location and severity of pain and confirm any findings made on other aspects of the physical exam. Palpation should always commence away from the area of greatest pain to prevent any voluntary guarding, which should be distinguished from the involuntary guarding that accompanies peritonitis. Palpation can produce various signs commonly associated with specific disease processes. These include Murphy's sign, characterized by an arrest in inspiration upon deep palpation of the RUQ in patients with acute cholecystitis, and Rovsing's sign, observed many times in patients with acute appendicitis in which pain is elicited at McBurney's point upon palpation of the left lower quadrant. Additionally, pain felt with hyperextension of the right hip, or iliopsoas sign, may indicate the presence of a retrocecal appendix, while a pelvic location of the appendix may be suspected in patients exhibiting Obturator sign, or pain created with internal rotation of a flexed right hip.

It is essential that all patients presenting with acute abdominal pain undergo a digital rectal exam as it may reveal the presence of a mass, the focal tenderness of a periappendiceal or peridiverticular abscess, and the presence of gross or occult blood. Finally, a pelvic examination should be performed in female patients presenting with lower quadrant pain to discern whether their pain has a gynecologic or obstetric source like pelvic inflammatory disease or a ruptured ectopic pregnancy. On exam, one should take note of any vaginal bleeding or discharge and any adnexal or cervical motion tenderness [4, 5].

Diagnosis Including Use/Value of Pertinent Diagnostic Studies

Laboratory Studies

Various laboratory studies can be used as adjuncts to help narrow down the differential, or to confirm or rule out a diagnosis. A complete blood count (CBC) with differential, for example, may help detect or confirm the presence of an infectious or inflammatory process by the demonstration of leukocytosis and/or a left shift. The accompanying hematocrit is also of value as it can provide information about one's plasma volume, altered in cases of dehydration and hemorrhage. In addition, serum electrolytes, blood urea nitrogen (BUN), and serum creatinine may provide clues to the extent of any fluid losses resulting from emesis, diarrhea, and third-spacing as can lactic acid levels and arterial blood gases. The latter two tests may also help to confirm the presence of any intestinal ischemia or infarction as well.

Liver function tests (LFTs) can help in determining whether conditions of the hepatobiliary tract are the source of the patient's symptoms, while measurements of serum amylase and lipase may implicate acute pancreatitis or its complications as the cause. Physicians should be mindful of the fact, however, that serum amylase levels may also be elevated in a variety of other acute abdominal conditions including intestinal obstruction, mesenteric thrombosis, ruptured ectopic pregnancy, and perforated PUD to name a few [7].

Urinary tests, namely, urinalysis, should be obtained in patients presenting with hematuria, dysuria, or flank pain to determine if their symptoms are genitourinary in origin. Urine samples can also be used to perform toxicology screens in those whose abdominal pain is thought to be the result of long-standing illegal drug use, as seen in the case of mesenteric ischemia that occurs with chronic cocaine abuse. Finally, human chorionic gonadotropin (Hcg) levels can help in determining whether complications of pregnancy, such as a ruptured ectopic pregnancy, are to blame. Regardless of whether or not it is the source of the patient's symptoms, Hcg levels should be obtained in all women of childbearing age as it may affect decision making, especially if additional studies or surgical intervention are deemed necessary [4]. Finally, depending on the clinical situation, blood may be obtained for typing and crossmatching.

Radiologic Studies

Radiologic imaging plays a key role in the evaluation and management of the acute abdomen (Table 2.1). Plain films, ultrasound (US), computed tomography (CT), and magnetic resonance imaging (MRI) are the most common imaging modalities employed in the diagnostic workup of these patients.

Table 2.1 Diagnostic imaging strategies and treatment options for common causes of acute abdominal pain based on age and gender

	Imaging strategy	Treatment options
Children/young adults		
Acute appendicitis	US, CT	Appendectomy (laparoscopic or open); percutaneous abscess drainage
Gastroenteritis	None	Supportive care
Functional constipation	XR	Manual or pharmacologic fecal disimpaction
Intussusception	XR, US, contrast enema	Contrast enema; operative reduction; resection of ischemic or perforated bowel
Abdominal trauma	FAST, DPL, CT	Exploratory laparotomy; IR
Older adults/elderly		
Acute cholecystitis	US	Cholecystectomy (laparoscopic or open); percutaneous cholecystostomy
Intestinal obstruction	XR, CT	Supportive care; exploratory laparotomy with adhesiolysis, resection of ischemic bowel
Perforated peptic ulcer	XR, CT or UGI with H_2O soluble contrast	Patch closure with *Helicobacter pylori* treatment if hemodynamic instability
Diverticulitis	CT	Supportive care; percutaneous abscess drainage; resection of involved bowel
Acute appendicitis	CT	Appendectomy (laparoscopic or open); percutaneous abscess drainage
Acute pancreatitis	US, CT	Supportive care; IR or operative pseudocyst drainage; debridement of infected necrosis
Mesenteric ischemia	CTA, MRA	Supportive care; IR; operative bypass, thrombectomy, resection of ischemic bowel
Women		
Acute appendicitis in pregnancy	US, CT, MRI	Appendectomy (laparoscopic or open)
Acute cholecystitis in pregnancy	US	Cholecystectomy (laparoscopic or open)
Ectopic pregnancy	US	Linear salpingostomy or salpingectomy (laparoscopic or open)
Ovarian torsion	US	Ovarian detorsion, possible oophorectomy (laparoscopic or open)
Pelvic inflammatory disease	US, MRI, CT	Supportive care; percutaneous or operative drainage of abscess

US ultrasound, *CT* computerized tomography, *XR* plain radiography, *FAST* focused abdominal sonography for trauma, *DPL* diagnostic peritoneal lavage, *UGI* upper gastrointestinal series, *IR* interventional radiology, *CTA, CT* computerized tomographic angiography, *MRA* magnetic resonance angiography, *MRI* magnetic resonance imaging

While plain films are less sensitive and specific compared to CT scanning, it is often the initial imaging study performed in patients presenting with acute abdominal pain. The advantages of their use include their rapidity and universal availability. Although patients are subject to ionizing radiation exposure, the dose is significantly lower than that of CT scans [8]. Plain films can be of greatest utility in patients suspected of a perforated viscus by the detection of a pneumoperitoneum, or the presence of free air beneath the right hemidiaphragm, as well as those with a suspected intestinal obstruction by the presence of dilated loops of bowel and air-fluid levels.

The advantages of abdominal US include the lower cost and the lack of ionizing radiation exposure [9], which is advantageous for the pediatric population and pregnant women. In addition, abdominal US is the imaging modality of choice for those patients presenting with suspected hepatobiliary pathology, with a sensitivity of 88% and specificity of 80% in the diagnosis of acute cholecystitis [10]. Features suggestive of acute cholecystitis on US include the presence of gallstones, gallbladder wall thickening, pericholecystic fluid, and an elicited Murphy's sign (Fig. 2.2).

If an obstetrical or gynecologic condition is suspected as the source of a patient's acute abdominal pain, pelvic and transvaginal US are the preferred imaging modalities to assess the uterus and adnexal structures. The presence of free fluid and an empty uterus on US in the setting of a positive pregnancy test is strongly suggestive of a ruptured ectopic pregnancy [11] while an enlarged and edematous ovary with an absence of blood flow is characteristic of a torsed ovary.

The CT scan has sensitivity of 96% overall for diagnosing most causes of the acute abdomen, compared to a 30% sensitivity for plain films [8]. As a result, the number of CT scans performed for patients presenting with acute abdominal pain has increased by 141% between 1996 and 2005 [12]. CT scanning has had a significant impact on the diagnosis of acute appendicitis as it has decreased the negative appendectomy rate from 24 to 3% [13]. Findings diagnostic of appendicitis on CT scan include an enlarged, nonopacified appendix, appendicoliths, and adjacent fat stranding while the presence of an abscess, phlegmon, and extraluminal gas points towards appendiceal perforation (see Fig. 2.2).

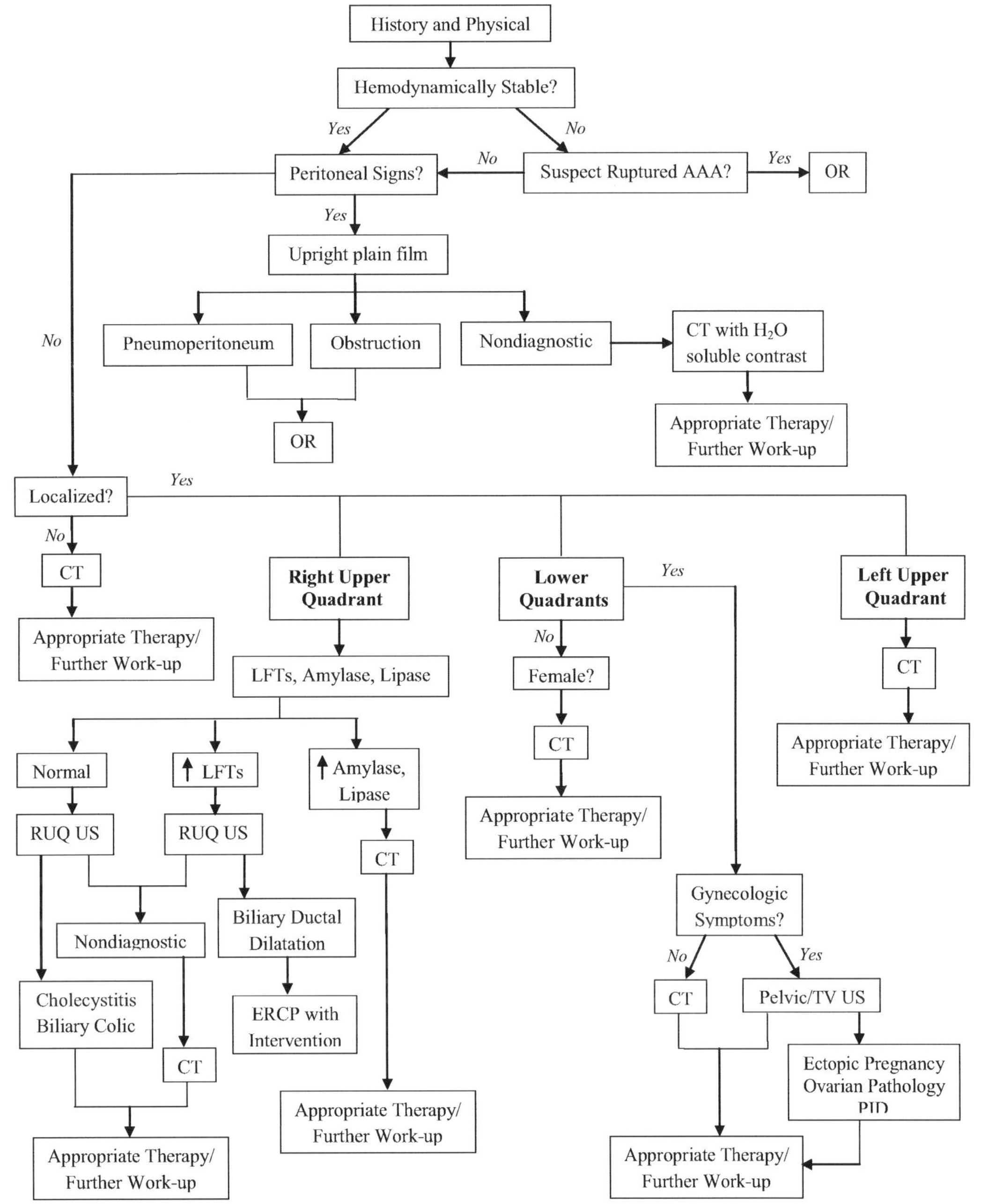

AAA, Abdominal Aortic Aneurysm; CT, Computerized Tomography; LFTs, Liver Function Tests; ERCP, Endoscopic Retrograde Cholangiopancreatography; RUQ, Right Upper Quadrant; US, Ultrasound; TV, Transvaginal; PID, Pelvic Inflammatory Disease.

Fig. 2.2 Algorithm for the treatment of the acute abdomen

Although MRIs provide excellent visualization of the intrabdominal organs without the need for ionizing radiation, their cost and lack of universal availability make them less ideal for use in the evaluation of the acute abdomen [14]. In addition, some patients have contraindications to undergoing an MRI or are simply unable to tolerate the test because of claustrophobia. MRI, however, may be of utility for pregnant women in the setting of acute abdominal pain with equivocal US findings [15].

Diagnostic Laparoscopy

Diagnostic laparoscopy may be of utility in the evaluation of acute abdominal pain, especially in situations in which the underlying etiology remains unclear despite a thorough clinical evaluation and radiologic imaging. The advantages of diagnostic laparoscopy include its ability to make a definitive diagnosis in 90–98% of cases and determine whether further intervention is necessary [16, 17]. A resultant decrease in the negative laparotomy rate—and the fact that if further treatment is indicated that many acute abdominal conditions can be treated laparoscopically—equates to a decrease in morbidity and mortality, a shorter length of stay, and decreased hospital costs [16].

Therapeutic Options

In the evaluation of patients presenting with acute abdominal pain, the physician must first determine whether operative intervention is necessary, and if so, whether it should be pursued on an immediate or emergent basis versus urgently or within a few hours of a patient's arrival. Treatment algorithms are beneficial in helping to make such decisions (see Fig. 2.2). In some cases, a short delay to fully correct any fluid and electrolyte abnormalities may prove to be beneficial, whereas in others, immediate operative intervention is necessary for stabilization of a patient's condition. This holds true in the presence of peritonitis, a pneumoperitoneum, intestinal ischemia or infarction, and continued hemodynamic instability despite aggressive resuscitative measures.

Specific treatment strategies for the acute abdomen are largely dependent upon the underlying etiology (see Table 2.1). In the case of acute appendicitis, patients should receive antibiotics and undergo urgent removal of their appendix through either an open or laparoscopic approach, unless their condition is complicated by a perforation with an associated abscess or phlegmon, for which initial nonoperative therapy with interval appendectomy is employed.

For those presenting with acute pancreatitis, however, treatment is largely supportive and includes bowel rest, aggressive fluid and electrolyte repletion, pain control, antibiotic therapy, and nutritional support. Surgery is reserved for the management of complications that may occur subsequently, including the development of infected pancreatic necrosis and large, symptomatic pseudocysts.

Lastly, for patients whose conditions do not warrant emergent surgery, but in whom the underlying etiology remains uncertain, treatment options include diagnostic laparoscopy as previously discussed or observation with frequent monitoring of their hemodynamic status and serial abdominal examinations. Studies have demonstrated that observation in properly selected patients is safe without an increased risk of complications [18].

Special Patient Populations

The Acute Abdomen in the Extremes of Age

Abdominal pain is one of the most common complaints among elderly patients presenting to the emergency department [19]. As the presentation is often different than what is seen in younger patients, the ability to accurately diagnose the underlying cause of their abdominal complaints can be challenging. Elderly patients may lack the febrile response, leukocytosis, and severity of pain expected in those suffering from serious intra-abdominal pathology as a result of the age-dependent decline in immune function [20] along with a well-documented delay in pain perception [21].

The atypical presentation commonly seen in these patients may also be attributed to the effects of other, coexisting medical conditions and medications. For example, beta blockers may blunt the normal tachycardic response to acute abdominal processes while nonsteroidal agents and acetaminophen may prevent the development of a fever. Finally, diagnostic accuracy may be difficult to achieve because of the inability to obtain an adequate history from elderly patients with memory and hearing deficits. Combined, these factors contribute to the increased incidence of complications and increased morbidity and mortality observed in elderly patients presenting with acute abdominal pain. For example, although the incidence of acute appendicitis is lower in this population compared to their younger counterparts, the rate of perforation is significantly higher, reaching almost 70% in some series [22]. Furthermore, complications of acute cholecystitis occur in more than 50% of patients aged 65 or older [23].

Although on the opposite end of the age spectrum, the diagnosis of the acute abdomen in children can be equally as challenging, particularly in children who are preverbal or uncooperative. Further adding to the difficulty is the fact that the etiologies of abdominal pain in children can range from trivial (e.g., constipation) to potentially life-threatening (e.g., malrotation with midgut volvulus) with little to no difference in their presentation [24]. As a result, there are higher rates of misdiagnosis and complications in the pediatric population as well. In fact, the rate of perforation in childhood cases of acute appendicitis is 30–65%, which is significantly higher than what is reported for adults [25].

Overall, physicians should be mindful of the potential challenges posed to them in the evaluation of acute abdominal pain in these extremes of age and adjust their diagnostic approach accordingly.

The Acute Abdomen in Immunocompromised Patients

The ability to make the diagnosis of an acute abdomen is often challenging for those patients who are immunocompromised as a result of conditions such as cancer requiring chemotherapy, transplantation, human immunodeficiency virus/acquired immunodeficiency syndrome (HIV/AIDS), renal failure, diabetes, and malnourishment to name a few.

As a result of their body's inability to launch a full inflammatory response, these patients may have a delayed onset of fever and other typical symptoms, experience less pain, and have an underwhelming leukocytosis [4]. As a result, a diagnosis may not be made until the development of overwhelming sepsis, multisystem organ failure, and death.

It is also important to consider that these patients may suffer from a variety of atypical infections—including ones that are viral (in particular, cytomegalovirus and Epstein–Barr virus infections), mycobacterial, fungal, and protozoal in origin—that may affect the pancreas and hepatobiliary, and gastrointestinal tracts. Furthermore, neutropenic enterocolitis is a common source of acute abdominal pain in patients with bone marrow suppression secondary to chemotherapy [26]. As a result of these challenges unique to this subset of patients, physicians should have a high index of suspicion for an acute abdominal process if such patients present with persistent abdominal complaints even if seemingly mild in intensity. These patients should undergo prompt diagnostic imaging and the possibility of operative intervention should be considered early on.

The Acute Abdomen in the Critically Ill

The acute abdomen in the critically ill presents a diagnostic challenge as even the history and physical exam are often unattainable or unhelpful, especially in those patients who are obtunded, sedated, or intubated. Physicians should therefore have a high index of suspicion and develop a strategy that will allow them to diagnose and treat acute abdominal illnesses in a timely fashion.

Physicians should initially take note of any recent abdominal surgery, the sudden onset of abdominal pain or distension, as well as any changes in laboratory studies or hemodynamic status as indicated by changes in vital signs, an increase in volume requirements, and the need for pressors.

If not contraindicated because of hemodynamic instability or physical constraints, radiologic imaging should be obtained to search for evidence of an acute abdominal process. As is the case for patients who are not critically ill, the sensitivity and specificity for diagnosing certain conditions may vary amongst imaging modalities.

If contraindicated, however, but clinical suspicion is high, then emergent laparotomy is indicated. If there are still doubts however, a less invasive technique such as diagnostic peritoneal lavage (DPL) may be used to assist in decision making. The advantages of DPL include the ability to perform the test at the bedside and the fact that it prevented unnecessary laparotomy in more than 60% of patients in a small series [27, 28]. Overall however, CT is the imaging modality of choice for most intra-abdominal processes, unless a biliary process is suspected for which US is the most sensitive and specific [10].

An acute abdominal condition of the biliary tract more commonly observed in the critically ill is that of acute acalculous cholecystitis. Although the exact etiology is unclear, biliary stasis and gallbladder ischemia with resultant bacterial colonization have been implicated in its development [29]. Such a scenario is common in critically ill patients who are typically not enterally fed and who are hemodynamically unstable.

Acalculous cholecystitis tends to have a more fulminant course and is therefore characterized by increased rates of gallbladder perforation and gangrene [29]. While cholecystectomy is the treatment of choice for this condition, for patients who are critically ill and unable to undergo surgery, percutaneous cholecystostomy is therapeutic until the patient is able to undergo cholecystectomy at a later time. Approximately 90% of patients experience significant improvement after percutaneous cholecystostomy [30].

Another acute abdominal process more prevalent in the critically ill population is that of abdominal compartment syndrome (ACS), which often occurs in the setting of abdominal sepsis coupled with aggressive fluid resuscitation [31]. Characterized by an increased intra-abdominal pressure (IAP) of 20 mmHg or higher, ACS can progress to hemodynamic compromise (due to impaired venous return), difficulties with ventilation and oxygenation (a result of elevated airway pressures), and oliguria (secondary to impaired venous return and renal vein compression) [32]. Treatment involves emergent abdominal fascial decompression.

The Acute Abdomen in the Morbidly Obese

It is often more challenging to diagnose the acute abdomen in morbidly obese patients as a result of the subtle changes in vital signs, atypical symptoms, and underwhelming physical exam findings these patients often present with. A mildly elevated heart rate, fever, nausea, and malaise may be the only indications to the presence of a serious intra-abdominal process. This is further complicated by the constraints created by an obese body habitus that make performing a physical exam and interpreting any exam findings more difficult. By the time the patient is found to have peritonitis, it is often a late finding with the patient at significant risk for the subsequent development of abdominal sepsis, multisystem organ failure, and death [33].

Physicians should also be aware of the fact that an obese body habitus may result in imaging studies being unattainable or more difficult to interpret. Weight limits may render some morbidly obese patients from being eligible to undergo CT or MRI scanning and large amounts of subcutaneous fat can result in poor radiographic and sonographic image quality [34]. As a result of these challenges, a high index of suspicion should be employed when making treatment decisions, in particular, whether to operate or not. Note that with the advent of laparoscopy and the development of bariatric laparoscopic ports and instruments less invasive measures may be taken to both diagnose and treat the source of the patient's symptoms [35].

The Acute Abdomen in Pregnant Patients

When evaluating a pregnant patient who presents with abdominal pain, one must keep in mind that delays in diagnosis and subsequent intervention can result in an increased risk of morbidity and mortality for both the patient and her unborn fetus.

Delays in presentation, diagnosis, and treatment may occur because many of the presenting signs and symptoms may mimic those normally observed in pregnancy, including abdominal pain, nausea, vomiting, and anorexia. In addition, vital signs and laboratory findings may be more difficult to interpret as they are routinely altered in pregnancy. There is notably a "physiologic anemia" in pregnancy in addition to mild leukocytosis. Additionally, there is typically a 10–15 bpm increase in pulse rate as well as relative hypotension as a result of hormone-mediated vasodilation [36].

The examining physician must also take into account that the presentation of certain disease processes and physical exam findings may differ in the pregnant patient as a result of the upward displacement of the gravid uterus. A classic example of this is seen in the case of acute appendicitis, in which tenderness may be palpated in the RUQ. Appendicitis is the most common nonobstetrical cause of the acute abdomen, complicating 1 in 1,500 births [37]. Although the overall incidence is similar to that of nonpregnant patients, the rate of perforation is higher at approximately 25%, presumably due to delays in diagnosis and intervention. If and when perforation occurs, the risk of both fetal and maternal mortality increases significantly [38].

Delays may occur because of hesitancy on the part of the physician to obtain certain radiologic studies like that of plain films or CT scans due to the concerns of the radiation exposure associated with these modalities. Ultrasound is therefore used as the initial imaging study in most evaluations of the pregnant acute abdomen [39]. In addition to fetal evaluation, ultrasound is the imaging study of choice for assessment of the biliary tract, pancreas, kidneys, and adnexa. In addition, multiple studies have shown that when paired with graded compression, ultrasound has a sensitivity between 67 and 100% and a specificity between 83 and 96% for diagnosing acute appendicitis in pregnancy [40].

If the diagnosis remains uncertain, CT scan is an acceptable alternative means of imaging the pregnant abdomen if used judiciously in order to minimize ionizing radiation exposure [41]. Although the estimated conceptus dose from a single CT acquisition is 25 mGy [42], as per the 1995 American College of Obstetricians and Gynecologists (ACOG) consensus statement, "Women should be counseled that X-ray exposure from a single diagnostic procedure does not result in harmful fetal effects. Specifically, exposure to less than 5 rad (50 mGy) has not been associated with an increase in fetal anomalies or pregnancy loss."[43] Ultimately, the use of CT scans as a secondary imaging tool in pregnancy can lead to a more timely diagnosis of acute appendicitis resulting in decreased rates of perforation. This along with the decreased rate of negative appendectomies observed in expectant women undergoing US followed by CT scan [44] likely reduces the risk of mortality for both the mother and fetus significantly.

MRI, which uses magnets instead of ionizing radiation, has also been shown recently to be of use in evaluating abdominal pain during pregnancy when ultrasonagraphy was deemed inconclusive [15]. Despite this however, MRI is not always readily available for emergent evaluations and the effects of using gadolinium-based contrast, which crosses the placenta, have yet to be determined and it is not approved for use in pregnancy, unlike iodinated CT contrast agents [14].

Once diagnosed, patients should undergo appendectomy. Despite initial concerns of the safety of such an approach, laparoscopy has been accepted as safe with the same advantages afforded for nonpregnant patients, including shorter hospitalizations and less narcotic medication needs [45]. Of course certain precautions should be taken to ensure safety, including using an open Hasson approach to enter the abdomen, a left tilted position, maintaining a CO_2 insufflation of 10–15 mmHg, and monitoring fetal heart tones during the procedure [46].

After appendicitis, the next most common nonobstetric cause of acute abdominal pain are disorders of the biliary tract, notably acute cholecystitis and gallstone pancreatitis. The incidence of acute cholecystitis ranges from 1 in 6,000 to 1 in 10,000 births [37]. Presenting symptoms, diagnostic workup, and treatment are similar to their nonpregnant counterparts. As previously stated, laboratory values may be more difficult to interpret, especially in the case of acute cholecystitis as white blood cell counts and alkaline phosphatase levels are normally elevated during pregnancy [37]. As is the case in nonpregnant patients, acute cholecystitis is usually treated conservatively early on with intravenous fluid hydration, bowel rest, pain control, and antibiotics. If the patient fails to respond to medical management, then surgery is indicated. Failing to operate on these patients in a timely fashion significantly increases the risk of preterm labor and fetal loss [47].

Regardless of whether patients respond appropriately to conservative management, the majority of surgeons still recommend surgery during pregnancy to prevent any recurrence or any complications that may pose a threat to the fetus [47].

In fact, the rate of fetal demise with gallstone pancreatitis has been reported to be as high as 60% [48]. As is the case with acute appendicitis, laparoscopic cholecystectomy has been deemed safe to perform during pregnancy without any increased risk of morbidity or mortality to the mother or fetus [49].

The Acute Abdomen from a Global Perspective

The acute abdomen can be especially concerning from a global health perspective. The low density of adequately trained physicians and quality treatment facilities in developing countries means long delays between symptom onset and treatment, resulting in worse outcomes [50, 51]. Proper management of the acute abdomen in these regions may be further complicated by the lack of modern radiographic and other diagnostic modalities, which may render contemporary treatment algorithms unusable. As a result, increased emphasis should be placed on careful history taking and physical exam skills. Findings of abdominal distension, abdominal masses, deranged vital signs, guarding, and a positive vaginal/rectal examination have been associated with worse outcomes in these regions, warranting further investigation [52]. In areas where advanced clinicians are unavailable, a standardized questionnaire may help in establishing a differential diagnosis in patients presenting with acute abdominal pain.

There is a lack of consensus on the overall incidence of the acute abdomen in the developing world, likely as a result of the range of locations which fall into this category (e.g., Southeast Asia, Sub-Saharan Africa, and Central America) in addition to various socioeconomic, dietary, cultural, and environmental differences. Despite this, some generalizations about the most common causes of the acute abdomen in impoverished regions can be made. Many are shared with those of developed nations, including acute appendicitis and intestinal obstruction, which account for up to 25 and 35% of all cases, respectively [52]. Other commonly shared causes of the acute abdomen include acute cholecystitis, gynecological disorders (e.g., ectopic pregnancy, uterine rupture, and tubo-ovarian abscesses), trauma (most commonly from gunshot wounds and car accidents), and perforated peptic ulcers [53, 54].

In addition to these conditions, physicians in developing countries must consider other exotic causes of acute abdominal pain, including typhoid enteritis, abdominal tuberculosis, and parasitic infections, which can themselves cause acute intestinal obstructions, appendicitis, cholangitis, and liver abscesses [55]. Typhoid, which usually presents with high fever, abdominal distension, and delirium, remains endemic in impoverished parts of the world [56]. Caused by the bacterium *Salmonella typhi*, typhoid fever is transmitted through fecal contamination of food or water supplies. If not identified and treated in a timely fashion with the appropriate antibiotics, typhoid can result in intestinal

hemorrhage or perforation—two potentially fatal causes of an acute abdomen requiring surgical intervention [56]. In one series, typhoid fever complicated by ileal perforation was diagnosed in 16% of patients in a region of West Africa, making it the second most common cause of the acute abdomen [51].

A large number of acute abdominal cases in developing countries are caused by parasitic infections, which like that of typhoid fever are typically acquired through fecal-oral transmission. In one study originating from West Africa, some 4% of acute abdominal cases necessitating emergency surgery were attributable to parasites [57]. The majority of these were secondary to infections with members of the amoeba family, which can cause colitis and hepatic abscesses, or *Ascaris lumbricoides*, a species of roundworms that can invade and overwhelm the gastrointestinal and hepatobiliary systems, resulting in intestinal obstruction, appendicitis, pancreatitis, and cholecystitis [58]. In addition to emergent surgical intervention, patients should be treated with antiparasitic medications to ensure complete eradication of disease.

Overall, the acute abdomen poses diagnostic challenges unique to the developing world given the limited access to resources and personnel required to sufficiently treat patients with potentially life-threatening abdominal conditions. Compounding this are the other exotic causes of acute abdominal pain prevalent in these regions that one must consider in their workup. Therefore, in addition to enhancing access to healthcare, health education, and sanitation, attention should be placed on the development of adequate history taking and physical exam skills to improve the outcomes of patients presenting with an acute abdomen in these regions of the world.

Potential Complications and Outcomes

The outcomes of patients presenting with an acute abdomen are influenced by the underlying etiology of their symptoms, age, comorbid conditions, and the time to diagnosis and treatment. In terms of etiology, one could assume that a patient with a noncontained hollow viscus perforation is likely to have higher rates of morbidity and mortality in the peri- and postoperative period compared to a patient presenting with acute, nonperforated appendicitis. With regard to age and health status, diminished physiologic reserve and an increased incidence of comorbidities place elderly patients at an elevated risk of complications and death compared to their younger counterparts. For example, the age-related decline in pulmonary function is associated with a prolonged need for mechanical ventilation and an increased risk of developing ventilator-associated pneumonias [59]. These issues are compounded by the fact that elderly patients tend to have delays in diagnosis and treatment, further contributing to their increased rates of morbidity and mortality. In the case of perforated PUD, older patients who underwent surgery more than 24 h after perforation were eight times more likely to die compared to those who were operated on within 4 h [60].

Morbidly obese patients with an acute abdomen are also at an increased risk of poor outcomes due to atypical presentations and the challenges posed by their body habitus that result in treatment delays [33]. Even in cases where surgery is indicated and performed in a timely manner, higher rates of postoperative complications including surgical wound infections and multisystem organ failure are experienced by morbidly obese patients [61].

In pregnant patients, the acute abdomen poses significant risks to both the mother and fetus. Atypical presentations and the inability to distinguish some acute abdominal symptoms from those normally experienced during pregnancy can result in treatment delays and an increased susceptibility for preterm labor and fetal loss [38].

In general, regardless of age or health status, patients presenting with an acute abdomen should undergo a thorough yet expeditious evaluation to help establish a diagnosis and initiate the therapeutic interventions necessary to help ensure positive outcomes for these patients.

References

1. Kamin RA, Nowicki TA, Courtney DS, Powers RD. Pearls and pitfalls in the emergency department evaluation of abdominal pain. Emerg Med Clin North Am. 2003;21(1):61–72. vi.
2. Leung AK, Sigalet DL. Acute abdominal pain in children. Am Fam Physician. 2003;67(11):2321–6.
3. Hendrickson M, Naparst TR. Abdominal surgical emergencies in the elderly. Emerg Med Clin North Am. 2003;21(4):937–69.
4. Sabiston DC, Townsend CM. Acute abdomen. Sabiston textbook of surgery: the biological basis of modern surgical practice. 18th ed. Philadelphia: Saunders/Elsevier; 2008. p. 1180–96.
5. Nagle A. Acute abdominal pain. In: Ashley S, Wilmore DW, Klingensmith ME, Cance WG, Napolitano LM, Jurkovich GJ, Pearce WH, Pemberton JH, Soper NJ, editors. ACS surgery: principles and practice 2011. BC Decker: Chicago, IL, 2011.
6. Newton E, Mandavia S. Surgical complications of selected gastrointestinal emergencies: pitfalls in management of the acute abdomen. Emerg Med Clin North Am. 2003;21(4):873–907. viii.
7. Chase CW, Barker DE, Russell WL, Burns RP. Serum amylase and lipase in the evaluation of acute abdominal pain. Am Surg. 1996;62(12):1028–33.
8. MacKersie AB, Lane MJ, Gerhardt RT, Claypool HA, Keenan S, Katz DS, et al. Nontraumatic acute abdominal pain: unenhanced helical CT compared with three-view acute abdominal series. Radiology. 2005;237(1):114–22.
9. Vasavada P. Ultrasound evaluation of acute abdominal emergencies in infants and children. Radiol Clin North Am. 2004;42(2):445–56.
10. Shea JA, Berlin JA, Escarce JJ, Clarke JR, Kinosian BP, Cabana MD, et al. Revised estimates of diagnostic test sensitivity and specificity in suspected biliary tract disease. Arch Intern Med. 1994;154(22):2573–81.
11. Frates MC, Laing FC. Sonographic evaluation of ectopic pregnancy: an update. AJR Am J Roentgenol. 1995;165(2):251–9.
12. Levin DC, Rao VM, Parker L, Frangos AJ, Sunshine JH. Ownership or leasing of CT scanners by nonradiologist physicians: a rapidly growing trend that raises concern about self-referral. J Am Coll Radiol. 2008;5(12):1206–9.
13. Raman SS, Osuagwu FC, Kadell B, Cryer H, Sayre J, Lu DS. Effect of CT on false positive diagnosis of appendicitis and perforation. N Engl J Med. 2008;358(9):972–3.
14. Singh A, Danrad R, Hahn PF, Blake MA, Mueller PR, Novelline RA. MR imaging of the acute abdomen and pelvis: acute appendicitis and beyond. Radiographics. 2007;27(5):1419–31.
15. Pedrosa I, Levine D, Eyvazzadeh AD, Siewert B, Ngo L, Rofsky NM. MR imaging evaluation of acute appendicitis in pregnancy. Radiology. 2006;238(3):891–9.
16. Majewski W. Diagnostic laparoscopy for the acute abdomen and trauma. Surg Endosc. 2000;14(10):930–7.
17. Salky BA, Edye MB. The role of laparoscopy in the diagnosis and treatment of abdominal pain syndromes. Surg Endosc. 1998; 12(7):911–4.
18. Thomson HJ, Jones PF. Active observation in acute abdominal pain. Am J Surg. 1986;152(5):522–5.
19. de Dombal FT. Acute abdominal pain in the elderly. J Clin Gastroenterol. 1994;19(4):331–5.
20. Martinez JP, Mattu A. Abdominal pain in the elderly. Emerg Med Clin North Am. 2006;24(2):371–88. vii.
21. Sherman ED, Robillard E. Sensitivity to pain in the aged. Can Med Assoc J. 1960;83(18):944–7.
22. Yamini D, Vargas H, Bongard F, Klein S, Stamos MJ. Perforated appendicitis: is it truly a surgical urgency? Am Surg. 1998; 64(10):970–5.
23. Rothrock SG, Greenfield RH, Falk JL. Acute abdominal emergencies in the elderly: clinical evaluation and management. Part II—diagnosis and management of common conditions. Emerg Med Rep. 1992;13:185–92.
24. Bundy DG, Byerley JS, Liles EA, Perrin EM, Katznelson J, Rice HE. Does this child have appendicitis? JAMA. 2007;298(4): 438–51.
25. McCollough M, Sharieff GQ. Abdominal pain in children. Pediatr Clin North Am. 2006;53(1):107–37. vi.
26. Scott-Conner CE, Fabrega AJ. Gastrointestinal problems in the immunocompromised host. A review for surgeons. Surg Endosc. 1996;10(10):959–64.
27. Amoroso TA. Evaluation of the patient with blunt abdominal trauma: an evidence based approach. Emerg Med Clin North Am. 1999;17(1):63–75. viii.
28. Walsh RM, Popovich MJ, Hoadley J. Bedside diagnostic laparoscopy and peritoneal lavage in the intensive care unit. Surg Endosc. 1998;12(12):1405–9.
29. Barie PS, Eachempati SR. Acute acalculous cholecystitis. Gastroenterol Clin North Am. 2010;39(2):343–57. x.
30. Patterson EJ, McLoughlin RF, Mathieson JR, Cooperberg PL, MacFarlane JK. An alternative approach to acute cholecystitis. Percutaneous cholecystostomy and interval laparoscopic cholecystectomy. Surg Endosc. 1996;10(12):1185–8.
31. Sugrue M, Buhkari Y. Intra-abdominal pressure and abdominal compartment syndrome in acute general surgery. World J Surg. 2009;33(6):1123–7.
32. Ertel W, Oberholzer A, Platz A, Stocker R, Trentz O. Incidence and clinical pattern of the abdominal compartment syndrome after "damage-control" laparotomy in 311 patients with severe abdominal and/or pelvic trauma. Crit Care Med. 2000;28(6):1747–53.
33. Byrne TK. Complications of surgery for obesity. Surg Clin North Am. 2001;81(5):1181–93. vii–viii.
34. Uppot RN, Sahani DV, Hahn PF, Gervais D, Mueller PR. Impact of obesity on medical imaging and image-guided intervention. AJR Am J Roentgenol. 2007;188(2):433–40.

35. Geis WP, Kim HC. Use of laparoscopy in the diagnosis and treatment of patients with surgical abdominal sepsis. Surg Endosc. 1995;9(2):178–82.
36. Stone K. Acute abdominal emergencies associated with pregnancy. Clin Obstet Gynecol. 2002;45(2):553–61.
37. Sharp HT. The acute abdomen during pregnancy. Clin Obstet Gynecol. 2002;45(2):405–13.
38. Cappell MS, Friedel D. Abdominal pain during pregnancy. Gastroenterol Clin North Am. 2003;32(1):1–58.
39. Glanc P, Maxwell C. Acute abdomen in pregnancy: role of sonography. J Ultrasound Med. 2010;29(10):1457–68.
40. Williams R, Shaw J. Ultrasound scanning in the diagnosis of acute appendicitis in pregnancy. Emerg Med J. 2007;24(5):359–60.
41. Patel SJ, Reede DL, Katz DS, Subramaniam R, Amorosa JK. Imaging the pregnant patient for nonobstetric conditions: algorithms and radiation dose considerations. Radiographics. 2007;27(6):1705–22.
42. McCollough CH, Schueler BA, Atwell TD, Braun NN, Regner DM, Brown DL, et al. Radiation exposure and pregnancy: when should we be concerned? Radiographics. 2007;27(4):909–17. discussion 17–8.
43. Guidelines for diagnostic imaging during pregnancy. The American College of Obstetricians and Gynecologists. Int J Gynaecol Obstet. 1995;51(3):288–91.
44. Wallace CA, Petrov MS, Soybel DI, Ferzoco SJ, Ashley SW, Tavakkolizadeh A. Influence of imaging on the negative appendectomy rate in pregnancy. J Gastrointest Surg. 2008;12(1):46–50.
45. Curet MJ, Allen D, Josloff RK, Pitcher DE, Curet LB, Miscall BG, et al. Laparoscopy during pregnancy. Arch Surg. 1996;131(5):546–50. discussion 50–1.
46. Yumi H. Guidelines for diagnosis, treatment, and use of laparoscopy for surgical problems during pregnancy: this statement was reviewed and approved by the Board of Governors of the Society of American Gastrointestinal and Endoscopic Surgeons (SAGES), September 2007. It was prepared by the SAGES Guidelines Committee. Surg Endosc. 2008;22(4):849–61.
47. Dixon NP, Faddis DM, Silberman H. Aggressive management of cholecystitis during pregnancy. Am J Surg. 1987;154(3):292–4.
48. Printen KJ, Ott RA. Cholecystectomy during pregnancy. Am Surg. 1978;44(7):432–4.
49. Jackson H, Granger S, Price R, Rollins M, Earle D, Richardson W, et al. Diagnosis and laparoscopic treatment of surgical diseases during pregnancy: an evidence-based review. Surg Endosc. 2008;22(9):1917–27.
50. Adamu A, Maigatari M, Lawal K, Iliyasu M. Waiting time for emergency abdominal surgery in Zaria, Nigeria. Afr Health Sci. 2010;10(1):46–53.
51. Ohene-Yeboah M. Acute surgical admissions for abdominal pain in adults in Kumasi, Ghana. ANZ J Surg. 2006;76(10):898–903.
52. Nega B. Pattern of acute abdomen and variables associated with adverse outcome in a rural primary hospital setting. Ethiop Med J. 2009;47(2):143–51.
53. Al-Gamrah A. Diagnostic and therapeutic management of acute abdomen in Hajah, Yemen. Chirurg. 2004;75(6):622–6.
54. McConkey SJ. Case series of acute abdominal surgery in rural Sierra Leone. World J Surg. 2002;26(4):509–13.
55. Asefa Z. Pattern of acute abdomen in Yirgalem Hospital, southern Ethiopia. Ethiop Med J. 2000;38(4):227–35.
56. Parry CM, Hien TT, Dougan G, White NJ, Farrar JJ. Typhoid fever. N Engl J Med. 2002;347(22):1770–82.
57. Essomba A, Chichom Mefire A, Fokou M, Ouassouo P, Masso Misse P, Esiene A, et al. Acute abdomens of parasitic origin: retrospective analysis of 135 cases. Ann Chir. 2006;131(3):194–7.
58. Khuroo MS. Ascariasis. Gastroenterol Clin North Am. 1996;25(3):553–77.
59. Nielson C, Wingett D. Intensive care and invasive ventilation in the elderly patient, implications of chronic lung disease and comorbidities. Chron Respir Dis. 2004;1(1):43–54.
60. Svanes C. Trends in perforated peptic ulcer: incidence, etiology, treatment, and prognosis. World J Surg. 2000;24(3):277–83.
61. Duchesne JC, Schmieg Jr RE, Simmons JD, Islam T, McGinness CL, McSwain Jr NE. Impact of obesity in damage control laparotomy patients. J Trauma. 2009;67(1):108–12. discussion 12–4.

Jacquelyn K. O'Herrin

Introduction

For patients who require emergency surgical intervention, the management of significant medical comorbidities requires rapid coordination between the surgeon, the anesthesiologist, and the primary medical team. Perioperative care is as important to the final outcome of the patient as the operation itself. Attention to detail and appropriate management of comorbidities is integral to optimizing outcomes for the acute surgical patient. An accurate preoperative assessment helps to avoid obvious pitfalls such as a critical medication allergy or a difficult airway.

The actual perioperative period is poorly defined, and surgical literature relating to the perioperative period is scarce compared to intraoperative and postoperative care; possibly due to that fact that a great deal of this care is provided by non-surgeons. However, the individual providing perioperative care must be knowledgeable and expert at the management of surgical physiology. It is therefore imperative that the surgeon be aware and involved in the perioperative care and decision making of each acute surgical patient in order to optimize outcomes and potentially avert complications.

Although there is not a standard definition of the perioperative period per se, it essentially begins at the time the decision is made to take a patient to surgery. This time period may be as brief as the few minutes required to take an unstable trauma patient to the operating room or for several weeks in the setting of an elective procedure in a patient with comorbidities. Obtaining an adequate medical history is always advantageous in the care of these patients. However, this is often difficult when the patients are compromised by their acute disease. They may also be elderly, poor historians, or residents of extended care facilities.

J.K. O'Herrin, M.D., F.A.C.S. (✉)
Department of Surgery, University of Oklahoma,
920 Stanton L Young Boulevard, WP Suite 2140,
Oklahoma City, OK 73126, USA
e-mail: jackie-oherrin@ouhsc.edu

Knowledge of a patient's baseline mental status is important as it allows the clinician to determine deviations from baseline in the postoperative period as an early indicator of potential complications. Knowledge of the patient's preoperative functional status is helpful in predicting ultimate recovery from the disease process, as well as the time frame for recovery. The effects of medication should be considered as these may block physiologic responses; for example, β (beta)-blockers mask tachycardia and are taken commonly in patients with hypertension or known coronary artery disease. Warfarin, aspirin, and clopidogrel are also common medications among the elderly that negatively impact surgical bleeding and postoperative renal function. In the acute general surgery patient, these factors must all be weighed in the decision to either proceed directly to the operating room, take time to resuscitate the patient and/or address comorbidities. In some cases, this period may identify factors or changes in a patient's condition that render an operative intervention.

Perioperative Cardiovascular Assessment

Recent studies [1, 2] suggest that more than 200 million patients worldwide have major noncardiac surgical procedures each year. Patients undergoing noncardiac surgery are at risk of major perioperative cardiac events such as cardiac death, myocardial infarction (MI), and nonfatal cardiac arrest. Aortic and peripheral vascular surgery, orthopedic surgery, and major intrathoracic or intraperitoneal procedures are more frequently associated with perioperative cardiac mortality than are other types of surgery [3]. Without a prior known history of cardiac disease, men are at increased risk for cardiac complications above age 35, whereas women are at increased risk above age 40. Mortality in both genders increases markedly over age 70.

Cardiac complications after noncardiac surgery reflect factors specific to the patient, the operation, and the circumstances surrounding the procedure. Perioperative

L.J. Moore et al. (eds.), *Common Problems in Acute Care Surgery*,
DOI 10.1007/978-1-4614-6123-4_3, © Springer Science+Business Media New York 2013

cardiac evaluation may lead to interventions that lower perioperative risk, decrease long-term mortality, or alter the surgical decision making process. Such alterations may include either choosing a lower risk, less invasive procedure, opting for a "damage control" rather than definitive procedure, or electing for nonoperative management. Although different procedures are associated with different cardiac risks (Table 3.1), these differences are most often a reflection of the context in which the patient undergoes surgery (stability or opportunity for adequate preoperative resuscitation or preparation), surgery specific factors such as fluid shifts, stress levels, the duration of the procedure or blood loss, or patient specific factors such as coronary artery disease and symptoms.

To minimize operative risk, the patient is ideally in optimal medical condition. In the acute care setting, however, the luxury of an elective preoperative cardiac evaluation is not often available. A careful history and physical exam in the emergency setting can alert the surgeon to opportunities to intervene and physiologically optimize the patient in order to decrease the risk of morbidity and mortality. Congestive heart failure, poorly controlled hypertension (diastolic blood pressure >110 mmHg), electrolyte imbalances, and hyperglycemia must be addressed prior to any operative intervention when possible. In general, cardiovascular medications should be continued through the perioperative period, as continuation of antihypertensive and beta-blocker therapy throughout the perioperative period does not typically contribute to postoperative hemodynamic instability. Discontinuation of antihypertensive therapy increases potential risks. Rebound hypertension may be precipitated if centrally acting α (alpha)-2 agonists such as clonidine are suddenly withheld. Congestive heart failure may recur or be exacerbated if angiotensin-converting enzyme inhibitors or angiotensin receptor blockades are stopped. β (beta)-blockade must be continued throughout the perioperative time period.

Patients who experience postoperative MI after noncardiac surgery have an estimated hospital mortality rate of 15–25%. Patients who have a cardiac arrest after noncardiac surgery have a hospital mortality rate of 65% [4]. Of these major vascular complications, MI is the most common [5]. The diagnosis of acute MI in the nonsurgical setting traditionally requires the presence of at least two of the following three elements: ischemic chest pain, evolutionary changes on the electrocardiogram (ECG), and rise and fall of cardiac biomarker levels (troponin). In the perioperative period, ischemic episodes are often silent (not associated with a patient complaint of chest pain) in up to 65% of patients with documented postoperative MI [2]. Additionally, many perioperative ECGs reflect nonspecific changes, and are therefore nondiagnostic. These nonspecific ECG changes, coupled with new onset dysrhythmias and

Table 3.1 Cardiac risk[a] stratification for noncardiac surgical procedures

Risk stratification	Procedure examples
Vascular (reported cardiac risk often more than 5%)	Aortic and other major vascular surgery
	Peripheral vascular surgery
Intermediate (reported cardiac risk generally 1–5%)	Intraperitoneal and intrathoracic surgery
	Carotid endarterectomy
	Head and neck surgery
	Orthopedic surgery
	Prostate surgery
Low[b] (reported cardiac risk generally less than 1%)	Endoscopic procedures
	Superficial procedure
	Cataract surgery
	Breast surgery
	Ambulatory surgery

Reprinted with permission from Fleisher LA, Beckman JA, Brown KA, et al. ACC/AHA 2007 guidelines on perioperative cardiovascular evaluation and care for noncardiac surgery: A Report of the American College of Cardiology/American Heart Association Task Force on Practice Guidelines. J Am Coll Cardiol. 2007;50(17):1707–1732

[a]Combined incidence of cardiac death and nonfatal myocardial infarction

[b]These procedures do not generally require further preoperative cardiac testing

noncardiac related hemodynamic instability, can further obscure the clinical picture of MI or acute coronary syndrome in the perioperative period.

In the perioperative setting, as in the nonoperative setting, an acute increase in troponin levels should be considered an acute MI. An increase in cardiac troponin is a marker of myocardial injury, and there is a good correlation between the duration of myocardial ischemia and the increase in cardiac-specific troponin [6, 7]. There is also a significant association between increased troponin levels and short- and long-term morbidity and mortality in surgical patients. This association exists for cardiac death, MI, myocardial ischemia, congestive heart failure, cardiac dysrhythmias, and cerebrovascular accident. Even relatively minor cardiovascular complications such as uncontrolled hypertension, palpitations, increased fatigue, or shortness of breath are correlated to increased levels of cardiac-specific troponins. An increase in troponin postoperatively, even in the absence of clear cardiovascular signs and symptoms, is an important finding that requires careful attention and further investigation and management.

Multiple physiologic triggers that have the potential to exacerbate underlying cardiac disease exist in the perioperative period (Fig. 3.1). Surgery, with its associated trauma, anesthesia, narcotics, intubation, extubation, pain, hypothermia, bleeding, and anemia is analogous to an extreme stress test. These variables all initiate inflammatory, hypercoagulable, stress, and hypoxic states, which are associated with perioperative elevations in troponin levels, arterial thrombosis, and morbidity/mortality [8–11].

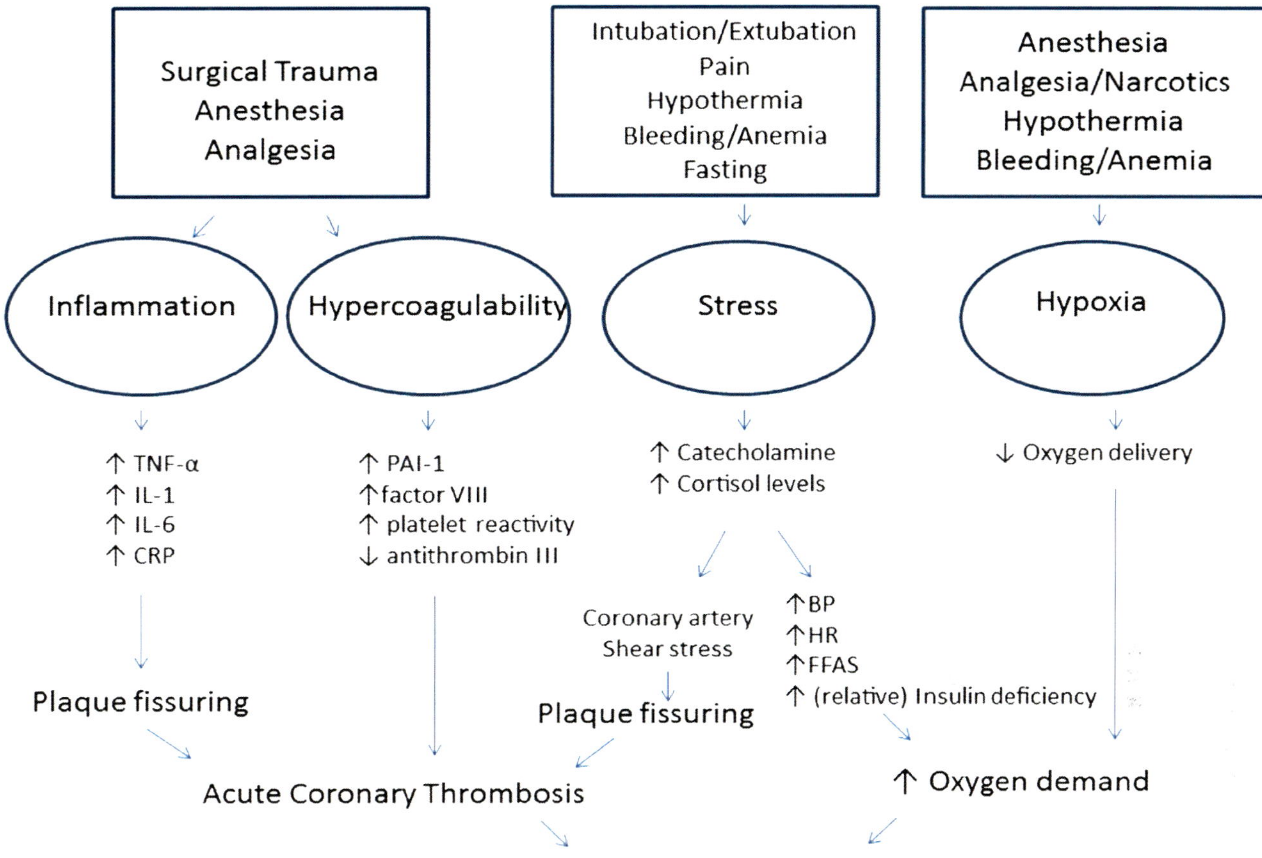

Fig. 3.1 Potential triggers of states associated with perioperative elevations in troponin levels, arterial thrombosis and fatal myocardial infarction. *TNF-α (alpha)* tumor necrosis factor α (alpha), *IL* interleukin, *CRP* C-reactive protein, *PAI-1* plasminogen activator inhibitor-1, *BP* blood pressure, *HR* heart rate, *FFAs* free fatty acids. Adapted from [4]

Lee et al. derived and validated a "simple index" for the prediction of cardiac risk for stable patients undergoing major non cardiac surgery [12]. Although this study was done in the setting of nonurgent major noncardiac surgery, the following risk factors can and should be assessed in the setting of acute or emergent surgical intervention. Five independent risk correlates were identified:

1. Ischemic heart disease (history of MI, history of positive treadmill test, use of nitroglycerin, current angina, or ECG with abnormal Q waves)
2. Congestive heart failure (history of heart failure, pulmonary edema, paroxysmal nocturnal dyspnea, peripheral edema, bilateral rales)
3. High-risk surgery (abdominal aortic aneurysm or other high-risk vascular, thoracic, abdominal, or orthopedic surgery—see Table 3.1)
4. Preoperative insulin dependence for diabetes mellitus, and
5. Preoperative creatinine greater than 2 mg/dL.

Increasing numbers of risk factors correlates with increased risk. This Revised Cardiac Risk Index has become one of the most widely used risk indices (Fig. 3.2).

Currently, there are no standard diagnostic criteria for perioperative MI in patients undergoing noncardiac surgery. The diagnosis of perioperative MI can be difficult as many are clinically silent, non transmural (non-Q-wave), and therefore have minimal accompanying ECG changes. On the basis of available literature, routine measurement of cardiac-specific troponin after surgery is more likely to identify patients without acute MI than with MI [13]. Additionally, studies of cardiac-specific troponin elevations neither consistently show associations with adverse cardiovascular outcomes at any time point nor provide insight into the effect of treatment on long-term or functional outcomes. Although it is known that patients with more extensive CAD are more likely to experience elevation in perioperative troponin levels, the role of revascularization in this population when no other manifestations of MI is unclear.

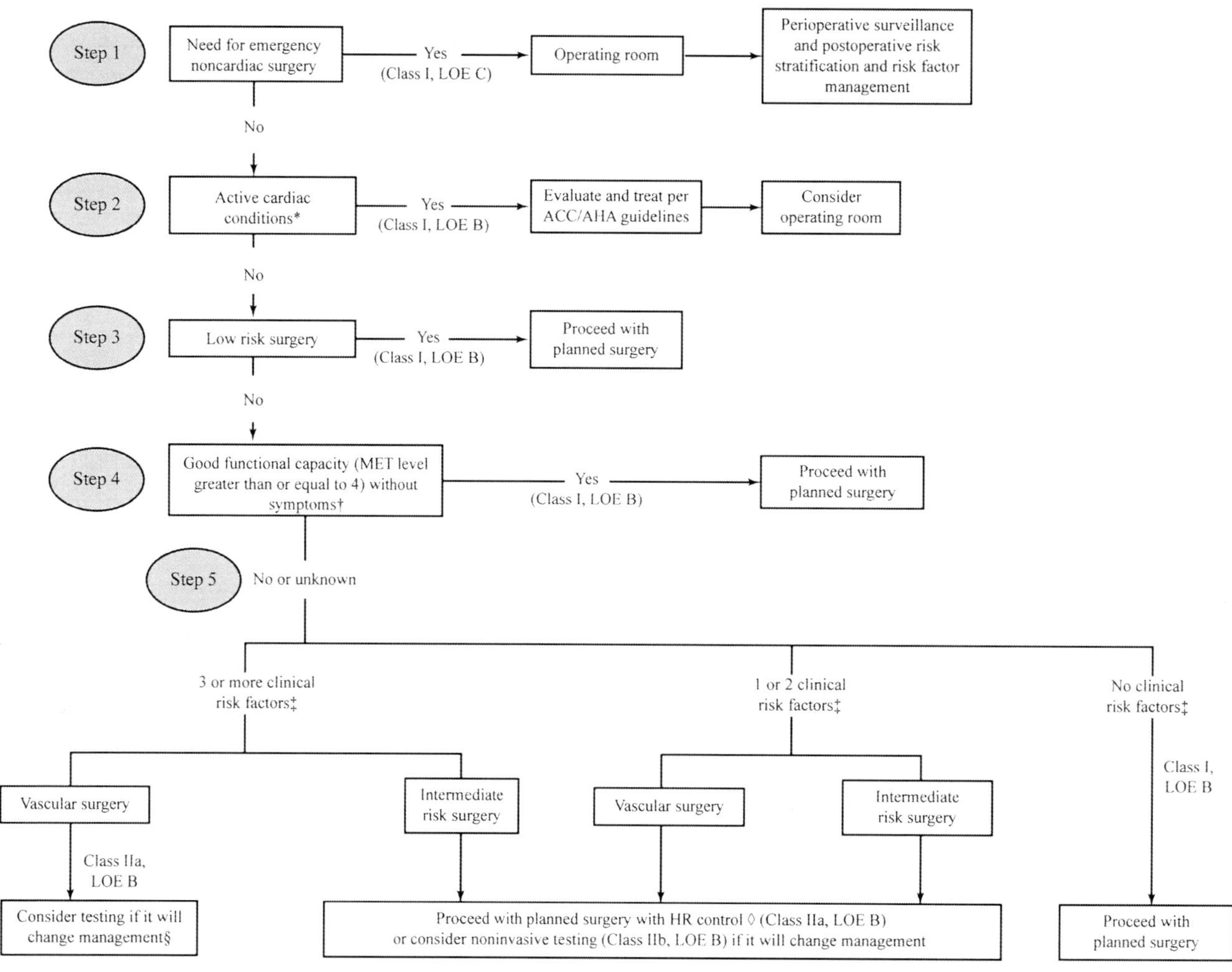

Fig. 3.2 Cardiac evaluation and care algorithm for noncardiac surgery. *Asterisk* Active clinical conditions: Unstable coronary syndromes, decompensated HF, significant arrhythmias, or severe valvular disease. *Dagger* Met 1 = Activities of Daily Living; Met 4 = heavy housework or climb a flight of stairs; Met 10 = strenuous exercise *Section* Noninvasive testing may be considered before surgery in specific patients with risk factors if it will change management. *Double dagger* Clinical risk factors include ischemic heart disease, compensated or prior heart failure, diabetes mellitus, renal insufficiency, and cerebrovascular disease. *Open diamond* Consider perioperative beta blockade. *ACC/AHA* American College of Cardiology/American Heart Association, *HR* heart rate, *LOE* level of evidence, *MET* metabolic equivalent. Modified with permission from Fleisher LA, Beckman JA, Brown KA, et al. ACC/AHA 2007 Guidelines on Perioperative Cardiovascular Evaluation and Care for Noncardiac Surgery: A Report of the American College of Cardiology/American Heart Association Task Force on Practice Guidelines. J Am Coll Cardiol. 2007;50(17): 1707–1732

Additionally, revascularization in this setting may lead to postoperative complications such as bleeding due to initiation of antiplatelet therapy. Until the aforementioned issues are adequately studied and addressed, perioperative surveillance for acute coronary syndromes with routine ECG and cardiac serum biomarkers is unnecessary in clinically low-risk patients undergoing low risk procedures [14].

The presence of intraoperative and postoperative ST-segment changes has been associated with cardiac morbidity and mortality in high-risk patients undergoing noncardiac surgery. Numerous studies have demonstrated the limited ability of physicians to detect significant ST-segment changes compared with computerized analysis, and allows for trending of the data. Because the algorithms used to measure ST-segment shifts are proprietary, variability in accuracy between different monitors has been evaluated in several studies [15–17]. ST-segment trending monitors were found to have an average sensitivity of 74% and specificity of 73%, compared to offline Holter ECG recordings [16].

Retrospective data from multiple studies suggest that ST-segment depression is an independent predictor of perioperative cardiac events in high-risk noncardiac surgery patients. Changes of prolonged duration (greater than 30 min per episode or greater than 2 h cumulative duration) are particularly associated with increased risk [18–21]. Postoperative ST-segment changes, particularly of a prolonged duration, have been shown to predict worse long-term survival in high-risk patients [22, 23]. However, because intraoperative

ST-segment changes may also be detected in the low-risk population, but are not associated with regional wall motion abnormality, ST-segment changes in this low-risk population may not be indicative of myocardial ischemia and CAD [24, 25]. Therefore, although there are data to support the use of ST-segment analysis to detect ischemia, no studies have yet addressed the issue of effect on patient outcome when therapy is based on these results alone. However, the general consensus of the American College of Cardiology (ACC) and the American Heart Association (AHA) is that early treatment, such as control of tachycardia, could lead to a reduction in cardiac morbidity [14].

Further evaluation regarding the optimal strategy for surveillance and diagnosis of perioperative MI is required. The current recommendations of the ACC/AHA, on the basis of current evidence, are for patients without documented coronary artery disease (CAD), surveillance should be restricted to those who develop perioperative signs of cardiovascular dysfunction. In patients with intermediate or high clinical risk who have known or suspected CAD and who are undergoing high- or intermediate-risk surgical procedures, the most cost effective strategy is to obtain a baseline (preoperative) ECG followed by an ECG in the immediate postoperative period and daily on the first and second postoperative day. If ECG changes are noted the use of cardiac-specific troponin measurements to supplement the diagnosis is warranted [15].

Once an intraoperative or postoperative MI has been correctly detected and diagnosed, it is important to recognize that the occurrence of a perioperative nonfatal MI carries a high risk for future cardiac events and cardiac related death [23, 26]. Patients who do sustain a perioperative MI should have evaluation of left ventricular function performed prior to hospital discharge, and standard post infarction medical therapy should be initiated. The use of pharmacological stress or dynamic exercise stress test should be obtained when feasible to assess risk stratification for possible coronary revascularization. In all cases, appropriate evaluation and management of complications and risk factors such as angina, heart failure, hypertension, hyperlipidemia, cigarette smoking, hyperglycemia or diabetes mellitus, and other cardiac abnormalities should occur prior to hospital discharge. Additionally, it is imperative to communicate these new observations and interventions to physician and nonphysician providers who will be responsible for the patient's subsequent care and follow-up.

In summary, the basic clinical evaluation obtained by patient history, physical examination, and review of the ECG usually provides the surgeon with sufficient data to estimate cardiac risk. In each situation, the surgeon must determine the urgency of the proposed surgical procedure and balance this with the noted cardiac risk factors assessed in the history, physical exam, laboratory and radiographic data.

In many instances, patient or surgery specific factors will dictate an obvious strategy (e.g., emergent surgery) that may not allow for further cardiac assessment or treatment. In these cases, the need for perioperative medical management and surveillance must be addressed. Selected postoperative risk stratification is often appropriate in patients with elevated coronary risk who have never undergone such assessment in the past. This should be initiated after the patient has recovered from any blood loss, deconditioning, and other postoperative complications that may confound interpretation of noninvasive test results, unless a perioperative MI has been diagnosed.

Preoperative Pulmonary Evaluation

Postoperative pulmonary complications (PPC) are equally prevalent as cardiac complications and contribute similarly to morbidity, mortality, and length of postoperative hospital stay. Late pulmonary complications are leading causes of morbidity and mortality after surgery, second only to cardiac complications. Pneumonia, respiratory failure, and atelectasis are the most commonly observed PPCs. However, multiple specific dysfunctions exist including laryngospasm, bronchospasm, airway obstructions, pulmonary embolism, reintubation or prolonged mechanical ventilation, pleural effusion, pneumothorax, and others.

PPCs are often multifactorial, and perioperative awareness and management of these factors can often help limit their occurrence. Procedural factors affecting pulmonary morbidity include upper abdominal and thoracic incisions, neurosurgical procedures, head and neck procedures, vascular procedures (particularly repair of abdominal aortic aneurysm), emergency operations, preoperative blood transfusion, use of nasogastric tubes, general anesthesia, and prolonged operative time (>3 h) [27–31]. Independent patient factors which contribute to postoperative pulmonary complications include older age (>60), severity of underlying pulmonary disease such as chronic obstructive pulmonary disease (COPD) or chronic bronchitis, American Society of Anesthesiologists (ASA) class II or greater (Table 3.2), functional dependence, alcohol abuse, cigarette smoking, and poor nutritional status (serum albumin <3.5 g/dL). Obesity and mild-to-moderate asthma have not been consistently shown to predict PPCs.

Until recently, no scoring systems existed for predicting PPCs similar to those used for cardiovascular risk stratification. Researchers with the Veterans' Administration National Surgical Quality Improvement Project (NSQIP) have now developed and prospectively validated a scoring system for predicting postoperative pneumonia and respiratory failure [31]. This system includes many of the above predictors in a numeric scoring system (Tables 3.3 and 3.4).

Table 3.2 American Society of Anesthesiologists (ASA) physical status classification

Classification	Description
1	Normal healthy patient; no organic, biochemical, or psychiatric disease
2	Mild systemic disease with no functional limitation
3	Severe systemic disease with functional limitation
4	Severe systemic disease that is a constant threat to life
5	Moribund patient equally likely to die in next 24 h with or without operation
6	Brain dead patient; organs are being removed for donor purposes
E	Emergency operation

Reprinted with permission from Stephen P. Fischer, Miller's Anesthesia, 7th Ed, Vol 34-1, Chapter 34 Preoperative Evaluation, pg. 1002, copyright Elsevier 2009

Table 3.3 Respiratory Failure Risk Index

Preoperative predictor	Point value
Type of surgery	
Abdominal aortic aneurysm	27
Thoracic	21
Neurosurgery	14
Upper abdominal surgery	14
Peripheral vascular	14
Neck	11
Emergency surgery	11
Albumin <3.0 g/dL	9
Blood urea nitrogen >3.0 mg/L	8
Partially or fully dependent functional status	7
History of chronic obstructive pulmonary disease	6
Age (years) ≥70	6
Age (years) 60–69	4

Adapted from: Arozullah AM, Daley J, Henderson WG, Khuri SF. Multifactorial risk index for predicting postoperative respiratory failure in men after major noncardiac surgery. The National Veterans Administration Surgical Quality Improvement Program. Ann Surg. 2000;232:242–253, with permission from Wolters Kluwer Health

Table 3.4 Risk index for postoperative pneumonia

Preoperative risk factor	Point value
Type of surgery	
Abdominal aortic	15
Thoracic	14
Upper abdominal	10
Neck	8
Neurosurgery	8
Vascular	3
Age	
>80	17
70–79	13
60–69	9
50–59	4
Functional status	
Totally dependent	10
Partially dependent	6
Weight loss >10% in past 6 months	7
History of chronic obstructive pulmonary disease	5
General anesthesia	4
Impaired sensorium	4
History of cerebrovascular accident	4
Blood urea nitrogen level	
<8 mg/dL	4
22–30 mg/dL	2
>30 mg/dL	3
Transfusion >4 units	3
Emergency surgery	3
Steroid use for chronic condition	3
Current smoker within 1 year	3
Alcohol intake >two drinks/day in past 2 weeks	2

Adapted from Arozullah AM, Khuri SF, Henderson WG, Daley J. Development and validation of a multifactorial risk index for predicting postoperative pneumonia after major noncardiac surgery. Ann Intern Med. 2001;135:847–857, with permission of American College of Physicians

Table 3.3 displays the point values assigned to each preoperative predictor used to calculate the respiratory failure risk index score. Based on the predicted probability associated with various scores, the NSQIP researchers then categorized the patients into five risk classes. Table 3.4 displays the point values assigned to each preoperative predictor used in calculating the pneumonia risk index score. Table 3.5 displays the five risk classes with associated point values, and the predicted probability of postoperative respiratory failure or pneumonia.

Decreases in functional residual capacity (FRC) and forced vital capacity (FVC) in the postoperative period can lead to atelectasis, decreased pulmonary compliance, increased work of breathing and tachypnea with low tidal volumes. Poor cough effort due to pain and impaired airway reflexes increase susceptibility to retained secretions, bacterial invasion and pneumonia. Aspiration of contaminated oropharyngeal secretions is thought to be a prominent mechanism leading to nosocomial and postoperative pneumonia [32]. Aspiration may occur during intubation, but undetected aspiration is probably frequent after surgery. Prolonged endotracheal intubation predisposes to aspiration of oropharyngeal material and puts the patient at risk for ventilator-associated pneumonia, a complication that doubles the risk for mortality [33]. Oropharyngeal and laryngeal protective mechanisms can be transiently decreased after surgery and may also predispose the nonintubated patient to pneumonia. Nasogastric intubation is likely to decrease airway protective mechanisms and predispose to occult aspiration. Residual subclinical muscle relaxation has been detected in patients who received long-acting muscle relaxants, and it was associated with an increased rate of pulmonary complications [34].

Table 3.5 Risk categories for respiratory failure and pneumonia

Class	Postoperative respiratory failure risk index (point total)	Probability of respiratory failure (%)	Postoperative pneumonia risk index (point total)	Probability of pneumonia (%)
1	0–10	0.5	0–15	0.2
2	11–19	2.2	16–25	1.2
3	20–27	5.0	26–40	4.0
4	28–40	11.6	41–55	9.4
5	>40	30.5	>55	15.3

Adapted from Arozullah AM, Khuri SF, Henderson WG, Daley J: Ann Intern Med 2001;135:847–857 with permission of American College of Surgeons; and Arozullah AM, Daley J, Henderson WG, Khuri SF. Multifactorial risk index for predicting postoperative respiratory failure in men after major noncardiac surgery. The National Veterans Administration Surgical Quality Improvement Program. Ann Surg. 2000;232:242–253, with permission from Wolters Kluwer Health

Perioperative fluid management and resuscitation in the acute surgical patient can impact cardiopulmonary function and may lead to PPCs. Because the acute surgical patient often presents in shock, overly aggressive resuscitation in the perioperative time frame may contribute to Acute Lung Injury (ALI) and PPCs. Large volume crystalloid resuscitation, particularly delayed resuscitation, may lead to undesirable extravascular pulmonary volume. Judicious resuscitation and ongoing clinical assessment by both the surgeon and anesthesia team is essential to reduce or minimize perioperative ALI.

The anesthetic and intraoperative ventilator strategy can influence the extent and course of perioperative lung injury. Kirkpatrick and Slinger recently examined the effects of perioperative mechanical ventilation, intraoperative lung protective ventilator strategies and their role in ventilator-induced lung injury [35]. The phenomenon of ventilator-induced lung injury (VILI) is well recognized. VILI involves a complex interaction of volutrauma, barotrauma, cyclic opening and closing of the alveoli (atelectotrauma), and inflammatory mediators (biotrauma). Although a degree of lung stretch is important for surfactant production, shear stress induces pro-inflammatory cytokines in endothelial, epithelial, and macrophage cells [35].

Atelectasis also plays a role in ALI. Atelectasis occurs frequently after open surgical procedures and in up to 90% of patients undergoing general anesthesia [36]. It is a pathologic state that has direct and indirect effects on the development or exacerbation of ALI. There is concern that the lower tidal volumes associated with lung protective ventilator strategies may predispose the lung to atelectasis and subsequent ALI. Unfortunately, there are conflicting data on the influence of tidal volume on atelectasis and recruitment [37, 38]. It is clear that the techniques to avoid or treat atelectasis,

including recruitment maneuvers and appropriate application of positive end expiratory pressure (PEEP), are effective in the setting of low tidal volumes. Therefore despite the lack of randomized controlled trials thus far to optimally define appropriate intraoperative tidal volume, PEEP and the use of intraoperative lung recruitment, it is reasonable to apply protective ventilator strategies in the intraoperative period based on our current understanding of mechanical ventilation and ALI.

Intraoperative factors may significantly affect the risk for PPCs. There is some evidence that suggests performing laparoscopic surgery rather than open abdominal surgery is associated with decreased pulmonary complications [39, 40], similar to endovascular interventions as opposed to open procedures [41]. The duration of anesthesia and of the surgery is probably one of the strongest predictors of PPCs. This association has been detected by more than one study [42–44]; however, it is not clear whether the duration or the complexity and type of the procedure itself is the cause of PPCs. Regarding to anesthetic technique, conflicting data exist. In the NSQIP studies, general anesthesia was associated with higher risk for respiratory failure and pneumonia [31]. In other studies, however, the use of general anesthesia had no correlation with risk for PPCs [27, 45]. The assessment of the type of anesthesia as a risk factor for PPCs through retrospective or observational studies is difficult in that the effect of anesthesia is not easily distinguishable from the effect of the site or complexity of the surgery itself. Additionally, general anesthesia is more frequently used in surgeries already at increased risk for PPCs, such as thoracoabdominal procedures, and relatively less frequently selected for lower risk or extremity procedures.

The use of a perioperative gastric tube is another important risk factor for the development of PPCs. Several studies have reported that the perioperative use of nasogastric tubes is an independent predictor of pulmonary complications [27, 28, 46]. This correlation has been confirmed by multivariate analysis, which suggests that gastric suctioning itself, and not simply the use of a nasogastric tube in higher risk procedures, causes the pulmonary complications. The mechanism is likely related to decreased airway protection and aspiration of pharyngeal secretions.

Preoperative pulmonary testing is only useful if it provides data that cannot be obtained from the history and physical examination, and if it helps determine the probability of a complication in patients who are known to have risk factors. Several studies have shown that pulmonary function tests (PFTs) results have no significant correlation with PPCs [28, 47]. Other studies also suggest that pulmonary and non-pulmonary data collected through clinical evaluation contain most of the information necessary to make a risk prediction.

Table 3.6 Evidence-based strategies to reduce the risk of PPCs

Factor	Clinical strategies	Evidence grade
Demonstrated benefit		
Lung expansion modalities	Incentive spirometry, chest physiotherapy, continuous positive airway pressure	A
Probable benefit		
Selective nasogastric decompression	Use nasogastric tube only for postoperative nausea/vomiting, abdominal distention	B
Shorter acting neuromuscular blockade	Use of vecuronium or atracurium vs. pancuronium	B
Possible benefit		
Laparoscopic vs. open operation	Choice of less invasive surgical approach	C
Uncertain benefit		
Smoking cessation[a]	Long term vs. short term (48 h)	I
Intraoperative regional block	Spinal or Epidural block	I
Postoperative epidural analgesia		I
Immunonutrition	Overall infections decreased; no data for PPCs	I
No benefit		
Pulmonary Artery Catheterization		D
Routine use of parenteral nutrition	? Exception for severely malnourished or prolonged decrease enteral intake	D[b]
Routine use of enteral nutrition	Overall infections and complications were lower however no difference in PPCs	D[b]

Data from Lawrence VA, Cornell JE, and Smetana GW. Strategies To Reduce Postoperative Pulmonary Complications after Noncardiothoracic Surgery: Systematic Review for the American College of Physicians. Ann Intern Med. 2006;144(8):596–608

EVIDENCE GRADE:

A—good evidence that PPCs are reduced and benefit outweighs risk

B—fair evidence that PPCs are reduced and that benefit outweighs risk

C—fair evidence that PPCs are reduced and but benefit between benefit and harm is too close to make a recommendation

D—fair evidence that PPCs are not reduced or that harm outweighs the benefit

I—Insufficient or conflicting data

[a]48 h cessation decreases carboxyhemoglobin level to that of nonsmoker; eliminates nicotine effect on cardiovascular system and improves mucociliary function. Sputum volume decreases after 1–2 weeks of abstinence, and spirometry improves after approximately 6 weeks

[b]Evidence remains uncertain (strength of evidence I) on total parenteral or enteral nutrition for severely malnourished patients or when a protracted time of inadequate nutrition is anticipated

The implication of these results is that no useful information is added by routinely performing PFTs as part of the clinical evaluation of patients undergoing nonthoracic surgery.

Arterial blood gas analysis has been used in the past for the preoperative evaluation of nonthoracic surgery patients despite the lack of evidence supporting its value. Hypercapnia with $PaCO_2$ (partial pressure of carbon dioxide in arterial blood) greater than 45 mmHg and arterial hypoxemia ($PO_2 <60$ mmHg) have in the past been considered important risk factors for PPCs and contraindications for surgery. These blood gas alterations may help in certain risk–benefit assessments for a given patient or procedure, as their presence is associated with a decreased life expectancy in patients with COPD. However, neither hypercapnia nor hypoxemia has been shown to be independent predictors of the risk for PPCs [27, 45].

Chest radiographs are still routinely performed preoperatively in older patients, in patients with known pulmonary disease, and in patients who smoke; however, there is little to no evidence that routine chest radiographs affect the perioperative management or outcomes in any way [48]. A reasonable use of chest radiology may be for patients with new or unexplained pulmonary symptoms, or for those with an acute process such as pneumonia or pneumothorax that will alter operative decision making and/or timing of surgery in the acute setting. Chest radiographs in asymptomatic patient are unlikely to add any information to the pulmonary risk stratification [48].

In summary, when assessing for pulmonary risk in the acute surgery setting, a thorough history and physical examination is essential, with particular attention to pulmonary and nonpulmonary factors that have been shown to be independent predictors of PPCs. Table 3.6 summarizes the aforementioned data and outlines risk reduction strategies for the prevention of PPCs. For patients with stable pulmonary symptoms who are undergoing a high-risk procedure (upper abdominal or thoracic surgery, major vascular surgery, duration longer than 3 h or the use of gastric suctioning), a further attempt at risk stratification using the postoperative pneumonia and respiratory failure risk indexes (Tables 3.3 and 3.4) can be performed. Those patients with a high score and therefore a high probability of PPCs can therefore be identified (Table 3.5), and the information used to guide not only preoperative counseling and consent but also in the implementation of risk-reduction strategies (Table 3.6), alternative surgical approaches, damage control procedure, or possibly nonoperative management. In patients with recent or ongoing respiratory infections, delay of surgery or nonsurgical management should be considered, if acceptable. Chest radiography with or without arterial blood gas measurement may be helpful in the acute setting to determine the presence,

Table 3.7 Levels of thromboembolism risk and recommended thromboprophylaxis in surgical patients

Level of risk	DVT risk without thromboprophylaxis	Suggested thromboprophylaxis options
Low risk Minor surgery in mobile patients	<10%	No specific thromboprophylaxis recommendation Early and "aggressive" ambulation
Moderate risk Most general, open gynecologic or urologic surgery patients	10–40%	LMWH (at recommended doses) LDUH bid or tid, fondaparinux
Moderate VTE risk with high bleeding risk		Mechanical thromboprophylaxis
High risk Hip or knee arthroplasty, hip fracture surgery, major trauma, SCI	40–80%	LMWH (at recommended doses), fondaparinux, warfarin (INR 2–3)
High VTE risk with high bleeding risk		Mechanical thromboprophylaxis[a]

Adapted from Geerts WH, Bergqvist D, Pineo GF, et al. Prevention of Venous Thromboembolism: American College of Chest Physicians Evidence-Based Clinical Practice Guidelines (8th Edition). Chest. 2008;133(6 Suppl):381S–453S with permission from American College of Chest Physicians

[a]Mechanical thromboprophylaxis includes intermittent pneumatic compression or venous foot pump and/or graduated compression stockings; consider switch or addition of anticoagulant thromboprophylaxis when increased bleeding risk decreases

absence or severity of any active pulmonary disease or infection.

Prophylaxis of Venous Thromboembolism

The morbidity and mortality of venous thromboembolism (VTE) makes consideration of prophylaxis mandatory for every major operation. In the acute care setting, multiple factors must be considered with regards to method and timing of initiation of chemical prophylaxis. Knowledge of risk factors for VTE in certain patient groups or in individual patients allows the most appropriate and cost effective use of prophylaxis. Multiple factors have been identified, including increasing age, prolonged immobility, obesity, prior VTE or history of pulmonary embolism, varicose veins, cancer, inflammatory bowel disease, nephrotic syndrome, pregnancy or estrogen use, indwelling central venous catheters, certain surgical procedures (in particular operations involving the abdomen, pelvis, or lower extremities), and trauma (especially pelvis or lower extremity fractures) [49–51]. These risk factors are often present in combination in hospitalized patients, and the risks are cumulative.

The 8th edition of the American College of Chest Physician (ACCP) guidelines (2008) recommends that every hospital develop a formal and active strategy to consistently identify medical and surgical patients at risk for VTE and to prevent VTE occurrence [52]. The Surgical Care Improvement Project (SCIP), a national partnership of organizations including the American Medical Association and the American College of Surgeons has been tasked with the goal to reduce surgical complications in the United States by 25% from 2005 to 2010. Two SCIP process mea-

sures have been developed in relation to improving VTE prophylaxis: (1) The proportion of surgical patients for whom recommended VTE prophylaxis is ordered, and (2) the proportion of surgical patients who actually receive appropriate VTE prophylaxis within 24 hours before or after surgery [53].

When considering the degree of VTE prophylaxis that a surgical patient may need, the surgeon must consider not only the individual specific risk factors but also the thromboembolic risk of the procedure itself (Table 3.7). A thorough preoperative assessment is essential to reveal any "hidden" risk factors such as thrombophilia or a family or personal history of VTE. The majority of patients who are hospitalized for surgery will fall into the moderate or high-risk categories in Table 3.7. Without thromboprophylaxis the incidence of hospital acquired deep vein thrombosis (DVT) is approximately 10–40% among medical or general surgical patients and 40–60% following major orthopedic surgery [53]. Patients who are at high risk for VTE require aggressive prophylaxis and multimodal therapy. The most common strategy is anticoagulation plus intermittent pneumatic compression.

Strategies for VTE prophylaxis range from nonpharmacologic for lower-risk patients to pharmacologic or combination strategies for higher-risk patients. Nonpharmacologic prophylaxis strategies include ambulation, mechanical devices such as graduated compression stockings, intermittent pneumatic devices, and vena caval interruption. Early ambulation offers many benefits to patients and should be encouraged but should not be considered VTE prophylaxis in and of itself. In contrast, multiple randomized controlled trials have been done evaluating the effectiveness of graduated compression or elastic stocking for preventing VTE in various groups of hospitalized patients, and have demonstrated effectiveness in diminishing the risk of VTE in hospitalized patients. Examination of the data suggests that graduated compression stockings used in combination with another method of prophylaxis is more effective than compression stocking prophylaxis on its own [54].

The 8th edition of the ACCP guidelines recommends that mechanical methods of VTE prophylaxis be used primarily in patients who are at high risk of bleeding and that careful attention be directed to ensuring their proper use and optimal adherence [52]. The importance of adherence cannot be emphasized enough, as mechanical compression devices have been shown to be not effective unless worn 18–20 h per day. Mechanical compression should be initiated prior to the induction of anesthesia, and continued intraoperative and in the post-anesthesia care unit.

Vena caval interruption involves placement of a retrievable vena cava filter ideally prior to surgery with removal sometime later; it offers the potential for VTE prophylaxis in patients who could not tolerate even minor bleeding, such as certain trauma patients. The Eastern Association for the Surgery of Trauma has put forth a consensus recommendation to consider vena caval interruption in high-risk trauma patients who cannot receive pharmacologic prophylaxis [55].

Pharmacologic strategies include low-dose unfractionated heparin (LDUH), low molecular weight heparin (LMWH), vitamin K antagonist (warfarin), and factor Xa specific inhibitors (fondaparinux). For general surgery patients, prophylaxis options that have proven beneficial in prospective trials include low-dose unfractionated heparin (LDUH), low molecular weight heparin (LMWH), intermittent pneumatic compression, and oral warfarin. Meta-analysis of more than 30 randomized controlled trials comparing LMWH to LDUH in general surgery patients demonstrated comparable efficacy for the prevention of thromboembolic phenomena but with a consequence of slightly higher incidence of minor wound bleeding [56]. LMWH, however, is not recommended for a patient following recent neurosurgery, gastrointestinal bleeding, or renal insufficiency and has been reported to cause spinal or epidural hematomas in patients with epidural catheters.

Although vitamin K antagonists (warfarin) still appear in the latest ACCP recommendations [52], LMWH is preferable. A 2004 meta-analysis assessing these two strategies demonstrated vitamin K antagonists were associated with more episodes of total deep venous thrombosis (DVT) and proximal DVT as compared to LMWH [57]. This finding is notable in that for these studies, warfarin was more likely administered correctly (to achieve an international normalized ration [INR] of 2.0 to 3.0 within 72 h after surgery) than the dosing for LMWH, which was likely not weight based or monitored at the time these data were reviewed.

The indirect factor Xa-specific inhibitor fondaparinux has been widely studied and has been found to be safe and effective [58]. It has a 17 h half-life, which raises concern about the length of time for effects to stop if a patient does begin to bleed while on this agent. Fondaparinux has been associated with increased bleeding events and transfusion requirements in the setting of knee replacement surgery [59].

Special considerations must be taken when considering pharmacologic VTE strategies in certain patient populations. In the 8th edition VTE guidelines, the ACCP added evidence-based recommendations for certain surgical procedures (Table 3.8). The guidelines additionally specified extended outpatient prophylaxis with LMWH for up to 28 days post-operatively in selected high-risk patients undergoing general or gynecologic surgery (for example those patients with cancer or a personal history of VTE) [52].

Renal function must be noted when considering LMWH, fondaparinux, and other antithrombotic agents that are renally cleared. Both fondaparinux and LMWH accumulate biologically in patients with renal insufficiency, increasing their risk for bleeding. Options for these patients include LDUH, using lower doses of these specific agents with close monitoring of the drug level or anticoagulant effect (such as monitoring factor Xa levels). Fondaparinux is explicitly contraindicated in patients with body weight <50 kg or creatinine clearance <30 mL/min.

The 8th edition of the ACCP guidelines recommends weight-based dosing of thromboprophylactic agents in obese patients, and specifically recommend higher dose LMWH or unfractionated heparin for bariatric procedures [52, 60]. Frederikson et al. measured the anticoagulant effect of a single fixed dose of LMWH using anti-factor Xa heparin activity levels. The anticoagulant effect of LMWH was found to be weight dependent [61]. Another observational study in bariatric patients reflected significantly fewer postoperative VTE complications in a higher dose LMWH regimen [62].

Newer therapies for pharmacologic prophylaxis are emerging, including direct factor Xa inhibitors. The antithrombotic effects of the therapeutic anticoagulants heparin and warfarin are mediated by indirect inhibition of coagulation serine proteases, including factor Xa and thrombin [63]. However, these anticoagulants also carry a bleeding liability, which highlights the central role of thrombin in both pathologic thrombosis and adaptive hemostasis. Thrombin is the final serine protease in the enzymatic cascade responsible for fibrin clot formation in blood, and it is also a strong activator of platelets. The serine protease factor Xa is essential for the conversion of prothrombin to thrombin. Inhibitors of factor Xa reduce thrombin generation and, by this mechanism, disrupt thrombotic vascular occlusion. In vitro studies suggest that factor Xa has a wider therapeutic window than thrombin [64]. Several emerging oral inhibitors of factor Xa are emerging as promising strategies for anticoagulation and VTE prophylaxis.

Table 3.8 Procedure-specific recommendations for VTE prophylaxis

Surgery type	Recommended options	Grade
Major vascular surgery (patient with risk factors)	LMWH, LDUH, or fondaparinux	1C
Major gynecologic surgery or laparoscopy (patient with risk factors)	LMWH, LDUH, intermittent pneumatic compression	1A
	Fonduparinux ± graduated compression stockings	1C
Major open urologic surgery	LDUH, intermittent pneumatic compression/graduated compression	1B
	LMWH, fonduparinux	1C
Bariatric surgery	Higher dose LMWH, LDUH tid, or fondaparinux	1C
Thoracic surgery	LMWH, LDUH, intermittent pneumatic compression	1C
CABG	LMWH over LDUH	2B

Adapted with permission from Geerts WH, Bergqvist D, Pineo GF, et al. Prevention of Venous Thromboembolism: American College of Chest Physicians Evidence-Based Clinical Practice Guidelines (8th Edition). Chest. 2008;133(6 Suppl):381S–453S with permission from American College of Chest Physicians

Guide to recommendation grades in the ACCP guidelines:

1A = strong recommendation, high quality evidence

1B = strong recommendation; moderate quality evidence

1C = strong recommendation; low or very low quality evidence

2B = weak recommendation; moderate quality evidence

Management of the Therapeutically Anticoagulated Patient

In the setting of acute care or emergency general surgery, it is often necessary to treat or operate on an anticoagulated patient. In such circumstances, it is preferable to reverse the patient's anticoagulation temporarily so that hemostasis can be optimized. Procoagulant therapy may sometimes obviate the need for surgery by stopping the bleeding (e.g., for gastrointestinal bleeding). The approach to the patient can be individualized, based on the urgency and magnitude of the surgery to be performed and the strength of the indication for anticoagulation.

Warfarin is commonly prescribed for patients with prosthetic heart valves and more commonly for chronic atrial fibrillation. Emergency reversal of warfarin anticoagulation may be required when a patient has major bleeding or needs an urgent procedure. Vitamin K should be given intravenously at the time of emergency reversal of anticoagulation. The recommended dose is 10 mg intravenously. The intravenous route acts more quickly than the oral route (6–12 h versus 18–24 h). Blood products, such as prothrombin complex concentrate or plasma, should be used only when the international normalized ratio (INR) is at least 1.5 and the patient either has major bleeding or needs a procedure within 6 h (e.g., repair of a ruptured aortic aneurysm or a perforated viscous). Although designed and licensed for the treatment of bleeding in hemophilia patients with inhibitors to factor concentrates, prothrombin complex concentrate and recombinant factor VIIa have been found to be useful but expensive treatments of uncontrolled intraoperative bleeding that is unresponsive to replacement of blood components. Prothrombin

complex concentrate contains variable concentrations of coagulation factors and may be associated with a high thrombotic risk [65, 66]. For elective reversal, guidelines support withholding warfarin or administering vitamin K [67] with or without a LMWH or full dose heparin "bridge" to surgery, depending on the underlying reason for the patient's anticoagulation.

In most circumstances, there is less physiologic urgency for restoration of anticoagulation than is generally appreciated. Protection of cardiac valve prosthesis and recently placed cardiac stents are the most urgent indications, but a metallic valve can be left without anticoagulation for at least 72 h, particularly in the aortic position; however, such a long interval is infrequently necessary. High-risk patients or those unable to resume their warfarin by mouth may be heparinized safely as early as 12 h after most procedures with secure hemostasis, except for neurosurgical procedures and some operations in severe trauma.

Clopidogrel and aspirin are commonly used for antiplatelet therapy. Percutaneous coronary interventions require antiplatelet therapy for 4 weeks to 12 months, depending on whether a bare metal stent or a drug-eluting stent has been inserted [68]. Drug-eluting stents effectively retard intimal hyperplasia but also delay formation of an antithrombotic intimal layer, rendering patients with these stents at risk for perioperative ischemic events if antiplatelet drugs are discontinued. For emergency procedures, negotiating the balance between risk of bleeding and risk of thrombosis (e.g., in the setting of recently placed cardiac stents) requires a multidisciplinary approach [69, 70]. After surgery the antiplatelet agents should be restarted as soon as safely possible, recognizing that clopidogrel is associated with postoperative bleeding complications for up to 2 weeks, and therefore should be resumed with caution.

Aspirin is commonly used to decrease risk of events in patients with known, or risk factors for, vascular disease, diabetes, renal insufficiency, or simply advanced age. Traditionally aspirin has been withdrawn in the perioperative period for 5–7 days because of concern of bleeding. However, this practice has recently come under scrutiny. A meta-analysis of almost 50,000 patients undergoing a variety of noncardiac surgeries (30% taking aspirin perioperatively) found that aspirin increased bleeding complications by a factor of 1.5, but not the severity, except in patients undergoing intracranial surgery and possibly transurethral resection of the prostate [71]. Surgeons blinded to aspirin administration could not identify patients taking or not taking aspirin based on bleeding [72].

There is, however, an increased risk of vascular events when aspirin taken regularly is stopped perioperatively [73]. There may be a rebound hypercoagulable state when aspirin is withdrawn [74]. Acute coronary syndromes occurred 8.5 ± 3.6 days and acute cerebral events occurred 14.3 ± 11.3 days after aspirin cessation, both time frames well within the typical duration of interruption for elective surgery. Events were twice as common in patients who had stopped taking aspirin in the previous 3 weeks when compared to those who continued aspirin [71]. Stopping aspirin for 3–4 days is usually sufficient, if aspirin is stopped at all, and dosing should be resumed as soon as possible. New platelets formed after aspirin is stopped (half-life of approximately 15 min) will not be affected. Normally functioning platelets at a concentration of more than $50,000/mm^3$ are adequate to control surgical bleeding. For many minor, superficial procedures such as cataract extraction, endoscopies, and peripheral procedures, the risk of withdrawing aspirin in at-risk patients is greater than the risk of bleeding [75]. Aspirin can safely be discontinued if taken only for primary prevention (no history of stents, strokes, MI). Aspirin administration should be continued if taken for secondary prevention (history of stents or vascular disease), except for procedures with a risk of bleeding in closed spaces (e.g., intracranial, posterior chamber of the eye or transurethral resection of the prostate) [76]. Neuraxial and peripheral anesthesia in patients taking aspirin is safe and endorsed by the American Society of Regional Anesthesia (ASRA) [77]. The risk of spinal hematoma with clopidogrel is unknown. Based on labeling and ASRA guidelines clopidogrel is discontinued 7 days before planned neuraxial blockade.

In the acute surgical setting, therefore, the bleeding risk specific to the procedure (e.g., intracranial or other closed spaced procedures) must be considered when assessing the need for perioperative platelet reversal and/or cessation versus resumption of antiplatelet agents in the postoperative period.

Hemoglobin Levels and Transfusion

There are currently no adequately powered clinical trials that examine different transfusion thresholds or outcomes in the perioperative setting. Clinical trials to date have focused on mortality rate but have not evaluated other important outcomes, such as myocardial infarction, central nervous system injury, or functional recovery. Prior to the late 1980s, the standard of care was to administer a perioperative transfusion whenever the hemoglobin level fell below 10 g/dL or the hematocrit fell below 30%. In 1988, a National Institutes of Health consensus conference on perioperative red blood cell transfusions concluded that there was no evidence to support a single criterion for transfusion [78]. Concerns at the time were raised due to the risks of transmission of serious viral illnesses such as HIV and hepatitis C [79]. In 1994, the American Society of Anesthesiologists established the Task Force on Blood Component Therapy in order to develop evidence based indications for transfusion. In general, the principle conclusion of the task force is that red blood cell transfusion should not be dictated by single hemoglobin "trigger" as previously established but rather be based on the patient's individual risk of developing complications of inadequate oxygenation [80]. The risk of bleeding in surgical patients is determined by the extent and type of surgery, the ability to control bleeding, and actual and anticipated rate of bleeding, and the consequences of uncontrolled bleeding. Additionally, the effects of anemia must be separated from those of hypovolemia, although both can interfere with oxygen transport and delivery.

The formal and current recommendations of the task force (updated in 1996), based on available data, are as follows: (1) transfusion is rarely indicated when the hemoglobin concentration is greater than 10 g/dL and is almost always indicated when it is less than 6 g/dL, especially when the anemia is acute; (2) the determination of whether intermediate hemoglobin concentrations (6–10 g/dL) justify or require RBC transfusion should be based on the patient's risk for complications of inadequate oxygenation; (3) the use of a single hemoglobin "trigger" for all patients and other approaches that fail to consider all important physiologic and surgical factors affecting oxygenation are not recommended; (4) when appropriate, preoperative autologous blood donation, intraoperative and postoperative blood recovery, acute normovolemic hemodilution, and measures to decrease blood loss (deliberate hypotension and pharmacologic agents) may be beneficial; and (5) the indications for transfusion of autologous RBCs may be more liberal than for allogeneic RBCs because of the lower (but still significant) risks associated with the former [80]. Ultimately, careful clinical assessment with thoughtful consideration of risks and benefits should guide the transfusion decision, not a specific hemoglobin concentration. No single set of guidelines will apply to every patient or disease process.

Steroid Administration

Traditionally, patients who present in need of acute care surgery who are on a maintenance glucocorticoid regimen, or who have received corticosteroids within the past 6 months receive supplemental "stress dose" steroids, due to presumed suppression of the hypothalamic–pituitary–adrenal (HPA) axis. In order to prevent potential adrenal crisis, large doses (hydrocortisone 100 mg IV every 8 h or equivalent) are commonly given for undefined periods with little to no monitoring, despite the deleterious effect that steroids have on wound healing, host defenses, carbohydrate metabolism, and other systems. Additionally, there has been no consideration for the variability of the stress response. Because the use of stress doses of corticosteroids has become routine, the true incidence of perioperative adrenal crisis is difficult to assess. Review of the available literature reveals very few cases in which death or hypotension could directly be attributed to perioperative adrenal crisis in these patients [81, 82]. This suggests that many patients receive unnecessary supplemental corticosteroid therapy. Recently, several smaller studies have suggested that the combination of the patient's baseline exogenous corticosteroid dose plus their endogenous steroid production is adequate to meet the demands of the physiologic stress of surgery [82]. Biochemical testing of the HPA axis in patients on glucocorticoid therapy may reveal a degree of adrenal insufficiency, however, these tests are extremely sensitive and do not predict the clinical outcome [83–85].

Management of Blood Glucose

Carbohydrate metabolism is inherently unstable during periods of surgical stress, and the stress of critical illness often induces hyperglycemia [86]. Several studies have clearly associated hyperglycemia with an increased risk for morbidity and mortality of critical illness. In 2001, Van den Berghe and colleagues published the first of two studies documenting a mortality benefit to tight glycemic control (blood glucose 80–110 mg/dL) [87, 88]. The benefit was observed in cohorts of both cardiac and noncardiac surgical patients. Postoperative morbidity was also reduced, including decreases in ventilator days, renal dysfunction, bloodstream infection, transfusion requirements, and polyneuropathy [87]. Intraoperative hyperglycemia has also been shown to have independent detrimental effects in cardiac surgical patients [89]. Defining an appropriate management strategy has recently been complicated by several prospective randomized studies of tight glycemic control demonstrating unacceptably high rates of hypoglycemia [90]. Severe or prolonged hypoglycemia can cause convulsions, coma, and irreversible brain damage as well as cardiac arrhythmias. While measured hypoglycemic events do increase with the implementation of intensive insulin therapy, these brief episodes of biochemical hypoglycemia have not been associated with any clinically significant sequellae [87, 91]. Additionally, in a recent case control study [92], no causal link was found between hypoglycemia in the intensive care unit (ICU) and death when case and control subjects were matched for baseline risk factors and time in the ICU before the hypoglycemic event. These observations support prior suggestions that hypoglycemia in ICU patients who receive intensive insulin therapy may merely identify patients at high risk of dying rather than representing a cause and effect [93]. Although there are few data on preoperative control of hyperglycemia in the emergency surgical patient, based on the currently available literature in other similar settings it would seem prudent to maintain blood glucose less than 150 mg/dL in accordance with the surviving sepsis campaign guidelines [94].

Fluids, Resuscitation and Intervention

Patients who require emergency or urgent operations often with severe metabolic derangements that require rapid intervention. These derangements commonly range from mild perfusion deficits to severe shock. Such shock may be hemorrhagic or multifactorial. The recommendations made by the authors of the surviving sepsis campaign guideline include early goal-directed resuscitation (EGDR) [94]. Many patients with emergency general surgical conditions present with septic physiology and should be resuscitated in a goal-oriented fashion. The timing of emergency operative intervention then becomes an important issue. EGDR can be successfully continued intraoperatively by anesthesia staff [95]. However, the completeness of preoperative resuscitation may be an important determinant in the outcome and the appropriate timing of an immediately necessary operation is often difficult to establish.

Many patients presenting with intra-abdominal catastrophes have sepsis and septic shock. In addition to aggressive resuscitation with fluids and correction of hypotension with vasopressors, these patients require source control as soon as their physiologic stability allows intervention. The most minimal procedure that achieves source control is generally appropriate Source control may be achievable at beside in the intensive care unit; for example, endoscopic biliary decompression in ascending cholangitis, or ultrasound-guided abdominal abscess or empyema drainage. In addition to source control, early institution of broad-spectrum antibiotics should if possible follow acquisition of cultures but should not be delayed solely for the purpose of obtaining culture material. Delay in initiation of effective antimicrobial therapy has a time-dependent effect on mortality for patients presenting with hypotension due to an infection [96].

Although patients with intra-abdominal emergencies often present with fever, some with severe sepsis may be hypothermic. Even mild hypothermia has multiple physiologic effects. Hypothermia has been associated with an increased incidence of wound infection and longer hospital stay [97]. Although this is a multifactorial problem, it has been noted that vasoconstriction secondary to hypothermia impairs healing by decreasing blood flow to the wound and therefore limiting bacterial killing by neutrophils. Hypothermia reduces platelet function and impairs activation of the coagulation cascade, which can increase intraoperative blood loss and transfusion requirements (which are also associated with an increase of surgical site infections) [98–100]. It is a key component in the lethal combination of the triad of hypothermia, acidosis, and coagulopathy frequently encountered in trauma and damage control surgery.

Because of the negative effects of hypothermia on coagulation and wound infection, it should be aggressively corrected preoperatively, as it will only be exacerbated by general anesthesia and ongoing fluid resuscitation. Correcting hypothermia is difficult in these patients as the most common methods such as gastric or bladder irrigation are difficult to accomplish intra-operatively. Preoperative warming using fluid warmers and ongoing intraoperative warming with forced air warming, increasing room temperature, and continuing the use of fluid warmers become key to regaining and maintaining normothermia.

Advanced Directives

Before proceeding with emergency surgical intervention, it is important to determine whether the patient has advanced directives. Patients presenting with surgical emergencies or urgencies are not infrequently elderly with multiple comorbidities or a terminal condition. These patients may have a preference for pain relief over extension of life [101]. The decision to pursue surgical therapy in a terminally ill patient will often involve the patient and family, the surgeon, the physician treating the terminal disease, and the emergency physician. Communication between the surgeon and the patient's physician is essential to establish a clear understanding of the risk of perioperative morbidity and mortality as well as the impact of the acute condition on the patient's chronic or terminal disease. The surgeon's autonomy is also important as adherence to the ethical principles of nonmaleficence and beneficence may guide the surgeon to elect not to perform an operation that he or she feels would not improve the patient's condition or alter the patient's outcome. Rarely, a conflict may arise between physicians or between physicians and family, a situation best avoided by open communication among all the individuals involved. If conflict should arise, it is acceptable and encouraged to seek a second opinion from a colleague or partner regarding treatment options. Ethics consults are often readily available in larger centers to assist with these decisions.

Once operative intervention has been agreed on, the status of any do-not-resuscitate (DNR) orders must be addressed. As recently as 1994 few institutions had policies governing DNR orders in the perioperative setting [102]. The American College of Surgeons (ACS), the American Society of Anesthesiologists (ASA) and the Association of Operating Room Nurses (AORN) have developed statements regarding DNR orders [103–105]. Patients exposed to anesthesia are at increased risk from transient insults that are reversible by resuscitation [106]. Should surgical intervention be selected by the patient and surgeon, in the presence of a preexisting DNR directive, a "required reconsideration" is recommended by the ACS, ASA, and AORN. Following DNR orders explicitly may result in potentially preventable death and is not endorsed [103–105]. "Required reconsideration" is a discussion between the patient (or surrogate) and the surgical and anesthesia team to clarify the goals and limits of care.

The patient with a DNR order may suspend it for a specified time after which the goals and limitations of care can be updated. However, the suspension of DNR orders denies patients autonomy of care and exposes them to procedures they would not otherwise accept. If a surgeon is uncomfortable with limitations on resuscitation, he or she is not obligated to perform the procedure but should offer to assist in alternative arrangements. For limitations on resuscitation, either goal-directed care or procedure based objectives can provide guidance. Procedure based limitations specify what is authorized and what is not (e.g., "may intubate," "no chest compressions"). Goal-based limitations identify a clinical end point (e.g., "comfort only," "keep patient alive until spouse returns to hospital"), which allows some flexibility for the providers as the patient or family will define their goals of care and the clinicians will provide procedures consistent with those goals. This strategy places more autonomy with the providers. Similarly, the ACS guidelines recommend customizing the advanced directive to remain consistent with the patient's goals during the perioperative period [106]. This should be clearly documented in the medical record and communicated to the entire operative team.

Conclusion

Patients presenting with general surgical emergencies can range from the simple appendectomy in a young healthy patient to florid sepsis from viscous perforation in a patient with multiple comorbidities. The surgeon and operative team are often faced with urgent risk versus benefit decisions in these patients in order to provide optimal intervention and minimize postoperative complications. These decisions must often be made in an expeditious manner with data available at the time of presentation. Attention to detail and appropriate management of comorbidities is essential to optimizing outcomes for the acute surgical patient.

References

1. Weiser TG, Regenbogen SE, Thompson KD, et al. An estimation of the global volume of surgery: a modeling strategy based on available data. Lancet. 2008;372:139–44.
2. Devereaux PJ, Xavier D, Pogue J, Guyatt G, Sigaman A, Garutti I, Leslie K, Rao-Melacini P, Chrolavicius S, Yang H, MacDonald C, Avezum A, Lanthier L, Hu W, Yusuf S, on behalf of the POISE (PeriOperative ISchemic Evaluation) Investigators. Characteristics and short-term prognosis of perioperative myocardial infarction in patients undergoing noncardiac surgery: a cohort study. Ann Intern Med. 2011;154:523–8.
3. Norton JA, Barie PS, Bollinger RR, Chang AE, Lowry S, Mulvihill SJ, Pass HI, Thompson RW. Surgery: basic science and clinical evidence. New York: Springer; 2008.
4. Devereaux PJ, Goldman L, Cook DJ, Gilbert K, Leslie K, Guyatt GH. Perioperative cardiac events in patients undergoing noncardiac surgery: a review of the magnitude of the problem, the pathophysiology of the events and methods to estimate and communicate risk. CMAJ. 2005;173(6):627–34.
5. Devereaux PJ, Yang H, Yusuf S, Guyatt G, Leslie K, Villar JC, POISE, et al. Effects of extended-release metoprolol succinate in patients undergoing non-cardiac surgery (POISE trial): a randomised controlled trial. Lancet. 2008;371:1839–47.
6. Kost GJ, Kirk JD, Omand K. A strategy for the use of cardiac injury markers (troponin I and T, creatine kinase-MB mass and isoforms, and myoglobin) in the diagnosis of acute myocardial infarction. Arch Pathol Lab Med. 1998;122(3):245–51.
7. Penttilä I, Penttilä K, Rantanen T. Laboratory diagnosis of patients with acute chest pain. Clin Chem Lab Med. 2000;38(3):187–97.
8. Shillinger M, Dumanovois H, Bayegan K, Holzenbein T, Grabenwoger M, Thonissen J, et al. C reactive protein and mortality in patients with acute aortic disease. Intensive Care Med. 2002;28:740–5.
9. Rosenfeld BA, Beattie C, Christopherson R, Norris EJ, Frank SM, Breslow MJ, et al. The effects of different anesthetic regimens on fibrinolysis and the development of postoperative arterial thrombosis. Anesthesiology. 1993;79:435–43.
10. Sametz W, Metzler H, Gries M, Porta S, Sadjak A, Supanz S, et al. Perioperative catecholamines in cardiac risk patients. Eur J Clin Invest. 1999;29:582–7.
11. Parker SD, Breslow MJ, Frank SM, Rosenfeld BA, Norris EJ, Christopherson R, et al. Catecholamine and cortisol responses to lower extremity revascularization; correlation with outcome variables. Crit Care Med. 1995;23:1954–61.
12. Lee TH, Marcantonio ER, Mangione CM, et al. Derivation and prospective validation of a simple index for prediction of cardiac risk of major noncardiac surgery. Circulation. 1999;100:1043–9.
13. Lee TH, Thomas EJ, Ludwig LE, et al. Troponin T as a marker for myocardial ischemia in patients undergoing major noncardiac surgery. Am J Cardiol. 1996;77:1031–6.
14. Fleisher LA, Beckman JA, Brown KA, et al. ACC/AHA 2007 guidelines on perioperative cardiovascular evaluation and care for noncardiac surgery: A Report of the American College of Cardiology/American Heart Association Task Force on Practice Guidelines. J Am Coll Cardiol. 2007;50(17):1707–32.
15. Ellis JE, Shah MN, Briller JE, Roizen MF, Aronson A, Feinstein SB. A comparison of methods for the detection of myocardial ischemia during noncardiac surgery: automated ST-segment analysis systems, electrocardiography, and transesophageal echocardiography. Anesth Analg. 1992;75:764–72.
16. Leung JM, Voskanian A, Bellows WH, Pastor D. Automated electrocardiograph ST segment trending monitors: accuracy in detecting myocardial ischemia. Anesth Analg. 1998;87:4–10.
17. Slogoff S, Keats AS, David Y, Igo SR. Incidence of perioperative myocardial ischemia detected by different electrocardiographic systems. Anesthesiology. 1990;73:1074–81.
18. Mangano DT, Browner WS, Hollenberg M, London MJ, Tubau JF, Tateo IM. Association of perioperative myocardial ischemia with cardiac morbidity and mortality in men undergoing noncardiac surgery. N Engl J Med. 1990;323:1781–8.
19. Raby KE, Barry J, Creager MA, Cook EF, Weisberg MC, Goldman L. Detection and significance of intraoperative and postoperative myocardial ischemia in peripheral vascular surgery. JAMA. 1992;268:222–7.
20. Fleisher LA, Nelson AH, Rosenbaum SH. Postoperative myocardial ischemia: etiology of cardiac morbidity or manifestation of underlying disease. J Clin Anesth. 1995;7:97–102.
21. Landesberg G, Luria MH, Cotev S, et al. Importance of long-duration postoperative ST-segment depression in cardiac morbidity after vascular surgery. Lancet. 1993;341:715–9.
22. Landesberg G, Mosseri M, Shatz V, et al. Cardiac troponin after major vascular surgery: the role of perioperative ischemia, preoperative thallium scanning, and coronary revascularization. J Am Coll Cardiol. 2004;44:569–75.
23. Mangano DT, Browner WS, Hollenberg M, Li J, Tateo IM. Long-term cardiac prognosis following noncardiac surgery. JAMA. 1992;268:233–9.
24. Mathew JP, Fleisher LA, Rinehouse JA, et al. ST segment depression during labor and delivery. Anesthesiology. 1992;77:632–41.
25. Fleisher LA, Zielski MM, Schulman SP. Perioperative ST-segment depression is rare and may not indicate myocardial ischemia in moderate-risk patients undergoing noncardiac surgery. J Cardiothorac Vasc Anesth. 1997;11:155–9.
26. McFalls EO, Ward HB, Santilli S, Scheftel M, Chesler E, Doliszny KM. The influence of perioperative myocardial infarction on long-term prognosis following elective vascular surgery. Chest. 1998;113:681–6.
27. McAlister FA, Bertsch K, Man J, et al. Incidence of and risk factors for pulmonary complications after nonthoracic surgery. Am J Respir Crit Care Med. 2005;171:514–7.
28. Mitchell CK, Smoger SH, Pfeifer MP, et al. Multivariate analysis of factors associated with postoperative pulmonary complications following general elective surgery. Arch Surg. 1998;133:194–8.
29. Hall JC, Tarala RA, Hall JL, Mander J. A multivariate analysis of the risk of pulmonary complications after laparotomy. Chest. 1991;99:923–7.
30. Arozullah AM, Khuri SF, Henderson WG, Daley J. Development and validation of a multifactorial risk index for predicting postoperative pneumonia after major noncardiac surgery. Ann Intern Med. 2001;135:847–57.
31. Arozullah AM, Daley J, Henderson WG, Khuri SF. Multifactorial risk index for predicting postoperative respiratory failure in men after major noncardiac surgery. The National Veterans Administration Surgical Quality Improvement Program. Ann Surg. 2000;232:242–53.
32. Ephgrave KS, Kleiman-Wexler R, Pfaller M, et al. Postoperative pneumonia: a prospective study of risk factors and morbidity. Surgery. 1993;114:819–21.
33. Safdar N, Dezfulian C, Collard HR, Saint S. Clinical and economic consequences of ventilator-associated pneumonia: a systematic review. Crit Care Med. 2005;33:2184–93.

34. Berg H, Roed J, Viby-Mogensen J, et al. Residual neuromuscular block is a risk factor for postoperative pulmonary complications: a prospective, randomised, and blinded study of postoperative pulmonary complications after atracurium, vecuronium and pancuronium. Acta Anaesthesiol Scand. 1997;41:1095–103.

35. Kilpatrick B, Slinger P. Lung protective strategies in anaesthesia. Br J Anaesth. 2010;105 Suppl 1:i108–16.

36. Richard JC, Maggiore SM, Jonson B, et al. Influence of tidal volume on alveolar entity. Anesthesiology. 2005;163:1609–13.

37. Cai H, Gong H, Zhang L, Wang Y, Tian Y. Effect of low tidal volume ventilation on atelectasis in patients during general anesthesia: a computed tomographic scan. J Clin Anesth. 2007;19:125–9.

38. Tusman G, Bohm SH, Suarez-Shipman F. Alveolar recruitment improves ventilatory efficiency of the lungs during anesthesia. Can J Anaesth. 2004;51(7):723–7.

39. Hall JC, Tarala RA, Hall JL. A case-control study of postoperative pulmonary complications after laparoscopic and open cholecystectomy. J Laparoendosc Surg. 1996;6(2):87–92.

40. Nilsson G, Larsson S, Johnsson F. Randomized clinical trial of laparoscopic versus open fundoplication: blind evaluation of recovery and discharge period. Br J Surg. 2000;87(7):873–8.

41. Prinssen M, Verhoeven EL, Buth J, et al. A randomized trial comparing conventional and endovascular repair of abdominal aortic aneurysms. N Engl J Med. 2004;351(16):1607–8.

42. Pereira ED, Fernandes AL, da Silva Ancao M, et al. Prospective assessment of the risk of postoperative pulmonary complications in patients submitted to upper abdominal surgery. Sao Paulo Med J. 1999;117(4):151–60.

43. Brooks-Brunn JA. Predictors of postoperative pulmonary complications following abdominal surgery. Chest. 1997;111(3):564–71.

44. Wong DH, Weber EC, Schell MJ, et al. Factors associated with postoperative pulmonary complications in patients with severe chronic obstructive pulmonary disease. Anesth Analg. 1995;80(2):276–84.

45. McAlister FA, Khan NA, Straus SE, et al. Accuracy of the preoperative assessment in predicting pulmonary risk after nonthoracic surgery. Am J Respir Crit Care Med. 2003;167(5):741–4.

46. Bullock TK, Waltrip TJ, Price SA, Galandiuk S. A retrospective study of nosocomial pneumonia in postoperative patients shows a higher mortality rate in patients receiving nasogastric tube feeding. Am Surg. 2004;70(9):822–6.

47. Lawrence VA, Dhanda R, Hilsenbeck SG, Page CP. Risk of pulmonary complications after elective abdominal surgery. Chest. 1996;110(3):744–50.

48. Joo HS, Wong J, Naik VN, Savoldelli GL. The value of screening preoperative chest x-rays: a systematic review. Can J Anaesth. 2005;52(6):568–74.

49. Claggett GP, Anderson Jr FA, Geerts W, et al. Prevention of venous thromboembolism. Chest. 1998;114(5 Suppl):531S–60.

50. Coon WW. Venous thromboembolism. Prevalence, risk factors, and prevention. Clin Chest Med. 1984;5(3):391–401.

51. Rosendaal FR. Risk factors for venous thrombotic disease. Thromb Haemost. 1999;82(2):610–9.

52. Geerts WH, Bergqvist D, Pineo GF, et al. Prevention of venous thromboembolism: American College of Chest Physicians Evidence-Based Clinical Practice Guidelines (8th edition). Chest. 2008;133(6 Suppl):381S–453.

53. Geerts WH, Pineo GF, Heit JA, et al. Prevention of venous thromboembolism: the seventh ACCP conference on antithrombotic and thrombolytic therapy. Chest. 2004;6(3 Suppl):338S–400.

54. Sachdeva A, Dalton M, Amaragiri SV, Lees T. Elastic compression stockings for prevention of deep vein thrombosis. Cochrane Database of Syst Rev. 2010;(7):CD001484.

55. Rogers FB, Cipolle MD, Velmahos G, et al. Practice management guidelines for the prevention of venous thromboembolism in trauma patients: the EAST Practice Management Work Group. J Trauma. 2002;53(1):142–64.

56. Palmer AJ, Schramm W, Kirchhof B, Bergemann R. Low molecular weight heparin and unfractionated heparin for prevention of thromboembolism in general surgery: a meta-analysis of randomised clinical trials. Haemostasis. 1997;27(2):65–74.

57. Mismetti P, Laporte S, Zufferey P, et al. Prevention of venous thromboembolism in orthopedic surgery with vitamin K antagonists: a metaanalysis. J Thromb Haemost. 2004;2(7):1058–70.

58. Turpie AG, Bauer KA, Eriksson BI, Lasssen MR. Fondaparinux vs enoxaparin for the prevention of venous thromboembolism in major orthopedic surgery: a meta-analysis of 4 randomized double-blind studies. Arch Intern Med. 2002;162(16):1833–40.

59. Bauer KA, Eriksson BI, Lassen MR, Turpie AG, Steering Committee of the Pentasaccaride in Major Knee Surgery Study. Fondaparinux compared with enoxaparin for the prevention of venous thromboembolism after elective major knee surgery. N Engl J Med. 2001;345(18):1305–10.

60. Hirsh J, Bauer KA, Donati MB, et al. Parenteral anticoagulants: American College of Chest Physicians Evidence-Based Clinical Practice Guidelines (8th edition). Chest. 2008;133(6 Suppl):160S–98. Erratum appears in Chest. 2008 Aug;134(2):473.

61. Frederiksen SG, Hedenbro JL, Norgren L. Enoxaparin effect depends on body-weight and current doses may be inadequate in obese patients. Br J Surg. 2003;90(5):547–8.

62. Scholten DJ, Hoedema RM, Scholten SE. A comparison of two different prophylactic dose regimens of low molecular weight heparin in bariatric surgery. Obes Surg. 2002;12(1):19–24.

63. Hirsh J, O'Donnell M, Eikelboom JW. Beyond unfractionated heparin and warfarin: current and future advances. Circulation. 2007;116(5):552–60.

64. Schumacher WA. Effect of the direct factor Xa inhibitor apixaban in rat models of thrombosis and hemostasis. J Cardiovasc Pharmacol. 2010;55(6):609–16.

65. Stratmann G. Hemostasis. In: Miller RD, Pardo MC, editors. Miller: basics of anesthesia. 6th ed. Philadelphia, PA: Saunders; 2011. p. 348–63.

66. Schick KS, Fertmann JM, Jauch KW, Hoffmann JN. Prothrombin complex concentrate in surgical patients: retrospective evaluation of vitamin K antagonist reversal and treatment of severe bleeding. Crit Care. 2009;13(6):R191.

67. Ansell J, Hirsh J, Hylek E, Jacobson A, Crowther M, Palareti G. Pharmacology and management of the vitamin K antagonists: American College of Chest Physicians Evidence-Based Clinical Practice Guidelines (8th edition). Chest. 2008;133(6 Suppl):160S–98.

68. O'Riordan JM, Margey RJ, Blake G, et al. Antiplatelet agents in the perioperative period. Arch Surg. 2009;144(1):69–76.

69. Rade JJ, Hogue Jr SW. Noncardiac surgery for patients with coronary artery stents: timing is everything. Anesthesiology. 2008;109(4):573–5.

70. Howard-Alpe GM, de Bono J, Hudsmith L, et al. Coronary artery stents and non-cardiac surgery. Br J Anaesth. 2007;98(5):560–74.

71. Burger W, Chemnitius JM, Kneissl GD, et al. Low-dose aspirin for secondary cardiovascular prevention—cardiovascular risks after its perioperative withdrawal versus bleeding risks with its continuation—review and meta-analysis. J Intern Med. 2005;257(5):399–414.

72. Berger PB, Bellot V, Bell MR, et al. An immediate invasive strategy for the treatment of acute myocardial infarction early after noncardiac surgery. Am J Cardiol. 2001;87(9):1100–2.

73. Albaladejo P, Geeraerts T, Francis F, et al. Aspirin withdrawal and acute lower limb ischemia. Anesth Analg. 2004;99(2):440–3.

74. Senior K. Aspirin withdrawal increases risk of heart problems. Lancet. 2003;362(9395):1558.

75. Eisen GM, Baron TH, Dominitz JA, et al. Guideline on the management of anticoagulation and antiplatelet therapy for endoscopic procedures. Gastrointest Endosc. 2002;55(7):775–9.

76. Chassot PG, Delabays A, Spahn DR. Perioperative antiplatelet therapy: the case for continuing therapy in patients at risk of myocardial infarction. Br J Anaesth. 2007;99(3):316–28.

77. Horlocker TT, Wedel DJ, Rowlingson JC, et al. Regional anesthesia in the patient receiving antithrombotic or thrombolytic therapy. American Society of Regional Anesthesia and Pain Medicine Evidence-Based Guidelines. Reg Anesth Pain Med. 2010;35(1): 64–101.

78. Consensus Conference. Perioperative red blood cell transfusion. JAMA. 1988;260:2700–3.

79. Hebert PC, Schweitzer I, Calder L, et al. Review of the clinical practice literature on allogeneic red blood cell transfusion. Can Med Assoc J. 1997;156:S9–26.

80. American Society of Anesthesiologists Task Force on Blood Component Therapy. Practice guidelines for blood component therapy. Anesthesiology. 1996;85:732–47.

81. Salem M, Trainsh Jr RE, Bromberg J, Loriaux DL, Chernow B. Perioperative glucocorticoid coverage: a reassessment 42 years after emergence of a problem. Ann Surg. 1994;219(4):416–25.

82. Marik PE, Varon J. Requirement of perioperative stress doses of corticosteroids. Arch Surg. 2008;143(12):1222–6.

83. Friedman RJ, Schiff CF, Bromberg JS. Use of supplemental steroids in patients having orthopaedic operations. J Bone Joint Surg Am. 1995;77(12):1801–6.

84. Glowniak JV, Loriaux DL. A double-blind study of perioperative steroid requirements in secondary adrenal insufficiency. Surgery. 1997;121(2):123–9.

85. Thomason JM, Girdler NM, Kendall-Taylor P, Wastell H, Weddel A, Seymour RA. An investigation into the need for supplementary steroids in organ transplant patients undergoing gingival surgery: a double-blind, split-mouth, cross-over study. J Clin Periodontol. 1999;26(9):577–82.

86. McCowen KC, Malhotra A, Bistrain BR. Stress-induced hyperglycemia. Crit Care Clin. 2001;17(1):107–24.

87. Van den Berghe G, Wouters P, Weekers F, et al. Intensive insulin therapy in critically ill patients. N Engl J Med. 2001;345(19): 1359–67.

88. Van den Berghe G, et al. Intensive insulin therapy in mixed medical/surgical ICU: benefit versus harm. Diabetes. 2006;55(11): 3151–9.

89. Gandhi GY, Nuttall GA, Abel MD, et al. Intraoperative hyperglycemia and perioperative outcomes in cardiac surgery patients. Mayo Clin Proc. 2005;80:862–6.

90. Vanhorebeek I, Langouche L, Van den Berghe G. Tight blood glucose control with insulin in the ICU facts and controversies. Chest. 2007;132(1):268–78.

91. Van den Berghe G, Wilmer A, Hermans G, et al. Intensive insulin therapy in medical intensive care patients. N Engl J Med. 2006;354(5):449–61.

92. Vriesendorp TM, DeVries JH, Van Santen S, et al. Evaluation of short-term consequences of hypoglycemia in an intensive care unit. Crit Care Med. 2006;34(11):2714–8.

93. Mackenzie I, Ingle S, Zaidi S, et al. Tight glycaemic control: a survey of intensive care practice in large English hospitals. Intensive Care Med. 2005;31(8):1136.

94. Dellinger RP, Levy MM, Carlet JM, et al. Surviving sepsis campaign: International guidelines for management of severe sepsis and septic shock. Crit Care Med. 2008;36(1):296–327.

95. Gan TJ, Soppitt A, Maroof M, et al. Goal-directed intraoperative fluid administration reduces length of hospital stay after major surgery. Anesthesiology. 2002;97(4):820–6.

96. Kumar A, Roberts D, Wood K, et al. Duration of hypotension before initiation of effective antimicrobial therapy is the critical determinant of survival in human septic shock. Crit Care Med. 2006;34(6):1589–96.

97. Kurz A, Sessler DI, Lenhardt R. Perioperative normothermia to reduce the incidence of surgical-wound infection and shorten hospitalization. N Engl J Med. 1996;334(19):1209–15.

98. Weber WP, Zwahlen M, Reck S, Misteli H, Rosenthal R, Buser AS, et al. The association of preoperative anemia and perioperative allogeneic blood transfusion with the risk of surgical site infection. Transfusion. 2009;49(9):1964–70.

99. Aslan S, Akinci M, Cetin B, Cakmak H, Pirhan Y, Cetin A. Postoperative changes related to intraoperative blood transfusions. Bratisl Lek Listy. 2001;112(10):575–8.

100. Bernard AC, Davenport DL, Chang PK, et al. Intraoperative transfusion of 1 U to 2 U packed red blood cells is associated with increased 30-day mortality, surgical-site infection, pneumonia, and sepsis in general surgery patients. J Am Coll Surg. 2009;208(5):931–9.

101. Somogyi-Zalud E, Zhong Z, Hamel MB, et al. The use of life-sustaining treatments in hospitalized persons aged 80 and older. J Am Geriatr Soc. 2002;50(5):930–4.

102. Margolis JO, McGrath BJ, Kussin PS, Schwinn DA. Do not resuscitate (DNR) orders during surgery: ethical foundations for institutional policies in the United States. Anesth Analg. 1995;80(4):806–9.

103. American College of Surgeons. [ST-19] Statement on Advance Directives by Patients: "Do Not Resuscitate" in the Operating Room. American College of Surgeons. [Online] Sept 1994. http://www.facs.org/fellows_info/statements/st-19.html.

104. American Society of Anesthesiologists. Ethical guidelines for the anesthesia care of patients with do-not-resuscitate orders or other directives that limit care; ASA Standards, Guidelines and Statements. Park Ridge, IL; 1999. p. 470–71.

105. Ball KA. Do-not-resuscitate orders in surgery: decreasing the confusion. AORN J. 2009;89:140–6.

106. Cohen CB, Cohen PJ. Do-not-resuscitate orders in the operating room. N Engl J Med. 1991;325:1879–82.

Additional Readings

Woods BD, Sladen RN. Perioperative considerations for the patient with asthma and bronchospasm. Br J Anaesth. 2009;103:157–65.

Ewanchuk M, Brindley PG. Ethics review: perioperative do-not-resuscitate orders—doing 'nothing' when 'something' can be done. Crit Care. 2006;10(4):219.

Detsky AS, Baker JP, O'Rourke K, Goel V. Perioperative parenteral nutrition: a meta-analysis. Ann Intern Med. 1987;107:195–203.

Committee on Ethics, American College of Surgeons. Statement on advance directives by patients: "Do Not Resuscitate" in the operating room. Bull Am Coll Surg. 1994;79:29.

Janku GV, Paiement GD, Green HD. Prevention of venous thromboembolism in orthopaedics in the United States. Clin Orthop Relat Res. 1996;325:313–21.

American College of Surgeons Continuous Quality Improvement. American College of Surgeons. [Online] 18 Dec 2011. http://www.facs.org/cqi/scip.html.

American Academy of Orthopedic Surgeons. Clearing up the confusion with venous thromboembolism and/or pulmonary embolism prophylaxis guidelines. [Online] 18 Dec 2011. http://www.aaos.org/news/aaosnow/jan08/clinical2.asp.

Lawrence VA, Cornell JE, Smetana GW. Strategies to reduce postoperative pulmonary complications after noncardiothoracic surgery: systematic review for the American College of Physicians. Ann Intern Med. 2006;144(8):596–608

Møller AM, Villebro N, Pedersen T, Tønnesen H. Effect of preoperative smoking intervention on postoperative complications: a randomised clinical trial. Lancet. 2002;359(9301):114–7.

Bluman LG, Mosca L, Newman N, Simon DG. Preoperative smoking habits and postoperative pulmonary complications. Chest. 1998; 113(4):883–9.

Sandham JD, Hull RD, Brant RF, Knox L, Pineo GF, Doig CJ, et al. A randomized, controlled trial of the use of pulmonary-artery catheters in high-risk surgical patients. N Engl J Med. 2003;348(1):5–14.

Moore FA, Feliciano DV, Andrassy RJ, McArdle AH, Booth FV, Morgenstein-Wagner TB, et al. Early enteral feeding, compared with parenteral, reduces postoperative septic complications. The results of a meta-analysis. Ann Surg. 1992;216(2):172–83.

Pacelli F, Bossola M, Papa V, Malerba M, Modesti C, Sgadari A, et al. Enteral vs parenteral nutrition after major abdominal surgery: an even match. Arch Surg. 2001;136(8):933–6.

Damage Control Laparotomy in Surgical Sepsis

Frederick A. Moore and Laura J. Moore

4

Introduction

Over the past decade tremendous efforts have been directed at defining and implementing evidence-based guidelines (EBGs) for sepsis in the intensive care unit (ICU) [1–6]. Given the magnitude and the complexity of this increasingly common ICU problem, these guidelines were badly needed [7–12]. However, these EBGs fail to distinguish surgical sepsis as a distinct entity. In August 2006, a new Division of Acute Care Surgery (ACS) was started at The Methodist Hospital (TMH) in Houston, Texas. The ACS group identified sepsis to be the major cause of mortality in the surgical intensive care unit (SICU). A multidisciplinary sepsis working group was developed and over the next year it created a comprehensive sepsis management protocol that included (a) routine sepsis screening, (b) computerized clinical decision support (CCDS) to consistently implement EBGs, and (c) selective use of damage control laparotomy (DCL) in patients presenting with an intra-abdominal infection and septic shock [6, 13, 14]. The purpose of this chapter is to review our rationale for the use of DCL in surgical sepsis, how DCL is implemented into comprehensive management of sepsis, and our ongoing experience with managing surgical sepsis with an emphasis on DCL.

Rationale for Damage Control Laparotomy in Surgical Sepsis

In the early 1980s, trauma surgeons recognized the high mortality associated with operating in the setting of "bloody viscous cycle" of acidosis, hypothermia, and coagulopathy [15]. This prompted the development of the concept of a truncated laparotomy using packing to stop bleeding with a temporary abdominal closure (e.g., towel clips closure of the skin) and triage to the ICU with the intent of optimizing physiology and then returning to the operating room (OR) after 24–48 h for definitive treatment of injuries and abdominal closure [16]. This concept was initially promoted for major liver injuries but was soon extended to all emergency laparotomies [17–19]. Over the next decade this concept evolved into "damage control," which was a major paradigm shift for trauma surgeons [20]. This practice has become standard of care worldwide and has saved the lives of many patients who previously exsanguinated on the operating room table. But how does this strategy relate to surgical sepsis?

As a group of acute care surgeons developing a comprehensive sepsis management protocol, it was natural to use DCL in the most physiologically deranged patients [21, 22]. However, this caused considerable consternation among the other members of medical staff. For several reasons they were confused. First, while they were aware of the "bloody viscous cycle," they appropriately noted that this is not a frequent fatal problem in surgical sepsis. Second, they did not appreciate that staying in the OR to perform a definitive operation often results in extended periods of hypovolemia and vasopressor therapy, which cause acute kidney injury (AKI). This sets the stage for multiple organ failure (MOF) and prolonged ICU stays [23]. In the laboratory, it has been demonstrated that AKI adversely affects the immune response (primarily T cell function) contributing to the compensatory anti-inflammatory response syndrome (CARS). Third, they mistakenly thought that the acute care surgeons were practicing "planned re-laparatomy." This strategy has been debated for more than 30 years. Reoperations are performed

F.A. Moore, M.D., F.A.C.S. (✉)
Department of Acute Care Surgery, Shands at the University of Florida, 1600 SW Archer Road, Box 100108, Gainesville, FL 32610, USA
e-mail: Frederick.Moore@surgery.ufl.edu

L.J. Moore, M.D., F.A.C.S.
Department of Surgery, The University of Texas Health Science Center, Houston, TX, USA

L.J. Moore et al. (eds.), *Common Problems in Acute Care Surgery*,
DOI 10.1007/978-1-4614-6123-4_4, © Springer Science+Business Media New York 2013

every 48 h for "washouts" until the abdomen is free of ongoing peritonitis and then the abdomen is closed. This supposedly prevents and/or provides early treatment for secondary infections, thus decreasing late MOF and deaths. The downside of the planned re-laparotomy approach is increased resource utilization and the increased potential risk for gastrointestinal fistulas and delayed hernias.

The alternative is referred to "laparotomy on demand" where re-laparotomy is performed for clinical deterioration or lack of improvement. The potential downside to this approach is harmful delays in diagnosing secondary abdominal infections and the presence of more dense adhesions if there is a need to reoperate. Over the years there have been eight case series that have offered conflicting results regarding the impact of this strategy on outcome. A meta-analysis of the data concluded "laparotomy on demand" was the preferred approach in patients with Acute Physiology and Chronic Health Evaluation II (APACHE II) scores <10 [24]. However, a recent prospective randomized trial by van Ruler et. al. in patients with APACHE II >10 indicates that the practice of "planned re-laparotomy" offered no clinical advantage over "laparotomy on demand" and was associated with substantial increases in expenditure of hospital resources [25].

To explain acute care surgeon's practice of DCL, Figs. 4.1–4.3 were developed. Fig. 4.1 emphasizes that an intra-abdominal infection is a progressive disease. As patients progress from sepsis with SIRS through severe sepsis with organ dysfunction into septic shock, the abdominal infection often turns into an abdominal catastrophe. Patients presenting with an abdominal catastrophe frequently present in full-blown septic shock. In these cases, the surgeon needs to recognize that the patient is in the "persistent septic shock cycle" (Fig. 4.2). This is characterized by excessive proinflammation, which causes vasodilation, hypotension, and myocardial depression. This combined with endothelial activation and diffused intravascular coagulopathy (DIC) causes ongoing endothelial leak, cellular shock, and microvascular thrombosis. The clinical manifestation is ongoing septic shock with progressive MOF. The crucial question is timing of the operative intervention for source control to break this persistent cycle. These patients are hemodynamically unstable and clearly not great candidates for operative interventions. The traditional approach has been to take the patient to the OR and perform a definitive operation (Fig. 4.3). However, this usually results in a hypovolemic septic shock patient being treated for prolonged periods in the OR with vasopressors. The end result is early deaths from fulminant MOF or AKI, which then sets the stage for ongoing MOF and prolonged ICU stays. However, with the recent EGBs recommending source control within 6 h, a paradigm shift was proposed [5]. The initial focus was preoperative optimization with administering antibiotics, placement of central venous and arterial lines, and optimizing resuscitation. This takes 2–3 h. The

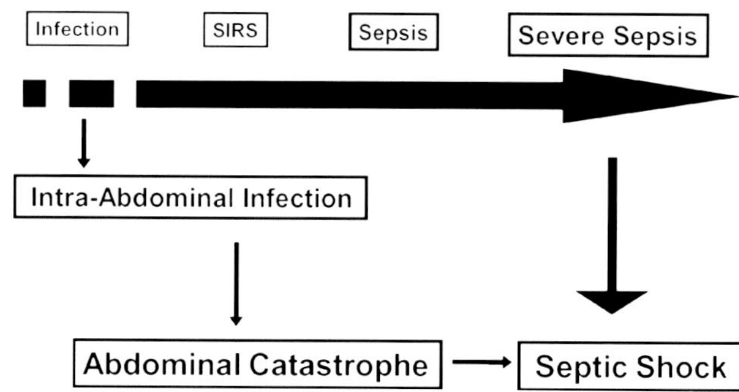

Fig. 4.1 The progression of an intra-abdominal infection

patient is taken to the OR for a truncated operation and is returned to the ICU for ongoing resuscitation with the intent of avoiding AKI. If this can be accomplished, it is surprising how quickly these very sick patients can recover.

Integrating Damage Control Laparotomy in Sepsis Management

Preoperative Optimization

This will take 2–3 h to accomplish. Patients are entered into the 24-h early sepsis management protocol. They are bolused with 20 ml/kg of ideal body weight of isotonic crystalloids and given rescue bolused norepinephrine as needed to maintain mean arterial pressure (MAP) greater than 65 mmHg. Broad-spectrum antibiotics are administered. At least two large-bore intravenous lines are needed. Given that the patient is in septic shock, a central line (via the internal jugular vein placed under ultrasound guidance) and an arterial line are placed. With ongoing volume loading, central venous pressure (CVP) is increased to above 10 cmH$_2$O. At this point the patient is intubated. Avoid etomidate as an induction agent as it is known to suppress the adrenal function and its use in critically ill patients is associated with increased mortality [26]. Use ketamine instead, because it does not adversely affect cardiac function and it down-regulates pro-inflammation [27]. Ventilation is then optimized. Norepinephrine is titrated to maintain MAP >65 mmHg, and if high doses are required, stress-dose steroids are administered. Electrolyte abnormalities are corrected and blood products are administered based on institutional guidelines. Lactate and mixed venous hemoglobin saturations are measured.

Laparotomy

The goal is to have this completed as soon as possible and the priority of this operative intervention is source control.

Fig. 4.2 The persistent septic shock cycle

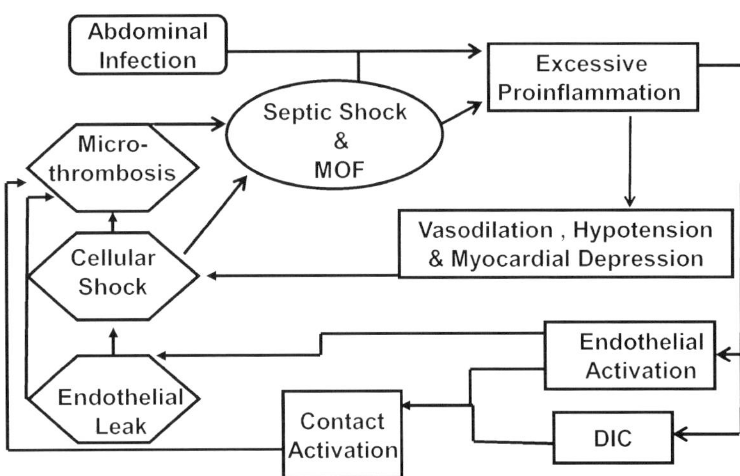

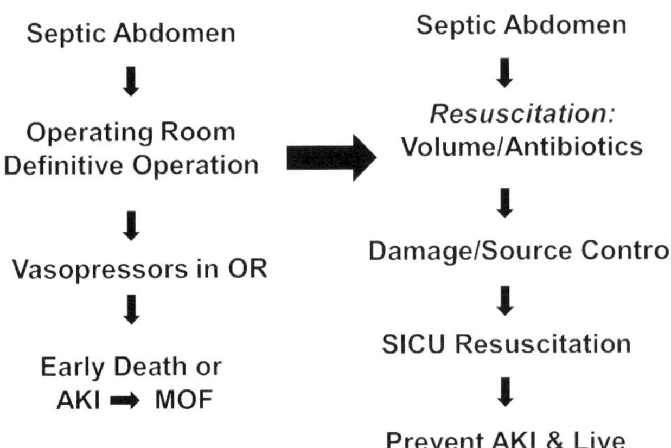

Fig. 4.3 Paradigm shift in management of patients with an abdominal infection and septic shock

At the beginning of the operation the surgeons assess the degree of physiologic derangement (i.e., vasopressor requirements, acidosis, and evidence of DIC). If the patient is judged to be physiologically deranged then proceed into "damage control" mode. The surgeon should announce to the operating room team his/her intent to perform DCL and specific supplies that are needed (e.g., staplers, temporary abdominal closure supplies) and that this is going to be a short operation. Dead bowel is resected and debrided. Holes in the bowel are stapled to limit contamination. Big dissections are avoided to minimize consequent bleeding. Bleeding is packed as needed. Limited irrigation is performed to ensure no ongoing contamination. Use vacuum-assisted temporary abdominal closure. The operation should last 30–45 min.

Postoperative Optimization

The primary focus is to optimize resuscitation. The patient is volume loaded to increase CVP to >10 cmH$_2$O and to decrease stroke volume variation to less than 13%.

Non-responding patients should have an echocardiogram to assess for the presence of myocardial dysfunction, which often occurs with severe sepsis and should prompt the use of inotropic agents [28]. During acute resuscitation, the patient is sedated and provided full ventilator support. A short course of neuromuscular blockade is administered if the patient is fighting the ventilator until the clinical course stabilizes (usually within 12 h). If the patient develops acute lung injury, paralysis should be continued for 48 h to facilitate lung-protective ventilation, which improves outcome [29]. The goals are to correct abnormal physiology (e.g., hypothermia, coagulopathy, and acidosis) to prepare for a definitive second operation. Bladder pressure should be monitored in patients who require high-volume crystalloid resuscitation. Avoid large volume of hetastarch as this has been shown to cause AKI [30].

Second Operation

The temporary abdominal closure device and packs are removed and the abdomen is explored. Further resection and/or debridement are performed as needed. Next the surgeon needs to decide whether to perform an anastomosis or an ostomy. A left colon anastomosis should only be performed when conditions are ideal [31, 32]. A nasojejunal tube should be placed to facilitate early enteral nutrition. If feasible the fascia is closed, but the skin is not closed. If the fascia cannot be closed, replace a temporary abdominal closure device.

Ongoing Supportive ICU Care

By now the patient has completed the 24-h early sepsis management protocol that is implemented by CCDS and will be managed by the surgical intensivist using standard

encounter: 10166 phase 1: ☐ MAP ☑ 55 mmHg lactate ☐ mM

protocol start: 2008-11-22 10:00 phase 2: ☑ 2008-11-22 10:00 UO ☐ mL/kg/hr GCS ☑ 3

hour	MAP	CVP	HR	RR	Temp	Scv02	pH	BD	Lactate	Creatinine	K	WBC	Hb	INR	LR	NS	Hextend	PRBC	FFP	Medications
0	55	10		17	40.3	65									2000					
1	58	10	151	24		70			3.9	2.5	3.0	6.6	12.9	1.70	2000					decadron/cefepime (maxipime)/levofloxacin/clindamycin
2	77	19	157	25	40.9	90														**norepinephrine (15 µg/min)**
3	82		151	17	41.1	91	7.24	7												**norepinephrine (10 µg/min)**
4	77	14	151	17		92														**vasopressin (0.04 units/min)**
5	73	15	146	15	40.8	92														
6	75	9	137	17	39.8	95									2000					**norepinephrine (15 µg/min)**
7	89	11	132	17	39.4	90	7.31	6	1.5	1.9	3.1	5.2	12.1		2000					**norepinephrine (10 µg/min)**
8	71		124		39.0	91														mycanine (micafungin)/decadron
9	70	11	123	16	39.2	90	7.26	5							2000					**norepinephrine (15 µg/min)**
10	84	12	125	16	38.9	96									2000					
11	86		116	16		90														
12	93		117	16	38.5	91	7.37	2												vancomycin/piperaillin-tazobactam/decadron/norepinephrine (l
13	84	15	117	16	38.7	90			2.1	1.2	3.4	3.5	10.6	1.50						
14	89	15	117	16		93														
15	87	15	120	16	38.9	94														
16	86	15	119	16		90														
17	87	14	117	16	38.8	90	7.39	0		1.0	3.5	4.0	10.6	1.50						
18	89	14	114	16	38.6	91									2000					dexamethasone
19	89		102	16	37.9	91														**norepinephrine (10 µg/min)**
20	88	15	97	16	37.8	90														piperacillin-tazobactam
21	88	14	95	15	37.7	91	7.43	−1	1.4	0.9	3.8	3.8	10.1	1.40						**norepinephrine (5 µg/min)**
22	94	14	107	16	37.4	96														**norepinephrine off**
23	78	9	99	14		92														
24	89	11	103	16	37.3	91	7.43	−2	1.2	0.9	3.7	3.4	9.9	1.40						vancomycin/piperacillin-tazobactam

Fig. 4.4 Early sepsis management

ICU protocols, including (a) sedation and analgesia, (b) lung-protective ventilation, (c) spontaneous breathing trials when indicated, (d) early enteral nutrition, (e) stress gastritis prophylaxis, (f) DVT prophylaxis, (g) tight glycemic control, (h) restrictive transfusions, and (i) early mobilization.

Recent Case Report

As part of the early sepsis management protocol hourly data are collected for 24 h. A flow sheet with these data is then given to the ICU team to review the next day on rounds so that they can see what happened during the sepsis resuscitation (see Fig. 4.4 as an example of one of these flow sheets). These data were collected from a 54 year old male that was undergoing chemotherapy for a brain tumor and experienced a sudden change in mental status and became short of breath on the floor. He was transferred to the SICU due to the fact that the neurosurgical ICU was full. He presented with a systolic blood pressure of 70 mmHg, heart rate of 160 beats per minute (BPM), and temperature of 40.3°C. He was volume resuscitated and bolused with norepinephrine. The patient was in full-blown septic shock but the etiology was unclear. A screening abdominal X-ray (see Fig. 4.5) was obtained and demonstrated a dilated colon. Given the clinical presentation, this was presumed to be dead. The patient had ongoing hypotension despite aggressive volume resuscitation and was now on high-dose norepinephrine, low-dose vasopressin, and stress-dose steroids. He was too unstable for transport to the operating room. The family and the patient's attending physician wanted to pursue all options. The ACS attending on call was notified and decided to perform a DCL in the ICU (see Figs. 4.6 and 4.7). The dead colon was removed and a temporary abdominal closure device was placed.

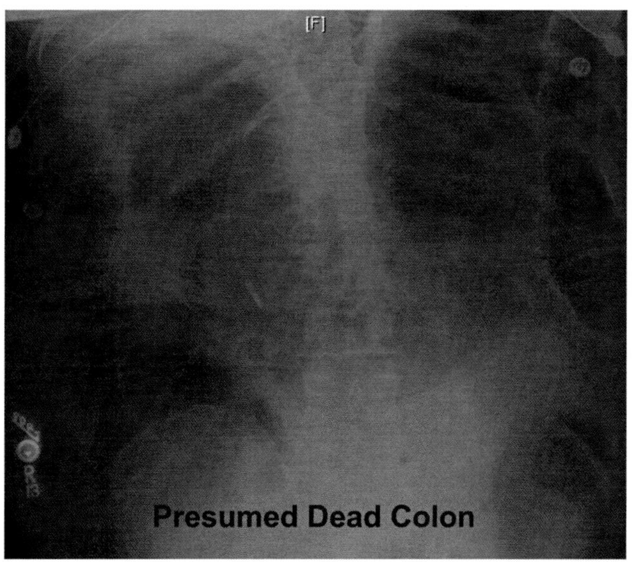

Fig. 4.5 Screening KUB X-ray

As can be seen in Fig. 4.4, this patient was gravely ill. He presented with a heart rate of 161 BPM, and he had a lactate of 3.9, and a creatinine of 2.5. With aggressive volume loading, the CVP was increased to 15 cmH$_2$O and the heart rate decreased to less than 100 BPM. He required 7 l of lactated Ringer's. Over the 24-h period, lactate levels normalized and the norepinephrine was weaned off. Of note, the creatinine levels normalized and there was no need for dialysis. The following day, the patient was taken to the OR where an ileostomy was performed and primary fascial closure was achieved. A nasojejunal tube was placed and the patient was placed on early enteral nutrition with an immune-enhancing diet. The patient underwent aggressive physical therapy and early mobilization. He was transferred to inpatient rehabilitation at day 11. His APACHE II score was 41 with a predicted mortality of 93%. This is an example of how DCL can salvage someone who would have previously died.

Our Recent Experience with an Early Sepsis Management Protocol in Surgical Sepsis

Over the last year a series of database analyses have been performed, some of which are relevant to this chapter. Fig. 4.8 depicts the 30-day mortality for severe sepsis/septic shock over 3 years of protocol development (2007–2009) [6]. Mortality data for 2006 and 2007 were collected by TMH Performance Improvement department as part of the Institute of Healthcare Improvement (IHI) Surviving Sepsis Campaign (SSC) [33]. The ACS group arrived in August 2006 and implemented a paper protocol in 2007 and 2008. Automated electronic medical record sepsis screening and

CCDS were fully implemented in 2009. The 2008 and 2009 mortality were collected as part of the ACS sepsis database. These mortality data are also compared to the reported mortality of a recently published analysis of the National Surgical Quality Improvement Project (NSQIP) database and the 8th quarter mortality reported by the IHI SSC [11, 32]. As can be seen there was a tremendous reduction in mortality from 35% in 2006 prior to protocol development to 14% in 2009 after full implementation of early sepsis management protocol. We believe this is primarily due to (a) early detection of sepsis prior to the development of septic shock, (b) rapid implementation of evidence-based care with CCDS, and (c) selective use of DCL in patients presenting with abdominal catastrophes and septic shock.

Recent Experience with Damage Control Laparotomy in Surgical Sepsis

In 2009, we reported at the American Association for the Surgery of Trauma annual meeting the results of the 2007–2008 ACS sepsis database analysis (Fig. 4.9). Our objective was to determine the actual mortality versus the predicted mortality for patients undergoing DCL for intra-abdominal infection who were in septic shock (Fig. 4.10). We queried our prospective database over a 2-year period to identify patients with (1) septic shock, (2) intra-abdominal infection, and (3) those who had undergone DCL. We identified 41 patients who met the criteria for septic shock. Twenty-one patients had an intra-abdominal infection and underwent DCL. Sources of infection included the colon in 13, small bowel in 6, stomach in 2, and primary peritonitis in 1. Their average APACHE II score was 31.8 (±11.3) with a predicted mortality of 76%. Their P-Possum score was 74.9±23.2 with a predicted mortality of 69.4%. The actual mortality was 27%, which is significantly lower ($p < 0.02$) than the predicted mortalities.

Benchmarking

More recently to assess the impact of the comprehensive sepsis management protocol, the 2005–2007 NSQIP database and the prospective ACS sepsis database were queried to identify patients (1) with severe sepsis/septic shock (using the same definitions) and (2) requiring emergency colon surgery [34]. The primary endpoint was 30-day mortality. Out of 363,897 general surgery patients in the NSQIP database, 1,101 patients were identified who met these criteria and out of 307 ACS database, 46 patients who met the same criteria were identified. Table 4.1 depicts the demographics, APACHE II scores, predicted mortality, and actual 30-day mortality.

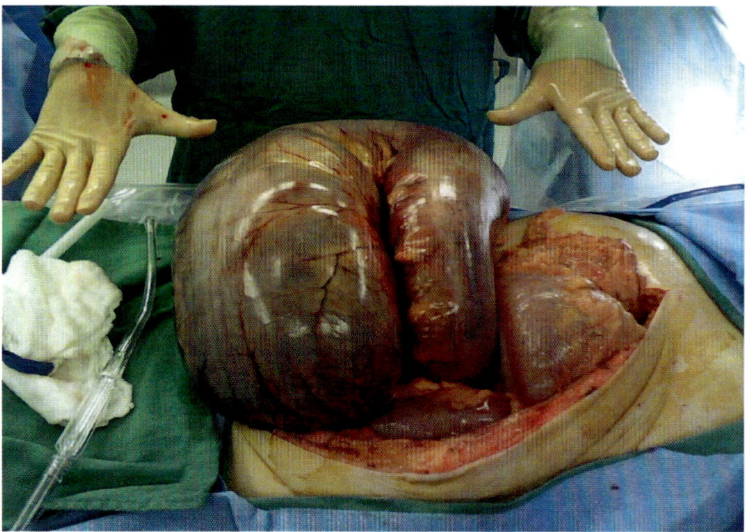

Fig. 4.6 Dilated colon found after opening the abdomen

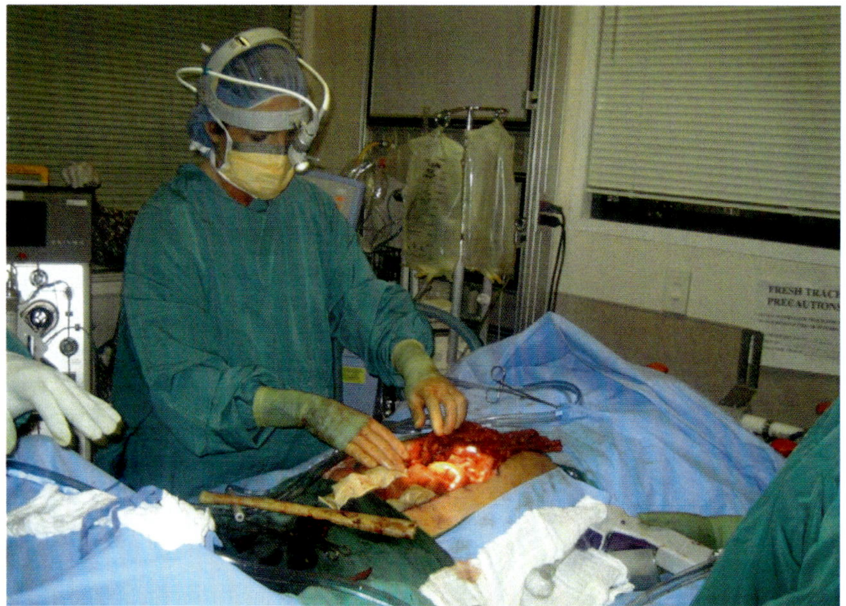

Fig. 4.7 Abdomen after colon was removed

The two cohorts had similar average ages and percent male gender. The ACS patients had a predicted mortality of 73%, which was significantly higher than the actual mortality of 28.3%. The actual NSQIP 30-day mortality was 40.4%, which was higher ($p = 0.06$) than the ACS actual 30-day mortality. Sixty-seven percent of the ACS database cohort had undergone DCL. It is unknown if any of the NSQIP patients underwent DCL.

Table 4.1 NSQIP benchmark study

	ACS ($n = 46$)	NSQIP ($n = 1{,}101$)
Average age	62.3 ± 17.9	68.5 ± 13.5
Male	45%	47.2%
APACHE II	31 ± 8.2	Not available
Predicted mortality (APACHE II)[a]	73%	Not available
Actual 30-day mortality[b]	28.3%	40.4%

[a]Actual versus predicted mortality $p < 0.0001$
[b]ACS versus NSQIP mortality $p = 0.06$

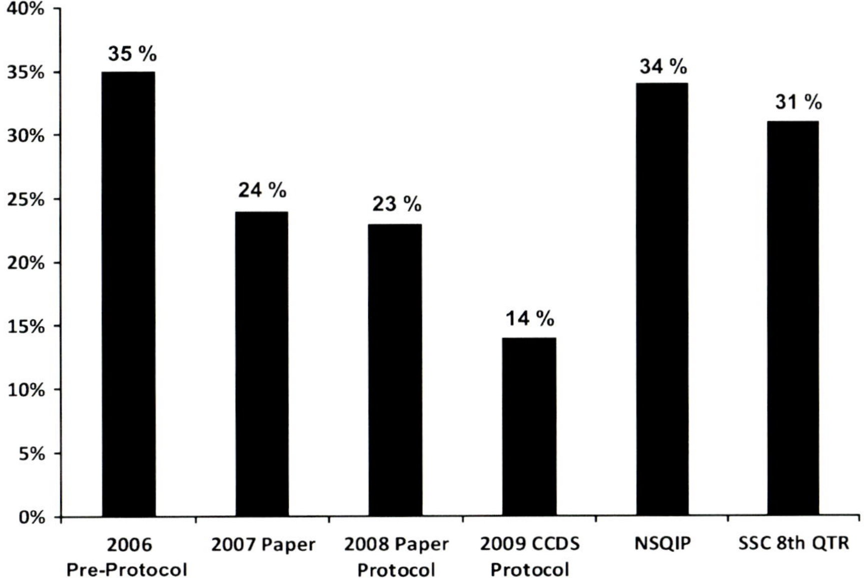

Fig. 4.8 Decreased mortality with comprehensive sepsis management

Fig. 4.9 AKI severity and mortality

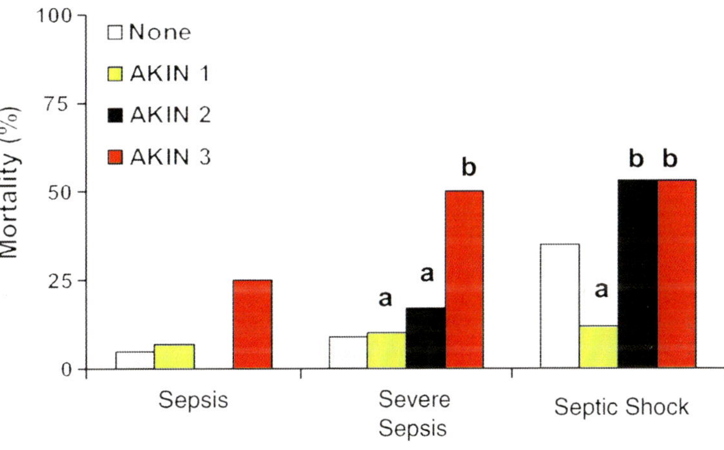

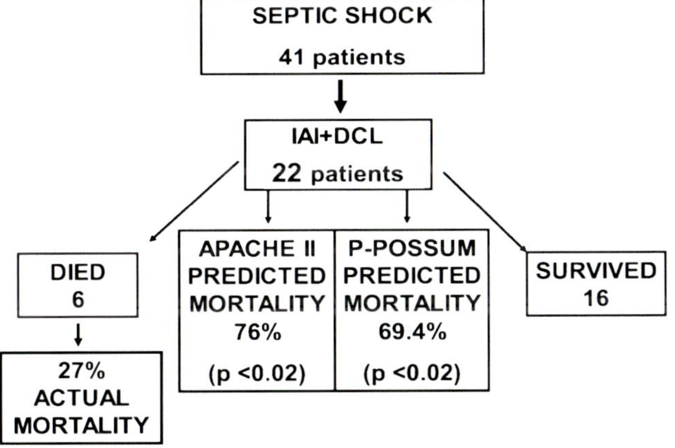

Fig. 4.10 Actual versus predicted mortality of DCL patients

Conclusion

Surgical sepsis is a complex and frequently deadly complication that requires complex processes of care to ensure survival. Routine screening helps identify septic patients early in the process before they progress to septic shock. CCDS is used to ensure high compliance with recommended interventions. Additionally, DCL is used in patients presenting an intra-abdominal infection and septic shock. The combination of routine screening, CCDS, and selective use of DCL can dramatically improve survival and appears to be better than the traditional methods of managing surgical sepsis.

References

1. Hollenberg SM, Ahrens TS, Annane D, Astiz ME, Chalfin DB, Dasta JF, Heard SO, Martin C, Napolitano LM, Susla GM, Totaro R, Vincent JL, Zanotti-Cavazzoni S. Practice parameters for hemodynamic support of sepsis in adult patients: 2004 update. Crit Care Med. 2004;32(9):1928–48.
2. Kortgen A, Niederprum P, Bauer M. Implementation of an evidence-based "standard operating procedure" and outcome in septic shock. Crit Care Med. 2006;34(4):943–9.
3. Nguyen HB, Corbett SW, Steele R, Banta J, Clark RT, Hayes SR, Edwards J, Cho TW, Wittlake WA. Implementation of a bundle of quality indicators for the early management of severe sepsis and septic shock is associated with decreased mortality. Crit Care Med. 2007;35(4):1105–12.
4. Thiel SW, Asghar MF, Micek ST, Reichley RM, Doherty JA, Kollef MH. Hospital-wide impact of a standardized order set for the management of bacteremic severe sepsis. Crit Care Med. 2009;37(3):819–24.
5. Dellinger RP, Levy MM, Carlet JM, Bion J, Parker MM, Jaeschke R, Reinhart K, Angus DC, Brun-Buisson C, Beale R, Calandra T, Dhainaut JF, Gerlach H, Harvey M, Marini JJ, Marshall J, Ranieri M, Ramsay G, Sevransky J, Thompson BT, Townsend S, Vender JS, Zimmerman JL, Vincent JL. Surviving sepsis campaign: international guidelines for management of severe sepsis and septic shock: 2008. Crit Care Med. 2008;36(1):296327.
6. McKinley BA, Moore LJ, Sucher JF, Todd SR, Turner KL, Valdivia A, Sailors RM, Moore FA. Computer protocol facilitates evidence-based care of sepsis in the surgical intensive care unit. J Trauma. 2011;70(5):1153–67.
7. Angus DC, Linde-Zwirble WT, Lidicker J, Clermont G, Carcillo J, Pinsky MR. Epidemiology of severe sepsis in the United States: analysis of incidence, outcome, and associated costs of care. Crit Care Med. 2001;29(7):1303–10.
8. Martin GS, Mannino DM, Eaton S, Moss M. The epidemiology of sepsis in the United States from 1979 through 2000. N Eng J Med. 2003;348:1546–54.
9. Dombrovskiy VY, Martin AA, Sunderram J, Paz HL. Rapid increase in hospitalization and mortality rates for severe sepsis in the United States: a trend analysis from 1993 to 2003. Crit Care Med. 2007;35(5):1244–50.
10. Moore LJ, Moore FA, Jones SL, Xu J, Bass BL. Sepsis in general surgery: a deadly complication. Am J Surg. 2009;198(6):868–74.
11. Moore LJ, Moore FA, Todd SR, Jones SL, Turner KL, Bass BL. Sepsis in general surgery. The 2005–2007 national surgical quality improvement program perspective. Arch Surg. 2010;145(7):695–700.
12. Moore LJ, McKinley BA, Turner KL, Todd SR, Sucher JF, Valdivia A, Sailors RM, Kao LS, Moore FA. The epidemiology of sepsis in general surgery patients. J Trauma. 2011;70(3):672–80.
13. Moore LJ, Turner KL, Jones SL, Kreiner LA, McKinley BA, Valdivia A, Todd SR, Moore FA. Validation of a screening tool for the early identification of sepsis. J Trauma. 2009;66(6):1539–47.
14. Moore LJ, Turner KL, Todd SR, McKinley BA, Moore FA. Computerized clinical decision support improves mortality in intra abdominal surgical sepsis. Am J Surg. 2010;200(6):839–44.
15. Kashuk JL, Moore EE, Millikan JS, Moore JB. Major abdominal vascular trauma—a unified approach. J Trauma. 1982;22:672–9.
16. Stone H, Strom PR, Mullins RJ. Management of the major coagulopathy with onset during laparotomy. Ann Surg. 1983;197(5):532–5.
17. Feliciano DV, Mattox KL, Burch JM, Bitondo CG, Jordan GL. Packing for control of hepatic hemorrhage. J Trauma. 1986;26:738–43.
18. Burch JM, Ortiz VB, Richardson RJ, Martin RR, Mattox KL, Jordan Jr GL. Abbreviated laparotomy and planned reoperation for critically injured patients. Ann Surg. 1992;215:476–84.
19. Morris JA, Eddy VA, Blinman TA, Rutherford EJ, Sharp KW. Management of the major coagulopathy with onset during laparotomy. Ann Surg. 1993;217(5):576–86.
20. Rotondo MF, Schwab CW, McGonigal MD, Phillips III GR, Fruchterman TM, Kauder DR, Latenser BA, Angood PA. 'Damage Control' an approach for improved survival in exsaguinating penetrating abdominal injury. J Trauma. 1993;35(3):375–82.
21. Finlay IG, Edwards TJ, Lambert AW. Damage control laparotomy. Br J Surg. 2004;91:83–5.
22. Stawicki SP, Brooks A, Bilski T, Scaff D, Gupta R, Schwab CW, Gracias VH. The concept of damage control: extending the paradigm to emergency general surgery. Injury. 2008;39:93–101.
23. White LE, Chaudhary R, Moore LJ, Moore FA, Hassoun HT. Surgical sepsis and organ crosstalk: the role of the kidney. J Surg Res. 2011;167(2):306–15.
24. Lamme B, Boermeester MA, Reitsma JB, Mahler CW, Obertop H, Gouma DJ. Meta-analysis of relaparotomy for secondary peritonitis. Br J Surg. 2003;90(3):369.
25. van Ruler O, Mahler CW, Boer KR, Reuland EA, Gooszen HG, Opmeer BC, de Graaf PW, Lamme B, Gerhards MF, Steller EP, van Till JW, de Borgie CJ, Gouma DJ, Reitsma JB, Boermeester MA, Dutch Peritonitis Study Group. Comparison of on-demand vs. planned relaporatomy strategy in patients with severe peritonitis. JAMA. 2007;298(8):865–72.
26. Albert SG, Ariyan S, Rather A. The effect of etomidate on adrenal function in critical illness: a systemic review. Intensive Care Med. 2011;37:901–10.
27. Takahashi T, Kinoshita M, Shono S, Habu Y, Ogura T, Seki S, Kazama T. The effect of ketamine anesthesia on the immune function of mice with postoperative septicemia. Anesth Analg. 2010;111(4):1051–8.
28. Turner KL, Moore LJ, Todd SR, Sucher JF, Jones SA, McKinley BA, Valdivia A, Sailors RM, Moore FA. Identification of cardiac dysfunction in sepsis with B-type natriuretic peptide. J Am Coll Surg. 2011;213(1):139–46. discussion 146–7. Epub 2011 Apr 21.
29. Papazian L, Forel JM, Gacouin A, Penot-Ragon C, Perrin G, Loundou A, Jaber S, Arnal JM, Perez D, Seghboyan JM, Constantin JM, Courant P, Lefrant JY, Guérin C, Prat G, Morange S, Roch A, ACURASYS Study Investigators. Neuromuscular blockers in early acute respiratory distress syndrome. N Engl J Med. 2010;363(12):11071116.
30. Bayer O, Reinhart K, Sakr Y, Kabisch B, Kohl M, Riedemann NC, Bauer M, Settmacher U, Hekmat K, Hartog CS. Renal effects of synthetic colloids and crystalloids in patients with severe sepsis: a prospective sequential comparison. Crit Care Med. 2011;39(6):13351342.
31. Ott MM, Norris PR, Diaz JJ, Collier BR, Jenkins JM, Gunter OL, Morris Jr JA. Colon anastomosis after damage control laparotomy: recommendations from 174 trauma colectomies. J Trauma. 2011;70(3):595–602.
32. Kashuk JL, Cothren CC, Moore EE, Johnson JL, Biffl WL, Barnett CC. Primary repair of civilian colon injuries is safe in the damage control scenario. Surgery. 2009;146(4):663–8.
33. Levy MM, Dellinger RP, Townsend SR, Linde-Zwirble WT, Marshall JC, Bion J, Schorr C, Artigas A, Ramsay G, Beale R, Parker MM, Gerlach H, Reinhart K, Silva E, Harvey M, Regan S, Angus DC, Surviving Sepsis Campaign. The surviving Sepsis Campaign: results of an international guideline-based performance improvement program targeting severe sepsis. Crit Care Med. 2010;38(2):367374.
34. Moore LJ, Turner KL, Jones SL, Fahy BN, Moore FA. The availability of acute care surgeons improves outcomes in patients requiring emergent colon surgery. Am J Surg. 2011;202(6):837–42. Epub 2011 Oct 19.

Surgical Procedures in the Intensive Care Unit

5

Linda A. Dultz, Vasiliy Sim, and S. Rob Todd

Introduction

Surgeons inherently favor performing procedures in the operating room. It is the obvious choice since it is a controlled, sterile environment, with the assistance of an anesthesiologist, surgical technician, and circulating nurse. However, through technological advances in the field of intensive care medicine, bringing the operating room to the bedside is becoming more feasible, cost-effective, efficient, and, most importantly, safe. Therefore, surgeons must adapt to this new operating venue if it will provide the best outcome for the patient. This chapter focuses on common procedures performed in the critically ill and the risks and benefits of performing these procedures at the bedside.

Background

In comparison to general, oncologic, and vascular surgeons whose time is equally split between the inpatient and outpatient settings, the majority of work by the acute care surgeon is conducted in the hospital, specifically in the intensive care unit (ICU) [1]. As ICUs continue to shift towards closed units due to the increasing evidence supporting lower morbidity and mortality [2–4], the acute care surgeon ultimately becomes the primary care physician during the patient's ICU period. It is important, therefore, for the surgeon to under-

stand what surgeries and procedures can benefit patients and be cost-effective if done at the bedside.

Common procedures such as central line placements, wound care, and tube thoracostomies, once the bread-and-butter of general surgery, have been taken over by the acute care surgeon [1]. While most of these procedures can obviously be performed at the bedside, controversy remains on topics such as tracheostomies, vena cava filters (VCFs), endoscopic procedures, and diagnostic laparoscopy/laparotomy. With so much of our work being transferred outside of the operating room, it is essential to understand what we are capable of doing safely at the bedside as technology advances.

Why the Bedside Instead of the Operating Room?

Critically ill patients are safest in the ICU. Here, they remain in a controlled environment, well equipped to handle any problem that arises. However, these patients frequently require trips to the computed tomography (CT) scanner, interventional radiology, and sometimes the operating room. The intra-hospital transport that accompanies these trips is often treacherous with adverse events occurring up to 70% of the time [5]. A few examples include arrhythmias, arterial hypotension/hypertension, elevated intracranial pressures, hypoxia, and hypercapnia.

Although inter- and intra-hospital transportation guidelines have been recommended by the American College of Critical Care Medicine and the Society of Critical Care Medicine [6], some institutions have simply tailored the procedure to be performed at the patient's bedside. Such examples include tracheostomies, percutaneous endoscopic gastrostomies, and VCFs. The advent of better technology, trained assistants, and better equipment has allowed surgeons to attempt these procedures in patients too critical to be transported. Now, with multiple centers publishing their outcomes, the question becomes what selection criteria are used to determine who is eligible for various bedside procedures? The remainder of this chapter reviews specific procedures that are performed in the ICU at the bedside.

L.A. Dultz, M.D., M.P.H. • S.R. Todd, M.D., F.A.C.S. (✉)
Division of Trauma, Emergency Surgery, and Surgical Critical Care,
Department of Surgery, New York University Langone
Medical Center, 550 First Avenue, New Bellevue 15 East 9,
10016, New York, NY, USA
e-mail: srtodd@nyumc.org; lindaann.dultz@nyumc.org

V. Sim, M.D.
Department of Surgery, Brookdale University Hospital
and Medical Center, One Brookdale Plaza, 11212, Brooklyn, NY, USA
e-mail: vasya_s_@yahoo.com

L.J. Moore et al. (eds.), *Common Problems in Acute Care Surgery*,
DOI 10.1007/978-1-4614-6123-4_5, © Springer Science+Business Media New York 2013

Tracheostomy

The word tracheostomy, first coined by Heister in 1739, is derived from two Greek words meaning, "I cut the trachea." Dating back to 2000 BCE, it has been suggested that the procedure was utilized by Homer, Hippocrates, and even Alexander the Great [7]. While initially being used as an emergent tool to relieve upper airway obstructions, the rise of positive pressure mechanical ventilation during the 1950s polio epidemic permanently changed how we manage respiratory failure [7].

The standard subcricoid technique that is used today was originally documented by Chevalier Jackson in 1909 [8]. This was modified in 1955 by Sheldon, [9] who proposed the first percutaneous dilatation tracheostomy (PDT). Sheldon found the traditional open method cumbersome and inefficient in times of placing an emergent tracheostomy. He therefore designed a kit consisting of only four parts. Using a needle to first puncture the trachea, he described how in less than 30 s he could successfully insert a tracheostomy tube attached to a cutting blade trocar over the needle to slide directly into the trachea [9]. Although not immediately catching on, a non-cutting, minimally invasive adaption by Ciaglia [10] in 1985 did. His method, with several other variations [11–14], is what we currently use today to perform PDTs.

Presently, respiratory failure is one of the most common reasons for ICU admissions. With prolonged intubation seen in several of these patients, tracheostomies are one of the most common ICU procedures. Current indications for tracheostomies consist of prevention of ventilator associated pneumonia, prevention of tracheo- and laryngomalacia from translaryngeal intubation, facilitation of weaning from mechanical ventilation, decreased dead space ventilation, improved oral care, pulmonary toilet, and patient comfort [15].

Choices for tracheostomies include location (bedside or operating room) and type of procedure (open versus percutaneous). Multiple studies have already been published supporting the safety and cost-effectiveness of performing elective tracheostomies at the bedside. However, opinions vary greatly regarding patient selection criteria and type of procedure to use [15–21]. Unfortunately many studies on this topic have been retrospective in nature or have inadequate sample sizes, making it difficult to conclusively side with one particular procedure. Furthermore, their sample groups range from comparing open bedside tracheostomy (OBT) to operating room tracheostomies (ORT) [19–21], OBT to PDT [22], or ORT to PDT [23, 24]. Few have actually described all three types of tracheostomies in one study for a true comparison [15, 16, 25].

In regard to performing a tracheostomy at the bedside versus the operating room, studies have shown similar rates of complications between OBTs and ORTs [19, 20]. However, most studies can demonstrate a cost savings with OBTs by sparing the use of the operating room and anesthesiologists [15, 16, 21]. Anesthesiology costs are bypassed by training respiratory therapists to manage the airway and critical care attendings to monitor sedation. Utilizing these resources has also led to a decrease in the waiting period for placement of a tracheostomy secondary to bypassing the operating room schedule, which is generally consumed with elective procedures [15]. Therefore, if possible, one can safely attempt a tracheostomy at the bedside without increasing the risk of complications.

Realistically, there are several variables that could conceivably decrease the likelihood of performing tracheostomies at the bedside. These include relying on a respiratory therapist and critical care attending to provide anesthesia, inferior lighting, wider and less maneuverable beds, and inferior equipment [15]. However, with careful planning, it is possible to create a tracheostomy cart similar to ones described in other studies [15, 21]. For example, Yoo et al. [15] designed a cart with the same headlights, electrosurgical unit, tracheotomy tray, drapes, gowns, and tracheotomy tubes used in the operating room. This group was able to successfully bring the operating room to the bedside in a controlled and efficient manor, thereby saving on operating room costs.

Once an infrastructure has been established to support tracheostomies at the bedside, the choice now becomes: which patients should receive an OBT and which should receive a PDT? This decision, for the most part, is ultimately surgeon preference. Multiple studies have now been published showing little to no difference in short- and long-term outcomes between OBTs and PDTs. Proponents of PDT argue that its benefits include minimal soft-tissue dissection to reduce the risk of infection and bleeding, a small stoma with decrease scar, and preservation of the cartilaginous rings, which can possibly minimizing the risk of developing subglottic stenosis [17, 26, 27]. However, when comparing short- and long-term complications of OBT to PDT, the only benefit shown to be reproducible in multiple studies is the smaller incision and subsequent scar, improving overall cosmesis of the procedure [22, 23].

Additionally, cost-savings analyses comparing these two procedures show PDTs to be slightly more expensive due to the disposable kit [25] and when adjunct modalities such as bronchoscopy are used [16]. However, bronchoscopy is not considered the standard of care when performing PDTs and can be performed based on surgeon preference [28]. While one may think that the routine use of bronchoscopy increases its safety by avoiding easily preventable complications such as threading the guide wire through the Murphy's eye of the endotracheal tube and avoiding the creation of false passages, only two studies [29, 30] have attempted to prove this true. Both, however, lacked control groups in their study and only analyzed PDTs with bronchoscopy. Therefore, although adding to the cost of the procedure without definitive evidence of its protective effects, bronchoscopy is ultimately at the discretion of the surgeon [28].

Relative contraindications to percutaneous tracheostomies that have been noted in the literature include positive-end expiratory pressure (PEEP) >10 cm H_2O, morbid obesity, enlarged or abnormal thyroid anatomy, calcified tracheal rings, unstable cervical spine injury, uncorrected coagulopathy, active cervical infection, and the need for an emergency airway [10, 21, 22, 27, 31]. However, some studies have shown that in experienced hands and with the improvement of dilator kits, many contraindications such as obesity and high ventilator requirements are simply surgeon preference [15, 16, 31]. For example, percutaneous dilatation was once considered dangerous in patients with a PEEP >10 cm H_2O because the technique involved serial dilations before placement of the tube. These serial dilations cause the trachea to remain open for a longer period of time causing a release of pressure and rapid alveolar collapse and hypoxia. However, the more recent single dilator kits allow surgeons to safely perform this operation with PEEPs up to 15 cm H_2O [27]. In fact, Kornblith [31] et al. recently published their experience of 1,000 bedside PDTs using the Ciaglia single dilator technique. Percutaneous dilatational tracheostomy is the standard of care at their institution and the only instances they actually recommend delaying PDT are in patients with abnormal neck anatomy, unstable or undetermined cervical spine injuries, patients requiring $FiO_2 \geq 80$, $PEEP \geq 15$ cm H_2O, and patients with supratherapeutic partial thromboplastin time levels on heparin drips that are not corrected. Using these guidelines, they published a 1.4% (14/1,000) complication rate for their experience with PDTs [31].

Overall, OBT and PDT are just as safe as ORT and have additional cost benefits. If a solid hospital infrastructure exists, the surgeon should attempt tracheostomies at the bedside in order to avoid intra-hospital transportation. Decision between OBT and PDT is surgeon preference, keeping in mind the relative contraindications in order to perform PDTs safely.

Inferior Vena Cava Filter

The treatment of thromboembolic disease has advanced tremendously over the twentieth and twenty-first century. Beginning in 1908 with Trendelenberg [32] proposing the first pulmonary embolectomy, Homans went on to suggest ligation of the femoral veins in 1934 [33] and then permanent ligation of the inferior vena cava (IVC) in 1944 [34] for prevention of fatal pulmonary emboli in critically ill patients. A revolution in treatment came in the 1950s and 1960s with

several novel studies [35–38] discussing positive outcomes with the placement of what they termed a VCF.

Today, there are several VCFs available; however, the Greenfield filter remains one of the most widely used filters on the market. Its introduction in 1973 [39] first described the technique as a cutdown procedure done solely in the operating room. However, reports of a percutaneous method for insertion published in 1984 [40] and 1985 [41] quickly made the procedure popular among surgeons. Today, VCFs are primarily placed under fluoroscopic or ultrasound guidance in the radiology suite, operating room, or at the bedside. These methods offer an overall reduction in morbidity, cost, and time compared to the days of Trendelenberg and Homan [42]. Additionally, performing VCF placements at the bedside provides the benefits of decreased transportation risks for critically ill patients and avoids delays and scheduling conflicts with the operating room [43].

Today, the gold standard for VCF placement is contrast venography, which requires the use of nephrotoxic contrast, radiation, and transportation to the operating room or angiography suite [43]. Using fluoroscopic guidance, successful VCF placement requires clear identification of the renal veins, an IVC diameter <28 mm, and assessment for anomalies and thrombus [44].

The disadvantages of the procedure include transporting critically ill patients outside of the ICU and the administration of nephrotoxic contrast to high risk patients. However, recent studies [45] have attempted to counteract these problems via two separate solutions. First, ICU rooms have been developed to accommodate fluoroscopy shields to protect against radiation exposure and specialized beds to allow C-arms for fluoroscopic insertion. This simple solution provides equal, if not better results than VCF insertion in the operating room [45] and avoids transporting patients in the critically ill setting. However, critics [43] argue that these specialized rooms come with a higher price tag and the complexity of performing contrast radiologic studies in the ICU limits the widespread use of this technique. Second, it has been suggested that the nephrotoxic contrast can be replaced with intravascular carbon dioxide (CO_2) injections [45] in patients at high-risk for renal failure. Originally tested in the 1940s, when injected, CO_2 is excreted via the lungs and does not affect renal function [46]. It has therefore been used in multiple imaging studies in the peripheral and central vasculature with the brain being the only exclusion. While it is still not commonly used, several studies [45–48] have confirmed CO_2's benefits when used in patients with renal disease. Specifically, in 2003, Holtzman [48] et al. reported no significant difference in the measurement of the supra- and infra-renal IVC when comparing measurements obtained via CO_2 and standard iodinated contrast. This study highlights that the use of CO_2 is equally effective in obtaining accurate cavagrams when compared to iodinated contrast.

While contrast venography is the gold standard for VCF placement, alternative methods include duplex-guided filter insertion (DGFI) and intravascular ultrasound (IVUS). The overall advantages with ultrasound include its increased portability making it an ideal bedside procedure and the avoidance of radiation exposure and iodinated contrast agents [42]. These features make it an appealing application to use during pregnancy, in renal failure, and in critically ill patients. However, differences exist between DGFI and IVUS that must be recognized by the surgeon in order to identify appropriate patients for each method [42, 43, 49]. For example, DGFI uses deep abdominal duplex imaging to evaluate the IVC, renal veins, and surrounding visceral structures. While this application has proven to successfully visualize the IVC in 85–95% [50–53] of patients, failures are predominately related to poor visualization secondary to obesity and intraluminal bowel gas. Critically ill patients are typically prone to anasarca and bowel ileus, making this technique difficult in these patients. The alternative therefore is IVUS. This technique emerged in 2000 [54] due to advancements in ultrasound technology. Several centers have experience with IVUS VCF placement, yet studies so far are limited [42, 43, 53, 54]. However, initial results have been promising with a success rate between 92 and 96% [43]. These studies cite the main advantage of IVUS over DGFI is the ability to perform VCF placement in obese patients and patients with intraluminal gas and anasarca [53]. The only true downside to ultrasound placement is its inability to pick up anomalies such as a duplicate IVC. However, proponents argue that the majority of critically ill patients have had a CT scan prior to VCF placement and it is suggested to review their imaging or obtain a pre-procedure transabdominal ultrasound before placement to assess for any anomalies.

Overall, several studies have confirmed the safety of placing VCFs at the bedside for the critically ill. Fluoroscopy, DGFI, and IVUS have all proven to be accurate and safe in the hands of experienced surgeons. Therefore, the options of fluoroscopy versus ultrasound guidance should depend on surgeon comfort, patient risk factors (i.e., renal failure, pregnancy), and equipment availability in the ICU.

Diagnostic Laparoscopy

Regardless of admitting diagnosis, acute intra-abdominal pathologies are a significant source of morbidity and mortality once a patient is in the ICU. Diseases plaguing this patient population include acalculous cholecystitis, diverticulitis, gastrointestinal bleeding, intestinal ischemia, intestinal perforation, peptic ulcer disease complications, pancreatitis, and pseudo-membranous colitis [55–58]. Specifically, acalculous cholecystitis has been documented in 0.5–1% of critically ill surgical and trauma patients [58–61]. Likewise,

intestinal ischemia is a significant risk following aortic procedures [62] and up to 1% of patients undergoing cardiopulmonary bypass procedures ultimately require surgical intervention for abdominal pathologies occurring post-bypass [63, 64].

Although these complications occur relatively infrequently, their associated morbidity and mortality cannot be overlooked [62, 65–67]. For example, if left undiagnosed and/or untreated, intra-abdominal sepsis may lead to multiple organ failure (MOF), with mortality rates approaching 100% [67, 68]. Furthermore, the reported mortality rates specific to acalculous cholecystitis and mesenteric ischemia range from 50 to 100% [65, 69, 70].

One significant contributor to the high morbidity and mortality rates is often a delay in diagnosis. These delays are multifactorial, including failure to consider the diagnosis, lack of accuracy of diagnostic modalities, and difficulty obtaining information due to patient neurological status.

Ultimately, challenges continue to exist in the diagnosis and treatment of intra-abdominal processes in the ICU. The diagnosis is frequently complicated by altered mental status, immunocompromization, recent abdominal surgery, corticosteroid utilization, traumatic spinal cord injury, hospital acquired infections, and preexisting comorbid conditions [71–75]. As such, surgical consultations in these patients are extremely difficult. Oft quoted requests for consultations include abdominal pain, abdominal distention, fever of unknown etiology, sepsis of unknown etiology, inexplicable acidosis, and enteral intolerance.

The diagnostic modalities to assess the abdomen in these critically ill patients include the physical examination, laboratory studies, plain radiography, CT scan, ultrasound, exploratory laparotomy, and increasingly so, diagnostic laparoscopy.

Contrary to the majority of patients where the differential diagnosis is highly reliant on the history and clinical examination, these tools are often inaccurate, unreliable, and difficult to obtain in the ICU patient. Secondary to this weakness, diagnostic emphasis has traditionally been placed on objective laboratory data. However, laboratory studies tend to add little to the diagnosis, as they are neither sensitive nor specific for intra-abdominal pathologies.

Plain radiography is generally non-diagnostic in the evaluation of the critically ill patient when considering an abdominal pathology. Additionally, studies have found that minor complications occur in up to 70% of ICU patients being transported for imaging studies; while life threatening complications (i.e., dysarrhythmias, hypotension, and respiratory distress) occur in up to 45% of patients [5, 76–78]. These disadvantages make plain radiography of rare utility in this patient population.

Computed tomography is the most commonly utilized modality in the evaluation of potential abdominal pathologies in the ICU; however, in patients who are unstable or have transport issues, CT scans are often difficult to obtain and/or interpret [79–82]. Statistically, CT scans have a 33–100% degree of accuracy for making a diagnosis [83]. For example, Norwood et al. [84] documented 40% sensitivity and 64% specificity in diagnosing intra-abdominal pathology in 53 critically ill surgical patients. More recently, Karasakalides et al. [83] published a 100% positive predictive value and a 52.94% negative predictive value for their critically ill patients that received CT scans during a workup for intra-abdominal pathologies. Therefore, while a positive finding on CT scan can reliably lead to a diagnosis, a negative CT scan provides little reassurance for the treating surgeon. Additional disadvantages of CT in the ICU population include the difficulty in differentiating postoperative changes from acute abdominal pathology, the inadequate bowel contrast secondary to ileus, renal dysfunction limiting the utilization of intravenous contrast mediums, requirement for transport, availability, and cost.

In contrast to CT, ultrasonography is easily portable and can be of particular usefulness in the evaluation of the biliary system in the ICU population with studies documenting accuracy rates of 60–94% in diagnosing acalculous cholecystitis [67, 81, 85]. However, ultrasound is of little utility for other intra-abdominal pathologies with one study documenting a 57% accuracy rate in diagnosing intra-abdominal sepsis in 72 ICU patients [86]. Ultrasonography also has limitations including operator dependency and diagnostic difficulties with large abdominal wounds, volume overload, and ascites (Table 5.1), often leading to nonspecific interpretations.

In patients with MOF, some authors advocate aggressive exploratory laparotomy (even at the bedside in the ICU) because of the unacceptably high morbidity and mortality rates associated with delays in the diagnosis of intra-abdominal sepsis [72, 86, 87]. However, in these studies the non-therapeutic laparotomy rate ranged from 9 to 26%. Unfortunately, the risks of a nontherapeutic laparotomy are not negligible, and include iatrogenic injuries, effects of general anesthesia, blood loss, fluid shifts, postoperative ileus, wound infection, and wound dehiscence [67, 88]. Following a nontherapeutic laparotomy, morbidity ranges from 5 to 22%, while mortality rates have been reported up to 90% [57, 89]. As such, the avoidance of nontherapeutic laparotomies is beneficial.

The introduction of laparoscopy is the newest tool in the surgeon's armamentarium that can substantially decrease morbidity and mortality as compared to exploratory laparotomy. Over the past three decades, it has proven itself an accurate diagnostic tool in a wide spectrum of clinical scenarios including the evaluation of acute and chronic abdominal pain, the evaluation of gynecological disorders, and cancer staging [86, 90–92]. It is now

Table 5.1 Ascites classification

Grade 1	Mild ascites visible by ultrasound only
Grade 2	Moderate ascites, evident by symmetrical distention
Grade 3	Large ascites, gross ascites with marked distention

considered an ideal adjunct in the care of ICU patients with potential intra-abdominal processes. Specifically, it is of great utility in diagnosing acalculous cholecystitis and intestinal ischemia [67]. Overall complication rates range from 1 to 9% [93–96].

There are several advantages to laparoscopy. First, it allows for the direct visualization and inspection of the intra-abdominal contents. Consequently, it is far superior in differentiating postoperative changes (i.e., free air, free fluid, inflammation) from acute abdominal pathologies in comparison to the other diagnostic modalities mentioned previously. Second, the direct visualization and inspection of the intra-abdominal contents allows the surgeon to limit unnecessary incisions and/or operative dissections that would otherwise be involved with an open surgical procedure. However, similar to exploratory laparotomy, it can also lead to a therapeutic intervention if indicated [67, 97] (i.e., perforated peptic ulcer disease, limited small bowel ischemia, and acalculous cholecystitis) [94, 98, 99]. Brandt et al. documented a change in clinical management in 36% of patients undergoing laparoscopy [67]. Finally, from a physiological perspective, the smaller incisions and minimal dissections associated with laparoscopy lead to less stress and a reduced acute phase response in comparison to laparotomy.

From an operational perspective, laparoscopy can be performed in the operating suite or at the bedside [72, 100]. Bedside laparoscopy initially seems cumbersome; however, once the team is comfortable, it is relatively simple and expedient. Given the level of sophisticated monitoring available in the ICU, it is an ideal location for the performance of laparoscopy [101]. Laparoscopy requires a limited set of instruments and may be performed under local anesthesia and/or conscious sedation. Advantages of bedside laparoscopy include decreased cost secondary to lack of requirement for the operating suite/anesthesia and the avoidance of transporting critically ill patients.

However, despite the significant advantages of laparoscopy, it is not without its disadvantages. The most concerning are the controversial detrimental physiological effects from insufflation with CO_2, specifically to the cardiovascular and pulmonary systems. Hemodynamic compromise has been demonstrated in experimental septic animals undergoing laparoscopy, usually secondary to the associated hypercarbia and acidosis [102]. Others document temporary myocardial insufficiency, with decreases in cardiac output up to 80% after only 20 min of CO_2 insufflation [103, 104]. However, many studies report no hemodynamic alterations during laparoscopy [67, 94, 97, 103–107]. Means of avoiding such outcomes include slow CO_2 insufflation, lower intra-abdominal pressures, the utilization of alternative gases for insufflation such as nitrous oxide, and ultimately desufflation if necessary [59, 101, 107–109]. Other potential disadvantages to laparoscopy include possible iatrogenic visceral and/or vascular injuries, a limited evaluation of the peritoneal cavity (specifically the deep pelvis, mesenteric root, pancreas, and retroperitoneum), and a great degree of operator dependency [94].

The final and most worrisome outcome is the detrimental effects laparoscopy can have on the pulmonary system. Within 15 min of insufflation, hypercarbia is present as a result of increased pulmonary dead-space and peritoneal absorption of the insufflated CO_2 [110]. This results in a 30% increase in CO_2 production, with a subsequent respiratory acidosis [111, 112]. The resultant hypercarbia is best prevented and/or managed via increased minute ventilation using mechanical ventilation [88, 101, 113]. The arterial CO_2 and pH may also be monitored by arterial blood gases and continuous capnometry [114].

In summary, the utilization of laparoscopy in the ICU continues to evolve. Laparoscopy is a safe and accurate means of evaluating (and possibly managing) critically ill patients with potential intra-abdominal processes. Furthermore, laparoscopy may help to avoid potential non-therapeutic laparotomies or confirm the need for operative intervention in complex clinical scenarios.

Bronchoscopy

Airway management is one of the most important tasks in the ICU. Proper care of endotracheal and tracheostomy tubes accelerates extubation and prevents the development of pneumonia. However, sometimes secretions are not cleared by patient's lungs sufficiently leading to the formation of mucous plugs and lobar collapse. This is one of the most common reasons that bronchoscopy is used in the ICU setting. Among other indications are performance of bronchial lavage, trans- or endo-bronchial biopsy, or for evaluation of a source of bleeding [115].

During the procedure the patient should have constant cardiac and oxygen saturation monitoring. This allows for early identification of arrhythmias and/or hypoxia and subsequent interruption of the procedure. Because of the possibility of arrhythmias, bronchoscopy should generally be postponed for 6 weeks if the patient has suffered from an acute myocardial infarction (unless it is deemed an emergency) [115]. There are two types of bronchoscopes available: rigid and flexible; however, the latter is used greater than 95% of the time [116]. A rigid bronchoscope is usually used for debulking of large tumors, insertion of stents, or removal of foreign objects [116]. A flexible bronchoscope is typically used for all other indications. Lidocaine injected through the endoscope to anesthetize the oropharynx and vocal cords can provoke asthmatic reaction and pretreatment with atropine is warranted in non-intubated asthmatics. Anticholinergics have an added benefit of decreasing bronchial secretions allowing for better visualization of the airway.

Mortality and morbidity rates associated with the procedure are 0.5 and 0.8%, respectively [117]. Some of the major complications that have been reported are respiratory depression, pneumothorax, airway obstruction, cardiorespiratory arrest, arrhythmias, and pulmonary edema. Severe bleeding is another complication which occurs in less than 5% of patients after biopsy. While the incidence of pneumothorax after biopsy is around 3%, it increases to 14% in mechanically ventilated patients [115].

Endoscopy

Nasoenteric Feeding Tubes

Malnutrition is frequently seen in critically ill patients. As long as there is a functional gastrointestinal tract, enteral nutrition is preferred over parenteral nutrition due to lower mucosal atrophy and decreased translocation of bacteria and toxins [118]. Several delivery methods are currently available for a variety of patients' conditions.

When supplemental feeding is expected to be needed for <30 days, nasogastric or nasoenteric tubes are the preferred delivery method. A nasogastric tube (NGT) is easy to place and can be performed bedside, but is associated with a high incidence of displacement, increased risk of aspiration, misplacement into the airway, and direct injury to the nasopharynx or oropharynx [119]. It is typically placed blindly at the bedside with radiologic verification of proper placement prior to the initiation of feeds. Despite its ease in placement, controversy persists as to the optimal site for enteral nutrition delivery (gastric versus small intestinal). Unlike the small intestine, the stomach commonly exhibits an ileus following surgery, major trauma, and during other critical illnesses. Ritz et al. demonstrated that 45% of mechanically ventilated patients showed delayed gastric emptying impeding adequate delivery of gastric enteral nutrition [120].

In order to avoid this, many clinicians advocate post-pyloric feeding. However, randomized, controlled trials comparing gastric to post-pyloric feeding have produced varying results [121–127]. A possible explanation for this is that most post pyloric feeding tubes are too short to go beyond the ligament of Treitz. Thus, enteral nutrition is being administered into the duodenum and studies have shown a high incidence of duodenogastric reflux in patients at risk for aspiration [122]. Heyland et al. documented an 80% rate of radioisotope-labeled reflux into the stomach, 25% into the esophagus, and 4% into the lung when radioisotope-labeled enteral formulas were fed through post-pyloric feeding tubes in mechanically ventilated ICU patients [125]. In postoperative patients, Tournadre et al. demonstrated gastroparesis and rapid discoordinated duodenal contractions with some 20% migrating in a retrograde fashion [128]. These studies provide compelling evidence that duodenogastric reflux is present in postoperative and critically ill patients. Thus, feeding into the duodenum is not significantly different than feeding into the stomach in these patients with regard to the aspiration risk.

The Canadian Critical Care Clinical Practice Guidelines Committee likewise studied this topic. They evaluated 11 Level 2 studies comparing enteral nutrition via the small intestine with gastric enteral nutrition [129]. The studies that reported nutritional delivery demonstrated more rapid and successful delivery in those patients fed via the small intestine. Nine studies documented infectious complications. When these were aggregated, small intestinal enteral nutrition was associated with a significant decrease in infectious complications (RR, 0.77; 95% CI, 0.60–1.00; $p = 0.05$). In respect to mortality, there was no difference between the two routes of delivery (RR, 0.93; 95% CI, 0.72–1.20; $p = 0.6$). Overall, the committee recommended small intestinal enteral nutrition when obtaining small bowel access was feasible. If this placement is unsuccessful blindly, a naso-jejunal feeding tube may be placed with endoscopic guidance.

Percutaneous Endoscopic Gastrostomy

A gastric tube has become the best alternative for enteral feeding in patients requiring nutrition for longer than 30 days. The major indication for gastric tube placement is the inability to maintain adequate oral nutritional intake as a result of a recent cerebrovascular accident, altered level of consciousness, dysphagia, oro-pharyngo-esophageal obstructing lesions, facial or esophageal trauma, or tracheal–esophageal fistula [130, 131].

Irrespective of the technique, gastrostomy tubes should not be placed in patients with rapidly progressing incurable diseases or those with a high likelihood of a rapid recovery [132]. Among other contraindications are signs of acute infection, peritonitis, coagulopathy, ulceration at future puncture site, and distal obstruction [133]. With percutaneous endoscopic gastrostomy (PEG), there are certain technique-specific contraindications that must be kept in mind. An absolute contraindication to PEG placement is any condition that prevents approximation of the stomach and anterior abdominal wall. Relative contraindications are obesity and hepatomegaly, which may prevent transillumination across the abdominal wall, as well as neoplastic and inflammatory diseases of the abdominal wall [131].

The primary techniques for gastrostomy tube placement are surgical and percutaneous. Surgical gastrostomies are performed in the operating room and require general anesthesia. With the introduction of PEGs, the surgical technique is now relegated to cases where the percutaneous option is unavailable, contraindicated, or unsuccessful. PEG tubes are the most common procedure performed in establishing an enteral route for nutrition due to their lower cost and faster recovery time [132]. They are often performed bedside utilizing either the "pull" or "push" method. The "pull" technique is more widely used due to a lower complication rate and cost [134]. That being said, more recent data documents the "push" technique to be safe with a lower insertion site infection rate [135–137].

During PEG placement via the "pull" technique, the anterior abdominal wall insertion site must meet certain criteria: (1) adequate transillumination via the endoscope within the stomach, and (2) appreciation of a distinct finger ballottement inside the stomach via the abdominal wall. The Seldinger technique is then utilized in inserting the guidewire into the stomach. It is snared and pulled retrograde through patient's mouth at which point the gastrostomy tube is attached to the guidewire. The guidewire (gastrostomy tube in tow) is then pulled into the stomach and through the anterior abdominal wall, where it is affixed to the abdominal wall [138].

The "push" technique starts with identification of the insertion site via transillumination with the endoscope. Next, a specially designed gastropexy device is used to pexy the stomach to the anterior abdominal wall. A trocar with an introducer sheath is then inserted through the anterior abdominal wall and into the stomach under endoscopic visualization. The trocar is withdrawn while the tip of the sheath remains inside the stomach and the gastric tube is inserted through the introducer sheath. The gastrostomy tube balloon is inflated and the peel away sheath is removed [135, 138]. The "push" technique should be considered in patients with a decreased oropharyngeal diameter that is insufficient for the gastrostomy tube's bumper (8–9 mm in diameter) to pass through if the "pull" technique were utilized. In such circumstances, the "pull" technique can still be used, but will often require dilatation with a bougie, which is associated with an added risk of perforation [136].

Procedure-related mortality for PEG tube placement is minimal, with a 30-day overall mortality rate of 19%. This has increased from 8% in the 1990s due to the significantly sicker patient population referred for PEGs [133]. PEG tube placement complications include PEG site leakage, PEG tube blockage or dislodgement, peri-stomal infection, necrotizing fasciitis, gastro-colic fistula, and peritonitis. The latter is most frequently secondary to separation of the stomach and anterior abdominal wall or injury to adjacent visceral organs [133]. The most common complication is peri-stomal infection with a reported rate of 5–30% [135, 139, 140].

A recent Cochrane analysis recommends administration of preoperative antibiotics to all patients undergoing "pull" gastrostomies [130]. Both penicillin-based and cephalosporin antibiotics have been used with significantly improved infection rates. Kulling et al. documented a favorable cost analysis for prophylactic antibiotics in "pull" gastrostomies; however, the antibiotics used as the comparison were not methicillin-resistant *Staphylococcus aureus* (MRSA) sensitive [141]. There are several other peri-stomal infection prevention strategies that proven useful. Radhakrishnan et al. showed that a combination of preoperative intravenous antibiotics with antiseptic spray decreased peri-stomal infection rate in comparison to antibiotic or antiseptic spray alone [142]. Another study showed that a single dose of trimethoprim/sulfamethoxazole per tube postoperatively had an equivalent peri-stomal infection rate to the group who received preoperative antibiotics [143]. MRSA-positive patients have a higher peri-stomal infection rate [139]. In an attempt to address this problem, Horiuchi et al. revealed that decolonization of MRSA positive patients with intranasal antibiotics significantly decreased the peri-stomal infection rate [144].

While it is clear that preoperative antibiotics should be administered to all "pull" gastrostomies, the same recommendation cannot be made for the "push" technique [130]. Shastri et al. recently reported an equivalent 7-day infection rate for "push" gastrostomy with and without prophylactic antibiotics [135]. As mentioned earlier, some data document a significantly lower infection rate with the "push" technique in comparison to the "pull" technique [137]. One of the theories is that during the "pull" technique, there is seeding of the gastrostomy tube as it passes through the heavily colonized oropharynx.

Percutaneous Endoscopic Gastrostomy/ Jejunostomy

One of the critical complications of enteral nutrition via a nasogastric or PEG tube is aspiration pneumonia as described earlier; therefore, small intestinal enteral nutrition is recommended when obtaining small bowel access was feasible. The placement of a percutaneous endoscopic gastrostomy/ jejunostomy (PEG/J) tube is only a slight modification of a PEG tube placement. A jejunal extension is necessitated with numerous techniques for placement.

Endoscopy for Upper Gastrointestinal Bleeding

Gastrointestinal bleeding is frequently seen in ICU patients and endoscopy has become the major diagnostic and therapeutic tool. Upper gastrointestinal bleeding is defined as bleeding proximal to the ligament of Treitz and can be broken down into two major categories: variceal and non-variceal.

The major cause of non-variceal bleeding is peptic ulcer disease with an incidence of 35–50% [145]. Another cause is transpapillary hemorrhage, which could be due to either hemobilia or pancreatic duct hemorrhage as a result of trauma, pancreatitis, malignancy, or arteriovenous malformation [145]. Variceal bleeding is one of the complications of portal hypertension and is associated with a mortality rate of 40% with an early re-bleed rate of 30–50% [146].

Characterization of upper gastrointestinal bleeding is best performed with endoscopy. In preparation for endoscopy, erythromycin has been shown by meta-analysis to be of benefit for emptying the stomach to allow better visualization of the bleeding area [147]. However, the International Consensus on Non-variceal Upper Gastrointestinal Bleeding recommends administration of promotility agents only to those patients suspected to have a large volume of blood in the stomach or those who have recently eaten [148].

While the general endoscopic technique for the management of variceal and non-variceal hemorrhage is similar, the medical treatment varies some. Meta-analyses have documented that octreotide, a somatostatin analog capable of decreasing portal hypertension, is comparable to sclerotherapy for control of variceal bleeding with fewer side-effects [149, 150]. Sclerotherapy involves endoscopic identification of the bleeding area and injection with sclerosing agents. Endoscopic variceal ligation, which involves placement of several bands over the varix, has previously been shown to be superior to 48-h somatostatin infusion in controlling acute variceal bleeding without increased complications [151]. However, more recent studies document that a combined treatment with endoscopic variceal ligation and somatostatin significantly improves initial control of variceal bleeding [151–153]. For non-variceal bleeding successfully placed hemoclips were equivalent to thermocoagulation and had significantly decreased re-bleeding rates and need for operation in comparison with injection of sclerosing agents alone [154].

If during endoscopic evaluation a clot is seen, attempts should be made to remove it in order to better visualize the area of concern. There is a controversy for appropriate treatment when the clot is not dislodged with irrigation. While some studies document that the incidence of re-bleeding from adherent clots is low, some authors recommend removal of the clot with a cold guillotine snare technique after pre-injecting the clot with epinephrine, especially in high risk patients [148]. If the bleeding cannot be controlled endoscopically, a clip can be left in the area of hemorrhage to serve as a guide for embolization by interventional radiology [155]. Transarterial embolization is considered equivalent to surgery in the case of failed endoscopic treatment with success rates of 60–90% [145, 148].

If endoscopy demonstrates bleeding esophageal varices, but the hemorrhage is too severe to manage endoscopically, balloon tamponade can be performed with a Sengstaken–Blakemore tube or one of its modifications. When properly placed, balloon tamponade has been reported to effectively control hemorrhage in 80–94% of patients; however, proper placement and maintenance are difficult and patients require close monitoring [156]. The tube is perfect for controlling variceal bleeding at the gastroesophageal junction, but will not be effective in distal gastric or duodenal bleeding.

In both variceal and non-variceal bleeding, recurrent hemorrhage is associated with increased mortality [157, 158]. Several factors have been identified that predict re-bleeding including hemodynamic instability, active bleeding (especially "spurting") on endoscopy, an ulcer size >2 cm, and a posterior duodenal wall bleed [159]. While routine repeat endoscopy is not warranted in all patients, if a combination of these factors is present, repeat endoscopy may be beneficial. Intravenous proton pump inhibitors are usually started prior to endoscopy in both variceal and non-variceal bleeding, which has been shown to decrease the necessity for endoscopic treatment and in some studies decreased the rate of re-bleeding [148, 160, 161]. In acute variceal bleeding, the addition of isosorbide mononitrate alone or in combination with beta-blockers to endoscopic variceal ligation did not affect the re-bleeding rate [162]. However, another meta-analysis definitively showed that a combination of beta-blockers and endoscopic variceal ligation significantly decreases re-bleeding and mortality rates in comparison to endoscopic therapy alone [163].

Endoscopy for Lower Gastrointestinal Bleeding

Lower gastrointestinal bleeding is defined as bleeding distal to the ligament of Treitz and accounts for 20% of all major gastrointestinal bleeds, diverticular disease representing the most common cause. Other causes of lower gastrointestinal bleeding in the ICU include inflammatory disease, vascular ectasia, post-polypectomy bleeding, malignancy, and anorectal disease [164–166]. Most diverticular bleeding (80%) will cease spontaneously; however, right-sided diverticular bleeding is often more severe and is more likely to require surgical intervention [167–170].

The patient's hemodynamic status and rate of bleeding determine the evaluation process in lower gastrointestinal bleeding. If the bleeding is moderate, the patient is hemodynamically stable, and can undergo appropriate bowel preparation, colonoscopy is the diagnostic modality of choice; however, very frequently the bleeding is intermittent and the source of bleeding may not be identified on colonoscopy. When the bleeding area is identified, thermocoagulation, sclerotherapy, epinephrine injection, or hemoclip application can be used to control the bleeding [171–173]. If the bleeding source is not identified and the patient remains hemodynamically stable, a tagged red blood cell scan, which can detect bleeding of at least 0.1 ml per minute, is the next diagnostic modality [167].

Colonoscopy has proven to be particularly helpful in minor and moderate lower gastrointestinal bleeding, while in severe hemorrhage, its value is limited, and angiography (standard or CT) should be performed [168]. If the bleeding is identified on angiogram, selective mesenteric embolization has been shown to have high success and low re-bleeding rates for diverticular bleeding [174]. Recurrent bleeding in patients embolized for non-diverticular bleeding has an incidence of >40%; however, it prevents emergent surgery and allows for proper resuscitation of the patient [174]. Emergent surgery for lower gastrointestinal hemorrhage has a mortality rate of 20–50% [175].

Conclusion

As technology and intensive care medicine advances continue, more and more procedures are being performed in the ICU that were once isolated to the operating suite. Acute care surgeons must adapt to this new operating venue and understand what surgeries and procedures can benefit patients and be cost-effective if done at the bedside.

References

 1. Galante JM, Phan HH, Wisner DH. Trauma surgery to acute care surgery: defining the paradigm shift. J Trauma. 2010;68(5):1024–31.
 2. Pronovost PJ, Angus DC, Dorman T, Robinson KA, Dremsizov TT, Young TL. Physician staffing patterns and clinical outcomes in critically ill patients: a systematic review. JAMA. 2002;288(17): 2151–62.
 3. Chittawatanarat K, Pamorsinlapathum T. The impact of closed ICU model on mortality in general surgical intensive care unit. J Med Assoc Thai. 2009;92(12):1627–34.
 4. Ghorra S, Reinert SE, Cioffi W, Buczko G, Simms HH. Analysis of the effect of conversion from open to closed surgical intensive care unit. Ann Surg. 1999;229(2):163–71.
 5. Waydhas C. Intrahospital transport of critically ill patients. Crit Care. 1999;3(5):R83–R9.
 6. Warren J, Fromm Jr RE, Robert E, Orr RA, Rotello LC, Horst HM. Guidelines for the inter- and intrahospital transport of critically ill patients. Crit Care Med. 2004;32(1):256–62.
 7. Pierson DJ. Tracheostomy from A to Z: historical context and current challenges. Respir Care. 2005;50(4):473–5.
 8. Jackson C. Tracheotomy. Laryngoscope. 1909;19:285–90.
 9. Shelden CH, Pudenz RH, Freshwater DB, Crue BL. A new method for tracheotomy. J Neurosurg. 1955;12(4):428–31.
10. Ciaglia P, Firsching R, Syniec C. Elective percutaneous dilatational tracheostomy. A new simple bedside procedure; preliminary report. Chest. 1985;87(6):715–9.
11. Byhahn C, Lischke V, Halbig S, Scheifler G, Westphal K. Ciaglia blue rhino: a modified technique for percutaneous dilatation tracheostomy. Technique and early clinical results. Anaesthesist. 2000;49(3):202–6.
12. Fantoni A, Ripamonti D. A non-derivative, non-surgical tracheostomy: the translaryngeal method. Intensive Care Med. 1997;23(4):386–92.
13. Frova G, Quintel M. A new simple method for percutaneous tracheostomy: controlled rotating dilation. Intensive Care Med. 2002;28(3):299–303.

14. Griggs WM, Worthley LI, Gilligan JE, Thomas PD, Myburg JA. A simple percutaneous tracheostomy technique. Surg Gynecol Obstet. 1990;170(6):543–5.

15. Yoo DB, Schiff BA, Martz S, et al. Open bedside tracheotomy: impact on patient care and patient safety. Laryngoscope. 2011;121(3):515–20.

16. Massick DD, Yao S, Powell DM, et al. Bedside tracheostomy in the intensive care unit: a prospective randomized trial comparing open surgical tracheostomy with endoscopically guided percutaneous dilational tracheotomy. Laryngoscope. 2001;111(3):494–500.

17. McHenry CR, Raeburn CD, Lange RL, Priebe PP. Percutaneous tracheostomy: a cost-effective alternative to standard open tracheostomy. Am Surg. 1997;63(7):646–51.

18. Hill BB, Zweng TN, Maley RH, Charash WE, Toursarkissian B, Kearney PA. Percutaneous dilational tracheostomy: report of 356 cases. J Trauma. 1996;41(2):238–43.

19. Futran ND, Dutcher PO, Roberts JK. The safety and efficacy of bedside tracheotomy. Otolaryngol Head Neck Surg. 1993;109(4):707–11.

20. Upadhyay A, Maurer J, Turner J, Tiszenkel H, Rosengart T. Elective bedside tracheostomy in the intensive care unit. J Am Coll Surg. 1996;183(1):51–5.

21. Wang SJ, Sercarz JA, Blackwell KE, Aghamohammadi M, Wang MB. Open bedside tracheotomy in the intensive care unit. Laryngoscope. 1999;109(6):891–3.

22. Silvester W, Goldsmith D, Uchino S, et al. Percutaneous versus surgical tracheostomy: a randomized controlled study with long-term follow-up. Crit Care Med. 2006;34(8):2145–52.

23. Gysin C, Dulguerov P, Guyot JP, Perneger TV, Abajo B, Chevrolet JC. Percutaneous versus surgical tracheostomy: a double-blind randomized trial. Ann Surg. 1999;230(5):708–14.

24. Bowen CP, Whitney LR, Truwit JD, Durbin CG, Moore MM. Comparison of safety and cost of percutaneous versus surgical tracheostomy. Am Surg. 2001;67(1):54–60.

25. Porter JM, Ivatury RR. Preferred route of tracheostomy—percutaneous versus open at the bedside: a randomized, prospective study in the surgical intensive care unit. Am Surg. 1999;65(2):142–6.

26. Ciaglia P, Graniero K. Percutaneous dilatational tracheostomy. Results and long-term follow-up. Chest. 1992;101(2):464–7.

27. Mittendorf EA, McHenry CR, Smith CM, Yowler CJ, Peerless JR. Early and late outcome of bedside percutaneous tracheostomy in the intensive care unit. Am Surg. 2002;68(4):342–6. discussion 346–347.

28. Al-Ansari MA, Hijazi MH. Clinical review: percutaneous dilational tracheostomy. Crit Care. 2006;10(1):202.

29. Marelli D, Paul A, Manolidis S, et al. Endoscopic guided percutaneous tracheostomy: early results of a consecutive trial. J Trauma. 1990;30(4):433–5.

30. Barba CA, Angood PB, Kauder DR, et al. Bronchoscopic guidance makes percutaneous tracheostomy a safe, cost-effective, and easy-to-teach procedure. Surgery. 1995;118(5):879 83.

31. Kornblith LZ, Burlew CC, Moore EE, et al. One thousand bedside percutaneous tracheostomies in the surgical intensive care unit: time to change the gold standard. J Am Coll Surg. 2011;212(2):163–70.

32. Trendelenberg F. Operative interference in embolism of the pulmonary artery. Ann Surg. 1908;48:772.

33. Homans J. Thrombosis of the deep veins of the lower leg, causing pulmonary embolism. N Engl J Med. 1934;221:993.

34. Homans J. Deep quiet venous thrombosis in the lower limb. Surg Gynecol Obstet. 1944;79:70.

35. Deweese MS, Hunter DC. A vena cava filter for the prevention of pulmonary embolism. A five-year clinical experience. Arch Surg. 1963;86:852–68.

36. De Weese MS, Hunter DC. A vena cava filter for the prevention of pulmonary emboli. Bull Soc Int Chir. 1958;17(1):17–25.

37. Patel J. Prevention of recurrent pulmonary embolism by means of a "filter" placed in the inferior vena cava. Presse Med. 1963;14(71):1776.

38. Stancanelli V, Motto G, Georgacopulo P, Fresu I. Ring-filter in the inferior vena cava. Experimental research. Minerva Chir. 1964;15(19):614–7.

39. Greenfield LJ, McCurdy JR, Brown PP, Elkins RC. A new intracaval filter permitting continued flow and resolution of emboli. Surgery. 1973;73(4):599–606.

40. Tadavarthy SM, Castaneda Zuniga W, Salomonowitz E, et al. Kimray-Greenfield vena cava filter: percutaneous introduction. Radiology. 1984;151(2):525–6.

41. Denny DF, Cronan JJ, Dorfman GS, Esplin C. Percutaneous Kimray-Greenfield filter placement by femoral vein puncture. AJR Am J Roentgenol. 1985;145(4):827–9.

42. Ebaugh JL, Chiou AC, Morasch MD, Matsumura JS, Pearce WH. Bedside vena cava filter placement guided with intravascular ultrasound. J Vasc Surg. 2001;34(1):21–6.

43. Ashley DW, Gamblin TC, McCampbell BL, Kitchens DM, Dalton Jr ML, Solis MM. Bedside insertion of vena cava filters in the intensive care unit using intravascular ultrasound to locate renal veins. J Trauma. 2004;57(1):26–31.

44. Hicks ME, Malden ES, Vesely TM, Picus D, Darcy MD. Prospective anatomic study of the inferior vena cava and renal veins: comparison of selective renal venography with cavography and relevance in filter placement. J Vasc Interv Radiol. 1995;6(5):721–9.

45. Paton B, Jacobs D, Heniford B, Kercher K, Zerey M, Sing R. Nine-year experience with insertion of vena cava filters in the intensive care unit. Am J Surg. 2006;192(6):795–800.

46. Kerns SR, Hawkins IF. Carbon dioxide digital subtraction angiography: expanding applications and technical evolution. AJR Am J Roentgenol. 1995;164(3):735–41.

47. Sing RF, Jacobs DG, Heniford BT. Bedside insertion of inferior vena cava filters in the intensive care unit. J Am Coll Surg. 2001;192(5):570–5. discussion 575–576.

48. Holtzman R. Comparison of carbon dioxide and iodinated contrast for cavography prior to inferior vena cava filter placement. Am J Surg. 2003;185(4):364–8.

49. Spaniolas K, Velmahos GC, Kwolek C, Gervasini A, Moya M, Alam HB. Bedside placement of removable vena cava filters guided by intravascular ultrasound in the critically injured. World J Surg. 2008;32(7):1438–43.

50. Corriere M, Passman M, Guzman R, Dattilo J, Naslund T. Comparison of bedside transabdominal duplex ultrasound versus contrast venography for inferior vena cava filter placement: what is the best imaging modality? Ann Vasc Surg. 2005;19(2):229–34.

51. Uppal B, Flinn WR, Benjamin ME. The bedside insertion of inferior vena cava filters using ultrasound guidance. Perspect Vasc Surg Endovasc Ther. 2007;19(1):78 84.

52. Sato DT, Robinson KD, Gregory RT, et al. Duplex directed caval filter insertion in multi-trauma and critically ill patients. Ann Vasc Surg. 1999;13(4):365–71.

53. Passman MA, Dattilo JB, Guzman RJ, Naslund TC. Bedside placement of inferior vena cava filters by using transabdominal duplex ultrasonography and intravascular ultrasound imaging. J Vasc Surg. 2005;42(5):1027–32.

54. Oppat WF, Chiou AC, Matsumura JS. Intravascular ultrasound-guided vena cava filter placement. J Endovasc Surg. 1999;6(3):285–7.

55. Liolios A, Oropello JM, Benjamin E. Gastrointestinal complications in the intensive care unit. Clin Chest Med. 1999;20(2):329–45. viii.

56. Martin RF, Flynn P. The acute abdomen in the critically ill patient. Surg Clin North Am. 1997;77(6):1455–64.

57. Ott MJ, Buchman TG, Baumgartner WA. Postoperative abdominal complications in cardiopulmonary bypass patients: a case-controlled study. Ann Thorac Surg. 1995;59(5):1210–3.

58. Brandt CP, Priebe PP, Jacobs DG. Value of laparoscopy in trauma ICU patients with suspected acute acalculous cholecystitis. Surg Endosc. 1994;8(5):361–4. discussion 364–365.

59. Iberti TJ, Salky BA, Onofrey D. Use of bedside laparoscopy to identify intestinal ischemia in postoperative cases of aortic reconstruction. Surgery. 1989;105(5):686–9.

60. Cornwell EE, Rodriguez A, Mirvis SE, Shorr RM. Acute acalculous cholecystitis in critically injured patients. Preoperative diagnostic imaging. Ann Surg. 1989;210(1):52–5.

61. Savino JA, Scalea TM, Del Guercio LR. Factors encouraging laparotomy in acalculous cholecystitis. Crit Care Med. 1985;13(5):377–80.

62. Hayward RH, Calhoun TR, Korompai FL. Gastrointestinal complications of vascular surgery. Surg Clin North Am. 1979;59(5):885–903.

63. Rosemurgy AS, McAllister E, Karl RC. The acute surgical abdomen after cardiac surgery involving extracorporeal circulation. Ann Surg. 1988;207(3):323–6.

64. Wallwork J, Davidson KG. The acute abdomen following cardiopulmonary bypass surgery. Br J Surg. 1980;67(6):410–2.

65. Barie PS, Eachempati SR. Acute acalculous cholecystitis. Gastroenterol Clin North Am. 2010;39(2):343–57.

66. Hessel E. Abdominal organ injury after cardiac surgery. Semin Cardiothorac Vasc Anesth. 2004;8(3):243–63.

67. Brandt CP, Priebe PP, Eckhauser ML. Diagnostic laparoscopy in the intensive care patient. Avoiding the nontherapeutic laparotomy. Surg Endosc. 1993;7(3):168–72.

68. Borzotta AP, Polk HC. Multiple system organ failure. Surg Clin North Am. 1983;63(2):315–36.

69. Stoney RJ, Cunningham CG. Acute mesenteric ischemia. Surgery. 1993;114(3):489–90.

70. McKinsey JF, Gewertz BL. Acute mesenteric ischemia. Surg Clin North Am. 1997;77(2):307–18.

71. Glenn J, Funkhouser WK, Schneider PS. Acute illnesses necessitating urgent abdominal surgery in neutropenic cancer patients: description of 14 cases and review of the literature. Surgery. 1989;105(6):778–89.

72. Ferraris VA. Exploratory laparotomy for potential abdominal sepsis in patients with multiple-organ failure. Arch Surg. 1983;118(10):1130–3.

73. Richardson JD, Flint LM, Polk HC. Peritoneal lavage: a useful diagnostic adjunct for peritonitis. Surgery. 1983;94(5):826–9.

74. Poole GV, Griswold JA, Muakkassa FF. Sepsis and infection in the intensive care unit: are they related? Am Surg. 1993;59(1):60–4.

75. Tibbs PA, Bivins BA, Young AB. The problem of acute abdominal disease during spinal shock. Am Surg. 1979;45(6):366–8.

76. Smith I, Fleming S, Cernaianu A. Mishaps during transport from the intensive care unit. Crit Care Med. 1990;18(3):278–81.

77. Braman SS, Dunn SM, Amico CA, Millman RP. Complications of intrahospital transport in critically ill patients. Ann Intern Med. 1987;107(4):469–73.

78. Waydhas C, Schneck G, Duswald KH. Deterioration of respiratory function after intra-hospital transport of critically ill surgical patients. Intensive Care Med. 1995;21(10):784–9.

79. Babb RR. Acute acalculous cholecystitis. A review. J Clin Gastroenterol. 1992;15(3):238–41.

80. Fig LM, Wahl RL, Stewart RE, Shapiro B. Morphine-augmented hepatobiliary scintigraphy in the severely ill: caution is in order. Radiology. 1990;175(2):467–73.

81. Mirvis SE, Vainright JR, Nelson AW, et al. The diagnosis of acute acalculous cholecystitis: a comparison of sonography, scintigraphy, and CT. AJR Am J Roentgenol. 1986;147(6):1171–5.

82. Indeck M, Peterson S, Smith J, Brotman S. Risk, cost, and benefit of transporting ICU patients for special studies. J Trauma. 1988;28(7):1020–5.

83. Karasakalides A, Triantafillidou S, Anthimidis G, et al. The use of bedside diagnostic laparoscopy in the intensive care unit. J Laparoendosc Adv Surg Tech A. 2009;19(3):333–8.

84. Norwood SH, Civetta JM. Abdominal CT scanning in critically ill surgical patients. Ann Surg. 1985;202(2):166–75.

85. Shuman WP, Rogers JV, Rudd TG, Mack LA, Plumley T, Larson EB. Low sensitivity of sonography and cholescintigraphy in acalculous cholecystitis. AJR Am J Roentgenol. 1984;142(3):531–4.

86. Sinanan M, Maier RV, Carrico CJ. Laparotomy for intra-abdominal sepsis in patients in an intensive care unit. Arch Surg. 1984;119(6):652–8.

87. Hinsdale JG, Jaffe BM. Re-operation for intra-abdominal sepsis. Indications and results in modern critical care setting. Ann Surg. 1984;199(1):31–6.

88. Desmond J, Gordon RA. Ventilation in patients anaesthetized for laparoscopy. Can Anaesth Soc J. 1970;17(4):378–87.

89. Memon MA, Fitztgibbons RJ. The role of minimal access surgery in the acute abdomen. Surg Clin North Am. 1997;77(6):1333–53.

90. Easter DW, Cuschieri A, Nathanson LK, Lavelle-Jones M. The utility of diagnostic laparoscopy for abdominal disorders. Audit of 120 patients. Arch Surg. 1992;127(4):379–83.

91. Callery MP, Strasberg SM, Doherty GM, Soper NJ, Norton JA. Staging laparoscopy with laparoscopic ultrasonography: optimizing resectability in hepatobiliary and pancreatic malignancy. J Am Coll Surg. 1997;185(1):33–9.

92. Lightdale CJ. Laparoscopy for cancer staging. Endoscopy. 1992;24(8):682–6.

93. Hackert T, Kienle P, Weitz J, et al. Accuracy of diagnostic laparoscopy for early diagnosis of abdominal complications after cardiac surgery. Surg Endosc. 2003;17(10):1671–4.

94. Orlando R, Crowell KL. Laparoscopy in the critically ill. Surg Endosc. 1997;11(11):1072–4.

95. Quasarano RT, Kashef M, Sherman SJ, Hagglund KH. Complications of gynecologic laparoscopy. J Am Assoc Gynecol Laparosc. 1999;6(3):317–21.

96. Saidi MH, Vancaillie TG, White AJ, Sadler RK, Akright BD, Farhart SA. Complications of major operative laparoscopy. A review of 452 cases. J Reprod Med. 1996;41(7):471–6.

97. Forde KA, Treat MR. The role of peritoneoscopy (laparoscopy) in the evaluation of the acute abdomen in critically ill patients. Surg Endosc. 1992;6(5):219–21.

98. Cueto J, Díaz O, Garteiz D, Rodríguez M, Weber A. The efficacy of laparoscopic surgery in the diagnosis and treatment of peritonitis. Experience with 107 cases in Mexico City. Surg Endosc. 1997;11(4):366–70.

99. Nathanson LK, Easter DW, Cuschieri A. Laparoscopic repair/ peritoneal toilet of perforated duodenal ulcer. Surg Endosc. 1990;4(4):232–3.

100. Barie PS, Fischer E. Acute acalculous cholecystitis. J Am Coll Surg. 1995;180(2):232–44.

101. Walsh RM, Popovich MJ, Hoadley J. Bedside diagnostic laparoscopy and peritoneal lavage in the intensive care unit. Surg Endosc. 1998;12(12):1405–9.

102. Greif WM, Forse RA. Hemodynamic effects of the laparoscopic pneumoperitoneum during sepsis in a porcine endotoxic shock model. Ann Surg. 1998;227(4):474–80.

103. Stuttmann R, Vogt C, Eypasch E, Doehn M. Haemodynamic changes during laparoscopic cholecystectomy in the high-risk patient. Endosc Surg Allied Technol. 1995;3(4):174–9.

104. Williams MD, Murr PC. Laparoscopic insufflation of the abdomen depresses cardiopulmonary function. Surg Endosc. 1993;7(1):12–6.

105. Rosin D, Haviv Y, Kuriansky J, et al. Bedside laparoscopy in the ICU: report of four cases. J Laparoendosc Adv Surg Tech A. 2001;11(5):305–9.

106. Bender JS, Talamini MA. Diagnostic laparoscopy in critically ill intensive-care-unit patients. Surg Endosc. 1992;6(6):302–4.

107. Rehm CG. Bedside laparoscopy. Crit Care Clin. 2000;16(1):101–12.

108. Gagné DJ, Malay MB, Hogle NJ, Fowler DL. Bedside diagnostic minilaparoscopy in the intensive care patient. Surgery. 2002;131(5):491–6.

109. Safran D, Sgambati S, Orlando R. Laparoscopy in high-risk cardiac patients. Surg Gynecol Obstet. 1993;176(6):548–54.

110. Wittgen CM, Andrus CH, Fitzgerald SD, Baudendistel LJ, Dahms TE, Kaminski DL. Analysis of the hemodynamic and ventilatory effects of laparoscopic cholecystectomy. Arch Surg. 1991;126(8):997–1000. discussion 1000–1001.

111. Leighton T, Pianim N, Liu SY, Kono M, Klein S, Bongard F. Effectors of hypercarbia during experimental pneumoperitoneum. Am Surg. 1992;58(12):717–21.

112. Puri GD, Singh H. Ventilatory effects of laparoscopy under general anaesthesia. Br J Anaesth. 1992;68(2):211–3.

113. Tan PL, Lee TL, Tweed WA. Carbon dioxide absorption and gas exchange during pelvic laparoscopy. Can J Anaesth. 1992;39(7):677–81.

114. Mullett CE, Viale JP, Sagnard PE, et al. Pulmonary CO2 elimination during surgical procedures using intra- or extraperitoneal CO2 insufflation. Anesth Analg. 1993;76(3):622–6.

115. British Thoracic Society Bronchoscopy Guidelines Committee, a Subcommittee Standards of Care Committee of British Thoracic Society. British Thoracic Society guidelines on diagnostic flexible bronchoscopy. Thorax. 2001;56 Suppl 1:i1–i21.

116. Prakash UB. Advances in bronchoscopic procedures. Chest. 1999;116(5):1403–8.

117. Pue CA, Pacht ER. Complications of fiberoptic bronchoscopy at a university hospital. Chest. 1995;107(2):430–2.

118. Hernandez G, Velasco N, Wainstein C, et al. Gut mucosal atrophy after a short enteral fasting period in critically ill patients. J Crit Care. 1999;14(2):73–7.

119. Rafferty GP, Tham TC. Endoscopic placement of enteral feeding tubes. World J Gastrointest Endosc. 2010;2(5):155–64.

120. Ritz MA, Fraser R, Edwards N, et al. Delayed gastric emptying in ventilated critically ill patients: measurement by 13 C-octanoic acid breath test. Crit Care Med. 2001;9:1744–9.

121. Kearns PJ, Chin D, Mueller L, Wallace K, Jensen WA, Kirsch CM. The incidence of ventilator-associated pneumonia and success in nutrient delivery with gastric versus small intestinal feeding: a randomized clinical trial. Crit Care Med. 2000;28:1742–6.

122. Kortbeek JB, Haigh PI, Doig C. Duodenal versus gastric feeding in ventilated blunt trauma patients: a randomized controlled trial. J Trauma. 1999;46:992–6.

123. Montejo JC, Grau T, Acosta J, et al. National and Metabolic working group of the Spanish Society of Intensive Care Medicine and Coronary Units. Multicenter, prospective, randomized, single-blind study comparing the efficacy and gastrointestinal complications of early jejunal feeding with early gastric feeding in critically ill patients. Crit Care Med. 2002;30:796–800.

124. Strong RM, Condon SC, Solinger MR, et al. Equal aspiration rates from postpylorus and intragastric-placed small-bore nasoenteric feeding tubes: a randomized, prospective study. JPEN J Parenter Enteral Nutr. 1992;16:59–63.

125. Heyland DK, Drover JW, MacDonald S, et al. Effect of postpyloric feeding on gastroesophageal regurgitation and pulmonary microaspiration: results of a randomized controlled trial. Crit Care Med. 2001;29:1495–500.

126. Davis AR, Froomes PRA, French CJ, et al. Randomized comparison of nasojejunal and nasogastric feeding in critically ill patients. Crit Care Med. 2002;30:586–90.

127. Montecalvo MA, Steger KA, Farber HW, et al. Nutritional outcome and pneumonia in critical care patients randomized to gastric versus jejunal tube feedings: the Critical Care Research Team. Crit Care Med. 1992;20:1377–87.

128. Tournadre JP, Barclay M, Fraser R, et al. Small intestinal motor patterns in critically ill patients after major abdominal surgery. Am J Gastroenterol. 2001;96:2418–26.

129. Heyland DK, Dhaliwal R, Drover JW, et al. Canadian clinical practice guidelines for nutrition support in mechanically ventilated, critically ill adult patients. JPEN J Parenter Enteral Nutr. 2003;27:355–73.

130. Lipp A, Lusardi G. Systemic antimicrobial prophylaxis for percutaneous endoscopic gastrostomy. Cochrane Database Syst Rev. 2006(4):CD005571.

131. Nicholson FB, Korman MG, Richardson MA. Percutaneous endoscopic gastrostomy: a review of indications, complications and outcome. J Gastroenterol Hepatol. 2000;15(1):21–5.

132. Tham TC, Taitelbaum G, Carr-Locke DL. Percutaneous endoscopic gastrostomies: are they being done for the right reasons? QJM. 1997;90(8):495–6.

133. Skelly RH, Kupfer RM, Metcalfe ME, et al. Percutaneous endoscopic gastrostomy (PEG): change in practice since 1988. Clin Nutr. 2002;21(5):389–94.

134. Akkersdijk WL, van Bergeijk JD, van Egmond T, et al. Percutaneous endoscopic gastrostomy (PEG): comparison of push and pull methods and evaluation of antibiotic prophylaxis. Endoscopy. 1995;27(4):313–6.

135. Shastri YM, Hoepffner N, Tessmer A, Ackermann H, Schroeder O, Stein J. New introducer PEG gastropexy does not require prophylactic antibiotics: multicenter prospective randomized double-blind placebo-controlled study. Gastrointest Endosc. 2008;67(4):620–8.

136. Dormann AJ, Wejda B, Kahl S, Huchzermeyer H, Ebert MP, Malfertheiner P. Long-term results with a new introducer method with gastropexy for percutaneous endoscopic gastrostomy. Am J Gastroenterol. 2006;101(6):1229–34.

137. Maetani I, Tada T, Ukita T, Inoue H, Sakai Y, Yoshikawa M. PEG with introducer or pull method: a prospective randomized comparison. Gastrointest Endosc. 2003;57(7):837–41.

138. Tucker AT, Gourin CG, Ghegan MD, Porubsky ES, Martindale RG, Terris DJ. 'Push' versus 'pull' percutaneous endoscopic gastrostomy tube placement in patients with advanced head and neck cancer. Laryngoscope. 2003;113(11):1898–902.

139. Hull M, Beane A, Bowen J, Settle C. Methicillin-resistant Staphylococcus aureus infection of percutaneous endoscopic gastrostomy sites. Aliment Pharmacol Ther. 2001;15(12):1883–8.

140. Gossner L, Keymling J, Hahn EG, Ell C. Antibiotic prophylaxis in percutaneous endoscopic gastrostomy (PEG): a prospective randomized clinical trial. Endoscopy. 1999;31(2):119–24.

141. Kulling D, Sonnenberg A, Fried M, Bauerfeind P. Cost analysis of antibiotic prophylaxis for PEG. Gastrointest Endosc. 2000;51(2):152–6.

142. Radhakrishnan NV, Shenoy AH, Cartmill I, et al. Addition of local antiseptic spray to parenteral antibiotic regimen reduces the incidence of stomal infection following percutaneous endoscopic gastrostomy: a randomized controlled trial. Eur J Gastroenterol Hepatol. 2006;18(12):1279–84.

143. Blomberg J, Lagergren P, Martin L, Mattsson F, Lagergren J. Novel approach to antibiotic prophylaxis in percutaneous endoscopic gastrostomy (PEG): randomised controlled trial. BMJ. 2010;341:c3115.

144. Horiuchi A, Nakayama Y, Kajiyama M, Fujii H, Tanaka N. Nasopharyngeal decolonization of methicillin-resistant Staphylococcus aureus can reduce PEG peristomal wound infection. Am J Gastroenterol. 2006;101(2):274–7.

145. Mirsadraee S, Tirukonda P, Nicholson A, Everett SM, McPherson SJ. Embolization for non-variceal upper gastrointestinal tract haemorrhage: a systematic review. Clin Radiol. 2011;66(6):500–9.

146. Garcia-Tsao G, Sanyal AJ, Grace ND, Carey WD. Prevention and management of gastroesophageal varices and variceal hemorrhage in cirrhosis. Am J Gastroenterol. 2007;102(9):2086–102.

147. Bai Y, Guo JF, Li ZS. Meta-analysis: erythromycin before endoscopy for acute upper gastrointestinal bleeding. Aliment Pharmacol Ther. 2011;34(2):166–71.

148. Barkun AN, Bardou M, Kuipers EJ, et al. International consensus recommendations on the management of patients with nonvariceal upper gastrointestinal bleeding. Ann Intern Med. 2010;152(2):101–13.

149. Corley DA, Cello JP, Adkisson W, Ko WF, Kerlikowske K. Octreotide for acute esophageal variceal bleeding: a meta-analysis. Gastroenterology. 2001;120(4):946–54.

150. D'Amico G, Pagliaro L, Pietrosi G, Tarantino I. Emergency sclerotherapy versus vasoactive drugs for bleeding oesophageal varices in cirrhotic patients. Cochrane Database Syst Rev. 2010(3):CD002233.

151. Chen WC, Lo GH, Tsai WL, Hsu PI, Lin CK, Lai KH. Emergency endoscopic variceal ligation versus somatostatin for acute esophageal variceal bleeding. J Chin Med Assoc. 2006;69(2):60–7.

152. Banares R, Albillos A, Rincon D, et al. Endoscopic treatment versus endoscopic plus pharmacologic treatment for acute variceal bleeding: a meta-analysis. Hepatology. 2002;35(3):609–15.

153. Lo GH. Management of acute esophageal variceal hemorrhage. Kaohsiung J Med Sci. 2010;26(2):55–67.

154. Sung JJ, Tsoi KK, Lai LH, Wu JC, Lau JY. Endoscopic clipping versus injection and thermo-coagulation in the treatment of nonvariceal upper gastrointestinal bleeding: a meta-analysis. Gut. 2007;56(10):1364–73.

155. Eriksson LG, Sundbom M, Gustavsson S, Nyman R. Endoscopic marking with a metallic clip facilitates transcatheter arterial embolization in upper peptic ulcer bleeding. J Vasc Interv Radiol. 2006;17(6):959–64.

156. Haddock G, Garden OJ, McKee RF, Anderson JR, Carter DC. Esophageal tamponade in the management of acute variceal hemorrhage. Dig Dis Sci. 1989;34(6):913–8.

157. Marmo R, Koch M, Cipolletta L, et al. Predicting mortality in nonvariceal upper gastrointestinal bleeders: validation of the Italian PNED Score and Prospective Comparison with the Rockall Score. Am J Gastroenterol. 2010;105(6):1284–91.

158. Chiu PW, Ng EK, Cheung FK, et al. Predicting mortality in patients with bleeding peptic ulcers after therapeutic endoscopy. Clin Gastroenterol Hepatol. 2009;7(3):311–6. quiz 253.

159. Garcia-Iglesias P, Villoria A, Suarez D, et al. Meta-analysis: predictors of rebleeding after endoscopic treatment for bleeding peptic ulcer. Aliment Pharmacol Ther. 2011;34(8):888–900.

160. Sreedharan A, Martin J, Leontiadis GI, et al. Proton pump inhibitor treatment initiated prior to endoscopic diagnosis in upper gastrointestinal bleeding. Cochrane Database Syst Rev. 2010(7):CD005415.

161. Hidaka H, Nakazawa T, Wang G, et al. Long-term administration of PPI reduces treatment failures after esophageal variceal band ligation: a randomized, controlled trial. J Gastroenterol. 2012;47(2):118–26.

162. Gluud LL, Langholz E, Krag A. Meta-analysis: isosorbide-mononitrate alone or with either beta-blockers or endoscopic therapy for the management of oesophageal varices. Aliment Pharmacol Ther. 2010;32(7):859–71.

163. Funakoshi N, Segalas-Largey F, Duny Y, et al. Benefit of combination beta-blocker and endoscopic treatment to prevent variceal rebleeding: a meta-analysis. World J Gastroenterol. 2010;16(47):5982–92.

164. Hendrickson RJ, Diaz AA, Salloum R, Koniaris LG. Benign rectal ulcer: an underground cause of inpatient lower gastrointestinal bleeding. Surg Endosc. 2003;17(11):1759–65.

165. Farrell JJ, Friedman LS. Gastrointestinal bleeding in the elderly. Gastroenterol Clin North Am. 2001;30(2):377–407. viii.

166. Bounds BC, Friedman LS. Lower gastrointestinal bleeding. Gastroenterol Clin North Am. 2003;32(4):1107–25.

167. Schuetz A, Jauch KW. Lower gastrointestinal bleeding: therapeutic strategies, surgical techniques and results. Langenbecks Arch Surg. 2001;386(1):17–25.

168. Zuckerman GR, Prakash C. Acute lower intestinal bleeding. Part II: etiology, therapy, and outcomes. Gastrointest Endosc. 1999;49(2):228–38.

169. Wong SK, Ho YH, Leong AP, Seow-Choen F. Clinical behavior of complicated right-sided and left-sided diverticulosis. Dis Colon Rectum. 1997;40(3):344–8.

170. Chen CY, Wu CC, Jao SW, Pai L, Hsiao CW. Colonic diverticular bleeding with comorbid diseases may need elective colectomy. J Gastrointest Surg. 2009;13(3):516–20.

171. Jensen DM. Diagnosis and treatment of patients with severe hematochezia: a time for change. Endoscopy. 1998;30(8):724–6.

172. Foutch PG, Zimmerman K. Diverticular bleeding and the pigmented protuberance (sentinel clot): clinical implications, histopathological correlation, and results of endoscopic intervention. Am J Gastroenterol. 1996;91(12):2589–93.

173. Binmoeller KF, Thonke F, Soehendra N. Endoscopic hemoclip treatment for gastrointestinal bleeding. Endoscopy. 1993;25(2):167–70.

174. Khanna A, Ognibene SJ, Koniaris LG. Embolization as first-line therapy for diverticulosis-related massive lower gastrointestinal bleeding: evidence from a meta-analysis. J Gastrointest Surg. 2005;9(3):343–52.

175. Vernava 3rd AM, Moore BA, Longo WE, Johnson FE. Lower gastrointestinal bleeding. Dis Colon Rectum. 1997;40(7):846–58.

Early Management of Sepsis, Severe Sepsis, and Septic Shock in the Surgical Patient

Laura A. Kreiner and Laura J. Moore

Introduction

Despite advances in surgical critical care, sepsis continues to be a common and serious problem. It is currently the leading cause of death in noncardiac intensive care units (ICUs) and the tenth leading cause of death in the United States [1]. It is estimated that in the United States, there are greater than 1.1 million cases of sepsis per year [2] at an annual cost of $24.3 billion [3]. The incidence of sepsis among hospitalized patients continues to increase as the population ages. The current incidence of severe sepsis among hospitalized patients in the United States is 208 cases/100,000 patients [4] with an associated mortality rate of greater than 30% [5]. But subsequent studies have shown this estimate to be low, with increases in sepsis rates subsequently reported to be as high as 10% per year [6, 7]. These epidemiologic studies document that severe sepsis remains a major challenge and an increasing burden on healthcare systems worldwide.

Among surgical patients, sepsis is a leading cause of morbidity and mortality. Surgical patients account for nearly one-third of sepsis cases in the United States, as determined in a large epidemiologic study from Angus et al. [5]. A recent analysis of the National Surgical Quality Improvement Project (NSQIP) Database determined that sepsis and septic shock are ten times more common than perioperative myocardial infarction and pulmonary embolism [8]. Risk factors for both the development of sepsis and death from sepsis included age older than 60 years, the need for emergency surgery, and the presence of comorbid conditions [9]. Colon perforation was the predominant source of sepsis, and the incidence of sepsis was highest among patients requiring emergency surgery. The development of septic shock was associated with a 39% mortality rate among emergent surgical patients and a 30% mortality rate among elective surgical patients.

Definition of Sepsis, Severe Sepsis, and Septic Shock

A clear and accurate definition of sepsis is essential for clinicians and researchers. A standard definition allows for the identification of patients, leads to a better understanding of the disease process, and facilitates clinical research. The sepsis syndrome was first defined in the literature by Roger Bone in 1989 [10]. Subsequently the American College of Chest Physicians and the Society of Critical Care Medicine Consensus Conference in 1991 defined the Systemic Inflammatory Response Syndrome (SIRS) (see Table 6.1) and Multiple Organ Dysfunction Syndrome (MODS) [11]. A second consensus conference was convened in 2001 to revise the original definitions in response to ongoing criticism from experts in the field. The updated consensus conference definitions included an expanded list of the signs and symptoms of sepsis [12]. While the definitions included in the 2001 update are widely accepted, they do not specifically define the concept of *surgical* sepsis. Additionally, the consensus conference definitions remain nonspecific and allow for some variability, especially with regard to defining organ dysfunction.

To better define the categories of sepsis, severe sepsis, and septic shock with regard to the surgical patient, we have modified the American College of Chest Physician/Society of Critical Care Medicine Consensus Conference definitions. We have defined surgical sepsis as systemic inflammatory response syndrome (SIRS) plus an infection requiring surgical intervention for source control or SIRS plus an infection within 14 days of a major surgical procedure. Major surgical procedure is defined as any procedure requiring general anesthesia for >1 h.

L.A. Kreiner, M.D. (✉) • L.J. Moore, M.D., F.A.C.S.
Department of Surgery, The University of Texas Health Science Center, Houston, TX, USA
e-mail: laura.a.kreiner@uth.tmc.edu

L.J. Moore et al. (eds.), *Common Problems in Acute Care Surgery*,
DOI 10.1007/978-1-4614-6123-4_6, © Springer Science+Business Media New York 2013

Table 6.1 SIRS criteria

Systemic inflammatory response syndrome (SIRS) criteria
Two or more of the following criteria must be present:
• Body temperature less than 36°C or greater than 38°C
• Heart rate greater than 90 beats per minute
• Tachypnea, with greater than 20 breaths per minute; or, an arterial partial pressure of carbon dioxide less than 4.3 kPa (32 mmHg)
• White blood cell count less than 4,000 cells/mm³ (4×10^9 cells/L) or greater than 12,000 cells/mm³ (12×10^9 cells/L); or the presence of greater than 10% immature neutrophils (band forms)

Severe sepsis is defined as SIRS plus infection plus acute organ dysfunction. Qualifications of acute organ dysfunction are defined as follows:

1. Neurologic: Glasgow Outcome Score (GCS) <13 upon recognition of sepsis or deteriorating GCS to <13 during first 24 h.
2. Pulmonary: PaO_2/FiO_2 ratio <250 (<200 if lung is primary site of infection) and pulmonary capillary wedge pressure (PCWP) (if available) not suggestive of fluid overload.
3. Renal (one of the following): urine output (UOP) <0.5 ml/kg for ≥1 h despite adequate volume resuscitation, increase in serum creatinine ≥0.5 mg/dl from baseline (measured within 24 h of starting sepsis resuscitation) despite adequate volume resuscitation or increase in serum creatinine ≥0.5 mg/dl during first 24 h of sepsis management despite adequate volume resuscitation. Adequate volume resuscitation is defined as a minimum intravenous fluid infusion of 20 ml/kg/ideal body weight (IBW) or central venous pressure (CVP) ≥8 mmHg or PCWP ≥12 mmHg.
4. Coagulation (one of following): INR >1.5, platelet count <80,000 or ≥50% decrease platelet compared to 24 h before instituting sepsis resuscitation or in the 24 h after starting sepsis resuscitation in the absence of chronic liver disease.
5. Hypoperfusion: lactate level >4 mmol/l. Septic shock is defined as SIRS plus infection plus acute cardiac dysfunction. Acute cardiac dysfunction is defined by the requirement of vasopressors to increase mean arterial pressure (MAP) ≥65 mmHg despite intravenous fluid (IVF) challenge ≥20 ml/kg/IBW of isotonic crystalloid infusion or CVP ≥8 mmHg or PCWP ≥12 mmHg.

Initial Assessment and Evaluation of the Septic Patient

Early Identification of Sepsis

Within our institution, we have identified sepsis to be a major cause of morbidity and mortality in our general surgery patients. Early signs of sepsis were often missed and interventions were delayed as bedside nurses and other team members focus on multiple priorities and tasks involved with patient care. Many of the early signs and symptoms of sepsis are often subtle and in the surgical population may be attributed to other problems. For example, oliguria is commonly seen in surgical patients and is often attributed to under resuscitation in the operating room or volume loss from the gastrointestinal tract. However, oliguria can also be an early finding in patients with sepsis. Alterations in mental status are often attributed to narcotic administration or ICU psychosis, but can also be an early warning sign off sepsis. Likewise, acute hypoxia on the surgical wards spurs a workup for pulmonary embolism but acute hypoxia may herald the onset of severe sepsis or septic shock.

Identifying patients in the early stages of sepsis is imperative. Progression to septic shock is associated with prohibitively high mortality (>30%) despite aggressive interventions. Considering the adverse outcomes associated with this progression, the benefit of routine, accurate screening of patients for sepsis quickly becomes apparent. In an attempt to increase the early identification of sepsis, we developed a sepsis screening tool for use in our SICU (see Fig. 6.1) [13]. Our initial experience with the implementation of this mandatory sepsis screening tool in our SICU showed promising results. The screening tool yielded a sensitivity of 96.5%, a specificity of 96.7%, a positive predictive value of 80.2%, and a negative predictive value of 99.5%. In addition, sepsis related mortality decreased from 35.1 to 23.3%. Subsequent expansion and statistical validation of the screening on the surgical floor yielded similar results [14]. Since implementing mandatory sepsis screening we have seen a significant decline in our severe sepsis and septic shock related mortality. Regardless of the method utilized to screen patients, all members of the patient care team must be aware and vigilant in the detection of the early signs and symptoms of sepsis.

Initial Assessment

A clinical suspicion for the presence of sepsis should prompt further evaluation of the patient. This initial evaluation should focus on determining the degree of physiologic derangement exhibited by the patient. It is especially important to assess for the presence and degree of tissue malperfusion. There are several clinical and laboratory variables that can be used to evaluate the state of tissue perfusion. The following are indicators that the patient is experiencing tissue hypoperfusion: (1) urine output <0.5 ml/kg of ideal body weight, (2) mean arterial pressure <65 mmHg, (3) Glasgow Coma Score <12, and (4) serum lactate ≥4 mmol/l. The detection of tissue hypoperfusion should prompt aggressive resuscitative measures focused on restoring tissue perfusion.

Based upon the definitions outlined previously those patients that do not have evidence of tissue hypoperfusion would fall into the category of sepsis. Those patients that do have evidence of tissue hypoperfusion would be categorized as having severe sepsis/septic shock. The initial resuscitation and management of these patients is discussed as follows.

Initial Resuscitation of Sepsis

The initial resuscitation phase of sepsis should begin immediately upon recognition of sepsis. Initiation of resuscitation should not wait until the patient is transferred to a higher level of care. The goals of the resuscitation include restoration of intravascular volume, diagnosis of the source of infection, initiation of broad spectrum antimicrobial therapy, and source control. Many institutions have developed order sets that specifically address each of these issues. The utilization of standardized protocols for the initial management of sepsis has been demonstrated to improve patient outcomes in multiple settings [15–20].

The major tenets of initial resuscitation can be initiated in any area of the hospital and should not be delayed pending transfer to the ICU. Establishing intravenous (IV) access is a critical first step as this allows for the administration of resuscitative intravenous fluid and antimicrobials. For those patients without evidence of tissue hypoperfusion, a large bore peripheral IV should be sufficient. In the event that peripheral IV access is not attainable, a central venous line should be inserted in a timely fashion.

Fluid resuscitation should be guided with the following goals in mind:

1. CVP (if available) of 8–12 mmHg in non-intubated patients and a target CVP of 12–15 mmHg in mechanically ventilated patients [21]
2. MAP of $\geq$65 mmHg [22]
3. Urine output of $\geq$0.5 ml/kg/h
4. Central venous ($ScvO_2$) oxygen saturation of $\geq$70% or mixed venous (SvO_2) oxygen saturation of $\geq$65%(if available) [23]

These endpoints of resuscitation should be achieved within 6 h of the recognition of sepsis. In addition a baseline serum lactate should be sent upon the identification of sepsis. A repeat serum lactate level should be sent 4 h later to monitor the progress of the initial resuscitation.

The initial resuscitation fluid of choice still remains extremely controversial. There are no prospective, randomized controlled trials evaluating crystalloid versus colloid resuscitation in surgical patients with sepsis. If colloids are given, the initial fluid bolus should be 300–500 ml of colloid over 30 min. If crystalloids are given, the initial fluid challenge

a

Current Heart Rate: _________

Temperature Minimum (prior 24 hours): _________

Temperature Maximum (prior 24 hours): _________

Current Respiratory Rate: _________

WBC (most recent): _________

Patient label

	0	1	2	3	4
Heart Rate	70-109		55-69 110-139	40-54 140-179	$\leq$ 39 $\leq$ 180
Temp (^{o}C)	36 – 38.4	34-35.9 38.5-38.9	32 – 33.9	30 – 31.9 39 – 40.9	$\leq$ 29.9 $\geq$ 41
Temp (^{o}F)	96.8 – 101.1	93.1-96.7 101.2-102.0	89.6-93.0	86 – 89.5 102.5 – 105.6	$\leq$ 85.9 $\geq$ 105.7
Respiratory Rate	12-24	10-11 25-34	6-9	35-49	$\leq$5 $\geq$50
Latest WBC Count	3-14.9	15-19.9	1 – 2.9 20-39.9		< 1 $\geq$ 40
Acute change in mental status	No	Yes			
SIRS Score (total points)		*If the SIRS Score is $\geq$ 4 please notify the mid level provider or resident physician to complete the assessment for infection.*			

Completed By: _________________________   Date/Time:_________

Fig. 6.1 Sepsis screening tool. (**a**) Sepsis screening score. (**b**) Midlevel/Physician sepsis screening assessment for source of infection

b

1. Vascular access?

type	dialysis	triple / quad	PICC	port	tunneled	other (IV, art)
date placed						
site						
local finding						
blood culture finding						

Suspicion of:

line infection?

Yes   No

2. Clinical pulmonary infection score (CPIS)

Variable	points	score
temperature (°C) time (hhmm)		
36.5 – 38.4	0	
38.5 – 38.9	1	
> 39.0 or < 36.0	2	
blood leukocyte count (# per mm^3) time (hhmm)		
4,000 – 11,000	0	
< 4,000 or > 11,000	1	
tracheal secretions time (hhmm)		
small	0	
moderate	1	
large	2	
purulent (add 1 point if purulent)	+1	
oxygenation (PaO$_2$/FiO$_2$) time (hhmm)		
≥ 240 or presence of ARDS	0	
< 240 and absence of ARDS	2	
chest radiograph time (hhmm)		
no infiltrate	0	
patchy or diffuse infiltrate	1	
localized infiltrate	2	

Intubated / mech vent support?

Yes   No

date intubated:

pneumonia?

Yes   No

3. Abdomen

recent abdominal surgery?	Yes	No
abdominal pain?	Yes	No
abdominal distention?	Yes	No
purulent drainage from surgical drains?	Yes	No
intolerance to enteral nutrition?	Yes	No

abdominal infection?

Yes   No

4. Skin / soft tissue

erythema / drainage from other surgical site?	Yes	No
site		

cellulitis / soft tissue infection?

Yes   No

5. Urinary tract

urinary catheter?	Yes	No
date placed		
latest urinalysis / urine culture results		

UTI?

Yes   No

6. Other site

site	

other infection?

Yes   No

Completed by: _________________________   Date / time: _____________

Fig. 6.1 (continued)

should be 1,000 cm^3 of crystalloid over 30 min. The patient's response to fluid bolus will dictate the need for additional resuscitation. The Saline versus Albumin Fluid Evaluation (SAFE) study randomized nearly 7,000 critically ill patients requiring fluid resuscitation to receive albumin or normal saline, and no difference in mortality was identified. Interestingly, a subgroup analysis of the 1,218 patients with severe sepsis documented that albumin was associated with a trend toward reduced mortality (relative risk of death 0.87; 95% confidence interval 0.74–1.02) [24]. Currently two randomized trials are ongoing to further investigate this finding: (1) Volume Replacement with Albumin in Severe Sepsis (ALBIOS) [25] (Italy) and (2) Early Albumin Resuscitation during Septic Shock (France) [26].

Initial Resuscitation of Severe Sepsis and Septic Shock

For those patients presenting with severe sepsis and septic shock the timely correction of tissue hypoperfusion is critical. The concept of early goal directed therapy (EGDT) in severe sepsis and septic shock was initially developed and validated in the emergency department (ED) setting in a single-center trial [23]. The ED is frequently the point of entry for many septic patients into the hospital. Unfortunately, many of these patients may wait for prolonged periods of time in the ED. The end result is often a delay in the implementation of early sepsis resuscitation.

The implementation of EGDT has been shown to improve survival in patient presenting with severe sepsis and septic shock [18, 23, 27, 28]. The basic principles of EGDT therapy are to recognize tissue hypoperfusion and initiate therapies to reverse global tissue hypoxia by optimizing oxygen delivery. Tissue perfusion can be monitored by measuring mixed venous hemoglobin oxygen saturation (SvO_2), central venous hemoglobin oxygen saturation ($ScvO_2$), or peripheral muscle hemoglobin oxygen saturation (StO_2). A SvO_2 of ≤65%, a $ScvO_2$ of ≤70%, or a StO_2 of ≤75% are considered indicators of tissue hypoperfusion. Once tissue hypoperfusion is identified, specific therapies should be instituted to reverse tissue hypoxia by restoring adequate perfusion. The factors affecting oxygen delivery are cardiac output (CO), hemoglobin ([Hb]), and percent arterial hemoglobin oxygen saturation (SaO_2). EGDT attempts to restore tissue perfusion by addressing these variables. The evidence-based Sepsis Resuscitation Bundle was established with a goal to accomplish all indicated tasks, 100% of the time, within 6 h of the diagnosis of sepsis was established, and is used to assist with the administration of prompt resuscitation efforts in the treatment of sepsis (Table 6.2).

To restore intravascular volume and enhance cardiac output, an initial crystalloid fluid bolus of 20 ml/kg of ideal body weight is recommended. This fluid bolus can be administered initially through existing peripheral IVs, however, placement of a central venous line for monitoring of CVP is recommended. An arterial line should be placed in patients with hypotension that do not rapidly respond to volume challenge. The use of noninvasive blood pressure monitoring for patients in septic shock often produces inaccurate measurements and should be avoided for titration of vasoactive medications. A Foley catheter should also be inserted to allow for close monitoring of urine output. Bladder pressures should be monitored in patients requiring aggressive volume loading.

The goals of resuscitation remain the same as those listed previously:

Table 6.2 Sepsis Bundles: The goal is to perform all indicated tasks 100% of the time within the first 6 h (Sepsis Resuscitation Bundle) or first 24 h (Sepsis Management Bundle) of the diagnosis of severe sepsis

Sepsis resuscitation bundle—(to be started immediately and completed within 6 h)

- Serum lactate measured
- Blood cultures obtained prior to antibiotic administration
- Broad-spectrum antibiotics administered within 3 h for ED admissions and 1 h for non-ED ICU admissions
- In the event of hypotension and/or lactate >4 mmol/L:
  - Deliver a minimum of 20 ml/kg of crystalloid (or colloid equivalent)
  - Apply vasopressors for hypotension not responding to initial fluid resuscitation to maintain mean arterial pressure (MAP) ≥65 mmHg
- In the event of persistent arterial hypotension despite volume resuscitation (septic shock) and/or initial lactate >4 mmol/L (36 mg/dl):
  - Achieve central venous pressure (CVP) of ≥8 mmHg
  - Achieve central venous oxygen saturation ($ScvO_2$) of ≥70%[a]

Sepsis management bundle—(to be started immediately and completed within 24 h)

- Low-dose steroids administered for septic shock in accordance with a standardized ICU policy
- Glucose control maintained ≥lower limit of normal, but <150 mg/dl (8.3 mmol/L)
- For mechanically ventilated patients inspiratory plateau pressures maintained <30 cmH$_2$O

[a]Achieving a mixed venous oxygen saturation of 65% is an acceptable alternative

1. A target CVP (if available) of 8–12 mmHg in non-intubated patients and a target CVP of 12–15 mmHg in mechanically ventilated patients [21]
2. MAP of ≥65 mmHg [22]
3. Urine output of ≥0.5 ml/kg/h, and
4. Central venous ($ScvO_2$) oxygen saturation of ≥70% or mixed venous (SvO_2) oxygen saturation of ≥65% [23].

In the event that a $ScvO_2$ of ≥70% or SvO_2 ≥65% cannot be achieved with restoration of intravascular volume and mean arterial pressure of 65–90 mmHg, red blood cells should be transfused to achieve of hematocrit of ≥30%.

Multiple international randomized controlled trials of early goal-directed therapy for patients with severe sepsis are underway to validate the findings of the single-center Rivers trial. These include ProCESS (Protocolized Care for Early Septic Shock), ARISE (Australian Resuscitation in Sepsis Evaluation), and ProMISe (Protocolized Management in Sepsis). The ProCESS trial will randomize 1950 patients who present to the emergency department in septic shock to three arms: (1) the EGDT Rivers protocol described previously, (2) a less complicated, less invasive protocol using esophageal Doppler monitor and no blood transfusion, and (3) usual care [29]. The ARISE trial will randomize 1,600 patients to EGDT versus standard care and assess 90-day mortality in patients presenting to the emergency department with severe sepsis [30]. The ProMISe trial will randomize 1,260 patients to EGDT versus standard care and assess 90-day mortality in patients presenting to the emergency department with septic shock [31]. Furthermore, an individual, patient data meta-analysis will be performed across the three trials.

Having achieved the goal CVP, the goal MAP, and the goal hematocrit, if there is still evidence of tissue hypoperfusion, inotropic agents should be administered to improve cardiac output. In patients presenting with septic shock, the initial fluid bolus may not restore their MAP to $\geq$65 mmHg. A repeat fluid bolus of 20 ml/kg of ideal body weight can be given to correct hypovolemia. However, transient vasopressors therapy may need to be initiated, even if volume resuscitation is still ongoing.

Vasopressor Therapy

Septic shock is primarily a vasodilatory shock, associated with a high cardiac output and a low systemic vascular resistance. Therefore, initial vasopressors therapy should be targeted at restoring vascular tone. Both norepinephrine and dopamine are acceptable first line agents for treatment of septic shock, and should be administered through a central venous catheter. Norepinephrine is primarily an α(alpha)-receptor agonist that promotes widespread vasoconstriction and has little effect on heart rate or stroke volume. Dopamine has dose dependent effects on α(alpha), β(beta), and dopaminergic receptors. The initial increase in blood pressure seen with dopamine is related to increasing cardiac output. At higher doses (>7.5 μ[mu]g/kg/min), dopamine does activate α(alpha)-receptors with resultant vasoconstriction.

In patients with septic shock that is refractory to first line vasopressors, the addition of vasopressin may be beneficial. Vasopressin is a stress hormone that has vasoactive effects. The use of vasopressin is supported by recent work by Landry et al. who suggest that in states of septic shock there is a relative deficiency of vasopressin [32]. The administration of vasopressin in this patient population has been shown to improve responsiveness to catecholamines and potentially reduce the amount of catecholamine needed to maintain blood pressure [33].

The Vasopressin and Septic Shock Trial (VASST) randomized 779 patients in septic shock requiring norepinephrine (5 μg/min) for at least 6 h and at least one organ system dysfunction present for <24 h to vasopressin (0.01–0.03 U/min) versus higher dose norepinephrine (5–15 μg/min) [34]. No difference in 28-day or 90-day mortality was identified. In the prospectively defined stratum of less severe septic shock, the mortality rate was lower in the vasopressin group

than in the norepinephrine group at 28 days (26.5% versus 35.7%, $p=0.05$), which persisted to 90-day mortality (35.8% versus 46.1%, $p=0.04$). In a post hoc analysis of the VASST study, it was identified that the combination of low-dose vasopressin and corticosteroids was associated with decreased mortality and organ dysfunction as compared with norepinephrine and corticosteroids [35]. Based on the results of studies to date, clinicians should consider the addition of low-dose continuous infusion vasopressin (up to 0.03 U/min) in individual septic shock patients who despite adequate resuscitation are still requiring high doses of vasopressors.

It is our current practice to initiate a vasopressin drip at a rate of 0.04 U/min in patients requiring norepinephrine infusion at $\geq$15 μg/min. The dose of vasopressin should not exceed 0.04 U/min because of the possibility of decreased cardiac output and myocardial ischemia at higher doses [36].

While most patients with sepsis initially present with increased cardiac output, a subset of patients will develop myocardial depression from sepsis. The exact mechanism for this reversible myocardial dysfunction is still under investigation. B-type natriuretic peptide (BNP) is secreted in response to stretching of myocardium and is used clinically to assess volume overload and predict death in acute congestive heart failure. More recently, BNP has been demonstrated to be elevated in early septic shock and likewise predict death. We have recently shown that BNP increases with initial sepsis severity and is associated with early left ventricular (LV) dysfunction that in itself is associated with later death. Monitoring BNP in early sepsis to identify occult LV dysfunction may prompt earlier use of inotropes which are not commonly used in early sepsis resuscitation.

For those patients with suspected or known cardiac dysfunction the addition of inotropic therapy is recommended. Dobutamine is the first line agent for treatment of cardiac dysfunction in patients with sepsis. The management of patients with a cardiac component to their shock state presents a unique challenge to the clinician since they require the titration of vasopressors and inotropic agents. In this subset of patients, the utilization of a pulmonary artery catheter can be extremely useful. This allows for the specific titration of vasopressors based upon systemic vascular resistance and inotropic agents based upon cardiac output. There is no evidence to support increasing cardiac index to predetermined supranormal levels.

Steroids in Septic Shock

The use of steroids for the management of septic shock has been debated for several decades. In recent years, the concept of relative adrenal insufficiency in septic shock has received renewed interest. Despite several large clinical trials addressing the issue of steroid use in patients with septic shock, the topic remains controversial. The ongoing debate is primarily surrounding the definition of relative adrenal insufficiency in critically ill patients and the "gold standard" for diagnosing adrenal insufficiency in this population.

It had previously been a common practice to perform a low dose ACTH (cosyntropin) stimulation test on all patients with septic shock as a means to identify those patients with relative adrenal insufficiency. To perform the cosyntropin stimulation test, a baseline serum cortisol is drawn which represents time zero (T_0). The patient is then given 250 µg of intravenous cosyntropin. Subsequent serum cortisol levels are measured at 30 (T_{30}) and 60 (T_{60}) minutes after the cosyntropin. If the delta cortisol is ≤ 9 µg/dl then the patient is considered to have relative adrenal insufficiency and steroids are initiated. Based on the current evidence to date, we now recognize that the ACTH stimulation test is not recommended to identify the subset of adults with septic shock who should receive hydrocortisone. A number of factors interfere with the ACTH stimulation test, and our current diagnostic tests are not accurate. The administration of etomidate causes a temporary suppression of the hypothalamic–pituitary–adrenal axis, resulting in transient adrenal insufficiency. In addition, patients that have received steroids at any time during the previous 6 months should not undergo testing of their adrenal function. Rather, these patients should be empirically initiated on steroid therapy. The current edition (2008) of the Surviving Sepsis Campaign Guidelines recommends that intravenous hydrocortisone should be considered for adult septic shock when hypotension responds poorly to adequate fluid resuscitation and vasopressors. The literature indicates that low dose corticosteroids decrease the time to cessation of vasopressors [37], increase the systemic vascular resistance and MAP [38], and decrease the risk of death [39]. The dose of hydrocortisone should be ≤ 300 mg/day. We currently give hydrocortisone 50 mg IV every 6 h. The duration of steroid administration also remains controversial. The current recommendation is that steroids be discontinued once vasopressors are no longer required.

Identifying the Source of Infection

Identifying the source of infection is essential to the initial management of sepsis. Whenever possible, cultures should be obtained prior to initiation of empiric antimicrobial therapy. Current recommendations include obtaining a minimum of two blood cultures, including one blood culture from each vascular access device and one blood culture from a peripheral puncture. Additional cultures from other sites (respiratory, urinary tract) and radiographic imaging should be dictated by clinical suspicion. In the surgical population this may include obtaining cultures from surgical drains and per-

forming pertinent imaging to identify an undrained abscess. Despite the importance of source identification, difficulty in the collection of cultures should not generate a significant delay in the administration of antimicrobial therapy.

In order to improve the chances of detecting bacteremia it is crucial to obtain the appropriate volume of blood for the culture medium. Several studies have demonstrated that the volume of blood cultured is the single most important factor in the detection of bacteremia [40–42]. The recommend volume of blood per culture tube is ≥ 10 ml. Obtaining blood cultures from all vascular access devices along with simultaneous collection of blood cultures from a peripheral site is beneficial in diagnosing catheter related infections. The concept of differential time to positivity has been well described in the literature [43, 44]. Differential time to positivity is defined as the difference in time necessary for blood cultured drawn simultaneously from a peripheral site and a central venous catheter to become positive. The differential time to positivity is considered to be positive if the blood culture that is drawn through the vascular access device becomes positive at least 120 min before the peripheral culture. If a patient has an indwelling vascular access device and the cultures drawn from that device become positive at least 120 min before the peripheral cultures become positive, it is recommended that the device be removed as it is likely infected [43].

Initiation of Empiric Antimicrobial Therapy

Another key component of the initial resuscitation of the septic patient is the administration of intravenous antimicrobial therapy. Antimicrobials should be administered after appropriate cultures have been collected but within 1 h of sepsis recognition. Difficulty with specimen collection should not delay the initiation of antibiotic therapy beyond the 1 h mark. The time to antimicrobial administration has been identified as a critical factor in survival of patients presenting with sepsis. A recent study by Kumar et al. found that each hour in delay of antimicrobials was associated with an average decrease in survival of 7.6% [45]. Delayed administration of antifungal therapy in patients with Candida bloodstream infections was an independent predictor of hospital mortality [46]. Maintaining a supply of commonly used antimicrobials in the ED and ICU can assist in the timely administration of these agents. The Surviving Sepsis guidelines recommend initiation of intravenous broad-spectrum antibiotics within the first hour of recognizing severe sepsis and septic shock.

The selection of antimicrobial therapy should take into account the patient's history (including drug allergies and recent antimicrobial exposure), suspected source of infection, and hospital specific antibiograms. Within our surgical

Table 6.3 Recommendations for source-specific Empiric Antibiotic Selection

Pneumonia	Antibiotic	Regimen
Community acquired (CAP)	1. Ceftriaxone + Levofloxacin 2. Aztreonam + Levofloxacin	1g IV q24h 750mg IV q24h 2gm IV q8h 750mg IV q24h
Aspiration (not chemical pneumonitis)	Piperacillin / Tazobactam	4.5g IV q6h
Ventilator associated (VAP)		
Early VAP (<5 day)	1. Cefepime 2. Ciprofloxacin	2g IV q12h 400mg IV q12h
Late VAP (≥5dy; pseudomonas risk: previous hosp or broad spectrum antibiotic exposure; +pseudomonas culture)	1. Cefepime + Vancomycin + Tobramycin 2. Ciprofloxacin + Vancomycin + Tobramycin	2g IV q8h 15mg/kg IV q12h 7mg/kg IV 400mg IV q8h 15mg/kg IV q12h 7mg/kg IV
Catheter related Infections		
Catheter-associated urinary tract infection (CAUTI)	1. Cefepime 2. Ciprofloxacin	1gm IV q12h 400mg IV q12h
IV, art cath; bloodstream	Vancomycin	1gm IV q12h
Candidemia high risk (TPN, steroid Tx, diabetes, hepatic failure)	Fluconazole	800mg IV q24h
Wound/Soft tissue Infections		
Necrotizing soft tissue infection (NSTI)	1. Piperacillin / Tazobactam + Vancomycin + Clindamycin 2. Ciprofloxacin + Vancomycin + Clindamycin	4.5g IV q6h 15mg/kg IV q12h 900mg IV q8h 400mg IV q8h 15mg/kg IV q12h 900mg IV q8h
Surgical Site Infection (SSI)	1. Ertapenem + Vancomycin 2. Ciprofloxacin + Vancomycin	1gm IV q24h 15mg/kg IV q12h 400mg IV q12h 15mg/kg IV q12h
Intra abdominal Infections		
Pseudomonas -low risk	1. Ertapenem + Vancomycin 2. Ciprofloxacin + Metronidazole + Vancomycin	1gm IV q24h 15mg/kg IV q12h 400mg IV q8h 500mg IV q8h 15mg/kg IV q12h
Pseudomonas- high risk (previous hospitalization or broad spectrum antibiotic exposure; positive pseudomonas culture)	1. Imipenem / Cilastatin + Vancomycin 2. Ciprofloxacin + Metronidazole + Vancomycin	500mg IV q6h 15mg/kg IV q12h 400mg IV q8h 500mg IV q8h 15mg/kg IV q12h
Candidiasis - high risk (TPN, steroid treatment, diabetes, hepatic failure, upper GI perforation ı H2 blocker, age ≥ 75, prolonged antibiotic, long term care)	consider Fluconazole	800mg IV q24h
Special Considerations		
1. indicates preferred therapy 2. alternative for severe β lactam allergy * dosing adjustments should be made if evidence of renal dysfunction * if Vancomycin allergy (not intolerance), then use Linezolid 600mg IV q12hr		

ICU, our multidisciplinary sepsis team has developed antimicrobial regimens based upon suspected source of infection and the current institution specific antibiogram (see Table 6.3). When choosing empiric antimicrobial therapy, a few general rules should be applied. Chiefly, the initial antimicrobial coverage should be broad enough to cover all potential pathogens. There is substantial evidence that administering inadequate initial antimicrobial coverage is associated with increased morbidity and mortality [47–50]. Any antimicrobial that the patient has recently received should be avoided. Vigilant monitoring of culture data and de-escalation of the antimicrobial regimen based upon culture results and sensitivities will reduce the risk of superinfection and the emergence of resistant organisms.

Obtaining Source Control

The final component of the initial resuscitation bundle is identification and control of the source of infection. This can be as simple as removing an infected vascular access device. However, in our experience, in surgical patients the abdomen is the site of infection in ≥50% of cases. These patients often require diagnostic imaging to identify the source and an operative procedure to attain source control. This includes, but is not limited to, emergent debridement of necrotic tissues, abscess drainage, removal of infected vascular access devices, and exploratory laparotomy. In the setting of septic shock, these procedures, although necessary, can present a unique challenge to the surgical team.

The concept of damage control laparotomy (DCL) was first recognized for the care of critically injured trauma patients [51–53]. Damage control is defined as rapid, initial control of hemorrhage and contamination followed by intraperitoneal packing as needed, and temporary abdominal closure. This concept was utilized on those patients that presented with severe physiologic derangements such as coagulopathy, acidosis, and hypothermia. Rather than persisting for hours performing the definitive operation, these patients have their critical surgical issues addressed in an abbreviated manner so they may be taken to the ICU for continued resuscitation. Once the physiologic derangements have been corrected the patient is taken back to the operating room for a definitive surgical procedure. The decision to utilize DCL should not be viewed as a bailout. Instead, it is a deliberate decision to truncate the surgical procedure in order to minimize the time away from the ICU. The decision to perform DCL is often made prior to arriving in the operating room and is based on the severity of the patient's physiologic derangements at the time of presentation.

The concept of DCL has now evolved to include critically ill patients with surgical sepsis. Like the trauma patient with the lethal triad of acidosis, hypothermia, and coagulopathy, many patients with septic shock present in a similar fashion. For those patients presenting with septic shock and an identified source of infection requiring surgical intervention, the utilization of DCL can be life saving.

The first priority is to initiate resuscitation. The patient needs to undergo preoperative optimization during which time the airway is secured, central venous and arterial lines are placed, volume resuscitation and broad spectrum antimicrobial agents are administered, and if needed, vasopressors are titrated to the appropriate endpoints. Within 6 h the patient is taken to the operating room for emergent laparotomy and potential damage control procedures. The surgeon needs to assess the degree of physiologic derangement early in the operation and if the severe physiologic derangements exist, then the operative interventions need to be abbreviated. The primary aim is to control the source of infection, e.g., resect dead bowel, manage bowel perforations (resection versus primary closure), drain abscesses, and wash out the abdomen. We do not create ostomies and bowel often is left in discontinuity at this first operation. The abdomen is then managed with a temporary abdominal closure device (via a variety of techniques) and the patient is rapidly returned to the ICU where they undergo continued physiologic optimization. This includes optimizing volume resuscitation and mechanical ventilation, correction of coagulopathy and hypothermia, and monitoring for abdominal compartment syndrome. Over the next 24–48 h abnormal physiology is corrected so that the patient can safely return to the OR for a definitive operation and abdominal closure. Septic shock is a formidable metabolic insult and it is very important to provide optimal nutritional support (this often requires combined enteral and parenteral nutrition) and early mobilization to prevent the loss of lean body mass and resultant impaired recovery.

One of the problems with this "damage control" strategy is that in some of the patients the midline abdominal fascia cannot be closed at the second operation because of bowel distention and edema and they require multiple additional laparotomies for definitive abdominal wall closure. The midline fascia is progressively closed with the use of a vacuum-assisted closure (VAC) device. For this technique to work it is important that the bowel not become adherent to peritoneum of the anterior abdominal wall out to the lateral paracolic gutters otherwise the abdomen becomes "frozen" and the fascia cannot be brought to midline. The VAC device actively removes fluid and decreases edema, provides medial tension which helps to minimize fascial retraction and loss of domain, and protects the abdominal contents by providing separation between abdominal wall and viscera, with no fascial damage since it does not require fascial suture placement. Traditionally, abdominal wall defects in these "frozen" abdomens were closed by mobilizing skin/subcutaneous tissue flaps to cover the defect (i.e., accepting a large hernia defect and need for delayed reconstruction) or by bridging the defect with mesh with later split thickness skin grafting once granulation tissue has developed. This is associated with a 20% gastrointestinal fistula rate, which is an extremely morbid complication. Additionally, many of these patients required delayed complex abdominal wall reconstructions. Recently, there has been significant enthusiasm for acute reconstruction with biological mesh. Unfortunately the long term follow up studies show that many of these patients still require delayed hernia repairs of large defects [54]. In our published experience of treating the open abdomen with the VAC device, we achieved primary fascia closure in 87% at a mean 7 days with a 2% fistula rate and no intra-abdominal abscesses [55, 56]. These results are nearly identical to the results reported by Miller et al. from Wake Forest University who taught us how to do this type of closure [57]. More recently, Cothren et al. have reported 100% primary fascial closure rate using a modified VAC device technique [58]. The long term outcomes are not known but in short term follow-up (mean 180 days) ventral hernia was 2.3%. However, as is true with all emergency laparotomies, this rate will without a doubt increase with time but the hernia defects will be small and more easily repaired.

In addition to "damage control" scenarios, there are other reasons that we leave the abdomen open and plan for a staged relaparotomy:

1. Patients with ischemic bowel that have undergone a resection will be taken back the next day to assess viability of the remaining bowel before attempts at anastomosis or ostomy creation. We have been quite successful in completing the small bowel to colon anastomosis at the second operation and thus these patients have avoided the need for a temporary ileostomy.

2. Patients with necrotizing pancreatitis. We attempt to avoid operative interventions in this group of patients but are occasionally forced to do so.

3. Patients who have massive bowel distention that cannot be closed without causing significant intra-abdominal hypertension (IAH) will undergo temporary abdominal closure. IAH sets the stage of abdominal compartment syndrome (ACS) which occurs with subsequent ICU resuscitation [59]. Avoiding ACS significantly improves survival.

4. Patients who develop ACS and require a decompressive laparotomy. As a result of advances in trauma care starting in the 1980s, this entity emerged as an epidemic in the mid 1990s in trauma centers worldwide. As we begin to understand this new entity, it has been increasingly recognized to occur in non-trauma ICU patients as well [60–62]. Unfortunately, if you do not look for ACS by monitoring bladder pressures, you will not diagnose it and these patients will die of refractory shock.

Within our SICU we have been utilizing DCL for our patients with septic shock. Over 2 years, we had 22 patients who underwent DCL for source control. Sources of intra-abdominal infection were colon (11 patients), small bowel (4), stomach (2), and pancreas (1). Four patients had peritonitis with no identified source. Of the 22 patients, 6 died from multiple organ failure, for an actual mortality rate of 27%. The mean P-POSSUM predicted mortality was significantly higher at 69.4% ($p<0.02$), as was the predicted mortality of 76% based on a mean APACHE II score of 31.8 ($p<0.02$) [63]. This data suggests that the implementation of DCL for patients with surgical sepsis is decreasing mortality and is a viable option for patients with septic shock and the need for immediate operative source control.

Activated Protein C for Severe Sepsis and Septic Shock

In the normal physiologic state, anticoagulation predominates. The major anticoagulant factors are protein C, protein S, antithrombin, and tissue factor pathway inhibitor. Protein C is activated by the binding of thrombin to thrombomodulin on the surface of the endothelium. Once activated, protein C directly inhibits factor Va and factor VIIIa in the clotting cascade. In patients with severe sepsis and septic shock there is a decreased expression of thrombomodulin on the vascular endothelium. As a result, there is decreased production of activated protein C (APC). This results in a shift toward the pro coagulant state. This shift to a pro coagulant state results in microvascular thrombosis, impaired fibrinolysis, and endothelial dysfunction. The microvasculature becomes occluded with resultant tissue hypoxia and direct tissue damage, which ultimately results in organ dysfunction/failure. The extent of coagulation disturbance ranges from mild laboratory abnormalities to disseminated intravascular coagulation (DIC). This underlying disruption of the intrinsic production of APC served as the physiologic impetus for the administration of APC as a means to reverse the pro coagulant state seen in severe sepsis and septic shock. In October, 2011 APC was withdrawn from the market after additional studies showed no change as compared to placebo in reducing mortality.

Discussion: Pathophysiology of Sepsis: A Complex Process

The clinical manifestations of sepsis are the result of a complex series of interactions between the inciting organism and the host's innate immune response. This intricate cellular interaction involves numerous signaling pathways as well as the production of cytokines and chemokines. A detailed discussion of each of these pathways is beyond the scope of this text; however, a few key elements are discussed.

Characteristics of the Pathogen

The host response to infection can be triggered by bacterial, viral, and/or fungal infection. The specific characteristics of the inciting organism have a role in the body's response to the infectious stimuli. Each organism has specific virulence factors that enable the organism to evade the host's defenses. These virulence factors include antigenic variation of surface molecules, inhibition of complement activation, resistance to phagocytosis, production of exotoxins, and scavenging of reactive oxygen intermediates [64]. Cell to cell communication between organisms allows for signaling and upregulation of virulence factors. Perhaps one of the best described virulence factors is lipopolysaccharide (LPS), also known as endotoxin, a component of the outer cell wall of all gram-negative bacteria. The presence of LPS provokes local and systemic inflammation, including proliferation of cytokines and activation of macrophages. The presence of LPS is essential to maintaining the integrity of the outer membrane of gram-negative bacteria, acting as a protective barrier against lysozymes, antimicrobial agents, and host phagocytic cells.

Characteristics of the Host

The human body is equipped with a variety of defense mechanisms against microorganisms. These include physical barriers such as the skin and mucosal surfaces, the innate immune response, and the adaptive immune response. Dysfunction of any of these components can lead to the development of sepsis. The recognition of pathogens by the innate immune response initiates a complex cascade of events with the intent of removing the pathogen from the host. This includes the release of reactive oxygen metabolites to destroy the pathogen, release of chemokines to recruit additional lymphocytes, and the generation of a variety of systemic cytokines to further activate the host immune response. We are just beginning to understand the potential impact of genetic polymorphisms and the impact on patient survival [65, 66].

Effect of Sepsis on Coagulation

Proper function of the coagulation system is of critical importance, particularly in the surgical patient as it plays an essential role in hemostasis. Extensive laboratory research has advanced our understanding of the relationship between inflammation and coagulation. In the septic patient, dysregulation of the coagulation system can result in derangements in laboratory tests of coagulation, increased bleeding risk, and DIC. A basic understanding of this relationship is important to understanding the pathophysiology of sepsis.

A key factor in the interaction between coagulation and inflammation is tissue factor (TF) expression. Under normal circumstances TF is found only on adventitial structures, myocytes, and fibroblasts. When tissue injury occurs, these subendothelial structures that express TF are exposed and the clotting cascade is initiated by TF binding with circulating factor VII. In a septic state, proinflammatory mediators induce the expression of TF on the endothelium. The expression of TF by the endothelium not only activates the coagulation cascade, but is a potent stimulus for excess thrombin generation. Thrombin is a procoagulant molecule that converts fibrinogen to fibrin and promotes platelet activation. The formation of fibrin is followed by consumption of clotting factors and the formation of fibrin clots in the microcirculation. These fibrin clots serve as filters, trapping platelets to form larger clots. All of these actions combined, shift the coagulation system into a procoagulant state. Additionally, there is a loss of anticoagulant factors such as thrombomodulin.

Proinflammatory cytokines downregulate the production of thrombomodulin on the surface of the endothelial cells. Thrombomodulin is an essential cofactor in the conversion of protein C into activated protein C. Clinically, this imbalance in the coagulation system is reflected as tissue hypoxia secondary to microvascular thrombosis. This disruption in the coagulation system and the resulting microvascular thrombosis has been the target of potential pharmacologic interventions.

Sepsis Screening: Increasing Awareness and Improving Outcomes

The early identification and management of sepsis remains a significant challenge to healthcare providers. In the recent past, multiple organizations have focused their efforts on providing evidence based guidelines in an attempt to decrease the morbidity and mortality associated with sepsis. Several recent studies in the literature have highlighted the correlation between early sepsis intervention and patient survival. The use of EGDT therapy as described by Rivers et al. has emphasized the importance of early intervention during the "golden hours" of sepsis [23]. A recently published study by Kumar et al. demonstrated a significant correlation between time to appropriate antimicrobial administration and patient survival [45]. In this study of 2,154 patients with septic shock, administration of effective antimicrobial therapy within the first hour of document hypotension was associated with a survival rate of 79.9%. Each hour of delay in administration of effective antimicrobial therapy was associated with an average decrease in survival of 7.6%.

Despite strong evidence that the early implementation of evidence based, sepsis specific interventions save lives, the early identification of sepsis remains a challenge. The signs and symptoms of sepsis are nonspecific, particularly in its early phases. As bedside nurses and other health care providers focus on multiple priorities and tasks, early signs of sepsis are often missed resulting in the delay of time critical interventions. Lack of awareness of the signs and symptoms of impending sepsis may contribute to the severity of the problem. In the surgical patient, the early signs of sepsis can often be attributed to other common postoperative problems. A recent audit of ward nurses' knowledge of sepsis demonstrated lack of awareness of the standard definitions of sepsis, severe sepsis and septic shock, the significance of increased blood lactate concentration as an indicator of severe sepsis, and the basic principles of early goal directed therapy [67]. The conclusion of this audit was that these deficits could result in the missed or delayed diagnosis of severe sepsis or septic shock, and seriously delayed therapy. This lack of awareness seems universal, as physicians too struggle with the early identification and evidence based management of sepsis. A recent international survey of physicians regarding their knowledge regarding sepsis reported that 83% of physicians surveyed had missed the diagnosis of sepsis [68]. The reasons listed for missing the diagnosis of sepsis included lack of monitoring, lack of a common definition for sepsis, and lack of knowledge. Of the 1,058 physicians surveyed, only 140 (13.2%) were able to provide the definition of sepsis as stated in the ACCP/SCCM consensus statement.

Our experience with the sepsis screening tool in the SICU has prompted us to expand our evaluation of sepsis in general surgery patients within our own institution. We conducted a quality improvement review of patients admitted to our SICU over a 5 month period with an admitting diagnosis of sepsis, severe sepsis, or septic shock. Of the 55 patients with these diagnoses, 26 (47%) were admitted to the SICU from an inpatient surgical ward. Of these, 26 patients admitted from the surgical ward, 15 (58%) presented to the SICU with severe sepsis or septic shock. Out of the 15 patients who presented to the SICU in severe sepsis/septic shock, 6 died (40%). There were no deaths among the 11 patients that presented with sepsis. For each of these 26 patients, the first step of our sepsis screening tool was performed in a retrospective fashion. Of the 26 patients, 20 (77%) had a positive retrospective SIRS screen (SIRS Score ≥4). On average, the screen became positive 25 h before the diagnosis of sepsis was made (range 30 min to 114.75 h, standard deviation 35.8, interquartile range 33.75). The Surviving Sepsis Campaign Guidelines place great emphasis on the speed with which sepsis specific interventions are initiated secondary to the impact this has on sepsis related mortality. This is supported by our data. The average delay of 25 h between the initial recognition of sepsis using this screening tool and the initiation of appropriate therapy is well beyond the recommended time for intervention. These findings would indicate that the use of this nurse initiated sepsis screening tool could significantly improve sepsis recognition and subsequent initiation of therapy on the inpatient surgical floor.

We subsequently implemented and validated our sepsis screening tool on the inpatient surgical ward [14]. The screening tool yielded a sensitivity of 99.9%, specificity of 91.3%, a positive predictive value of 16.3%, and a negative predictive value of 99.9%. The sepsis related mortality in those patients that screened positive for sepsis was 6.3%. Of the 16 patients that developed sepsis, 4 (25%) required transfer to the SICU. Of the 16 true positive screens, 14 (87.5%) had sepsis, and 2 (12.5%) had severe sepsis at the time of the screen. These results underscore the importance of sepsis screening in order to identify sepsis before the patient progresses into septic shock.

Implementing Evidence Based Guidelines: The Use of Computerized Clinical Decision Support

In the recent past, multiple organizations have focused on providing evidence based guidelines (EBGs) in an attempt to decrease the sepsis associated morbidity and mortality [69–71]. These EBGs provide a comprehensive list of therapies and include several time sensitive interventions. Despite strong evidence that the early implementation of evidence based, sepsis specific therapies saves lives, the complexity of these recommendations makes bedside implementation difficult and compliance poor. A recent study by McGlyn et al. which evaluated compliance with implementation of evidence based care in a variety of acute and chronic health conditions found that only 55% of patients currently receive appropriate evidence based care [72]. This failure of health care providers to consistently implement evidence based care is multifactorial. Busy clinicians struggle to keep up with the information overload that has resulted from the recent explosion in health care related guidelines. As a result, it often takes 15–20 years for a newly proven therapy to become standard of care [73]. Additionally, guidelines are often difficult to implement at the local level because they are not patient specific and rarely provide explicit directions for use at the bedside. These factors result in a significant hurdle that clinicians must overcome in order to provide current, evidence based care.

In the case of EBGs for sepsis management, the number and complexity of the recommendations makes it difficult to consistently implement these interventions. In addition, many of the interventions are time sensitive and require prioritization. Patients with an intra-abdominal source of surgical sepsis are at particularly high risk due to severity of illness and treatment complexity. These patients often require emergent operation for source control, with damage control techniques employed for the most severely ill. Integration of surgical intervention with ICU resuscitation introduces even more variables in sepsis management paradigm. This necessitates a system which ensures adequate and timely resuscitation, adherent to EBGs for sepsis.

Our previous experience with computerized clinical decision support (CCDS) has proven valuable in implementing other complex EBGs for critically ill patients [74]. A computer-based algorithm has the ability to accurately and precisely manage clinical interventions, frequently more consistent than the bedside clinician. Prior studies evaluating the use of CCDS in implementing EBGs for ARDS management and hemorrhagic shock resuscitation have demonstrated that the utilization of CCDS improves compliance with EBGs at the bedside [75–78]. Based upon this experience we developed a CCDS protocol for the management of sepsis. This bedside CCDS program includes an algorithm for goal-directed volume resuscitation, with subsequent real-time prompts for specific therapies such as antimicrobials, vasopressors, and further modalities within the initial 24 h after sepsis identification (Fig. 6.2). Acknowledgement of administered therapies allows the computer logic to proceed to the next step, ensuring compliance with all aspects of the EBGs.

Implementation of CCDS for the management of sepsis has significantly improved our ability to consistently implement EBGs in our SICU. Since implementing our CCDS sepsis management protocol we have increased our compliance with all components of the 6 h resuscitation bundle has increased from 29 to 79%. In addition, our overall severe sepsis/septic shock mortality has declined from 24 to 12%. We attribute this significant decrease in sepsis related mortality to increased compliance with the EBGs, a finding which is consistent with other reports in the literature [17, 23, 45, 79, 80].

Fluid Resuscitation: Crystalloid Versus Colloid

Since the early 1940s, the restoration of intravascular volume has been embraced as a pivotal intervention in shock resuscitation. Considerable controversy has persisted since this time concerning the optimal resuscitation fluid to use, largely due to conflicted evidence within the literature. No large randomized trials addressing the issue exist, however, a number of meta-analyses have been performed. One large meta-analysis of 1,419 patients by the Cochrane Injuries Group Albumin Reviewers revealed an increased risk of death in those patients resuscitated with albumin as compared to those resuscitated with crystalloid [81]. Another large meta-analysis of by Wilkes et al. revealed no difference in mortality between patients resuscitated with albumin as compared to those resuscitated with crystalloid [82].

The SAFE trial was a large, multicenter, randomized controlled trial that compared the effect of colloid as compared to crystalloid fluid resuscitation on mortality in patients admitted to the ICU [24]. The results of the study revealed similar outcomes for patients in both groups, suggesting there is no advantage to the use of either resuscitation fluid. A subgroup analysis of patients with severe sepsis showed a slight improvement in survival among patients that received albumin but this difference was not statistically significant as this study was not specifically designed to evaluate patients with sepsis.

There are several essential differences between crystalloid (lactated ringers, normal saline) and colloid (albumin, hydroxyethyl starch, hypertonic saline) as resuscitation fluid. The volume of distribution of crystalloids is significantly larger than that of colloids. Because of this, the ratio of crystalloid to colloid infusion is approximately three to one. Proponents of crystalloid resuscitation cite improved expansion of the extracellular compartment, minimal risk of anaphylactoid reaction, replacement of volume loss with physiologically balanced solution, and decreased costs. Proponents of colloid resuscitation cite faster restoration of intravascular volume due to the decrease in volume required and reduced risk of interstitial edema secondary to the high oncotic pressure. If colloids are used for resuscitation, one must be particularly vigilant about monitoring cardiac filling pressures and avoiding fluid overload. Additionally, the expense and availability of albumin may be a factor dissuading use in some settings. The utilization of hydroxyethyl starch solutions is associated with alterations of the coagulation cascade and therefore great caution should be heeded in surgical patients. In addition, hydroxyethyl starch solutions have been associated with renal dysfunction and higher rates of acute renal failure in sepsis [83].

The Use of Steroids in Septic Shock

The administration of steroids in septic shock has been debated for decades. In the 1960s, high dose steroid replacement therapy was found to improve survival in animal models of septic shock. A clinical study by Bennet et al. found no benefit to the use of steroids in sepsis and the practice was largely abandoned. In the 1970s, high dose steroids were widely used for patients with septic shock. Schumer et al. demonstrated significant improvement in survival among patients that received high dose steroids. This practice continued into the 1980s, at which point new evidence emerged suggesting that high dose steroids were associated with an increased risk of death and a higher frequency of secondary infections. Because of these discrepancies in the medical literature regarding the use of steroids in sepsis there was no clear consensus at the time. The 1990s produced several meta-analyses evaluating the use of high dose steroids in septic shock. The conclusion of these studies was that high dose steroids provided no survival benefit and in fact they were associated with increased mortality. As a result of these studies the use of high dose steroids for patients with septic shock has been largely abandoned. However, the use of low dose steroids for the management of septic shock remains a topic of intense discussion.

The concept of relative adrenal insufficiency in septic shock has been the focus of several recent clinical studies. In order to better understand the debate, a basic understanding of the role of the adrenal glands is required. The adrenal gland produces several substances including sympathetic hormones and glucocorticoids, including cortisol. Cortisol has immunologic and anti-inflammatory effects including inhibition of many pro-inflammatory cytokines (IL-1, IL-2,

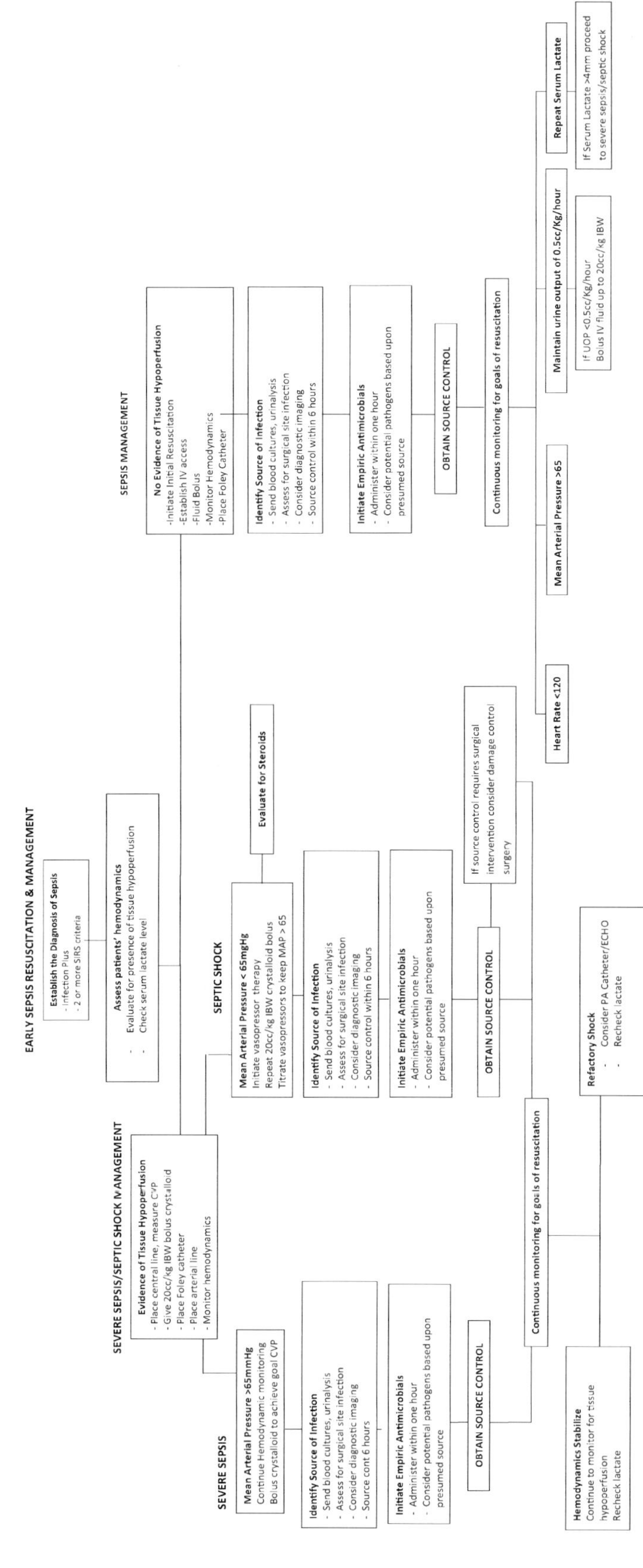

Fig. 6.2 Treatment algorithm for early sepsis resuscitation and management, severe sepsis/septic shock management, and severe sepsis

IL-3, IL-6, INF-γ[gamma], and TNF-α[alpha]). Cortisol also stimulates the production of anti-inflammatory mediators such as IL-10 and decreases the local inflammatory reaction. Cortisol plays a vital role in maintaining vascular tone and endothelial integrity. Additionally, cortisol augments the vasoconstrictor effect of catecholamines. During critical illness, the normal physiologic response stimulates the adrenal glands resulting in a nearly sixfold increase in cortisol production. During sepsis, the adrenal glands ability to increase cortisol production may be impaired. Multiple factors contribute to this including high levels of circulating inflammatory cytokines, decreased glucorticoid sensitivity of receptors, and suppression of the hypothalamic–pituitary–adrenal axis by various medications. The end result is a state of relative adrenal insufficiency.

Recently, numerous trials have been undertaken to evaluate the use of low dose steroids in sepsis. Low dose steroid use is defined as ≤300 mg of hydrocortisone (or an equivalent steroid) over long duration ≤5 days. In 2002, Annane published the results of a multicenter, randomized, double-blind, placebo-controlled trial evaluating the use of low dose steroids in patients with septic shock [39]. All patients with septic shock were randomized within 3 h of the onset of septic shock to either the treatment arm or the placebo arm. Patients underwent a low dose cosyntropin stimulation test and relative adrenal insufficiency was defined as a delta cortisol of ≤9 μg/dl or less. Patients in the treatment arm received hydrocortisone 50 mg IV every 6 h and 50 μg of fludrocortisone PO daily or matching placebos. Patients receiving low dose steroids showed a decreased time to shock reversal and a decreased mortality compared to placebo. Since that time, two smaller trials and two meta-analyses demonstrated similar results [84, 85]. These findings suggest that low dose steroid use in patients with relative adrenal insufficiency significantly improves time to shock reversal and 28-day mortality. However, a follow up study published in 2008 brought the use of low dose steroids in septic shock back into question. The CORTICUS trial was a multicenter, randomized, double-blind, placebo-controlled trial that also evaluated the use of low dose steroids in patients with septic shock [86]. Patients with septic shock underwent a low dose cosyntropin stimulation test with a delta cortisol of ≤9 μg/dl used to define relative adrenal insufficiency. Unlike the Annane study, patients in the CORTICUS trial were randomized up to 72 h after the diagnosis of septic shock to receive either hydrocortisone 50 mg IV every 6 h or placebo. No difference in 28-day all-cause mortality was identified, however earlier shock resolution was confirmed in the steroid group (median time to reverse shock 3.1 versus 5.7 days, $p=0.003$). However, it is important to note that the patients enrolled in this trial had a lower placebo group mortality (63% in Annane study; 31% in CORTICUS trial). The Annane study enrolled only patients with vasopressor-dependent septic shock, while the CORTICUS trial enrolled all patients with septic shock. In the Annane study, patients were randomized within 3 h of the onset of septic shock. In the CORTICUS trial, patients were randomized up to 72 h after the onset of septic shock. Additionally, patients in the Annane study received both hydrocortisone and fludrocortisones as opposed to only hydrocortisone in the CORTICUS trial. The CORTICUS trial patients differed as well, with more abdominal sepsis and more surgical patients, and fewer patients diagnosed with pneumonia. The CORTICUS trial documented that 46.7% of patients did not have a response to corticotropin-stimulation test, and these patients had a higher mortality rate. CORTICUS was however, underpowered for the primary outcome measure, death within 28 days in patients who did not respond to corticotropin. Therefore considerable controversy still remains. An important contribution of the CORTICUS trial was the identification that hospital-based immunoassays are not accurate for cortisol measurements in critically ill patients.

Despite the ongoing debate over the optimal use of low dose steroids in patients with septic shock, the Surviving Sepsis Campaign Guidelines still recommend consideration of hydrocortisone in patients with septic shock not responsive to volume resuscitation and vasopressor therapy. The dose of hyrdrocortisone given should not exceed 300 mg/day and should be administered in divided doses. The use of fludrocortisone is still considered optional. Optimal duration of steroids also remains in question, however most would agree that steroid administration should continue until the patient is weaned from vasopressor therapy.

Importance of Early Broad Spectrum Antimicrobials

The timely administration of empiric antimicrobial therapy is perhaps the most beneficial pharmacologic intervention in patients with sepsis. While antimicrobial therapy has always been a mainstay in the treatment of infection, not until recently has the importance of antimicrobial choice and rapid administration been demonstrated to significantly impact patient mortality. In a landmark study by Kumar et al. the relationship between time to antimicrobial administration and patient mortality was clearly illustrated [45]. This multicenter, retrospective study evaluated 2,154 patients with septic shock over a 15 year period. The primary objective was to determine the prevalence of delays in antimicrobial administration from initial onset of septic shock and its impact on mortality. The results of this study demonstrated a 7.6% decrease in survival for each hour of delay in antimicrobial administration after the onset of shock [45]. In addition, patients that received effective antimicrobial therapy within 1 h of the onset of septic shock had the highest survival rate at 79.9%. The results of this study have subsequently been corroborated by other studies [87, 88].

Despite convincing evidence that early antimicrobial administration significantly improves outcomes in patients with sepsis, compliance with this recommendation remains problematic. In Kumar's previously mentioned study, >50% of septic shock patients experienced a delay in antimicrobial administration of at least 6 h. A recent multicenter prospective analysis of compliance with antimicrobial administration revealed that only 60% of patients were receiving antimicrobials within 1 h [89]. After a 2 year educational campaign for performance improvement programs compliance only reached 67%. Clearly, there exist significant clinical hurdles that we must overcome in order to implement this seemingly straightforward intervention.

Several barriers to the timely administration of antimicrobials have been identified. One critical issue is the availability of intravenous access in a timely manner. During active sepsis resuscitation intravenous access is needed for fluid administration as well as antimicrobial therapy. In addition, appropriate cultures, typically from various sites, must be sent prior to antimicrobial administration. Many antimicrobials are not readily available in patient care areas and must be transported from the pharmacy to the bedside. Most patients receive at least two empiric antimicrobials, which can result in additional delays if adequate IV access is not available. Performing this multitude of tasks, particularly in an unstable septic shock patient can quickly overwhelm the clinical team. The end result is a significant delay in antimicrobial administration.

While each institution has their own specific barriers to implementation, it is important to recognize the importance of administering IV antimicrobials within 1 h. This one simple task of administering antimicrobial agents can significantly improve patient survival. In order to minimize the time to antimicrobial administration, there are a few basic clinical practices that can be implemented to help overcome these barriers. Rapidly establishing IV access is critical to the success of the initial resuscitation. If peripheral IV access is not easily attainable, central venous access should be secured promptly. Central venous access has the benefit of providing the clinical team with multiple infusion ports as well as a means of monitoring central venous pressure. Working in conjunction with pharmacy to establish a rapidly available, pre mixed supply of commonly administered antimicrobials will also help to minimize delays. Many institutions have developed a "sepsis toolbox" containing IV fluids, culture materials, blood tubes for measuring serum lactate, and a pre mixed supply of antimicrobials. This toolbox can be taken to the bedside of sepsis patient at any location in the hospital, avoiding potential delays in the initiation of resuscitation.

The choice of empiric antimicrobial therapy is equally as important as administering antimicrobials within 1 h.

Antimicrobial selection can be a complex process and should take into include consideration of the patient's history and comorbid conditions, recent antimicrobial exposure, and probable source of infection. With the recent emergence of several virulent, drug resistant pathogens, the length of the patient's hospital course and the potential for infection with such organisms should be considered. Failure to provide effective antimicrobial coverage for the causative organism significantly increases the risk of death from sepsis. The best practice is to provide broad coverage initially and de-escalate antimicrobial therapy based upon culture data as it becomes available.

Planned Laparotomy for Established Peritonitis Is Not Damage Control

The treatment strategy for patients with established peritonitis has been debated for three decades. After an initial emergent laparotomy, relaparotomy is frequently necessary to eliminate persistent peritonitis or a newly developed infectious focus. There are two widely used strategies for relaparotomy including relaparotomy when the patient's condition demands it ("on-demand") and "planned" relaparotomy. In the planned strategy, a relaparotomy is performed every 48 h for inspection, drainage, and peritoneal lavage of the abdominal cavity until findings are not suspicious for ongoing peritonitis. The "planned" strategy may lead to early detection of persistent peritonitis or a new infectious focus which reduces the risk for MOF but harbors the risk of potentially unnecessary reexplorations in critically ill patients. The on-demand strategy, while minimizing the number of surgical interventions, harbors the risk of a potentially harmful delay in the detection of intra-abdominal infection with increased risk for MOF. Additionally there is a risk that the need for a delayed laparotomy will occur at a time when intra-abdominal adhesions (day 10–14) create a hostile operative environment. Over the years, there have been number of case series that have offered conflicting results. The consensus and meta-analysis conclusion is that for the non-critically ill patient (APACHE II <10) use of the "on demand" strategy is preferred. Newer developments in CT scan technology can accurately detect intra-abdominal infections in patients who clinically deteriorate or fail to improve. With aggressive interventional radiology greater than 95% of the infections can be successfully treated without a repeat laparotomy. More recently, Ruler et al. have performed a prospective randomized controlled trial (PRCT) in patients with severe peritonitis (defined as APACHE II >10) which confirmed that the practice of "planned" relaparotomy was associated with no difference in outcome compared with "on demand" laparotomy and was associated with increased expenditure of hospital resources and length of hospital stay [90]. It is important to emphasize that this recent PRCT is not relevant to the previous discussion of "damage control" in patients with septic shock. Patients randomized into this PRCT had a mean APACHE II score of 15 (with predicted mortality of <25%) while the patients we described had a mean APACHE II score of 32 (with a predicted mortality of >75%). We use damage control in patients in the "persistent septic shock cycle," who require an expedient procedure to attain source control, and continued resuscitation prior to the definitive procedure. Its rationale is to appropriately time and limit the duration of source control to break the cycle and then optimize resuscitation in the ICU. Planned and on demand laparotomy are considered in the case of patients requiring surgical source control, who are not exhibiting severe metabolic derangements.

Conclusion

Sepsis continues to be a common and potentially lethal problem for surgical patients. The early identification and management of surgical patients with sepsis presents a significant challenge to the surgical team. The implementation of rapid, evidence based care in conjunction with timely surgical source control improves survival.

References

1. Dombrovskiy VY, Martin AA, Sunderram J, Paz HL. Rapid increase in hospitalization and mortality rates for severe sepsis in the United States: a trend analysis from 1993 to 2003. Crit Care Med. 2007;35(5):1244–50.
2. Hall MJ, Williams SN, Defrances CJ, Golosinskiy A. Inpatient care for septicemia or sepsis: a challenge for patients and hospitals. NCHS Data Brief. 2011;62:1–8.
3. Lagu T, Rothberg MB, Shieh M-S, et al. Hospitalizations, costs, and outcomes of severe sepsis in the United States 2003 to 2007. Crit Care Med. 2012;40(3):754–61. Available at http://www.ncbi.nlm.nih.gov/pubmed/21963582. Accessed 5 Jan 2012.
4. Dombrovskiy VY, Martin AA, Sunderram J, Paz HL. Facing the challenge: decreasing case fatality rates in severe sepsis despite increasing hospitalizations. Crit Care Med. 2005;33(11):2555–62.
5. Angus DC, Linde-Zwirble WT, Lidicker J, et al. Epidemiology of severe sepsis in the United States: analysis of incidence, outcome, and associated costs of care. Crit Care Med. 2001;29(7):1303–10.
6. Martin GS, Mannino DM, Eaton S, Moss M. The epidemiology of sepsis in the United States from 1979 through 2000. N Engl J Med. 2003;348(16):1546–54.
7. McBean M, Rajamani S. Increasing rates of hospitalization due to septicemia in the US elderly population, 1986–1997. J Infect Dis. 2001;183(4):596–603.
8. Moore LJ, Moore FA, Todd SR, et al. Sepsis in general surgery: the 2005–2007 National Surgical Quality Improvement Program Perspective. Arch Surg (Chicago, Ill: 1960). 2010;145(7):695–700.
9. Moore LJ, Moore FA, Jones SL, Xu J, Bass BL. Sepsis in general surgery: a deadly complication. Am J Surg. 2009;198(6):868–74.
10. Balk RA, Bone RC. The septic syndrome. Definition and clinical implications. Crit Care Clin. 1989;5(1):1–8.
11. Anon. American College of Chest Physicians/Society of Critical Care Medicine Consensus Conference: definitions for sepsis and organ failure and guidelines for the use of innovative therapies in sepsis. Crit Care Med. 1992;20(6):864–74.
12. Levy MM, Fink MP, Marshall JC, et al. 2001 SCCM/ESICM/ACCP/ATS/SIS International Sepsis Definitions Conference. Intensive Care Med. 2003;29(4):530–8.
13. Moore LJ, Jones SL, Kreiner LA, et al. Validation of a screening tool for the early identification of sepsis. J Trauma. 2009;66(6):1539–46. discussion 1546–7.
14. Moore LJ, Jones SL, Turner KL, et al. A concise instrument for sepsis screening in general surgery patients. Surg Infect. 2010;11(2):215.
15. Sebat F, Johnson D, Musthafa AA, et al. A multidisciplinary community hospital program for early and rapid resuscitation of shock in nontrauma patients. Chest. 2005;127(5):1729–43.
16. Shorr AF, Micek ST, Jackson WL, Kollef MH. Economic implications of an evidence-based sepsis protocol: can we improve outcomes and lower costs? Crit Care Med. 2007;35(5):1257–62.
17. Nguyen HB, Corbett SW, Steele R, et al. Implementation of a bundle of quality indicators for the early management of severe sepsis and septic shock is associated with decreased mortality. Crit Care Med. 2007;35(4):1105–12.
18. Shapiro NI, Howell MD, Talmor D, et al. Implementation and outcomes of the Multiple Urgent Sepsis Therapies (MUST) protocol. Crit Care Med. 2006;34(4):1025–32.
19. Micek ST, Roubinian N, Heuring T, et al. Before-after study of a standardized hospital order set for the management of septic shock. Crit Care Med. 2006;34(11):2707–13.
20. Moore LJ, Turner KL, Todd SR, et al. Computerized clinical decision support improves survival in intra abdominal surgical sepsis. Am J Surg. 2010;200(6):839–43.
21. Bendjelid K, Romand J-A. Fluid responsiveness in mechanically ventilated patients: a review of indices used in intensive care. Intensive Care Med. 2003;29(3):352–60.
22. Varpula M, Tallgren M, Saukkonen K, Voipio-Pulkki L-M, Pettilä V. Hemodynamic variables related to outcome in septic shock. Intensive Care Med. 2005;31(8):1066–71.
23. Rivers E, Nguyen B, Havstad S, et al. Early goal-directed therapy in the treatment of severe sepsis and septic shock. N Engl J Med. 2001;345(19):1368–77.
24. Finfer S, Bellomo R, Boyce N, et al. A comparison of albumin and saline for fluid resuscitation in the intensive care unit. N Engl J Med. 2004;350(22):2247–56.
25. Anon. Volume replacement with albumin in severe sepsis (ALBIOS). NCT00707122. Available at http://www.clinicaltrials.gov/ct2/show/NCT00707122?term=albumin+sepsis&rank=1.
26. Anon. Early albumin resuscitation during septic shock. NCT00327704. Available at http://www.clinicaltrials.gov/ct2/show/NCT00327704?term=albumin+sepsis&rank=10.
27. Kortgen A, Niederprüm P, Bauer M. Implementation of an evidence-based "standard operating procedure" and outcome in septic shock. Crit Care Med. 2006;34(4):943–9.
28. Trzeciak S, Dellinger RP, Abate NL, et al. Translating research to clinical practice: a 1-year experience with implementing early goal-directed therapy for septic shock in the emergency department. Chest. 2006;129(2):225–32.
29. Anon. ProCESS. Available at https://crisma.upmc.com/process-trial/index.asp; http://clinicaltrials.gov/ct2/show/NCT00510835.
30. Anon. ARISE trial. Available at http://www.anzicrc.monash.org/process.html; http://clinicaltrials.gov/ct2/show/NCT00975793.
31. Anon. ProMISe trial. Available at http://www.icnarc.org; https://www.icnarc.org/documents/ProMISe%20Information%20Sheet.pdf.
32. Landry DW, Levin HR, Gallant EM, et al. Vasopressin deficiency contributes to the vasodilation of septic shock. Circulation. 1997;95(5):1122–5.

33. Russell JA. Vasopressin in vasodilatory and septic shock. Curr Opin Crit Care. 2007;13(4):383–91.

34. Russell JA, Walley KR, Singer J, et al. Vasopressin versus norepinephrine infusion in patients with septic shock. N Engl J Med. 2008;358(9):877–87.

35. Russell JA, Walley KR, Gordon AC, et al. Interaction of vasopressin infusion, corticosteroid treatment, and mortality of septic shock. Crit Care Med. 2009;37(3):811–8.

36. Holmes CL, Walley KR, Chittock DR, Lehman T, Russell JA. The effects of vasopressin on hemodynamics and renal function in severe septic shock: a case series. Intensive Care Med. 2001;27(8):1416–21.

37. Oppert M, Schindler R, Husung C, et al. Low-dose hydrocortisone improves shock reversal and reduces cytokine levels in early hyperdynamic septic shock. Crit Care Med. 2005;33(11):2457–64.

38. Keh D, Boehnke T, Weber-Cartens S, et al. Immunologic and hemodynamic effects of "low-dose" hydrocortisone in septic shock: a double-blind, randomized, placebo-controlled, crossover study. Am J Respir Crit Care Med. 2003;167(4):512–20.

39. Annane D, Sébille V, Charpentier C, et al. Effect of treatment with low doses of hydrocortisone and fludrocortisone on mortality in patients with septic shock. JAMA. 2002;288(7):862–71.

40. Arpi M, Bentzon MW, Jensen J, Frederiksen W. Importance of blood volume cultured in the detection of bacteremia. Eur J Clin Microbiol Infect Dis. 1989;8(9):838–42.

41. Mermel LA, Maki DG. Detection of bacteremia in adults: consequences of culturing an inadequate volume of blood. Ann Intern Med. 1993;119(4):270–2.

42. Bouza E, Sousa D, Rodríguez-Créixems M, Lechuz JG, Muñoz P. Is the volume of blood cultured still a significant factor in the diagnosis of bloodstream infections? J Clin Microbiol. 2007;45(9):2765–9.

43. Blot F, Schmidt E, Nitenberg G, et al. Earlier positivity of central-venous- versus peripheral-blood cultures is highly predictive of catheter-related sepsis. J Clin Microbiol. 1998;36(1):105–9.

44. Blot F, Nitenberg G, Chachaty E, et al. Diagnosis of catheter-related bacteraemia: a prospective comparison of the time to positivity of hub-blood versus peripheral-blood cultures. Lancet. 1999;354(9184):1071–7.

45. Kumar A, Roberts D, Wood KE, et al. Duration of hypotension before initiation of effective antimicrobial therapy is the critical determinant of survival in human septic shock. Crit Care Med. 2006;34(6):1589–96.

46. Morrell M, Fraser VJ, Kollef MH. Delaying the empiric treatment of candida bloodstream infection until positive blood culture results are obtained: a potential risk factor for hospital mortality. Antimicrob Agents Chemother. 2005;49(9):3640–5.

47. Kreger BE, Craven DE, McCabe WR. Gram-negative bacteremia. IV. Re-evaluation of clinical features and treatment in 612 patients. Am J Med. 1980;68(3):344–55.

48. Ibrahim EH, Sherman G, Ward S, Fraser VJ, Kollef MH. The influence of inadequate antimicrobial treatment of bloodstream infections on patient outcomes in the ICU setting. Chest. 2000;118(1):146–55.

49. Leibovici L, Shraga I, Drucker M, et al. The benefit of appropriate empirical antibiotic treatment in patients with bloodstream infection. J Intern Med. 1998;244(5):379–86.

50. Fitousis K, Moore LJ, Turner KL, et al. Evaluation of emperic antibiotic use in surgical sepsis. Am J Surg. 2010;200(6):776–82.

51. Cué JI, Cryer HG, Miller FB, Richardson JD, Polk HC. Packing and planned reexploration for hepatic and retroperitoneal hemorrhage: critical refinements of a useful technique. J Trauma. 1990;30(8):1007–11. discussion 1011–3.

52. Rotondo MF, Schwab CW, McGonigal MD, et al. "Damage control": an approach for improved survival in exsanguinating penetrating abdominal injury. J Trauma. 1993;35(3):375–82. discussion 382–3.

53. Burch JM, Ortiz VB, Richardson RJ, et al. Abbreviated laparotomy and planned reoperation for critically injured patients. Ann Surg. 1992;215(5):476–83. discussion 483–4.

54. de Moya MA, Dunham M, Inaba K, et al. Long-term outcome of acellular dermal matrix when used for large traumatic open abdomen. J Trauma. 2008;65(2):349–53.

55. Garner GB, Ware DN, Cocanour CS, et al. Vacuum-assisted wound closure provides early fascial reapproximation in trauma patients with open abdomens. Am J Surg. 2001;182(6):630–8.

56. Suliburk JW, Ware DN, Balogh Z, et al. Vacuum-assisted wound closure achieves early fascial closure of open abdomens after severe trauma. J Trauma. 2003;55(6):1155–60. discussion 1160–1.

57. Miller PR, Thompson JT, Faler BJ, Meredith JW, Chang MC. Late fascial closure in lieu of ventral hernia: the next step in open abdomen management. J Trauma. 2002;53(5):843–9.

58. Cothren CC, Moore EE, Johnson JL, Moore JB, Burch JM. One hundred percent fascial approximation with sequential abdominal closure of the open abdomen. Am J Surg. 2006;192(2):238–42.

59. Balogh Z, McKinley BA, Cox Jr CS, et al. Abdominal compartment syndrome: the cause or effect of postinjury multiple organ failure. Shock. 2003;20(6):483–92.

60. Cothren CC, Moore EE, Johnson JL, Moore JB. Outcomes in surgical versus medical patients with the secondary abdominal compartment syndrome. Am J Surg. 2007;194(6):804–7. discussion 807–8.

61. McNelis J, Marini CP, Jurkiewicz A, et al. Predictive factors associated with the development of abdominal compartment syndrome in the surgical intensive care unit. Arch Surg. 2002;137(2):133–6.

62. Malbrain ML, Chiumello D, Pelosi P, et al. Incidence and prognosis of intraabdominal hypertension in a mixed population of critically ill patients: a multiple-center epidemiological study. Crit Care Med. 2005;33(2):315–22.

63. Turner KL, Moore LJ, Sucher JF, et al. *Damage Control Laparotomy: Beyond Trauma* - Presented at the 68th Annual Meeting of the American Association for the Surgery of Trauma; Pittsburg, PA October 1–3, 2009.

64. Abbas AK, Lichtman AH. Cellular and molecular immunology. 5th ed. Philadelphia, PA: Elsevier Saunders; 2005.

65. Arcaroli J, Fessler MB, Abraham E. Genetic polymorphisms and sepsis. Shock. 2005;24(4):300–12.

66. Namath A, Patterson AJ. Genetic polymorphisms in sepsis. Crit Care Clin. 2009;25(4):835–56. x.

67. Robson W, Beavis S, Spittle N. An audit of ward nurses' knowledge of sepsis. Nurs Crit Care. 2007;12(2):86–92.

68. Poeze M, Ramsay G, Gerlach H, Rubulotta F, Levy M. An international sepsis survey: a study of doctors' knowledge and perception about sepsis. Crit Care. 2004;8(6):R409–13.

69. Dellinger RP, Carlet JM, Masur H, et al. Surviving Sepsis Campaign guidelines for management of severe sepsis and septic shock. Crit Care Med. 2004;32(3):858–73.

70. Dellinger RP, Levy MM, Carlet JM, et al. Surviving Sepsis Campaign: international guidelines for management of severe sepsis and septic shock: 2008. Crit Care Med. 2008;36(1):296–327.

71. Hollenberg SM, Ahrens TS, Annane D, et al. Practice parameters for hemodynamic support of sepsis in adult patients: 2004 update. Crit Care Med. 2004;32(9):1928–48.

72. McGlynn EA, Asch SM, Adams J, et al. The quality of health care delivered to adults in the United States. N Engl J Med. 2003;348(26):2635–45.

73. Institute of Medicine. Crossing the quality chasm: a new health system for the 21st century. Washington, DC: National Academies Press; 2001.

74. Sucher JF, Moore FA, Todd SR, Sailors RM, McKinley BA. Computerized clinical decision support: a technology to implement and validate evidence based guidelines. J Trauma. 2008;64(2):520–37.

75. McKinley BA, Moore FA, Sailors RM, et al. Computerized decision support for mechanical ventilation of trauma induced

ARDS: results of a randomized clinical trial. J Trauma. 2001;50(3):415–24. discussion 425.

76. Moore FA, McKinley BA, Moore EE. The next generation in shock resuscitation. Lancet. 2004;363(9425):1988–96.

77. Santora RJ, McKinley BA, Moore FA. Computerized clinical decision support for traumatic shock resuscitation. Curr Opin Crit Care. 2008;14(6):679–84.

78. Thomsen GE, Pope D, East TD, et al. Clinical performance of a rule-based decision support system for mechanical ventilation of ARDS patients. Proc Annu Symp Comput Appl Med Care. 1993; 339–43.

79. Gao F, Melody T, Daniels DF, Giles S, Fox S. The impact of compliance with 6-hour and 24-hour sepsis bundles on hospital mortality in patients with severe sepsis: a prospective observational study. Crit Care. 2005;9(6):R764–70.

80. Levy MM, Dellinger RP, Townsend SR, et al. The Surviving Sepsis Campaign: results of an international guideline-based performance improvement program targeting severe sepsis. Intensive Care Med. 2010;36(2):222–31.

81. Anon. Human albumin administration in critically ill patients: systematic review of randomised controlled trials. Cochrane Injuries Group Albumin Reviewers. BMJ. 1998;317(7153):235–40.

82. Wilkes MM, Navickis RJ. Patient survival after human albumin administration. A meta-analysis of randomized, controlled trials. Ann Intern Med. 2001;135(3):149–64.

83. Brunkhorst FM, Engel C, Bloos F, et al. Intensive insulin therapy and pentastarch resuscitation in severe sepsis. N Engl J Med. 2008;358(2):125–39.

84. Annane D, Bellissant E, Bollaert PE, et al. Corticosteroids for severe sepsis and septic shock: a systematic review and meta-analysis. BMJ. 2004;329(7464):480.

85. Minneci PC, Deans KJ, Banks SM, Eichacker PQ, Natanson C. Meta-analysis: the effect of steroids on survival and shock during sepsis depends on the dose. Ann Intern Med. 2004;141(1):47–56.

86. Sprung CL, Annane D, Keh D, et al. Hydrocortisone therapy for patients with septic shock. N Engl J Med. 2008;358(2):111–24.

87. Gaieski DF, Mikkelsen ME, Band RA, et al. Impact of time to antibiotics on survival in patients with severe sepsis or septic shock in whom early goal-directed therapy was initiated in the emergency department. Crit Care Med. 2010;38(4):1045–53.

88. Kumar A, Ellis P, Arabi Y, et al. Initiation of inappropriate antimicrobial therapy results in a fivefold reduction of survival in human septic shock. Chest. 2009;136(5):1237–48.

89. Levy MM, Dellinger RP, Townsend SR, et al. The Surviving Sepsis Campaign: results of an international guideline-based performance improvement program targeting severe sepsis. Crit Care Med. 2010;38(2):367–74.

90. van Ruler O, Mahler CW, Boer KR, et al. Comparison of on-demand vs. planned relaparotomy strategy in patients with severe peritonitis: a randomized trial. JAMA. 2007;298(8):865–72.

Stephanie Gordy and Martin A. Schreiber

Introduction

While traumatic brain injury and uncontrolled hemorrhage remain the leading causes of death after trauma, sepsis followed by multiple organ failure (MOF) are leading contributors to mortality in critically ill surgical and trauma patients. MOF is the leading cause of morbidity in the intensive care unit (ICU) following trauma and represents the endpoint of the spectrum of SIRS and sepsis [1]. Despite the identification of this disease process in the early 1970s, our understanding of the pathophysiology and the ensuing treatment of this syndrome remains a perplexing entity to which entire books have been dedicated. This chapter provides a brief overview of the evolution of the disease, the clinical presentation, and discusses the epidemiology and salient pathophysiology, as well as current treatment options and future considerations of this disease.

Historical Perspective

Military conflicts have historically been the impetus for knowledge advancement in the arena of care of the critically injured patient. The evolution of the medical communities' knowledge of morbidity and mortality from a single organ injury to MOF is an example of such a process. In World War I, death of the injured was primarily due to hemorrhagic shock and infections. During World War II (WWII) the lessons learned from prior conflicts, including control of hemorrhagic shock and expeditious evacuation to a surgical treatment facility, greatly reduced the immediate death rate

S. Gordy, M.D., F.A.C.S. (✉)
Department of Trauma, Acute Care Surgery and Surgical
Critical Care, Oregon Health and Science University,
3181 SW Sam Jackson Park Road, L-611, Portland, OR 97239, USA
e-mail: gordys@ohsu.edu

M.A. Schreiber, M.D., F.A.C.S.
Professor of Surgery, Chief of Trauma Surgery, Oregon Health and
Science University, USA

to half of what it had been for the US Army in early WWII [2–4]. Transfusions in WWII aided resuscitation in stabilizing hemodynamic parameters but delayed renal failure was a significant morbidity. In the Korean War, delayed deaths in resuscitated patients were most often as a result of acute renal failure [5]. The increased resuscitation with crystalloid improved the renal failure but resulted in acute lung injury. This emerging constellation of symptoms is now known as Acute Respiratory Distress Syndrome (ARDS) [6]. These serial improvements were beneficial in the understanding of resuscitation of severely injured patients. However, the survival of these patients revealed the damage that multiple end organs had sustained as manifested in a new syndrome now known as MOF. MOF is at the severe end of the severity of illness spectrum of both systemic inflammatory response syndrome (SIRS) and sepsis.

The term "multiple organ failure" (MOF), was used by Shoemaker in a 1973 editorial to describe the circulatory, respiratory, renal, cerebral and cardiac complications that ensued after the initial resuscitation of a trauma patient [7]. Around the same time, Tilney described a similar syndrome of sequential organ failure in 18 patients following surgical repair of their abdominal aortic aneurysms [8]. In 1975, Baue expanded on the organ systems affected and recognized that when more than one organ system failed, the knowledge and ability to care for the patient was stretched. Additionally, Baue offered suggestions (Table 7.1) to prevent further damage as well as potential therapeutic options which included prevention of respiratory failure, volume resuscitation, early vasopressor use, source control, and early nutrition. It is salient to point out that these principles are still very central to the treatment of this disease process. Currently, the terms multiple organ dysfunction syndrome (MODS) and MOF are often used interchangeably [9]. The nuances of the two words effectively describe the syndrome of organ impairment at the point where expeditious treatment might prevent overt organ failure (MODS) versus established coexisting MOF as described in numerous organ failure scores [10]. Effectively, MOF is the end of a continuum that ranges from SIRS to severe organ dysfunction.

L.J. Moore et al. (eds.), *Common Problems in Acute Care Surgery*,
DOI 10.1007/978-1-4614-6123-4_7, © Springer Science+Business Media New York 2013

Table 7.1 Goals to prevent MOF identified in 1975

Goals to prevent MOF
- Prevent ventilatory failure by early support, not allowing the lungs to fail and produce hypoxemia.
- Avoid fluid overload, maintaining a urine output of 25–50 ml/h and no more.
- Avoid excess sodium and sodium bicarbonate.
- Filter blood before transfusion.
- Insist on sighing and deep breathing during operation, during resuscitation, and afterward.
- Maintain adequate cardiac output by circulatory support using inotropic agents early such as isoproterenol, dopamine, and epinephrine.
- Empty the stomach, keep it empty and instill antacids after operation or injury.
- Continue controlled ventilation after operation if ventilatory problems are anticipated.
- Follow a sigh-suction-sit treatment program for ventilation.
- Prevent renal failure by maintaining renal blood flow and urine output.
- Use diuretics or dialysis early.
- Provide for early nutritional support of such patients.
- With tissue injury, use antibiotics before operation to reduce invasive sepsis.
- Drain septic foci and eliminate continuing peritoneal contamination.

Table 7.2 Definitions of SIRS, sepsis, severe sepsis, and multiple organ dysfunction

SIRS
- Two or more of the following conditions and can result from infectious or noninfectious causes:
- Temperature >38°C or <36°C
- Heart rate > than 90 beats per minute
- Respiratory rate > than 20 breaths per minute or $paCO_2$ < than 32 mmHg
- White blood cell count >12,000 or <4,000, or >10% bands

Sepsis
- SIRS in conjunction with an infection is termed sepsis

Severe sepsis
- Sepsis associated with organ dysfunction
- May include hypotension, elevated lactate, acute renal failure, liver failure, altered mental status, and/or hematologic abnormality

Septic shock
- Subset of severe sepsis with the addition of hypotension manifested by
- Systolic blood pressure (SBP) <90 mmHg
- Mean arterial pressure (MAP) <70 mmHg
- Decrease in systolic blood pressure (SBP) >40 mmHg from baseline

Multiple organ dysfunction (MODS)
- Presence of altered organ function in an acutely ill patient such that homeostasis cannot be maintained without intervention

Definitions

In the mid 1980s, after the recognition of sequential organ failure as a syndrome was recognized, multiple terms were used inconsistently by the medical community [11]. These disparate definitions attempting to describe the same physiologic phenomena led to the 1991 consensus conference. The societies of the American College of Chest Physicians (ACCP) and the Society of Critical Care Medicine (SCCM) were present. The goal of this conference was to establish a definition to describe what is now known as the spectrum of physiologic response to infection and/or inflammation. The term "systemic inflammatory response syndrome" (SIRS) was introduced at this conference. Additionally the terms sepsis, severe sepsis, septic shock and multiple organ dysfunction were defined as a result of this meeting (Table 7.2). The term "SIRS" was established to differentiate sepsis from a noninfectious, inflammatory state [12]. SIRS was defined as two or more of the following conditions:
- Core body temperature >38°C or <36°C
- Heart rate > than 90 beats per minute
- Respiratory rate > than 20 breaths per minute
- $paCO_2$ <32 mmHg
- White blood cell count >12,000 or <4,000, or >10% bands.

SIRS could represent the symptoms from an infectious or noninfectious source. Infection was described as the invasion of normally sterile tissue by organisms. The term "sepsis" was defined as SIRS in conjunction with a confirmed infection. "Severe sepsis" was defined as sepsis associated with organ dysfunction, hypotension or hypoperfusion as evidenced by: elevated lactate, acute renal failure, liver failure, altered mental status and/or hematalogic abnormalities. "Septic shock" was the term established as a subset of severe sepsis with the added additional clinical information of persistent hypotension, despite adequate fluid resuscitation. Hypotension was defined as systolic blood pressure (SBP) <90 mmHg, mean arterial pressure (MAP) <70 mmHg, or a decrease in SBP >40 mmHg from baseline.

MODS was defined as the presence of altered organ function in an acutely ill patient such that homeostasis cannot be maintained without intervention and is the culmination of septic shock and multiple end-organ failure [13]. The 2001 Consensus Conference further expanded on these definitions [14]. A problem similar to the disparate use of the word "sepsis" in the early 1980s remains a problem in regard to the definition of MOF. This is evidenced by a lack of consensus with regard to the innumerable scoring systems available to assess mortality.

Epidemiology

Sepsis, severe sepsis, septic shock, and MOF are commonplace in intensive care units and afflict 1.1 million people annually. Moreover, MOF results in 215,000 deaths in the

United States alone. Mortality from the spectrum of sepsis is estimated to be 9.3% of all deaths in the United States [15]. The individual costs of treating a single patient with MOF can be upwards of $150,000 per patient [16]. In the United States alone the costs of treating sepsis and its related sequelae is approximately $24 billion annually [17]. Additionally, the cost of critical care can account for as much as 1% of the gross national product of some countries. The resultant morbidity from this disease and consequent loss of wages and quality of life are difficult to quantify. These costs illustrate the substantial financial and societal burden this disease process inflicts. The irony of MOF is that it emerged as a result of improvements in critical care but that it has remained a substantial encumbrance in terms of morbidity, mortality, and cost despite numerous improvements made in critical care in regard to resuscitation and supportive measures.

The overall mortality ranges between 40 and 60% for MOF in all patients and this mortality increases as more organ systems are affected [18, 19]. The incidence of any organ failure in all ICUs ranges from 30 to 60% [20]. In a 1985 study of intensive care patients by Knaus, single organ failure occurred in approximately one-third of all patients at some point during their ICU stay and MOF occurred in 15% of these patients [21]. MOF following septic shock remains the leading contributor to mortality in ICU patients. In a study by Mayr that looked at causes of death in 3,700 ICU patients, the most common cause of death in a single ICU was MOF (47%) [20]. Specifically regarding trauma patients, traumatic brain injury and uncontrolled hemorrhage remain the leading causes of early death after trauma. MOF is, however, the number one cause of late deaths in trauma patients [22]. Despite our improved understanding of the pathophysiology of this disease, the use of antibiotic agents, and more innovative therapies, there continues to be a high mortality rate for MOF.

Regarding the demographics of sepsis and organ failure, a study by Martin et al. in 2003 elucidated some important differences. This study revealed that men are more likely to have sepsis and are more frequently enrolled in clinical trials despite the predominance of women in the population of the United States. Additionally, African-American men had the youngest age of onset in this study as well as the highest mortality. The reason for these demographic differences is not known; however, genetic differences and socioeconomic factors most likely contribute to these disparities [23]. Recently, research has confirmed a lower overall incidence of MOF [24]. The incidence of early single organ dysfunction has not changed but there has been a decrease in early MOF from 22 to 7%. The incidence of MOF in 1992 was 1.8 times the incidence in 2002 [25, 26]. A similar study of trauma patients by Durham also revealed a lower overall mortality for single organ failure as well as a decrease in the overall incidence of MOF [27].

Risk Factors for the Development of Organ Failure

MOF resides at the most severe end of a spectrum of illness that includes SIRS, sepsis, severe sepsis and septic shock. Any point along this constellation of criteria puts the patient at risk for MOF. The risks of organ failure are multiple and due to lack of consensus regarding a scoring system, it is difficult to ascertain which risk factors are most specific. MOF was originally thought to be catalyzed by an infectious process. While the majority of patients with MOF will have an infectious source, it is also known that MOF occurs without an infection, per se, and can be solely due to unregulated inflammation, as occurs with severe pancreatitis, trauma or burns [28]. Immunosuppression, pneumonia, blood transfusions and bacteremia are all associated with increased risk for developing sepsis, severe sepsis, or septic shock and therefore also increases a patient's risk for MOF [29, 30].

A demographic risk factor for MOF includes advanced age. Advanced age, defined as greater than 65, has likewise been associated with worse quality of life indicators in survivors of sepsis. These patients more often require extensive rehabilitation as well as skilled nursing facility admission upon their hospital discharge from their acute septic event [31]. In a multivariate analysis, adjusted for age, sex, and severe head injury, patients with MOF had four times greater odds of requiring assistance from others in activities of daily living more than 2 years after trauma as compared to trauma patients without organ failure. There was no statistically significant difference regarding self-care between patients who did not have a history of organ failure when compared with those patients who had a history of a single organ failure [32]. Obese patients, in general, have been found to have higher post-traumatic morbidity and mortality. Obesity is defined as body mass index (BMI) >30 kg/m and as the BMI goes up, the incidence of MOF increases as well [33]. Moreover, when age, injury severity score (ISS), and transfusions are adjusted for, obesity is associated with an 80% increased risk of MOF [22, 34]. This is likely associated to the pro-inflammatory state that obesity confers to patients [35]. Additionally, patients with nonoperative diagnoses—for example, patients admitted postacute myocardial infarction—have also been found to have a higher likelihood of developing MOF [21].

In trauma patients, Balk and colleagues aptly identified several major risk factors for the development of postinjury MOF. These included prolonged periods of hypotension, trauma, bowel infarction, hepatic insufficiency, advanced age, and alcohol abuse [36]. Additionally, ISS, number of units of packed red blood cells transfused, base deficit, and lactate levels are all associated with an increased risk of developing MOF [37, 38]

Table 7.3 MOF risk factors

Risk factors for MOF
- Hypotension
- Trauma
- Ischemic bowel
- Pancreatitis
- Advanced age >65
- Shock
- Infection
- Obesity
- Alcohol abuse
- Transfusion of blood products
- Injury severity score ISS >25
- Immunosuppression
- Base deficit >8
- Genetic factors
- Lactate >2.5

(Table 7.3). Blood transfusions have independently been shown to be predictors of SIRS, MODS and mortality [39]. Furthermore, Durham et al. also validated that total blood products infused in the first 24 h after injury in addition to higher Acute Physiology and Chronic Health Evaluation (APACHE) III scores, amplified the risk for MOF occurrence [27].

Genetic factors also play a role in determining the severity and progression of organ failure. Genetic variants, particularly single-nucleotide polymorphisms (SNPs), are critical determinants for individual differences in both inflammatory responses as well as clinical outcomes in trauma patients [40]. Individuals who possess specific genetic polymorphisms in genes controlling the synthesis of cytokines or toll like receptors (TLR) may be predisposed to excessive inflammatory response to sepsis which increases their risk for the development of MODS [41]. For example, toll-like receptor 9 (TLR9) signaling plays an important role in the innate immune response. Trauma patients with SNPs of TLR9 have been found to have a greater responsiveness of their peripheral blood leukocytes as well as a higher risk of sepsis and multiple organ dysfunction [42]. Henckaerts and colleagues furthermore showed that these functional polymorphisms involved in innate immunity predispose patients to severe infections and death. Further study and elucidation could contribute to formation of a risk model where patients could be stratified as to who could benefit from specific preventative or therapeutic options [43].

Scoring Systems

MOF does not have a consensus definition and there are a variety of scoring systems used to categorize the severity of organ dysfunction. Trending these scores during a patient's hospital course enables physicians to prognosticate the patient's risk of mortality [44]. There is also a direct relationship between the number of organ failures and ICU mortality. Moreover, improvements in cardiovascular, respiratory and renal function during an ICU course can predict a better survival [45].

Scoring systems like the Acute Physiology and Chronic Health Evaluation (APACHE) score are based on measured laboratory values that enable staging of the severity of organ dysfunction. One of the most commonly used scoring systems is the Sequential Organ Failure Assessment Score (SOFA) (Table 7.4). Clinical and laboratory variables in six organ systems (respiratory, hematologic, liver, cardiovascular, central nervous system, renal) are utilized to calculate a total score [46]. Patients with no organ failure defined by a SOFA score below or equal to two for each organ at admission have an ICU mortality rate of 6% compared to 65–100% for those with four or more organ failures [34]. The Denver MOF score is also a frequently used and well validated score. It is defined as two or more organ systems failing greater than 48 h after injury. The Denver score looks at dysfunction in the cardiac, respiratory, renal and hepatic systems [47] (Table 7.5). When comparing the Denver postinjury MOF score with the SOFA score, the SOFA score is very sensitive but not as specific as the Denver MOF score, whereas the Denver postinjury MOF score is more specific and less sensitive than the SOFA score when dealing with the trauma population. This distinction is important when analyzing epidemiologic data as more sensitive scores will have a higher incidence of MOF, while a more specific score will have a higher mortality rate [48–50]. Regardless of what score is used to evaluate the various physiologic and clinical parameters, it is an underlying theme in all organ failure scores, that as the number of organ systems that are affected increase, so does the mortality [51, 52]. Moreover, these scoring systems were developed to quantify the severity of illness and the risk of mortality in ICU patients. These prognostic scores will not tell how a patient will respond to therapy and are best utilized to predict outcomes in certain homogenous groups of patients. Additionally, these scores are unable to provide details regarding how a patient will respond to treatment. However, they can be repeatedly assessed to evaluate a patient's progress and used to identify patients for enrollment and to assess morbidity in clinical trials [53].

Clinical Presentation, Evaluation, and Diagnosis

The common clinical manifestations leading to multiple organ dysfunction are included in the ACCP-SCCM guidelines and can fall anywhere within the continuum of SIRS to MOF. These most commonly include alterations in body temperature (hyper or hypothermia), tachypnea or hypocarbia, tachycardia, leukocytosis, leukopenia or bandemia, hypotension, thrombocytopenia or coagulopathy, and

Table 7.4 SOFA score. MOF is defined as a score ≥4 with involvement of ≥2 organ systems

SOFA score					
System	Grade 0	Grade 1	Grade 2	Grade 3	Grade 4
Respiratory PaO2/FiO2	>400	<400	<300	<200 with respiratory support	<100 with respiratory support
Coagulation platelets (Ā-103/mm³)	>150	<150	<100	<50	<20
Liver bilirubin (mol/l)	<20	20–32	33–101	102–204	>204
Cardiovascular	No hypotension	MAP <70 mmHg	Dopamine >5 or any dobutamine dose	Dopamine >5 or epi_0.1	Dopamine >15 or epi >0.1
Renal creatinine (mol/l)	<110	110–170	171–299	300–440	>440
Central nervous system Glasgow Coma Scale	15	13–14	10–12	6–9	<6

Table 7.5 Denver postinjury multiple organ failure score

Denver postinjury multiple organ failure score				
Dysfunction	Grade 0	Grade 1	Grade 2	Grade 3
Pulmonary PaO2/FiO2 ratio	>250	250–200	200–100	<100
Renal creatinine (mol/l)	<159	160–210	211–420	>420
Hepatic total bilirubin (mol/l)	<34	34–68	68–137	>137
Cardiac	No inotropes	Only 1 ionotrope at small dose	Any ionotrope at moderate dose or >1 agent at small dose	Any ionotrope at large dose or >2 agents at moderate doses

The MOF score is the addition of the worst value for the day for each organ system. MOF is defined as score >3

alterations in mental status [54]. Fever is the most common presenting symptom of sepsis and should be an impetus for further evaluation the patient as well as identification of a source. Elderly patients with sepsis or those that are immunosuppressed may not mount a febrile response or conversely may be hypothermic [55]. In sepsis, common sites of infection are the pulmonary, gastrointestinal, and urinary tract systems. Other nosocomial causes of sepsis are intravenous catheter infections, ventilator-associated pneumonia, and sinusitis. As approximately 20% of patients will not have an identifiable source, noninfectious etiologies for SIRS should be considered [56]. These may include surgery, trauma, hematoma, subarachnoid hemorrhage, venous thrombosis, pancreatitis, myocardial infarction, transplant rejection, thyroid storm, acute renal or adrenal insufficiency, lymphoma, tumor lysis syndrome, transfusion reaction, opiates, benzodiazepines, anesthetic related malignant hyperpyrexia, and neuroleptic malignant syndrome [57].

A thorough physical examination should include a head-to-toe exam as well as inspection of indwelling catheters, a rectal exam, and examination of all wounds, including those under casts/fixation devices. Potential atypical causes of sepsis should be given consideration when an obvious source is identified. These potential causes of sepsis include sinusitis, meningitis, septic joint, acalculous cholecystitis, septic thrombophlebitis, deep muscular abscess, or a viral infection. Corresponding laboratory values based on the suspected differential diagnoses should be obtained.

Infections leading to sepsis can also arise in surgical sites from the skin to the deep muscle layers. Physical examination should be repeated if no source is identified. An investigation of all organ systems should be thorough and systematic. Subtle findings of end organ hypoperfusion such as altered mental status, tachypnea, hypoxia, hypotension, oliguria may be missed if the physician does not have a high index of suspicion and an incomplete exam is performed; i.e., failure to remove a dressing to inspect a wound. Failure to investigate thoroughly can lead to a delay in diagnosis and increased morbidity and mortality. Physical examination should include a rapid review of the patient's hemodynamic condition and should include continuous monitoring. Patients in shock should have arterial catheters placed for blood pressure monitoring. Persistent clinical signs of SIRS may suggest ongoing inflammation or infection. In addition to the patient's hemodynamic status, clinical signs of poor end organ perfusion, such as change in mental status, low urine output, mottling, and poor capillary refill, should be taken into consideration and used to guide resuscitation [58]. Initiation of resuscitation should take place immediately upon recognition of SIRS or sepsis symptoms and should not wait for transport to the next level of care.

Laboratory Evaluation

While no laboratory value will diagnose sepsis or MOF, they may assist in narrowing the differential diagnosis, localizing the source and guiding appropriate antibiotic therapy. Laboratory studies should include a complete blood count with differential, chemistry profile, arterial blood gas with lactic acid, prothrombin time and partial thromboplastin time, fibrinogen, and urinalysis [59]. Utilizing lactic acid level trends to guide resuscitation has been shown to be helpful in septic patients. For prognostication purposes, resolution of lactic acidosis with resuscitation efforts is associated with improved outcomes [60].

Pan cultures of the urine, blood, and sputum should be collected. The SCCM guidelines recommend that one pair of blood cultures be obtained at the onset of symptoms and another set obtained again at 24 h [12]. When taking blood cultures, two sets of blood cultures should be drawn from peripheral sites. If this is not possible, then one set should be drawn peripherally and the other from a recently inserted central catheter after careful cleansing of the port site. Every effort must be made to draw the first cultures before the initiation of antimicrobial therapy. They can be drawn consecutively or simultaneously, unless there is suspicion of an endovascular infection, in which case separate peripheral blood draws separated by timed intervals can be drawn to demonstrate continuous bacteremia [61].

Based on physical exam, additional body fluids may be sampled if the patient exhibits localized symptoms of infection. For example, cerebrospinal fluid, pleural fluid, joint aspiration, and ascites can all be sampled to localize the source of infection and help guide antibiotic therapy. Radiographic images should be tailored to the most likely source. If plain films are nondiagnostic, CT scans can assist in elucidating a suspected source and used to guide therapy, for example abscess drainage.

Pathophysiology

The pathophysiology of MOF is at best a nebulous interaction of multiple inflammatory mediators. Our understanding of this process and the innumerable interactions is in its infancy. A complete discussion of the immunology of this process is beyond the scope of this chapter as entire books have been dedicated to this task [62–64]. This section highlights some salient points regarding the pathophysiology of MOF.

Initially, SIRS was thought to be an overwhelming, uncontrolled response to infection. While MOF frequently is the end point of the spectrum of SIRS and severe sepsis, severe inflammation is also a mitigating factor and can result in the same endpoint of organ failure. This indicates overlap in the pathophysiology between inflammation and infection. The progression to MOF from SIRS from either cause is likely the result of an unbalanced interaction between the

Table 7.6 Risk factors for early and late MODS

Risk factors for early MODS <72 h of injury	Risk factors late MODS >72 h after injury
• ISS > 24	• Age > 55
• SBP < 90	• >6 units of blood transfused within 12 h of injury
• >6 units of blood transfused within 12 h of injury	• Base deficit >8 mEq/l within first 12 h of injury
• Lactate > 2.5	• Lactate > 2.5 mmol/l within 12–24 h of injury

pro and anti inflammatory mediators. In most patients, the initial SIRS response is physiologically followed by a compensatory anti-inflammatory response syndrome (CARS). This acts to limit the SIRS response so that it is not counterproductive. The subsequent balance between the pro-inflammatory (SIRS) and anti-inflammatory (CARS) response has been referred to as the mixed antagonistic response syndrome or MARS [36]. If the balance of these two systems is disturbed the inflammatory response becomes systemic and deregulated. The result is whole-body activation of the inflammatory response, with resultant disruption of normal cellular metabolism and microcirculatory perfusion. Both of these responses, if unchecked can result in complications, the former leading to MOF and the later secondary infections. At the site of injury, endothelial cells and leukocytes coordinate the local release of mediators of the inflammatory response, including cytokines interleukins, interferons, leukotrienes, prostaglandins, nitric oxide, reactive oxygen species, and products of the classic inflammation pathway. It is this usually functional biologic response that becomes unregulated and leads to MOF [65].

In 1996, Moore and colleagues recognized MOF is not necessarily related to an infectious process and follows a bimodal distribution. Early MOF is now defined as organ failure that develops within 72 h of the initial diagnosis of sepsis (Table 7.6). Late MOF was defined as organ failure that develops after 72 h after the initial diagnosis of sepsis [66]. When compared to the late MOF group, patients with early organ failure died sooner, had more cardiac dysfunction and had greater evidence of hyper inflammation. In contrast, patients with late MOF were older, had greater evidence of hepatic failure, and were more likely to have an infection as a "second hit" [67].

Multiple theories exist regarding the cause for MOF and it is likely that these pathways overlap to cause initially organ insufficiency that, unless reverses, ultimately leads to failure. Four overlapping categories have been proposed to the complex pathophysiology of MOF. These are the cytokine hypothesis, the microcirculatory hypotheses, the gut hypothesis and the two-hit hypothesis [63].

The Cytokine Hypothesis of MOF

In the cytokine hypothesis, the immune response to infection or inflammation results in excessive or prolonged activation or stimulation of mediators. These include interactions between polymorphonuclear neutrophils (PMNs), endothelial cells, and macrophages. PMN stimulation results in "priming" of the neutrophil and can lead to overzealous production, surface expression, and liberation of cytokines [68]. These mediators often have an exaggerated response and the products of these cascades exert damaging local and systemic effects. A temporal relationship between cytokine production and time of injury was recognized. Cytokines predictive of MOF in trauma patients include inducible protein (IP)-10, macrophage inflammatory protein (MIP)—1B, interleukin (IL) IL-10, IL-6, IL-1Ra, and eotaxin [69]. Several lines of evidence support the central role of inflammatory cells in the pathogenesis of lung and systemic organ injury. Tumor necrosis factor (TNF) has been considered one of the most potent pro-inflammatory cytokines identified in SIRS and sepsis. Administration of TNF to experimental animals creates the hemodynamic and metabolic observations consistent with SIRS. Analysis of cytokine serum biomarkers has shown that patients with MOF show a biphasic elevation of IL-6 and significantly higher soluble TNF receptor (sTNF-R) concentrations [70]. Activation of leucocytes and their subsequent inappropriate sequestration in organs appears to additionally be one of the key events in the development of early MOF. Once activated, leukocytes have the capacity to release their cytotoxic factors including nitric oxide and lysosomal granules, which aid in polymicrobial killing. These factors can cause necrosis and inflammation of organs such as the lung despite a lack of an infectious stimulus [71]. Additionally, PMN stimulation provokes endothelial and epithelial injury through up-regulation of adhesion molecules on these cells. This prompts changes in the cell wall, increased permeability cell swelling and culminates in cellular dysfunction. Neutrophil elastase is a key marker of severity of injury and has also been found to be a prognostic marker [72].

The Microcirculatory Hypothesis of MOF

The microcirculatory hypothesis proposes that organ injury is related to ischemia or vascular endothelial injury [73]. Some authors have speculated that even though adequate blood flow may reach the various tissue beds, there may be an inability of the mitochondria or cells to take up or use the delivered oxygen and substrate. Although prolonged tissue hypoperfusion and hypoxia leads to inadequate adenosine triphosphate (ATP) generation and potentially irreversible cell damage, this shock period is not long enough in most clinical conditions for that to occur. This damage is relieved by reperfusion and thus pro-inflammatory factors and oxygen radicals are introduced and lead to injury [74]. In vitro studies have found that nitric oxide (NO) up-regulates the production of pro-inflammatory cytokines (TNF-alpha, IL-8 and prostaglandins) and can lead injury of the lung, and intestine. Additionally, the superoxide anion and hydrogen peroxide can interact with NO and form peroxynitrite, which is toxic to cells [72]. During shock, these mediators, such as reactive oxygen species, are released to destroy the offending bacteria and to inactivate toxins. The unintended effects are that when unregulated, they also result in damaging the patient's organ systems [75].

Gut Hypothesis of MOF

The gut is considered an immunologically active organ and a main in the burden of infection-induced systemic inflammation [76]. Gut barrier dysfunction can occur for a variety of reasons including trauma, shock, infection, and malnutrition. It is proposed that, as a result of the loss of the gut barrier function, intestinal bacteria and endotoxin cross the mucosal barrier and lead to exposure of the intestinal immune cells. The production of gut-derived toxins and inflammatory products reach the systemic circulation through the intestinal lymphatics, leading to SIRS, ARDS, and MOF [68]. These translocating bacteria are phagocytosed by intestinal immune cells and contribute to the intestinal inflammatory response. Some of these translocating bacteria or their toxic products are trapped in the intestinal lymph nodes, causing inflammatory reaction [72]. This hypothesis is supported by the demonstration of circulating levels of endotoxin in the peripheral blood of critically ill patients with sepsis and SIRS. Reports of endotoxemia in these critically ill patients, even without clinical or microbiologic evidence of infection with gram-negative organisms supports the potential role of translocation in the production of MODS/ MOF [36]. The phenomenon of bacterial translocation, however, is not sufficient to explain the development of MODS in ICU patients. The development of MODS in these high-risk patients is likely due to intestinal injury and the resultant inflammatory cascade that reaches the systemic circulation via the intestinal lymphatics [77].

Two-Hit Phenomenon in MOF

The phrase "two-hit phenomenon in MOF" is used to describe the biologic phenomenon in which an initial insult primes the host such that on a second or subsequent insults, the host's response is greatly amplified. Primers to the subsequent insult can be infection, shock, inflammation, or trauma.

Despite the decreasing incidence of MOF, the rate of PMN priming has not changed. PMN priming increases elastase release, IL-8 production, L-selectin expression, and CD-18 expression, and delays apoptosis. This is evident by a lack of change in the incidence of early lung dysfunction postinjury, which is a surrogate marker of PMN priming [78]. The timing of the second hit phenomenon was shown in laboratory experiments evaluating abdominal compartment syndrome (ACS). If subjects had early decompressive laparotomy (<2 h) or late (>18 h), they had a lower mortality than those having a decompressive laparotomy at 8 h. This correlates with the clinically identified time frame of the development of postinjury ACS, which manifests 8–12 h window after trauma. Severely injured patients who develop ACS have a fourfold increase in their chance of developing MOF compared to the non-ACS patients with similar demographics, shock parameters and injury severity [24]. These insults prime the immune system to mount an exaggerated response when exposed to a second physiologic insult. Botha described the observation that the first hit primes and activates PMNs within 3–6 h after injury. This primer creates a vulnerable window during which a second insult activates excessive cytokine release. This second hit results in an elevated risk of developing MOF [79]. This exaggerated immune response then results in end organ injury [80]. In summary, MOF results from an excessive host response to an infectious or inflammatory stimulus. Any or all of the aforementioned hypotheses can coexist and each overlaps with the other. The cytokine, endovascular, and systemic storm that ensues thereafter, predisposes to additional infections and can lead to organ failure [45].

The temporal series of events in MOF is usually predictable and is independent of the etiology. Multiple studies have demonstrated that the respiratory system is usually the first to fail and is the most commonly affected [15]. This is typically followed by hepatic, intestinal, and renal failure, in that order. As the number of organ systems affected increases from 1 to 4, the mortality increased from 21 to 100% [81]. Hematologic and myocardial failures are usually later manifestations of MOF, whereas the onset of central nervous system alterations can occur either early or late [24]. Physiologically, these patients are hyper metabolic and they have a hyper dynamic circulation, which is characterized by an increased cardiac output and a decreased systemic vascular resistance. This classical sequential pattern of organ failure may be modified, however, by the presence of preexistent disease or by the nature of the precipitating clinical event. For example, renal failure may precede hepatic or even pulmonary failure in patients with intrinsic renal disease or in patients who have sustained prolonged periods of shock, whereas hepatic or myocardial failure may be an early or even the initial manifestation of this syndrome in the patient

with cirrhosis or myocardial damage [82]. The exact sequence of organ failure, however, is not always predictable and can be influenced by the patient's preexisting morbidities as well as their acute process. However, as the number of organs that fails increases from one to four, the mortality rate progressively increases from 30 to 100% [27].

Multiple Organ Failure by System

Pulmonary Dysfunction

The sequence of organ dysfunction is predictable and the lung is usually the first organ to show signs of failure. Initial pulmonary insufficiency and renal impairment are followed by circulatory failure and then metabolic dysfunction and liver failure. Respiratory failure can range from mild hypoxia and tachypnea to ARDS [83]. ARDS is defined as a P_aO_2/F_iO_2 ratio lower than 200 mmHg in association with bilateral fluffy pulmonary infiltrates and a pulmonary capillary wedge pressure lower than 18 mmHg [84]. Increased capillary permeability and neutrophil influx are the earliest pathologic events in ARDS. As the acute inflammatory process resolves, further lung injury results both from the process of repair, which involves fibrosis and the deposition of hyaline material, and from further lung trauma, resulting from positive pressure mechanical ventilation [85]. ARDS may occur within a few days of admission or after the development of SIRS and sepsis. Sepsis-induced ARDS is associated with the highest mortality rates. Additionally, the data suggests that approximately 40% of patients with severe sepsis develop ARDS. Historically, 10–12 ml/kg tidal volumes were commonplace and resulted in alveolar damage due to over distention. Parenchymal injury appears to be due primarily to oxidative damage from the activated neutrophils in the lung. Endotracheal intubation and a controlled mode of ventilation are the mainstays of support for respiratory failure. Lung protection ventilation strategies, with low tidal volumes (4–6 ml/kg) for patients with ARDS, are recommended and showed a decreased mortality from 40 to 31%. Due to the smaller tidal volumes, patients typically will have a rise in carbon dioxide [86]. This permissive hypercapnia has been shown to have a protective effect in critically ill patients [87]. Some patients with refractory hypoxemia may require alternative therapies such as extracorporeal membrane oxygenation (ECMO), high-frequency oscillation, or inhaled nitrous oxide.

Gastrointestinal and Hepatic Dysfunction

The gastrointestinal tract is a crucial component of the SIRS response. Shock is associated with obligatory gut ischemia due to vasoconstriction. With resuscitation efforts, reperfusion results in a local inflammatory response that can set the stage for ACS. ACS is a syndrome that occurs either primarily or secondarily [88]. Primary ACS occurs in patients undergoing damage control laparotomy. The presence of laparotomy pads, blood products and resuscitation fluid increases the pressure in the abdomen to a tipping point, usually 25 mmHg. Secondary ACS occurs after a non-abdominal injury that requires massive transfusion. The products of resuscitation result in edematous bowel and fluid sequestration and the same impaired end-organ perfusion [89]. This pressure elevation is higher than the mesenteric and splanchnic arterial beds resulting in ischemia. Respiratory physiology is impaired due to elevated peak pressures and vena cava compression results in impaired cardiac filling. This constellation of symptoms requires an investigative clinician. Once the diagnosis is made, the abdominal pressure is usually relieved by emergent laparotomy. Clinical studies have clearly documented the poor outcome of patients developing ACS and the frequent association of ACS and MOF [90].

Risk factors for hepatic insufficiency include perfusion deficits, persistent foci of dead or injured tissue, an uncontrolled focus of infection, the presence of the respiratory distress syndrome, and preexisting fibrotic liver disease [91]. In patients with septic shock, transaminitis is a common laboratory finding in patients. The catecholamine, norepinephrine induces injury to hepatocytes by activating adrenergic receptors on Kupffer cells. In turn, norepinephrine enhances chemokine and NO production, resulting in mitochondrial damage [50]. This process is usually transient and limited to a laboratory abnormality that corrects once the patient is resuscitated. However, if hemodynamics are not restored, a secondary hepatic dysfunction may occur and can lead to bacterial product spillover, amplified inflammation and may lead to MOF and death [92].

Renal Dysfunction

Acute renal failure is a common dysfunction in patients with sepsis. It confers its own mortality risk and when it develops in association with MOF [93]. In a recent review by Wohlauer et al. early acute kidney injury was present in 2.13% of severely injured patients and was associated with a 78% MOF incidence and 27% mortality. Both rates were higher than those associated with early heart, lung, or liver failure [94]. The causes of renal dysfunction are multifactorial and can be due to inadequate perfusion, nephrotoxic medications, acute tubular necrosis, contrast induced nephropathy, ACS, and obstruction. Activation of the renin–angiotensin system may contribute to reduced perfusion as vasoconstriction

exacerbates ischemia. This is clinically manifested as oliguria (<30 ml/h) or anuria and as an increased serum concentration of creatinine and urea [83]. The vasoconstrictive shunting due to compensatory mechanisms or concomitant vasopressors agents can exacerbate the injury and results in further nephron ischemia. Additionally, TNF has been shown to be directly injurious to nephrons by inducing apoptosis [50]. Treatment is aimed at identifying the source and provision of supportive care. Moreover, up to 70% of patients with severe sepsis require some form of renal replacement therapy [57]. While intermittent and continuous hemodialyses are equivalent, continuous dialysis avoids the hemodynamic instability often seen with intermittent dialysis [95]. The typical indications for dialysis are volume overload, refractory acidosis, uremia, and electrolyte derangements.

Cardiovascular Dysfunction

Myocardial depression is a well-recognized manifestation of organ dysfunction in sepsis. Due to the lack of a generally accepted definition and the absence of large epidemiologic studies, its frequency is uncertain. Cardiac dysfunction in sepsis is characterized by decreased contractility, impaired ventricular response to fluid therapy, and ventricular dilatation. Cardiac echocardiograms suggest that 40–50% of patients with prolonged septic shock develop myocardial depression, as defined by a reduced systolic and diastolic ejection fraction. Additionally, peroxynitrite has a direct damaging effect on myocyte mitochondria and causes reduced contractility [96]. Troponin elevation is also seen and correlates to the severity of illness and dysfunction [50]. Sepsis-related changes in circulating volume and vessel tone inevitably affect cardiac performance. The principle hemodynamic profile shows elevated cardiac output, but substantially reduced systemic vascular resistance [97]. Mitochondrial dysfunction, another feature of sepsis-induced organ dysfunction, will also place the cardiac myocytes at risk of ATP depletion. However, clinical studies have demonstrated that myocardial cell death is rare and that cardiac function is fully reversible in survivors. Hence, functional rather than structural changes seem to be responsible for intrinsic myocardial depression during sepsis [98]. Current studies support that myocardial depression is due to a complex underlying physiopathology with a multiple overlapping pathways. Cytokine release and circulation such as TNF-alpha, IL-1, and endothelin-1 directly inhibit myocyte contractility contributing to the overall cardiac dysfunction [99]. Nitric oxide production additionally has a complex role in sepsis-induced cardiac dysfunction and may have a deleterious as well as a beneficial role [100].

Endocrine Dysfunction

Endocrine abnormalities are common during sepsis and MOF and include hyperglycemia and insulin resistance. Hyperglycemia is common in critically ill patients, with approximately 90% of patients treated in an ICU developing blood glucose concentrations >110 mg/dl [101]. Historically, hyperglycemia was not treated until the blood glucose level rose above 200 g/dl. In a randomized controlled study, Van den Berge and colleagues used insulin infusions to maintain tight control of blood sugars in critically ill surgical patients. The strictly controlled group had their blood glucose maintained between 80 and 110 g/dl. The more liberal threshold was only treated at >180 g/dl. A mortality benefit, from 8 to 4.6%, was identified in the surgical patients that had strict control of their blood sugar. This survival benefit was largely related to a reduction in deaths due to MOF [102]. Due to tighter control utilizing insulin drips, patients were noted to more episodes of hypoglycemia requiring treatment. Subsequently, follow-up studies have shown that hypoglycemia is an increased risk factor for mortality [103]. Conversely, the Normoglycemia in Intensive Care Evaluation-Survival Using Glucose Algorithm Regulation (NICE-SUGAR) study reported increased mortality with a tight blood sugar control approach [104]. Recent meta-analyses do not support intensive glucose control for critically ill patients and more moderate recommendations to target a blood glucose concentration between 144 and 180 mg/dl (8–10 mmol/l) are now in effect [105].

In addition to hyperglycemia, a relative state of adrenal insufficiency is common in critically ill patients [50]. This is defined as an abnormally low level of the patient's endogenous cortisol at the time of physiologic stress. In response to hypotension and following trauma or surgery, circulating cortisol concentrations should exceed 25 μ(mu)g/dl. Marik et al. discovered that 70% of ICU patients had inappropriately low levels of cortisol. This low level of cortisol can result in a blunted response to hypoglycemia and hypotension [106]. The Surviving Sepsis Campaign suggests giving intravenous hydrocortisone to adult septic shock patients after their hypotension is identified to be poorly responsive to fluid resuscitation and vasopressor therapy. If one suspects adrenal insufficiency, corticosteroids should be administered without waiting on results of a cosyntropin stimulation test [107].

Hematalogic Dysfunction

Thrombocytopenia is the most common hematalogic dysfunction and is present in 20% of patients and is associated with an increased mortality [108]. The causes are multifactorial but include bone marrow suppression from sepsis, sequestration, consumption and heparin induced thrombocytopenia (HIT). As critically ill patients are often immobilized and mechanically ventilated, they are at elevated risk for deep vein thromboses. If no contraindication exists, critically ill patients should be on daily chemical thromboprophylaxis. This chemical prophylaxis can lead to HIT by production of antibodies against the heparin-platelet factor 4 complex. The antibody-platelet complex is then removed prematurely from the circulation leading to thrombocytopenia [109].

Anemia is also a common finding in patients who are critically ill. The etiology is usually multifactorial and can result from direct inhibition by cytokines, deficiency of erythropoietin, blunted erythropoietic response, acute blood loss, nutritional deficiencies, as well as renal insufficiency [110]. Leukocytosis is also common within hours after injury or the onset of sepsis. Typically, the number of leukocytes markedly increases and the number of lymphocytes and monocytes decreases. This post injury leukocytosis is primarily due to increased PMN numbers, and several studies have shown a link between high number of PMNs during the first hours after injury and an increased risk of organ failure and mortality [79].

Neurologic Dysfunction

Central nervous system (CNS) dysfunction occurs in as many as 70% of critically ill patients. The brain plays a pivotal role in sepsis, acting as both a mediator of the immune response and a target for the pathologic process. Sepsis-associated encephalopathy is associated with increased mortality and morbidity [111]. Its pathophysiology remains insufficiently elucidated, although there is evidence for a neuroinflammatory process sequentially involving endothelial activation, blood–brain barrier alteration and cellular dysfunction and alteration in neurotransmission [112]. Increased permeability to cytokines, neuroamines, and endotoxemia have all been implicated in septic encephalopathy [113]. It is difficult to quantify neurologic impairment as there are no specific biomarkers of neuronal injury and bedside evaluation of cognitive performance is difficult in an ICU [114]. The Glasgow Coma Scale is frequently utilized by organ failure scoring systems to evaluate the severity of a patient's neurologic failure but sedatives and analgesics can make this score unreliable. New delirium in a critically ill patient should raise the suspicion of the physician to the possibility that this is the first presentation of infection.

Treatment

Initial Resuscitation

Current strategies are aimed at preventing organ failures and supporting failing organ systems in critically ill patients. Once MOF has developed, therapies are aimed at supporting failed organ systems and preventing secondary example infection. Currently there is no specific pharmacotherapy for ARDS or MOF.

A crucial component in preventing the progression of septic shock to MOF is early recognition and expeditious implementation of goals of therapy. Initial resuscitation should include establishing intravenous access and prompt initiation of fluid resuscitation. Rivers et al. in a study of patients with severe sepsis and septic shock found that early goal-directed therapy, directed toward attaining a SvO_2 >70%, conferred a substantial reduction in mortality from 46.5 to 30.5%. This study also demonstrated the importance of the urgency of resuscitation and that it should be started as soon as it is recognized, whether it is in the emergency department or the hospital ward. Studies in which aggressive resuscitation was delayed until after transfer to the ICU failed to show improved outcome or a reduction in MODS [115]. Patients should be admitted to an ICU that is conducive for invasive hemodynamic monitoring and frequent reassessment.

Vascular access with two large bore intravenous (IV) catheters is adequate for initiating resuscitation but if hemodynamic compromise is present, central venous access should be established. The optimal type of fluid is an ongoing controversy in the critical care literature, but crystalloid should be given at an initial bolus of 20 ml/kg of ideal body weight. Fluids should be bolused to attain a goal central venous pressure (CVP) of 8–12 mmHg, MAP >65 mmHg, urine output >0.5 ml/kg/h, and a SvO_2 >70% (Table 7.7). Recognition of the sequelae of each IV fluid should be recognized and tailored to the patient's specific pathophysiology, i.e., resultant hyperchloremic acidosis with normal saline administration [50]. If hypotension is still present after the CVP goals are attained, vasopressor assistance should also be initiated.

The Surviving Sepsis Campaign established resuscitation and management bundles that emphasize the prompt initiation of therapy for sepsis. The resuscitation bundle describes tasks that should begin immediately, and must be accomplished within the first 6 h of presentation for patients with severe sepsis or septic shock (Table 7.8).

Some items may not be completed if the clinical conditions described in the bundle do not apply, but clinicians should assess their patients for them. The goal is to perform all of the indicated tasks 100% of the time within the first 6 h of identification of severe sepsis. The management bundle provides evidence-based goals that similarly must be completed within 24 h for patients with severe sepsis, septic shock and/or lactate >4 mmol/l (36 mg/dl) (Table 7.9). For patients with severe sepsis, as many as four bundle elements must be accomplished within the first 24 h of presentation. Again, some items may not be completed if the clinical conditions described in the bundle do not apply but a high index

Table 7.7 Endpoints of resuscitation

Endpoints of resuscitation
• Central venous pressure (CVP) of 8–12 mmHg
• Mean arterial pressure (MAP) >65 mmHg
• Urine output >0.5 ml/kg/h
• SvO2 >70%

Table 7.8 Sepsis resuscitation bundle: must be completed within the first 6 h of presentation

Sepsis resuscitation bundle
• Measure serum lactate
• Obtain blood cultures prior to antibiotic administration
• Administer broad-spectrum antibiotic within 3 h of ED admission and within 1 h of non-ED admission
• Treat hypotension and/or elevated lactate with fluids
• In the event of hypotension and/or serum lactate >4 mmol/l:
– Deliver an initial minimum of 20 ml/kg of crystalloid or an equivalent
– Apply vasopressors for hypotension not responding to initial fluid resuscitation to maintain mean arterial pressure (MAP) >65 mmHg
• In the event of persistent hypotension despite fluid resuscitation (septic shock) and/or lactate >4 mmol/l:
– Achieve a central venous pressure (CVP) of >8 mmHg
– Achieve a central venous oxygen saturation (ScvO2) >70% or mixed venous oxygen saturation (SvO2) >65%

Table 7.9 Sepsis management bundle: must be completed within 24 h

Sepsis management bundle
• Administer low-dose steroids for septic shock in accordance with a standardized ICU policy.
• The prior Drotrcogin alfa (rhAPC) recommendation is discontinued
• Maintain glucose control lower limit of normal, but <180 mg/dl (10 mmol/l)
• Maintain a median inspiratory plateau pressure (IPP) <30 cm H_2O for mechanically ventilated patients

of suspicious by physicians should exist to rule them out. The goal is to perform all indicated management tasks, 100% of the time, within the first 24 h of presentation [12].

Along with the aforementioned endpoints of resuscitation, measurement of blood lactate has also been used as a means to assess prognosis and is inversely proportional to survival [116]. As the lactate concentration increased from 2.1 to 8 mM/l, the estimated probability of survival decreased from 90 to 10% [117]. Abramson et al. also revealed the importance of lactate clearance and survival following traumatic injury. If a patient's lactate normalized (lactate <2 mmol/l) within 24 h their survival rate was 75% versus 14% if the lactate level did not return to normal by 48 h [118].

Vasopressors

Once fluid resuscitation has been initiated and hemodynamic monitoring established, if the patient's MAP remains <65 mmHg, vasopressor therapy should be initiated. The Surviving Sepsis Campaign Guidelines (SSCG) recommends norepinephrine or dopamine as the first line vasopressor agents. Due to a relative deficiency of vasopressin in septic shock, consideration should be given to adding a low dose vasopressin drip (0.04 units/min), which may assist in correcting refractory hypotension [119]. Additionally, the SSCG guidelines regarding vasopressors also recommend using epinephrine as an alternative if blood pressure is poorly responsive but it should not be used as a first line agent. Volume resuscitation should be occurring simultaneously but if hypotension is refractory, vasopressors should be initiated to maintain MAP>65.

Source Control and Antibiotic Therapy

Once the suspicion for SIRS or sepsis is present, a thorough physical exam, laboratory studies and radiographic evaluation of the patient should ensue to identify the causative agent. Ongoing sources of infection are known to "prime" the host immune system so that a second insult can cause an exaggerated systemic inflammation ultimately culminating in MOF [53]. Laboratory values that should be sent were mentioned earlier. Indwelling catheters should be inspected for signs of infection or outright removed if the clinical suspicion is high. A positive blood culture from a centrally placed catheter is considered infected if the culture becomes positive at least 2 h before the peripherally obtained culture does [120]. Antibiotics should be administered within 1 h of suspicion of sepsis and the urgency should be conveyed to the ICU pharmacist to assist in expediting the administration of the antibiotics to the patient. A study by Kumar et al. demonstrated that patients had a survival rate of 79% if antibiotics were given within 1 h of the development of hypotension. Conversely, the same study showed a decrease in survival of 7.6% for every hour antibiotic administration was delayed [121]. This illustrates the importance of having a high index of suspicion and initiating antimicrobial therapy. According to the SSCG antibiotics should be broad spectrum and active against bacterial/fungal pathogens. Therapy should be limited to 7–10 days unless a mitigating circumstance is present and once susceptibilities return, de-escalation of therapy is appropriate.

Should a surgical source of infection be identified, utilization of damage control techniques is appropriate to prevent further injury. Originally described in trauma patients as an abbreviated laparotomy, this involves making a decision, to address only the critical issues at the first surgery and to return the patient to the ICU for further resuscitation [122].

Depending on the intracavitary findings, a conscious decision to leave bowel in discontinuity or to leave the abdominal wall open may be made with a planned returned once the patient is further resuscitated. This technique has been used in trauma and emergency general surgery and should be considered for any surgical patient with ongoing resuscitation needs or who has preexisting or is at risk for, acidosis, coagulopathy and hypothermia.

Corticosteroids

Relative adrenal insufficiency is often seen in septic shock due to what is hypothesized as suppression of the hypothalamic-pituitary-adrenal axis. The debate regarding the benefit of giving corticosteroids is ongoing and multiple studies have had conflicting results. Annane et al. performed a multicenter, double-blind, placebo-controlled trial study that administered hydrocortisone plus fludrocortisone to patients with septic shock [123]. This landmark study showed improved survival in patients and decreased vasopressor requirements. In contrast, the Corticosteroid Therapy of Septic Shock (CORITCUS) trial was a multicenter, randomized, double-blind, placebo-controlled trail that also evaluated the use of hydrocortisone in patients with septic shock. This study failed to show a mortality benefit but did show a statistically significant benefit of faster shock reversal [124]. Despite the ongoing controversy and presence of multiple conflicting studies, the current Surviving Sepsis Guidelines recommendations include administering corticosteroids to septic patients if hypotension is refractory to fluid resuscitation and vasopressor initiation. Cosyntropin (ACTH) stimulation test is not required and clinical suspicion of adrenal insufficiency should be the impetus to start steroids rather than waiting on the stimulation test to be resulted. Once the patient's vasopressor requirements have subsided, the steroid therapy may be weaned [105].

Activated Protein C

Activated protein C (APC) directly inhibits clotting factors Va and VIIIa and restores the fibrinolytic system by blocking plasminogen activator inhibitor. In sepsis, there is decreased production of APC resulting in a procoagulant state [125]. APC also has anti-inflammatory effects that include limiting leukocyte chemotaxis and reducing thrombin production. However, the levels of endogenous APC are depleted during sepsis [50, 126]. In 2001, the protein c worldwide evaluation in severe sepsis (PROWESS) study found that when patients with APACHE scores >25 received activated protein C for sepsis; they had a relative and absolute risk reduction of 19.4 and 6.1%, respectively [127]. The PROWESS study also demonstrated that patients that received APC had a statistically significant increase in serious bleeding events. (3.5%

vs. 2.0%) In 2004, the first SSCG included the use of dretrecogin alfa on patients at high risk of death, APACHE II ≥25, sepsis-induced MOF, septic shock, or sepsis-induced ARDS and no absolute contraindication related to bleeding risk or relative contraindication that outweighs the potential benefit of activated protein C [128]. The 2008 guidelines suggested that consider its use in the patients that met the previous criteria but that it should not be used on patients with a low risk of death. Of note in 2011, a Cochrane review in 2011 and 2012 found no evidence to suggest that APC reduced the risk of death in any patient [129]. Moreover, heightened risk of bleeding precluded its use and the drug was pulled from the market [130].

Nutrition

The past few decades have led to considerable interest regarding nutritional support of critically ill patients. Sepsis and organ failure are hypermetabolic states and increase the patient's metabolic demand. If the caloric needs are not met by supplemental nutrition, muscle breakdown and weakness can ensue. The intestinal tract is now recognized as an immune organ and the intact intestinal wall acts as a barrier. It has been recognized that loss of this barrier can potentially lead to bacterial translocation, progressive shock and ultimately organ failure. The use of enteral nutrition is known to reduce infectious complications in subpopulations of patients with trauma and burns [131]. No single formula matches every patient's needs thus formulas should be tailored to match the pathophysiology of the individual patient. Formulas containing linoleic acid, antioxidants, and omega-3 fatty acids may reduce the incidence of organ failure in patients with acute lung injury and may reduce mortality rates in mechanically ventilated patients [132, 133]. Arginine and glutamine containing formulas have shown benefit in trauma and burn patients [134, 135]. Arginine containing formulas, however, may be detrimental to patients with septic shock [136].

Current guidelines strongly recommend early use of enteral nutrition, with parenteral nutrition being reserved for patients in whom enteral nutrition fails to provide sufficient nutrition [137]. While enteral feeding is preferred, ileus due to ongoing infection or inflammation may prohibit enteral feeding. In these patients, parenteral nutrition is the preferred option.

Innovative Therapies

The overlap of inflammatory cells, cytokines, endothelial cells, and organ systems offers numerous potential locations to intervene by enhancing or blocking specific receptors and halt the damaging effects of the deregulated immune system. Potential targets for therapy have been anti-endotoxin antibodies, anti-tumor necrosis factor monoclonal antibodies, interleukin-1 receptor antagonists, antioxidants, dialysis, and activated protein C [82]. A better understanding of the dynamic of interactions at the cellular level is needed to direct therapy and more research is ongoing. Thus far, supportive care is the mainstay once sepsis has progressed to MOF.

Conclusion

MOF remains a major cause of morbidity and mortality in the trauma and surgical ICUs. Due to improvements in recognition of sepsis and early institution of therapy, the incidence of MOF has decreased. Further research is needed to obtain a better understanding of the pathophysiology of this disease and how the inciting event progresses to organ failure. This understanding will afford more potential targets for therapy. Thus far there is not one "magic bullet" therapy and the mainstay of critical care should be prompt recognition of SIRS and the sequelae of sepsis, expeditious treatment, and prevention of end organ damage.

References

1. Stewart RM. Injury prevention: why so important? J Trauma. 2007;62:112–9.
2. Champion HR, Bellamy RF, Roberts P, et al. A profile of combat injury. J Trauma. 2003;54:S13–S9.
3. Bellamy RF. Combat trauma overview. In: Zajtchuk R, Grande CM, editors. Textbook of military medicine, anesthesia and perioperative care of the combat casualty. Falls Church, VA: Office of the Surgeon General, United States Army; 1995. p. 1–42.
4. Bellamy RF. The causes of death in conventional land warfare: implications for combat casualty care research. Mil Med. 1984;149:229–30.
5. Howard JM, ed. Battle casualties in Korea: Studies of the Surgical Research Team. Vol. 4:Post-traumatic renal insufficiency. Army Medical Service Graduate School, Walter Reed Army Medical Center, Washington, DC. US Government Printing Office, 1955.
6. Ciesla DJ, Moore FA, Moore EE. Chapter 68. Multiple organ failure. In: Moore EE, Feliciano DV, Mattox KL, editors. Trauma. 6th ed. New York: McGraw-Hill; 2008. p. 1316–77.
7. Shoemaker WC. Editorial: multiple injuries and multiple organ failure. Crit Care Med. 1973;1(3):157.
8. Tilney NL, Bailey GL, Morgan AP. Sequential system failure after rupture of abdominal aortic aneurysms: an unsolved problem in postoperative care. Ann Surg. 1973;178:117–22.
9. Marshall JC, Cook DJ, Christou NV. Multiple organ dysfunction syndrome score: a reliable descriptor of a complex clinical outcome. Crit Care Med. 1995;23:1638–52.
10. Baue AE. Multiple, progressive, or sequential systems failure. A syndrome of the 1970s. Arch Surg. 1975;110(7):779–81.
11. Baue AE. MOF, MODS, and SIRS: what is in a name or an acronym? Shock. 2006;26(5):438–49.
12. ACCP-SCCM Consensus Conference: definitions of sepsis and multiple organ failure and guidelines for the use of innovative therapies in sepsis. Crit Care Med. 1992;20:864–74.

13. Vincent JL, Martinez EO, Silva E. Evolving concepts in sepsis definitions. Crit Care Clin. 2009;25:665–75.

14. Levy MM, Fink MP, Marshall JC, et al. 2001 SCCM/ESICM/ACCP/ATS/SIS International Sepsis Definitions Conference. Crit Care Med. 2003;31(4):1250.

15. Angus DC, Linde-Zwirble WT, Lidicker J, et al. Epidemiology of severe sepsis in the United States: analysis of incidence, outcome and associated costs of care. Crit Care Med. 2001;29:1303–10.

16. Marshall JC. Inflammation, coagulopathy, and the pathogenesis of multiple organ dysfunction syndrome. Crit Care Med. 2001;2(7 Suppl):S99–S106. Review.

17. Lagu T, Rothberg MB, Shieh M-S, et al. Hospitalizations, costs, and outcomes of severe sepsis in the United States 2003 to 2007. Crit. Care Med. 2011. http://www.ncbi.nlm.nih.gov/pubmed/21963582. Accessed 5 Jan 2012.

18. Balk R. A outcome of septic shock: location, location, location. Crit Care Med. 1998;26(6):1020–4.

19. Baue AE, Durham R, Faist E. Systemic inflammatory response syndrome (SIRS), multiple organ dysfunction syndrome (MODS), multiple organ failure (MOF): are we winning the battle? Shock. 1998;10(2):79–89.

20. Mayr VD, Dunser MW, Greil V, et al. Causes of death and determinant of outcome in critically ill patients. Crit Care. 2006;10:R154.

21. Knaus WA, Draper EA, Wagner DP, et al. Prognosis in acute organ-system failure. Ann Surg. 1985;202(6):685–93.

22. Sauaia A, Moore FA, Moore EE, et al. Epidemiology of trauma deaths: a reassessment. J Trauma. 1995;38(2):185–93.

23. Martin GS, Mannino DM, Moss M. The effect of age on the development and outcome of adult sepsis. Crit Care Med. 2006;34(1):15.

24. Dewar D, Moore FA, Moore EE, Balogh Z. Postinjury multiple organ failure. Injury. 2009;40(9):912–8.

25. Aldrin S, Koenig F, Weniger P, et al. Characteristics of polytrauma patients between 1992 and 2002. Injury. 2007;3:1059–64.

26. Dewar C, Mackay P, Balogh Z. Postinjury multiple organ failure: the Australian context. ANZ J Surg. 2009;79:434–9.

27. Durham RM, Moran JJ, Mazuski JE, et al. Multiple organ failure in trauma patients. J Trauma. 2003;55(4):608–16.

28. Raghavan M, Marik PE. Management of sepsis during the early "golden hours". J Emerg Med. 2006;31(2):185–99.

29. Jones GR, Lowes JA. The systemic inflammatory response syndrome as a predictor of bacteremia and outcome from sepsis. QJM. 1996;89(7):515.

30. Neviere R. Sepsis and the systemic inflammatory response syndrome: definitions, epidemiology, and prognosis. In: Parsons P, editor. UpToDate. http://www.uptodate.com/. Accessed 28 March 2012.

31. Dremsizov T, Clermont G, Kellum J, et al. Severe sepsis in community-acquired pneumonia: when does it happen, and do systemic inflammatory response syndrome criteria help predict course? Chest. 2006;129(4):968.

32. Ulvik A, Kvåle R, Wentzel-Larsen T, et al. Multiple organ failure after trauma affects even long-term survival and functional status. Crit Care. 2007;11(5):R95.

33. Edmonds RD, Cuschieri J, Minei JP, et al.; Inflammation the Host Response to Injury Investigators. Body adipose content is independently associated with a higher risk of organ failure and nosocomial infection in the nonobese patient postinjury. J Trauma. 2011;70(2):292–8.

34. Nast-Kolb D, Aufmkolk M, Rucholtz S, et al. Multiple organ failure still a major cause of morbidity but not mortality in blunt multiple trauma. J Trauma. 2001;51:835.

35. Ciesla DJ, Moore EE, Johnson JL. Obesity increases risk of organ failure after severe trauma. J Am Coll Surg. 2006;203(4):539–45.

36. Balk RA. Pathogenesis and management of multiple organ dysfunction failure in severe sepsis and septic shock. Crit Care Clin. 2000;16(2):337–52.

37. Sauaia A, Moore FA, Moore EE, et al. Early risk factors for postinjury multiple organ failure. World J Surg. 1996;20:392.

38. Moore FA, Moore EE, Sauaia A. Blood transfusion. An independent risk factor for postinjury multiple organ failure. Arch Surg. 1997;132(6):620–4. discussion 624–5.

39. Dunne JR, Malone DL, Tracy JK, et al. Allogenic blood transfusion in the first 24 hours after trauma is associated with increased systymic inflammatory response syndrome (SIRS) and death. Surg Infect. 2004;5:395–404.

40. Jiang JX. Genomic polymorphisms and sepsis. Chin J Traumatol. 2005;21:45–9.

41. Villar J, Macao-Meyer N, Perez-Mendez L, et al. Bench-to-bedside review: understanding genetic predisposition to sepsis. Crit Care. 2004;8:180–9.

42. Chen KH, Zeng L, Gu W. Polymorphisms in the toll-like receptor 9 gene associated with sepsis and multiple organ dysfunction after major blunt trauma. Br J Surg. 2011;98(9):1252–9.

43. Henckaerts L, Nielsen KR, Steffensen R, et al. Polymorphisms in innate immunity genes predispose to bacteremia and death in the medical intensive care unit. Crit Care Med. 2009;37(1):192–201. e1–3.

44. Marshall JE, Cook DJ, Christou NV, et al. Multiple organ dysfunction score: a reliable descriptor of a complex clinical outcome. Crit Care Med. 1995;23:1638–52.

45. Gustot T. Multiple organ failure in sepsis: prognosis and role of systemic inflammatory response. Curr Opin Crit Care. 2011;17(2):153–9.

46. Vincent JL, Moreno R, Takala J, et al. The SOFA (sepsis-related organ failure assessment) score to describe organ dysfunction/failure. Intensive Care Med. 1996;22:707–10.

47. Dewar DC, Butcher NE, King KL, Balogh ZJ. Post injury multiple organ failure. J Trauma. 2011;13:81–91.

48. Zygun DA, Fick KK, Sandham GH, et al. Limited ability of SOFA and MOD scores to discriminate outcome: a prospective evaluation in 1436 patients. Can J Anaesth. 2005;52:302–8.

49. Sauaia A, Moore EE, Johnson JL, et al. Validation of post injury multiple organ failure scores. Shock. 2009;31:438–47.

50. Mizock BA. The multiple organ dysfunction syndrome. Dis Mon. 2009;55:476–526.

51. Vincent JL, Ferreira F, Moreno R. Scoring systems for assessing organ dysfunction and survival. Crit Care Clin. 2000;16(2):353–66.

52. Ferreira AM, Sakr Y. Organ dysfunction: general approach, epidemiology, and organ failure scores. Semin Respir Crit Care Med. 2011;32(5):543–51.

53. Carrico C, Meakins JL, Marshall JC, Fry D, Maier RV. Multiple-organ-failure syndrome. Arch Surg. 1986;121(2):196–208.

54. Bone RC, Balk RA, Cerra FB, et al.; ACCP/SCCM Consensus Conference Committee. Definitions for sepsis and organ failure and guidelines for the use of innovative therapies in sepsis. The ACCP/SCCM Consensus Conference Committee. American College of Chest Physicians/Society of Critical Care Medicine. Chest. 2009;136(5 Suppl):e28.

55. Tiruvoipati R, Ong K, Gangopadhyay H, et al. Hypothermia predicts mortality in critically ill elderly patients with sepsis. BMC Geriatr. 2010;10:70.

56. Balk RA. Severe sepsis and septic shock. Definitions, epidemiology, and clinical manifestations. Crit Care Clin. 2000;16(2):179–92.

57. Wahl WL. SIRS, sepsis and multi-system organ dysfunction. Chapter 61. In: Flint L, Meredith JW, Schwab CW, et al., editors. Trauma: contemporary principles and therapy. 1st ed. Philadelphia: Lippincottt Williams & Wilkins; 2008.

58. Llewelyn M, Cohen J. Diagnosis of infection in sepsis. Intensive Care Med. 2001;27(Suppl):S10–S214.

59. Balk RA, Ely EW, Goyette RE. General principles of sepsis therapy. Sepsis Handbook: Nashville, TN, Vanderbilt University Press; 2003.

60. Wanner GA, Keel M, Steckholzer U. Relationship between procalcitonin plasma levels and severity of injury, sepsis, organ failure, and mortality in injured patients. Crit Care Med. 2000;28:950–7.

61. O'Grady NP, Barie PS, Bartlett JG, et al. Guidelines for evaluation of new fever in critically ill adult patients: 2008 update from the American College of Critical Care Medicine and the Infectious Diseases Society of America. Crit Care Med. 2008;36(4):1330–49.

62. Fry DE, Pearlstein L, Fulton RL, et al. Multiple system organ failure. The role of uncontrolled infection. Arch Surg. 1980;115(2):136–40.

63. Deitch EA. Multiple organ failure: pathophysiology and potential future therapy. Ann Surg. 1992;216:117–34.

64. Beal AL, Cerra FB. Multiple organ failure syndrome in the 1990s: systemic inflammatory response and organ dysfunction. JAMA. 1994;271:226–33.

65. Mundy LM, Doherty GM. Chapter 8. Inflammation, infection, and antimicrobial therapy. In: Doherty GM, editor. Current diagnosis and treatment: surgery. 13th ed. New York: McGraw-Hill; 2010.

66. Moore FA, Sauaia A, Moore EE, et al. Postinjury multiple organ failure: a bimodal phenomenon. J Trauma. 1996;40:501–12.

67. Ciesla DJ, Moore EE, Johnson JL, et al. Multiple organ dysfunction during resuscitation is not postinjury multiple organ failure. Arch Surg. 2004;139:590–5.

68. Deitch EA. Bacterial translocation or lymphatic drainage of toxic products from the gut: what is important in human beings? Surgery. 2002;131:241–4.

69. Jastrow KM, Gonzalex EA, McGuire MF, et al. Early cytokine production risk stratifies trauma patients for multiple organ failure. J Am Coll Surg. 2009;209:320–31.

70. Maier B, Lefering R, Lehnert M, et al. Early versus late onset of multiple organ failure is associated with differing patterns of plasma cytokine biomarker expression and outcome after severe trauma. Shock. 2007;28(6):668–74.

71. Giannoudis PV. Current concepts of the inflammatory response after major trauma: an update. Injury. 2003;34:397–404.

72. Tsukamoto T, Chanthaphavong RS, Pape HC. Current theories on the pathophysiology of multiple organ failure after trauma. Injury. 2010;41:21–6.

73. Deitch EA. What's new in general surgery? Ann Surg. 1992;216(2):117–24.

74. Watkins A, Deitch EA. Systemic inflammatory response syndrome and multiple-organ dysfunction syndrome: definition, diagnosis, and management. In: Asensio J, Trunkey DD, editors. Current therapy of trauma and surgical critical care. 1st ed. Philadelphia: Mosby; 2008. p. 663–9.

75. Werdan K. Pathophysiology of septic shock and multiple organ dysfunction syndrome and various therapeutic approaches with special emphasis on immunoglobulins. Ther Apher. 2001;5(2):115–22.

76. Dewar D, Moore FA, Moore EE, et al. Postinjury multiple organ failure. Injury. 2009;40(9):912–8.

77. Deitch EA. Gut-origin sepsis: evolution of a concept, the surgeon. 2012. http://www.sciencedirect.com/science/article/pii/S1479666X12000339. Accessed 15 May 2012.

78. Adams CA, Hauser CJ, Adams JM, et al. Trauma-hemorrhage-induced neutrophil priming is prevented by mesenteric lymph duct ligation. Shock. 2002;18(6):513–7.

79. Botha AJ, Moore FA, Moore EE, et al. Postinjury neutrophil priming and activation states: therapeutic challenges. Shock. 1995;3(3):157–66.

80. Deitch EA. Multiple organ failure. Pathophysiology and potential future therapy. Ann Surg. 1992;216(2):117–34.

81. Vincent JL, Sakr Y, Sprung CL, et al. Sepsis in European intensive care units: results of the SOAP study. Crit Care Med. 2006;34:344–53.

82. Fry DE. Sepsis, systemic inflammatory response, and multiple organ dysfunction: the mystery continues. Am Surg. 2012;78(1):1–8.

83. Windsor JA, Schweder P. Chapter 37. Complications of acute pancreatitis (including pseudocysts). In: Ashley SW, Zinner MJ, editors. Maingot's abdominal operations. 11th ed. New York: McGraw-Hill; 2007.

84. Bernard GR, Artigas A, Brigham KL, et al. The American-European consensus conference on ARDS. Definitions, mechanisms, relevant outcomes and clinical trial coordination. Am J Respir Crit Care Med. 1994;149:818.

85. Marshall JC. Multiple organ dysfunction syndrome. In: ACS surgery: principles and practice. Chapter 13. http://www.acssurgery.com/acs/pdf/ACS0813.pdf. Accessed 13 April 2012.

86. The Acute Respiratory Distress Syndrome Network. Ventilation with lower tidal volumes for acute lung injury and the acute respiratory distress syndrome. N Engl J Med. 2000;342:1301–8.

87. Curley G, Hayes M, Laffey JG. Can 'permissive' hypercapnia modulate the severity of sepsis-induced ALI/ARDS? Crit Care. 2011;15(2):212.

88. Kozar RA, Weisbrodt NW, Moore FA. Chapter 64. Gastrointestinal failure. In: Moore EE, Feliciano DV, Mattox KL, editors. Trauma. 6th ed. New York: McGraw-Hill; 2008.

89. Balogh Z, McKinley BA, Cocanour CS, et al. Both primary and secondary abdominal compartment syndrome can be predicted early and are harbingers of multiple organ failure. J Trauma. 2003;54:848.

90. Raeburn CD, Moore EE, Biffl WL, et al. The abdominal compartment syndrome is a morbid complication of postinjury damage control surgery. Am J Surg. 2001;182:542.

91. Cerra FB, West M, Billiar TR, Holman RT, et al. Hepatic dysfunction in multiple systems organ failure as a manifestation of altered cell–cell interaction. Prog Clin Biol Res. 1989;308:563–73.

92. Dhainaut JF, Marin N, Mignon A, et al. Hepatic response to sepsis: interaction between coagulation and inflammatory processes. Crit Care Med. 2001;29(7 Suppl):S42–S7.

93. Schiffl H, Lang SM, Fischer R. Daily hemodialysis and the outcome of acute renal failure. N Engl J Med. 2002;346(5):305–10.

94. Wohlauer MV, Sauaia A, Moore EE, et al. Acute kidney injury and posttrauma multiple organ failure: the canary in the coal mine. J Trauma Acute Care Surg. 2012;72(2):373–8.

95. Vinsonneau C, Camus C, Combes A, et al.; Hemodiafe Study Group. Continuous venovenous haemodiafiltration versus intermittent haemodialysis for acute renal failure in patients with multiple-organ dysfunction syndrome: a multicentre randomised trial. Lancet. 2006;368(9533):379–85.

96. Flierl MA, Rittirsch D, Huber-Lang MS, et al. Molecular events in the cardiomyopathy of sepsis. Mol Med. 2008;14(5–6):327–36.

97. Lorts A, Burroughs T, Shanley T. Elucidating the role of reversible protein phosphorylation in sepsis-induced myocardial dysfunction. Shock. 2009;32(1):49–54.

98. Rudiger A, Singer M. Mechanisms of sepsis-induced cardiac dysfunction. Crit Care Med. 2007;35(6):1599–608.

99. Zanotti-Cavazzoni SL, Hollenberg SM. Cardiac dysfunction in severe sepsis and septic shock. Curr Opin Crit Care. 2009;15(5):392–7.

100. Flynn A, Chokkalingam Mani B, Mather PJ. Sepsis-induced cardiomyopathy: a review of pathophysiologic mechanisms. Heart Fail Rev. 2010;15(6):605–11.

101. Treggiari MM, Karir V, Yanez ND, et al. Intensive insulin therapy and mortality in critically ill patients. Crit Care. 2008;12:R29.

102. Van den Berghe G, Wouters P, Weekers F, et al. Intensive insulin therapy in critically ill patients. N Engl J Med. 2001;345:1359–67.

103. Van den Berghe G, Wilmer A, Hermans G, et al. Intensive insulin therapy in the medical ICU. N Engl J Med. 2006;354:449–61.

104. Egi M, Finfer S, Bellomo R. Glycemic control in the ICU. Chest. 2011;140(1):212–20.

105. Dellinger RP, Levy MM, Carlet JM, Bion J, Parker MM, Jaeschke R, et al. Surviving sepsis campaign: international guidelines for management of severe sepsis and septic shock: 2008. Crit Care Med. 2008;36:296–327.

106. Marik PE. The diagnosis of adrenal insufficiency in the critically ill patient: does it really matter? Crit Care. 2006;10(6):176.

107. Dellinger RP, Levy MM, Carlet JM, Bion J, et al. Surviving sepsis campaign: international guidelines for management of severe sepsis and septic shock: 2008. Crit Care Med. 2008;36:296–327.

108. Warkentin TE. Heparin-induced thrombocytopenia in critically ill patients. Crit Care Clin. 2011;27(4):805–23.

109. Warkentin TE, Greinacher A, Koster A et al.; American College of Chest Physicians. Treatment and prevention of heparin-induced thrombocytopenia: American College of Chest Physicians Evidence-Based Clinical Practice Guidelines (8th Edition). Chest. 2008;133(6 Suppl):340S.

110. Asare K. Anemia of critical illness. Pharmacotherapy. 2008;28(10):1267–82.

111. Eidelman LA, Putterman D, Putterman C, Sprung CL. The spectrum of septic encephalopathy. Definitions, etiologies, and mortalities. JAMA. 1996;275:470–3.

112. Sharshar T, Polito A, Checinski A. Septic-associated encephalopathy—everything starts at a microlevel. Crit Care. 2010;14(5):199.

113. Mizock BA, Sabelli HC, Dubin A, et al. Septic encephalopathy. Evidence for altered phenylalanine metabolism and comparison with hepatic encephalopathy. Arch Intern Med. 1990;150(2):443–9.

114. Zampieri FG, Park M, Machado FS, et al. Sepsis-associated encephalopathy: not just delirium. Clinics. 2011;66(10):1825–31.

115. Rivers E, Nguyen B, Havstad S, et al. Early goal-directed therapy in the treatment of severe sepsis and septic shock. N Engl J Med. 2001;345:1368–77.

116. Bakker J, Gris P, Coffernils M, et al. Serial blood lactate levels can predict the development of multiple organ failure following septic shock. Am J Surg. 1996;171:221–6.

117. Manikis P, Jankowski S, Zhang H, et al. Correlation of serial blood lactate levels to organ failure and mortality after trauma. Am J Emerg Med. 1995;13:619–22.

118. Abramson D, Scalea TM, Hitchcock R, et al. Lactate clearance and survival following injury. J Trauma. 1993;35:584–9.

119. Landry DW, Levin HR, Gallant EM, et al. Vasopressin deficiency contributes to the vasodilation of septic shock. Circulation. 1997;95:1122–5.

120. Blot F, Schmidt E, Nitenberg G, et al. Earlier positivity of central venous versus peripheral blood cultures is highly predictive of catheter-related sepsis. J Clin Microbiol. 1998;36:105–9.

121. Kumar A, Roberts D, Wood KE, et al. Duration of hypotension before initiation of effective antimicrobial therapy is the critical determinant of survival in human septic shock. Crit Care Med. 2006;34:1589–96.

122. Burch JM, Ortiz VB, Richardson RJ, et al. Abbreviated laparotomy and planned reoperation for critically injured patients. Ann Surg. 1992;215:476–83.

123. Annane D, Sebille V, Charpentier C, Bollaert PE, et al. Effect of treatment with low doses of hydrocortisone and fludrocortisone on mortality in patients with septic shock. J Am Med Assoc. 2002;288:862–71.

124. Sprung CL, Annane D, Keh D, et al. Hydrocortisone therapy for patients with septic shock. N Engl J Med. 2008;358:111–24.

125. Moore LJ, Moore FA. Early management of sepsis, severe sepsis, and septic shock in the surgical patient. In: ACS surgery: principles and practice. Chapter 4. http://www.acpmedicine.com/bcdecker/pdfs/acs/part08_ch04.pdf. Assessed 10 April 2012.

126. Casserly B, Gerlach H, Phillips GS, et al. Evaluating the use of recombinant human activated protein C in adult severe sepsis: results of the Surviving Sepsis Campaign. Crit Care Med. 2012;40(5):1417–26.

127. Bernard GR, Vincent JL, Laterre PF, et al. The recombinant human activated protein C worldwide evaluation in Severe Sepsis (PROWESS) Study Group. N Engl J Med. 2001;344:699–709.

128. Toussaint S, Gerlach H. Activated protein C for sepsis. N Engl J Med. 2009;361:2646–52.

129. Martí-Carvajal AJ, Solà I, Lathyris D, et al. Human recombinant activated protein C for severe sepsis. Cochrane Database Syst Rev. 2011;(4):CD004388.

130. Martí-Carvajal AJ, Solà I, Lathyris D, et al. Human recombinant activated protein C for severe sepsis. Cochrane Database Syst Rev. 2012;3:CD004388.

131. Vincent JL. Metabolic support in sepsis and multiple organ failure: more questions than answers. Crit Care Med. 2007;35(9 Suppl):S436–S40.

132. Artinian V, Krayem H, DiGiovine B. Effects of early enteral feeding on the outcome of critically ill mechanically ventilated medical patients. Chest. 2006;129:960–7.

133. Gadek JE, DeMichele SJ, Karlstad MD, et al. Effect of enteral feeding with eicosapentaenoic acid, gamma-linolenic acid, and antioxidants in patients with acute respiratory distress syndrome. Enteral Nutrition in ARDS Study Group. Crit Care Med. 1999;27:1409–20.

134. Galban C, Montejo JC, Mesejo A, et al. An immune-enhancing enteral diet reduces mortality rate and episodes of bacteremia in septic intensive care unit patients. Crit Care Med. 2000;28:643–8.

135. Bertolini G, Iapichino G, Radrizzani D, et al. Early enteral immunonutrition in patients with severe sepsis: results of an interim analysis of a randomized multicentre clinical trial. Intensive Care Med. 2003;29:834–40.

136. Marik PE. Arginine: Too much of a good thing may be bad! Crit Care Med. 2006;34:2844–7.

137. Kreymann KG, Berger MM, Deutz NE, et al. ESPEN guidelines on enteral nutrition: intensive care. Clin Nutr. 2006;25:210–23.

Brittany Busse and Christine S. Cocanour

Introduction

Acute lung injury (ALI) is a spectrum of pulmonary insufficiency ranging from minor and easily correctable hypoxemia to severe refractory respiratory failure or acute respiratory distress syndrome (ARDS). The American-European Consensus Conference on ARDS in 1994 defined ALI as "a syndrome of inflammation and increased permeability that is associated with a constellation of clinical, radiologic, and physiologic abnormalities that cannot be explained by, but may coexist with, left atrial or pulmonary capillary hypertension" [1]. The resultant pulmonary insufficiency can be an indirect result of a systemic inflammatory state (circulating inflammatory mediators causing reactivity and edema in the lung parenchyma), or a direct result of a localized release of inflammatory mediators from a process affecting the lung parenchyma such as blunt chest trauma, toxic inhalation, aspiration, or pneumonia. Factors increasing a patient's likelihood of developing ALI are those that predispose a patient to massive inflammation, as well as increasing age, preexisting need for mechanical ventilation, smoke inhalation, massive transfusion, and drug overdose.

Pulmonary insufficiency of shock, trauma, and sepsis can be a frustrating challenge for physicians caring for postsurgical or post-trauma patients. The overall incidence of ALI in hospitalized patients is estimated to be 86.2 cases per 100,000 person years. Its development leads to increased immediate and long-term health care costs. In the acute period, the associated costs of ALI are the result of an increase in ventilator days, and both intensive care unit (ICU) and hospital lengths of stay. Patients with ALI spend a median of 5.3 days on the mechanical ventilator, 7.8 days in the ICU, and 14.0 days in the hospital [2]. Long-term costs are those associated with disability following severe ALI including those related to the care of post-traumatic stress disorder, asthma, and impairment in pulmonary function, cognitive dysfunction, and prolonged rehabilitation. Although mortality from severe acute respiratory failure is decreasing, it remains substantial with estimates ranging from 34 to 64% and it is often secondary to multi-organ failure (MOF) rather than a direct result of pulmonary insufficiency [3].

Clinical Presentation

ALI is a disease of acute, diffuse lung inflammation that can arise secondary to a variety of clinical insults. It can be the direct result of local pulmonary injury such as lung contusion, aspiration of gastric contents, or pneumonia, or it can result indirectly from an extra-pulmonary process such as gram-negative sepsis, shock, or acute pancreatitis. A combination of atelectasis and the physiologic response of the lung parenchyma to inflammation results in mild to severe pulmonary insufficiency. Surgical patients are especially at risk for respiratory insufficiency due to a combination of hypoventilation (either due to over-narcotization or splinting secondary to postoperative pain) and a pro-inflammatory state. Whatever the inciting factor, the progression of ALI begins with infiltration and sequestration of inflammatory cells within the lung interstitial and alveolar spaces. These inflammatory cells, as well as the pulmonary parenchymal cells, release a variety of inflammatory mediators, cytokines, and toxic metabolites which result in the manifestations of ALI—vascular leakage of proteinaceous exudate, fibrin deposition, coagulation, and atelectasis. Further discussion of the inflammatory mediators and clinical phases of ALI is provided in the "Pathophysiology" section of this chapter.

The primary pulmonary pathology associated with the clinical presentation is atelectasis and acute, non-cardiogenic pulmonary edema. Atelectasis results initially from hypoventilation and then progresses due to both decreased compliance and increased fibroproliferation of collagen and scarring of the lung parenchyma. Secondarily, decreased surfactant production leads to poor gas exchange, decreased compliance, and

B. Busse, M.D. • C.S. Cocanour, M.D., F.A.C.S., F.C.C.M. (✉)
Department of Surgery, University of California Davis Medical School, 2315 Stockton Blvd., Sacramento, CA 95818, USA
e-mail: christine.cocanour@ucdmc.ucdavis.edu

L.J. Moore et al. (eds.), *Common Problems in Acute Care Surgery*,
DOI 10.1007/978-1-4614-6123-4_8, © Springer Science+Business Media New York 2013

a tendency towards atelectasis. Pulmonary edema is a result of the increased permeability of the alveolar-capillary membrane secondary to the localized and systemic release of inflammatory mediators. In combination, edema and atelectasis lead to worsening pulmonary compliance resulting in the restriction of oxygenation and ventilation.

Following the establishment of edema and atelectasis within the lung parenchyma, clinical signs and symptoms of ALI begin to develop. The clinical presentation of ALI is one of the hypoxemic respiratory failures as compared to hypercapnic respiratory failure. There are five broad categories of hypoxemic respiratory failure: decreased FiO_2, hypoventilation, shunt, ventilation/perfusion (V/Q) mismatch, and diffusion limitation. The hypoxemia of ALI is primarily that of shunt with a component of diffusion limitation. Hypoxemia stimulates the carotid body chemoreceptors resulting in the activation of the sympathetic nervous system. This leads to a constellation of clinical signs including tachycardia, diaphoresis, systemic vasoconstriction, and tachypnea, which causes the initial hypocapnia. As inflammation increases, airway resistance increases and lung compliance decreases secondary to edema and airway constriction. This leads to decreased expiratory flow, decreased functional residual capacity, and increased intrinsic positive end-expiratory pressure (PEEP). The patient increases his or her work of breathing in order to compensate for the increased airway resistance and decreased pulmonary compliance. Eventually, the patient begins to suffer respiratory muscle fatigue which results in the propagation of atelectasis and air-trapping. As carbon dioxide (CO_2) is trapped in the alveoli and the patient hypoventilates due to fatigue, this results in the hypercapnia characteristic of progressive pulmonary insufficiency. Therefore, in ALI, hypercapnia is a secondary problem that arises late in the course of respiratory failure.

Pathophysiology

Inflammation is part of the body's normal response to pathogens or injury that results in leukocyte recruitment and activation, vasodilatation, and increased vascular permeability. The clinical presentation of atelectasis and diffuse non-cardiogenic pulmonary edema that is characteristic of ALI and ARDS results from excessive activation and dysregulation of the physiologic inflammatory response. Increased transcription and release of inflammatory mediators from sites of injury or infection as well as from within the lung parenchyma lead to the progression of ALI to ARDS. This section provides a discussion of factors that contribute to the clinical presentation of ALI, an overview of certain molecular compounds that have been shown to play a role in the progression of ALI, as well as a short overview of the inciting factors in transfusion-related acute lung injury (TRALI)—a similar but distinctly different entity in the spectrum of ALI.

Atelectasis

Postsurgical patients and patients who have sustained traumatic injury are at a significant risk for atelectasis because of their impaired ability to maintain adequate inspiratory volumes. Alveolar collapse leads to activation of alveolar macrophages and the release of locally and systemically acting cytokines such as interleukin-1 (IL-1). Collapse of alveoli also results in a pro-coagulant state within the lung parenchyma and the development of microthrombi within the pulmonary vasculature. Tissue factor is present in alveolar macrophages and endothelial cells and increased production is readily induced by bacterial endotoxin in a model of sepsis and ALI [4]. Tissue factor is the initiator of the extrinsic pathway of coagulation, the end product of which is fibrin. Alveolar fibrin deposition is characteristic of ALI and represents a derangement of normal wound healing and a loss of fibrinolytic function. Increased translocation of pro-coagulant factors and infiltration of fibroblasts into the interstitial and alveolar space lead to increased collagen deposition. Examination of the bronchoalveolar lavage (BAL) fluid in patients with ARDS demonstrates increased amounts of fibrin and pro-coagulant factors that remain elevated for several weeks following the initial injury [4].

Accelerated remodeling of intracellular and extracellular fibrin deposits results in impaired gas exchange and decreased pulmonary compliance. Coagulation and fibroproliferation with collagen deposition result in scarring of the lung parenchyma and the propagation of atelectasis. This response is usually transient but organization and remodeling can occur, leading to permanent scarring of the lung parenchyma, and chronic impairment in lung function.

Inflammatory Cytokines

The body's response to injury and infection involves the transcription and release of numerous cytokines that act both locally and systemically leading to acute inflammation. Several of these cytokines have been shown to play a specific role in the pathophysiology of ALI. These cytokines include IL-1, interleukin-8 (IL-8), tissue necrosis factor-alpha (TNF-α), transforming growth factor-beta (TGF-β), thromboxane A2, and thrombin (Table 8.1).

The predominant form of IL-1 in humans is IL-1β. Interleukin-1β is released from alveolar macrophages in response to atelectasis and acts locally on endothelial and vascular epithelial cells to promote inflammation, increased vascular permeability, and apoptosis. IL-1β is considered to be the central mediator of inflammatory injury in ALI.

IL-8 is a neutrophil chemoattractant and activating agent that results in neutrophil degranulation, increased respiratory burst activity, and increased neutrophil aggregation by up regulation of adhesion molecules [5]. In response to IL-8 and cytokine induction, neutrophils readily cross into the pulmonary parenchyma during many types of inflammatory states

Table 8.1 Cytokines in acute lung injury

Cytokine	Action
IL-1β (beta)	Increased vascular permeability and apoptosis of epithelial cells
IL-8	Increased neutrophil aggregation and activation
TNF-α (alpha)	Induction of inflammation, cachexia, and increased transcription of cytokines
TGF-β (beta)	Increased transcription of pro-inflammatory cytokines and integrins
TXA2	Increased aggregation and activation of platelets
Thrombin	Increased vascular permeability, increased expression of cytokines, increased recruitment of inflammatory cells

including sepsis, ischemia/reperfusion injury, hemorrhage, and hypovolemic shock. The aggregation and activation of neutrophils within the lung parenchyma is an important contributor to the development of ALI. The necessity of neutrophil activation to the development of ALI has been demonstrated by experiments in which neutrophils are eliminated before injury occurs [6]. It is further demonstrated by the attenuation of the severity of ALI in neutropenic patients as compared to patients with normal leukocytes. Acute neutrophilic alveolitis is defined as an increased concentration of neutrophils in the alveolar fluid leading to inflammation and increased leakage of fluid between epithelial tight junctions [6]. Neutrophils also release proteases into the alveolar fluid that in normal wound healing function in cell growth, remodeling, and repair; however, in ALI excessive activity can result in cell death and tissue injury. One of these proteases, neutrophil elastase, degrades collagen and elastin resulting in the breakdown of the endothelial vascular barrier.

TNF-α is released from both macrophages and endothelial cells of the lung in response to bacterial endotoxin and IL-1. Its systemic effects include the induction of fever and up regulation of catabolic processes resulting in cachexia. The primary action of TNF-α in ALI is the regulation of immune cells and induction of inflammation through the increased transcription and release of other inflammatory mediators such as IL-1 and nuclear factor-kappa B (NF-κB [kappa beta]). NF-κB is a transcription factor that acts on enhancer/promoter regions that are located on genes known to produce cytokines as well as other immunoregulatory molecules [6].

TGF-β is generated in response to tissue injury. Of its three isoforms, it is TGF-β1 that is present in its inactive form in endothelial cells and contributes to the progression to fibrosis in ALI. The activation of TGF-β signaling pathways results in induction of many genes including those that contribute to fibrosis after lung injury, increased endothelial cell permeability, and decreased ion and fluid transport contributing to increased pulmonary edema [7, 8]. All cells in the body have receptors for TGF-β and activation of these receptors results in a signaling pathway that modulates the transcription of genes for pro-inflammatory factors such as

TNF-α and IL-1 by a protein kinase-linked mechanism. Other functions of TGF-β include the increased transcription and expression of integrins that result in increased transmigration of fibroblasts, macrophages, and neutrophils into sites of inflammation [8].

Platelets play a key role in inflammation associated with ALI. Neutrophil activation results in the sequestration of platelets within the lungs. These activated platelets release thromboxane A2, which is a pro-inflammatory cytokine. Thromboxane A2 is a derivative of arachidonic acid through the action of cyclooxygenase that contributes to thrombosis of the microvasculature by increasing the activation and aggregation of platelets. Activated platelets also release prostaglandins, prostacyclins, and leukotrienes—all of which play a role in acute inflammation and increased vascular permeability.

Thrombin is not only a pro-coagulant factor but also acts to propagate lung injury in ALI by regulation of cellular contraction, thus increasing vascular permeability, increasing the expression of inflammatory mediators, and increasing chemotaxis and transendothelial migration of neutrophils and other inflammatory cells [9].

Non-cardiogenic Pulmonary Edema and Endothelial Layer Disruption

Development of pulmonary edema results from changes in oncotic pressure across the endothelial–epithelial membrane. An increase in the leakage of proteins into the interstitial and alveolar space results in fluid shifts and the accumulation of exudative edema fluid within the airways. The usual barrier function is maintained by a single layer of vascular endothelial cells that are joined together by proteins called adherens that form tight junctions between cells. This single cell layer forms the basis for gas exchange as well as regulates permeability to water and electrolytes. Inflammatory mediators cause dysfunction in this barrier by disrupting adherens.

Calcium diffusion across the cell membrane and through disrupted tight junctions results in propagation of inflammatory signals across gap junctions and also functions in the activation of myosin light-chain kinase (MLCK). Increased expression of MLCK contributes to the rearrangement of actin and increased actin–myosin interactions that result in contraction of cells, increased permeability to proteins and fluids, and increased transmigration of neutrophils into the alveoli. MLCK knockout models result in decreased pulmonary edema and reduced nitric oxide, reactive oxygen species, and vascular permeability implicating an interaction between MLCK and paracrine signaling pathways in ALI [10].

Nitric oxide release from endothelial cells and neutrophils is also increased in response to inflammation. Nitric oxide is a potent vasodilator and at high concentrations is toxic to endothelial cells. Nitric oxide synthase expression is increased in response to pulmonary inflammation and sepsis [11].

Apoptosis

Endothelial cell dysfunction alone does not result in pulmonary edema, but a combination of endothelial dysfunction with disruption of the epithelial cell layer results in massive pulmonary edema characteristic of ARDS and life-threatening hypoxemia. The epithelial layer provides a substantial barrier to the accumulation of fluid within the airspace and also functions in the active clearance of fluid by the up regulation of Na/K-ATPase. In the acute inflammatory phase several factors favor apoptosis of epithelial cells including decreased surfactant, increased TGF-β, and increased activity of angiotensin-converting enzyme leading to increased production of angiotensin II.

Normally there is a balance between pro-apoptotic and anti-apoptotic factors within the lungs. Fas and fas ligand (FasL) are regulators of apoptosis in epithelial cells. Increases in the expression of Fas have been demonstrated in experimental models of lung inflammation secondary to exposure to endotoxin. Increases in the amount of FasL in the BAL fluid of patients with ALI are associated with a poor prognosis [12] and survivors of ALI have been demonstrated to have significantly lower levels of FasL in BAL fluid samples compared to non-survivors [13]. Caspase-3 is an executioner protein that is upregulated in Fas-mediated apoptosis [13]. Jo2 is a potentiator of Fas that favors epithelial cell apoptosis, neutrophilic inflammation, and increased permeability in experimental models of ALI [12].

The over-expression of Her 2, a tyrosine kinase receptor expressed in pulmonary epithelial cells, has also been shown to play an active role in epithelial cell barrier disruption. Activation of Her 2 through interactions with IL-1 by A disintegrin and metalloproteinase 17 (ADAM 17) and neuroregulin-1-dependent mechanism during inflammation results in barrier disintegration in an experimental model of ALI [14].

Injury to the epithelial barrier has three direct consequences: (1) it contributes to alveolar fluid accumulation through loss of barrier function; (2) the damage to type II pneumocytes leads to loss of adequate surfactant production; (3) and disorganized repair leads to fibrosis and scarring [8]. Loss of the epithelial layer through apoptosis results in edema, hemorrhage, and increase in proteinaceous fluid accumulation within the remaining alveoli.

Transfusion-Related Acute Lung Injury

Although the clinical presentation of TRALI is nearly identical to other forms of ALI there are a few key differences in the pathophysiology. Patient-related risk factors for TRALI include recent surgery, active infections, and hematologic malignancies. A two-hit theory of inflammatory response to transfusion has been proposed as a mechanism for TRALI [15]. The first event involves priming of neutrophils to induce ALI in response to the major histocompatability complex (MHC) class I antibody by bacterial endotoxin, sepsis, or even stress of surgery. The second hit develops in response to anti-leukocyte antibodies contained within the blood products

Table 8.2 Diagnostic criteria for ARDS

American-European consensus committee diagnostic criteria for ALI and ARDS
PaO_2/FiO_2 <300 (ALI) or <200 (ARDS)
Absence of cardiogenic pulmonary edema
Diffuse bilateral patchy infiltrates on chest radiograph

with resultant activation of neutrophils and aggregation within the lung parenchyma in a manner similar to other forms of ALI. This theory is supported by the fact that donor-related risk factors include plasma from donors exposed to class I antibodies, including plasma from female donors who may have been exposed to antibodies during pregnancy. For this reason most blood banking centers restrict plasma donations to male donors and as a result, the incidence of TRALI has significantly decreased.

Diagnosis

The diagnosis of ALI is made based on the consensus criteria established by the American-European Consensus Committee shown in Table 8.2. Additionally, for TRALI, the patient must develop ALI within 6 hours of receiving blood products.

Experimentally, researchers have utilized positron emission tomography (PET) in the diagnosis of ALI. PET scanning has been shown to be useful in delineation of several of the pathophysiologic characteristics of ALI and can be used to elucidate the heterogeneity of diseased lung parenchyma. Currently there are three areas of pathophysiologic interest that have been elucidated using PET scanning: the aggregation of activated neutrophils within the diseased lung parenchyma, fluid movement and vascular permeability, and ventilation and perfusion. Because the metabolic activity of neutrophils can be measured using fluorodeoxyglucose (^{18}F) [16], PET scanning can be used to localize aggregates of activated neutrophils within the lung parenchyma in patients with ALI. Fluid movement and vascular permeability can be measured using radiolabeled transferrin. Finally, ventilation and perfusion can be measured using radiolabeled nitrogen (inspired and intravenous, respectively) [17]. Although it is of significant interest to investigational researchers, PET scanning is not currently utilized clinically.

Management

When managing ALI, it is important to have a systematic approach with the goal of improving oxygenation and pulmonary compliance while diminishing morbidity and ultimately improving survivability. The management of ALI in surgical patients begins with the prevention of the causative factors that contribute to its development, most notably atelectasis and systemic inflammatory response syndrome (SIRS).

Basic Principles

As noted previously, atelectasis is a common problem in surgical patients due to the compounding effects of preoperative pulmonary conditions and postoperative pain. Thus adequate management of postoperative pain is of paramount importance, as is maintaining adequate lung volumes for oxygenation but without inducing barotrauma. Appropriate pain control includes early identification of patients who may benefit from epidural analgesia, appropriate usage of patient-controlled analgesia, and early transition to oral analgesia to provide steady-state pain control. Other conditions that can limit chest wall excursion and exacerbate atelectasis include abdominal compartment syndrome, rib fractures, and burns to the thorax. Appropriate intervention would include early decompressive laparotomy, rib fracture plating, and escharotomy as indicated. Prevention of atelectasis in surgical patients can also be accomplished through appropriate training in incentive spirometry (IS) and early involvement of the respiratory therapist for patients determined to be at high risk based on the type of surgery and preoperative pulmonary comorbidities. Respiratory therapists can provide additional recruitment maneuvers to awake, spontaneously breathing patients that result in improvement in the functional residual capacity (FRC) with improved oxygenation and ventilation. These maneuvers serve as an adjunct to IS or as a replacement in patients unable to adequately perform IS due to cognitive or physical limitations. Intermittent positive pressure breathing (IPPB) with systems including the Acapella valve (Smith Medical, St. Paul, MN) and EZPAP (Smith Medical, St. Paul, MN) makes IPPB easier for patients to perform and tolerate. These devices each contains an inspiratory valve and expiratory resistance dial and results in hyperinflation of the lungs, thus increasing lung capacity. Respiratory therapists can also provide chest physiotherapy with the goals of improving respiratory efficiency, expansion of the lungs, strengthening of the respiratory muscles, and elimination of secretions.

Trauma and sepsis are the most common causes of SIRS in the acute care surgery patient. Early goal-directed therapy for sepsis is paramount in preventing ARDS. Risk factors for the development of ALI in patients with sepsis due to infectious extra-pulmonary processes are delayed goal-directed resuscitation and delayed antibiotic treatment. Appropriate identification of the etiology of sepsis and therapy tailored to provide adequate source control is of utmost importance. Identification of patients presenting with clinical signs and symptoms of systemic inflammation and appropriate initiation of treatment at the earliest time point has been associated with improved outcomes. The definition of SIRS is outlined in Table 8.3. The treatment of SIRS is directed at the inciting cause as well as appropriate supportive care that may

Table 8.3 Systemic inflammatory response syndrome (SIRS)

Diagnosis of the systemic inflammatory response syndrome
Any two of the following:
Temperature <36 °C or >38 °C
Heart rate >90 bpm
Respiratory rate >20 bpm
WBC <4,000/mm^3 or <12,000/mm^3
Or >10% bands

include broad-spectrum antibiotics, appropriate fluid resuscitation, and close cardiac monitoring as indicated whether by invasive means (pulmonary artery catheterization) or noninvasive means (cardiac and inferior vena cava ultrasound, impedance…), as well as early, appropriate source control.

The prevention of MOF is the main indicator of survivability in ARDS. Numerous studies have concluded that death in ARDS is directly attributable to MOF rather than refractory hypoxemia, and that improvement in oxygenation does not necessarily predict a better outcome. A large international study determined that disease severity and MOF were the strongest independent predictors of death from ARDS [18].

In patients presenting with mild hypoxemia and risk factors for ALI, appropriate administration of noninvasive ventilatory support is indicated. This can include continuous positive airway pressure (CPAP) and bilevel positive airway pressure (BiPAP) as appropriate. However careful monitoring of patients undergoing these interventions is important as rapidly progressive and treatment-refractory hypoxemia is most often imminent. These interventions may also be contraindicated in patients with recent upper gastrointestinal anastomoses if nasogastric decompression cannot be adequately maintained.

Standard Mechanical Ventilation Using a Lung Protective Strategy

Paramount to the treatment of ALI and ARDS is support with mechanical ventilation. Although invasive mechanical ventilation is often necessary for adequate oxygenation in cases of ALI and ARDS, it can exacerbate pulmonary parenchymal injury and complicate the care of patients. Shear forces associated with high-lung-volume ventilation cause damage to alveolar epithelial cell membranes leading to disruption and necrosis. Spillage of intracellular contents into the extracellular milieu potentiates the influx of inflammatory cells and cytokines in the pulmonary parenchyma. This repeated overdistention of the alveolar units and shearing injury due to volutrauma and barotrauma is known as ventilator-induced lung injury (VILI), which can exacerbate both ALI and MOF by increasing the release and dissemination of inflammatory mediators within the body and may increase translocation of

Table 8.4 ARDS network lung-protective ventilation

ARDS network lung-protective ventilation criteria
Tidal volume 6 ml/kg
FiO_2 <60 mmHg
PEEP at an adequate level to keep PaO_2 between 50 and 80 mmHg
Inspiratory plateau pressures <30 mmHg

bacteria from the lungs into the systemic circulation. The prevention of VILI has become the cornerstone of what is known as lung-protective ventilation for patients with ALI (Table 8.4). Lung-protective ventilation as described by the ARDS Net lung protective strategy [19] is defined by low tidal volumes, limited inspiratory plateau and peak pressures, and adequate PEEP to prevent cyclic opening and closing of lung units, thus ameliorating lung stretch and resultant shear injury. PEEP and FiO_2 should be adjusted to keep the PaO_2 between 50 and 80 mmHg. The fraction of inspired oxygen should ultimately be kept below 60% to prevent absorption atelectasis and oxygen toxicity with resultant free radical injury.

Low Tidal Volume

The reduction in tidal volumes for patients on mechanical ventilation in order to prevent complications from ARDS was initially resisted by many clinicians. This was due to concern for patient comfort (compensatory tachypnea), as well as the resultant hypercapnia and respiratory acidosis. The ARDS Net trial definitively demonstrated the morbidity- and mortality-reducing benefits of a low-tidal-volume ventilatory strategy. This was a multicenter randomized controlled trial examining the outcomes of 6 ml/kg tidal volumes versus 12 ml/kg tidal volumes. Overall, patients treated with the lower tidal volume strategy had decreased mortality, increased ventilator free days, and a decreased rate of MOF than their cohorts treated with the higher tidal volume. The reduction in tidal volume also seems to be associated with improvement in the function of the sodium/potassium adenosine triphosphate (Na/K ATPase) transporter [20]. This results in improved Na and water transport across the epithelial–endothelial cell junction and out of the pulmonary parenchyma, resulting in a reduction in pulmonary edema.

Limited Inspiratory Peak and Plateau Pressures

Mechanical ventilation can be based on either volume or pressure controlled parameters. For both strategies, the maintenance of plateau pressures below lung injury thresholds is important for the prevention of barotrauma. The upper limit of inspiratory plateau pressures should be maintained below 30 mmHg. Complications of barotrauma include migration of air into the extra-pulmonary space leading to pneumothorax, pnuemomediastinum, pneumoperitoneum, subcutaneous emphysema, and air embolism [21].

Management of Positive End-Expiratory Pressure

Cyclic recruitment/derecruitment of alveoli can lead to increased activation of neutrophils, promote additional edema secondary to lung epithelial cell injury, and lead to increasing loss of FRC [20]. An open lung strategy focuses on the reduction of cyclic recruitment/derecruitment and atelectrauma. This is accomplished by utilizing optimal levels of PEEP to prevent collapse of alveoli during exhalation. Determination of optimal levels of PEEP using the open lung strategy is based on a curve with two inflection points: the lower inflection point is the theoretical critical opening pressure, also known as P_{flex}, and the higher inflection point is the loss of elastic properties due to overdistention. Setting the PEEP just above the P_{flex} should theoretically maintain the constant opening of alveoli during exhalation. This will result in improvement in the FRC, decreased intrapulmonary shunting, and increased oxygenation capacity.

Salvage Strategies for Mechanical Ventilation

Acute respiratory distress syndrome with refractory hypoxemia affects 7–26% of patients with ARDS and may require interventions in addition to the standard lung-protective ventilatory strategy. When patients fail to improve their oxygenation on standard lung-protective ventilation, there are additional rescue therapies that should be attempted. These include but are not limited to alveolar recruitment maneuvers, prone positioning, inverse inspiratory/expiratory (I:E) ratios, and airway pressure release ventilation (APRV). These interventions should only be undertaken at centers with the availability of adequate treatment modalities, and by physicians and ancillary staff who are comfortable with these modalities.

Before initiation of other strategies it is important to address all other factors that may be complicating oxygen delivery in the patient. Because adequate oxygen delivery is based on maintaining cardiac output and an adequate hemoglobin level, these measures should be addressed prior to instituting any potentially dangerous or costly interventions, especially considering that the data related to these interventions is inconclusive. Efforts should also focus on reducing the overall oxygen demand by addressing systemic inflammation and oxygen consumption.

Alveolar recruitment maneuvers are postulated to assist in the prevention of atelectasis and atelectrauma, thus improving oxygenation/ventilation and preventing VILI by keeping regions of the lung open that would otherwise be collapsed. Specific protocols for recruitment maneuvers vary between institutions but can include increased PEEP or sustained inflation at increased pressure (>40 mmHg) for time periods of about 20–30 seconds or incremental increases in PEEP over a period of several minutes. Studies have shown a clear improvement in oxygenation but no benefit in mortality. Additionally, these benefits do not appear to be sustained over time with progressive declines in oxygenation in the minutes to hours following the maneuver. As of yet, no study has compared recruitment maneuvers to determine which protocol is optimal for improving oxygenation.

Prone positioning, or kinetic therapy, is thought to improve oxygenation by dependent positioning of involved portions of the lungs to improve oxygenation. This allows gravity to redistribute perfusion/ventilation to the dependent portions of the lung. An additional proposed benefit of prone positioning is less compression of the lungs by the heart and abdominal organs, and thus less overall lung collapse. The greatest benefit in oxygenation has been shown in patients who are proned for less than 17 hours a day with frequent repositioning between the prone and supine positions (every few hours), but the benefits tend to diminish as patients are returned to the supine position. Although oxygenation may improve with prone positioning, mortality has not improved. There are also risks associated with prone positioning that include inadvertent extubation, pressure ulcers, and difficulty with positioning. Prone positioning is typically accomplished using a specialized bed such as the Rotoprone ™ (KCI, San Antonio, TX) and availability of this device may be limited.

Inverse I:E ratios of 2:1 can improve oxygenation in mechanically ventilated patients. It is postulated to do so by increasing the intrinsic PEEP and preventing alveolar collapse during exhalation. In its classic form, it was poorly tolerated by spontaneously breathing, awake patients, and therefore required sedation and sometimes neuromuscular blockade. Numerous clinical studies have examined the results of inverse I:E ratios as a salvage maneuver for patients unresponsive to conventional lung-protective ventilatory strategy, and so far the results have been variable with no clear benefit shown.

APRV is a pressure-limited, time-cycled mode of ventilation that results in short periods of reduction in pressure to allow for CO_2 clearance. It is a mode based on spontaneous breathing against a continued high pressure. This continuous recruitment pressure is provided throughout 85–90% of the ventilatory cycle. It is equivalent to inverse I:E ratios but is useful for patients who are spontaneously breathing and prevents the need for sedation and neuromuscular blockade. It can also be used as an alternative to the open lung strategy and is felt to allow for more continuity in recruitment.

High-Frequency Oscillatory Ventilation

High-frequency oscillatory ventilation (HFOV) is considered a rescue strategy for patients unable to adequately oxygenate using conventional modes of mechanical ventilation. Severity criteria for ARDS can be used to determine which patients may benefit from HFOV and include the following:

- FiO_2 >60% and SpO_2 <88% on conventional mechanical ventilation with:
  - PEEP >15 mmHg
  - Plateau pressures >30 mmHg
  - Mean airway pressures >24 mmHg
  - APRV high pressure >35 mmHg
- High-frequency oscillatory ventilation uses a piston-pump oscillating between 3 and 10 Hz to provide inspiratory biased flow at 30–60 l/min. The four variables that can be manipulated to improve oxygenation are mean airway pressure, frequency (lower frequency=increased tidal volume), inspiratory time (typically 33% total cycle), and finally amplitude, which effects chest wall excursion and adequate elimination of CO_2. Oxygenation on HFOV is postulated to occur by Taylor dispersion and molecular diffusion as molecules move at differing velocities in and out of alveoli. The Multi-Center Oscillatory Ventilation for Acute Respiratory Distress Syndrome Trial (MOAT) demonstrated improvement in PaO_2/FiO_2 ratio but the difference did not persist past 24 h [22]. They also demonstrated a reduction in 30-day all-cause mortality but no difference in ventilator-free days or overall liberation from ventilatory support. An additional systematic review completed by Young and colleagues determined that although there is improved oxygenation and ventilation with HFOV in severely hypoxemic patients refractory to conventional ventilatory management, the improvements are transient, lasting only 24–48 h. Additional trials have failed to duplicate the results of the MOAT trial.

Extracorporeal Membrane Oxygenation

Extracorporeal membrane oxygenation (ECMO) or extracorporeal life support (ECLS) is indicated in cases of acute, severe, but potentially reversible cases of ARDS in patients who have failed all other methods to improve oxygenation. It is based on venovenous or venoarterial life support with membrane oxygenation to replace the function of the injured lung. Patients on ECMO are continued on mechanical ventilation using conventional lung protective strategy. The goal is to be able to wean ECMO to moderate ventilator settings. The 2009 CESAR trial (Conventional Ventilatory Support versus Extracorporeal Membrane Oxygenation for Severe Adult Respiratory Failure) documented decreased mortality for patients with refractory hypoxemia and ARDS [23]. Overall, 67% of patients were successfully weaned from ECMO, with an overall 52% survival rate. Prior to this study, ECMO in adult patients was considered a treatment of last resort as survival in adult patients was based solely on case reports. Current survival rates for infants, pediatric, and adult patients on ECMO are stated to be 85%, 74%, and 52%, respectively. It is necessary for patients on ECMO to undergo systemic anticoagulation with heparin. For this reason, the risk of ECLS is primarily associated with uncontrolled bleeding and the potential of hemorrhagic stroke. Newer, smaller, more efficient devices have ameliorated these risks by allowing for less profound anticoagulation. Improved results are also associated with early identification of patients who may benefit from ECMO and careful transport of these patients to centers capable of providing ECMO [24].

Pharmacologic Adjuncts

Numerous pharmacologic adjuncts have been evaluated in ARDS including alprostadil [25], acetylcysteine [26], corticosteroids [27], inhaled nitric oxide [28], and surfactant [29] with only limited mortality benefit [30].

Inhaled nitric oxide results in selective pulmonary vasodilation in well-ventilated segments of the lung. This improves perfusion to less diseased portions of the lung and subsequently improves oxygenation. A large-scale, randomized, placebo-controlled trial carried out in the United States demonstrated improved oxygenation but failed to demonstrate any improvement in mortality or decrease in duration of mechanical ventilation [28]. A follow-up study of ARDS patients surviving low-dose inhaled nitric oxide did show significantly better values for several pulmonary function tests at 6 months post treatment than placebo-treated patients [31].

Similar to nitric oxide, sildenafil is associated with selective pulmonary vasodilation but did not improve oxygenation in ARDS [32].

Trials of NSAIDS to prevent the conversion of arachidonic acid to thromboxane A2 and ameliorate inflammation in the lung parenchyma produced no benefit in patients with ARDS [25].

Corticosteroid administration was thought to be beneficial in combating the inflammation that is the predominant causative factor of lung damage in ALI. It was felt that early mitigation of the inflammatory process should halt the progression of injury. Currently there is no evidence to support this theory. The ARDS Network trial failed to show any improvement in all-cause mortality after a short course of high-dose steroid administration, but it did result in improved oxygenation and improved pulmonary compliance with a resultant increase in ventilator-free days [27]. This was, however, complicated by an overall increase in 60-day and 180-day all-cause mortality in relation to an increase in long-term negative effects and infectious complications. Another study further demonstrated no benefit in all-cause mortality in patients with ARDS due to viral pneumonia who received corticosteroids, and also found that administration of steroids was correlated with an increase in all-cause mortality [33].

Surfactant deficiency is concomitant with ARDS and exacerbates atelectasis and atelectrauma. Exogenous surfactant replacement therapy is a standard of care in infants with neonatal lung disease, but this has been shown to be of little benefit in adult patients. So far no surfactant studies have shown an improvement in mortality in an adult population with ARDS but it is still considered as part of salvage therapy for patients who are failing to improve despite maximization of other strategies [34].

Because ARDS is associated with microthrombi and a pro-coagulant state with resultant fibrin deposition and fibrosis, fibrinolytic therapy has been investigated as a possible intervention to improve outcomes in ARDS. The PROWESS trial (Recombinant Human Activated Protein C Worldwide Evaluation in Severe Sepsis) demonstrated benefit to activated protein C administration in patients with severe sepsis, but did not specifically address effects on ALI [35]. The results of this trial have since been repudiated.

Intravenous beta-adrenergic agonists are currently under investigation for treatment of patients with ARDS. The results of the BALTI-1 trial (Beta-agonist in lung injury) showed improved clearance of extracellular water in the lungs with administration of salbutamol at 15 μg/kg/h over 7 days [36]. Results of the BALTI-2 clinical trial are still pending [37].

The role of enteral nutrition in patients with ALI has been investigated in one of the most recent publications by the ARDS Network, known as the EDEN trial [38]. The EDEN trial investigated the difference in outcomes between patients with ARDS who received full enteral feedings versus trophic feedings. Trophic feedings for up to 6 days did not increase the number of ventilator-free days, improve mortality, or decrease the number of infectious complications. They were associated with less gastrointestinal intolerance (i.e., diarrhea). It must be noted that what was considered full enteral feedings in this study was only 1,300 kcal per day.

The supplementation of enteral nutritional therapy with omega-3 fatty acids was considered potentially beneficial as omega-6 fatty acids are the precursors to pro-inflammatory cytokines, eicosanoids and leukotrienes, while omega-3 fatty acids favor anti-inflammatory molecule production. It was postulated that a diet rich in omega-3 fatty acids would provide lung-protective, anti-inflammatory, and mortality-reducing benefits. So far several studies have reported reduction in all-cause mortality related to reduced pulmonary capillary leakage and reduced neutrophils and pro-inflammatory cytokines in BAL fluid; however, a large multicenter, randomized trial did not support these findings and found no significant difference in MOF, nosocomial infections, reduction in ventilatory support days, or all-cause mortality [39].

Potential Complications

A lung-protective ventilation strategy is associated with hypercapnia and resultant hypercapnic respiratory acidosis (pH 7.20–7.30). Permissive hypercapnia may in and of itself be lung protective in that it reduces pro-inflammatory cytokines and neutrophil chemotactic activation, as well as an attenuation of in vivo apoptosis [40]. Acidosis with a pH <7.15 is managed medically with infusions of bicarbonate or tromethamine (THAM). Complications of hypercapnia can include depressed cardiac contractility and increased intracranial pressure. In patients with concomitant head injury or who are unable to have their mental status assessed due to sedation or neuromuscular blockade, intracranial pressure monitoring may be warranted.

The management of patients with ALI centers around prevention of VILI-associated complications by the judicious and correct use of mechanical ventilation. The adherence to a lung protective strategy prevents most cases of further pulmonary compromise by volutrauma, barotrauma, or atelectrauma. The most common complication from barotrauma is pneumothorax. This is not seen just when ARDS is worsening, but more often as ARDS is improving and both PEEP and FiO_2 are being decreased. Other complications of VILI include increased tendency towards fibrosis and scarring. Extreme cases of VILI can result in bronchopleural fistula. This can be extremely difficult to manage in the setting of ALI and results in continuous air leak into the pleural space. The treatment often necessitates the reduction of airway pressures to reduce air leak and favor closure; however, this can compromise attempts at improved oxygenation. Another rare complication of ALI is pulmonary ossification. This is diagnosed as a formation of dense calcifications in the lung parenchyma that is fibrosed and is usually seen as bilateral reticulonodular pulmonary infiltrates on chest radiographs. This is likely a complication related to hemorrhage into the airspace and diffuse fibrosis.

In patients who require prolonged ventilatory support, tracheostomy should be considered. The optimal timing of tracheostomy is debatable, with some physicians favoring placement as soon as the need for prolonged ventilator support is identified. This is based on the fact that edema and injury to the trachea from endotracheal intubation begin to become apparent within 3–7 days with scarring evident after 7 days of intubation. However, since this is an elective procedure in most ALI patients, it should not be considered until it can be done safely. Patients that require high levels of PEEP and/or FiO_2 may not have the reserve necessary to tolerate tracheostomy placement. For each patient, the risks and benefits of the procedure must be weighed carefully. For most patients tracheostomy is a well-tolerated procedure that results in improved patient comfort, ability to communicate, and better oral care potentially resulting in a lower rate of ventilator-associated pneumonia [41].

Ventilator-associated pneumonia should be identified and treated early with broad-spectrum antibiotics with de-escalation of antibiotic coverage when the causative agent is identified in order to prevent exacerbation of acute lung injury and improve oxygenation.

Conclusion

ARDS is a highly morbid disease but with improved goal-directed and systematic care more patients are surviving the acute phase of the disease. Current use of lung-protective ventilation strategy with permissive hypercapnia has reduced overall mortality from 53 to 26%. The majority of patients who achieve liberation from mechanical ventilation can expect a full and complete recovery of the respiratory system.

Some patients with mild to moderate pulmonary fibrosis caused by the fibroproliferative stage of ALI, or any patient with bronchopleural fistula, or pulmonary ossification should receive follow-up monitoring of pulmonary function tests. Up to 35% of patients with pulmonary fibrosis become disabled and are unable to return to work for a period of 24 months following ARDS [42].

Patients with ARDS may have other chronic problems related to neuromuscular weakness and psychological maladjustment. Prevention of physical disability should be a goal of clinicians and ancillary staff. Physical therapy intervention with the goal of early mobilization is important in maintaining and improving strength necessary to achieve liberation from ventilatory support.

References

1. Bernard GR, Artigas A, Brigham KL, Carlet J, Falke K, Hudson L, et al. The American-European consensus conference on ARDS. Definitions, mechanisms, relevant outcomes, and clinical trial coordination. Am J Respir Crit Care Med. 1994;149:818–24.
2. Rubenfeld GD, Caldwell E, Peabody E, Weaver J, Martin DP, Neff M. Incidence and outcomes of acute lung injury. N Engl J Med. 2005;353(16):1685–93.
3. Del Sorbo L, Slutzky AS. Acute respiratory distress syndrome and multiple organ failure. Curr Opin Crit Care. 2011;17:1–6.
4. Ruf W, Riewald M. Tissue factor dependent coagulation protease signaling in acute lung injury. Crit Care Med. 2003;31(4):S231–7.
5. Moraes TJ, Chow C-W, Downey G. Proteases and lung injury. Crit Care Med. 2003;31(4):S189–94.
6. Abraham E. Neutrophils and acute lung injury. Crit Care Med. 2003;31(4):S195–9.
7. Wesselkamper SC, Case LM, Henning LN, Borchers MT, Tichelaar JW, Mason JM, et al. Gene expression changes during the development of acute lung injury—the role of transforming growth factor β (beta). Am J Respir Crit Care Med. 2005;172:1399–411.
8. Dhainaut J-F, Charpentier J, Chiche J-D. Transforming growth factor β (beta): a mediator of cell regulation in acute respiratory distress syndrome. Crit Care Med. 2003;31(4):S258–64.
9. Idell S. Coagulation, fibrinolysis, and fibrin deposition in acute lung injury. Crit Care Med. 2003;31(4):S213–20.
10. Maniatis NA, Orfanos SE. The endothelium in acute lung injury/acute respiratory distress syndrome. Curr Opin Crit Care. 2008;14:22–30.
11. Lange M, Connelly R, Traber DL, Hamahata A, Nakano Y, Esechie A, et al. Time course of nitric oxide synthases, nitrosative stress, and poly(ADP ribosylation) in an ovine sepsis model. Crit Care. 2010;14:R129.
12. Martin TR, Nakamura M, Mutute-Bello G. The role of apoptosis in acute lung injury. Crit Care Med. 2003;31(4):S184–8.
13. Perl M, Chung CS, Perl U, Thakkar R, Lomas-Neira J, Ayala A. Therapeutic accessability of caspase-mediated cell-death as a key pathomechanism in indirect acute lung injury. Crit Care Med. 2010;38(4):1176–86.
14. Finigan JH, Faress JA, Wilkinson E, Mishra RS, Nethery DE, Wyler D, et al. Neuroregulin-1-human epidermal recptor-2 signaling is a central regulator of pulmonary epithelial permeability and acute lung injury. J Biol Chem. 2011;286(12):10660–70.
15. Looney MR, Gilliss BM, Matthay MA. Pathophysiology of tranfusion-related acute lung injury. Curr Opin Hematol. 2010;17(4):418–23.

16. Musch G. Positron emission tomography: a tool for better understanding ventilator-induced and acute lung injury. Curr Opin Crit Care. 2011;17:7–12.

17. Bellani G, Amigoni M, Pesenti A. Positron emission tomography in ARDS: a new look at an old syndrome. Minerva Anesthesiol. 2011;77(4):439–47.

18. Ferguson ND, Frutos-Vivar F, Esteban A, Anzueto A, Alía I, Brower RG, et al. Airway pressures, tidal volumes, and mortality in patients with acute respiratory distress syndrome. Crit Care Med. 2005;33:21–30.

19. The ARDS Network. Ventilation with lower tidal volumes as compared with traditional tidal volumes for acute lung injury and the acute respiratory distress syndrome. N Engl J Med. 2000;342:1301–8.

20. Dada LA, Sznajder JI. Mechanisms of pulmonary edema clearance during acute hypoxemic respiratory failure: role of Na, K-ATPase. Crit Care Med. 2003;31(4):S248–52.

21. Hemmila MR, Napolitano LM. Severe respiratory failure: advanced treatment options. Crit Care Med. 2006;34(9):S278–90.

22. Derdak S, Mehta S, Stewart TE, Smith T, Rogers M, Buchman TG, et al. Multi-center oscillatory ventilation for acute respiratory distress syndrome trial (MOAT) Study Investigators. High frequency oscillatory ventilation for acute respiratory distress syndrome in adults: a randomized controlled trial. Am J Respir Crit Care Med. 2002;166(6):801–8.

23. Peek GJ, Mugford M, Tiruvoipati R, Wilson A, Allen E, Thalanany MM, The CESAR trial collaboration, et al. Efficacy and economic assessment of conventional ventilatory support vs extracorporeal membrane oxygenation for severe adult respiratory failure (CESAR): a multicentre randomized controlled trial. Lancet. 2009;374:1351–63.

24. Müller T, Philipp A, Lubnow M, Weingart C, Pfeifer M, Riegger GA, et al. First application of a new portable miniaturized system for extracorporeal membrane oxygenation. Perfusion. 2011;26(4):284–8.

25. Bone RC, Slotman G, Maunder R, Silverman H, Hyers TM, Kerstein MD, Ursprung JJ. Randomized double-blind, multicenter study of prostaglandin E1 in patients with adult respiratory distress syndrome Prostaglandin E1 Study Group. Chest. 1989;96:114–9.

26. Suter PM, Domenighetti G, Schaller MD, Laverrière MC, Ritz R, Perret C. N-acetylcysteine enhances recovery from acute injury in man. A randomized, double-blind, placebo-controlled clinical study. Chest. 1994;105:190–4.

27. Steinberg KP, Hudson LD, Goodman RB, Hough CL, Lanken PN, Hyzy R, et al. Efficacy and safety of corticosteroids for persistent acute respiratory distress syndrome. N Engl J Med. 2006;354:1671–84.

28. Taylor RW, Zimmerman JL, Dellinger RP, Straube RC, Criner GJ, Davis Jr K, et al. Low-dose inhaled nitric oxide patients with acute lung injury: a randomized controlled trial. JAMA. 2004;291:1603–9.

29. Spragg RG, Lewis JF, Walmrath HD, Johannigman J, Bellingan G, Laterre PF, et al. Effect of recombinant surfactant protein C-based surfactant on the acute respiratory distress syndrome. N Engl J Med. 2004;351:884–92.

30. Adhikari N, Burns KE, Meade MO. Pharmacologic treatments for acute respiratory distress syndrome and acute lung injury: systematic review and meta-analysis. Treat Respir Med. 2004;3:307–28.

31. Dellinger RP, Trzeciak SW, Criner GJ, Zimmerman JL, Taylor RW, Usansky H, et al. Association between inhaled nitric oxide treatment and long-term pulmonary function in survivors of acute respiratory distress syndrome. Crit Care. 2012;16(2):R36.

32. Cornet AD, Hofstra JJ, Swart EL, Girbes AR, Juffermans NP. Sildenafil attenuates pulmonary arterial pressure but does not improve oxygenation during ARDS. Intensive Care Med. 2010;36:758–64.

33. Brun-Buisson C, Richard JC, Mercat A, Thiébaut AC, Brochard L. REVA-SRLF A/H1N1v 2009 Registry Group. Early corticosteroid in severe influenza A/H1N1 pneumonia and acute respiratory distress syndrome. Am J Respir Crit Care Med. 2011;183:1200–6.

34. Lewis JF, Brackenbury A. Role of exogenous surfactant in acute lung injury. Crit Care Med. 2003;31(4):S324–8.

35. Bernard GR, Vincent JL, Laterre PF, LaRosa SP, Dhainaut JF, Lopez-Rodriguez A, Recombinant human protein C Worldwide Evaluation in Severe Sepsis (PROWESS) study group, et al. Efficacy and safety of recombinant human activated protein C for severe sepsis. N Engl J Med. 2001;344:699–709.

36. Perkins GD, McAuley DF, Thickett DR, Gao F. The beta-agonist lung injury trial (BALTI): a randomized, placebo-controlled clinical trial. Am J Respir Crit Care Med. 2006;173(3):281–7.

37. Perkins GD, Gates S, Lamb SE, McCabe C, Young D, Gao F. Beta-agonist lung injury trial-2 (BALTI-2) trial protocol: a randomized, double-blind placebo-controlled clinical trial of intravenous infusion of salbutamol in the acute respiratory distress syndrome. Trials. 2011;12:113.

38. The ARDS clinical trial network. Initial trophic versus full enteral feeding in patients with acute lung injury: the EDEN randomized trial. JAMA. 2012;307(8):E1–9.

39. Grau-Carmona T, Morán-García V, García-de-Lorenzo A, Heras-de-la-Calle G, Quesada-Bellver B, López-Martínez J, et al. Effect of enteral diet enriched with eicosapentaenoic acid, gamma-linolenic acid and anti-oxidants on the outcome of mechanically ventilated, critically ill, septic patients. Clin Nutr. 2011;30(5):578–84. doi:10.1016/j.clnu.2011.03.004.

40. Ishmaiel NM, Henzler D. Effects of hypercapnia and hypercapnic acidosis on attenuation of ventilator-induced lung injury. Minerva Anesthesiol. 2011;77(7):723–33.

41. Durbin CG. Indications for and timing of tracheosotomy. Respir Care. 2005;50(4):483–7.

42. Hall JB, Kress JP. The burden of functional recovery from ARDS. N Engl J Med. 2011;364(14):1358–9.

Rosemary Kozar and Diane A. Schwartz

Introduction

Nutrition in the surgical patient is a multifactorial, complex subject. Beyond the decision to feed enterally or parenterally, a surgeon must consider specific patient characteristics that interfere with the delivery of nutrients for useful and purposeful digestion and metabolism. The patient with postoperative ileus, a previous bowel obstruction, short gut, the trauma open, damage-controlled abdomen, or discontinuous bowel, to mention only a few special circumstances, has energy requirements beyond what is provided by maintenance or resuscitative fluids, and these examples comprise situations in which early feeding would inherently be of benefit. Certainly the patient with fistulization to the skin deserves focused discussion as this patient population, more than the standard surgical patient or the disaster, damage-controlled abdomen, has the additional complexity of nutrient and digestive component loss.

Attention should also be given to the consideration of nutritional access as many patients with these special circumstances do not have the ability to take food orally. Surgeons must decide how they will provide nutrition to their patients and many times this requires surgical or endoscopic placement of lines and tubes that can be used to conduct nutrients into the body. Timing of feeding and location of feed entry into the body are further decisions that the surgeon faces. This chapter serves to discuss and present data regarding the differences in parenteral, enteral, gastric, and post-pyloric feeding, and includes algorithms for instituting early nutritional support in the acute and traumatic patient populations.

R. Kozar, M.D., Ph.D. (✉)
Department of Surgery, The University of Texas Medical
School at Houston, 6431 Fannin, Suite 4.284,
Houston, TX 77030, USA
e-mail: Rosemary.A.Kozar@uth.tmc.edu

D.A. Schwartz, M.D.
Department of Surgery, John Hopkins School of Medicine,
4940 Eastern Ave, 5th block A building,
Baltimore, MD 21224
e-mail: dschwa37@jhmi.edu

Rationale for Nutritional Support

The rationale for providing nutritional support is to prevent acute protein malnutrition, to modulate the immune response, and to promote normal gut function [1].

Types of Nutritional Support

Enteral Versus Parenteral

In the 1970s total parenteral nutrition (TPN) was introduced, but despite its availability, enteral nutrition (EN) was still more economical and convenient to provide. However, the practice at that time was to hold enteral nutrition until the gut proved to be completely functional, which could take days, even more than a week, for surgical and trauma patients. By the 1980s enough data had been collected to support the use of enteral nutrition in these surgical populations. Enteral nutrient provisions were functional and processed effectively in the critically ill patient with mal-adapted gut mucosa [2, 3]. In fact it was shown in multiple studies that introducing enteral feeds into the gut stimulated immunologic response and competence [4–7]. The 1990s introduced data that TPN may be harmful in patients who could otherwise tolerate enteral feeds. There were more infections, including catheter-related sepsis, seen in the parenteral group [8, 9]. Meta-analyses confirmed that early enteral feeding, compared to parenteral nutrition, reduced postoperative infections and complications [10, 11].

Enteral Nutrition

Enteral nutrition is the preferred form of nutritional supplementation in surgical patients who have enteral access [12–14]. Absolute contraindications to enteral feeds include functional complications such as bowel obstruction, peritonitis, progressive ileus, massive gastrointestinal hemorrhage, and gastrointestinal ischemia associated with shock and vasopressors.

L.J. Moore et al. (eds.), *Common Problems in Acute Care Surgery*,
DOI 10.1007/978-1-4614-6123-4_9, © Springer Science+Business Media New York 2013

Relative contraindications include proven intolerance to enteral nutrition and intolerance associated with short gut syndrome, high-output fistula, pancreatitis, and inflammatory bowel disease.

Early enteral feeding supports gastrointestinal structure and function, and in the critically ill surgical patient can reduce gut hyper-permeability, enhance gut blood flow, promote gastric emptying, and stimulate gut-associated immunity. Multiple studies have shown tolerance of trophic feeds in critically ill and mechanically ventilated patients, and in patients with recent bowel surgery [15]. While there are studies that show some increased infectious complications with early goal enteral feeds, there is more convincing data to the contrary [13, 14, 16]. Based on 14 Level 2 studies, early enteral nutrition was shown to reduce infectious complications and mortality and is overwhelmingly recommended in mechanically ventilated patients after adequate resuscitation [17, 18].

Parenteral Nutrition

Total parenteral nutrition is appropriate in situations in which enteral feeds cannot be used. Its disadvantages include need for vascular access, infection of vascular access and associated bloodstream infection, sepsis, cost, need to monitor electrolytes and adjust formula, and hyperglycemia. Several types of amino acid-specific formulas for TPN are available and there is evidence to support the use of glutamine for both enteral and parenteral nutrition, regardless of the formula used [19, 20]. Glutamine shows decreased complications and increased survival when added as a supplement to TPN [21].

Whenever possible, the gastrointestinal track should be utilized for nutritional support. The algorithm (Fig. 9.1) reviews the decision process for starting enteral nutrition and for the administration of TPN. In general, TPN should be started by 7–10 days postoperatively if the patient is well nourished at baseline and unable to tolerate a regular diet. Critically ill patients should be started on TPN if they are unable to achieve adequate enteral caloric intake by postoperative days 6–8. Unlike enteral feeding, there is no clear benefit to early TPN. There is equally no difference in outcomes for patients who take enteral and parenteral nutrition in combination [22]. Patients with persistent ileus, bowel obstruction, short gut, high-output fistulas, and malabsorption may all benefit from TPN. Additionally, patients unable to tolerate enteral nutrition or who are at risk for nonocclusive bowel necrosis (hypoperfusion, vasopressor, or paralytic requirements) may benefit from TPN.

Determining Caloric Needs

Caloric needs can be calculated using one of many formulas such as the Harris–Benedict equation, or measured with indirect calorimetry.

Harris–Benedict Equation

The Harris–Benedict equation estimates basal energy expenditure (BEE) to determine caloric requirements. The Harris–Benedict equations are specific to men and women based on weight, body mass index (BMI), and height and are as follows:

$$\text{Men}: \quad \text{BEE} = 66 + \left(13.7 \times \text{weight}\right)$$
$$+ \left(5 \times \text{height}\right) - \left(6.8 \times \text{age}\right)$$

$$\text{Women}: \quad \text{BEE} = 665 + \left(9.6 \times \text{weight}\right)$$
$$+ \left(1.9 \times \text{height}\right) - \left(4.7 \times \text{age}\right).$$

Weight is in kilograms (kg), height in centimeters (cm), and age in years. The BEE represents energy requirements in the fasting, resting, and non-stressed state, so it may not be completely accurate in trauma or surgical patients. In the presence of metabolic stress, the BEE must be multiplied by an empirically derived stress factor; this factor may grossly overestimate the true caloric needs of the individual and remains the source of controversy in using this formula in the critically ill. Overestimation of caloric needs results in complications such as overfeeding, hypercapnia, hyperglycemia, and hepatic steatosis. The new multiplication constants to estimate the stressed caloric needs range from 1.2 to 1.6 times the BEE. These new recommendations better estimate the caloric needs of even the most stressed patient scenarios, such as burns.

Indirect Calorimetry

Indirect calorimetry is a tool used to measure resting energy expenditure (REE) and relies on the relationship of oxygen consumption and carbon dioxide production. Because of the components necessary to calculate the REE, patients should be ventilated for best accuracy, although there is support to use it even in spontaneously breathing patients. It is recommended that steady state be achieved, defined as a change in either parameter of less than 10% over 5 min or more [23]. The REE obtained should then be used to estimate the patient's baseline nutritional goal. Indirect calorimetry may be helpful when overfeeding would be undesirable (as in diabetes, obesity, or chronic obstructive pulmonary disease), underfeeding would be especially detrimental (renal failure, large wounds), physical or clinical factors promote energy expenditure that deviates from normal, drugs are used that may significantly alter energy expenditure (paralytic agents, beta-blockers, corticosteroids), patient response to calculated regimens is suboptimal, or body habitus makes energy expenditure predictions challenging (morbid obesity, quadriplegia).

The respiratory quotient is another derivative from the components of the indirect calorimetry. The formula is below:

$$\text{Respiratory quotient (RQ)} = V_{O2}/V_{CO2} = CO_2 \text{ production}/ O_2 \text{ consumption.}$$

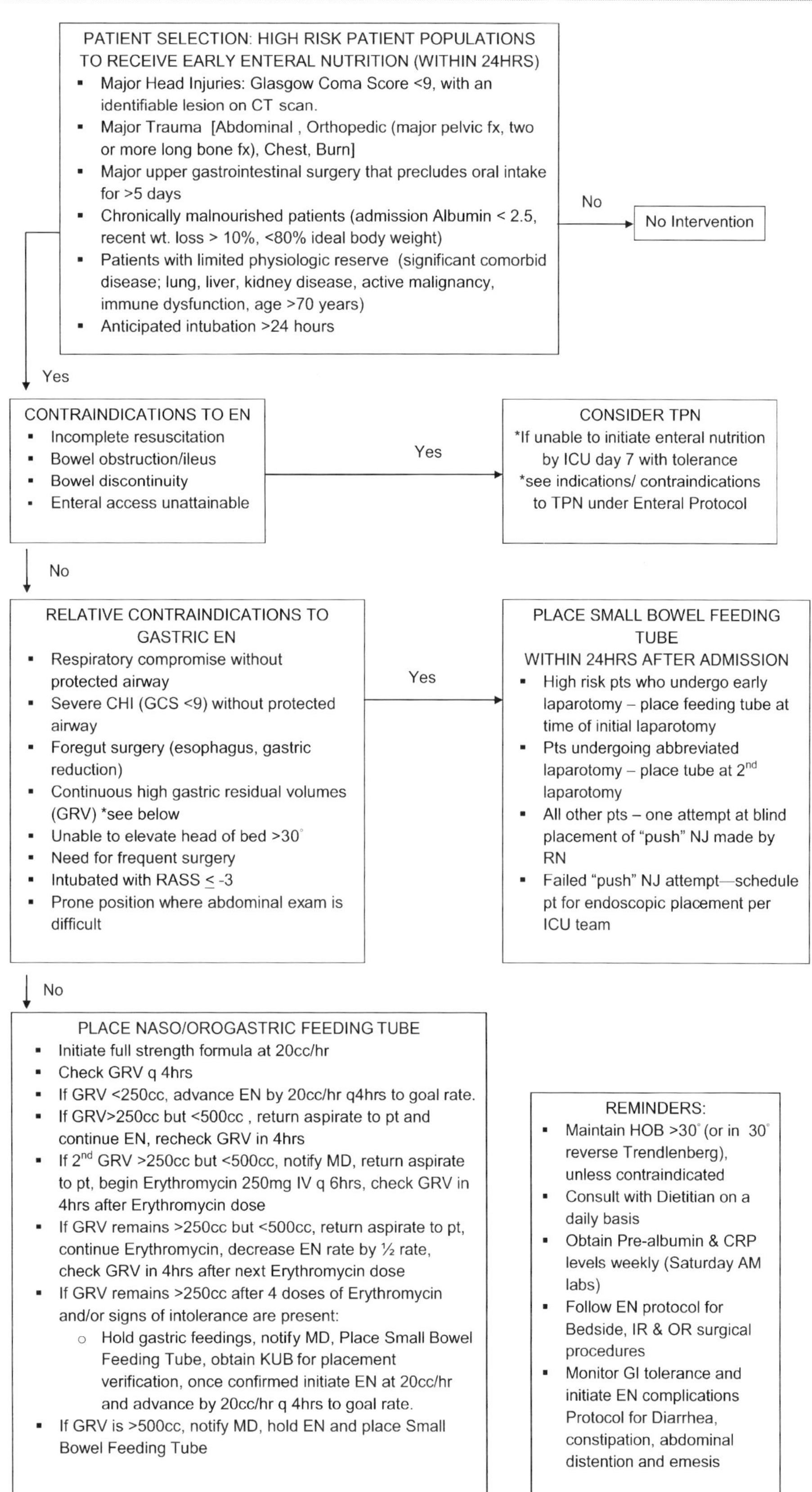

Fig. 9.1 Enteral nutrition protocol algorithm

The RQ is a gross measurement of substrate utilization [24]. When an RQ value ≥ 1 is obtained, CO_2 production may be increased by one of the two mechanisms: either a high proportion of nonprotein calories are being supplied as glucose (carbohydrates have RQ of 1) or less commonly, the patient is being provided excess calories. Failure to wean with a persistently elevated PCO_2 on an arterial blood gas should prompt measurement of the RQ. An RQ of 0.85 provides optimal utilization, while <0.7 suggests gross underfeeding and ketone utilization.

Calculating TPN

Components of TPN include dextrose, fatty acids, amino acids, electrolytes, vitamins, and trace minerals. Dextrose is the carbohydrate at a caloric density of 3.4 kcal/g. Dextrose solutions of 50 or 70% dextrose are readily available, but any carbohydrate percentage and volume can be mixed according to the patient's need. Protein provides 4 kcal/g and is provided as amino acids. Standard amino acid solutions contain a balance of essential and nonessential amino acids and are available as either 10 g/100 ml or 15 g/100 ml. Fat emulsions are 2.0 $kcal/cm^3$ of 20% lipid and are the source of essential fatty acids, linoleic, linolenic, and arachidonic acids. The electrolyte cations, which include sodium, potassium, magnesium, phosphorus, and calcium, are mixed into the TPN solution using one of several anions. Acid–base status may be affected by the amount of chloride or acetate used in providing sodium and potassium. The concentrations of calcium and phosphorus are limited to avoid precipitation of a calcium phosphate salt. Vitamins included are A, C, D, E, and B vitamins, including folate, but not vitamin K, which must be added separately. Mineral product is added to provide copper, chromium, manganese, zinc, and selenium. The basic steps in calculating TPN are as follows: (1) establish the kilocalories and protein desired, (2) select the appropriate amino acid formula and quantity, (3) calculate 10% of kcal as lipid emulsion, and (4) tally the kcal from amino acids and fat and subtract from goal, which is the amount of dextrose kcal needed. Divide this number by 3.4 to get the grams of dextrose required [25].

Types of Formulas

The primary categories of enteral formulas include polymeric, elemental, immune-enhancing, and specialty formulas.

Standard Enteral Diet Versus Immune-Enhancing Diets

Both basic and clinical research suggests that the beneficial effects of enteral nutrition can be amplified by supplementing formulas with specific nutrients that exert immune-enhancing effects, including glutamine, arginine, nucleotides, and omega-3 fatty acids. There are numerous prospective randomized controlled trials comparing immune-enhancing enteral diets to standard enteral diet and most, but not all, demonstrate improved outcomes. The majority of trials are in trauma and cancer patients, though a few trials include mixed intensive care unit (ICU) and septic ICU patients.

Pharmaconutrition

The concept of pharmaconutrition allows the separation of nutritional support from the provision of key nutrients that may modulate the inflammatory and immune response associated with critical illness. This came about after the realization that the greatest benefit in clinical outcomes was from studies utilizing specific nutrients [16]. This is likely due to their effects on the enteric inflammatory response and the way in which they work to block inflammatory stimulation. Any event that stimulates a gastrointestinal inflammatory response and a change in gut perfusion alters the way that the gastrointestinal tract utilizes nutrients. Providing intraluminal alimentation to stressed mucosa of the gut improves intestinal transit [26]. Pharmaconutrients alone or as supplementation have been shown to decrease infectious complications and complication-associated length of hospital stay [27].

Glutamine is the primary fuel source for the enterocyte and is preferred to glucose as a fuel source in times of stress [28]. It is released from muscle during the stress response and then exploited as a signal mechanism, promoting immune regulation and cellular protection, and as a nutrient and source of energy [29]. But in addition, glutamine has anti-catabolic and antioxidant properties that enhance its use and its receipt at enterocytes. Furthermore it increases plasma concentration of arginine [30], which will be addressed later. Although glutamine can be provided both enterally and parenterally, it demonstrates the most benefit of barrier to infection and control of the immune response when given enterally [30]. Meta-analysis and prospective randomized trials for trauma and burn patients showed benefit of glutamine in these patient populations in terms of decreasing infectious complications and enhancing the gut's use of other enteric nutrients [31–35]. Based on the available data, glutamine, despite the administration route, appears to lower infectious complications, decrease hospital length of stay, and enhance nutrient use in the critically ill patient [36, 37]. Heat-shock proteins, which serve as molecular regulators of denatured proteins, are induced by glutamine, which may be another way in which glutamine modulates the cyto-protection and inflammatory response [38–40]. Equally important is the lack of data showing adverse effect of using glutamine in either form.

Arginine is another modulator of immune response of the enteric system. It is produced both endogenously from glutamine and the urea cycle, and obtained from the diet. When there is normal physiology without ongoing stress response, arginine serves to enhance immune function, contribute to wound healing, and stimulate anabolic hormones. L-arginine is a substrate for nitric oxide, which itself enhances the inflammatory response. L-arginine and its pathway to creating nitric oxide is a potential target for modification of immune activation. Specifically in trauma patients it has been shown that the release of IL-4, IL-10, and transforming growth factor beta increases arginase I expression, which corresponds to increased immune cell arginase activity and decreased plasma arginine and citrulline levels [41, 42]. By shunting arginine use in this way, it can no longer be used as a substrate for nitric oxide synthase dimerization and nitric oxide production. Therefore, administration of supplemental arginine in the critically ill patient may reduce the amount of nitric oxide produced in the post-injury period. Arguing against this data is work from another group suggesting that arginine supplementation increases nitric oxide production, thereby amplifying the systemic inflammatory response syndrome (SIRS) response and increasing mortality in the trauma or critically ill patient [43, 44]. There exists data supporting and refuting the use of arginine supplementation for both enteral and parenteral routes of administration [45–48]. It is clear, however, that arginine supplementation in elective surgical patients is beneficial. A recent meta-analysis by Drover et al. demonstrated a significant decrease in postoperative complications and hospital length of stay when patients undergoing gastrointestinal surgery received pre-, peri-, or postoperative arginine supplementation [49]. The effect was greatest when the supplementation included arginine as well as omega-3 fatty acids and nucleotides.

Nucleotides play an active role in cellular proliferation and immune modulation and are building blocks for several intrinsic cellular molecules. They are produced de novo and by salvage pathways. T cell proliferation and appropriate recognition of antigen are thought to be dependent on the presence of nucleotide because it has been shown that artificial decrease in interleukin-2 is corrected by addition of supplemental nucleotide [50]. They are either purine or pyridimine derived with a ribose and one or more phosphate groups [51]. Similar to glutamine and arginine, intravenous (IV) and enteral forms are available. Infusions of nucleotides decrease bacterial translocation and decrease graft rejection [50, 52]. These references also show that parenteral doses of nucleotides, administered with TPN, decrease associated gut atrophy.

Omega-3 fatty acids are the active components of fish oils and have significant anti-inflammatory properties [53], the mechanism of which is likely a combination of functions including arachidonic acid displacement from cellular membranes, production of prostaglandins, and reduced activation of various nuclear factors [54]. Specifically, they target and down-regulate NF-κB and AP-1 [54] on the nuclear membrane and they down-regulate iNOS, thereby reducing production of nitric oxide. While there are no studies of critically ill patients who received only omega-3 fatty acid and no additional supplementation, there are three prospective randomized studies that included omega-3 fatty acid in the supplementation package and had a significant improvement in respiratory function of their critically ill patients [55–57].

Beyond activation of the immune system, the critically ill and traumatic patient suffers damage at the cellular level secondary to the effects of oxidation-induced injury. Antioxidants have been found to catalyze the breakdown of the substances that are implicated in causing this damage [58]. Superoxide dismutase, catalase, and glutathione peroxidase have been identified as antioxidants; cofactors include selenium, zinc, manganese, and iron. Supplementation of these substances decreases the inflammatory response and halts oxidative stress [59–61]. Similar to nucleotides, it has been shown that the number of days on mechanical ventilation and overall mortality can be reduced by supplementation of antioxidants and their cofactors [61–63]. The REDOX trial, a prospective randomized trial comparing enteral and parenteral glutamine and antioxidants in critically ill patients with organ failure, has just been completed. Thus far no adverse effects have been identified [58, 64].

Optimal Route of Delivery of Enteral Nutrition

Access can be divided into gastric (and duodenal) and jejunal with push, endoscopic, radiologic, and surgical options all available. For patients to be fed gastrically, a soft, non-sump nasogastric tube can be placed. There are also blindly placed nasojejunal tubes. If blind placement is unsuccessful, an endoscopically placed nasojejunal tube is an option. Nasojejunal feeding may be done indefinitely, but if the need for long-term access becomes apparent, either a percutaneous endoscopic gastrostomy (PEG) or a PEG with a jejunal extension limb (PEG-J) can be placed. For those patients identified as candidates for jejunal feeds and undergoing laparotomy, either a standard open jejunostomy or a needle catheter jejunostomy (NCJ) can be placed.

The largest study examining the safety of needle catheter jejunostomies in patients undergoing major elective and emergency abdominal operations documented an incidence of major complications of 1% and minor complications of 1.7% [65]. When feeding jejunostomy-related complications in trauma patients were reviewed by Holmes et al. [66] the overall major complication rate was 4%. However, the majority of complications occurred in patients with a Witzel tube jejunostomy (10%), with only a 2% rate with NCJs. In fact, the only difference between patients with and without major complications was the type of feeding access. Major complications included small bowel perforation, volvuli with infarction, intraperitoneal leaks, and nonocclusive small bowel necrosis. The first three of these complications can be minimized by improved technique and the latter minimized by more judicious feeding.

Gastric Versus Small Bowel Feeding Controversy

While gastric and post-pyloric nutrition have been compared, statistically no difference is noted in the time to reach caloric goal, length of stay in the ICU, or length of ventilator time between the two [67]. There is a consistent delay in initiating gastric feeds when compared to post-pyloric feeds in surgical patients, but again, the ultimate outcomes data do not differ. In fact gastric feeds and post-pyloric feeds can achieve the same caloric supplementation in the same amount of time in the critically ill patients [68]. It has also been shown that initiating early enteric feeds (within 36 h) improves survival and decreases infectious complications [69].

If feeds are provided past the ligament of Treitz, enteral feeds do not require a hold for return to the operating room [70]. This is important in the surgical population where frequent trips to the operating room might otherwise greatly hamper uninterrupted full caloric nutrition in these patients. Aspiration during intubation remains a risk for patients who have been gastrically fed [71]. This same risk does not appear as evident even for patients who have continuous jejunal tube feeds running during their operations. There is no difference in aspiration risk in gastric or post-pyloric feeds with respect to aspiration risk or residuals [72].

Additionally the question of gastrointestinal prophylaxis in the patient who is ventilated and fed into the small bowel is significant. Gastric pH must be addressed in any patient intubated more than 48 h and undergoing non-gastric nutritional support. This is to prevent stress ulceration, which is a known complication of ICU patients. Because gastric tubes can be placed nasally and blindly by push technique easier than jejunal tubes, the natural tendency is toward placing nasogastric (NG) tubes for decompression and to pass a nasojejunal tube and feed it even if gastric. There may be a need for recommendations on post-pyloric feeds in ICU-level patients secondary to their frequent trips to the operating room, need for continuous uninterrupted feeds to prevent malnutrition, and prevention of aspiration. Equally one could argue for gastric feeds with head of bed elevation, which might cut the number of stress ulcers and reduce the number of procedures and sedation that ICU patients are getting for placement of endoscopic tubes.

Effectiveness of Nutritional Delivery

Once the provision of nutrition has been started at goal, it is equally important to measure the effectiveness of that nutrition. Several ways of assessing caloric use in the critically ill and surgical patient have been described. Updated BMI, 12-h urinary urea nitrogen, prealbumin, and C-reactive protein (CRP) levels are obtained weekly after recording a baseline measurement and starting nutrition. Indirect calorimetry is also available as required for further assessment. The urinary urea nitrogen serves to estimate the protein need and loss in patients who have a creatinine clearance greater than 50 ml/min. A normal range is 6–24 g/day. A negative result indicates excessive muscle shunting for energy. (Total urinary nitrogen is more accurate in the critically ill, but is less readily available [73]. In addition, exclude spinal cord-injured patients because loss is tremendous and ongoing [74].)

CRP is an acute-phase protein that directly correlates with injury and ongoing inflammatory states. Elevation above 15 mg/dl indicates that the liver is unable to synthesize other types of proteins such as albumin, prealbumin, and transferrin. It therefore can be used to measure whether there is still acute inflammatory response preventing anabolism, appropriate, expected use of nutrients, and healing.

Prealbumin has a 2–4-day half-life, and its level indicates anabolic activity. Normal response during the critical phase would be an increase of 0.5–1 mg/dl/day.

Indirect calorimetry measures expired carbon dioxide to extrapolate energy consumption in the ventilated patient. Patients must be on an FiO_2 of less than 60% with a peep of less than ten. The usefulness of the measurement is apparent for patients where over- or underfeeding would be clinically undesirable based on their known medical comorbidities [75].

Consequences of Inadequate Feeding

Though the precise caloric requirements for critically ill patients is not well defined and is dependent on numerous factors, it is well recognized that adequate caloric intake is important. In a prospective observational study of critically ill patients, an increase of 1,000 cal/day significantly reduced mortality, with the most pronounced effects in those patients with a body mass index less than 25 or greater than 35 [17]. In a recent study of more than 7,000 ICU intubated patients, there was a significant association between the percent of prescribed calories received, and 60-day mortality [76]. Patients receiving more than two-thirds of prescribed calories were less likely to die than those receiving less than one-third of prescribed calories. The optimal percent of prescribed calories was approximately 80–85%.

Early delivery of adequate calories to critically ill surgical patients, however, can prove challenging. Vasopressor use, bowel in discontinuity after damage control surgery, and ileus can all impede adequate early delivery of feeds.

Nutritional adequacy is defined as the actual 24-h caloric or protein intake/prescribed 24-h caloric or protein intake and has been studied in the trauma adult and pediatric populations [77]. For both patient age groups, adequacy was ≤60%. Therefore early placement of feeding access and a focus on the importance of early nutritional delivery are paramount.

Open abdomens and recent bowel anastomosis are not contraindications to early feeding [78]. In a recent meta-analysis of early versus traditional postoperative feeding in patients with bowel anastomosis, there was a significant reduction in total postoperative complications in patients receiving some type of nutritional support (either enteral feeds or diets) within 24 h of surgery, even if it was provided proximal to the anastomosis [79]. The use of enteral glutamine during shock may also be safe and is worthy of consideration [80].

In an attempt to improve nutritional adequacy, the PEP uP Protocol has been proposed by Heyland et al. [18, 81]. In a single center feasibility trial, enteral feeds were started at 25 ml/h, motility and protein supplements were started immediately, and the target was a 24-h volume of enteral nutrition rather than an hourly rate. If a patient missed feeds, "makeup" feeds were provided. They found a significant improvement in caloric and protein delivery, with no increase in complications.

Parenteral Supplementation of Enteral Nutrition

If critically ill patients are not receiving adequate enteral nutrition and adequate delivery of calories and protein is important, the question arises as to whether supplemental TPN should be added until full needs are met by the enteral route. This was recently investigated by Casaer et al. in a prospective randomized multicenter trial [82]. All patients received early enteral nutrition but were randomized to either early (<48 h) or late (>day 7) parenteral nutrition. Survival was equal between groups but the late parenteral group had fewer ICU infections and a greater likelihood of being discharged alive. Though the study demonstrated that the early use of supplemental TPN is not beneficial, there were several limitations of the study. The majority of patients were not malnourished at ICU admission, the severely malnourished were excluded, the patient population was that requiring primary cardiac surgery, and approximately half the patients were extubated by day 2, suggesting that those patients who may have benefited from supplemental nutrition were not included in the study. However, until the time supplemental TPN is shown to have proven benefit, it is not recommended in the surgical patient when enteral nutrition can be used.

Complications of Nutritional Support

Refeeding

The refeeding syndrome can occur in any nutritionally deplete individual regardless of the manner in which he or she is being fed. The syndrome is most frequently seen in patients who are alcoholics, have eating disorders, suffer from hyperemesis gravidarum, or who have experienced excessive, rapid weight loss following bariatric surgery. Symptoms are not limited to cardiac arrhythmias, organ failure, and death. The crux of the syndrome is that fat metabolism, which predominated in the unstressed, starved state, now with refeeding, switches to a primarily carbohydrate-based metabolism. The carbohydrate-based metabolism is responsible for a rapid uptake of electrolytes causing intra- and extracellular levels to drop quickly creating disturbances and related effects. Prevention is by recognizing inherent risks and repleting electrolytes before the syndrome can ensue. An additional strategy is to start feeds at one-third to one-half of goal and increase gradually. Electrolytes should be serially checked in high-risk patients.

Nonocclusive Mesenteric Ischemia

There does not seem to be any decisive data regarding feeding the gut for patients on pressor therapy. Based on observational data, it appears that if vasopressors are being used for indications other than fulminant non-septic shock (such as phenylephrine for spinal perfusion), it is of little detriment to feed the gut. A nonocclusive pattern would be expected to involve the entire length of the bowel, and, if it were from feeds, would be expected to begin wherever feeds were initiated. For example, if the stomach is the point of nutritional entry, then any nonocclusive bowel necrosis would be expected to involve the stomach, even despite its robust blood supply. Patchy areas may result if the period of ischemia were short. However, the data appear to be lacking for definitive recommendations in such situations. The mortality for fulminant nonocclusive bowel necrosis approaches 50% [83].

Nutritional Support in Specific Surgical Patients

Pancreatitis

Pancreatitis demands special attention. There is some debate in the literature of whether post-ligament of Treitz feeding prevents continued inflammation. Placement of endoscopic or push nasojejunal tubes has allowed the patient with pancreatitis to be fed enterally. There are several well-documented populations where outcomes have shown a positive benefit to enteral feeds as compared to nutrition provided by TPN [84, 85]. Despite previous concern that small bowel enteral feeds would still have some, even if minimal, effect on pancreatic stimulation, this has proven to be unfounded [86].

Chylothorax/Chyloperitoneum

Although an uncommon phenomenon, chylothorax and even chyloperitoneum do require special attention. While overall this complication is more likely seen as a result of malignancy or operative management of malignancy, at our institution these are more often seen in the trauma population, after central line placements, with lumbar spine fractures, and iatrogenic. Recommendations include attempting nonoperative management with dietary modification and TPN, chest tube drainage to quantify the volume, followed by surgical ligation if the output continues of 1,500 ml/24-h periods or for more than 2 weeks [87]. When the volume of this problem is uncontrollable, TPN or enteral feeds with medium-chain fatty acids seem to be most effective in decreasing the output. We typically use elemental formulas, such as Vivonex, for several weeks to ensure adequate seal of the lymphatic chain. Because the majority of chylothoraces seen on our service are secondary to traumatic insult, we are less hasty to perform operative management if patients show response to dietary modification. Substantial loss of protein and albumin occurs during the leak and this can lead to significant malnutrition and immunologic derangement [88, 89].

Enterocutaneous Fistulas

Enterocutaneous fistulas drain bowel content to the atmosphere and are the bane of surgical complication. They are thought to be caused by anastomotic failure and breakdown, intra-abdominal abscesses, foreign body erosion (for example, drains), malignancy, or inflammatory processes, and there is some data that they can be due to prolonged wound vac usage [90, 91]. They additionally can occur without identifiable cause. The biggest problems associated with them are damage and excoriation to the skin, loss of electrolytes and fluid with dehydration risk, and understanding how to provide effective and usable nutritional support [92]. Spontaneous closure is more likely if the output is low, the surrounding bowel is healthy, and the fistula resulted as a postoperative complication [93]. There is no definitive data in the literature regarding medications or supplements that will decrease fistula output and promote ultimate closure; glutamine, use of TPN with avoidance of enteral nutrition, and specific dressings have all been credited with enabling closure [94–98]. Spontaneous

closure does not occur often, and if does not occur, indicates need for planned, delayed, surgical closure [99–101]. Mortality is directly correlated with output volume and additional related complications [93]. High-output fistula is defined as volume loss greater than 500 ml per 24-h period. This fluid contains significant electrolytes, mimicking the makeup of the specific fluid in that part of the gastrointestinal system. These electrolytes must be accounted for and appropriately replaced to prevent dehydration and complications related to specific electrolyte loss [102, 103]. Significant albumin wasting is associated with increased morbidity and mortality [104, 105].

Short Gut

Short bowel is more associated with the clinical outcomes of having insufficient length to perform effective digestion, than defined by the actual length, since there is evidence that the bowel has some ability to adapt function over time [106, 107]. Providing long- and short-chain fatty acids, immunomodulators, and trophic feeds or elemental formulas may play a role in gut adaptation [108–110]. It should be noted that the adaptation of the bowel includes adaptation of each of the enterocytes, overall function, motility, secretion, and absorption [111, 112]. Short bowel implies inadequate length to enable all the necessary components of digestion without the ability to maintain nutritional support. It is a spectrum, with some patients still able to maintain some degree of enteral support. Less than 100 cm of missing length of small bowel is extremely well tolerated; total remaining lengths of less than 100 cm are poorly tolerated and typically require complete replacement of nutrition by parenteral route [113]. Those with true short bowel are TPN dependent, which of course introduces the risks of line sepsis, intra-abdominal sepsis from gut overgrowth, and bowel disuse. There is also increased cost of the TPN itself and of hospitalization necessary for placement of lines and treatment of infections. The most likely cause of short bowel is from resection, the majority of these cases resulting from resections in childhood [114, 115]. Treatment focuses on nutrition; surgical management includes preserving any remaining length, reversing small segments to enhance absorption and motility, and intestinal transplants [116–122]. No surgical intervention has been shown to have overwhelming benefit.

Conclusion

The delivery of early, appropriate nutritional support is a critical component of the comprehensive care of the surgical patient. An understanding of the various options for enteral nutrition, the indications for enteral versus parenteral nutrition, and the complications of the various modalities of nutrition delivery are fundamental for delivering optimal care.

References

1. Jolliet P, Pichard C, Biolo G, Chioléro R, Grimble G, Leverve X, Nitenberg G, Novak I, Planas M, Preiser JC, Roth E, Schols AM, Wernerman J. Enteral nutrition in intensive care patients: a practical approach. Working Group on Nutrition and Metabolism, ESICM. European Society of Intensive Care Medicine. Intensive Care Med. 1998;24(8):848–59.
2. Piccone VA, LeVeen HH, Glass P. Prehepatic hyperalimentation. Surgery. 1980;87:263–71.
3. Enrione EB, Gelfand MJ, Morgan D, et al. The effects of rate and route of nutrient intake on protein metabolism. J Surg Res. 1986;40:320–8.
4. McArdle AH, Palmason C, Morency I. A rationale for enteral feeding as the preferred route for hyperalimentation. Surgery. 1981;90:616–23.
5. Mochizuki H, Trocki O, Dominioni L. Mechanism of prevention of postburn hypermetabolism and catabolism by early enteral feeding. Ann Surg. 1984;200:297–306.
6. Kudsk KA, Carpenter G, Peterson SR. Effect of enteral and parenteral feeding in malnourished rats with hemoglobin—E. coli adjuvant peritonitis. J Surg Res. 1981;31:105–11.
7. Alverdy J, Chi HS, Sheldon GF. The effect of parenteral nutrition on gastrointestinal immunity. Ann Surg. 1985;202:681–90.
8. Kudsk KA, Li J, Renegar KB. Loss of upper respiratory tract immunity with parenteral feeding. Ann Surg. 1996;223:629–35.
9. Moore FA, Moore EE, Jones TN, McCroskey BL, Peterson VM. TEN vs. TPN following major abdominal trauma reduced septic morbidity. J Trauma. 1989;29(7):916–24.
10. Mazaki T, Ebisawa K. Enteral versus parenteral nutrition after gastrointestinal surgery: a systematic review and meta-analysis of randomized controlled trials in the English literature. J Gastrointest Surg. 2008;12(4):739–55.
11. Moore FA, Feliciano DV, Andrassy RJ, McArdle AH, Booth FV, Morgenstein-Wagner TB, Kellum Jr JM, Welling RE, Moore EE. Early enteral feeding, compared with parenteral, reduces postoperative septic complications. The results of a meta-analysis. Ann Surg. 1992;216(2):172–83.
12. Jansen JO, Turner S, Johnston AM. Nutritional management of critically ill trauma patients in the deployed military setting. J R Army Med Corps. 2011;157(3 Suppl 1):S344–9.
13. Heyland DK, Dhaliwal R, Drover JW, Gramlich L, Dodek P, Canadian Critical Care Clinical Practice Guidelines Committee. Canadian clinical practice guidelines for nutrition support in mechanically ventilated, critically ill adult patients. JPEN J Parenter Enteral Nutr. 2003;27(5):355–73.
14. Gramlich L, Kichian K, Pinilla J, Rodych NJ, Dhaliwal R, Heyland DK. Does enteral nutrition compared to parenteral nutrition result in better outcomes in critically ill adult patients? A systematic review of the literature. Nutrition. 2004;20(10):843–8.
15. Rice TW, Mogan S, Hays MA, Bernard GR, Jensen GL, Wheeler AP. Randomized trial of initial trophic versus full-energy enteral nutrition in mechanically ventilated patients with acute respiratory failure. Crit Care Med. 2011;39(5):967–74.
16. Ibrahim EH, Mehringer L, Prentice D, Sherman G, Schaiff R, Fraser V, Kollef MH. Early versus late enteral feeding of mechanically ventilated patients: results of a clinical trial. JPEN J Parenter Enteral Nutr. 2002;26(3):174–81.
17. Alberda C, Gramlich L, Jones N, Jeejeebhoy K, Day AG, Dhaliwal R, Heyland DK. The relationship between nutritional intake and clinical outcomes in critically ill patients: results of an international multicenter observational study. Intensive Care Med. 2009;35(10):1728–37.
18. Heyland DK, Dhaliwal R, Drover JW, Gramlich L, Dodek P, for the Guidelines Committee. Clinical practice guidelines for nutrition support in the adult critically ill patient. JPEN J Parenter Enteral Nutr. 2003;27:355–73.
19. Weitzel LR, Wischmeyer PE. Glutamine in critical illness: the time has come, the time is now. Crit Care Clin. 2010;26(3):515–25. ix–x.
20. Lu CY, Shih YL, Sun LC, Chuang JF, Ma CJ, Chen FM, Wu DC, Hsieh JS, Wang JY. The inflammatory modulation effect of glutamine-enriched total parenteral nutrition in postoperative gastrointestinal cancer patients. Am Surg. 2011;77(1):59–64.
21. Giffiths RD, Jones C, Palmer TE. Six-month outcome of critically ill patients given glutamine-supplemented parenteral nutrition. Nutrition. 1997;13:295–302.
22. Dhaliwal R, Jurewitsch B, Harrietha D, Heyland DK. Combination enteral and parenteral nutrition in critically ill patients: harmful or beneficial? A systematic review of the evidence. Intensive Care Med. 2004;30(8):1666–71.
23. McClave SA, Spain DA, Skolnick JL, Lowen CC, Kieber MJ, Wickerham PS, Vogt JR, Looney SW. Achievement of steady state optimizes results when performing indirect calorimetry. JPEN J Parenter Enteral Nutr. 2003;27(1):16–20.
24. Wooley JA, Sax HC. Indirect calorimetry: application to practice. Nutr Clin Pract. 2003;18:434–9.
25. Chen-Maynard D. http://health.csusb.edu/dchen/368%20stuff/tpn%20calculation.htm. Accessed 1 Jun 2012.
26. Grossie Jr VB, Weisbrodt NW, Moore FA, Moody F. Ischemia/reperfusion-induced disruption of rat small intestine transit is reversed by total enteral nutrition. Nutrition. 2001;17(11–12):939–43.
27. Moore F. Effects of immune enhancing diets on infectious morbidity and multiple organ failure. JPEN J Parenter Enteral Nutr. 2001;25(2 suppl):S36–43.
28. Kles KA, Tappenden KA. Hypoxia differentially regulates nutrient transport in rat jejunum regardless of luminal nutrient present. Am J Physiol Gastrointest Liver Physiol. 2002;283:G1336–42.
29. Wischmeyer PE. The glutamine story: where are we now? Curr Opin Crit Care. 2006;12:142–8.
30. Houdijk AP, Rijnsburger ER, Jansen J, et al. Randomised trial of glutamine-enriched enteral nutrition on infectious morbidity in patients with multiple trauma. Lancet. 1998;352:772–6.
31. Novak F, Heyland DK, Avenell A, Drover JW, Su X. Glutamine supplementation in serious illness: a systematic review of the evidence. Crit Care Med. 2002;30:2022–9.
32. Houdijk APJ, Rijnsburger ER, Jansen J, Wesdorp RIC, Weiss JK, McCamish MA, Teerlink T, Meuwissen SGM, Haarman HJ, Thijs LG, Van Leeuwen PAM. Randomized trial of glutamine-enriched enteral nutrition on infectious morbidity in patients with multiple trauma. Lancet. 1998;352:772–6.
33. Garrel D, Patenaude J, Nedelec B, Samson L, Dorais J, Champoux J, D'Elia M, Bernier J. Decreased mortality and infectious morbidity in adult burn patients given enteral glutamine supplements: a prospective, controlled, randomized clinical trial. Crit Care Med. 2003;31:2444–9.
34. Zhou Y, Jiang Z, Sun Y, Wang X, Ma E, Wilmore D. The effect of supplemental enteral glutamine on plasma levels, gut function, and outcome in severe burns: a randomized, double-blind, controlled clinical trial. JPEN J Parenter Enteral Nutr. 2003;27:241–5.
35. Conejero R, Bonet A, Grau T, Esteban A, Mesejo A, Montejo JC, Lopez J, Acosta JA. Effect of a glutamine-enriched enteral diet on intestinal permeability and infectious morbidity at 28 days in critically ill patients with systemic inflammatory response syndrome: a randomized, single-blind, prospective, multicenter study. Nutrition. 2002;18:716–21.
36. Estivariz CF, Griffith DP, Luo M, et al. Efficacy of parenteral nutrition supplemented with glutamine dipeptide to decrease hospital infections in critically ill surgical patients. JPEN J Parenter Enteral Nutr. 2008;32(4):389–402.

37. Griffiths RD, Allen KD, Andrews FJ, Jones C. Infection, multiple organ failure, and survival in the intensive care unit: influence of glutamine-supplemented parenteral nutrition on acquired infection. Nutrition. 2002;17(7–8):546–52.

38. Wischmeyer PE, Kahana MD, Wolfson R, Hongyu R, et al. Glutamine induces heat shock protein and protects against endotoxin shock in the rat. J Appl Physiol. 2001;90:2403–10.

39. Hartl F. Molecular chaperones in cellular protein folding. Nature. 1996;381:571–80.

40. Musch MW, Hayden D, Sugi K, Strasu D, Chang EB. Cell-specific induction for hsp72-mediated protection by glutamine against oxidant injury in IEC 18 cells. Proc Assoc Am Physicians. 1998;110(2):136–9.

41. Ochoa JB, Bernard AC, O'Brien WE, Griffen MM, et al. Arginase 1 expression and activity in human mononuclear cells after injury. Ann Surg. 2001;233:393–9.

42. Popovic P, Zeh HJ, Ochoa JB. Arginine and immunity. J Nutr. 2007;137:1681S–6.

43. Heyland DK, Samis A. Does immunonutrition in patients with sepsis do more harm than good? Intensive Care Med. 2003;29:667–71.

44. Sato N, Moore FA, Kone BC, Zou L. Differential induction of PPAR-γ by luminal glutamine and iNOS by luminal arginine in the rodent post ischemic small bowel. Am J Physiol Gastrointest Liver Physiol. 2006;290:G616–23.

45. Hua TC, Moochhala SM. Influence of L-arginine, aminoguanidine, and NG-nitro-L-arginine methyl ester (L-name) on the survival rate in a rat model of hemorrhagic shock. Shock. 1999;11:51–7.

46. Daughters K, Waxman K, Nguyen H. Increasing nitric oxide production improves survival in experimental hemorrhagic shock. Resuscitation. 1996;31:141–4.

47. Fukatsu K, Ueno C, Maeshima Y, Hara E, Nagayoshi H, Omata J, Mochizuki H, Hiraide H. Effects of L-arginine infusion during ischemia on gut perfusion, oxygen tension, and circulating myeloid cell activation in murine gut ischemia/reperfusion model. JPEN J Parenter Enteral Nutr. 2004;228:224–31.

48. Jacob TD, Ochoa JB, Udekwu AO, Wilkinson J, Murray T, Billiar TR, Simmons RL, Marion DW, Peitzman AB. Nitric oxide production is inhibited in trauma patients. J Trauma. 1993;35:590–7.

49. Drover JW, Dhaliwal R, Weitzel L, et al. Arginine supplementation in surgical patients. J Am Coll Surg. 2011;212:385.

50. Kulkarni AD, Rudolph FB, Van Buren CT. The role of dietary sources of nucleotides in immune function: review. J Nutr. 1994;124(8 Suppl):1442S–6.

51. Cosgrove M. Perinatal and infant nutrition. Nucleotides. Nutrition. 1998;14(10):748–51.

52. Iwasa Y, Iwasa M, Ohmori Y, Fkutomi T, Ogoshi S. The effect of the administration of nucleosides and nucleotides for parenteral use. Nutrition. 2000;16:598–602.

53. Furst P, Kuhn KS. Fish oil emulsions: what benefits can they bring? Clin Nutr. 2000;19(1):7–14.

54. Razzak A, Aldrich C, Babcock TA, Saied A, et al. Attenuation of iNOS in an LPS-stimulated macrophage model by omega-3 fatty acids is independent of COX-2 derived PGE2. J Surg Res. 2008;145:344–50.

55. Singer P, Theilla M, Fisher H, et al. Benefit of an enteral diet enriched with eicosapentaenoic acid and gamma-linolenic acid in ventilated patients with acute lung injury. Crit Care Med. 2006;34(4):1033–8.

56. Pontes-Arruda A, Aragao AM, Albuquerque JD. Effects of enteral feeding with eicosapentaenoic acid, gamma-linolenic acid, and antioxidants in mechanically ventilated patients with severe sepsis and septic shock. Crit Care Med. 2006;34:2325–33.

57. Gadek JE, DeMichele SJ, Karlstad MD, et al. Effect of enteral feeding with eicosapentaenoic acid, gamma-linolenic acid, and antioxidants in patients with acute respiratory distress syndrome. Enteral Nutrition in ARDS Study Group. Crit Care Med. 1999;27:1409–20.

58. Heyland DK, Dhaliwal R, Day AG, Muscedere J, et al. Reducing Deaths due to Oxidative Stress (The REDOXS Study): rationale and study design for a randomized trial of glutamine and antioxidant supplementation in critically-ill patients. Proc Nutr Soc. 2006;65:250–63.

59. Forceville X, Vitoux D, Gauzit R, Combes A, et al. Selenium, systemic immune response syndrome, sepsis and outcome in critically ill patients. Crit Care Med. 1998;26:1536–44.

60. Goode HF, Cowley HC, Walker BE, Howdle PD, Webster NR. Decreased antioxidant status and increased lipid peroxidation in patients with septic shock and secondary organ dysfunction. Crit Care Med. 1995;23:646–51.

61. Nathens AB, Neff MJ, Jurkovich GJ, et al. Randomized, prospective trial of antioxidant supplementation in critically ill surgical patients. Ann Surg. 2002;236:814–22.

62. Collier BR, Giladi A, Dossett LA, et al. Impact of high-dose antioxidants on outcomes in acutely injured patients. JPEN J Parenter Enteral Nutr. 2008;32:384–8.

63. Heyalnd DK, Dhaliwal R, Suchner U, Berger M. Antioxidant nutrients: a systemic review of trace elements and vitamins in the critically ill patient. Intensive Care Med. 2005;31:327–37.

64. Heyland DK, Dhaliwalm R, Day A, et al. Optimizing the dose of glutamine dipeptides and antioxidants in critically ill patients: a phase I dose-finding study. JPEN J Parenter Enteral Nutr. 2007;31:109–18.

65. Myers JG, Page CP, Stewart RM, Schwesinger WH, Sirinek KR, Aust JB. Complications of needle catheter jejunostomy in 2,002 consecutive applications. Am J Surg. 1995;170(6):547–51.

66. Holmes JH, Brundage SI, Hall RA, Maier RV, Jurkovich GJ. Complications of surgical feeding jejunostomy in trauma patients. J Trauma. 1999;47(6):1009–12.

67. Marik PE, Zaloga GP. Gastric versus post-pyloric feeding: a systematic review. Crit Care. 2003;7(3):R46–51.

68. Boivin MA, Levy H. Gastric feeding with erythromycin is equivalent to transpyloric feeding in the critically ill. Crit Care Med. 2001;29(10):1916–9.

69. Marik PE, Zaloga GP. Early enteral nutrition in acutely ill patients: a systematic review. Crit Care Med. 2001;29:2264–70.

70. Moncure M, Samaha E, Moncure K, et al. Jejunostomy tube feedings should not be stopped in the perioperative patient. JPEN J Parenter Enteral Nutr. 1999;23(6):356–9.

71. Heyland DK, Drover JW, MacDonald S, Novak F, Lam M. Effect of postpyloric feeding on gastroesophageal regurgitation and pulmonary microaspiration: results of a randomized controlled trial. Crit Care Med. 2001;29:1495–501.

72. Esparza J, Boivin MA, Hartshorne MF, Levy H. Equal aspiration rates in gastrically and transpylorically fed critically ill patients. Intensive Care Med. 2001;27(4):660–4.

73. Konstantinides FN, Konstantinides NN, Li JC. Urinary urea nitrogen: too sensitive for calculating nitrogen balance studies in surgical clinical nutrition. JPEN J Parenter Enteral Nutr. 1991;15:189–93.

74. Rodriguez DJ, Clevenger FW, Osler TM, et al. Obligatory negative nitrogen balance following spinal cord injury. JPEN J Parenter Enteral Nutr. 1991;15(3):319–22.

75. McClave SA, Snider HL. Understanding the metabolic response to critical illness: factors that cause patients to deviate from the expected pattern of hypermetabolism. New Horiz. 1994;2(2):139–46.

76. Heyland DK, Cahill N, Day AG. Optimal amount of calories for critically ill paitents: depends on how you slice the cake. Crit Care Med. 2011;39(12):2619–26.

77. Kozar RA, Dyer C, Bulger E, Mourtzakis M, Wade CE, Heyland DK. Elderly trauma patients: highest risk, fewest calories. JPEN J Parenter Enteral Nutr. 2011;35:S26.

78. Kozar RA, McQuiggan MM, Moore EE, Kudsk K, Jurkovich G, Moore FA. Postinjury enteral tolerance is reliably achieved by a standardized protocol. J Surg Res. 2002;104(1):70–5.

79. Osland E, Yunus RM, Khan S, Memon MA. Early versus traditional postoperative feeding in patients undergoing resectional gastrointestinal surgery: a meta-analysis. JPEN J Parenter Enteral Nutr. 2011;35(4):473–87.

80. McQuigan M, Kozar RA, Moore FA. Enteral glutamine during active shock resuscitation is safe and enhances tolerance. JPEN J Parenter Enteral Nutr. 2008;32(1):28–35.

81. Heyland DK, Cahill NE, Dhaliwal R, Wang M, Day AG, Ahmed A, Aris F, Muscedere J, Drover JW, McClave SA. Enhanced protein-energy provision via the enteral route in critically ill patients: a single center feasibility trial. Crit Care. 2010;14:R78.

82. Casaer MP, Mesotten D, Hermans G, et al. Early versus late parenteral nutrition in critically ill adults. N Engl J Med. 2011;365(6):506–17.

83. Marvin RG, McKinley BA, McQuiggan M, Cocanour CS, Moore FA. Nonocclusive bowel necrosis occurring in critically ill trauma patients receiving enteral nutrition manifests no reliable clinical signs for early detection. Am J Surg. 2000;179(1):7–12.

84. Banks PA, Freeman ML, And the Practice Parameters Committee of the American College of Gastroenterology. Practice guidelines in acute pancreatitis. Am J Gastroenterol. 2006;101:2379–400.

85. Kumar A, Singh N, Prakash S, Saraya A, Joshi YK. Early enteral nutrition in severe acute pancreatitis: a prospective randomized controlled trial comparing nasojejunal and nasogastric routes. J Clin Gastroenterol. 2006;40(5):431–4.

86. Corcoy R, Ma Sanachez J, Domingo P, et al. Nutrition in patients with severe acute pancreatitis. Nutrition. 1988;4:269–75.

87. Marts BC, Naunheim KS, Fiore AC, Pennington DG. Conservative versus surgical management of chylothorax. Am J Surg. 1992;164:532–5.

88. Bell JD, Marshall GD, Shaw BA, et al. Alterations in human thoracic duct lymphocytes during thoracic duct drainage. Transplant Proc. 1983;15:677–80.

89. Machleder HI, Paulus H. Clinical and immunological alterations observed in patients undergoing long-term thoracic duct drainage. Surgery. 1978;84:157–65.

90. Medeiros AC, Aires-Neto T, Marchini JS, Brandao-Neto J, Valenca DM, Egito ES. Treatment of postoperative enterocutaneous fistulas by high-pressure vacuum with a normal oral diet. Dig Surg. 2004;21:401–5.

91. Berry SM, Fischer JE. Classification and pathophysiology of enterocutaneous fistulas. Surg Clin North Am. 1996;76:1009–18.

92. Lloyd DA, Gabe SM, Windsor AC. Nutrition and management of enterocutaneous fistula. Br J Surg. 2006;93(9):1045–55.

93. Campos AC, Andrade DF, Campos GM, Matias JE, Coelho JC. A multivariate model to determine prognostic factors in gastrointestinal fistulas. J Am Coll Surg. 1999;188:483–90.

94. Meguid MM, Campos AC. Nutritional management of patients with gastrointestinal fistulas. Surg Clin North Am. 1996;76:1035–80.

95. Hyon SH, Martinez-Garbino JA, Benati ML, Lopez-Avellaneda ME, Brozzi NA, Argibay PF. Management of a high-output postoperative enterocutaneous fistula with a vacuum sealing method and continuous enteral nutrition. ASAIO J. 2000;46:511–4.

96. Spiliotis J, Vagenas K, Panagopoulos K, Kalfarentzos F. Treatment of enterocutaneous fistulas with TPN and somatostatin, compared with patients who received TPN only. Br J Clin Pract. 1990;44:616–8.

97. Haffejee AA. Surgical management of high output enterocutaneous fistulae: a 24-year experience. Curr Opin Clin Nutr Metab Care. 2004;7:309–16.

98. Ysebaert D, Van Hee R, Hubens G, Vaneerdeweg W, Eyskens E. Management of digestive fistulas. Scand J Gastroenterol Suppl. 1994;207:42–4.

99. Reber HA, Roberts C, Way LW, Dunphy JE. Management of external gastrointestinal fistulas. Ann Surg. 1978;188:460–7.

100. Lynch AC, Delaney CP, Senagore AJ, Connor JT, Remzi FH, Fazio VW. Clinical outcome and factors predictive of recurrence after enterocutaneous fistula surgery. Ann Surg. 2004;240:825–31.

101. Hill GL. Operative strategy in the treatment of enterocutaneous fistulas. World J Surg. 1983;7:495–501.

102. Foster III CE, Lefor AT. General management of gastrointestinal fistulas. Recognition, stabilization, and correction of fluid and electrolyte imbalances. Surg Clin North Am. 1996;76:1019–33.

103. Gonzalez-Pinto I, Gonzalez EM. Optimising the treatment of upper gastrointestinal fistulae. Gut. 2001;49 Suppl 4:iv21–31.

104. Altomare DF, Serio G, Pannarale OC, Lupo L, Palasciano N, Memeo V, et al. Prediction of mortality by logistic regression analysis in patients with postoperative enterocutaneous fistulae. Br J Surg. 1990;77:450–3.

105. Fischer JE. The pathophysiology of enterocutaneous fistulas. World J Surg. 1983;7:446–50.

106. Jeppesen PB. Clinical significance of GLP-2 in short bowel syndrome. J Nutr. 2003;133:3721–4.

107. Wilmore DW, Byrne TA, Persinger RL. Short bowel syndrome: new therapeutic approaches. Curr Probl Surg. 1997;34:389–444.

108. Jeppesen PB. Glucagon-like peptide-2: update of the recent clinical trails. Gastroenterology. 2006;130(2 Suppl 1):S127–31.

109. Wilmore DW, Lacey JM, Soultanakis RP, Bosch RL, Byrne TA. Factors predicting a successful outcome after pharmacologic bowel compensation. Ann Surg. 1997;226:288–93.

110. Seetharam P, Rodrigues G. Short bowel syndrome: a review of management options. Saudi J Gastroenterol. 2011;17(4):229–35.

111. Thompson JS, Quingley EM, Adrian TE. Factors affecting outcome following proximal and distal intestinal resection in the dog: an examination of the relative roles of mucosal adaptation, motility, luminal factors and, enteric peptides. Dig Dis Sci. 1999;44:63–74.

112. Schmidt T, Pfeiffer A, Hackelsberger N, Widmer R, Meisel C, Kaess H. Effect of intestinal resection on human small bowel motility. Gut. 1996;38:859–63.

113. Niv Y, Charash B, Sperber AD, Oren M. Effect of octreotide on gastrostomy, duodenostomy, and cholecystostomy effluents: a physiological study of fluid and electrolyte balance. Am J Gastroenterol. 1997;92:2107–11.

114. Thompson JS. Comparison of massive vs. repeated resection leading to the short bowel syndrome. J Gastrointest Surg. 2000;4:101–4.

115. DiBaise JK, Young RJ, Vanderhoof JA. Intestinal rehabilitation and the short bowel syndrome: Part 1. Am J Gastroenterol. 2004;99:1386–95.

116. Grant D, Abu-Elmagd K, Reyes J, Tzakis A, Langnas A, Fishbein T, et al. 2003 Report of the intestine transplant registry: a new era has dawned. Ann Surg. 2005;241:607–13.

117. Thompson JS, Pinch LW, Young R, Vanderhoof JA. Long term outcome of intestinal lengthening. Transplant Proc. 2000;32:1242–3.

118. Thompson JS, Langnas AN. Surgical approaches to improving intestinal function in the short bowel syndrome. Arch Surg. 1999;134:706–11.

119. Thompson JS, Langnas AN, Pinch LW, Kaufman S, Quigley EM, Vanderhoof JA. Surgical approach to short bowel syndrome. Experience in a population of 160 patients. Ann Surg. 1995;222:600–7.

120. Thompson JS. Surgical approach to the short bowel syndrome: procedures to slow intestinal transit. Eur J Pediatr Surg. 1999;9:263–6.

121. Thompson JS. Strategies for preserving intestinal length in short bowel syndrome. Dis Colon Rectum. 1987;30:208–13.

122. Panis Y, Messing B, Rivet P, Coffin B, Hautefeuille P, Matuchansky C, et al. Segment reversal of the small bowel as an alternative to intestinal transplantation in patients with short bowel syndrome. Ann Surg. 1997;225:401–7.

Chang-I Wu, Vasiliy Sim, and S. Rob Todd

Introduction

One of the primary roles of the kidneys is to filter waste material from the blood. The inability of the kidneys to do this leads to renal failure. Acute renal insufficiency (ARI) is defined as the sudden onset (<48 h) of impaired kidney function. This is represented by a rise in the serum creatinine or a decrease in the urine output. The serum creatinine serves as a useful biomarker for measuring the flow rate of fluids through the kidneys, termed the glomerular filtration rate (GFR). As the clearance of creatinine and GFR decrease, the serum creatinine correspondingly increases signifying impaired renal function. The most common formula used to estimate GFR is the Cockcroft–Gault formula:

$$\text{GFR} = \frac{(140 - \text{Age}) \times \text{Weight (kg)}}{72 \times \text{Serum creatinine (mg/dL)}} \times [0.85 \text{ if Female}]$$

Classification

Initial classification systems simply divided ARI into two groups: oliguric or non-oliguric. Oliguric ARI is defined as having a urine output of less than 0.5 mL/kg/h or 5 mL/kg/day. While ARI with an elevated serum creatinine and

C.-I. Wu, M.D.
Columbia University Mailman School of Public Health,
722 West 168ᵗʰ Street, New York, NY 10032
e-mail: cw2623@columbia.edu

V. Sim, M.D.
Department of Surgery, Brookdale University Hospital
and Medical Center, One Brookdale Plaza, Brooklyn, NY 11212, USA
e-mail: vasya_s_@yahoo.com

S.R. Todd, M.D., F.A.C.S. (✉)
Division of Trauma, Emergency Surgery, and Surgical Critical Care,
Department of Surgery, New York University Langone Medical Center, 550 First Avenue, New Bellevue 15 East 9,
New York, NY 10016, USA
e-mail: srtodd@nyumc.org

near-normal urine output is called non-oliguric. Patients with non-oliguric ARI generally fair better and have a lower mortality rate than patients with oliguric ARI [1]. In an attempt to better differentiate the various stages of ARI, the Acute Dialysis Quality Initiative (ADQI) group developed the RIFLE criteria (Table 10.1) [2]. RIFLE stands for risk, injury, failure, loss, and end-stage renal disease, and represents progression of the disease. The staging is based on changes in the serum creatinine or urine output. Another similar classification system for acute renal failure also based on the serum creatinine and urine output is the Acute Kidney Injury Network (AKIN) criteria. While some studies have shown no difference between the two systems, others show that the RIFLE criteria are more robust and have an increased sensitivity of ARI detection during the first 48 hours in the intensive care unit (ICU) [3, 4].

Epidemiology

Acute renal insufficiency usually presents as a complication of other disease processes and not as the primary disease. The reported incidence of ARI is 5–10% in all hospitalized patients and ~30% in critically ill patients [3, 5]. Some identified risk factors for developing ARI include the following:

1. Elderly (>65 years of age)
2. Male gender
3. Comorbid conditions (i.e., obesity, chronic obstructive pulmonary disease [COPD])
4. Infection
5. Major surgeries, especially cardiac surgery
6. Cardiogenic shock
7. Hypovolemia
8. Nephrotoxic medications
9. Cirrhosis

Since ARI is most commonly a secondary injury, its mortality rate varies widely, and therefore reflects the mortality rate of the underlying primary disease. In general, two organs failing have a 50% mortality rate, three organs—80%, and five

L.J. Moore et al. (eds.), *Common Problems in Acute Care Surgery*,
DOI 10.1007/978-1-4614-6123-4_10, © Springer Science+Business Media New York 2013

Table 10.1 The RIFLE criteria

RIFLE criteria for ARI		
	GFR criteria	Urine output criteria
Risk	1.5× baseline serum creatinine or GFR decreased >25%	<0.5 mL/kg/h×6 h
Injury	2× baseline serum creatinine or GFR decreased >50%	<0.5 mL/kg/h×12 h
Failure	3× baseline serum creatinine or GFR decreased >75% or serum creatinine >4 mg/dL or acute rise of >0.5 mg/dL	<0.3 mL/kg/h×24 h or anuria×12 h
Loss	Loss of kidney function×4 weeks	
ESRD	Loss of kidney function×3 months	

RIFLE risk, injury, failure, loss, and end-stage renal disease

organs—100% [6]. A large multicenter prospective study reported a 60% mortality rate in ICU patients who developed ARI [7]. Several studies have documented an association between the RIFLE classification of ARI and in-hospital mortality: 9–27% in the at risk group, 11–30% in the injury group, and 26–40% in the failure group [8, 9]. Some identified risk factors for mortality in ARI include the following:

1. Elderly (>65 years of age)
2. Male gender
3. Comorbid conditions (i.e., obesity, chronic obstructive pulmonary disease [COPD])
4. Oliguric ARI
5. Sepsis
6. Non-renal organ failure (heart, lungs, liver…)
7. Mechanical ventilation

Etiology

The pathophysiology of ARI can be divided into three categories based on anatomy: prerenal, renal (parenchymal), and postrenal (obstructive). A combination of imaging and serum and urine studies can be utilized to differentiate between these categories. The urine sodium concentration and fractional excretion of sodium (FE_{Na}) are particularly useful in differentiating renal parenchymal injury from prerenal and postrenal pathologies, which is further discussed later in this chapter. The FE_{Na} formula is:

$$FE_{Na} = \left(U_{Na} \times P_{Cr} \right) / \left(U_{Cr} \times P_{Na} \right) \times 100$$

where U_{Na} = urine sodium, P_{Cr} = plasma creatinine, U_{Cr} = urine creatinine, and P_{Na} = plasma sodium.

Prerenal Etiologies

Prerenal azotemia is caused by a decrease in renal perfusion and accounts for 30–60% of inpatient ARI [10]. There is no intrinsic renal disease but rather a systemic factor that decreases GFR. Most prerenal causes involve low flow states or shunting of the blood flow away from the kidneys (Table 10.2). A decrease in

renal perfusion results in activation of the renin-angiotensin-aldosterone system. Angiotensin II increases glomerular filtration pressure by constricting the efferent arteriole, and also increases the proximal reabsorption of sodium, while aldosterone increases the distal reabsorption of sodium. Actions of these hormones not only preserve renal blood flow, but also help with the diagnosis since they decrease urine sodium concentration to less than 20 mmol/L and the FE_{Na} to less than 1%. Once prerenal pathophysiology is established, clinical suspicion should guide the further differentiation between the numerous causes of prerenal ARI. Treatment includes reversing the underlying cause of renal hypoperfusion and is discussed later in this chapter.

Renal (Parenchymal) Etiologies

Primary renal azotemia is caused by injury to the renal parenchyma either by ischemia or cytotoxic drugs and occurs in ~50% of inpatient ARI [10]. Some of the causes of renal parenchymal injury are presented in Table 10.2. The most common cause of renal (parenchymal) disease is acute tubular necrosis (ATN), which is also the most common cause of ARI in general. As the name suggests, tubular function is impaired due to death and sloughing off of the renal tubular epithelial cells. The sloughed off cells obstruct the renal tubules reducing GFR, the process known as tubule-glomerular feedback. Tubular sodium reabsorption is also reduced, increasing the urine sodium concentration to greater than 40 mmol/L and the FE_{Na} to greater than 2%.

A urinalysis is most helpful in differentiation of renal azotemia from prerenal and postrenal causes of ARI. Tubular epithelial cells and casts in the urine are pathognomonic for ATN. Urine sediments with red cells and red cell casts are suggestive of glomerulonephritis or vasculitis. White cell casts are suggestive of acute interstitial nephritis (AIN) or infection. Finally, pigmented casts suggest myoglobinuria. Renal biopsy can be used to determine the cause of renal insufficiency, but due to its invasive nature should only be used if other methods are inconclusive and identification of a specific cause is necessary to direct treatment.

Table 10.2   Acute renal insufficiency etiologies

Pre-renal	Parenchymal	Post-renal
Hypovolemia	ATN	Prostatic disease
Hypotension	AIN	Urethral stricture
Decreased cardiac output	Glomerulonephritis	Pelvic or retroperitoneal mass
Raised intra-abdominal pressure	Vasculitis	Nephrolithiasis (rare)
Aortic stenosis	Nephrotoxins (aminoglycosides, amphotericin, cisplatin…)	Crystals (ethylene glycol, uric acid, light chain disease…)
Mechanical ventilation	Sepsis	
Medications (Ketorolac, ACEi, ARB…)	Trauma	
	Major surgery (AAA repair)	
	Renal allograft rejection	
	Contrast	

ACEi angiotensin converting enzyme inhibitors, *ARB* angiotensin II receptor blockers, *ATN* acute tubular necrosis, *AIN* acute interstitial nephritis, *AAA* abdominal aortic aneurysm

Postrenal (Obstructive) Etiologies

Postrenal (obstructive) azotemia is caused by the obstruction of urine flow distal to the renal tubules. Just like in prerenal azotemia, there is no intrinsic kidney disease, which leads to a similar urine sodium concentration and FE_{Na} as in prerenal disease. Postrenal azotemia accounts for ~10% of inpatient ARI [10]. Obstruction can either be renal or extrarenal in origin (Table 10.2). Renal obstruction includes crystal formation from ethylene glycol poisoning, uric acid nephropathy from tumor lysis syndrome, and light chain diseases including multiple myeloma. Nephrolithiasis rarely causes obstructive azotemia unless there is only one functioning kidney. Extrarenal causes include prostatic disease, urethral stricture, and pelvic or retroperitoneal masses. Renal and pelvic ultrasound are the mainstay imaging studies for the diagnosis of postrenal azotemia. Consultation with a urologist may be warranted to discuss treatment options.

Diagnosis and Management

The initial diagnostic evaluation involves identifying prerenal and reversible causes of ARI. Commonly, ARI first presents as low urine output in a patient who recently had a significant systemic injury such as surgery, trauma, infection, or shock. Decreased urine output is not seen in patients with non-oliguric ARI and while they have better outcomes, they are also not detected as often. Clinical suspicion based on known risk factors should lead a clinician to follow the serum creatinine. An acute rise in serum creatinine (>0.5 mg/dL) suggests ARI and the need to investigate and treat the cause. A sudden onset of anuria in a patient with a urinary catheter suggests obstruction of the catheter. Flushing or changing the catheter may resolve the anuria. After a confirmed report of oliguria, the initial diagnostic tests that should be ordered include the following:

1. Urinalysis
2. Serum creatinine concentration
3. Serum sodium concentration
4. Urine creatinine concentration
5. Urine sodium concentration
6. Basic electrolytes

A FE_{Na} less than 1% signifies prerenal or postrenal disease, while a value greater than 2% signifies a renal cause, as previously mentioned. The exception is seen with myoglobinuria, where the FE_{Na} is less than 1%, while still being a renal parenchymal cause. Another caveat is that the recent use of loop diuretics (i.e., furosemide) makes the FE_{Na} calculation inaccurate. Microscopic analysis of urine sediments can help to further classify causes of renal azotemia. More specific testing can be done based on clinical suspicion.

Since early treatment is so important with ARI, the diagnosis and management often occur simultaneously. Fluid support is the first option for most causes of ARI. This typically involves a 500–1,000 mL crystalloid bolus or a 250–500 mL albumin containing bolus. This should occur while diagnostic testing is underway. The purpose of fluid support and resuscitation is to flush out toxins and prevent further renal injury. While a euvolemic state is preferred, if the fluid status of a patient is not known it may be better to be volume overloaded. This avoids end-organ hypoperfusion that may lead to irreversible ischemia. Volume overload does have its sequelae, including pulmonary edema and its associated risks. It is also relatively contraindicated in patients with critical aortic stenosis where additional volume may lead to heart failure.

A large variety of resuscitation fluids is available for use in the hypovolemic patient. Colloids may be more effective in keeping fluids in the intravascular space and therefore may be preferred. However, several studies have documented that some colloid solutions may be harmful to the kidneys. A meta-analysis evaluating nephrotoxicity of colloid solutions revealed that several hydroxyethyl starch (HES) containing solutions are nephrotoxic, while albumin containing colloids are not [11]. Furthermore, several subsequent meta-analyses have revealed that both starches and dextrans can exacerbate a renal insult [12, 13]. Therefore, crystalloids should be the first choice of resuscitation fluids until we gain a better understanding of colloid related renal injury.

Response to the fluid challenge needs to be assessed. If the patient responds with an appropriate increase in urine output but remains under-resuscitated, fluid boluses should be continued until the patient is euvolemic. If more invasive monitoring of the volume status is needed, central venous pressure (CVP) monitoring can be performed. In addition to patients with renal hypoperfusion, fluid resuscitation has also been shown beneficial in myoglobinuria, contrast-induced nephropathy, and in patients exposed to nephrotoxic drugs and drugs that cause tubular crystal precipitation [8]. If a patient is euvolemic but is hypotensive with a mean arterial pressure (MAP) of less than 65 mmHg, inotropes such as norepinephrine may be used to improve cardiac output and renal perfusion. Historically, low dose ("renal dose") dopamine (2 µg/kg/min) was used to increase urine output by serving as a renal vasodilator. More recent evidence suggests that it is not effective, may actually be harmful, and thus should not be used [14, 15].

Once the cause of ARI is determined and the patient is fluid resuscitated, specific management of the underlying cause, especially in reversible conditions, should be addressed. Some of the specific management options include stopping offending agents such as ketorolac, angiotensin converting enzyme (ACE) inhibitors, angiotensin II receptor blockers (ARB), and antibiotics such as aminoglycosides and amphotericin. The use of loop diuretics such as furosemide was once thought to be beneficial by delaying the need for renal replacement therapy (RRT). Now RRT is not viewed as being a failure of medical therapy, but as merely another treatment option. Even though loop diuretics have been shown to convert oliguria to diuresis, allowing for improved control of electrolyte abnormalities and volume overload without increased mortality, there is still a lack of strong evidence for the role of diuretics in critically ill patients [16, 17]. Furthermore, several studies suggest that diuretic use might actually delay proper RRT leading to worse outcomes [17–19]. Therefore, a nephrologist should be consulted early in the process to reduce complications of ARI and to quickly initiate RRT when necessary.

Renal Replacement Therapy

Early RRT is now considered to be an effective strategy in managing ARI. It takes over the kidneys' function by removing toxins and establishing electrolyte, acid–base, and fluid balances. Indications for RRT include the following:

1. Volume overload refractory to medical therapy
2. Metabolic acidosis
3. Severe hyperkalemia (>6.5 mmol/L)
4. Uremia (encephalopathy, pericarditis, myopathy, neuropathy…)
5. Dialyzable toxins (salicylate, ethylene glycol…)

In critically ill patients, ARI has been associated with increased mortality [20]. However, the optimal RRT has not yet been established. Renal replacement therapy has different modes, intensity, and even timing. The choice of RRT mode, intermittent hemodialysis (IHD) versus continuous renal replacement therapy (CRRT), is determined by the needs of the patient. Intermittent hemodialysis is preferred either in stable or recovering patients or in those who cannot tolerate the anticoagulation required for CRRT. Continuous renal replacement therapy on the other hand is for patients who cannot tolerate fluid shifts such as hemodynamically unstable patients or those with intracranial swelling [8, 21, 22].

The intensity of CRRT is also debatable with some studies documenting improved survival with high dose, while others showing no benefit [23–25]. A recent meta-analysis identified five studies that compared low dose (<35 ml/kg/h) versus high dose (35–45 ml/kg/h) CRRT. The combined results show no difference in 28 day survival [26]. However, when looked at individually, two studies showed improved survival in the high dose group and three showed no survival benefit.

The timing of the initiation of RRT is similarly unclear. A recent systematic review identified 15 studies that had a wide range of definitions of "early" and "late" RRT initiation periods based on the onset of oliguria, increasing blood urea levels, RIFLE criteria, hyperkalemia, or simply ICU admission [27]. While the conclusion of the systematic review was that early RRT might be beneficial, a wide heterogeneity in definitions and poor quality of studies does not allow for any concrete recommendations.

Nutrition in Acute Renal Insufficiency

As with any injury, renal insults cause the secretion of catabolic factors; therefore, in order to facilitate recovery, adequate nutritional support is required. While there is a lack of strong evidence, the American Society for Parenteral and Enteral Nutrition (ASPEN) guidelines recommend the use of enteral nutrition when possible [28]. If parenteral nutrition is required, a standard amino acid formulation should be used in ARI.

Due to a high catabolic state in ARI, the protein needs are usually in the 1.8–2.5 g/kg/day range and should be replaced accordingly to avoid a negative protein balance [28–30].

Specific Etiologies and Their Management

Hepatorenal Syndrome

Acute renal insufficiency from hepatorenal syndrome (HRS) is typically seen in advanced cirrhosis or acute liver failure. The exact reason why liver failure causes prerenal azotemia is not fully appreciated, but may be partially due to the reduced ability of the liver to metabolize vascular mediators including prostaglandins and endotoxin that result in renal hypoperfusion. Hepatorenal syndrome presents in a typical prerenal fashion with oliguria, a rise in the serum creatinine, and a normal urinalysis. These patients typically have a low albumin secondary to their liver failure. Numerous studies have shown improved outcome in patients treated with vasopressin analog and albumin containing solutions [31, 32]. Ultimately improving hepatic function, up to and including liver transplant, is the only way to resolve the associated ARI.

Contrast-Induced Nephropathy

Radiocontrast dye is recognized as the third leading cause of ARI and the leading iatrogenic cause in hospitalized patients. A meta-analysis of 40 studies documented an incidence of 6% following contrast computed tomography (CT) scans, with 1% of all patients who received a CT scan having persistent decline in renal function [33]. Risk factors to contrast-induced nephropathy include preexisting renal disease, diabetes mellitus, and the use of large volumes of dye. Clinically, patients present with an acute rise in the serum creatinine within 48 h of the contrast exposure. Levels peak after 5 days before returning to baseline in 7–10 days. Some patients, especially the ones with risk factors, experience permanent reduction in kidney function. Besides supportive care with fluids to prevent further kidney injury, there is no proven treatment option. There are several agents that have been used in an attempt to prevent contrast-induced nephropathy such as N-acetylcysteine, statins, and adenosine receptor antagonists. While all three agents have been shown to be beneficial in numerous meta-analyses, the studies used in the analyses had significant weaknesses [34–36]. In addition, in the case of N-acetylcysteine, when studies analyzed were limited to those that had allocation concealment, double blinding, and were intention-to-treat, there was no benefit in pretreatment [36].

Rhabdomyolysis

The causes of muscle injury leading to rhabdomyolysis include major trauma, especially crush injuries with compartment syndrome, vascular embolism with reperfusion injury, medications (i.e., statins), prolonged seizures, and many other mechanisms that can cause damage to muscle tissue. The breakdown of muscle cells releases myoglobin, which is toxic to the renal tubules causing azotemia. Clinically, the urine appears reddish brown with pigmented granular casts. Creatine kinase (CK) is also released from damaged muscle cells along with myoglobin and is markedly elevated in the serum. Electrolyte imbalances include hyperphosphatemia and hyperkalemia secondary to their release from injured muscle cells. Treatment includes aggressive fluid resuscitation to achieve urine outputs of more than 100–200 mL/h if tolerated by the patient. Bicarbonate can be used to alkalinize the urine to reduce renal toxicity by improving solubility of the myoglobin. Electrolyte imbalances should be corrected. If supportive therapy is not enough, RRT should be considered.

Complications and Outcomes

Complications usually stem from not recognizing ARI. The kidneys serve many functions, and loss of those functions can result in dire and acute consequences including:
1. Uremia from the buildup of waste nitrogen compounds
2. Metabolic acidosis from the failure to reabsorb bicarbonate and excrete hydrogen ions
3. Electrolyte imbalance and the loss of osmolality regulation
4. Loss of blood pressure regulation from the failure of the renin-angiotensin-aldosterone system
5. Loss of hormone regulation including erythropoietin

Conclusion

After ARI is recognized and the cause is identified, treating the underlying cause and fluid support to prevent further kidney injury are the goals of management. If the insult was transient, the kidneys should be able to recover most of their pre-insult function. However, renal function may take weeks to months to recover requiring long-term supportive care including RRT and nutritional support in the meantime. The risk factors for permanent loss of kidney function are the same as the risk factors for mortality. The result is end stage kidney disease requiring life-long RRT or renal transplant.

Algorithm

1. Clinical presentation of low urine output (<0.5 mL/kg/h) after a major systemic insult
2. Confirm oliguria and initiate a crystalloid (500–1,000 mL) or colloid (250–500 mL) fluid bolus

3. Check urinalysis, serum and urine sodium concentrations, serum and urine creatinine concentrations, and basic electrolytes
4. Calculate the FE_{Na} and determine the volume status of the patient, and correct the electrolytes if necessary
5. Assess the response to the fluid bolus, continue fluid resuscitation if necessary
6. If euvolemic but hypotensive, initiate inotropes to maintain the MAP greater than 65 mmHg
7. Identify the etiology of the ARI: prerenal, renal, or postrenal

   (a) Prerenal
   - Identify the underlying cause of ARI and correct if possible (stop offending agents, treat hypovolemia/hypotension, reverse non-renal organ failure)
   - Supportive care with normalization of the electrolytes and acid–base balance
   - RRT as needed

   (b) Renal
   - Identify the underlying cause of ARI with further diagnostic studies and treat (stop offending agents, pretreat with N-acetylcysteine for radiocontrast dye, antibiotics for sepsis…)
   - Supportive care with normalization of the electrolytes and acid–base balance
   - RRT as needed (including dialyzable toxins such as salicylates or ethylene glycol)

   (c) Postrenal
   - Identify the underlying cause with renal and pelvic ultrasound
   - Consult urology if necessary
   - Supportive care with normalization of the electrolytes and acid–base balance
   - RRT as needed

8. Long term supportive care including nutritional support and RRT
9. Acute renal insufficiency conversion to ESRD leads to life-long RRT and evaluation for renal transplant

References

1. Morgan DJ, Ho KM. A comparison of nonoliguric and oliguric severe acute kidney injury according to the risk injury failure loss end-stage (RIFLE) criteria. Nephron Clin Pract. 2010;115(1):c59–65 [Comparative Study].
2. Bellomo R, Ronco C, Kellum JA, Mehta RL, Palevsky P. Acute renal failure—definition, outcome measures, animal models, fluid therapy and information technology needs: the Second International Consensus Conference of the Acute Dialysis Quality Initiative (ADQI) Group. Crit Care. 2004;8(4):R204–12 [Consensus Development Conference Guideline Practice Guideline Review].
3. Joannidis M, Metnitz B, Bauer P, Schusterschitz N, Moreno R, Druml W, et al. Acute kidney injury in critically ill patients classified by AKIN versus RIFLE using the SAPS 3 database. Intensive Care Med. 2009;35(10):1692–702 [Research Support, Non-U.S. Gov't].
4. Bagshaw SM, George C, Bellomo R. A comparison of the RIFLE and AKIN criteria for acute kidney injury in critically ill patients. Nephrol Dial Transplant. 2008;23(5):1569–74 [Comparative Study Multicenter Study Research Support, Non-U.S. Gov't].
5. Hou SH, Bushinsky DA, Wish JB, Cohen JJ, Harrington JT. Hospital-acquired renal insufficiency: a prospective study. Am J Med. 1983;74(2):243–8 [Research Support, U.S. Gov't, P.H.S.].
6. Liano F, Junco E, Pascual J, Madero R, Verde E. The spectrum of acute renal failure in the intensive care unit compared with that seen in other settings. The Madrid Acute Renal Failure Study Group. Kidney Int Suppl. 1998;66:S16–24 [Comparative Study Research Support, Non-U.S. Gov't].
7. Uchino S, Kellum JA, Bellomo R, Doig GS, Morimatsu H, Morgera S, et al. Acute renal failure in critically ill patients: a multinational, multicenter study. JAMA. 2005;294(7):813–8 [Multicenter Study Research Support, Non-U.S. Gov't].
8. Brochard L, Abroug F, Brenner M, Broccard AF, Danner RL, Ferrer M, et al. An official ATS/ERS/ESICM/SCCM/SRLF statement: prevention and management of acute renal failure in the ICU patient: an international consensus conference in intensive care medicine. Am J Respir Crit Care Med. 2010;181(10):1128–55 [Consensus Development Conference].
9. Chen YC, Jenq CC, Tian YC, Chang MY, Lin CY, Chang CC, et al. Rifle classification for predicting in-hospital mortality in critically ill sepsis patients. Shock. 2009;31(2):139–45 [Research Support, Non-U.S. Gov't].
10. Nolan CR, Anderson RJ. Hospital-acquired acute renal failure. J Am Soc Nephrol. 1998;9(4):710–8 [Review].
11. Wiedermann CJ, Dunzendorfer S, Gaioni LU, Zaraca F, Joannidis M. Hyperoncotic colloids and acute kidney injury: a meta-analysis of randomized trials. Crit Care. 2010;14(5):R191 [Meta-Analysis].
12. Brunkhorst FM, Engel C, Bloos F, Meier-Hellmann A, Ragaller M, Weiler N, et al. Intensive insulin therapy and pentastarch resuscitation in severe sepsis. N Engl J Med. 2008;358(2):125–39 [Comparative Study Multicenter Study Randomized Controlled Trial Research Support, Non-U.S. Gov't].
13. Celik I. Renal dysfunction after hydroxyethyl starch. Anesth Analg. 2004;99(1):309–10. Author reply 10 [Comment Letter].
14. Lauschke A, Teichgraber UK, Frei U, Eckardt KU. 'Low-dose' dopamine worsens renal perfusion in patients with acute renal failure. Kidney Int. 2006;69(9):1669–74 [Randomized Controlled Trial].
15. Friedrich JO, Adhikari N, Herridge MS, Beyene J. Meta-analysis: low-dose dopamine increases urine output but does not prevent renal dysfunction or death. Ann Intern Med. 2005;142(7):510–24 [Meta-Analysis Research Support, Non-U.S. Gov't Review].
16. Bagshaw SM, Bellomo R, Kellum JA. Oliguria, volume overload, and loop diuretics. Crit Care Med. 2008;36(4 Suppl):S172–8 [Review].
17. Uchino S, Doig GS, Bellomo R, Morimatsu H, Morgera S, Schetz M, et al. Diuretics and mortality in acute renal failure. Crit Care Med. 2004;32(8):1669–77 [Multicenter Study Research Support, Non-U.S. Gov't].
18. Townsend DR, Bagshaw SM. New insights on intravenous fluids, diuretics and acute kidney injury. Nephron Clin Pract. 2008;109(4):c206–16 [Review].
19. Liangos O, Rao M, Balakrishnan VS, Pereira BJ, Jaber BL. Relationship of urine output to dialysis initiation and mortality in acute renal failure. Nephron Clin Pract. 2005;99(2):c56–60 [Research Support, N.I.H., Extramural Research Support, Non-U.S. Gov't Research Support, U.S. Gov't, P.H.S.].
20. Uchino S, Bellomo R, Goldsmith D, Bates S, Ronco C. An assessment of the RIFLE criteria for acute renal failure in hospitalized patients. Crit Care Med. 2006;34(7):1913–7 [Research Support, Non-U.S. Gov't].
21. Pannu N, Klarenbach S, Wiebe N, Manns B, Tonelli M. Renal replacement therapy in patients with acute renal failure: a system-

atic review. JAMA. 2008;299(7):793–805 [Research Support, Non-U.S. Gov't Review].

22. Rabindranath K, Adams J, Macleod AM, Muirhead N. Intermittent versus continuous renal replacement therapy for acute renal failure in adults. Cochrane Database Syst Rev. 2007(3):CD003773 [Meta-Analysis Review].

23. Ronco C, Bellomo R, Homel P, Brendolan A, Dan M, Piccinni P, et al. Effects of different doses in continuous veno-venous haemofiltration on outcomes of acute renal failure: a prospective randomised trial. Lancet. 2000;356(9223):26–30 [Clinical Trial Randomized Controlled Trial].

24. Palevsky PM, Zhang JH, O'Connor TZ, Chertow GM, Crowley ST, Choudhury D, et al. Intensity of renal support in critically ill patients with acute kidney injury. N Engl J Med. 2008;359(1):7–20 [Multicenter Study Randomized Controlled Trial Research Support, N.I.H., Extramural Research Support, U.S. Gov't, Non-P.H.S.].

25. Bellomo R, Cass A, Cole L, Finfer S, Gallagher M, Lo S, et al. Intensity of continuous renal-replacement therapy in critically ill patients. N Engl J Med. 2009;361(17):1627–38 [Multicenter Study Randomized Controlled Trial Research Support, Non-U.S. Gov't].

26. Negash DT, Dhingra VK, Copland M, Griesdale D, Henderson W. Intensity of continuous renal replacement therapy in acute kidney injury in the intensive care unit: a systematic review and meta-analysis. Vasc Endovascular Surg. 2011;45(6):504–10 [Meta-Analysis Review].

27. Karvellas CJ, Farhat MR, Sajjad I, Mogensen SS, Leung AA, Wald R, et al. A comparison of early versus late initiation of renal replacement therapy in critically ill patients with acute kidney injury: a systematic review and meta-analysis. Crit Care. 2011;15(1):R72 [Comparative Study Meta-Analysis Review].

28. Brown RO, Compher C. A.S.P.E.N. clinical guidelines: nutrition support in adult acute and chronic renal failure. JPEN J Parenter Enteral Nutr. 2010;34(4):366–77 [Practice Guideline].

29. Scheinkestel CD, Kar L, Marshall K, Bailey M, Davies A, Nyulasi I, et al. Prospective randomized trial to assess caloric and protein needs of critically Ill, anuric, ventilated patients requiring continuous renal replacement therapy. Nutrition. 2003;19(11–12):909–16 [Clinical Trial Randomized Controlled Trial Research Support, Non-U.S. Gov't].

30. Scheinkestel CD, Adams F, Mahony L, Bailey M, Davies AR, Nyulasi I, et al. Impact of increasing parenteral protein loads on amino acid levels and balance in critically ill anuric patients on continuous renal replacement therapy. Nutrition. 2003;19(9):733–40 [Research Support, Non-U.S. Gov't].

31. Arroyo V, Fernandez J, Gines P. Pathogenesis and treatment of hepatorenal syndrome. Semin Liver Dis. 2008;28(1):81–95 [Review].

32. Moreau R, Durand F, Poynard T, Duhamel C, Cervoni JP, Ichai P, et al. Terlipressin in patients with cirrhosis and type 1 hepatorenal syndrome: a retrospective multicenter study. Gastroenterology. 2002;122(4):923–30 [Multicenter Study Research Support, Non-U.S. Gov't].

33. Kooiman J, Pasha SM, Zondag W, Sijpkens YW, van der Molen AJ, Huisman MV, et al. Meta-analysis: serum creatinine changes following contrast enhanced CT imaging. Eur J Radiol. 2012;81(10): 2554–61.

34. Dai B, Liu Y, Fu L, Li Y, Zhang J, Mei C. Effect of theophylline on prevention of contrast-induced acute kidney injury: a meta-analysis of randomized controlled trials. Am J Kidney Dis. 2012;60(3): 360–70.

35. Li Y, Liu Y, Fu L, Mei C, Dai B. Efficacy of short-term high-dose statin in preventing contrast-induced nephropathy: a meta-analysis of seven randomized controlled trials. PLoS One. 2012;7(4): e34450.

36. Acetylcysteine for prevention of renal outcomes in patients undergoing coronary and peripheral vascular angiography: main results from the randomized Acetylcysteine for Contrast-induced nephropathy Trial (ACT). Circulation. 2011;124(11):1250–9 [Comparative Study Meta-Analysis Randomized Controlled Trial Research Support, Non-U.S. Gov't].

Vanessa P. Ho, Soumitra R. Eachempati,
and Philip S. Barie

Introduction

Infections of surgical incisions are a common complication of surgery, occurring in about 3% of all surgical procedures and in up to 20% of patients who undergo emergency intra-abdominal operations [1]. In 1992, the US Centers for Disease Control and Prevention (CDC) changed the terminology from wound infection to surgical site infection (SSI) to differentiate infections of surgical incisions from infections of traumatic wounds [2]. Surgical site infections can cause substantial morbidity to patients by failure of incisions to heal, incisional hernias, fistulae, recurrent pain, and disfiguring scars; additionally, SSIs may bring about further infectious complications such as bacteremia. This morbidity also creates a substantial financial burden to hospitals and patients [3]. The development of SSIs is also used increasingly as a performance measure in recent government and insurance "pay for performance" initiatives, such that surgeons and hospitals with higher rates of SSI will be receiving lower reimbursements. For all of these reasons, surgeons must be aware of all measures to prevent and treat SSI effectively.

Surgical site infections have been occurring since the inception of surgery. The first description of purulent drainage from incisions or wounds was from Hippocrates, who described operations performed for both elective and emergency indications. Early surgeons considered the discharge of pus from wounds ("laudable pus") as the beginning of a healing process that was allowed to occur by secondary intention. Progress in this field started in the mid-nineteenth century, when Pasteur, Semmelweis, and Lister became pioneers of infection control by introducing bacteriology and the germ theory of disease, asepsis, and antiseptic surgery,

respectively. Ignaz Semmelweis, who practiced obstetrics in Vienna in the mid-nineteenth century, was the first to recognize the importance of hand hygiene, especially when going from dissecting cadavers to examining parturient women. He also was the first to soak his instruments in an antiseptic solution. Although his peers failed to adopt these measures, the rate of postpartum endometritis ("child-bed fever"), which was extremely high for other practitioners, decreased markedly in his patients to an estimated 5% [4]. Because deep or extensive soft tissue infections carried mortality rates as high as 70–80%, elective surgery did not become a practical option until the mid-twentieth century, when developments in the fields of microbiology and pharmacology led to major advancements in perioperative care [5]. Whereas SSIs are no longer prohibitive for elective surgery, they remain among the most common complications in surgical patients and create undue morbidity and cost [6].

Clinical Presentation

Surgical site infections are defined by the CDC as infections of surgical sites that occur within 30 days of the operation (within 1 year if implants are emplaced). These are classified into superficial incisional, deep incisional, and organ/space infections (Table 11.1). Superficial incisional SSI involves the skin and subcutaneous tissue of the incision down to (but not including) muscle fascia. Deep incisional SSI involves the fascia and the immediate sub-fascial space but not include intra-cavitary spaces. Organ/space infections are intra-cavitary and affect organs or spaces that are related to the operation performed. An individual infection is classified by its deepest extent. Numerous factors determine whether a patient will develop an SSI, and understanding the pathophysiology of the infection process is fundamental to understanding the diagnosis, prevention, and treatment of SSIs.

Every surgical incision, no matter the wound class, has bacteria that are present and can be cultured at the conclusion of the procedure. Inoculation of the surgical site occurs

V.P. Ho, M.D., M.P.H., (✉) • S.R. Eachempati, M.D.,
• P.S. Barie, M.D., M.B.A.
Department of Surgery, New York-Presbyterian Hospital-Weill
Cornell Medical Center, 525 East 68 Street, P713A,
New York, NY 10065, USA
e-mail: vanpho@gmail.com

L.J. Moore et al. (eds.), *Common Problems in Acute Care Surgery*,
DOI 10.1007/978-1-4614-6123-4_11, © Springer Science+Business Media New York 2013

Table 11.1 Centers for Disease Control and Prevention definitions of surgical site infection (SSI)

Superficial incisional SSI

Infection occurs within 30 days after the operation

- *and* infection involves only skin or subcutaneous tissue of the incision
- *and* at least *one* of the following:
  - Purulent drainage, with or without laboratory confirmation, from the superficial incision
  - Organisms isolated from an aseptically obtained culture of fluid or tissue from the superficial incision
  - At least one of the following signs or symptoms of infection: pain or tenderness, localized swelling, redness, or heat *and* superficial incision is deliberately opened by surgeon, *unless* incision is culture-negative
  - Diagnosis of superficial incisional SSI by the surgeon or attending physician

Deep incisional SSI

Infection occurs within 30 days after the operation if no implant is left in place or within 1 year if implant is in place and the infection appears to be related to the operation

- *and* infection involves deep soft tissues (e.g., fascial and muscle layers) of the incision
- *and* at least *one* of the following:
  - Purulent drainage from the deep incision but not from the organ/space component of the surgical site
  - A deep incision spontaneously dehisces or is deliberately opened by a surgeon when the patient has at least one of the following signs or symptoms: fever (>38°C), localized pain, or tenderness, unless site is culture-negative
  - An abscess or other evidence of infection involving the deep incision is found on direct examination, during reoperation, or by histopathologic or radiologic examination
  - Diagnosis of a deep incisional SSI by a surgeon or attending physician

Organ/space SSI

Infection occurs within 30 days after the operation if no implant is left in place or within 1 year if implant is in place and the infection appears to be related to the operation

- *and* infection involves any part of the anatomy (e.g., organs or spaces), other than the incision, which was opened or manipulated during an operation
- *and* at least *one* of the following:
  - Purulent drainage from a drain that is placed through a stab wound into the organ/space.
  - Organisms isolated from an aseptically obtained culture of fluid or tissue in the organ/space.
  - An abscess or other evidence of infection involving the organ/space that is found on direct examination, during reoperation, or by histopathologic or radiologic examination.
  - Diagnosis of an organ/space SSI by a surgeon or attending physician.

inevitably during surgery, either inward from the skin or outward from the tissues being operated on (e.g., surgery upon a hollow viscus). However, the presence of bacteria does not predict infection by itself, and other clinical parameters amplify microbial effects. The pathophysiology of SSIs is related to several factors, including the following: the inoculum, the presence of adjuvants (e.g., suture material, prosthetic devices, devitalized tissue, blood), bacterial virulence factors, the microenvironment of the surgical site (e.g., oxygenation, perfusion), antibiotic prophylaxis, and host factors.

The Inoculum

Surgical site infections are nearly always the consequence of contamination that occurs at the time of the operation, and infection is most closely linked to the number of bacteria that contaminate the surgical site. Classic studies have demonstrated that greater numbers of bacteria, the greater the likelihood of infection; the "magic number" of 10^5 organisms/g of tissue has been the commonly recognized threshold [7]. However, this threshold is not valid across all types of microorganisms or different strata of host responses and can be reduced dramatically by the presence of adjuvants, and therefore is not practical for routine monitoring or everyday decision making.

Contamination of the surgical site with bacteria occurs from multiple sources, including the patient's skin, the organ or tissue being operated upon, airborne organisms, and even the surgical team. Wounds are classified by the amount of contamination of the incision into clean, clean-contaminated, contaminated, and dirty (Altemeier classification). Clean surgical procedures involve the skin and subcutaneous and musculoskeletal soft tissues (e.g., breast, hernia, orthopedic joint replacement procedures), and have the lowest incidence of SSIs. Clean-contaminated procedures involve the controlled opening of a hollow viscus, including the respiratory, genitourinary, or gastrointestinal tract. In contaminated procedures, bacteria are introduced into a normally sterile tissue or body cavity, but are not present for a long enough time to establish an infection (e.g., penetrating abdominal trauma, unintentional enterotomy, open extremity fractures). Dirty procedures are performed to control an established infection (e.g., colon resection for complicated diverticulitis), and have the highest rate of SSI. Contaminated and dirty procedures carry an independent risk of SSI.

Operative procedures that enter a normally colonized area of the body allow contamination of the surgical site with organisms that are specific to the area's colonizing flora. Procedures involving only the skin and subcutaneous tissues result in lower inocula because the mechanical preparation of the surgical site should minimize the number of bacteria present. However, colonic bacterial density may exceed 10^{10} organisms/g of feces. Bacterial contamination occurs of the surgical site even with meticulous preparation and surgical technique. Hence, colon operations have clearly higher rates of SSI than inguinal hernia procedures. A classic technique to decrease SSIs following high-risk procedures is to leave the incision open at the original procedure and then allow the wound to heal by secondary intention or attempt delayed primary closure in a few days (usually on or after the fourth day). Small randomized trials have demonstrated that delayed primary closure decreases the SSI rate, but this tactic should only be employed in dirty or infected cases as it increases the time to wound closure and, if the wound cannot be closed, may subject the patient to delayed wound healing and prolonged postoperative care [8–10].

Bacteria and Virulence Factors

The microbiology of SSI depends on the nature of the operation. Most SSI are caused by gram-positive cocci that are commensal skin flora [11], including *Staphylococcus aureus*, coagulase-negative staphylococci (usually *S. epidermidis*), and *Enterococcus* spp.; antibiotic prophylaxis for most cases should emphasize coverage of these organisms. The likelihood of gram-negative bacilli causing SSI is increased after head and neck surgery (if pharyngo-esophageal structures are entered), thoracic surgery (if tracheobronchial or esophageal structures are entered), gastrointestinal surgery, or infra-inguinal surgery of any type. Colorectal surgery and surgery of the female genital tract are at risk for SSI caused by obligate anaerobic bacteria (e.g., *Bacteroides fragilis*), as well as some gram-positive colonists (e.g., *Enterococcus* spp., *Streptococcus* spp.). The biliary tract harbors *Escherichia coli*, *Klebsiella* spp., and enterococci. Any of these potential pathogens may contaminate the surgical site, and infection occurs commonly with microbes that are most likely to contaminate a given procedure.

Patients who are chronic carriers of *S. aureus* are at increased risk of SSI [12], and surgeons who harbor *S. aureus* have increased rates of SSI among their patients. The staphylococcal carrier state may afflict as many as 30% of normal individuals [13], but nearly all carriers are colonized with relatively sensitive strains. The methicillin-resistant carrier state has also been described but remains unusual (<5% of the US population) [13]. Topical 2% mupirocin ointment applied to the nares of patients who are chronic carriers of *S. aureus* may reduce the increased incidence of SSI that is characteristic of chronic staphylococcal carriage, and may be useful in patients with previous methicillin-resistant *Staphylococcus aureus* (MRSA) infection [14], but is ineffective when applied to the general population. In a recent randomized trial of cardiac surgery patients, decontamination of the nasopharynx and oropharynx with 0.12% chlorhexidine gluconate reduced significantly the proportion of patients with *S. aureus* nasal colonization ($p < 0.001$) [15]. Topical chlorhexidine reduced the overall postoperative infection rate by 6.4% (95% confidence interval [CI] 1.1–11.7%, $p < 0.01$), lower respiratory tract infections by 6.5% (95% CI 2.3–10.7%, $p < 0.01$), and the risk of deep incisional SSI by 3.2% (95% CI 0.9–5.5%, $p < 0.01$). The benefit of pharyngeal decontamination has not been replicated in abdominal surgery.

Virulence factors vary among bacterial species, such that organisms with more potent virulence characteristics may require smaller inocula to cause infection. Virulence factors include structural components of the bacterial cell, secreted products of bacteria, and resistance of bacteria to antibiotics that shield the pathogen from prevention and treatment. The prototypical virulence factor of gram-negative bacteria is lipopolysaccharide (LPS), or endotoxin. Endotoxin is located in the outer membrane of gram-negative bacteria, and contains a potent Lipid A moiety that stimulates many components of the innate and adaptive host responses [16]. It is toxic to host tissues and generally enhances virulence by activating several mediator cascades. The Enterobacteriacae are the most common endotoxin-associated bacteria.

Other bacterial species elaborate specific virulence features. The peptidoglycans of gram-positive bacterial cell walls activate host immunity in a manner analogous to LPS. Gram-positive cocci also elaborate exotoxins and numerous proteases that destroy tissue and facilitate invasion. *Streptococcus pyogenes* has a cell surface M-protein capsule that resists phagocytosis by neutrophils [17]. A number of different M-proteins exert differential effects upon virulence; strains lacking the M-protein component lose the potential to cause infection [18]. *Bacteroides fragilis* has a polysaccharide capsule that retards phagocytosis [19]. This capsular material appears to still incite abscess formation even when the bacterium itself has been heat-killed. Because *Bacteroides* spp. are obligate anerobes, they are usually associated in a synergistic relationship to cause infection with aerobic pathogens (well documented, in the case of enterococci), which consume oxygen from the microenvironment and thereby promote strict anaerobiosis.

Other virulence factors are exotoxins, products secreted by gram-positive bacteria. For example, *S. aureus* elaborates the exotoxin coagulase [20]. Coagulase activates the coagulation cascade and creates a fibrin-rich local environment in soft tissue, which protects the organism from phagocytosis by host neutrophils. Another much-discussed exotoxin is the Panton–Valentine leukocidin (PVL), which is associated with community-associated methicillin-resistant *S. aureus* (CA-MRSA) [21]. The PVL exotoxin is a potent leukocidin. Interplay among the bacteria, the exotoxin, and the liquefactive necrosis of neutrophils results most commonly in a dramatic local soft tissue infection with a black central eschar (Fig. 11.1). Infection with this organism will likely be observed with SSIs in addition to community-acquired soft tissue infections [22]. Other examples of exotoxins include streptococcal superantigens associated with necrotizing soft tissue infections and toxic shock-like syndrome [23]. Toxic shock toxins produced by some strains of *S. aureus* may

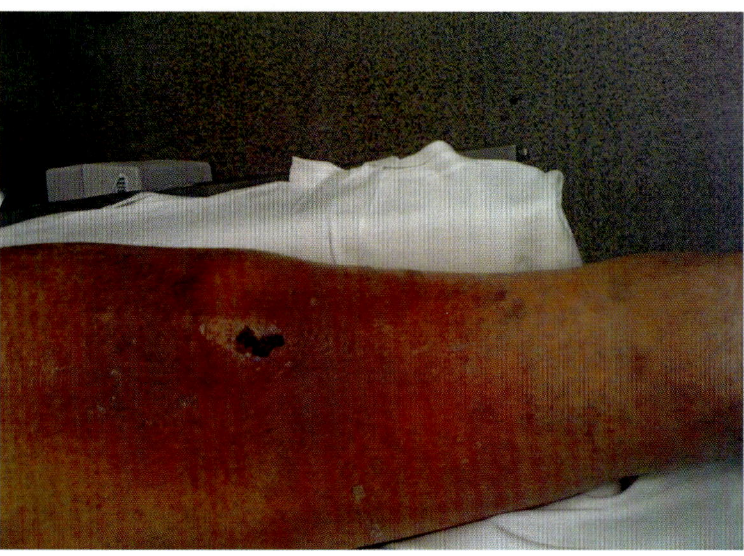

Fig. 11.1 A local soft tissue infection with a black central eschar

cause a fulminant shock syndrome associated with surgical packing in open wounds [24].

Antibiotic resistance should also be considered a virulence factor, as the increasing prevalence of resistant organisms in both the community and the hospital become a larger problem in SSI prevention and management. Beta-lactamase production has reduced dramatically the susceptibilities of vast numbers of bacteria. Mutations change the bacterial cellular phenotype with changes in porin proteins [25] and other structural changes of the cell that mediate resistance. Carbapenemase activity has been detected in a variety of organisms, including *E. coli*, *Acinetobacter baumannii*, *K. pneumoniae*, and other Enterobacteriaceae. Of note, MRSA, although usually not resistant per se to vancomycin, may be associated with treatment failures due to inability to reach high-enough concentrations when the minimum inhibitory concentration (MIC) exceeds 1 mcg/mL. Isolates of MRSA with vancomycin MIC 1 mcg/mL are at high risk for treatment failure, and MRSA with MIC$\geq$2 mcg/mL should be treated routinely with an alternative agent to vancomycin because bactericidal drug concentrations cannot be achieved with nontoxic doses [26, 27].

Microenvironment of the Surgical Site

The foundation of any strategy to decrease the risk of SSI is proper patient preparation and sound surgical technique [28]. Disruption of skin integrity provides a portal of entry for pathogenic organisms and represents the most important etiologic factor for most skin and soft tissue infections [29]. Local factors predisposing to infection within the surgical incision also affect the ability of bacteria to overcome host defenses. Local factors predisposing to infection include soft tissue trauma (including thermal injury from exuberant use of electrocautery), animal or human bites, burns, wound contamination, diminished perfusion (e.g., peripheral vascular disease), obesity, poor hygiene, presence of a foreign body, or venous insufficiency and stasis [30].

Surgeons have attempted to decrease the inoculum size at the site of surgery by hair removal and antiseptic showering. The routine removal of hair has been questioned as a potential cause of SSIs by causing unnecessary breaks in the skin (by shaving in particular). Several randomized controlled trials (RCTs) have examined hair removal with clipping, shaving, or depilatory agents, and no hair removal. In a meta-analysis, shaving with razors increased SSIs over clipping (relative risk [RR] 2.02, 95% CI 1.21–3.36) or depilatories (RR 1.54, 95% CI 1.05–2.24) [31]. By contrast, neither dispensing with hair removal altogether nor hair removal immediately prior to surgery had an effect on SSIs. Antiseptic showering has been studied in two prospective, randomized, controlled trials [32, 33]. Although bacterial counts were reduced, there was no lowering of the rate of SSI in those who showered with the antiseptic. Showering might be useful in certain high-risk patients or where the institutional SSI rate is high; if done they should be repeated, as cumulative benefit may accrue.

Surgeon hand antisepsis has been studied as a potential way to decrease SSIs, whether by alcohol hand-rub or traditional surgical scrub techniques with soap and water. Most studies have examined bacterial load (colony-forming units, CFUs) as the endpoint rather than the clinical endpoint of SSI [34]. One equivalence study, which examined SSI rates as the primary endpoint after aqueous alcohol hand rub versus traditional hand scrub in 4,387 patients [35], found no difference in SSI rates between groups (hand-rubbing 2.44% versus hand-scrubbing 2.48%, for a difference of 0.04%, 95% CI −0.88% to +0.96%). Compliance is better and cost is lower for hand-rubbing solutions [35, 36], which is now the primary method of hand antisepsis for many centers. Chlorhexidine–

alcohol preparations for hand scrubbing are superior to povidone–iodine for reducing CFUs recovered from skin.

Chlorhexidine–alcohol also appears to be superior to iodine-based preparations for patient skin preparation. A RCT of preoperative skin preparation with chlorhexidine–alcohol scrub versus povidone–iodine in clean-contaminated surgery found that the rates of superficial and deep incisional SSIs were significantly lower in the chlorhexidine–alcohol group (4.2% versus 8.6% for superficial SSIs, $p = 0.008$; 1% versus 3% for deep incisional SSIs, $p = 0.05$) [37]. There was no difference in organ-space SSIs. A meta-analysis, which included the aforementioned study in addition to eight other randomized controlled trials comparing povidone–iodine and chlorhexidine ($n = 3,614$ patients), concurred with these observations [38]. A cost–benefit model in the same study estimated a net cost savings of \$16–26 per case [38].

Incisional hematoma is another important local risk factor for SSIs. In addition to being impenetrable to neutrophils, hemoglobin is a rich source of ferric iron, making the hematoma a fertile environment for bacterial growth [39]. Foreign bodies provide a nonbiological surface for adherence of microbes, and pose a functional challenge to phagocytosis. In addition, foreign bodies such as mesh, drains, and other implants are potential nidi for infection and formation of difficult-to-treat biofilms. The classic studies of Elek and Conen [40] have demonstrated the dramatic reduction in inoculum size that is required to cause soft tissue infection when a mere silk suture is present. Tissue ischemia or damage from electrocautery becomes a haven for contaminants from the surgical procedure. Dead space within the incision accumulates serum and provides a locale where microbes are inaccessible by neutrophils. These adjuvant effects enhance microbial proliferation, reduce the inoculum necessary, and inhibit host defenses, which in turn result in clinical infection.

Antibiotic Prophylaxis

Antimicrobial prophylaxis is a key step in the prevention of SSI, but not a panacea. Prophylaxis was shown by Polk and Lopez-Mayor in their seminal 1969 RCT to reduce the SSI rate following colectomy from more than 30% to 5% [41]. However, prophylaxis only protects the incision itself, and only during the period of time when it is open. If not administered properly, antibiotic prophylaxis is ineffective and puts the patient at risk for other complications, such as drug reactions or superinfection such as *Clostridium difficile* infection (CDI). Four principles guide the administration of the appropriate antimicrobial agent for prophylaxis: (1) safety, (2) an appropriate narrow spectrum that covers relevant pathogens, (3) little or no reliance upon the agent for therapy of infection so that resistance is not promoted, and (4) administra-

tion within 1 h before surgery and for a defined, brief period of time thereafter (ideally a single dose, but no more than 24 h) [42]. According to these principles, fluoroquinolones or carbapenems should not be used for surgical prophylaxis. However, in prophylaxis for colon surgery, fluoroquinolones have been endorsed by the Surgical Care Improvement Project (SCIP) for penicillin-allergic patients, and ertapenem has also been recommended [43].

Antibiotic prophylaxis is indicated for most clean-contaminated and contaminated (or potentially contaminated) operations. An example of a clean-contaminated operation where antibiotic prophylaxis is usually not indicated is elective laparoscopic cholecystectomy [44–46]. Three separate meta-analyses have been performed examining antibiotic prophylaxis for elective laparoscopic cholecystectomy [44–46]. The most recent of these, by the Cochrane collaboration, included 11 randomized clinical trials (1,664 patients) at low anesthesia risk, with few comorbidities and low risk of infection. There was no difference between antibiotic prophylaxis and no prophylaxis in the proportion of SSIs (odds ratio [OR] 0.87, 95% CI 0.49–1.54), or extra-abdominal infections (OR 0.77, 95% CI 0.41–1.46) [46]. However, antibiotic prophylaxis is indicated for high-risk biliary surgery; high risk is conferred by age >70 years, diabetes mellitus, or a recently instrumented biliary tract (e.g., bile duct stent).

Elective colon surgery is a clean-contaminated procedure where preparatory practices are in evolution [47, 48]. The use of antibiotic prophylaxis in colorectal surgery has been shown consistently to be beneficial in RCTs when the antibiotic is administered prior to the incision and the regimen demonstrates appropriate activity against colonic flora [41, 49–52]. A Cochrane meta-analysis of prophylaxis of colorectal surgery reported results of 182 trials, including 11 RCTs comparing any regimen to placebo, clearly showing a decrease in risk of SSI with any appropriate prophylaxis regimen (RR 0.30, 95% CI 0.22–0.41) [53]. However, there is no consensus as to which regimen is best. Oral antibiotic regimens, standardized in the 1970s by the administration of nonabsorbable neomycin and erythromycin base in addition to mechanical cleansing, reduced the risk of incisional SSI further to its present rate of approximately 4–8% [48]. Currently, oral antibiotic prophylaxis is often omitted, due to the belief that no additive benefit exists beyond parenteral antibiotic prophylaxis. Current SCIP guidelines for antibiotic prophylaxis of elective colon surgery recommend regimens including oral prophylaxis alone, parenteral prophylaxis alone, or the combination [47]. However, oral prophylaxis alone likely is not as effective as parenteral prophylaxis. Song and Glenny [54] examined oral antibiotics alone compared with oral/systemic antibiotic prophylaxis (five trials), and found a higher SSI rate with oral prophylaxis alone (OR 3.34, 95% CI 1.66–6.72), although the CI was wide. However, there may be benefit to the combined use of oral and parenteral prophylaxis; Lewis et al. performed a meta-analysis of 13 RCTs of systemic versus combined oral and systemic prophylaxis, and showed significant benefit for the combined approach (RR 0.51, 95% CI 0.24–0.78) [48]. Mechanical bowel preparation in colon surgery is also currently controversial. A 2009 Cochrane meta-analysis of 13 RCTs compared bowel preparation to no bowel preparation for 4,777 participants undergoing elective colorectal surgery. Patients received no benefit from mechanical bowel preparation, as the rates of anastomotic leak and SSI were similar in both groups [55].

Antibiotic prophylaxis of clean surgery has been also been controversial. Where bone is incised (e.g., craniotomy, sternotomy) or a prosthesis is inserted, antibiotic prophylaxis is generally indicated. Some controversy persists with clean surgery of soft tissues such as breast or hernia. Meta-analysis of RCTs shows some benefit of antibiotic prophylaxis of breast cancer surgery without immediate reconstruction [56, 57]. The use of antibiotic prophylaxis for elective open groin hernia surgery with or without mesh has also been controversial. A variety of small studies have been performed which showed no benefit of antibiotics [58–60]. However, a 2007 meta-analysis suggested that there may be a benefit to antibiotic prophylaxis in elective groin hernia repairs if mesh is used, with infection rates of 1.4% and 2.9% in the prophylaxis and control groups, respectively (OR 0.48, 95% CI 0.27–0.85). If mesh was not used, the difference was less pronounced (3.5% versus 4.9%, OR 0.71, 95% CI 0.51–1.00) [61].

Arterial reconstruction with prosthetic graft is an example of clean surgery where the antibiotic prophylaxis is warranted because the susceptibility to infection is high. These cases are high-risk due to the presence of ischemic tissue and the infrainguinal location of many incisions. One recent meta-analysis [62] identified 35 RCTs for prevention of infection after peripheral arterial reconstruction, with 23 specifically examining prophylactic systemic antibiotics. Prophylaxis reduced the risk of SSI by approximately 75%, and early graft infection by about 69%. There was no benefit to prophylaxis for more than 24 h, of antibiotic bonding to the graft material itself, or preoperative bathing with an antiseptic agent compared with un-medicated bathing. Placement of closed suction drains also does not decrease the rate of SSIs [63].

Given that most SSIs are caused by gram-positive cocci, the antibiotic chosen should be directed primarily against staphylococci for clean cases and high-risk clean-contaminated biliary and gastric surgery. A first-generation cephalosporin is preferred almost always; clindamycin may be used in cases of penicillin allergy [42]. If gram-negative or anaerobic coverage is required, a second-generation cephalosporin or a combination of a first-generation agent plus metronidazole is the regimen of first choice. Single agent prophylaxis is often preferred in institutions due to ease of administration. Vancomycin prophylaxis is generally appropriate only in institutions where the incidence of MRSA infection is high (>20% of all SSIs caused by MRSA) or if a patient is a known carrier of MRSA.

Parenteral antibiotic prophylaxis should be given within 30–60 min prior to incision [64]. Antibiotics given sooner are ineffective, as are agents that are given after the incision is closed. However, compliance with this guideline in the USA has been poor. A 2001 nationwide audit of prescribing practices in the USA indicated that only 56% of patients who received prophylactic antibiotics did so within 1 h prior to the skin incision [42]; timeliness was documented in only 76% of cases in a 2005 audit in US Department of Veterans Affairs (VA) hospitals [43]. Most inappropriately timed first doses of prophylactic antibiotic occur too early [42, 43]; changing institutional processes to administer the drug in the operating room can improve compliance with best practices [43]. Even though SCIP specifies a 24-h limit for prophylaxis, preoperative single-dose prophylaxis (with intraoperative re-dosing, if indicated) is equivalent to multiple doses for the prevention of SSI [65]. Antibiotics with short half-lives (e.g., cefazolin or cefoxitin) should be re-dosed every 3 (for cefoxitin) to 4 h (for cefazolin) during surgery if the operation is prolonged or bloody [66]. As SCIP reporting becomes linked to hospital payments, compliance with these guidelines has improved, but there is no definitive evidence that SSI rates have declined as a result.

Prolonged antibiotic prophylaxis is both pervasive and potentially harmful. Antibiotics should not be given to "cover" indwelling drains or catheters, in irrigation fluid, or as a substitute for poor surgical technique. As a result of ischemia caused by surgical hemostasis, antibiotic penetration into the incision immediately after surgery is questionable until neovascularization occurs (24–48 h). However, recent US data show that only 40% of patients who receive antibiotic prophylaxis do so for less than 24 h [42]. *Clostridium difficile* infection follows disruption of the normal balance of gut flora, resulting in overgrowth of the enterotoxin-producing *C. difficile* [67]. Although virtually any antibiotic may cause CDI (even a single dose), prolonged antibiotic prophylaxis increases the risk. Prolonged prophylaxis also increases the risk of nosocomial infections unrelated to the surgical site, and encourages the emergence of multi-drug-resistant (MDR) pathogens. Both pneumonia and vascular catheter-related infections have been associated with prolonged prophylaxis [68, 69], as has the emergence of SSI caused by MRSA [70].

Host Factors

In the majority of procedures, the host manages effectively the inoculum of bacteria and all of the other parameters that favor infection. It is almost certain that genetic variability among patients leads to increased susceptibility to infection: an intrinsic difference in the capacity to generate an inflammatory response, differences in phagocytic efficiency, or differences in specific immune response. Whereas the exact mechanisms of host defense impairment are not defined, it is clear that each host variable is impactful in some way on the probability of infection. However, quantifying the risk of individual patients and the risk associated with each variable has remained elusive.

The relationships among the surgical site, microbes, and host defenses describe the overall risk of SSI. Acquired problems of host defense have been associated by statistical inference in subpopulations of patients that appear to have higher rates of SSIs than others. These variables include age, obesity, corticosteroids, systemic chronic illness, or immunocompromised states, malnutrition, low serum albumin concentration, tobacco smoking, uncontrolled diabetes mellitus, and ischemia secondary to vascular disease or irradiation [71–79]. Scott et al. showed that age and albumin concentration were most predictive of SSI in a cohort of more than 9,000 patients from a single community hospital [80]. A low serum albumin concentration is a surrogate marker for a wide range of comorbid conditions that render the patient immunocompromised or impaired nutritionally. Patients who are malnourished should be considered for preoperative enteral feeding or, if necessary, total parenteral nutrition (TPN) if extensive surgery is planned. The Veterans Affairs Cooperative study on preoperative nutritional support demonstrated fewer complications other than catheter-related infections in those patients who were malnourished and given an average of 9 days of preoperative TPN [81]. More recently, supplemental enteral nutrition reduced the risk of SSI in malnourished patients [82, 83]. Impaired lymph flow may also be a potential risk factor for SSI, with axillary or inguinal lymphadenectomy. These are now used less commonly for the regional treatment of cancer, having been supplanted by sentinel node biopsy. Transitory physiological states may also increase the risk of SSI; examples include severe injury, shock, blood transfusion, hypothermia, hypoxia, and hyperglycemia.

The length of the preoperative hospital stay was considered historically a risk factor for SSI, but has become less so as outpatient surgery is performed increasingly. Bacterial colonization with often-MDR nosocomial organisms occurs routinely within 72 h of hospitalization. Such patients should have their microbiologic history reviewed prior to an operation so that a rational decision can be made about the choice of agent for prophylaxis. In patients who have had infections with MDR microbes, antibiotics should be used that are potent against the bacteria demonstrated previously. Existing infection should be treated before elective surgery is undertaken, as the presence of a concomitant infection even at a remote site increases the risk of SSI. Colonization by MRSA often leads to infection by the same organism, especially in elderly patients, dialysis patients, and nursing home residents. These patients should be given an antibiotic active against MRSA for prophylaxis. Use of agents with treatment efficacy against MRSA may also be helpful in institutions with a high rate of MRSA SSIs.

Risk Stratification for Surgical Site Infections

It is important to consider these factors (bacteria, host, and surgical site factors) to stratify an individual's risk for SSI. The CDC guidelines formulate the risk of SSI as the size of the bacterial inoculum (contamination) multiplied by bacterial virulence, the product being divided by host resistance; however, this is not of much use clinically [84]. The Study on Efficacy of Nosocomial Infection Control (SENIC) assessed the effectiveness of various measures in the years 1976–1988 [85]. Four parameters were independent markers of a higher risk of SSI: Abdominal surgery, surgery lasting longer than 2 h, a contaminated or dirty procedure, and more than three diagnoses at the time of discharge. This predictive method proved to be more accurate than the long-standing practice of surgeons of making risk predictions on the basis of their clinical experience. A similar attempt to identify factors predictive of SSI was the National Nosocomial Infection Surveillance (NNIS) study [86–88], begun in 1970 and continuing to the present time as the National Healthcare Safety Network (NHSN). This risk factor index score remains in wide usage. The three important factors identified were an American Society of Anesthesiologists (ASA) score of 3 or more on a 5-point scoring system, a contaminated or dirty procedure, and an operation lasting longer than the 75th percentile of the average duration for that procedure. The NNIS system may be used to formulate a risk categorization index ranging from 0 to 3, where 1 point each is assigned for an ASA score of 3 to 5 points, a contaminated or dirty incision, and prolonged operating time [87, 88]. The risks for SSI associated with different index scores are: $0 = 1.5\%$; $1 = 2.9\%$; $2 = 6.8\%$; and $3 = 13\%$ [87]. A modification subtracts one point for laparoscopic procedures, so that the final index score ranges from -1 to 3 points [89].

Diagnosis

Despite their often nonspecific appearance and paucity of symptoms, SSIs remain a clinical diagnosis based on history and physical examination. Infection is the result of microbial proliferation in tissue, which in turn activates the inflammatory cascade. This local inflammatory response produces the classic clinical findings of rubor (erythema), dolor (pain), calor (heat), and tumor (swelling). These manifestations of inflammation provide the physical evidence for the diagnosis of infection, and are often accompanied by increasing wound pain, lack or stagnation of clinical recovery, or malaise. Surgical control of the infectious source remains the crucial diagnostic and therapeutic maneuver. Often times, this can be achieved by simply opening and draining the infected incision in superficial incisional SSIs. However, deep incisional SSIs may require thorough surgical debridement and open wound care to resolve the infectious process, whereas organ/space SSIs usually require percutaneous drainage of formal intracavitary reoperation. In select cases, a small intracavitary abscess (<5 cm diameter) may respond to antibiotic therapy alone, but the clinical response must be adjudged with diligence.

The presenting complaints depend on the depth of infection. Typical complaints include localized pain that worsens upon physical activity and contact to the affected area. Instead of steady clinical improvement postoperatively, patients with a developing SSI often begin to worsen clinically on postoperative day 4 or 5. Rare early SSIs include infections caused by beta-hemolytic streptococci or *Clostridium* spp., and may manifest as early as postoperative day 1 or 2. Streptococcal infections cause pain and local wound erythema, whereas clostridial infections drain a grey-colored thin fluid and lack the characteristic inflammatory skin changes.

The incision itself is usually the source of increasing pain and erythema prior to the discharge of pus. The presenting symptoms may appear out of proportion to the clinical findings, especially in deep or necrotizing infections [90]. Probing the wound after partial removal of sutures is simple and allows diagnosis and treatment of a superficial incisional SSI. Alternatively, if the infection only involves the organ/space, symptoms specific to that body cavity will usually predominate, such as prolonged postoperative ileus, persistent respiratory distress, neurologic deficit, or altered mental status.

Culturing the wound by the swab method has been shown experimentally to be reliable. Recovery of 10^5 CFU of bacteria/g of tissue or mL of fluid has been the traditional indicator of local infection, whether of the lung, the urinary tract, or the surgical incision [91]. Intraoperative cultures of high-risk incisions may also be considered, and the results may be used later to guide treatment; these cultures must not be utilized as justification to prolong prophylaxis. In a study of 52 open fractures, patients with intraoperative quantitative bacterial counts $>10^5$ CFU/mL had an SSI rate of 50%, whereas patients with $<10^5$ CFU/mL had an SSI rate of 5% [91]. Among patients who underwent abdominal hysterectomy, recovery of $>10^4$ CFU/mL from pelvic fluid was associated with a subsequent SSI rate of 42%, whereas only 12% of patients had an SSI when $<10^3$ CFU/mL were recovered at operation [92]. In the case of deep incisional SSIs, tenderness may extend beyond the margin of erythema, or

crepitus and cutaneous vesicles or bullae may manifest [93]. With ongoing infection, signs of systemic inflammation such as fever, tachycardia, hypotension, and altered mental status manifest the clinical picture of sepsis/severe sepsis (sepsis with organ dysfunction). These clinical findings usually portend a worse clinical prognosis and are often observed with more severe infections that will require surgical intervention in order to resolve.

Laboratory analysis should include basic hematologic and chemistry parameters. Leukocytosis >15,400/microliter with simultaneous hyponatremia <135 mEq/L has been shown to predict necrotizing infections [94]. Measurement of serum creatine phosphokinase (CPK) concentration can be helpful, effectively ruling out myonecrosis if normal, and indicating ongoing tissue destruction and the need for further debridement if elevated concentrations persist following resection of established myonecrosis [93].

Computed tomography (CT) and magnetic resonance imaging (MRI) are more sensitive in detecting small amounts of free air and suspicious fluid collections in soft tissues than plain radiographs, and can be of diagnostic value in cases of suspected necrotizing infections, although plain X-rays are obtained more easily [95] The use of intravenous contrast may be helpful to differentiate infected fluid collections with rim enhancement from simple fluid collections, although this must be weighed against the risk of contrast-related toxicity for the individual patient. The value gained from these sophisticated, but time-consuming imaging studies must be judged against the risk of rapid clinical deterioration and higher mortality [96]. Suspicion of deep incisional SSI should prompt timely transfer to the operating room if necrotizing infection is suspected. Treatment for deteriorating patients should never be delayed to obtain imaging.

Management

In general, early clinical recognition, correct assessment of the severity of infection and prompt initiation of surgical and adjunctive antibiotic therapies are the tenets of appropriate treatment (Fig. 11.2). The decision to initiate outpatient treatment or to admit the patient for more intensive treatment with intravenous antibiotics and formal surgical exploration under anesthesia is a common clinical challenge. Thorough and repetitive clinical examination over time may be acceptable in the outpatient setting, particularly of compliant patients. Inpatient admission or early surgical exploration may reduce the risk for sudden clinical deterioration and increased morbidity and mortality caused by delayed definitive therapy.

When faced with a potentially infected incision, the first steps are to remove the sutures, open and examine the suspicious-looking parts of the incision, and decide about

Fig. 11.2 SSI treatment algorithm

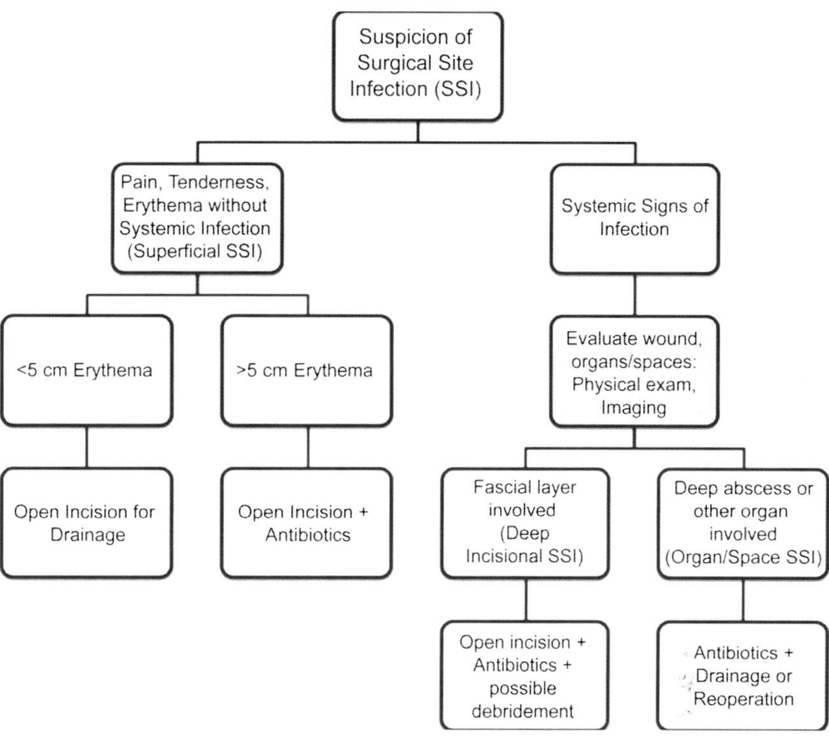

further surgical treatment. Partial wound opening with healing by secondary intention is adequate for most cases of superficial incisional SSIs. If the infection is not confined to the skin and subcutaneous tissue, urgent formal surgical exploration and debridement is essential to obtain local control of the infection, remove necrotic tissue, and establish aerobic conditions. The presence of SSI must also be considered in incisions with delayed or failed healing, and promote the same decisions as described previously [4]. More severe soft tissue infections with abscess formation usually require complete opening of the incision to examine adequately the integrity of the underlying fascia and to determine if there is a deep incisional SSI such as fasciitis or myositis. Formal surgical exploration for debridement or open drainage is often required for deep incisional SSIs or organ/space infection.

Escalating resistance among common nosocomial pathogens often complicates resolution of apparently simple infectious complications in the postoperative period, and represents a growing challenge for practicing surgeons today [97]. This is particularly true for those patients have had a prolonged hospital stay prior to elective surgery, such as those who have been trauma victims and require antimicrobial therapy for antecedent or concomitant infections [98]. These patients are often colonized with MDR organisms, highlighting again the importance of careful choice of antibiotic for prophylaxis.

Superficial Incisional SSIs

Superficial incisional SSIs cause local discomfort, but lead to systemic infection only rarely. Superficial incisional SSIs may be regarded functionally as subcutaneous abscesses, and clinical resolution is achieved routinely by opening, draining, and irrigating the surgical incision, allowing healing by secondary intention. Loculations should be broken up mechanically and the incision should be packed with moist saline dressings. Stronger emoluments (e.g., acetic acid, sodium hypochlorite) are toxic to fibroblasts and impair wound healing. Adequate opening of the incision is the single crucial component in this therapy, and must not be compromised for cosmetic reasons; ultimately, incisions may be more likely to form disfiguring scars if they are drained inadequately, due to prolonged time to healing and continued inflammation at the site. Antibiotic therapy is not indicated for superficial incisional SSI without systemic signs of infection or incisions with limited erythema. Antibiotics may be added for associated cellulitis beyond 5 cm away from the incision. Surgical intervention is limited to complicated infections defined by frank abscess formation, skin or subcutaneous tissue necrosis, or formation of bullae. Adequate antibiotic therapy will lead to clinical resolution in most forms of cellulitis, and therefore, debridement should be limited to necrotic areas in most circumstances.

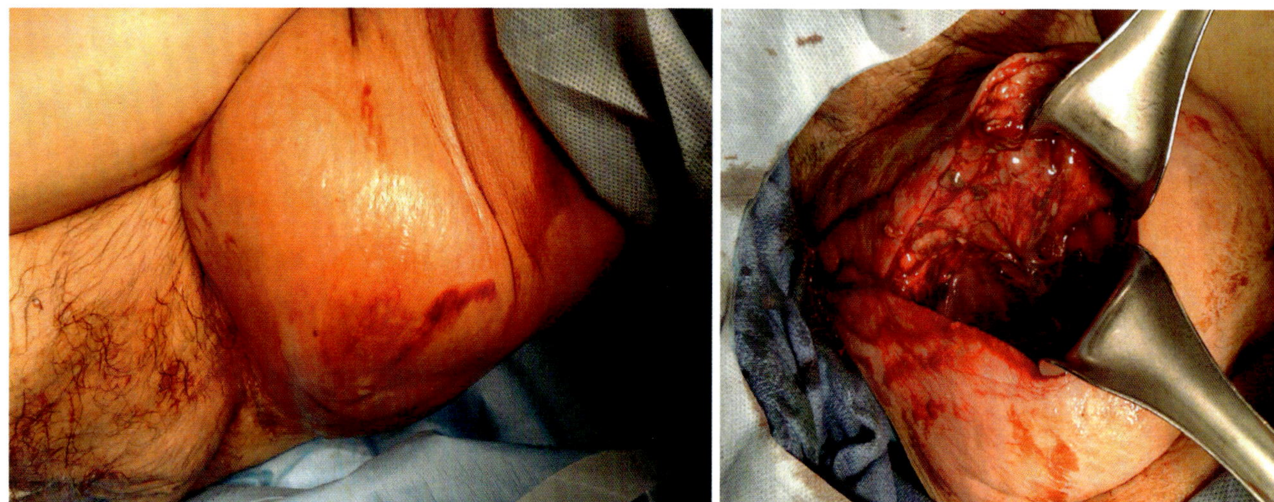

Fig. 11.3 A case of necrotizing fasciitis of the thigh. (**a**) The skin appears tense and erythematous but could be mistaken for cellulitis. (**b**) Incision of this lesion revealed necrotic infected tissue that required wide debridement

Deep Incisional SSIs

In contrast to superficial SSIs, which are rather benign, deep incisional SSIs are considerably more problematic. Patients present with extensive discomfort and usually show systemic signs of sepsis. The diagnosis is made clinically in patients in whom the infection extends to or below the superficial fascia. Deep incisional SSI may cause extensive liquefactive necrosis of fascia and muscle. Underlying tissue necrosis often extends far beyond the obvious limits of cutaneous involvement. If this is suspected, the patient should be explored in the operating room to resect all necrotic tissue. Necrotizing soft tissue infection (referred to often as *necrotizing fasciitis*) can be a rare, severe variant of deep incisional SSIs and is a dreaded complication with mortality rates of up to 50% [99]. Necrotizing fasciitis is a rapidly progressive infection, usually with widespread necrosis of the superficial fascia. Although risk factors include diabetes mellitus, older age, chronic skin infection, and intravenous drug abuse, necrotizing fasciitis also occurs frequently in young, previously healthy patients. Necrotizing fasciitis is often mistaken with cellulitis, as it the early stages may only manifest the nonspecific signs of erythema, edema, and fevers (Fig. 11.3). According to its pathogenesis, necrotizing fasciitis is categorized as type I (poly-microbial) or type II (mono-microbial). Therapy consists of urgent surgical exploration and debridement beyond necrotic areas until viable tissue is found. Affected patients should be monitored closely on a surgical intensive care unit (ICU), and surgical debridement repeated on a daily basis until the incision is entirely viable. In the setting of SSI, the two organisms associated with early, necrotizing infections are *Streptococcus pyogenes* and *C. perfringens*.

Severe SSIs, especially their most dangerous forms of necrotizing fasciitis or clostridial myonecrosis, are true emergencies and need immediate surgical attention. Even modest delays can increase patient mortality substantially. In a study by Freischlag et al., mortality increased from 32% to 70% when therapy was delayed more than 24 h [100]. With a suspected diagnosis of necrotizing infection, immediate and widespread operative debridement must be undertaken without waiting for precise identification of the causative pathogen or even that infection is present. These patients often require planned, sequential, repetitive surgical debridements to achieve source control. Empiric broad-spectrum antimicrobial therapy is given to cover likely pathogens upon initial diagnosis, and the antibiotic regimen should be reassessed following receipt of culture and sensitivity analysis. Hyperbaric oxygen therapy has been proposed by several authors to decrease mortality in patients suffering from necrotizing fasciitis, particularly those from whom clostridia are isolated. However, the results of studies on the use of hyperbaric oxygen are inconsistent and its use is not recommended routinely [101].

Commercially available vacuum-assisted closure (VAC) devices have gained popularity for the treatment of large open or problematic wounds. Experimentally, its value was first appraised by Morykwas and Argenta in a swine model in 1997 [102]. These and further animal studies have shown that VAC closure optimizes blood flow, decreases local tissue edema, and removes excessive fluid from the wound bed, thereby facilitating the removal of bacteria from the wound. Two general mechanisms of action have been proposed: Removal of fluid, which decreases interstitial edema and shortens the distance of diffusion, and mechanical deformation, which promotes tissue expansion to cover the defect [102]. Moreover, the cyclical application of subatmospheric pressure has been suggested to affect the cytoskeleton of cells in the wound bed, triggering a cascade of intracellular signals that increases the rate of cell division and subsequent formation of granulation tissue [103].

The value of VAC systems has been described only in small case series and cohort studies that relate predominantly to sternal infections following thoracotomy, abdominal wall dehiscence, the management of complex perineal wounds, or as a method to secure skin grafts [104, 105]. Despite their use for a variety of indications, a lack of well-designed RCTs precludes more general recommendations. Future RCTs in patients with deep incisional or even superficial incisional SSIs are needed to delineate better the benefits and cost-effectiveness of VAC therapy over standard wound management options. In the long term, these patients will often develop large abdominal wall defects secondary to debridement of abdominal wall fascia and muscle. Temporary abdominal closure with an absorbable synthetic mesh followed by skin grafting over large defects may be performed. Biologic mesh can be used, but may degrade if not covered immediately by skin. Enterocutaneous fistula is a risk if temporary abdominal closure is delayed or not achieved, which can substantially impair wound healing and delay or complicate definitive abdominal wall reconstruction, in addition to local skin irritation and the potential for malnutrition. Abdominal wall reconstruction, when the patient is ready, is usually a complex undertaking.

Organ/Space SSIs

Infections occurring intra-cavitary that are related directly to a surgical procedure are categorized separately as organ/space SSIs. This group comprises a multitude of different infections, ranging from intra-abdominal or intra-pleural infections to spinal abscesses, intracranial infections, or osteomyelitis following orthopedic interventions. These complications may present with few symptoms other than fever, and may mimic incisional SSIs initially and lead to inadequate initial treatment. They may also remain occult for prolonged periods of time and become apparent only when patients resume their previous everyday activities, or their normal diet. Diagnostic evaluation usually requires some form of imaging to confirm the site and extent of infection, in addition to empiric broad-spectrum antimicrobial therapy. To ensure adequate source control of the infection, surgical therapy is usually required to drain infected organs or body cavities. However, advances in interventional radiology, which has become the standard of treatment for a variety of such infections, provide equivalent source control while reducing interventional risk, length of hospital stay, and discomfort.

Patients with contained or discrete infected collections may benefit from CT-guided aspiration or drainage for diagnosis or therapy. In some instances of discrete organ/space SSIs where the incision per se is not involved, percutaneous drainage may serve as definitive source control. Reoperation is usually indicated in cases of anastomotic leak and clinical deterioration.

Exudates or drainage specimens from deep incisional SSI and organ/space SSI should be sent routinely for cultures (including fungi in immune-compromised patients) and susceptibility testing. However, specimen collection and testing may not be indicated (except for epidemiologic purposes) for superficial incisional SSI if there is no plan to treat with an antibiotic (as is usual).

Potential Complications

Surgical site infections cause considerable morbidity to patients as well as a substantial financial burden to hospitals and society. Patients may have disfiguring scars, recurrent complex abdominal wall hernias, and enterocutaneous fistulas following SSIs [106, 107]. Afflicted patients are subjected to additional radiographic procedures and antibiotic treatment, with risk of side effects, notably CDI. Patients who require long-term antibiotics and venous access are at risk for phlebitis, catheter-related infections, and superinfections. The patient's overall quality of life may be degraded. One case–control study of orthopedic surgery patients with and without SSIs [108] found that SSI prolonged hospitalization by a median of 2 weeks, doubled the rehospitalization rate, and increased cost by more than 300%. Using the Medical Outcome Study Short Form 36 (SF-36), a standardized quality of life survey, patients reported significant reductions in physical functioning and role-physical domains 1 year after the diagnosis of SSI. Another case–control study showed that patients with SSI are twice as likely to die, 60% more likely to spend time in the intensive care unit, and five times more likely to be readmitted [109]. Patients and family members also suffer loss of productivity during the time that they are ill and hospitalized.

The cost of SSIs to patient, institution, and society is noteworthy. One review suggested that healthcare cost for a patient with SSI is, on average, approximately twice the cost for a patient without SSI [110]. However, not all SSIs are the same. Whereas many less complex SSIs are associated with relatively low cost, the deeper the extent of infection, the more costly. One study estimated that superficial incisional SSIs cost approximately $400, whereas serious organ/space infections could cost $30,000 [111]. A study of the Healthcare Utilization Project National Inpatient Sample (HCUP NIS) in 2009 showed that for 723,490 hospitalizations, 6,891 (1%) developed SSI. In this patient population, the length of stay increased by 9.7 days and cost increased by approximately $20,842 per admission. In addition, 91,613 patients were readmitted for SSI treatment [112]. If this patient sample is extrapolated nationally, this would account for over 400,000

Table 11.2 Surgical Care Improvement Project (SCIP) [119–121]

Title	Process measure
SCIP-Inf 1	Prophylactic antibiotic received within 1 h prior to incision
SCIP-Inf 2	Prophylactic antibiotic selection for surgical patients • Measure added in 2007
SCIP-Inf 3	Prophylactic antibiotics discontinued within 24 h after surgery end time (48 h for cardiac patients)
SCIP-Inf 4	Cardiac surgery patients with controlled 6 AM postoperative serum glucose (≤200 mg/dL) • Measure added in 2008
SCIP-Inf 5	Postoperative wound infection diagnosed during index hospitalization • Outcome measure
SCIP-Inf 6	Surgical patients with appropriate hair removal • Added in 2008 • Retired in 2011due to high overall compliance
SCIP-Inf 7	Colorectal surgical patients with immediate postoperative normothermia • Proposed for 2009 but not endorsed
SCIP-Inf 8	Short half-life prophylactic administered preoperatively re-dosed within 4 h after preoperative dose • Proposed for 2010 but not endorsed
SCIP-Inf 9	Removal of postoperative urinary catheter removal by day 1 or 2 • Newly added for 2011
SCIP-Inf 10	Perioperative temperature management • Newly added for 2011

additional hospital days and incremental hospital cost exceeding $900 million.

Most experts in this field believe that vigilant patient care and systematic quality improvement protocols can decrease the incidence and national burden from SSIs. As a result, attempts to create a clinically useful and effective "SSI bundle" are underway. In the National Surgical Infection Prevention Collaborative [113], infection rates were analyzed in approximately 35,000 surgical patients at 56 hospitals over a 12-month period. Infection risk in the first 3 months was compared with that in the last 3 months, during which time, antimicrobial prophylaxis was supervised closely and normothermia, proper oxygenation, and euglycemia were maintained carefully. Appraisal of prophylaxis took into account the particular antimicrobial agent chosen and the timing and duration of administration. In addition, hair clipping replaced preoperative shaving. The initial infection rate of 2.3% decreased to 1.7% in the last 3 months of the study. Although this may seem trivial, it is a substantial benefit considering the large number of patients at risk and the large reduction in cost of treating SSI. A program initiated at the Mayo Clinic decreased SSIs by 57% with systematic institutional interventions such as protocol-driven order sets, a standard preoperative evaluation clinic, compliance monitoring, and reporting of outcomes [114]. Interestingly, the implementation of a World Health Organization (WHO) 19-item perioperative checklist decreased SSIs in eight distinctive institutions from 6.2% to 3.4% ($p < 0.001$), even though SSI was not the primary target of the checklist [115].

Historically, compliance with prophylaxis guidelines in the USA has been poor and variable across hospitals. In 2005, a study examining the practices of 2,965 acute care hospitals noted that only 55.7% of patients received antibiotics within 1 h of incision, and only 40.7% of prophylaxis regimens were discontinued within 24 h of surgery end time [116]. A national quality initiative entitled the Surgical Care Improvement Project (SCIP) was developed as an effort to standardize quality across hospitals and reduce surgical complications through performance measurement and quality improvement. The SCIP focuses on prevention of potentially preventable events: cardiovascular events, SSIs, postoperative pneumonia, and venous thromboembolism [117]. When considering SSI prevention measures, SCIP examined a variety of performance measures and mandates reporting with financial incentives for compliance, with a plan for future penalties for noncompliance [118]. Each year in the Federal Register, updates are made as to which SCIP measures will be reported as quality control indicators (Table 11.2) [119–121].

The goal of implementing SCIP measures is to improve outcomes by focusing on improving compliance with defined process measures. To this end, implementation of the SCIP has led to improved compliance with processes [113]. This initial study examined 44 hospitals reporting on 35,543 cases over a 1-year period, and noted improvement in all SCIP process measures studied and a significant decrease in SSI rate from 2.3% to 1.7% from the first 3 to the last 3 months. However, subsequent follow-up studies examining whether improved compliance leads to fewer SSIs show mixed results. Initial study results are mixed, and five studies have reported that the incidence of SSI has not changed as a result of SCIP or SCIP-like interventions despite improved compliance [122–126]. Currently, there is strong concern among experts that the notion that improved processes lead to improved outcomes is misplaced.

Healthcare payers are determined to improve quality and lower costs. "Pay for performance" and "value-based purchasing" are payment models that reward physicians and hospitals for meeting certain quality measures. On the other hand, disincentives are also being used increasing, meaning that hospitals with poor outcomes receive lower payments. In a proposal addressing value-based purchasing in 2011, the Centers for Medicare and Medicaid Services (CMS) suggested that SCIP performance measures be linked to Medicare payments so that hospitals with poor performance would receive lower payments [127]. Clearly, such a proposal is flawed considering that there may be no relationship between process improvement and better outcomes. In addition, the

CMS has deemed that SSIs following certain elective operations are "hospital-acquired conditions" for which hospitals would not be reimbursed. Currently, these conditions include SSI following coronary artery bypass grafting, certain orthopedic procedures, and bariatric surgery for weight loss [128], but the list of operations is likely to grow.

Conclusion

Patients who develop SSIs should be monitored carefully until the resolution of infection. Patients with open incisions may be discharged home with dressing changes supervised by visiting nurses and examined in the outpatient setting until healed. Once healed, patients with superficial or deep incisional SSIs involving the abdomen should be examined periodically to check for hernias at the site of the infection (the risk is 10–20%, even if the fascia is intact initially). Patients with organ/space infections who improved with percutaneous drainage should have the drains studied with contrast after the output decreases to ensure collapse of the cavity before removal of the drains (usually at 10–14 days). Patients who develop abdominal wall hernias should be evaluated for feasibility of abdominal wall reconstruction when stable. Risk and benefits and the patient's overall quality of life and medical health should be considered carefully, as these operations are often complex and have considerable recovery considerations.

In conclusion, SSI is a common complication; probably more than 3% of surgical patients are affected. Although many incisional infections are controlled easily, deeper and more extensive infections may have devastating long-term consequences for the patient's quality of life. Patient factors, including immune function, body temperature, oxygenation, glycemic control, the particular surgical procedure performed, and the infecting organism, all interact and eventually determine whether an SSI develops. Antimicrobial prophylaxis should be utilized carefully and appropriately to maximize benefit and minimize risk. Additionally, good surgical technique should be emphasized; simple local measures such as antisepsis, minimal use of electrocautery and implanted foreign bodies (e.g., nonabsorbable sutures), and prevention of hematoma are also important. Surgeons should be vigilant in addressing modifiable risk factors to help prevent of the development of SSI for every patient.

References

1. Barie PS. Surgical site infections: epidemiology and prevention. Surg Infect (Larchmt). 2002;3 Suppl 1:S9–21.
2. Horan TC, Gaynes RP, Martone WJ, Jarvis WR, Emori TG. CDC definitions of nosocomial surgical site infections, 1992: a modification of CDC definitions of surgical wound infections. Infect Control Hosp Epidemiol. 1992;13(10):606–8.
3. Fry DE. The economic costs of surgical site infection. Surg Infect (Larchmt). 2002;3 Suppl 1:S37–43.
4. Turina M, Cheadle WG. Management of established surgical site infections. Surg Infect (Larchmt). 2006;7 Suppl 3:s33–41.
5. Altemeier WA. Sepsis in surgery. Presidential address. Arch Surg. 1982;117(2):107–12.
6. Cheadle WG. Risk factors for surgical site infection. Surg Infect (Larchmt). 2006;7 Suppl 1:S7–11.
7. Robson MC, Krizek TJ, Heggers JP. Biology of surgical infection. Curr Probl Surg. 1973:1–62.
8. Velmahos GC, Vassiliu P, Demetriades D, et al. Wound management after colon injury: open or closed? A prospective randomized trial. Am Surg. 2002;68(9):795–801.
9. Duttaroy DD, Jitendra J, Duttaroy B, et al. Management strategy for dirty abdominal incisions: primary or delayed primary closure? A randomized trial. Surg Infect (Larchmt). 2009;10(2):129–36.
10. Cohn SM, Giannotti G, Ong AW, et al. Prospective randomized trial of two wound management strategies for dirty abdominal wounds. Ann Surg. 2001;233(3):409–13.
11. National Nosocomial Infections Surveillance (NNIS) report, data summary from October 1986–April 1996, issued May 1996. A report from the National Nosocomial Infections Surveillance (NNIS) System. Am J Infect Control. 1996;24(5):380–8.
12. Wertheim HF, Melles DC, Vos MC, et al. The role of nasal carriage in Staphylococcus aureus infections. Lancet Infect Dis. 2005;5(12):751–62.
13. Graham III PL, Lin SX, Larson EL. A U.S. population-based survey of Staphylococcus aureus colonization. Ann Intern Med. 2006;144(5):318–25.
14. Perl TM, Cullen JJ, Wenzel RP, et al. Intranasal mupirocin to prevent postoperative Staphylococcus aureus infections. N Engl J Med. 2002;346(24):1871–7.
15. Segers P, Speekenbrink RG, Ubbink DT, van Ogtrop ML, de Mol BA. Prevention of nosocomial infection in cardiac surgery by decontamination of the nasopharynx and oropharynx with chlorhexidine gluconate: a randomized controlled trial. JAMA. 2006;296(20):2460–6.
16. Trent MS, Stead CM, Tran AX, Hankins JV. Diversity of endotoxin and its impact on pathogenesis. J Endotoxin Res. 2006;12(4):205–23.
17. Courtney HS, Hasty DL, Dale JB. Molecular mechanisms of adhesion, colonization, and invasion of group A streptococci. Ann Med. 2002;34(2):77–87.
18. Bessen DE, Veasy LG, Hill HR, Augustine NH, Fischetti VA. Serologic evidence for a class I group A streptococcal infection among rheumatic fever patients. J Infect Dis. 1995;172(6):1608–11.
19. Onderdonk AB, Kasper DL, Cisneros RL, Bartlett JG. The capsular polysaccharide of Bacteroides fragilis as a virulence factor: comparison of the pathogenic potential of encapsulated and unencapsulated strains. J Infect Dis. 1977;136(1):82–9.
20. Kawabata S, Morita T, Iwanaga S, Igarashi H. Enzymatic properties of staphylothrombin, an active molecular complex formed between staphylocoagulase and human prothrombin. J Biochem (Tokyo). 1985;98(6):1603–14.
21. Melles DC, van Leeuwen WB, Boelens HA, Peeters JK, Verbrugh HA, van Belkum A. Panton-Valentine leukocidin genes in Staphylococcus aureus. Emerg Infect Dis. 2006;12(7):1174–5.
22. Fridkin SK, Hageman JC, Morrison M, et al. Methicillin-resistant Staphylococcus aureus disease in three communities. N Engl J Med. 2005;352(14):1436–44.
23. Proft T, Sriskandan S, Yang L, Fraser JD. Superantigens and streptococcal toxic shock syndrome. Emerg Infect Dis. 2003;9(10):1211–8.
24. Fry D. Toxic shock syndromne. In: Fry D, editor. Surgical infections. Boston: Little, Brown and Co.; 1995:569–75.

25. Chevalier J, Pages JM, Mallea M. In vivo modification of porin activity conferring antibiotic resistance to Enterobacter aerogenes. Biochem Biophys Res Commun. 1999;266(1):248–51.

26. Liu C, Bayer A, Cosgrove SE, et al. Clinical practice guidelines by the infectious diseases society of america for the treatment of methicillin-resistant Staphylococcus aureus infections in adults and children: executive summary. Clin Infect Dis. 2001;52(3): 285–92.

27. Rybak MJ, Lomaestro BM, Rotschafer JC, et al. Vancomycin therapeutic guidelines: a summary of consensus recommendations from the infectious diseases Society of America, the American Society of Health-System Pharmacists, and the Society of Infectious Diseases Pharmacists. Clin Infect Dis. 2009;49(3): 325–7.

28. Barie PS, Eachempati SR. Surgical site infections. Surg Clin North Am. 2005;85(6):1115–35. viii–ix.

29. Turina M, Cheadle W. Clinical challenges and unmet needs in the management of complicated skin and soft tissue infections. Surg Infect. 2005;6:s23–36.

30. DiNubile MJ, Lipsky BA. Complicated infections of skin and skin structures: when the infection is more than skin deep. J Antimicrob Chemother. 2004;53 Suppl 2:ii37–50.

31. Tanner J, Woodings D, Moncaster K. Preoperative hair removal to reduce surgical site infection. Cochrane Database Syst Rev. 2006;3:CD004122.

32. Hayek LJ, Emerson JM, Gardner AM. A placebo-controlled trial of the effect of two preoperative baths or showers with chlorhexidine detergent on postoperative wound infection rates. J Hosp Infect. 1987;10(2):165–72.

33. Rotter ML, Larsen SO, Cooke EM, et al. A comparison of the effects of preoperative whole-body bathing with detergent alone and with detergent containing chlorhexidine gluconate on the frequency of wound infections after clean surgery. The European Working Party on Control of Hospital Infections. J Hosp Infect. 1988;11(4):310–20.

34. Tanner J, Swarbrook S, Stuart J. Surgical hand antisepsis to reduce surgical site infection. Cochrane Database Syst Rev. 2008(1):CD004288.

35. Parienti JJ, Thibon P, Heller R, et al. Hand-rubbing with an aqueous alcoholic solution vs traditional surgical hand-scrubbing and 30-day surgical site infection rates: a randomized equivalence study. JAMA. 2002;288(6):722–7.

36. Weight CJ, Lee MC, Palmer JS. Avagard hand antisepsis vs. traditional scrub in 3600 pediatric urologic procedures. Urology. 2010;76(1):15–7.

37. Darouiche RO, Wall Jr MJ, Itani KM, et al. Chlorhexidine-alcohol versus povidone-iodine for surgical-site antisepsis. N Engl J Med. 2010;362(1):18–26.

38. Lee I, Agarwal RK, Lee BY, Fishman NO, Umscheid CA. Systematic review and cost analysis comparing use of chlorhexidine with use of iodine for preoperative skin antisepsis to prevent surgical site infection. Infect Control Hosp Epidemiol. 2010;31(12):1219–29.

39. Polk Jr HC, Miles AA. Enhancement of bacterial infection by ferric iron: kinetics, mechanisms, and surgical significance. Surgery. 1971;70(1):71–7.

40. Elek SD, Conen PE. The virulence of Staphylococcus pyogenes for man; a study of the problems of wound infection. Br J Exp Pathol. 1957;38(6):573–86.

41. Polk Jr HC, Lopez-Mayor JF. Postoperative wound infection: a prospective study of determinant factors and prevention. Surgery. 1969;66(1):97–103.

42. Bratzler DW, Houck PM. Antimicrobial prophylaxis for surgery: an advisory statement from the National Surgical Infection Prevention Project. Am J Surg. 2005;189(4):395–404.

43. Hawn MT, Gray SH, Vick CC, et al. Timely administration of prophylactic antibiotics for major surgical procedures. J Am Coll Surg. 2006;203(6):803–11.

44. Al-Ghnaniem R, Benjamin IS, Patel AG. Meta-analysis suggests antibiotic prophylaxis is not warranted in low-risk patients undergoing laparoscopic cholecystectomy. Br J Surg. 2003;90(3):365–6.

45. Choudhary A, Bechtold ML, Puli SR, Othman MO, Roy PK. Role of prophylactic antibiotics in laparoscopic cholecystectomy: a meta-analysis. J Gastrointest Surg. 2008;12(11):1847–53. discussion 1853.

46. Sanabria A, Dominguez LC, Valdivieso E, Gomez G. Antibiotic prophylaxis for patients undergoing elective laparoscopic cholecystectomy. Cochrane Database Syst Rev. 2010(12):CD005265.

47. Bodden C. SDPS memorandum: Center for Medicare and Medicaid Services; 2006.

48. Lewis RT. Oral versus systemic antibiotic prophylaxis in elective colon surgery: a randomized study and meta-analysis send a message from the 1990s. Can J Surg. 2002;45(3):173–80.

49. Bernard HR, Cole WR. The prophylaxis of surgical infection: the effect of prophylactic antimicrobial drugs on the incidence of infection following potentially contaminated operations. Surgery. 1964;56:151–7.

50. Coppa GF, Eng K, Gouge TH, Ranson JH, Localio SA. Parenteral and oral antibiotics in elective colon and rectal surgery. A prospective, randomized trial. Am J Surg. 1983;145(1):62–5.

51. Fry DE. Preventive systemic antibiotics in colorectal surgery. Surg Infect (Larchmt). 2008;9(6):547–52.

52. Stone HH, Hooper CA, Kolb LD, Geheber CE, Dawkins EJ. Antibiotic prophylaxis in gastric, biliary and colonic surgery. Ann Surg. 1976;184(4):443–52.

53. Nelson RL, Glenny AM, Song F. Antimicrobial prophylaxis for colorectal surgery. Cochrane Database Syst Rev. 2009(1):CD001181.

54. Song F, Glenny AM. Antimicrobial prophylaxis in colorectal surgery: a systematic review of randomized controlled trials. Br J Surg. 1998;85(9):1232–41.

55. Guenaga KK, Matos D, Wille-Jorgensen P. Mechanical bowel preparation for elective colorectal surgery. Cochrane Database Syst Rev. 2009(1):CD001544.

56. Cunningham M, Bunn F, Handscomb K. Prophylactic antibiotics to prevent surgical site infection after breast cancer surgery. Cochrane Database Syst Rev. 2006(2):CD005360.

57. Tejirian T, DiFronzo LA, Haigh PI. Antibiotic prophylaxis for preventing wound infection after breast surgery: a systematic review and metaanalysis. J Am Coll Surg. 2006;203(5):729–34.

58. Othman I. Prospective randomized evaluation of prophylactic antibiotic usage in patients undergoing tension free inguinal hernioplasty. Hernia. 2011;15(3):309–13.

59. Perez AR, Roxas MF, Hilvano SS. A randomized, double-blind, placebo-controlled trial to determine effectiveness of antibiotic prophylaxis for tension-free mesh herniorrhaphy. J Am Coll Surg. 2005;200(3):393–7. discussion 397–8.

60. Sanabria A, Dominguez LC, Valdivieso E, Gomez G. Prophylactic antibiotics for mesh inguinal hernioplasty: a meta-analysis. Ann Surg. 2007;245(3):392–6.

61. Sanchez-Manuel FJ, Lozano-Garcia J, Seco-Gil JL. Antibiotic prophylaxis for hernia repair. Cochrane Database Syst Rev. 2007(3):CD003769.

62. Stewart A, Eyers PS, Earnshaw JJ. Prevention of infection in arterial reconstruction. Cochrane Database Syst Rev. 2006;3:CD003073.

63. Stewart AH, Eyers PS, Earnshaw JJ. Prevention of infection in peripheral arterial reconstruction: a systematic review and metaanalysis. J Vasc Surg. 2007;46(1):148–55.

64. Classen DC, Evans RS, Pestotnik SL, Horn SD, Menlove RL, Burke JP. The timing of prophylactic administration of antibiotics

and the risk of surgical-wound infection. N Engl J Med. 1992;326(5):281–6.

65. McDonald M, Grabsch E, Marshall C, Forbes A. Single-versus multiple-dose antimicrobial prophylaxis for major surgery: a systematic review. Aust N Z J Surg. 1998;68(6):388–96.

66. Zanetti G, Giardina R, Platt R. Intraoperative redosing of cefazolin and risk for surgical site infection in cardiac surgery. Emerg Infect Dis. 2001;7(5):828–31.

67. Magann EF, Chauhan SP, Rodts-Palenik S, Bufkin L, Martin Jr JN, Morrison JC. Subcutaneous stitch closure versus subcutaneous drain to prevent wound disruption after cesarean delivery: a randomized clinical trial. Am J Obstet Gynecol. 2002;186(6): 1119–23.

68. Fukatsu K, Saito H, Matsuda T, Ikeda S, Furukawa S, Muto T. Influences of type and duration of antimicrobial prophylaxis on an outbreak of methicillin-resistant Staphylococcus aureus and on the incidence of wound infection. Arch Surg. 1997;132(12):1320–5.

69. Namias N, Harvill S, Ball S, McKenney MG, Salomone JP, Civetta JM. Cost and morbidity associated with antibiotic prophylaxis in the ICU. J Am Coll Surg. 1999;188(3):225–30.

70. Manian FA, Meyer PL, Setzer J, Senkel D. Surgical site infections associated with methicillin-resistant Staphylococcus aureus: do postoperative factors play a role? Clin Infect Dis. 2003;36(7): 863–8.

71. Banbury MK, Brizzio ME, Rajeswaran J, Lytle BW, Blackstone EH. Transfusion increases the risk of postoperative infection after cardiovascular surgery. J Am Coll Surg. 2006;202(1):131–8.

72. de Oliveira AC, Ciosak SI, Ferraz EM, Grinbaum RS. Surgical site infection in patients submitted to digestive surgery: risk prediction and the NNIS risk index. Am J Infect Control. 2006;34(4): 201–7.

73. Dunne JR, Malone DL, Tracy JK, Napolitano LM. Abdominal wall hernias: risk factors for infection and resource utilization. J Surg Res. 2003;111(1):78–84.

74. Furnary AP, Zerr KJ, Grunkemeier GL, Starr A. Continuous intravenous insulin infusion reduces the incidence of deep sternal wound infection in diabetic patients after cardiac surgical procedures. Ann Thorac Surg. 1999;67(2):352–60. discussion 360-2.

75. Greif R, Akca O, Horn EP, Kurz A, Sessler DI, Outcomes Research Group. Supplemental perioperative oxygen to reduce the incidence of surgical-wound infection. N Engl J Med. 2000;342(3): 161–7.

76. Imperatori A, Rovera F, Rotolo N, Nardecchia E, Conti V, Dominioni L. Prospective study of infection risk factors in 988 lung resections. Surg Infect (Larchmt). 2006;7 Suppl 2:S57–60.

77. Kaye KS, Sloane R, Sexton DJ, Schmader KA. Risk factors for surgical site infections in older people. J Am Geriatr Soc. 2006; 54(3):391–6.

78. Kurz A, Sessler DI, Lenhardt R. Perioperative normothermia to reduce the incidence of surgical-wound infection and shorten hospitalization. Study of Wound Infection and Temperature Group. N Engl J Med. 1996;334(19):1209–15.

79. Schwartz SR, Yueh B, Maynard C, Daley J, Henderson W, Khuri SF. Predictors of wound complications after laryngectomy: a study of over 2000 patients. Otolaryngol Head Neck Surg. 2004;131(1):61–8.

80. Scott NB, Turfrey DJ, Ray DA, et al. A prospective randomized study of the potential benefits of thoracic epidural anesthesia and analgesia in patients undergoing coronary artery bypass grafting. Anesth Analg. 2001;93(3):528–35.

81. Perioperative total parenteral nutrition in surgical patients. The Veterans Affairs Total Parenteral Nutrition Cooperative Study Group. N Engl J Med. 1991;325(8):525–32.

82. Gianotti L, Braga M, Nespoli L, Radaelli G, Beneduce A, Di Carlo V. A randomized controlled trial of preoperative oral supplementation with a specialized diet in patients with gastrointestinal cancer. Gastroenterology. 2002;122(7):1763–70.

83. Tepaske R, Velthuis H, Oudemans-van Straaten HM, et al. Effect of preoperative oral immune-enhancing nutritional supplement on patients at high risk of infection after cardiac surgery: a randomised placebo-controlled trial. Lancet. 2001;358(9283): 696–701.

84. Mangram AJ, Horan TC, Pearson ML, Silver LC, Jarvis WR. Guideline for prevention of surgical site infection, 1999. Hospital Infection Control Practices Advisory Committee. Infect Control Hosp Epidemiol. 1999;20(4):250–78.

85. Hughes JM. Study on the efficacy of nosocomial infection control (SENIC Project): results and implications for the future. Chemotherapy. 1988;34(6):553–61.

86. National Nosocomial Infections Surveillance (NNIS) System Report, data summary from January 1992 through June 2004, issued October 2004. Am J Infect Control. 2004;32(8):470–85.

87. Culver DH, Horan TC, Gaynes RP, et al. Surgical wound infection rates by wound class, operative procedure, and patient risk index. National Nosocomial Infections Surveillance System. Am J Med. 1991;91(3B):152S–7.

88. Horan TC, Culver DH, Gaynes RP, Jarvis WR, Edwards JR, Reid CR. Nosocomial infections in surgical patients in the United States, January 1986-June 1992. National Nosocomial Infections Surveillance (NNIS) System. Infect Control Hosp Epidemiol. 1993;14(2):73–80.

89. Gaynes RP, Culver DH, Horan TC, Edwards JR, Richards C, Tolson JS. Surgical site infection (SSI) rates in the United States, 1992-1998: the National Nosocomial Infections Surveillance System basic SSI risk index. Clin Infect Dis. 2001;33 Suppl 2:S69–77.

90. Fry D. Infections of the skin and soft tissues. In: Chorpenning N, editor. Surgical infections. Boston/New York/Toronto/London: Little, Brown and Co.; 1994. p. 145–226.

91. Moore TJ, Mauney C, Barron J. The use of quantitative bacterial counts in open fractures. Clin Orthop Relat Res. 1989;248:227–30.

92. Houang ET, Ahmet Z. Intraoperative wound contamination during abdominal hysterectomy. J Hosp Infect. 1991;19(3):181–9.

93. Lewis RT. Soft tissue infections. World J Surg. 1998;22(2): 146–51.

94. Wall DB, Klein SR, Black S, de Virgilio C. A simple model to help distinguish necrotizing fasciitis from nonnecrotizing soft tissue infection. J Am Coll Surg. 2000;191(3):227–31.

95. Ahrenholz DH. Necrotizing soft-tissue infections. Surg Clin North Am. 1988;68(1):199–214.

96. Anaya DA, McMahon K, Nathens AB, Sullivan SR, Foy H, Bulger E. Predictors of mortality and limb loss in necrotizing soft tissue infections. Arch Surg. 2005;140(2):151–7. discussion 158.

97. Raghavan M, Linden PK. Newer treatment options for skin and soft tissue infections. Drugs. 2004;64(15):1621–42.

98. Franklin GA, Moore KB, Snyder JW, Polk Jr HC, Cheadle WG. Emergence of resistant microbes in critical care units is transient, despite an unrestricted formulary and multiple antibiotic trials. Surg Infect (Larchmt). 2002;3(2):135–44.

99. Seal DV. Necrotizing fasciitis. Curr Opin Infect Dis. 2001;14(2): 127–32.

100. Freischlag JA, Ajalat G, Busuttil RW. Treatment of necrotizing soft tissue infections. The need for a new approach. Am J Surg. 1985;149(6):751–5.

101. Jallali N, Withey S, Butler PE. Hyperbaric oxygen as adjuvant therapy in the management of necrotizing fasciitis. Am J Surg. 2005;189(4):462–6.

102. Morykwas MJ, Simpson J, Punger K, Argenta A, Kremers L, Argenta J. Vacuum-assisted closure: state of basic research and physiologic foundation. Plast Reconstr Surg. 2006;117(7 Suppl):121S–6.

103. Venturi ML, Attinger CE, Mesbahi AN, Hess CL, Graw KS. Mechanisms and clinical applications of the vacuum-assisted closure (VAC) device: a review. Am J Clin Dermatol. 2005;6(3):185–94.

104. Heller L, Levin SL, Butler CE. Management of abdominal wound dehiscence using vacuum assisted closure in patients with compromised healing. Am J Surg. 2006;191(2):165–72.

105. Schaffzin DM, Douglas JM, Stahl TJ, Smith LE. Vacuum-assisted closure of complex perineal wounds. Dis Colon Rectum. 2004;47(10):1745–8.

106. Burger JW, Luijendijk RW, Hop WC, Halm JA, Verdaasdonk EG, Jeekel J. Long-term follow-up of a randomized controlled trial of suture versus mesh repair of incisional hernia. Ann Surg. 2004;240(4):578–83. discussion 583–5.

107. Luijendijk RW, Hop WC, van den Tol MP, et al. A comparison of suture repair with mesh repair for incisional hernia. N Engl J Med. 2000;343(6):392–8.

108. Whitehouse JD, Friedman ND, Kirkland KB, Richardson WJ, Sexton DJ. The impact of surgical-site infections following orthopedic surgery at a community hospital and a university hospital: adverse quality of life, excess length of stay, and extra cost. Infect Control Hosp Epidemiol. 2002;23(4):183–9.

109. Kirkland KB, Briggs JP, Trivette SL, Wilkinson WE, Sexton DJ. The impact of surgical-site infections in the 1990s: attributable mortality, excess length of hospitalization, and extra costs. Infect Control Hosp Epidemiol. 1999;20(11):725–30.

110. Broex EC, van Asselt AD, Bruggeman CA, van Tiel FH. Surgical site infections: how high are the costs? J Hosp Infect. 2009;72(3):193–201.

111. Urban JA. Cost analysis of surgical site infections. Surg Infect (Larchmt). 2006;7 Suppl 1:S19–22.

112. de Lissovoy G, Fraeman K, Hutchins V, Murphy D, Song D, Vaughn BB. Surgical site infection: incidence and impact on hospital utilization and treatment costs. Am J Infect Control. 2009;37(5):387–97.

113. Dellinger EP, Hausmann SM, Bratzler DW, et al. Hospitals collaborate to decrease surgical site infections. Am J Surg. 2005;190(1):9–15.

114. Thompson KM, Oldenburg WA, Deschamps C, Rupp WC, Smith CD. Chasing zero: the drive to eliminate surgical site infections. Ann Surg. 2011;254(3):430–6. discussion 436–7.

115. Haynes AB, Weiser TG, Berry WR, et al. A surgical safety checklist to reduce morbidity and mortality in a global population. N Engl J Med. 2009;360(5):491–9.

116. Bratzler DW, Houck PM, Richards C, et al. Use of antimicrobial prophylaxis for major surgery: baseline results from the National Surgical Infection Prevention Project. Arch Surg. 2005;140(2):174–82.

117. Fry DE. Surgical site infections and the surgical care improvement project (SCIP): evolution of national quality measures. Surg Infect (Larchmt). 2008;9(6):579–84.

118. Barie PS. No pay for no performance. Surg Infect (Larchmt). 2007;8(4):421–33.

119. Federal Register: Fiscal Year 2011, final rule. http://www.gpo.gov/fdsys/pkg/FR-2010-08-16/pdf/2010-19092.pdf. Accessed 10 Aug 2011.

120. Federal Register: Fiscal Year 2009, final rule. http://edocket.access.gpo.gov/2008/pdf/E8-17914. Accessed 10 Aug 2011.

121. Federal Register: Fiscal Year 2010, final rule. http://edocket.access.gpo.gov/2009/pdf/E9-18663.pdf. Accessed 10 Aug 2011.

122. Ingraham AM, Cohen ME, Bilimoria KY, et al. Association of surgical care improvement project infection-related process measure compliance with risk-adjusted outcomes: implications for quality measurement. J Am Coll Surg. 2010;211(6):705–14.

123. Stulberg JJ, Delaney CP, Neuhauser DV, Aron DC, Fu P, Koroukian SM. Adherence to surgical care improvement project measures and the association with postoperative infections. JAMA. 2010;303(24):2479–85.

124. Nicholas LH, Osborne NH, Birkmeyer JD, Dimick JB. Hospital process compliance and surgical outcomes in medicare beneficiaries. Arch Surg. 2010;145(10):999–1004.

125. Anthony T, Murray BW, Sum-Ping JT, et al. Evaluating an evidence-based bundle for preventing surgical site infection: a randomized trial. Arch Surg. 2011;146(3):263–9.

126. Hawn MT, Vick CC, Richman J, et al. Surgical site infection prevention: time to move beyond the surgical care improvement program. Ann Surg. 2011;254(3):494–501.

127. Patterson P. SCIP measures to weigh in Medicare pay starting in 2013. OR Manager. 2011;27(3):1, 7–10.

128. Hospital-Acquired Conditions (HAC) in Acute Inpatient Prospective Payment System (IPPS) Hospitals. https://www.cms.gov/HospitalAcqCond/downloads/HACFactsheet.pdf. 2010. Accessed 7 Aug 2011.

Agathe Streiff and Bryan A. Cotton

Introduction

Hemorrhage is the leading cause of intraoperative deaths. Many cardiovascular and hepatobiliary procedures result in massive hemorrhage and postpartum hemorrhage events in labor and delivery place the patient at a high risk for mortality. Gastrointestinal bleeding from diverticulosis, varices, and ulcer disease can result in significant blood loss requiring massive transfusion and resuscitation from hemorrhagic shock. Timely and effective transfusion of blood products is of critical in these scenarios. The frequency in which blood component products are transfused in surgical patients begs for a greater understanding of them. The aim of this chapter is to provide clinicians with a discussion of the current literature on the various blood component products, their indications, and unique hemostatic conditions in the surgical patient. While the majority of data concerning optimal management of acquired coagulopathy and hemorrhagic shock resuscitation is based on trauma patients, many of the principles can and should be applied to the surgical patient (or likely any patient) with profound hemorrhage.

The Lethal Triad of Acute Resuscitation

The concept of the lethal triad—hypothermia, acidosis and coagulation—was first promoted in the trauma population in those undergoing emergency surgery. In an effort to combat its development (or at least attenuate its effects), several authors began advocating for Damage Control Surgery [1, 2]. However, the principles of Damage Control have spread through the trauma centers and into the operating theaters and intensive care units [3]. Central to this concept is

A. Streiff, B.S. • B.A. Cotton, M.D., M.P.H. (✉)
Department of Surgery and The Center for Translational Injury Research, The University of Texas Health Science Center, 6410 Fannin, 1100 UPB, Houston, TX 77030, USA
e-mail: bryan.a.cotton@uth.tmc.edu

aggressively and rapidly addressing all three components simultaneously, as each greatly affects the other.

Hypothermia, a core body temperature of $34-36°C$, in the trauma patient primarily results from reflexive peripheral vasoconstriction in the hypovolemic patient. This phenomenon is further exacerbated by rapid infusion of unwarmed crystalloid fluid during initial resuscitation. This condition impairs coagulation factor activity and platelet function, such as their ability to produce thromboxane, and must be rapidly reversed [4]. Crystalloid and colloid fluids also contribute to hemodilution of clotting factors, further promoting ongoing bleeding. Hence, in this situation, early plasma therapy and platelets have been shown to improve outcomes [5].

Acidosis has been hypothesized to result from hypoperfusion and excess administration of ionic chloride in normal saline administration. The acidosis disturbs platelet function and morphology, reduces coagulation factor complex activity, and degrades fibrinogen. Approximately 25% of trauma patients present with abnormal coagulation parameters, and these have been associated with poorer outcomes in these patients. The three conditions previously mentioned contribute to poor clot formation and aggravated coagulopathy [4].

Evidence exists supporting increased survival upon rapid treatment of initial coagulopathy [5, 6]. Preemptive strategies have been shown to actually reduce coagulopathy and the number of overall transfusions required to treat the patient [7, 8]. However, challenges to implementation include time limitations of laboratory-guided component therapy since the results of the tests are not immediate. Another difficulty is that once it has been determined that the patient should receive plasma, it may take another 30–45 min to thaw and deliver the products [5]. As such, hospitals should have in place a thawed plasma program, keeping adequate numbers of "universal" and type-specific thawed plasma available for immediate release. Plasma thawing protocols exist to avoid this issue and are discussed in later sections. In acutely bleeding patients, massive transfusion protocols are often activated in order to efficaciously restore blood volume and hemostasis and thawed plasma is critical to their success [5, 6].

L.J. Moore et al. (eds.), *Common Problems in Acute Care Surgery*,
DOI 10.1007/978-1-4614-6123-4_12, © Springer Science+Business Media New York 2013

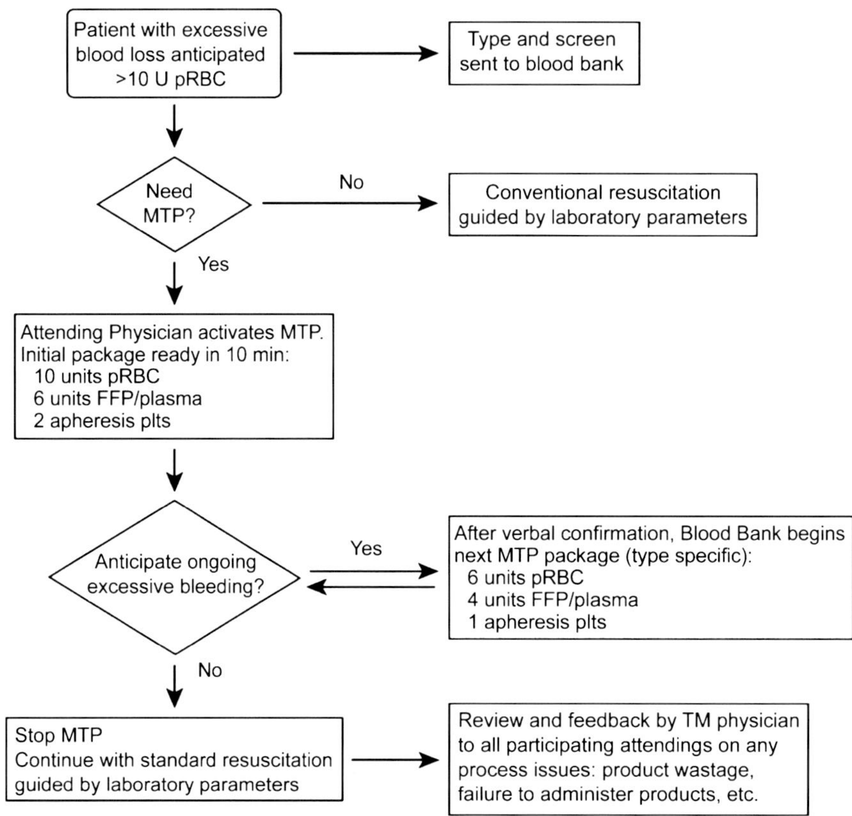

Fig. 12.1 An example of a massive transfusion protocol. Adapted from reference [5]

Massive Transfusion Protocols

A massive transfusion (MT) is defined as more than ten units of red blood cells (RBC) in 24 h [5]. A massive transfusion protocol (MTP) is the standardization of the delivery and transfusion of RBC, plasma, and platelets in predetermined and predefined ratios as facilitated by a surgical or medical team. In the patient requiring immediate resuscitation, a typical MTP will call for six to ten units of RBC, with a ratio of RBC to plasma and platelets in 1:1:1 to 1:1:2 fashion. This protocol and release of products will continue based on ongoing bleeding (Fig. 12.1). These assessments are generally implemented "blind," with subsequent releases guided by routine coagulation laboratory studies as well as thromboelastography (TEG) [9].

Even before the transfusions take place, MTPs call for the rapid mobilization of blood components by having AB thawed plasma and group O RBC [10]. A type and screen should be drawn as soon as possible to allow for the transition from universal products to type-specific ones. The efficacy of an MTP also lies in its early implementation as well as identification of patients who would benefit from such an intervention. Criteria for activation include laboratory values, anatomic injuries, and mechanism of injury. Several authors have demonstrated that the transfusion of uncross-matched RBCs is an independent predictor of substantial hemorrhage and the transfusion of multiple units of RBC, plasma, and platelets [10, 11]. As such, when one is requesting uncross-matched product for transfusion, the institution's MTP should be activated.

Prior to the advent of MTPs, resuscitation protocols for severely injured patients began with large volumes of crystalloid followed by RBC transfusions. Later on, plasma, platelets, and cryoprecipitate were administered if the patient had survived the operating theater and then only based on laboratory values and the opinion of anesthesiologists and transfusion specialists. These guidelines recommended transfusions at prothrombin time ratio of >1.5, platelet counts of $<50 \times 10^9$/L, fibrinogen level <1.5–2.0 g/L or after a predetermined volume loss. This approach relied on a reactive strategy where the clinician was constantly "catching up" with values representing an earlier hemodynamic state of the patient [12].

While this standard resuscitation method is adequate for patients who are not in shock or not bleeding, studies have demonstrated that it does not suffice for the subset of patients who have sustained serious injuries, are coagulopathic or in shock [5]. One reason is that the coagulopathy is addressed after a time lapse since the original laboratory values were obtained. Other reasons for the suboptimal results of this method are due to the ratios of each blood component product infused. Specifically, evidence exists that demonstrates that large volume of crystalloid fluids is associated with increased hemorrhage and lower survival rates [13]. It has been hypothesized that this effect is due to insufficient replenishing of hemostasis factors, and the complex coagulopathy of dilution, consumption of factors, and fibrinolysis is not adequately addressed. MTPs also offer the advantage of reducing intraoperative crystalloid use and hence, reducing opportunities for hemodilution.

Damage control resuscitation (DCR) expands on the MTP process and calls for low-volume resuscitation, sparing the patient of resuscitation with fluids such as crystalloids and colloids that are low in hemostasis factors [14]. Instead, DCR adheres to transfusion of blood products in a ratio of plasma and platelets to red blood cells consistent with that which is being lost to hemorrhage. It also involves more permissive hypertension, and acting preemptively on the hypovolemic, hemorrhaging patient. DCR is also supported by findings from the US Army's Institute of Surgical Research, which demonstrated improvement in outcomes in severely bleeding patients who were transfused in ratios of products similar to whole blood. Civilian trauma data has also shown that RBC to plasma ratio between 3:2 and 1:1 lead to reduced 30-day mortality and increased odds of survival [5]. Fox et al. found that patients undergoing vascular surgery with DCR had improved revascularization and graft patency. Their results demonstrated that recombinant VIIa, whole blood, fresh frozen plasma (FFP), platelets, cryoprecipitate and minimal crystalloid prevented early graft failures [15].

While there is a wealth of data in the trauma population, less data is available regarding coagulopathy in the severely bleeding patient in other surgical specialties. It is, however, important to consider the underlying pathology responsible for exsanguination, such as in obstetric patients, as well as related comorbidities, such as uremia, pharmacologic anticoagulation, in assessing for need of blood products [5]. For instance, Kılıç et al.'s review of resuscitation in patients with gastrointestinal bleeding found that 1:1:1 ratios of pRBCs, FFPs, and platelets reduced dilutional coagulopathy, similarly to trauma patients [16]. Patients undergoing open thoracoabdominal aortic aneurysm repair are also vulnerable to coagulopathy due to systemic heparinization, hypothermia, and left-heart bypass with a centrifugal pump [17]. As well, several authors have noted its benefit in the vascular population [15, 18, 19]. Mell evaluated 168 patients with ruptured abdominal aortic aneurysm who had massive hemorrhage in the perioperative period. Their findings showed reduced 30-day mortality in patients who were transfused 1:1 RBC to plasma ratios. These patients also experienced lower rates of colonic ischemia. The value of this study is that the average age of patients was 73 years, much older than the average trauma patient, demonstrating applicability of MTPs in different patient age populations [19].

Lastly, evidence on MTPs has focused on the acutely bleeding surgical patient, and less is known about patients in other surgical settings. Due to the less emergent nature of such settings, it is likely that MTPs are activated more reactively, and it may have a different effect on patient outcome [5]. However, some groups have shown that those patients receiving less than massive transfusion levels may still benefit from higher plasma to red blood cell ratios [20]. Wafaisade and colleagues demonstrated decreased mortality rates in such patients.

Thawed Plasma Protocols

Because of the nature of frozen plasma, transfusion delays of 45 min occur as units are thawed and prepared. Young and colleagues surveyed members of the University Health System Consortium, consisting of 107 academic medical centers and 232 affiliated hospitals and found that only 60% of participating hospitals had thawed plasma sufficient for the first cycle of their MTP. This problem delays the critical availability of plasma in the initial phase of resuscitation. Reviews of plasma, cryoprecipitate and platelet transfusions alongside massive blood transfusion protocols have demonstrated that earlier use of plasma and platelets in trauma patients have decreased the incidence of coagulopathy [21]. Unfortunately, by the time one or more blood volumes have been lost, plasma may still be unavailable in the absence of a thawed or liquid plasma program. Hence, protocols have been established to reduce wastage of products and use them for patients in an efficacious manner [22].

Blood Component Products: Red Blood Cells

Red blood cells are the component of choice used to restore hemoglobin levels in resuscitation. More than 30% of intensive care unit (ICU) patients receive RBC transfusions and more than 40% are transfused during hospitalization [23]. The Cardiovascular Health Study found that anemia is associated with increased mortality in elderly patients, emphasizing the importance of treatment [24]. However, correction of anemia in surgical patients has not been readily studied, and its benefits remain controversial.

In their review, Englesbe et al. note that there is not yet a consensus of in what degree of anemia can RBC transfusions offer a benefit [25]. They discuss the current findings by various studies, which have found that survival was not increased when postoperative patients were transfused to correct a hematocrit of 25%, and similarly, while studies favor transfusion in cardiac patients with a hematocrit of 33% or less, a true benefit remains to be seen. Hence, they recommend making the decision to transfuse using a host of physiological measures and evaluation of the patient's compensatory ability, not only the hematocrit. They have used a trigger of a hematocrit of 16% for initiating transfusion when the patient has excellent compensatory ability, and 21% when this is not the case [25]. The 21% trigger should also be employed in stable elderly patients without tachycardia or hypoxia. Otherwise, their investigations have not yet shown benefits in stratification of surgical patients by specialty or procedures. One surgical population that has been studied with regards to transfusion is patients undergoing infrarenal abdominal aortic aneurysm surgery. A meta-analysis of randomized controlled trials demonstrated that intraoperative autotransfusion in these patients decreased the allogeneic blood transfusion requirement [26].

High quality evidence, notably Hébert et al.'s, exists to support conservative triggers for RBC transfusion in critically ill patients [27]. This multicenter randomized, controlled, clinical trial of 838 critically ill patients compared the outcomes of patients who were transfused at hemoglobin levels of less than 7.0 g/dL and those who were transfused at hemoglobin levels below 10.0 g/dL. Their study ultimately found that the more restrictive trigger of 7.0 g/dL was superior to the liberal one and patients experienced improved 30-day survival rates. Of note, of the various patient populations studied, this improvement was not found to be significant in patients with acute myocardial infarction and unstable angina [27].

It is important to be mindful of false triggers for transfusion, such as anemia due to hemodilution, commonly seen in patients receiving fluids during prolonged hospital stays. A peripheral hematocrit is not enough to determine the patient's red blood cell levels, and calculations of total blood volume, red blood cell volumes, and normalized hematocrit are necessary [28]. Van et al. report that relying on peripheral hematocrit alone resulted in overdiagnosis of anemia in 23.8% of analyses, and this finding can lead to unnecessary transfusions. Blood Volume Analyzers are one option that has been shown to separate anemia due to hemodilution compared to other sources such as surgical bleeding [28].

In patients with prolonged hospital stays and critically ill patients, it is important to keep in mind anemia due to phlebotomy for various laboratory testing and other needs [23]. Between 40 and 240 ml of blood per day is collected from ICU patients, with surgical patients generally on the higher end. Hence, the conservation of blood and reducing unnecessary blood draws is key to preventing a need for pRBC transfusions.

Erythropoetin

Because RBC transfusions are associated with certain risks that are discussed in a later section, it is important to also consider possible alternatives or treatments that reduce transfusion requirements, such as epoetin alfa.

Silver et al.'s randomized, double-blind, placebo-controlled trial investigated the role of epoetin alfa, a recombinant erythropoietin, in reducing the RBC transfusion requirement of long-term acute care patients, thereby reducing risks associated with transfusions[29]. Their findings showed that treatment with epoetin alfa significantly increased hemoglobin concentration and the odds ratio for receiving an RBC transfusion compared to patients on the placebo arm was 0.28 [29]. Additionally, Vincent et al.'s randomized, double-blind, placebo-controlled study demonstrated that a once weekly dose of epoetin alfa augmented the erythropoietin response [30]. Knight et al.'s review found that patients with cancers of various organs who did not have anemia, most due to correction with epoetin alfa, required less transfusions and experienced more quality of life [31]. However, epoetin alfa is limited by its delayed onset at 5–7 days. As for its effects on mortality, Corwin et al. conducted a prospective, randomized, placebo-controlled trial of 1,460 medical, surgical, or trauma patients [32]. Weekly injections of epoetin alfa were shown to decrease mortality at day 29 and day 140, especially in trauma patients compared to placebo. However, epoetin alfa was associated with an increase in thrombotic events, and did not affect the number of patients who received a transfusion of RBCs [32].

Iron Supplementation

Iron sucrose has also been investigated as a possible adjunct to RBC transfusions in order to reduce transfusion requirements. To answer this question in colorectal cancer surgery patients, Edwards et al. conducted a randomized prospective blinded placebo-controlled trial of 60 patients [33]. Patient outcomes, which were assessed using change in hemoglobin levels, serum iron markers, transfusion rate, length of hospital stay and perioperative events, were found to be unchanged by the addition of 600 mg of iron sucrose [33].

Blood Component Products: Plasma

Plasma is an acellular blood product consisting of clotting factors involved in coagulation and fibrinolysis, as well as proteins involved in immune reactions and maintenance the oncotic balance of blood. Plasma can be obtained from separation of whole blood or unique plasma donations from a donor using plasmapheresis. Common indications for plasma are reversal of warfarin-induced anticoagulation, massive transfusion in trauma and surgery, procedures with limited bleeding or risk thereof, liver disease with coagulation factor deficiencies, single coagulation factor deficiency, and thrombotic thrombocytopenic purpura (TTP) [34].

Historically, plasma transfusions have been associated with various side effects including transfusion related acute lung injury (TRALI) [35]. However, these complications have been dramatically reduced with blood donation centers transitioning to male only and/or nulliparous female donors [36].

Norda et al. studied two types of plasma: thawed plasma and liquid plasma (never frozen). Liquid plasma is an AABB approved product and may be stored at 2–6°C for up to 26 days. Both of these types of plasma have been considered clinically equivalent. As for their individual components, liquid plasma has been shown to contain levels of Factor V and von Willebrand factor at levels 70% or greater. However, studies have noted that C1 esterase inhibitor (C1INH) was consumed by day 14 in 22% of plasma products due to cold-induced contact activation [37]. In order to avoid this effect that places patients at risk for inadequate perfusion, some institutions have introduced a maximum storage time of 7 days for nonfrozen plasma [37].

Murad et al.'s meta-analysis of 37 studies on adults transfused with plasma compared with nontransfused controls demonstrated that in the setting of massive transfusions in trauma patients, transfusion may be associated with increased survival and decreased multiorgan failure. However, they also noted increased mortality in patients who received plasma not part of a massive transfusion protocol. This finding may be due to the unbalanced ratio of transfusion of products, unlike in mass transfusion protocols, which call for 1:1 transfusion of RBCs and plasma. In addition, plasma transfusion was associated with increased risk of developing TRALI, and by itself did not reduce transfusion requirements [34]. Their findings, in the first comprehensive meta-analysis and systematic review of plasma transfusion outcomes, highlight the need of assessing each patient's indications for plasma. The maturation of this field will be needed to strengthen the findings, which the authors did note were subject to survivor biases in some studies. However, none of these studies involved the use of plasma in patients with hemorrhagic shock. In this population of patients, the incidence of multi-organ failure has been shown to be lower than comparison cohorts (most likely as a result of less overall transfusions in the higher plasma group) [13, 14].

Blood Component Products: Platelets

The purpose of platelet transfusions is to avoid spontaneous hemorrhage, which can occur at very low platelet levels, especially in patients who are already hemorrhaging or have various platelet deficiencies and abnormalities of function. Along with plasma and fibrinogen, platelets are key in achieving hemostasis in the obstetric patient with post-partum hemorrhage [38]. Approximately 50,000 cells/L of platelets are necessary in order to achieve adequate hemostasis.

In addition to the total number of platelets, their quality is also important to overall hemostatic function. A patient's platelets must be efficacious, that is, remaining in circulation and completing its physiological role in clot formation [39]. This efficacy can be assessed by various modalities, from the traditional laboratory coagulation studies to the more recent thrombelastograms (TEG), also known as thromboelastography, and this topic is covered in the last section.

Blood Component Products: Cryoprecipitate

Cryoprecipitate consists of von Willebrand factor/VIII complex, factor XIII, and fibrinogen. It is used to supplement plasma transfusions with fibrinogen, especially in patients with fibrinogen levels of less than 100 mg/dL, the level at which hypofibrinogenemia results in bleeding [5]. It is named cryoprecipitate because single units of plasma are rapidly frozen to −30°C and are slowly thawed overnight to 4°C, causing many clotting factors such as fibrinogen to precipitate out of the solution [35]. Indications for cryoprecipitate include factor VII deficiency, congenital or acquired hypofibrinogenemia, disseminated intravascular coagulation, and massive transfusion.

Unlike plasma, virus-inactivated cryoprecipitate is not yet available, and studies on the efficacy of SD FFP and MB FFP have not shown a benefit [35]. The complications of cryoprecipitate are similar to those of plasma, with a slightly lower occurrence of complications associated with higher volumes of plasma, such as TRALI and hemolysis [35].

Blood Component Products: Whole Blood

The practice of using whole blood is largely uncommon due to the separation of blood components for targeting specific deficiencies currently supported by evidence-based medicine. Decision-making for each transfusion requires laboratory testing, and each product must carefully be stored and transported to the site of need. When this is not possible, such as in acute settings with limited resources, whole blood transfusions can adequately resuscitate certain patients. Grosso et al. recount a case of collecting whole blood from hospital personnel donors in a US field surgical hospital in Kosovo [40]. This whole blood was used to treat exsanguinating coagulopathy in an acutely bleeding patient. The advantage of whole blood is its ability to increase hemoglobin levels, similarly to red blood cells, and its ability to restore blood volumes, similarly to crystalloids [40]. Because of its physiological ratios of each blood component, it may hold an advantage over individual blood component transfusions, but more work is necessary to substantiate this idea.

Blood Component Products: Recombinant Activated Factor VII

Recombinant activated factor VII (rFVIIa), originally developed for use in hemophilia A and B patients, has recently been explored in various off-label uses, such as stemming acute bleeding alongside standard replacement therapy. Mayo et al. demonstrate the use of a coagulopathy score that they found to be statistically correlated to rFVIIa response and survival in 13 trauma patients in Israel [41]. This finding was a turning point in the understanding of rFVIIa indications due to its previous contraindication in coagulopathy. Other uses for rFVIIa are factor VII deficiency, thrombocytopenia, functional platelet disorders, von Willebrand disease, intracranial bleeding, and reversal of warfarin overdose, liver disease, and transplantation. However, little evidence is currently available to support these uses [41].

Transfusion-Related Complications

Before entering the discussion on complications related to transfusions, the difficulty of study design to answer such questions must be appreciated. There are ethical obstacles to randomizing patients to transfusion and non-transfusion arms. Hence, many trials show patients who received more blood component transfusions fared worse than patients who did not, but this may be entirely because of the condition of the patients that necessitated the transfusions [25]. Khorana et al.'s retrospective cohort study of 504,208 patients hospitalized with cancer demonstrated that RBC and platelet transfusions were associated with increased mortality, as well as venous and arterial thrombotic events [42]. However, it is unclear if this is a causal relationship.

As with large-scale introduction of exogenous elements to the body, immune reactions can develop, a sequela that is notorious in blood products. This complication is particularly devastating in severely ill patients. The most notorious of these immune reactions are hemolytic reactions. In order to prevent this event, it is important to cross-match patient and donor blood whenever possible. The most common cause of hemolytic reactions due to transfusion of an incorrect match is clerical error. Hemolytic reactions in blood transfusions occur because each individual carries antibodies against the blood group (A or B) that it does not express endogenously. Hence, when products containing anti-A or anti-B antibodies in plasma, such as plasma, are transfused to patients of A, B, or both blood groups, the donor antibodies stage an attack on the patient's red blood cells. Allergic reactions are another common immune-mediated complication of transfusions. Severely anaphylactic reactions are more common after plasma compared to RBC transfusion

[35]. Patients present with wheeze, hypotension, tachycardia, laryngeal edema, and urticarial rash.

TRALI is defined as acute lung injury occurring within 6 h of transfusion with a blood product, with most commonly reported cases occurring due to FFP [43]. TRALI is the most common cause of death due to transfusion [35]. TRALI is characterized by respiratory insufficiency, not limited to but including tachypnea, cyanosis, dyspnea, and acute hypoxemia [43]. Unfortunately, the occurrence of TRALI in critically ill patients who received a blood transfusion is estimated to be around 25% and increases with each subsequent transfusion, has a mortality rate of approximately 40%, and it is the most common transfusion-related complication [16]. Eighty-five percent of patients with bleeding varices receive blood transfusions, and the trigger for transfusions is much debated. In patients with gastrointestinal bleeding, TRALI is further exacerbated by the presence of end-stage liver disease. Proposed mechanisms for this phenomenon have included antibody-mediated reactions, but these findings are not definitive and many are subject to selection bias due to no screening in the asymptomatic population [43]. Autopsies and animal models have suggested hyperactive PMN involvement, since mass infiltration was noted [43]. A two-event model has also been proposed, with the first event dictated by the clinical health of the patient and the second event by the quality (affected by storage, donor immunologic components) of the blood product [43]. The treatment of TRALI is aggressive respiratory support and ventilation in more severe cases, such as in critically ill patients [43]. Practices to reduce the risk of TRALI include prestorage leukoreduction as well as avoiding the use of old blood products, defined as older than 14 days for RBCs and older than 2 days for platelet concentrates. Another prevention strategy is using only male donors or donors who have never been pregnant due to look back studies showing fewer TRALI events in blood donations from those populations [16]. Eder et al. demonstrated that preferential distribution of plasma from male donors reduced the reported number of TRALI cases [44].

Transfusion-associated immunomodulation refers to the immunosuppression resulting from the introduction of foreign antigens via blood products to the host [25]. The exact mechanism of this effect has not yet been elucidated, but plasma components, white blood cells (WBCs), metabolic products from storage processes are thought to play a role. This effect may be responsible for the immunosuppressive effects of transfusions on severely ill patients.

Transfusions can cause sensitization to HLA antigens, creating a unique problem in potential kidney transplant patients. Studies have demonstrated increased sensitization of patients on a kidney transplant waiting list after transfusion, rendering them unsuitable candidates for living donation. Their only remaining alternative once this has occurred is to wait for a cadaveric graft, which takes up to four times longer, and may never receive a transplant.

Hence, non-life-sustaining transfusions should be avoided in potential kidney transplant recipients [25].

Red blood cell transfusion is an independent predictor of systemic inflammatory response syndrome (SIRS), ICU admission, mortality, and length of hospital stay, and the development of multiple organ failure (MOF) [45]. In particular, the age of the blood plays an important role, with increased age of RBCs resulting in increased instances of MOF. RBCs are not alone in this adverse event. A multicenter prospective cohort study demonstrated that FFP was independently associated with increased risk of MOF and acute respiratory distress syndrome (ARDS) of 2.1% and 2.5% [46]. The same study found, however, decreased risk of MOF per unit of cryoprecipitate, and platelets were not found to be associated with MOF or ARDS [46].

In addition to MOF, blood transfusions are notorious in lay media for their association with infectious agents. In their review of the current literature, Englesbe et al. found that patients who received transfusions compared to those who did not experienced significant increase nosocomial infection rates, and each additional pRBC transfused correlated to increased infection risk [25]. *Staphylococcus aureus* is the most commonly transmitted bacterial pathogen [16]. Bacterial pathogen in blood products arise mainly from donor skin, and platelets are especially prone to these contaminants [35]. However, bacterial infections are less common than viral infections in blood transfusions.

Despite increased screening and testing, each RBC transfusion is associated with a risk for viral infections such as hepatitis [29]. Virus risks in the UK in FFP have been estimated at 1 in 8 million for HIV, 1 in 30 million for HCV and 1 in 900,000 for HBV [35]. Since up to 50% of adult donors are cytomegalovirus (CMV) carriers, there is a risk of transmission of this virus to patients, especially the immunosuppressed, transplant patients and neonates [35]. Compared to viral causes, bacterial, endotoxin and prion contamination rates are more rare [35]. In order to avoid this deleterious complication, virus-inactivated preparations of plasma exist, such as methylene blue and solvent-detergent treated products. While these options may offer increased viral protection, they have been associated with loss of clotting factors [35]. The most stringent testing protocols and sensitive tests may not ever eradicate the risk of infectious agent transmission due to several reasons. First, new pathogens of unknown methods of spread are constantly emerging and may not actively be screened for in its early emergence, such as human immunodeficiency virus (HIV) and West Nile virus. Another obstacle in prevention is the incubation period of pathogens before seroconversion of blood [29].

Prion diseases transmitted by transfusion has been a concern in the UK, following the bovine spongiform encephalopathy (BSE) epidemic. Unfortunately, no screening test for this condition has been established, and the occurrence of prion diseases in blood products in the UK is largely unknown. In order to avoid transfusions with prion disease, plasma has been imported from the USA since 2002 for pediatric transfusions [35].

Another concerning complication is the loss of efficacy in stored blood, and the adverse effects it causes. These consequences of the storage process are known as a storage lesion. With current technology, the shelf life of red blood cells cannot be extended further than its physiological shelf life of 120 days, and 35 and 42 days is the limit of viability in whole blood and adenine-saline preservation, respectively [29]. Even this length of shelf-life results in counterproductive transfusions. Specifically, RBC products older than 2 weeks have been shown to not improve oxygen uptake in septic patients. In fact, RBCs of that age have been associated with higher mortality, increased adverse events, extended hospital stay, and electrolyte imbalances. This reduction in efficacy may be due to decreased ability of the older RBCs to unload oxygen [29]. Another proposed mechanism is that since stored RBCs have depleted nitric oxide, this may have a vasoconstrictive effect, leading to thrombosis and the observed increases in venous and arterial thrombotic events in patients with increased pRBC and platelet transfusions [42]. The question is how realistic it is to maintain strict storage age in a finite and scarce resource such as blood. A double-blind, prospective randomized pilot study demonstrated that controlling the storage age of RBCs in transfusion compared to the current standard of care is feasible and results in decreased exposure to older blood [47]. More evidence is needed to determine precisely the cut off age of RBCs in their efficacy and availability. In stored platelets, it has been estimated that the recovery rate of 5-day old platelets is about 50%, with many nonviable platelets being sequestered into the spleen [21]. For these reasons, there is some concern that platelet counts performed immediately after transfusion do not provide an accurate picture of platelet function [21].

Given the complications listed previously, a discussion of known preventative measures is warranted. Transfusion with RBCs that have not been leukoreduced has been associated with increased risk of multiple organ failure and degenerating leukocytes may cause RBC toxicity. Furthermore, nationwide leukoreduction protocols in Canada were shown to lower mortality rates [29]. Currently, in the USA, leukoreduction is not a standard practice despite evidence of benefit, and additional work is required to determine effects on outcome in various patient populations, such as ICU patients [29].

Hospitalized patients receiving transfusions are already in a vulnerable state of health, and when transfusion-related adverse events occur, it is most regrettable. With institutional triage protocols and transfusion guidelines, such unnecessary harm can be avoided, and cost reduction of a limited and precious resource can be achieved [48]. Protocols and scoring systems, such as the Emergency Transfusion Score (ETS), have been successfully shown to triage patients in need of transfusions and those for whom it would be unnecessary [49].

Special Populations

The Anticoagulated Patient and the Patient Receiving Platelet Inhibitors

There are many considerations to address in the management of an anticoagulated surgical patient, such as reversing anticoagulation fully before operation, in order to avoid bleeding complications. In the nonelective setting, such as life-threatening hemorrhage or emergent surgical indications, this process must be sped up, using prothrombin complex concentrate (PCC) [50]. Unlike FFP, PCC can be administered without the need for cross-matching or thawing, has more predictable concentrations of clotting factors, and has been shown to reverse warfarin-related coagulopathy. The clotting factors are also in high concentrations, approximately 25 times that of plasma, decreasing the volume of PCC needed. In addition, the INR is rapidly corrected, taking about 15 min [50].

Anticoagulated patients and patients using antiplatelet agents are especially vulnerable to coagulopathies, which may develop during resuscitation. Kılıç et al.'s findings recommend using individualized treatment, providing the deficient blood component as per laboratory value deficiency [16]. In addition, patients who are overly anticoagulated with warfarin may also be treated with PCC containing vitamin K dependent factors [16].

Due to the teratogenocity of warfarin, pregnant patients requiring anticoagulation receive heparin as the preferred drug for preventing pulmonary embolism or in thromboprophylaxis in atrial fibrillation [51]. Insertion of a venal caval filter is another option.

In the surgical patient, it is important to discontinue aspirin and reversible platelet inhibitors such as clopidogrel 10 and 7 days respectively before an operation to avoid bleeding complications [50]. However, risks of thrombotic events in discontinuation of these agents in cardiovascular surgeries have been noted [50]. Because of these risks with anticoagulated patients and patients receiving antiplatelet agents, it is important to weigh the benefits of the surgery against these risks, among others.

Obstetrical and Gynecological Patients

Obstetric patients are one subpopulation of actively bleeding surgical patients that can easily confuse the provider. Their generally young age may lead one to dismiss some vital sign changes or lab values, while alterations of their physiology in response to pregnancy often results in the misinterpretation of critical findings. During pregnancy, blood becomes less viscous in order to increase oxygen carrying capacity while minimizing increased cardiac load as much as possible. Intravascular volume, and more specifically, plasma volume increases proportionately more than red cell volume, creating a "physiologic anemia of pregnancy" [51]. Fibrinogen, von Willebrand factor and factors VII, VIII, IX, X, XII are synthesized more frequently while levels of factors XI and XIII and platelets decrease [38]. Levels of factor II decrease, yet interestingly, prothrombin time (PT) and partial thromboplastin time (PTT) remain unaffected [51]. Mechanical obstruction of the uterus on the inferior vena cava and other vessels encourage stasis and the formation of thrombi. The summation of these effects result in a net hypercoagulable state [51].

The utero-placental circulation has increased activity of both coagulation and fibrinolysis, contributing to increased levels of fibrin degradation products such as D-dimer, especially in the third trimester [38]. This effect may contribute to the hemostatic challenges in obstetric patients. Antifibrinolytics such as tranexamic acid and aminocaproic acid can be used to treat hyperfibrinolysis. In fact, tranexamic acid has been shown to reduce blood loss after elective caesarean section and vaginal delivery [38]. Plasma and cryoprecipitate contain fibrinogen and may be used to replenish fibrinogen in states of hypofibrinogenemia (<180 mg/dL).

Post-partum hemorrhage (PPH) is a major cause of obstetric mortality that may require peripartum hysterectomy and is the most common cause of maternal mortality worldwide. PPH, in general, is not associated with underlying coagulation disorders but rather acute events related to placenta abnormalities, trauma from large births or instrumentation, or uterine atony [38]. In addition to rapid surgical intervention, hematologic management of PPH includes rapid volume replacement and blood transfusions. These patients are likely to benefit from management strategies similar to that for acutely injured patients who are in shock from hemorrhage.

In obstetrical patients, rFVIIa has also been found to control and decrease hemorrhage. Segal et al.'s observation of three patients with PPH, hypovolemic shock, and DIC who received massive transfusions suggests that rFVIIa may be beneficial adjunctive therapy after the completion of hysterectomy [52]. The therapeutic effect of rFVIIa may be due to its binding of tissue factor at the site of vessel injury and forming a complex, activating platelets and facilitating fibrin clot formation [52]. However, these findings have not been consistent in the current literature, and especially because of the expense of rFVIIa, the decision to administer this to the patient must involve a thorough consideration of the benefits, if any [38].

The Non-hemorrhaging Surgical Patient

Intensive care unit (ICU) patients are another patient population that frequently receives blood transfusions in order to correct their anemia, which has been shown by a large body of work to indicate worse prognosis [29]. These patients are anemic due to sepsis, occult blood loss, hemorrhage, decreased production and functional iron deficiency. ICU patients with low hemoglobin levels are more likely to suffer from complications such as sepsis, and they are more likely to experience delayed weaning from ventilator support. The decision to transfuse such patients should weigh the benefits and the risks of blood transfusions, especially given the patients' increased susceptibility to infections, iatrogenic events and increased metabolic demands [53]. Vincent et al.'s multicenter prospective observational study of 1,136 patients demonstrated that ICU patients frequently received transfusions, with a transfusion rate of 37% during their stay. The patients who received transfusions also experienced a higher mortality rate, prolonged hospital stay, and decreased organ function [53]. There is also evidence suggestive of increased transfusions in patients with hemoglobin levels higher than the generally accepted trigger value of 8 g/dL. Specifically, Vincent et al. found that in under 30% of cases, patients with hemoglobin levels greater than 9 g/dL received blood transfusions [53]. Hence, future work is needed to recommend strict hemoglobin cut offs for transfusion.

Thrombelastography and TEG-Guided Therapy

In the acute trauma setting, conventional coagulation testing (CCT), which consists of prothrombin time, international normalized ratio (INR), partial thromboplastin time, and platelet count, is used to assess coagulation status. This approach, however, is limited by slow results, incomplete characterization of the coagulation abnormality, and poor prediction of patient outcome. Furthermore, CCTs, which are riddled with delays from time to arrival in the laboratory and duration of testing, end up reflecting the coagulation state of the patient after 30–45 min of interventions and resuscitation [54]. Since CCT only examines plasma factors, the integral role of platelets and their function is ignored. In addition, the CCT assesses only the extrinsic pathway, intrinsic pathway, and platelet count, painting an incomplete picture of the pathologies of clotting in the severely exsanguinating patient. These deficiencies are addressed by thrombelastography (TEG), a test that creates a dynamic, graphical representation of the coagulation characteristics of a blood sample from initial clot formation to fibrinolysis. Since specific coagulation components have specific disturbances on TEG, this test reveals diagnostic as well as therapeutic information [55].

The procedure involves obtaining an uncitrated whole blood sample, activation of the specimen with kaolin and spinning the sample in a thrombelastograph machine within 4–5 min in order to avoid clotting [55]. If this timeframe cannot be achieved, a "reversal" method can be used, where citrate is used to avoid clotting until the sample has arrived at the laboratory, at which point, the citrate will be "reversed" using calcium chloride as per manufacturer instructions. While this method has been shown to affect TEG results, it has not been shown to be inferior to the standard

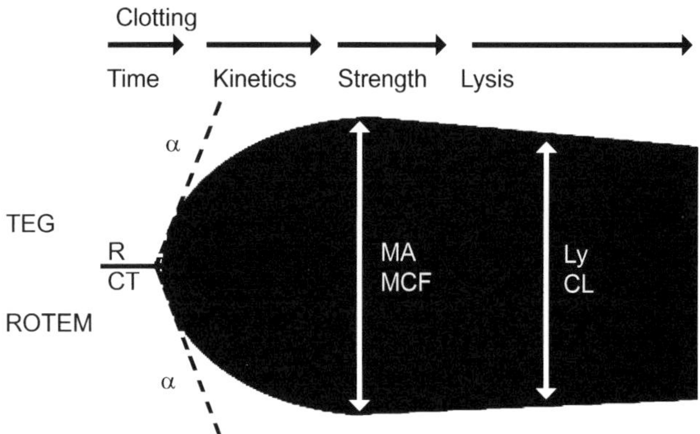

Fig. 12.2 The various sequential and parallel measurements of TEG and ROTEM [4]

method and may be used in centers where 4–5 min from sample collection to running the TEG is not realistic [55].

Rapid TEG differs from conventional TEG in its addition of tissue factor to the blood sample and kaolin, accelerating activation of the clotting cascade. This modification makes it well suited for the trauma setting since its results are available much earlier, namely under 20 min, compared to kaolin TEG and CCTs, which can take over 30 min, without sacrificing accuracy [55].

Interpreting the results involves analyzing each of the sequential measurements (Fig. 12.2). Reaction time, or R-time, in TEG is the time until initial clot formation. It is also known as activated clotting time (ACT) in r-TEG in order to denote intentional anticoagulant agents in the sample. Factor deficiency or severe hemodilution can prolong reaction time or ACT. Next, k-time represents the time needed to reach 20-mm clot strength, and has a normal range of 1–2 min. The -angle, normally between 66 and 82°, represents the rate of clot formation. In platelet deficiency or hypofibrinogenemia, where one of the two key components of clots are missing, the k-time is increased and the -angle is decreased. Oshita et al.'s linear regression analysis of 36 samples from healthy individuals reported that MA and k-time were linearly related to platelet count [56]. The maximal amplitude (MA) of the tracing represents platelet contribution to clot strength (normal range 54–72 mm). It is decreased in states of platelet dysfunction and hypofibrinogenemia. The G-value represents overall clot strength, including platelet function as well as enzymatic, and is decreased in hypocoagulable states (normal 5.3–12 K dynes/cm^2). The LY30 is the percent of amplitude reduction at 30 min after the MA, and is elevated in hyperfibrinolytic states (normal range 0.0–7.5%) [55] (Figs. 12.3 and 12.4).

The use of r-TEG is further facilitated by advanced software that displays the r-TEG tracing as the test is being performed, providing physicians with "real time" results. Cotton et al. report that early r-TEG parameter tracings (ACT, k-time and r-value) appeared within 5 min while later values (-angle, MA) were seen within 15 min, compared to CCT panels,

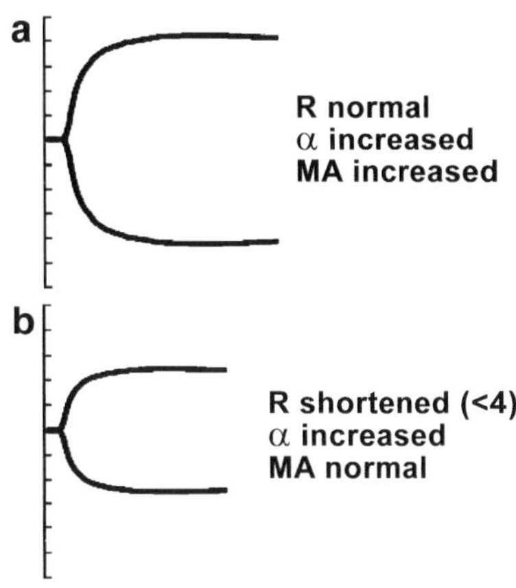

Fig. 12.3 TEG tracings in hypercoagulation abnormalities. (**a**) Platelet hypercoagulability. (**b**) Cascade hypercoagulability. Adapted from reference [62]

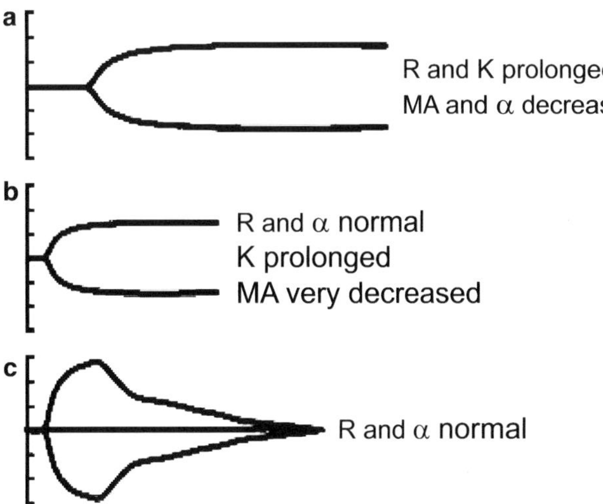

Fig. 12.4 TEG tracings in hypocoagulation abnormalities. (**a**) Decreased coagulation factors or heparin (**b**). Thrombocytopenia or decreased platelets (**c**). Fibrinolysis. Adapted from reference [62]

Table 12.1 Thrombelastography treatment algorithm for actively bleeding patients implemented at Rigshospitalet, University of Copenhagen, Denmark [4]

TEG parameter	Treatment
R (11–14 min)	2× plasma or 10 ml/kg
$R > 14$ min	4× plasma or 20 ml/kg
MA (46–50 mm)	1 PC or 10 ml/kg
MA < 46 mm	2 PC or 20 ml/kg
Angle < 52°	2× plasma or fibrinogen
Ly30 > 8%	Tranexamic acid

R reaction time, *alpha angle* clot dynamics, *MA* maximal amplitude, *Ly30* lysis in percent 30 min after MA is reached, *plasma* fresh frozen plasma, *PC* platelet concentrate

Treatment algorithm based on r-TEG values implemented at the Texas Trauma Institute, University of Texas Health Science Center-Houston [63]

ACT >128 sec	Plasma and RBCs
k-time >2.5 min	Cryoprecipitate (or fibrinogen) and plasma
α-angle <60 deg	Cryoprecipitate (or fibrinogen) and plasma
mA <55 mm	Platelets and cryoprecipitate (or fibrinogen)
LY30 >3%	Tranexamic acid (or aminocaproic acid)

which were not available until 48 min [55]. Installation of graphical software in the trauma bay, operating room and shock-trauma intensive care unit computers can further facilitate the rapid access to TEG results [55].

TEG data results compare well to the previous standard, CCTs. In 2011, Cotton et al. conducted a pilot study of 272 patients to investigate the role of rapid thrombelastography (r-TEG) in (1) assessing speed of results, (2) correlation with CCT findings, and (3) predictability of early transfusions of pRBCs, plasma, and platelets [55]. Their findings demonstrated that graphical r-TEG is available within minutes, an improvement compared to CCTs. They also demonstrated that ACT, *r*-value and *k*-time strongly correlated with PT, INR, and PTT. MA and -angle strongly correlated with platelet count, and ACT, *r*-value, -angle and MA were predictive of pRBC, plasma and platelet transfusions within the first 2 h of arrival. In fact, an ACT > 128 predicted massive transfusion in the first 6 h and

an ACT < 105 predicted patients that did not receive transfusions in the first 24 h [55]. In addition, comparison of TEG and CCT in cardiopulmonary bypass patients found that TEG measures were useful surrogates for CCT values [57]. Because of the speed of their availability and predictive ability, integrating TEG results in MTPs can strengthen decision-making and management of patients and improve patient outcomes.

A wide array of evidence exists in surgical patients in support of TEG's ability to predict prognosis, and in some instances, guide therapy that improves it. Table 12.1 is an example of TEG-guided protocol with such an aim. Platelet dysfunction in cardiopulmonary bypass patients has been attributed to microvascular bleeding, and TEG has been used in the setting of cardiac surgery as a predictor of worsening patient outcomes due to this mechanism [17]. Solomon et al. demonstrated that fibrinogen clot elasticity assessed by TEG correlated to fibrinogen concentration in cardiopulmonary bypass patients [58]. TEG has been found to predict the risk of postoperative bleeding, and has been used to direct desmopressin therapy and FFP transfusion requirement in cardiopulmonary bypass patients [17].

TEG has been shown to be useful in liver surgery, especially in transplantation. Unlike other surgeries, liver surgery poses the additional problem of increased risk of coagulation factor deficiencies due to hepatic dysfunction and lack of synthesis. TEG-guided transfusion algorithms in this area have been shown to reduce the transfusion requirements in such patients [17].

However, Ogawa et al.'s prospective observational study of 26 patients undergoing cardiac surgery did not find a significant correlation between TEG measures and volume of intraoperative and total transfusions. Despite these findings,

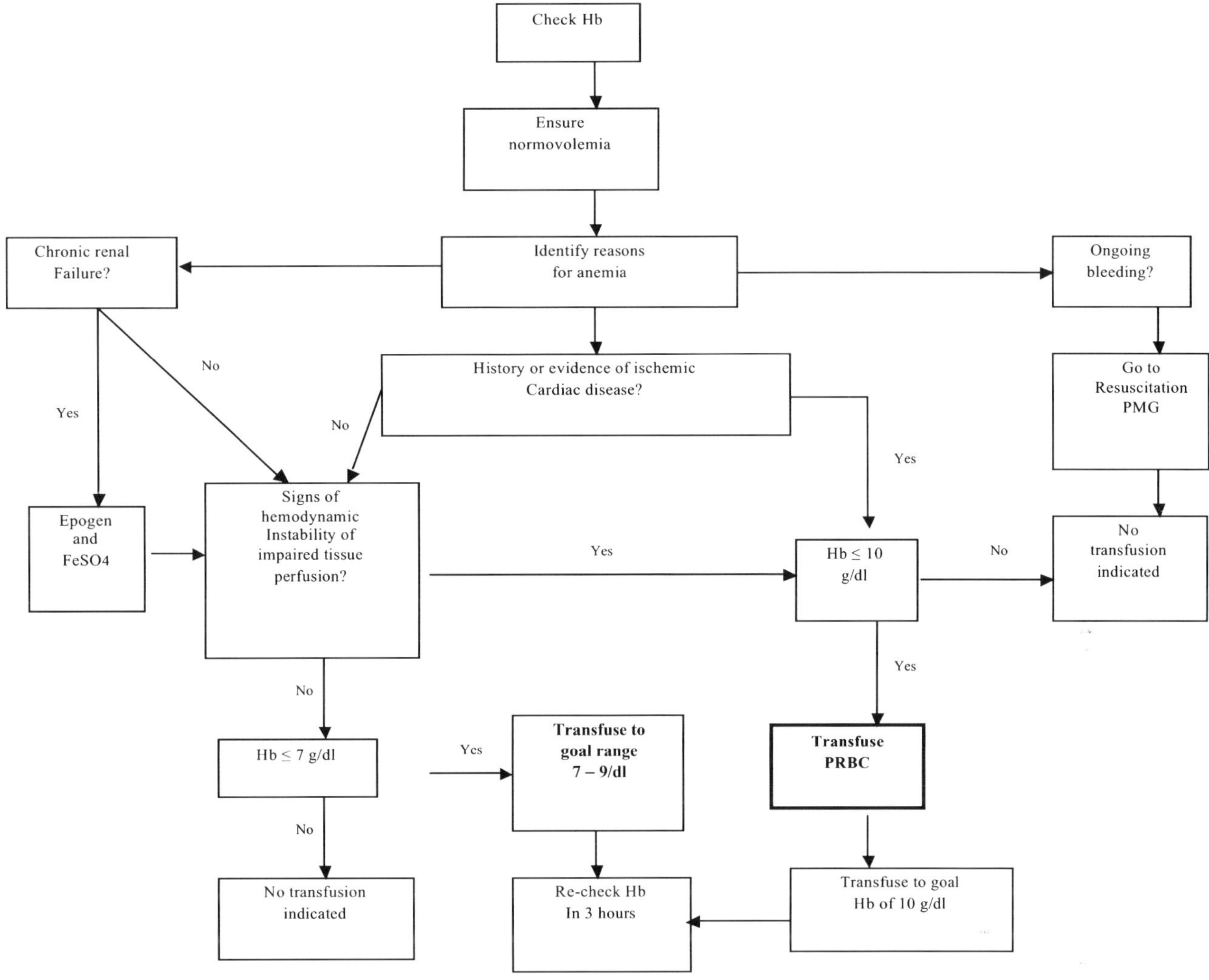

Fig. 12.5 Example of a practice management guideline for managing anemia in the ICU patient

Ronald et al.'s literature search and appraisal of 170 studies on the topic found otherwise [59]. They investigated thromboelastography in cardiac surgery patients and found 14 studies that provided the best evidence. Their synthesis concluded that TEG can guide transfusion therapy algorithms and result in decreased blood component requirements.

In orthopedic surgery patients, TEG was used in a prospective study to identify disturbed fibrin polymerization as a pathological mechanism in dilutional coagulopathy, and to rescue this state with fibrinogen administration [60].

However, TEG has been found to be less sensitive for certain categories of platelet inhibition. In addition, hemostatis point of care tests such as PFA-100 and TEG are affected by nonopiod analgesic drugs. Scharbert et al.'s crossover, double-blinded, placebo controlled study demonstrated that in low back pain patients scheduled for invasive pain therapy, cytochalasin D-modified thromboelastometry had a low sensitivity for detecting platelet inhibition by diclofenac [61].

Conclusion

There are hemostatic states unique to the surgical patient as a result of medications such as warfarin, perioperative bleeding especially in high bleeding risk surgeries, and emergent surgical indications such as trauma. Various mechanisms affect coagulation cascades in these patients, and techniques from the standard coagulation tests to TEG are currently available. These have shown mostly success in predicting the course of the patient and guiding therapy. The therapeutic options include various blood product components, ranging from whole blood to concentrations of individual factors. Using physiological ratios of pRBCs, FFP, and platelets have improved patient survival in the massively hemorrhaging patient. However, like all powerful therapy, they are associated with adverse effects. Preventative options, such as decreasing storage lengths and screening for infectious agents have drastically reduced these risks. Lastly, administering these products in a rapid and directed fashion would not be feasible without in-house triage and massive transfusion protocols. These algorithms include steps that must be taken to smooth out logistics of urgent transfusions, such as anticipating adequate thawing times of FFPs and collaborating with blood banks to cross-check appropriateness of each order (Fig. 12.5).

References

1. Rotondo MF, Schwab CW, McGonigal MD, et al. 'Damage control': an approach for improved survival in exsanguinating penetrating abdominal injury. J Trauma. 1993;35:375–82.

2. Stone HH, Strom PR, Mullins RJ. Management of the major coagulopathy with onset during laparotomy. Ann Surg. 1983;197:532–5.

3. van Ruler O, Mahler CW, Boer KR, on behalf of The Dutch Peritonitis Study Group. Comparison of on-demand versus planned relaparotomy strategy in patients with severe peritonitis. JAMA. 2007;298(8):865–73.

4. Johansson PI, Ostrowski SR, Secher NH. Management of major blood loss: an update. Acta Anaesthesiol Scand. 2010;54:1039–49.

5. Young PP, Cotton BA, Goodnough LT. Massive transfusion protocols for patients with substantial hemorrhage. Transfus Med Rev. 2011;25(4):293–303. Epub 2011 Jun 12.

6. Cotton BA, Au BK, Nunez TC, Gunter OL, Robertson A, Young PP. Predefined massive transfusion protocols are associated with a reduction in organ failure and post-injury complications. J Trauma. 2009;66:41–9.

7. Cotton BA, Gunter OL, Isbell J, et al. Damage control hematology: the impact of a trauma exsanguination protocol on survival and blood product utilization. J Trauma. 2008;64:1177–82. discussion 82–3.

8. O'Keeffe T, Refaai M, Tchorz K, et al. A massive transfusion protocol to decrease blood component use and costs. Arch Surg. 2008;143:686–90. discussion 90–1.

9. Kashuk JL, Moore EE, Wohlauer M, Johnson JL, Pezold M, Lawrence J, Biffl WL, Burlew CC, Barnett C, Sawyer M, Sauaia A. Initial experiences with point-of-care rapid thrombelastography for management of life-threatening postinjury coagulopathy. Transfusion. 2012;52(1):23–33. doi:10.1111/j.1537-2995.2011.03264.x. Epub 2011 Jul 25.

10. Nunez TC, Dutton WD, May AK, Holcomb JB, Young PP, Cotton BA. Emergency department blood transfusion predicts early massive transfusion and early blood component requirement. Transfusion. 2010;50:1914–20.

11. Inaba K, Teixeira PG, Shulman I, Nelson J, Lee J, Salim A, Brown C, Demetriades D, Rhee P. The impact of uncrossmatched blood transfusion on the need for massive transfusion and mortality: analysis of 5166 uncross-matched units. J Trauma. 2008;65:1222–6.

12. Reed MJ, Lone N, Walsh TS. Resuscitation of the trauma patient: tell me a trigger for early haemostatic resuscitation please! Crit Care. 2011;15:126.

13. Cotton BA, Dossett LA, Au BK, Nunez TC, Robertson AM, Young PP. Room for performance improvement: provider-related factors associated with poor outcomes in massive transfusion. J Trauma. 2009;67:1004–12.

14. Cotton BA, Cotton BA, Reddy N, Hatch QM, Podbielski J, McNutt MK, Albarado R, Gill BS, Wade C, Kozar RA, Holcomb JB. Damage control resuscitation reduces resuscitation volumes and improves survival in 390 damage control laparotomy patients. Ann Surg. 2011;254:598–605.

15. Fox CJ, Gillespie DL, Cox ED, Kragh JF, Mehta SG, Salinas J, Holcomb JB. Damage control resuscitation for vascular surgery in a combat support hospital. J Trauma. 2008;65:1–9.

16. Kılıç YA, Konan A, Kaynaroglu. Resuscitation and monitoring in gastrointestinal bleeding. Eur J Trauma Emerg Surg. 2011;1–9.

17. Dickinson KJ, Troxler M, Homer-Vanniasinkam S. The surgical application of point-of-care haemostasis and platelet function testing. Br J Surg. 2008;95:1317–30.

18. Johansson PI, Stensballe J, Rosenberg TL, Hilsløv LJ, Jorgensen L, Secher NH. Proactive administration of platelets and plasma for patients with a ruptured abdominal aortic aneurysm: evaluating a change in transfusion practice. Transfusion. 2007;47:593–8.

19. Mell MW, O'Neil AS, Callcut RA, Acher CW, Hoch JR, Tefera G, Turnipseed WD. Effect of early plasma transfusion on mortality in patients with ruptured abdominal aortic aneurysm. Surgery. 2010;148:955–62.

20. Wafaisade A, Maegele M, Lefering R, Braun M, Peiniger S, Neugebauer E, Bouillon B, Trauma Registry of DGU. High plasma to red blood cell ratios are associated with lower mortality rates in patients receiving multiple transfusion (4 ≤ red blood cell units < 10) during acute trauma resuscitation. J Trauma. 2011;70:81–9.

21. Ketchum L, Hess JR, Hiippala S. Indications for early fresh frozen plasma, cryoprecipitate, and platelet transfusion in trauma. J Trauma. 2006;60:S51–8.

22. Wehrli G, Taylor NE, Haines AL, Brady TW, Mintz PD. Instituting a thawed plasma procedure: it just makes sense and saves cents. Transfusion. 2009;49:2625–30.

23. Fowler RA, Rizoli SB, Levin PDL, Smith T. Blood conservation for critically ill patients. Crit Care Clin. 2004;20:313–24.

24. Zakai NA, Katz R, Hirsch C, Shlipak MG, Chaves PHM, Newman AB, Cushman M. A prospective study of anemia status, hemoglobin concentration, and mortality in an elderly cohort. Arch Intern Med. 2005;165:2214–20.

25. Englesbe MJ, Pelletier SJ, Diehl KM, Sung RS, Wahl WL, Punch J, Bartlett RH. Transfusions in surgical patients. J Am Coll Surg. 2005;200:249–54.

26. Takagi H, Sekino S, Kato T, Matsuno Y, Umemoto T. Intraoperative autotransfusion in abdominal aortic aneurysm surgery. Arch Surg. 2007;142:1098–101.

27. Hébert PC, Wells G, Blajchman MA, Marshall J, Martin C, Pagliarello G, Tweeddale M, Schweitzer I, Yetisir E, Transfusion Requirements in Critical Care Investigators for the Canadian Critical Care Trials Groups. A multicenter, randomized, controlled clinical trial of transfusion requirements in critical care. N Engl J Med. 1999;340:409–17.

28. Van PY, Riha GM, Cho D, Underwod SJ, Hamilton GJ, Anderson R, Ham LB, Schreiber MA. Blood volume analysis can distinguish true anemia from hemodilution in critically ill patients. J Trauma. 2011;70:646–51.

29. Silver M. Anemia in the long-term ventilator-dependent patient with respiratory failure. Chest. 2005;128:568S–75.

30. Vincent JL, Spapen HD, Creteur J, Piagnerelli M, Hubloue I, Diltoer M, Roman A, Stevens E, Vercammen E, Beaver JS. Pharmacokinetics and pharmacodynamics of once-weekly subcutaneous epoetin alfa in critically ill patients: results of a randomized, double-blind, placebo-controlled trial. Crit Care Med. 2006; 34: 1661–7.

31. Knight K, Wade S, Balducci L. Prevalence and outcomes of anemia in cancer: a systematic review of the literature. Am J Med. 2004; 116:11S–26.

32. Corwin HL, Gettinger A, Fabian TC, May A, Pearl RG, Heard S, An R, Bowers PJ, Burton P, Klausner MA, Corwin MJ, For the EPO Critical Care Trials Group. Efficacy and safety of epoetin alfa in critically ill patients. N Engl J Med. 2007;357:1–12.

33. Edwards TJ, Noble EJ, Durran A, Mellor N, Hosie KB. Randomized clinical trial of preoperative intravenous iron sucrose to reduce blood transfusion in anaemic patients after colorectal cancer surgery. Br J Surg. 2009;96:1122–8.

34. Murad MH, Stubbs JR, Gandhi MJ, Wang AT, Paul A, Erwin PJ, Montor VM, Roback JD. The effect of plasma transfusion on morbidity and mortality: a systematic review and meta-analysis. Transfusion. 2010;50:1370–83.
35. MacLennan S, Williamson LM. Risks of fresh frozen plasma and platelets. J Trauma. 2005;60:S46–50.
36. Damiani G, Pinnarelli L, Sommella L, Farelli V, Mele L, Menichella G, Ricciardi W. Appropriateness of fresh-frozen plasma usage in hospital settings: a meta-analysis of the impact of organizational intervations. Transfusion. 2010;50:139–44.
37. Norda R, Tynell E. Utilisation de plasma: indications médicales et préparation de plasma en Suède [Use of plasma: clinical indications and types of plasma components in Sweden]. Transfus Clin Biol. 2007;14:560–3.
38. Ahonen J, Stefanovic V, Lassila R. Management of post-partum haemorrhage. Acta Anaesthesiol Scand. 2010;54:1164–78.
39. Vostal JG. Efficacy evaluation of current and future platelet transfusion products. J Trauma. 2006;60:S78–82.
40. Grosso SM, Keenan JO. Whole blood transfusion for exsanguinating coagulopathy in a U.S. field surgical hospital in postwar Kosovo. J Trauma. 2000;49:145–8.
41. Mayo A, Misgav M, Kluger Y, Geenberg R, Pauzner D, Klausner J, Ben-Tal O. Recombinant activated factor VII (NovoSeven): addition to replacement therapy in acute, uncontrolled and life-threatening bleeding. Vox Sang. 2004;87:34–40.
42. Khorana AA, Francis CW, Blumberg N, Culakova E, Refaai MA, Lyman GH. Blood transfusions, thrombosis, and mortality in hospitalized patients with cancer. Arch Intern Med. 2008;168:2377–81.
43. Silliman CC, Fung YL, Ball JB, Khan SY. Transfusion-related acute lung injury (TRALI): current concepts and misconceptions. Blood Rev. 2009;23:245–55.
44. Eder AF, Herron RM, Strupp A, Dy B, White J, Notari EP, Dodd RY, Benjamin RJ. Effective reduction of transfusion-related acute lung injury risk with male-predominant plasma strategy in the American Red Cross (2006–2008). Transfusion. 2010;50:1732–42.
45. Napolitano L. Cumulative risks of early red blood cell transfusion. J Trauma. 2006;60:S26–34.
46. Watson GA, Sperry JL, Rosengart MR, Minei JP, Harbrecht BG, Moore EE, Cuschieri J, Maier RV, Billiar TR, Peitzman AB, Inflammation and the Host Response to Injury Investigators. Fresh frozen plasma is independently associated with a higher risk of multiple organ failure and acute respiratory distress syndrome. J Trauma. 2009;67:221–30.
47. Bennett-Guerrero E, Stafford-Smith M, Waweru PM, Bredehoeft SJ, Campbell ML, Haley NR, Phillips-Bute B, Newman MK, Bandarenko N. A prospective, double-blind, randomized clinical feasibility trial of controlling the storage age of red blood cells for transfusion in cardiac surgical patients. Transfusion. 2009;49:1375–83.
48. Sarode R, Refaai MA, Matevosyan K, Burner JD, Hampton S, Rutherford C. Prospective monitoring of plasma and platelet transfusions in a large teaching hospital results in significant cost reduction. Transfusion. 2010;50:487–92.
49. Kuhne CA, Zettl RP, Fischbacher M, Lefering R, Ruchholtz S. Emergency transfusion score (ETS): a useful instrument for prediction of blood transfusion requirement in severely injured patients. World J Surg. 2008;32:1183–8.
50. Thachil J, Gatt A, Martlew V. Management of surgical patients receiving anticoagulation and antiplatelet agents. Br J Surg. 2008;95:1437–48.
51. Naylor DF, Olson MM. Critical care obstetrics and gynecology. Crit Care Clin. 2003;19:127–49.
52. Segal S, Shemesh IY, Blumenthal R, Yoffe B, Laufer N, Ezra Y, Levy I, Mazor M, Martinowitz U. Treatment of obstetric hemorrhage with recombinant activated factor VII (rFVIIa). Arch Gynecol Obstet. 2003;268:266–7.
53. Vincent JL, Baron JF, Reinhart K, Gattinoni L, Thijs L, Webb A, Meier-Hellmann A, Nollet G, Peres-Bota D, the ABC Investigators. Anemia and blood transfusion in critically ill patients. JAMA. 2002;288:1499–507.
54. Riordan WP, Cotton BA. All bleeding stops: how we can help…. Crit Care. 2010;14:146.
55. Cotton BA, Faz G, Hatch QM, Radwan ZA, Podbielski J, Wade C, Kozar RA, Holcomb JB. Rapid thromboelastography delivers real-time results that predict transfusion within 1 hour of admission. J Trauma. 2011;71:407–17.
56. Oshita K, Az-ma T, Osawa Y, Yuge O. Quantitative measurement of thromboelastography as a function of platelet count. Anesth Analg. 1999;89:296–9.
57. Ogawa S, Szlam F, Chen EP, Nishimura T, Kim H, Roback JD, Levy JH, Tanaka KA. A comparative evaluation of rotation thromboelastometry and standard coagulation tests in hemodilution-induced coagulation changes after cardiac surgery. Transfusion. 2012;52(1):14–22. doi:10.1111/j.1537-2995.2011.03241.x. Epub 2011 Jul 14.
58. Solomon C, Cadamuro J, Ziegler B, Schöchl H, Varvenne M, Sørensen B, Hochleitner G, Rahe-Meyer N. A comparison of fibrinogen measurement methods with fibrin clot elasticity assessed by thromboelastometry, before and after administration of fibrinogen concentrate in cardiac surgery patients. Transfusion. 2011;8:1695–706.
59. Ronald A, Dunning J. Can the use of thromboelastography predict and decrease bleeding and blood and blood product requirements in adult patients undergoing cardiac surgery? Interact Cardiovasc Thorac Surg. 2005;4:456–63.
60. Mittermayr M, Streif W, Haas T, Fries D, Velik-Salchner C, Klinger A, Oswald E, Bach C, Schnapka-Koepf M, Innerhofer P. Hemostatic changes after crystalloid or colloid fluid administration during major orthopedic surgery: the role of fibrinogen administration. Anesth Analg. 2007;105:905–17.
61. Scharbert G, Gebhardt K, Sow Z, Duris M, Deusch E, Kozek-Langenecker S. Point-of-care platelet function tests: detection of platelet inhibition induced by nonopioid analgesic drugs. Blood Coagul Fibrinolysis. 2007;18:775–80.
62. Kroll MH. Thromboelastography: theory and practice in measuring hemostasis. Clinical Laboratory News. 2010;36(12).
63. Holcomb JB, Minei KM, Scerbo ML, Radwan ZA, Wade CE, Kozar RA, Gill BS, Albarado R, McNutt MK, McCarthy JJ, Cotton BA. Admission rapid thrombelastography (r-TEG) can replace conventional coagulation tests in the emergency department: experience with 1974 consecutive trauma patients. Ann Surg. 2012;256(3):476–86.

Part II

Common Diseases in Acute Care Surgery

Obtaining a Surgical Airway

13

Tanner Baker, Spencer Skelton, Krista Turner,
and Hassan Aijazi

Introduction

An understanding of airway management skills and concepts is essential for any clinician. Maintaining a patent airway is a prerequisite for successful ventilation and oxygenation, and even a temporary lapse in airway patency can lead to permanent, potentially fatal consequences. The first successful attempt at creating an artificial airway dates to 1667, when Robert Hooke inserted a narrow-lumen tube into a dog's trachea and then manually insufflated the dog's lungs using a bellows. The need for airway proficiency combined with technological advancement in fields such as laryngoscopy allowed physicians to improve the standard of care in airway management after World War I, and by the mid-1920s, most patients were intubated under direct laryngoscopic vision. The basic fundamentals of airway management have remained largely unchanged since that time. This chapter discusses basic airway skills such as proper patient positioning and mask ventilation. It will also describe how to conduct a focused airway examination and give a short overview of how to proceed if a difficult airway is encountered. Surgical airway techniques and their complications will also be covered in detail.

T. Baker, M.D. (✉)
Department of General Surgery, University of Texas Health Science Center, Houston, TX, USA

S. Skelton, M.D.
Department of General Surgery, The Methodist Hospital, Houston, TX, USA

K. Turner, M.D., F.A.C.S. (✉)
Department of Surgery, Weill Cornell Medical College, The Methodist Hospital, 6550 Fannin St, SM 1661A, Houston, TX 77030, USA
e-mail: kristaturnermd@hotmail.com

H. Aijazi, M.B.B.S.
Department of Anesthesiology, University of Texas at Houston Medical School, Houston, TX, USA

Airway Anatomy

It is important to have a clear understanding of the functional anatomy of the airway, as illustrated in Fig. 13.1. The airway begins with the mouth and nasal cavity. The tongue fills the floor of the oral cavity and extends posteriorly into the oropharynx. In unconscious and/or paralyzed patients, the tone of these attaching tongue muscles can become impaired, allowing the tongue to fall back into the pharynx and obstruct the airway. Anteriorly, the palate divides the oral and nasal cavities into two distinct entities; these cavities merge posteriorly to form the pharynx. The pharynx acts as a conduit connecting the oral and nasal cavities to the esophagus and larynx inferiorly. The pharynx serves as part of both the digestive and respiratory systems, and has two inferior openings: the esophageal opening and the laryngeal opening. For the purposes of securing an airway, there are three specific anatomic considerations:

1. *The size and orientation of the pharyngeal openings.* The laryngeal opening is the smaller of the two hypopharyngeal openings, and lies on the anterior aspect of the pharynx. Conversely, the esophageal opening is larger and closer to the terminal, inferior aspect of the hypopharynx. This arrangement of the two openings allows pharyngeal contents to more naturally progress down into the esophagus as opposed to the larynx. Thus, a tube blindly inserted into a patient's mouth is more likely to enter the esophagus than the airway.

2. *The epiglottis.* The epiglottis is a cartilaginous flap that is attached to the entrance of the larynx. Its function is to cover the laryngeal opening during swallowing and protect against aspiration. During normal respiration, the epiglottis points upwards and out of the way of the laryngeal opening, allowing air to pass easily into the larynx. During swallowing, elevation of the hyoid bone draws the larynx upwards, rolling the epiglottis into a more horizontal position. In this position, the epiglottis covers the laryngeal opening and protects against aspiration. During laryngoscopy, the practitioner uses the laryngoscope to "lift"

L.J. Moore et al. (eds.), *Common Problems in Acute Care Surgery*,
DOI 10.1007/978-1-4614-6123-4_13, © Springer Science+Business Media New York 2013

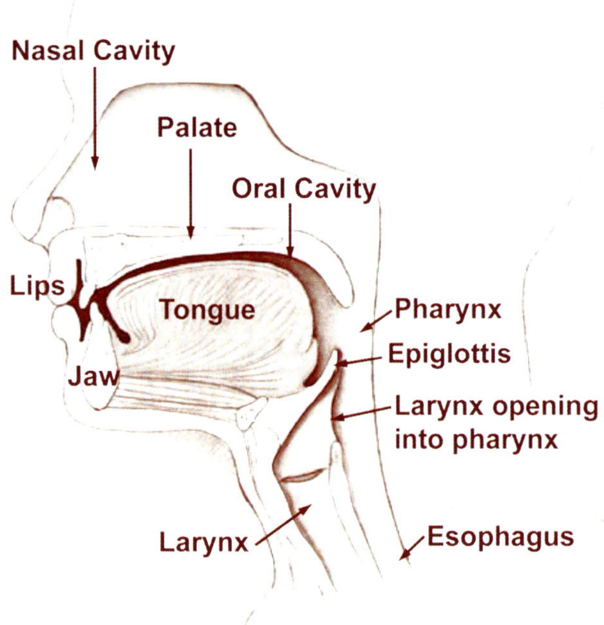

Fig. 13.1 Upper airway anatomy. Reproduced with permission from http://training.seer.cancer.gov/head-neck/anatomy/overview.html

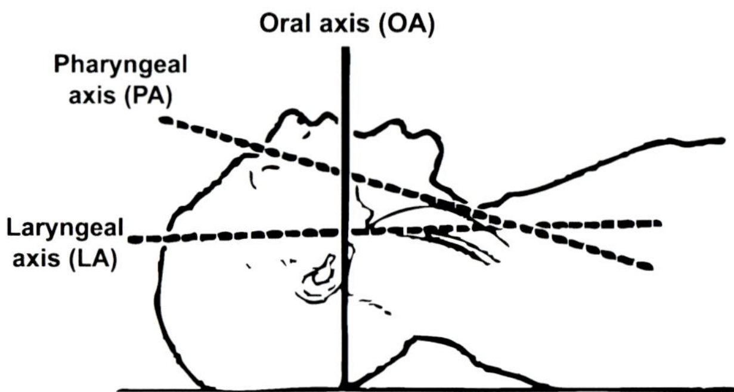

Fig. 13.2 This picture shows the misaligned axes of the oral cavity (OA), pharynx (PA), and larynx (LA). Stone DJ, Gal TJL. Airway management. In: Miller RD, editor: Anesthesia. 4th ed. New York: Churchill Livingstone; 1994, p. 1408

the epiglottis out of the way, allowing direct visualization of the glottic opening.

3. *The axes of the oral cavity in relation to the pharynx and larynx.* The orientation of the axes of the oral cavity, pharynx, and larynx, as seen in Fig. 13.2, is misaligned with respect to each other. In order to successfully visualize the vocal cords, the three axes must be maximally aligned, allowing the airway practitioner to see directly from the mouth to the glottis. This is done by positioning the patient in the "sniffing" position, which is discussed later in the chapter.

Airway Assessment

Just as it is important to conceptualize what a "normal" airway looks like, it is important to recognize that the airway is subject to anatomical variation. Patients with such "difficult airways" are a significant cause of anesthesia-related morbidity and mortality [1]. It is important to attempt to predict which patients might present difficult airways, and to take extra precautionary measures in these patients.

History

Airway assessment begins with a solid history of potential airway-related concerns. The patient and or family should be questioned regarding history of previous difficult intubation

or history of sleep apnea or snoring. If previous anesthetic records are available, they should be referenced for any indication of a difficult intubation or airway.

The Airway Examination

After taking a detailed history, the next step is to complete a detailed airway examination. Some of the more important points to assess are described as follows.

1. *Visibility of uvula.* The most commonly used method of assessing airway difficulty is the modified Mallampati test (MMT) as denoted in Fig. 13.3. Dr. Seshagiri R. Mallampati created the original Mallampati test in 1983, which was later modified by Samsoon and Young in 1987. Mallampati hypothesized that the size of the base of the tongue is an important factor in predicting difficult laryngoscopy and that a large tongue would cramp the oropharyngeal space. The MMT is conducted while the patient is sitting upright with his or her mouth fully open and tongue extended as far as possible. Intubation becomes progressively more difficult as the score increases. MMT scores of I–II generally indicate a good chance of being able to easily visualize the glottic opening, while MMT scores of III–IV predict a more difficult laryngoscopy.

2. *Thyromental distance.* This is the distance measured from the superior aspect of the thyroid cartilage to the mentum while the neck is fully extended. A thyromental distance of greater than 7 cm generally predicts a straightforward intubation, whereas a distance of less than 6 cm may predict difficulty. A short thyromental distance is associated with an anterior larynx, meaning that it is at a more acute angle to the hypopharynx. This can make aligning the axes of the larynx and the pharynx more difficult. A shorter thyromental distance also allows for less mandibular space for the tongue to be compressed into by the laryngoscope blade.

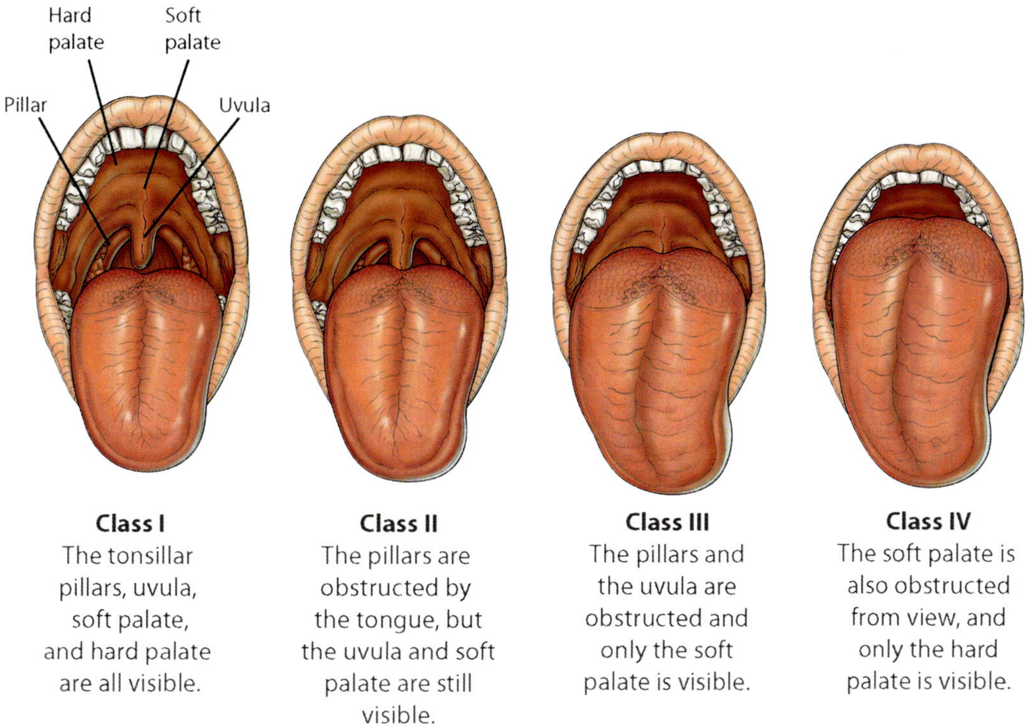

Class I
The tonsillar pillars, uvula, soft palate, and hard palate are all visible.

Class II
The pillars are obstructed by the tongue, but the uvula and soft palate are still visible.

Class III
The pillars and the uvula are obstructed and only the soft palate is visible.

Class IV
The soft palate is also obstructed from view, and only the hard palate is visible.

Fig. 13.3 Mallampati classifications. Modified with permission from Finucane BT, Tsui BCH, Santora AH (eds). Principles of airway management. 4th ed. (ISBN: 978-0-387-09557-8). New York, NY: Springer; 2011

3. *Range of motion of head and neck.* The ideal position for intubation is with the neck flexed and the head extended at the atlanto-occipital joint. Any restriction in neck movement or contraindication to moving the neck can prevent optimal neck positioning and greatly affect the ease of laryngoscopy. Normal neck mobility is assessed by asking the patient to sit with his or her head upright and mouth open as wide as possible. At this point the maxillary teeth should be parallel to the floor. The patient is then asked to tilt his or her head back as far as it goes. The angle that the maxillary teeth make to their original position is measured, and should be 35° or greater. The patient is then asked to fully flex his or her neck, at which point his or her chin should touch his or her chest wall.

4. *Neck length and thickness.* In general, patients with longer and slimmer necks have greater neck mobility and present easier subjects for laryngoscopy. Conversely, patients with shorter, thicker, and more muscular necks present greater difficulty. While the neck is being examined, other indications of difficult airway can be assessed, such as discoloration (which could indicate previous neck radiation and tissue scarring) and stigma of a previous tracheostomy (which could indicate tracheal stenosis).

5. *Length of upper incisors, interincisor distance.* The length of the upper incisors should be compared to the surrounding teeth. The examiner should then ask the patient to open his mouth as wide as possible, and the distance between the upper and lower incisors measured. An interincisor distance of less than 4.5 cm (or about three fingerbreadths) signifies a potentially difficult intubation. Long upper incisors and a narrow interincisor gap restrict the laryngoscope's range of movement within the mouth. A small interincisor gap can also present a greater risk of complications such as tooth injury and bleeding.

6. *Relation of maxillary and mandibular incisors during normal jaw closure.* In this test, the patient is asked to close his or her mouth while the practitioner observes the relationship of the upper and lower incisors. Normally the upper and lower incisors should be mostly opposed, or at least very close to each other. The more anteriorly the upper incisors lie in relation to the lower incisors, the more likely it is that difficulty will be encountered during intubation.

7. *Foreign bodies.* Foreign objects include dentures, tongue rings, and loose teeth that can be damaged or dislodged during airway manipulation. If dislodged, these objects can aspirate into the airway and cause obstruction or infection. Try to remove any such foreign objects prior to attempts at intubation. If they cannot be removed (for example a loose tooth), document the object and confirm its presence after the airway maneuver is performed. If the object is missing after intubation, perform a chest X-ray to confirm its location.

Basic Airway Skills

These basic airway skills can be useful whether preparing to intubate a patient for surgery or attempting to ventilate a patient with an emergently compromised airway. This part of the chapter is dedicated to explaining these skills and the concepts behind them.

Head Tilt–Jaw Lift Maneuver

The basic goal of this technique is to manipulate the patient's airway to provide the clearest path for airflow. With the patient supine, place one hand on the patient's forehead and the other hand under the patient's chin. The hand on the patient's forehead should be used to tilt the patient's head back so that it is extended at the neck as well as the atlanto-occipital joint. Use your second hand to protrude the patient's mandible upward and away from the head. This position widens the pharyngeal openings and helps to move the tongue out of the pharynx and back into the oral cavity. It is important to note that *this technique should be avoided in any patient with a possible C-Spine injury*. It is important to have a high suspicion of C-Spine injury, because moving an injured C-Spine may further damage the spinal cord and cause permanent debilitation. When a C-Spine injury is possible, it is better to open the airway using a jaw thrust maneuver instead.

Jaw Thrust Maneuver

This has a similar effect as the head tilt–chin lift maneuver in terms of widening the airway and ensuring that the tongue does not occlude the oropharynx. Instead of tilting the head, both hands are focused on protruding the mandible. Use your hands to grip the angles of patient's mandible, with one hand on either side of the mandible. Your thumbs should be on the patient's chin, positioned slightly below his or her lower lip. Your other four fingers should be at the angle of the mandible. Use these four fingers to push the patient's mandible upward and away from his or her head. Use your thumbs to pull the patient's chin out slightly so that his or her mouth is partially open.

Foreign Body Obstruction

If the head tilt–chin lift and jaw thrust techniques fail at establishing a patent airway, then a foreign body may be obstructing the airway. In a partial obstruction the patient will still be passing some air, but a whistling or wheezing sound might be heard with each breath, and the patient might be coughing. If the airway is only partially obstructed and the patient is still moving some air, do not interfere. Let the patient try to cough and allow the body's natural reflexes to expel the foreign body.

Patients presenting with complete obstruction will not be able to cough or make any sound. They will often present with the "universal choking sign," clutching at their throat to indicate they are choking. Perform the Heimlich maneuver until the foreign body is expelled or the patient loses consciousness. If the patient is unconscious, it is important *not* to blindly stick a finger into his or her mouth to search for a foreign body, as this could lodge a foreign body deeper into the pharynx. Instead, carry out chest compressions and give breaths as you would during normal cardiopulmonary resuscitation (CPR). After each round of compressions and breaths, open the patient's mouth to look for a foreign object. If a foreign object is visible, then attempt to use a finger to carefully remove it from the patient's mouth. If nothing is visible, then proceed with another round of CPR.

Airway Equipment and Techniques

The following equipment is available in most operating rooms and in an increasing number of intensive care settings.

Oropharyngeal and Nasopharyngeal Airways

These are small, often soft plastic or rubber devices that can be used to maintain an airway once it has been established by the preferred techniques of repositioning, head tilt–chin lift and jaw thrust. Occasionally oropharyngeal (OP) and nasopharyngeal (NP) airway devices are used to supplement these airway-opening maneuvers if the initial maneuvers prove unsuccessful at maintaining a patent airway.

The OP airway is inserted upside down into the mouth, with the peak of the device's arch facing downwards towards the tongue. Once it has been inserted about halfway into the mouth, it is flipped 180° and simultaneously inserted deeper into the pharynx. This maneuver helps to lodge the tip of the airway behind the tongue, securing it in place. It is important to note that *OP airways are only indicated in unconscious patients.* This is because they commonly elicit the gag reflex, which can lead to vomiting or aspiration. If an artificial airway is indicated in a conscious patient, a nasal airway should be used instead, as it does not elicit the gag reflex.

The nasopharyngeal airway (or nasal trumpet) is a thinner device that has a horn or a ring shape at its proximal end. Nasal trumpets also come in a variety of sizes. Nasal trumpets are usually 2–4 cm longer than the OP airway indicated in the same patient. Before a nasal trumpet is used it should be well lubricated. Continuous, gentle pressures should be applied to slowly guide the trumpet along the floor of the nasal cavity. Although nasal trumpets are better tolerated in conscious patients, they also present a higher risk of bleeding and epistaxis. NP airways are contraindicated in patients presenting with basal skull fractures, as there is a risk of penetrating through the fracture directly into the cranial vault. It is also important to note that most patients have at least mild deviations in their nasal septums, which means that the nasal cavity on one side is wider than the other. If resistance is encountered while placing a nasal trumpet, attempt to insert it into the other nostril, or change to a smaller diameter tube.

Mask Ventilation

If a patient can be adequately ventilated using a face mask, they are at very little risk of becoming hypoxic and the practitioner is afforded time to determine how to establish a more secure airway. It is important to note that *mask ventilation is contraindicated in patients with airway obstruction*. These patients require more invasive measures to secure a patent airway. Face masks are designed to create an airtight seal over the nose and mouth. Different sized masks are available, the best mask being the one that creates the best seal over the patient's face. An appropriately sized mask covers the patient's nose and mouth in a way that the nasal bridge is covered superiorly but the mask does not go over the chin inferiorly. It is important to keep a "best-fitting" mask next to a patient's bed so that it is immediately available in emergent situations.

There are two different mask ventilation techniques: ventilating with one person, and ventilating with two people when the assistant knows how to perform a jaw thrust. With one-person ventilation, the patient is positioned so the head is semi-flexed at the neck and the ear is in the same plane as the sternal notch. This is possible by placing the patient's head on a towel or a pillow. The mask is gently placed over the patient's nose and mouth and held in position using the non-dominant hand, whereas the dominant hand is used to ventilate. The best seal is created using the "E-C technique," named as the thumb and index are held in a C shape over the mask, while the three remaining fingers form an E on the angle of the patient's mandible. This technique allows you to use all five fingers to accomplish three seal-creating goals simultaneously: push the mask onto the patient's face, tilt his or her head back slightly, and lift his or her jaw. When two people are available for ventilation and the airway assistant is adept at using the jaw thrust maneuver, the role of the primary airway manager is similar to what they would do on their own. The nondominant hand is placed on the mask, and the dominant hand used to squeeze the bag. The role of the airway assistant is to use both of his or her hands to assist in lifting the jaw to open the airway. This allows the primary ventilator to focus more on creating a seal than lifting the jaw.

Difficult Mask Ventilation

Difficult mask ventilation (DMV) is defined as inability to maintain $SpO_2 > 92\%$, or reverse signs of inadequate ventilation. It can be due to an inadequate mask seal, excessive gas leak, excessive resistance to the flow of gas, or mechanical obstruction. The MOANS mnemonic can be remembered to predict difficulties in mask ventilation:

- *M*ask seal: The main problems leading to a difficult seal are facial deformities such as nasal or mandibular fractures, or micrognathia. Patients with facial hair present difficulties in creating an adequate seal.
- *O*besity: Patients with body mass index (BMI) of greater than 26 are more difficult to ventilate. It is critical to optimize positioning in these patients.
- *A*ge: Patients older than 55 years may have problems due to decreasing neck mobility.
- *N*o teeth: Edentulous patients pose difficulties due to distortion of normal facial contours. This can often be overcome by placing an OP airway to give the mouth more structure.
- *S*noring: Patients with obstructive sleep apnea are likely to have obstruction at the hypopharynx and base of tongue. OP, NP, and supraglottic airways should be immediately available for these patients.

If good ventilation is not possible using two people, an OP or NP airway should be considered. A mask ventilation attempt should not be considered failed until it is performed by two people with the use of sufficiently large artificial airways, especially since any subsequent step in such a patient would be much more invasive.

Endotracheal Intubation

Although mask ventilation commonly ensures adequate ventilation and oxygenation, it is not a feasible option to use over-prolonged periods of time. Endotracheal intubation is considered the gold standard of maintaining an airway as it is secure, accessible, and much less invasive than a surgical airway. Although endotracheal intubation has become a routine part of the management of patients in the operating room (OR), emergency room (ER), and intensive care unit (ICU), it is not a procedure free of complications. Visualizing the vocal cords to insert a tube through them requires certain measures of training and skill. The task becomes easier with a proper understanding of the underlying principles.

Preparation

Before a patient is put under general anesthesia and given a muscle relaxant, the physician should be fully prepared for intubation. This means checking that all the necessary equipment is available and functioning, and that backup equipment is available in case of equipment failure.

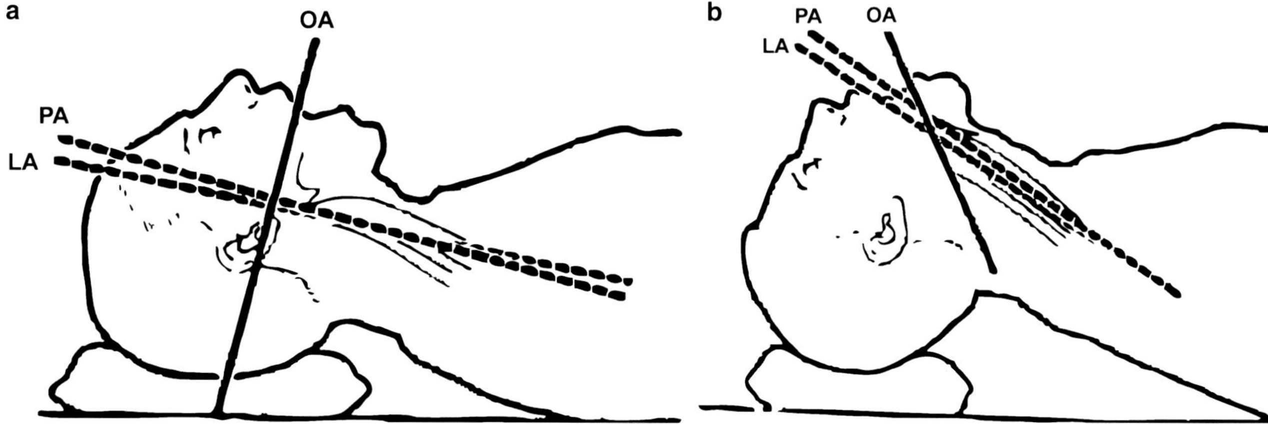

Fig. 13.4 (**a**) Flexing the neck aligns the pharyngeal and laryngeal axes more closely. This is usually accomplished by putting a pillow under the patient's head. (**b**) Extending the patient's head at the atlanto-occipital joint serves to align the oral axis with the two other axes. Stone DJ, Gal TJL. Airway management. In: Miller RD, editor. Anesthesia. 4th ed. New York: Churchill Livingstone: 1994, p. 1408

The physician must consider potential difficulties in intubating a particular patient and plan backup strategies in case intubation proves difficult. When performing an intubation the following equipment should be available:

- Two laryngoscope handles.
- A variety of laryngoscope blades including curved and straight blades of the required size, a size above required, and a size below.
- Endotracheal (ET) tubes of an appropriate size, a size above required, and a size below. Generally, size 7 ET tubes are appropriate for women and size 8 tubes for men.
- Oxygen supply.
- Stylet.
- Oral and nasal airways.
- Functioning suction apparatus.

Both laryngoscopes should be checked to ensure functionality, including battery power and bulb function. The endotracheal tubes should be assessed to ensure that the lumen is patent and the cuff is functioning. The patient should be given 100% oxygen via face mask for 3–5 min, or three maximal inhalation breaths. Appropriate drugs should be drawn and labeled.

Positioning

Positioning should be accomplished before preoxygenation is begun. The patient should be laid supine, with the head towards the top of the head and on a shallow pillow. The practitioner should be positioned at the top of the bed. Adjust the bed according to your height so that you are at a comfortable level and not hunched over the patient. A comfortable level for intubation is when the patient's head is at the level of your xiphoid process. One of the obstacles to intubation is the misalignment of the axes of the oral cavity, pharynx, and larynx. In order to create a direct line of sight from the mouth to the glottis, the practitioner must place the patient in the "sniffing" position. This is accomplished by flexing the patient's neck, and then extending the head at the atlanto-occipital joint as demonstrated in Fig. 13.4.

Direct Laryngoscopy

Once the equipment has been checked and the patient pre-oxygenated, administer sedation and a muscle relaxant. Once the patient is properly positioned, pick up the laryngoscope with your left hand. With the laryngoscope in your left hand, slightly open the patient's mouth using your right hand. Insert your right hand between the patient's teeth at the right angle of the mouth, and use your thumb and middle finger to pry the patient's mouth wide open. This is called the scissors technique. Introduce the laryngoscope into the right side of the oral cavity and gently move the laryngoscope blade to the left side of the mouth, sweeping the tongue to the left. Advance the blade until you see the white epiglottic cartilage. The laryngoscope is now positioned according to which blade is being used: curved blades (Macintosh) should be lodged into the vallecula, between the epiglottis and the root of the tongue; straight blades (Miller) are positioned posteriorly to the epiglottis.

Once the blade is appropriately positioned, lift the patient's tongue and mandible using the laryngoscope. This is done by lifting the entire laryngoscope up and away from you at a 45° angle. Imagine you are lifting towards the opposite side of the room, where the roof meets the wall. If done correctly, the patient's head may lift slightly from the table. Take care not to hurt the teeth as you carry out this maneuver. You should now be able to see the vocal cords. Slide the ET tube between the vocal cords once visualized. Advance the tube 2–3 cm after crossing the glottic opening. If a stylet was in place, ask an assistant to remove the stylet while you hold the laryngoscope and tube in place. Slowly withdraw the laryngoscope from the patient's mouth, taking care to avoid the teeth and hold the tube in place. Now inflate the cuff on the tube using a 10 ml syringe, and attach the connector piece of the tube to the ventilator's circuit.

Ensuring Tube Placement

Once the cuff has been inflated, it is essential to assess correct tube placement. Observe the patient's chest to see if it rises and falls with each breath. Then use a stethoscope to auscultate the patient's chest to make sure that breath sounds are equal on both sides. If breath sounds are present on the right side only, suspect right main stem bronchial intubation; deflate the tube's ET cuff, pull the tube back 1 cm, reinflate the cuff, and reassess ventilation. The gold standard of checking for correct tube placement is observing CO_2 waveforms on a capnograph. An esophageal intubation is easy to miss, and the practitioner must remain vigilant and use multiple means of detecting error to make sure that correct positioning is established.

Surgical Airway

Long-term endotracheal intubation carries an increased incidence of acute and chronic complications such as an increased rate of ventilator-associated pneumonias, as well as injury to the mucosal surface of the trachea and larynx leading to post-intubation stenosis. Tracheotomy originates from Greek and translates into "cutting the trachea," such that tracheostomy is the surgical creation of an opening in the trachea through the anterior neck bringing the tracheal mucosa in continuation with the skin [2]. While prolonged respiratory failure is probably the most common reason for performing a tracheostomy, other indications such as decreased level of consciousness, impaired protective reflexes, and trauma victims with severe physiologic derangements are also indications.

Tracheostomy affords several advantages over traditional endotracheal intubation such as (1) easier oral care, (2) earlier patient mobilization, (3) improved patient comfort, (4) reduced need for sedation, (5) more effective cough reflex and pulmonary toilet, (6) lower airway resistance and decreased work of breathing, (7) enhanced patient communication efforts, (8) reduced long-term complications from translaryngeal intubation, (9) less sinusitis, and (10) reduced incidence of accidental extubation [3–5]. Unfortunately, tracheostomy too has associated risk and complications, the most common of these being tracheal stenosis and hemorrhage, in addition to stomal infections, and pneumothorax. Additional disadvantages include (1) the invasive nature of the operation, (2) procedural cost, and (3) occasional severe long-term complications such as tracheomalacia, tracheal stenosis, and tracheoinnominate fistula (TIF). The incidence of these procedure-related complications has been reported to be anywhere between 3.5 and 36% [6, 7]. Only about 10–25% of patients requiring ventilator support ever receive a tracheostomy as part of their critical care management [8]. Proposed indications for tracheostomy include the following: (1) failed trials of extubation/weaning attempts, (2) requiring prolonged mechanical ventilation, (3) need for tracheal access to remove thick pulmonary secretions, (4) airway protection and prevention of aspiration, (5) upper airway obstruction bypass, and (6) trauma or surgery to the face and neck region [5].

Early Versus Late Tracheostomy

The timing of tracheostomy in a ventilator-dependent patient has been a subject of debate, and there is considerable variation in the timing and incidence of tracheotomy. A consensus conference on artificial airways management in mechanically ventilated patients made recommendations that tracheostomy should be performed after 3 weeks of endotracheal intubation [9]. While this timetable is still in practice, observational studies have reported earlier tracheostomy to be associated with better patient outcomes [6, 10]. However, there is a discrepancy in results obtained from randomized trials comparing early versus late tracheotomy and the duration of mechanical ventilation, incidence of ventilator-associated pneumonias, and mortality. The definition of "early" in these studies has been reported as performing a tracheotomy procedure anywhere within 2–16 days ventilator dependency [4, 11]. Currently common practice dictates that tracheotomy should be performed after 2 weeks of endotracheal intubation or in patients clinically suspected to require longer than 2 weeks of ventilator support. This has been supported by the American College of Chest Physicians guidelines on ventilator weaning [12].

Open Versus Percutaneous Tracheostomy

Open surgical tracheostomy (ST) has traditionally been the only technique available, but within the last 15 years numerous methods of percutaneous tracheostomy have come into clinical practice. Currently, there are six different methods of performing percutaneous tracheostomy with the Ciaglia percutaneous tracheostomy (PT) being the most commonly utilized [13] (William). The percutaneous technique offers several advantages over the open approach, such as smaller skin incisions, less tissue trauma, and a lower incidence of wound infection and bleeding. Percutaneous tracheostomies can also be performed in the ICU by nonsurgical staff, adding additional benefits in not having to transfer patients to the operating room. The debate whether ST is better than PT is hindered by the paucity of good randomized trials, many of which lack sufficient power, clearly defined criteria for complications, and poor long-term follow-up. A recent meta-analysis comparing the two techniques showed significantly fewer wound infections and scarring in the percutaneous group but was associated with more decannulation complications [13]. No differences were seen in terms of false passage, hemorrhage, or death. Considering all complications, there was a trend towards favoring percutaneous tracheostomy over the open approach. Similar comparison between the two methods performed between 1985 and 1996 revealed more perioperative complications in the percutaneous groups (10% vs. 3%) and more postoperative complications with the open technique (10% vs. 7%) [14]. In contrast, Freeman et al. showed no significant differences in overall complication rates but with less perioperative complications such as bleeding and infection in patients who received a percutaneous tracheostomy [6].

Cricothyroidotomy

Less commonly performed, cricothyroidotomy can be a lifesaving maneuver when faced with the scenario when orotracheal or nasotracheal intubation is unsuccessful in a patient who is otherwise not able to ventilate or oxygenate. This procedure essentially involves placing a tube through a surgically created incision in the cricothyroid membrane. While this procedure only accounts for 1% of all intubations in the emergency room setting, it continues to be a lifesaving intervention for failed airway treatment [15]. Certain conditions may necessitate cricothyroidotomy such as massive hemorrhage, obstructing lesions, and an array of traumatic injuries. No absolute contraindications exist as maintaining oxygenation is the primary goal; however, traumatic tracheal or laryngotracheal injury should be viewed with caution. The procedure is not recommended in children. Cricothyroidotomies are rarely kept in place, but serve as a bridge to oxygenate/ventilate critical patients until more definitive airway management can be achieved. Several early complications have been observed such as bleeding, laceration to the tracheal cartilage, cricoid cartilage, and tracheal rings, perforation of the posterior trachea, extratracheal passage of the tube into a false tract, and infection.

Procedural Description

Before attempting any airway maneuver, the essential equipment must be readily available. The airway cart should consist of the necessary drugs for induction and sedation as well as paralytic agents. The mainstay of the cart however is the ET tube and should be available in several different sizes. Both Miller (straight) and Macintosh (curved) laryngoscopes should be included in any set as well as additional bulbs and handles with well-charged batteries. While endotracheal intubation will suffice in many situations, the need for a surgical airway may eventually become necessary or even needed emergently.

Open Tracheostomy

Performing an open tracheostomy requires proper patient positioning, where the shoulders are elevated with a shoulder roll and extension of the neck (unless there is cervical spine instability).

The skin of the anterior neck is sterilely prepped and any hair is removed with clippers. A vertical incision, 2–3 cm in length, is made over the second tracheal ring just below the cricoid cartilage. Care is taken not to violate anterior neck veins or the thyroid isthmus. The platysma is divided and any bleeding is controlled with ties and electrocautery. The strap muscles of the neck are displaced laterally, parallel to the long axis of the trachea. If the thyroid isthmus overlies the second and third tracheal rings, it must be mobilized to clear space for tracheostomy placement. Blunt dissection is used to clear the pre-tracheal fascia off of the second and third tracheal rings.

Tracheal entry is facilitated by either complete removal of the anterior tracheal ring, creating a stoma, or creation of a rectangular flap with a portion of the tracheal ring still intact. When the ring is removed, stay sutures are placed laterally on the trachea at the level of the stoma to provide countertraction as the tracheostomy tube is inserted. These sutures can then be used to secure the tracheostomy tube in position. The newly created fistula is considered unstable for several days and dislodgement of the tube frequently results in the inability to reinsert it. If the flap method is used, the inferior anterior ring is incised in a U-shaped fashion and the flap is sutured to the skin. This is done by sharp dissection of the pre-tracheal fascia, entering the trachea along its inferior margin of the second ring. Two lateral incisions are made creating an inverse U-shaped flap that can then be sutured to the skin. This method is believed to be superior to the ring resection technique in recanulation; however no studies have confirmed this.

Cricothyroidotomy

This procedure can be performed with as little as a #11 scalpel, tissue forceps, and a hemostat or Trousseaus dilator. Additionally, adequate lighting and a good suctioning device are paramount to performing a successful emergent cricothyroidotomy as it is essentially a blind operation in many instances and bleeding can profuse. With the aforementioned equipment and experience, cricothyroidotomy is greater than 90% effective in establishing an adequate airway [16]. The greatest impediment to the procedure is delayed recognition that it should be performed in the first place.

The procedure is initiated by prepping the skin of the anterior neck and identification of external landmarks such as the thyroid and cricothyroid cartilages. The site of endotracheal tube insertion occurs between these two cartilaginous structures, within the cricothyroid membrane. Using the nondominant hand, the trachea and larynx are stabilized followed by making generous vertical incision over the area between the thyroid and cricothyroid. Sharp dissection is continued down through the pre-tracheal fascia and the cricothyroid membrane is entered through a horizontal incision. The membrane incision can then be dilated with forceps of a hemostat to facilitate easier endotracheal tube passage. To assist in inserting the tube, tracheal hooks can be used to elevate the trachea. Care should be taken to avoid inadvertent puncture of the balloon cuff as the hooks have sharp points. The index finger of the stabilizing hand is used to guide ET insertion to a depth of 5 cm over a rigid stylet. Alternatives to traditional surgical cricothyroidotomies have become commercially available which employee the use of a guidewire passed through the membrane by needle puncture. The ET can then be passed by the Seldinger technique over a dilator into the airway. These maneuvers may expedite airway securement and lessen the degree of expertise required in performing such critical airway management.

Needle Cricothyroidotomy

In a last effort to provide temporarily lifesaving oxygenation and ventilation after failed tracheal intubation or when surgical expertise is lacking, transtracheal jet ventilation can be performed through a needle cricothyroidotomy. Identification of external landmarks is the same as when performing a surgical cricothyroidotomy. A large-bore catheter (14–16 gauge) is attached to a syringe filled with saline. The cricothyroid membrane is then cannulated with the catheter in a caudal direction. Air bubbles upon aspiration of the syringe confirm tracheal position. The needle is removed and the catheter is attached to a jet ventilation system using a Luer lock. Jet insufflation should occur at 1 s of inspiration for every 3 s of expiration. This is, however, only a temporizing measure as ventilation is not occurring and the partial pressure of CO_2 will rise. It does provide roughly an additional 30 min until a definitive airway can be achieved once the necessary personnel and equipment become available.

Complications

Tracheostomy can be associated with numerous acute complications such as hemorrhage, surgical suite infections, pneumothorax, and accidental decannulation. While these complications are not limited to the acute setting, several unique late complications can occur as well. The most common of these late complications is the development of granulation tissue, which may manifest as failure to wean from the ventilator or upper airway obstruction with respiratory failure after decannulation [17]. While other complications occur less frequently, up to 65% of patients receiving a tracheostomy experience some form of tracheostomy-related complication [18]. Complications may be directly related to the procedure itself, delayed healing of the stoma site, cuff pressure, or chemical exposure to gastric juice as occurs with gastroesophageal reflux and polling of secretions above the tracheostomy cuff. These complications may not be readily identifiable due to confounding factors such as multi-organ failure, sepsis, shock, loss to follow-up when transferred to long-term care facilities, or lack of postmortem identification. Separating out the effects of prolonged endotracheal intubation may also contribute to the development of long-term complications in that intubation may be the contributing factor that leads to such entities such as tracheal stenosis and tracheomalacia [19]. Complication rates, comparing open versus percutaneous techniques, have shown a lower incidence of long-term complications with the percutaneous approach; however, the percutaneous approach was associated with higher perioperative complications [14, 20].

Tracheal Stenosis

Tracheal stenosis results in narrowing of the tracheal lumen at or above the stoma site as well as at the site of cuff inflation. Stomal granulation tissue frequently develops in nearly all patients with the result of tracheal narrowing; however, only 3–12% demonstrates clinically significant narrowing that requires intervention [21]. This granulation tissue initially is soft and vascular and may bleed at the time of tube exchange. As it matures, it becomes fibrous and epithelialized. With the development of fibrosis, the tracheal wall becomes narrowed. Risk factors associated with stenosis include stomal infection, sepsis, hypotension, advanced age, male sex, use of steroids, prolonged placement, and disproportionate excision of anterior tracheal cartilage during the creation of the tracheostomy. Diagnosis requires a high index of suspicion. Tracheal stenosis may present early in patients still undergoing ventilator support, which may present as failure to wean successfully or weeks to months after decannulation as dyspnea. In fact, tracheal stenosis may not produce any symptoms until the lumen has been reduced by 50–75% as exertional dyspnea and eventually stridor at rest [19]. Diagnostic modalities include radiography such as chest X-ray/computed tomography (CT)/ magnetic resonance imaging (MRI), endoscopic visualization, and flow–volume curves showing obstructed patterns.

Suprastomal stenosis has particularly been reported to occur after percutaneous dilatational techniques, related to guidewire injury to the posterior tracheal wall and subsequent development of granulation tissue and protrusion into the lumen [22, 23]. Additionally, dilation causes injury to the anterior tracheal cartilage/ring fracture with invagination and narrowing of the lumen. Stenosis seemed to be less common following the Ciaglia technique versus the Griggs technique [20].

The tracheal cuff also serves as a site for potential tracheal stenosis as a result of ischemic mucosal injury. This occurs from high cuff pressure that exceeds capillary perfusion pressure of the tracheal wall as well as from shearing forces of the tube/cuff. Prolonged ischemia leads to chondritis and necrosis with the development of fibrous granulation tissue similar to other forms of tracheal stenosis. Risk factors for cuff site stenosis include female sex, older age, prolonged tube placement, and excess cuff pressure.

Numerous strategies exist to treat tracheal stenosis such as laser excision of granulation tissue and bronchoscopic dilatation. Suprastomal granulation tissue can be excised using sharp dissection. Other options included tracheal stents and tracheal segment resection with primary anastomosis. Despite all these therapeutic approaches, the recurrence rate can be up to 90%, especially if there is a lengthy stenotic segment that requires large amounts of dissection or excision [24].

Tracheomalacia

Tracheomalacia is the weakening of the tracheal wall that results from ischemic injury with resultant chondritis and necrosis of tracheal cartilage leading to airway collapse following expiration. The trachea is also susceptible to external compression. Patients frequently exhibit failure to wean from the ventilator or with dyspnea. Again a high index of suspicion is required to diagnose and can be appreciated by bronchoscopic visualization of airway collapse. Treatment depends on the extent of airway collapse and airway obstruction. It may require placing a longer tube to bypass the affected segment, stenting, tracheal resection, or tracheoplasty.

Tracheoinnominate Fistula

This uncommon yet life-threatening complication only occurs in 0.1–1% of tracheostomies performed, usually around 7–14 days post procedure. TIF has been reported to occur following surgical and percutaneous tracheotomies. It is usually fatal if not recognized immediately. Risk factors for its development include excessive movement of the tube, high pressure in the cuff, excessive neck extension, and placement of the tracheostomy below the third tracheal ring as it can erode into the innominate artery as it courses near the trachea. The innominate artery is the first branch off the aortic arch, which divides into the right common carotid and right subclavian arteries 3–4 cm lateral to the trachea.

Two main mechanisms are capable of producing pressures sufficient to cause an erosive process. First, a fistula can occur between the anterior tracheal wall secondary to mechanical force generated by the tube cuff of tube tip. The second mechanism involves pressure generated beneath the angulated neck of the tracheostomy tube, which can erode through the mucosa and into the artery. Low-lying placement is the most obvious cause, but even well-placed tubes between the second and third tracheal do not prevent TIF occurrence.

Diagnosis is based on lag time between tracheostomy placement and onset of bleeding. Early bleeding within 48 h is typically a result of traumatic puncture of anterior jugular and inferior thyroid veins, coagulopathy, local trauma from tracheal suctioning, and bronchopneumonia. Massive hemorrhage or hemoptysis occurring 3 days to 6 weeks post procedure is TIF until proven otherwise. A sentinel bleed is reported to occur in more than 50% who later go on to develop a TIF [25]. Bleeding occurring greater than 6 weeks is not typically a result of TIF but from granulation tissue or malignancy.

Management of a TIF first involves minimizing its risk for occurring and whether there is active bleeding hindering adequate ventilation. Rigid bronchoscopy can be used to determine the extent and source of bleeding as well as exclude other sources of bleeding and to obtain a blood-free airway. If a self-terminating sentinel bleed occurs and the main bronchi are blood free, then immediate intervention can be delayed to further investigate the source of bleeding. If active bleeding is ongoing, the potential for airway compromise is imminent. Attempts to manipulate the tube should be discouraged as this can precipitate loss of the airway. Acute management of active bleeding includes overinflation of the cuff. If this maneuver fails to halt bleeding, one should proceed to endotracheal intubation below the site of bleeding to protect the airway followed by digital compression of the artery against the posterior manubrium. Bleeding can be temporized in 90% of occurrences and allows time to plan surgical intervention [26]. This complication is a surgical emergency and carries a 100% mortality without surgery. A median sternotomy allows access where proximal and distal control can be achieved and the arterial lumen ligated. No evidence suggests significant neurological or vascular compromise with this maneuver [27].

Tracheoesophageal Fistula

An even more unusual complication is that of a tracheoesophageal fistula (TEF), which involves the development of a connection between the trachea and esophagus. This iatrogenic complication results from injury to the posterior wall of the trachea from excessive cuff pressures or from unknown perforation of the posterior wall during placement of percutaneous tracheostomies. Patients have an abundance of copious secretions as well as recurrent aspiration of food, dyspnea, persistent cuff leak, and gastric distension. Repair is surgical if patients' condition allows it; otherwise esophageal stents allow for less invasive means to control the fistula.

Conclusion

Airway management is one of the crucial skills required of the acute care surgeon. A thorough understanding of the anatomy, as well as familiarity with advanced airway techniques, can help ease anxiety when in a pressing situation and potentially prevent disastrous results. Appropriate timing and method for tracheostomy placement should also be considered by the acute care surgeon, as this decision often falls to the intensivist caring for the patient. Complications of this otherwise straightforward procedure can be devastating, so careful technique and planning are paramount.

References

1. McNicol L, Mackay P. Anaesthesia-related morbidity in Victoria: a report from 1990 to 2005. Anaesth Intensive Care. 2010;38(5):837–48.
2. McWhorter AJ. Tracheotomy: timing and techniques. Curr Opin Otolaryngol Head Neck Surg. 2003;11(6):473–9.
3. Nathens AB, Rivara FP, Mack CD, Rubenfeld GD, Wang J, Jurkovich GJ, et al. Variations in rates of tracheostomy in the critically ill trauma patient. Crit Care Med. 2006;34(12):2919–24.
4. Rumbak MJ, Newton M, Truncale T, Schwartz SW, Adams JW, Hazard PB. A prospective, randomized, study comparing early percutaneous dilational tracheotomy to prolonged translaryngeal intubation (delayed tracheotomy) in critically ill medical patients. Crit Care Med. 2004;32(8):1689–94.
5. Mallick A, Bodenham AR. Tracheostomy in critically ill patients. Eur J Anaesthesiol. 2010;27(8):676–82.
6. Freeman BD, Isabella K, Lin N, Buchman TG. A meta-analysis of prospective trials comparing percutaneous and surgical tracheostomy in critically ill patients. Chest. 2000;118(5):1412–8.
7. Melloni G, Muttini S, Gallioli G, Carretta A, Cozzi S, Gemma M, et al. Surgical tracheostomy versus percutaneous dilatational tracheostomy. A prospective-randomized study with long-term follow-up. J Cardiovasc Surg (Torino). 2002;43(1):113–21.
8. Clec'h C, Alberti C, Vincent F, Garrouste-Orgeas M, de Lassence A, Toledano D, et al. Tracheostomy does not improve the outcome of patients requiring prolonged mechanical ventilation: a propensity analysis. Crit Care Med. 2007;35(1):132–8.
9. Plummer AL, Gracey DR. Consensus conference on artificial airways in patients receiving mechanical ventilation. Chest. 1989;96(1):178–80.
10. Scales DC, Thiruchelvam D, Kiss A, Redelmeier DA. The effect of tracheostomy timing during critical illness on long-term survival. Crit Care Med. 2008;36(9):2547–57.
11. Blot S, Rello J, Vogelaers D. What is new in the prevention of ventilator-associated pneumonia? Curr Opin Pulm Med. 2011;17(3):155–9.
12. MacIntyre NR, Cook DJ, Ely Jr EW, Epstein SK, Fink JB, Heffner JE, et al. Evidence-based guidelines for weaning and discontinuing ventilatory support: a collective task force facilitated by the American College of Chest Physicians; the American Association for Respiratory Care; and the American College of Critical Care Medicine. Chest. 2001;120(6 Suppl):375S–95S.
13. Higgins KM, Punthakee X. Meta-analysis comparison of open versus percutaneous tracheostomy. Laryngoscope. 2007;117(3):447–54.
14. Dulguerov P, Gysin C, Perneger TV, Chevrolet JC. Percutaneous or surgical tracheostomy: a meta-analysis. Crit Care Med. 1999;27(8):1617–25.
15. Erlandson MJ, Clinton JE, Ruiz E, Cohen J. Cricothyrotomy in the emergency department revisited. J Emerg Med. 1989;7(2):115–8.
16. Wright MJ, Greenberg DE, Hunt JP, Madan AK, McSwain Jr NE. Surgical cricothyroidotomy in trauma patients. South Med J. 2003;96(5):465–7.
17. Wood DE, Mathisen DJ. Late complications of tracheotomy. Clin Chest Med. 1991;12(3):597–609.
18. Heffner JE, Miller KS, Sahn SA. Tracheostomy in the intensive care unit. Part 2: complications. Chest. 1986;90(3):430–6.
19. Sue RD, Susanto I. Long-term complications of artificial airways. Clin Chest Med. 2003;24(3):457–71.
20. Leonard RC, Lewis RH, Singh B, van Heerden PV. Late outcome from percutaneous tracheostomy using the Portex kit. Chest. 1999;115(4):1070–5.
21. Streitz Jr JM, Shapshay SM. Airway injury after tracheotomy and endotracheal intubation. Surg Clin North Am. 1991;71(6):1211–30.
22. Benjamin B, Kertesz T. Obstructive suprastomal granulation tissue following percutaneous tracheostomy. Anaesth Intensive Care. 1999;27(6):596–600.
23. Koitschev A, Graumueller S, Zenner H-P, Dommerich S, Simon C. Tracheal stenosis and obliteration above the tracheostoma after percutaneous dilational tracheostomy. Crit Care Med. 2003;31(5):1574–6.
24. Noppen M, Schlesser M, Meysman M, D'Haese J, Peche R, Vincken W. Bronchoscopic balloon dilatation in the combined management of postintubation stenosis of the trachea in adults. Chest. 1997;112(4):1136–40.
25. Courcy PA, Rodriguez A, Garrett HE. Operative technique for repair of tracheoinnominate artery fistula. J Vasc Surg. 1985;2(2):332–4.
26. Grant CA, Dempsey G, Harrison J, Jones T. Tracheo-innominate artery fistula after percutaneous tracheostomy: three case reports and a clinical review. Br J Anaesth. 2006;96(1):127–31.
27. Brewster DC, Moncure AC, Darling RC, Ambrosino JJ, Abbott WM. Innominate artery lesions: problems encountered and lessons learned. J Vasc Surg. 1985;2(1):99–112.

Esophageal Perforation

14

James Wiseman and Shanda H. Blackmon

Introduction

The esophagus is a critical component of the human alimentary tract, traversing three domains of the body: the neck, chest, and abdomen. It differs from other elements of the digestive system in that it lacks an outside serosal layer, and is thus both more susceptible to leakage and less tolerant of surgical repair. Additionally, with the increasing use of endoscopy for both diagnostic and therapeutic purposes, the incidence of esophageal perforation is on the rise. As such, the management of perforations demands experience and proficiency with its anatomic features, surgical approaches, and a growing array of available endoscopic modalities.

Esophageal leaks are broadly classified as acute or chronic and contained or uncontained. The mortality associated with acute extravasation increases with every hour of delay in treatment, and carries an overall mortality of 3–67% [1]. This condition is particularly lethal when associated with mediastinitis, empyema, or intra-abdominal sepsis, which occurs more frequently with perforation of the thoracic or abdominal esophageal segments.

Etiology

Nearly 60% of all cases of esophageal perforation are iatrogenic in etiology [2]. A smaller percentage (15%) occur spontaneously due to foreign body ingestion (12%), or traumatic injury (9%). Table 14.1 presents a full listing of the causes and

clinical findings associated with esophageal perforations of various etiologies. No definitive correlation between the etiology of the perforation and mortality rate has been established; however, all ruptures must be promptly addressed. The majority of iatrogenic perforations are the result of endoscopic procedures, with those undertaken for therapeutic purposes harboring a greater risk. Furthermore, those patients undergoing pneumatic dilation for stricture or achalasia appear to be particularly vulnerable. The overall rate of perforation associated with endoscopy remains less than 0.1% [3]. Other iatrogenic causes include surgical procedures involving the esophagus and the use of Sengstaken–Blakemore or Linton tubes.

Spontaneous esophageal perforation, commonly known as Boerhaave's syndrome, results from abrupt increases in intraesophageal pressure. It was originally described by Herman Boerhaave in 1724, in a pamphlet detailing his post-mortem observations of Baron de Wassenaer, the Grand Admiral of Holland. Though Boerhaave's syndrome has historically come to be linked with violent emesis following unrestrained imbibition or food consumption, the Baron suffered a fatal esophageal rupture as a result of self-induced vomiting in an attempt to relieve the discomfort of indigestion [4]. Spontaneous perforations associated with weight lifting, childbirth, seizures, and defecation have been reported, and likely bear a similar physiologic origin.

The superficial course of both the cervical and thoracic esophagus renders them susceptible to injury from penetrating trauma. Additionally, gunshot wounds can also inflict indirect thermal injury easily missed at initial examination that can subsequently become the site of a rupture. Esophageal disruption can likewise occur in the setting of blunt traumatic injuries. Putative mechanisms include torsive and stretching forces, as well as rapid acceleration with injury occurring at fixed points. Ingestion of caustic materials, broadly classified as acidic or alkaline, can also result in esophageal perforation. This is most common with alkaline consumption, as these agents are both more palatable and cause a liquefactive necrosis with a propensity for transmural progression of the

J. Wiseman, M.D.
Department of General Surgery, The Methodist Hospital, Weill
Cornell Medical College, Houston, TX, USA

S.H. Blackmon, M.D., M.P.H, F.A.C.S (✉)
Section of Thoracic Surgery, Department of Surgery, Weill Cornell
Medical College, 6550 Fannin Street, Smith Tower 1661,
Houston, TX 77030, USA
e-mail: Shblackmon@tmhs.org

L.J. Moore et al. (eds.), *Common Problems in Acute Care Surgery*,
DOI 10.1007/978-1-4614-6123-4_14, © Springer Science+Business Media New York 2013

Table 14.1 Etiologies of esophageal perforations

Type	Causes	Clinical findings
Anatomic	External compression from an aberrant right subclavian artery	
Pyriform sinus	Singing, yelling, trumpet playing, recent endoscopy	Marked mediastinal and cervical subcutaneous emphysema
Anastomotic	Leakage at or near the site of a surgical anastomosis	History of surgically created esophageal anastomosis
Boerhaave's	Vomiting, straining, retching, weight lifting, hyperemesis, seizures causing a full-thickness tear at the gastroesophageal junction	Characteristic longitudinal tear on the left side of the esophagus, typically in the distal 1/3 segment Mucosal defect typically longer than muscular defect
Iatrogenic	Endoscopic: Ablation, dilation, sclerotherapy, instrumentation Surgical: Esophageal surgery, foregut cyst decortication, spine surgery	Recent history of surgery or endoscopy
Traumatic	Penetrating or blunt trauma to neck or torso	Strong association with neck hyperextension
Cancer	Perforation of an esophageal tumor Erosion of surrounding tumor through esophageal wall	Gas near or abutting the tumor on imaging
Paraesophageal hernia	Incarceration with necrosis of the distal esophagus	Evidence of left pleural effusion or abdominal fluid on imaging studies
Foreign body	Ingestion of a substance (i.e., chicken bone) that becomes lodged Impaction at a stricture Esophageal webs Eosinophilic esophagitis	Upper esophageal impaction at the sphincter
Esophagitis	Inflammation and erosion of ulceration Zollinger–Ellison syndrome Barrett's ulcer Infection (Candida, Herpes simplex, viruses, CMV)	Immunocompromised patient
Ingestion	Ingestion of caustic substance Drug ingestion/impaction	Tetracycline Potassium Quinidine NSAIDS Sustained-release formulations

CMV—cytomegalovirus
NSAIDS—nonsteroidal anti-inflammatory drugs

injury. Although acid ingestion results in a coagulative necrosis with less potential for penetration, perforation can occur.

Acute inflammation and infection can also lead to perforation of a weakened esophageal wall, particularly in the immunocompromised patient. One noteworthy etiology is eosinophilic esophagitis, characterized by unexplained focal penetration of eosinophils. Multiple reports of spontaneous perforation in this setting exist [5, 6].

Presentation

The clinical signs and symptoms of esophageal perforation are largely dependent upon the anatomic location of the defect. Fever, tachycardia, tachypnea, dyspnea, shock, and leukocytosis are frequently present regardless of the site of the injury. Crepitus, indicative of underlying subcutaneous emphysema, suggests a perforation in the neck or pyriform sinus. Additionally, these patients may describe neck pain of varying severity, vocal disturbances classically described as a prominent "nasal" tonality, dysphagia, or bleeding through the mouth. Perforations of the thoracic or abdominal esophagus often result in vomiting, chest and/or back pain, dyspnea, dysphagia, and bleeding. In addition, defects of the intra-abdominal esophagus commonly cause abdominal pain and distention. "Mackler's Triad" denotes the classic presenting syndrome of patients with spontaneous esophageal rupture, and includes vomiting, lower chest pain, and subcutaneous emphysema. The Anderson Triad, likewise suggestive of spontaneous esophageal rupture, includes subcutaneous emphysema, rapid respirations, and abdominal rigidity.

Evaluation

Evaluation of the patient with suspected esophageal perforation begins with a detailed history and physical examination. Particular attention should be given to any recent history of instrumentation or trauma to the neck or torso, quantitative and qualitative assessment of recent food and liquid consumption, evidence of malignancy such as recent weight loss or dysphagia, or any signs of progressing sepsis. Hemodynamic instability should be immediately addressed with placement of large-bore intravenous catheters and fluid administration. Once esophageal perforation is suspected, antero-posterior and lateral upright chest and abdominal radiographs should be obtained without delay. Radiographic findings suspicious for perforation include subcutaneous emphysema, the

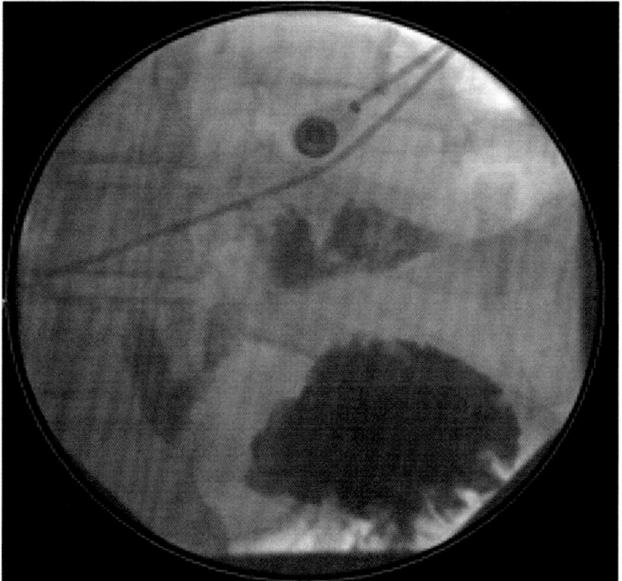

Fig. 14.1 Contrast esophagram of a Boerhaave perforation of the esophagus at the gastroesophageal junction resulting in left pleural contamination

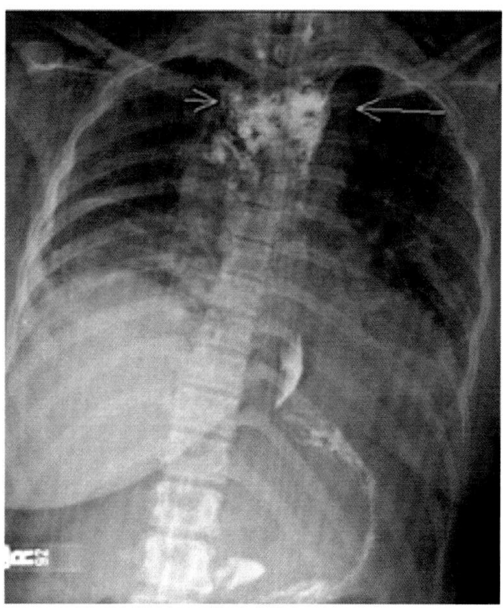

Fig. 14.2 Contrast esophagram of a fish bone perforation of the cervical esophagus resulting in mediastinal contamination

presence of pleural effusions, pneumomediastinum, hydro/pneumothorax, and pleural thickening. Radiographs are particularly useful in the setting of suspected iatrogenic perforation, as they may prove diagnostic in up to 80% of these patients. Furthermore, radiographs have utility in terms of localization of the defect; a right pleural effusion suggests a mid-esophageal perforation, while a left effusion portends a lower esophageal lesion.

The gold standard for diagnosis of perforation is a contrast swallow study, done in the presence of the treating surgeon. Performed fluoroscopically, the patient should be oriented obliquely relative to the source and remain in a standing, semierect position, which will facilitate the detection of small leaks (Fig. 14.1 through Fig. 14.5). Given the risk of severe pneumonitis associated with gastrograffin aspiration, angiography agents are preferred. Barium use can complicate future imaging in the patient due to persistence of the substance in the esophagus for several days, and should only be used if an obvious perforation is not detected on initial swallow evaluation with a water-soluble contrast agent. Although essential in the initial evaluation of suspected esophageal perforation, the false negative rate of contrast radiography approaches thirty percent.

Computed tomography (CT) is useful in cases where perforation remains suspected in the setting of a non-diagnostic swallow study. Additionally, it is the primary diagnostic modality in intubated patients or in those in whom a swallow evaluation is otherwise not possible, impractical, or negative. It is essential to ensure that the endotracheal or tracheostomy cuff is inflated prior to contrast administration to prevent

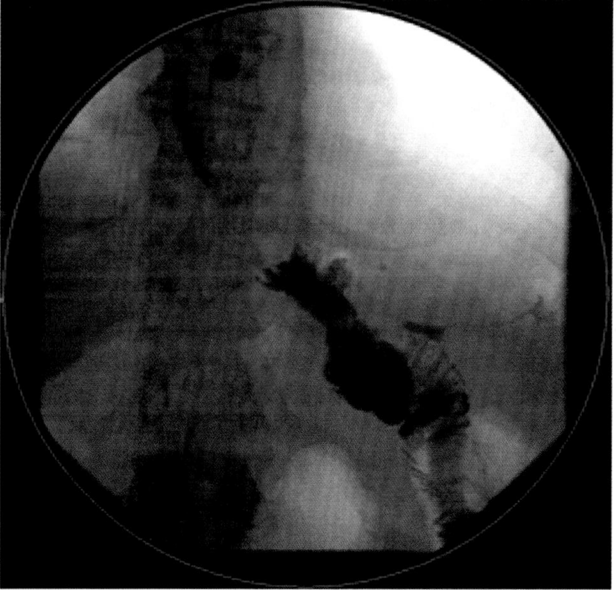

Fig. 14.3 Contrast esophagram of a gastric bypass leak resulting in left pleural and abdominal contamination

aspiration. Computed tomography offers the advantage of more reliable identification of associated abscesses or fluid collections. A further consideration is that some contrast agents must be diluted prior to CT scan imaging to prevent artifact interference with image interpretation.

Endoscopy is also a valuable adjunct to diagnosis, and can facilitate irrigation and drainage of large perforations prior to intervention. As is discussed below, endoscopy is

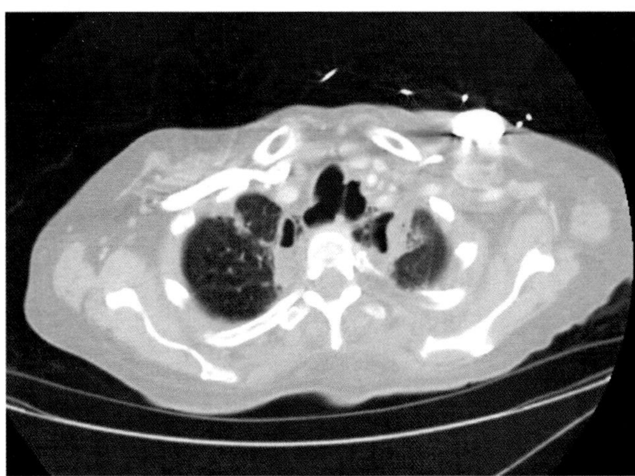

Fig. 14.4 CT scan of a tracheo-esophageal fistula after chemotherapy and radiation therapy for esophageal squamous cell carcinoma

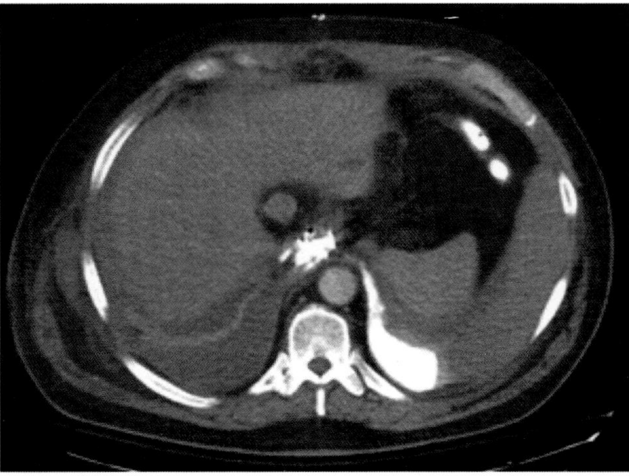

Fig. 14.5 CT scan of an intrathoracic anastomotic leak after esophagectomy resulting in left pleural contamination

increasingly being used for definitive management of some perforations. When being employed in the evaluation for esophageal perforation, endoscopy should only be performed by an experienced practitioner under general anesthesia in an operating room with the patient's airway protected.

Management

The principal goals in the management of esophageal perforation are as follows: complete drainage of extraluminal infection, prevention of progressive contamination, restoration of visceral integrity, and provision of nutritional support (Fig. 14.6). The first successful surgical repair of an esophageal perforation was reported in 1944 [7]. Since then, surgery has become the mainstay of definitive treatment, although this paradigm is being increasingly challenged by the advent of esophageal stents [8–10]. The primary surgical task is to achieve drainage of all contaminated spaces and

repair leakage when clinically appropriate. Soilage of the pleural cavity can be addressed via decortication through an open thoracotomy incision or with the use of video-assisted thoracoscopic surgery (VATS). Cervical esophageal perforations are accessed via a left oblique neck incision just anterior to sternocleidomastoid (Fig. 14.7, #1). In the upper two-thirds of the thoracic esophagus, a right posterolateral (often muscle-sparing) thoracotomy in the fourth or fifth intercostal space is required (Fig. 14.7, #2). If an intercostal muscle flap is planned for repair of the esophagus, it can be harvested during the exposure. A muscle-sparing approach is often preferred when performing open thoracotomy in the interest of preserving chest wall musculature for potential use later. Perforations in the lower third of the esophagus are best accessed through a left posterolateral thoracotomy in the sixth or seventh intercostal space (Fig. 14.7, #3). A vertical midline celiotomy incision or laparoscopic approach should be used for perforations of the intra-abdominal esophagus (Fig. 14.7, #4). Video-assisted thoracoscopic surgery should be reserved for early perforations and in those patients in whom adequate debridement of infected tissue can be ensured utilizing this technique [11]. Furthermore, thorough decortication allowing full expansion of the lung will augment healing. Tube thoracostomies with a minimum caliber tube of 32-french should be placed generously to achieve optimum postoperative drainage. Smaller caliber tubes are vulnerable to obstruction and should be avoided.

Most uncontained esophageal defects, particularly when detected early, are amenable to primary repair. This is done by closing the esophageal mucosa and muscularis in separate layers using 3–0 vicryl or similar absorbable suture. It may be necessary to separate the outer components of the inner circular and outer longitudinal muscle layers in order to gain adequate exposure to the underlying mucosal disruption. The thoracic cavity is then filled with saline and the esophagus insufflated using an endoscope to assess the integrity of the repair, which may be buttressed using a flap. We commonly use a pedicled intercostal muscle flap for this purpose, although the latissimus dorsi, serratus muscle, pericardial fat pad, diaphragm, omentum, or gastric fundus flap are alternate options [12]. The sternocleidomastoid, rhomboid, or pectoralis muscles are available for use in the repair of cervical esophageal perforations; however, these typically respond well to open drainage and often close spontaneously. Additionally, some authors have advocated for the use of reinforcing fibrin tissue patches at the time of primary repair, although research into the longevity of this approach is ongoing [13]. Our practice is to bridle a nasogastric tube into position with the distal end just above the level of the perforation at the time of operation.

Defects deemed not amenable to repair should be resected or stented. These include perforations encompassing more than fifty percent of the circumference of the esophageal wall, or those longer than three centimeters

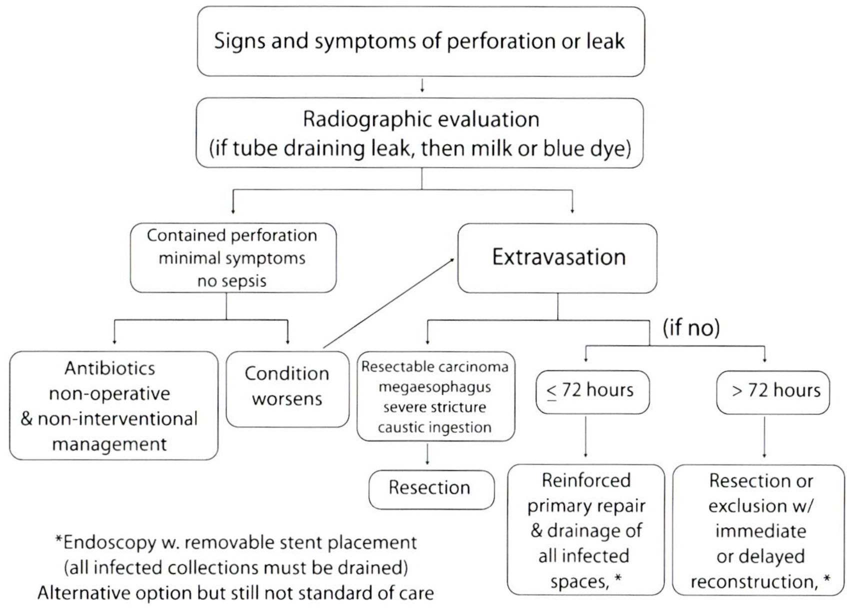

Fig. 14.6 Algorithm for the management of esophageal perforations

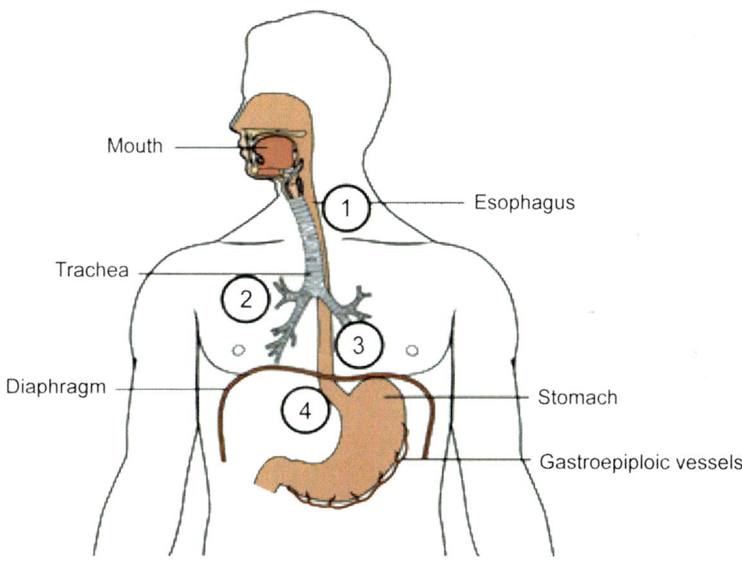

Fig. 14.7 Common locations of esophageal perforation

as they bear an unacceptable risk of stricture formation. Additionally, attempts at surgical repair are not recommended in those patients with a delayed presentation (>48 h). Alternative management strategies that can be considered for delayed perforations include hybrid approaches for complicated perforations. These include surgical debridement to place buttressing muscle flaps over the perforation, debride the contaminated area, provide wide local drainage of infected spaces, and complement the internal coverage achieved with stenting. It is important in this highly selected population for the surgeon to monitor for adequate drainage of infected spaces and competent sealage of the perforation postoperatively, and to proceed immediately to alternate therapy such as diversion oft an unsalvageable esophagus when either of these is compromised. T-tubes can be used to drain perforations deemed irreparable, but are an unreliable means of ensuring fistula control. High cervical defects with insufficient length for a diverting esophagostomy may require placement of a salivary bypass drainage tube.

Placement of a surgical gastrostomy tube at the time of operation should be considered in diverted patients and in those in whom the need for prolonged gastric drainage is anticipated. Additionally, either a gastrostomy or jejunostomy tube offers access for enteral feeding. Considering future needs for reconstruction, the gastrostomy tube should be placed in such a way that the gastroepiploic artery is not injured in an effort to prevent conduit complications.

Laparoscopic placement of the enteral tubes is preferred for this reason. If possible, esophagostomies should be created on the left anterior chest wall just below the clavicle rather than out of the neck incision, as this improves the fit and function of the ostomy appliance.

Postoperatively, the patient must be under continuous daily monitoring to ensure continued durability of the intervention. Daily vigilance must be exercised in securing all lines and tubes, and these authors advocate the use of bridling for all trans-nasal tubes to minimize inadvertent removal. Nutritional support either orally or through a feeding tube is always preferred. Additionally, patients should be continued on broad-spectrum antibiotics until they have recovered fully from the current infection, typically two weeks. Narrowing the spectrum of antibiotic coverage, as is typical for any infection, is recommended after a few days or once the sensitivities of the offending agent(s) are known. Microbes responsible for infections associated with esophageal perforations include *Staphylococcus*, *Pseudomonas*, *Streptococcus*, and *Bacteroides*, and adequate coverage for each of these species should be provided.

Conclusion

Re-perforation following complete healing is rare. Persistence of a leak after what is considered to be otherwise standard therapy should prompt an investigation for the presence of cancer or other impediments to normal wound healing. These include epithelialization, steroids, retained foreign body, poor nutritional status, radiation damage, persistent undrained infection, or distal obstruction. Patients who develop any symptoms, such as dysphagia, odynophagia, regurgitation, or noncardiac chest pain following hospital discharge should undergo a contrast swallow evaluation to assess for stricture, which occurs in up to 33% of patients [14].

References

1. Eroglu A, Turkyilmaz A, Aydin Y, Yekeler E, Karaoglanoglu N. Current management of esophageal perforation: 20 years experience. Dis Esophagus. 2009;22:374–80.
2. Brinster CJ, Singhal S, Lee L, Marshall MB, Kaiser LR, Kucharczuk JC. Evolving options in the management of esophageal perforation. Ann Thorac Surg. 2004;77:1475–83.
3. Kavic SM, Basson MD. Complications of endoscopy. Am J Surg. 2001;181:319–32.
4. Barrett NR. Spontaneous perforation of the oesophagus: review of the literature and report of three cases. Thorax. 1946;1:48–70.
5. Lucendo AJ, Friginal-Ruiz AB, Rodriguez B. Boerhaave's syndrome as the primary manifestation of adult eosinophilic esophagitis. Two case reports and a review of the literature. Dis Esophagus. 2011;34:E11–5.
6. Cohen MS, Kaufman A, DiMarino AJ, Cohen S. Eosinophilic esophagitis presenting as spontaneous esophageal rupture. Clin Gastroenterol Hepatol. 2007;5:24.
7. Olson AM, Clagget OT. Spontaneous rupture of the esophagus: report of a case with immediate diagnosis and successful surgical repair. Postgrad Med. 1947;2:417–21.
8. Blackmon SH, Santora R, Schwarz P, et al. Utility of removable esophageal covered self-expanding metal stents for leak and fistula management. Ann Thorac Surg. 2010;89(3):931–6.
9. David EA, Kim MP, Blackmon SH. Esophageal salvage with removable covered self-expanding metal stents in the setting of intrathoracic esophageal leakage. Am J Surg. 2011;202:796–801.
10. Freeman RK, Van Woerkom JM, Vyverberg A, Ascioti AJ. Esophageal stent placement for the treatment of spontaneous esophageal perforations. Ann Thorac Surg. 2009;88(1):194–8.
11. Nguyen NT, Hinojosa MW, Fayad C, Wilson SE. Minimally invasive management of intrathoracic leaks after esophagectomy. Surg Innov. 2007;14(2):96–101.
12. Martin LW, Hofstetter W, Swisher SG, Roth JA. Management of intrathoracic leaks following esophagectomy. Adv Surg. 2006;40:173–90.
13. Erdogan A, Gurses G, Keskin H, Demircan A. The sealing effect of a fibrin tissue patch on the esophageal perforation area in primary repair. World J Surg. 2007;31:2199–203.
14. Iannettoni MD, Vlessis AA, Whyte RI, Orringer MB. Functional outcome after surgical treatment of esophageal perforation. Ann Thorac Surg. 1997;34(6):1606–10.

Heena P. Santry and Bruce J. Simon

Introduction

Pneumothorax (PTX), hemothorax (HTX), and empyema are the most common pleural-based problems encountered by the acute care surgeon. Timely recognition and intervention can usually abort what would otherwise be highly morbid disease processes. This chapter discusses the presentation, diagnostic features, and current treatment strategies for these entities.

Pneumothorax

Epidemiology

Most PTX presenting to the emergency department are due to trauma. The incidence of PTX in the trauma population is as high as 20% in patients who arrive alive at the trauma center [1]. While penetrating trauma is a source of PTX, the mechanism of injury is more often blunt [2]. PTX is one of the most common injuries seen following blunt vehicular trauma where it is usually secondary to displaced rib fractures. Air leaking out of the punctured or lacerated lung decreases the negative pressure generated upon inhalation and causes the lung to collapse. In penetrating trauma, the PTX may also be caused by direct injury to the lung from the penetrating object causing air leakage. Alternatively, there may be entrance of air into the pleural space from the outside through the wound yielding an open PTX. If a one-way valve is created by a flap of lung or chest wall tissue preventing air egress on exhalation, positive pressure may build up shifting the mediastinum and impairing cardiac filling resulting in a tension PTX.

H.P. Santry, M.D. • B.J. Simon, M.D. (✉)
Trauma and Surgical Critical Care, Department of Surgery,
Umass Memorial Medical Center, 55 Lake Avenue North,
Worcester, MA 01655, USA
e-mail: Bruce.Simon@umassmemorial.org

The second most common cause of PTX, commonly referred to as spontaneous PTX, seen in the emergency room is a ruptured bleb. The age-adjusted incidence of spontaneous PTX is reported to range from 1 to 18 cases per 100,000 population per year [3]. Young adults will present with the rupture of an apical congenital bleb, an area of thinned lung tissue with abnormal interstitial development. This is far more common among young males and is rarely seen after age forty. In the middle-aged and older population, blebs result from long-standing emphysematous changes related to chronic obstructive pulmonary disease (COPD) due to tobacco use [4]. The risk of spontaneous PTX in the smoking population is reported to be 20 times higher than the non-smoking population and is dose dependent [3].

In the inpatient setting, acute care surgeons may be consulted for iatrogenic PTX. These are most commonly due to an attempted central venous catheter placement or other invasive procedure. The incidence of PTX after subclavian catheterization is reported to be 2.2% and after all invasive procedures is reported to be 1.4% [5].

Clinical Presentation and Diagnosis

The trauma victim with PTX will, of course, have an appropriate history of exposure to an injury mechanism. Complaints may relate to pain from associated rib fractures or may localize to extra-thoracic injuries. The young, otherwise healthy individual may not identify primary respiratory symptoms while the older person with less pulmonary reserve and possible co-morbidities may be in extremis from a unilateral simple PTX. Vital signs may be relatively normal or reveal sinus tachycardia. Pulse oximetry may be normal or decreased depending upon preexisting conditions, extent of PTX and other injuries, and splinting due to rib fractures. If a tension PTX is present, the patient may be hypotensive due to the impaired cardiac filling and demonstrate distended neck veins and a shift of the trachea to the contralateral side. Figure 15.1 shows the mediastinal shift that occurs with a tension PTX. It should be

L.J. Moore et al. (eds.), *Common Problems in Acute Care Surgery*,
DOI 10.1007/978-1-4614-6123-4_15, © Springer Science+Business Media New York 2013

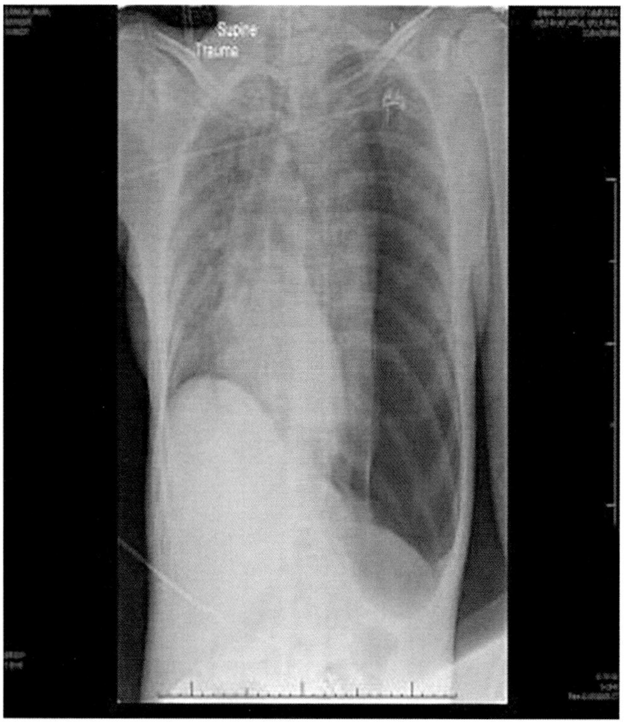

Fig. 15.1 A 43-year-old blunt trauma patient presenting with hypotension. Tension pneumothorax was not clinically diagnosed as the cause of hypotension and this chest radiograph was obtained. The image shows left-sided pneumothorax with mediastinal shift to the right causing vena cava compression and life-threatening hypotension. The patient's vital signs normalized after left-sided needle thoracostomy. A chest tube was subsequently placed. Image courtesy of Dr. Timothy Emhoff, University of Massachusetts Medical School

The diagnosis of PTX in the trauma setting has traditionally been made on a supine anterior–posterior (AP) chest radiograph [9]. Recently the extended focused assessment with sonography for trauma (FAST) exam has been promoted as a more sensitive modality for the identification of PTX, especially smaller ones. A recent meta-analysis revealed that ultrasound was 86–97% sensitive for detecting traumatic PTX as opposed to 28–75% for supine chest radiograph [9, 10]. The normal chest ultrasound will show visceral and pleural surfaces "sliding" over one another during respiration. Absence of "sliding" is a sensitive and specific indicator of PTX. In some trauma centers, ultrasound has supplanted initial supine radiograph for the diagnosis of PTX [9, 11]. Stable trauma patients without concern for spine injury should have an upright posterior–anterior (PA) chest radiograph. Many smaller PTX in trauma are seen only on computed tomography (CT) scan of the chest. These are termed occult PTX. Stable patients suspected of a non-traumatic PTX should still have conventional upright PA and lateral radiographs in the radiology suite.

Because it is immediately life-threatening, the conventional teaching for tension PTX is that if it is suspected on clinical grounds, it should be treated without confirmatory radiography [12]. The increasing availability of immediate bedside ultrasound may alter this practice in the future as more information on the efficacy of this modality emerges [13, 14].

Management

noted, however, that the absence of these two findings does not rule out a tension PTX. For example, if there is significant concurrent blood loss from other injuries, distended neck veins may be absent despite the presence of a tension PTX.

The teenager or young adult with a spontaneous rupture of a congenital bleb can usually identify the onset of acute pain. As these individuals are healthy, they usually complain of minimal to no dyspnea [6–8]. They are rarely hypoxic. Conversely, the middle-aged smoker with COPD and rupture of an emphysematous bleb will usually be dyspneic due to the acute loss of lung volume on the background of borderline pulmonary function. Physical examination will reveal absent breath sounds on the affected side. Auscultation should always be performed in the axilla as transmitted contralateral breath sounds may be falsely interpreted as ipsilateral aeration. The examiner may note chest wall tenderness and crepitus due to subcutaneous emphysema. This occurs when air leaking from the lung insinuates into the chest wall through a tear in the parietal pleura. It is classically manifest on exam as "Rice Krispies crunching" under the skin, and, if widespread, may cause the patient to appear like the "Stay Puft marshmallow man" due to subcutaneous emphysema involving the neck and face.

All patients who are being seen in consultation for a traumatic chest injury should have an appropriate overall trauma evaluation commensurate with the Advanced Trauma Life Support (ATLS) practices of the American College of Surgeons and in accordance with local institutional practices [12]. The traditional initial treatment for all symptomatic traumatic PTX has been, and for the most part remains, the placement of a large tube thoracostomy tube (32–36 French) in the fifth intercostal space at the anterior or mid-axillary line with the application of suction through a water seal drainage system [12]. Recently, however, there has been a trend to place smaller percutaneous tubes by the Seldinger technique in the second intercostal space at the anterior axillary line for the evacuation of smaller PTX. Though seemingly less traumatic, the use of these so-called pigtail catheters remains controversial. Small amounts of concurrent pleural blood, often unappreciated on semi-upright chest radiographs after injury, may clog these tubes. Fig. 15.2a shows a subtle left-sided HTX as visualized on the initial chest radiograph taken in the trauma bay. However, as seen in Fig. 15.2b, the patient had a sizeable posteriorly layering left HTX. Additionally, pigtail catheters do not have the diameter to evacuate large-volume air leaks and often require a second tube [15].

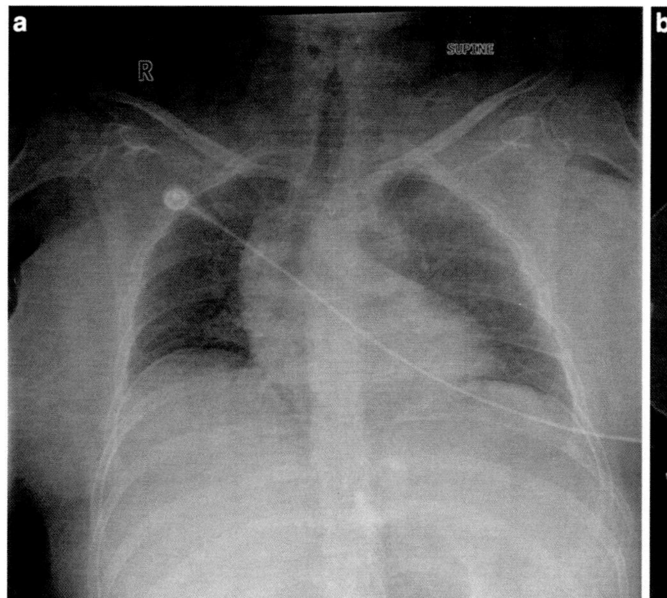

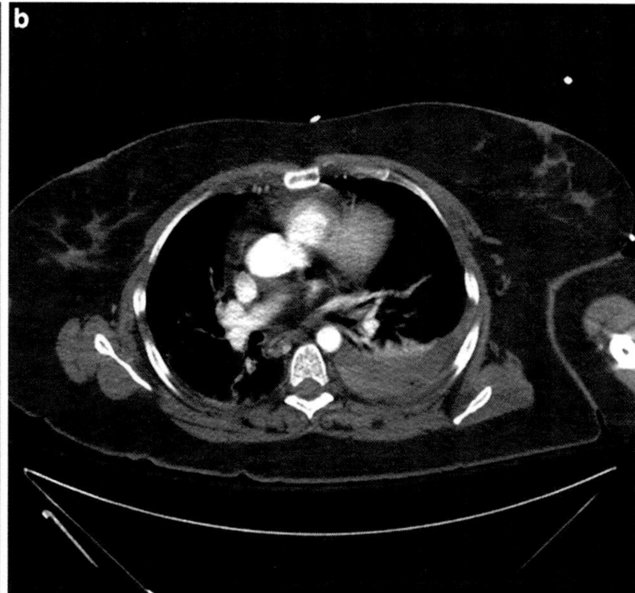

Fig. 15.2 (**a**) This supine radiograph shows slightly increased opacity on the left side. The size of hemothorax was not appreciated until subsequent CT imaging was obtained. (**b**) This CT scan of the chest corresponds to Fig. 15.2a and shows a sizeable left-sided hemothorax that was missed on initial supine chest radiograph. Images courtesy of Dr. Dennis Coughlin, University of Massachusetts Medical School

Patients who have hemodynamic or respiratory instability felt due to a tension PTX should have needle decompression of the pleural space using a 14 gauge 2-in. angiocatheter in the second intercostal space at the mid-clavicular line while preparations are made for thoracostomy tube placement. This is an immediate life-threatening condition and should be diagnosed on clinical grounds rather than radiographic findings as demonstrated in Fig. 15.1. Decompression will release positive pressure, allowing the mediastinum to return to midline and the patient to re-compensate. If the diagnosis of tension PTX was correctly made, the patient will improve in color and blood pressure almost immediately. A tube thoracostomy is then required as previously mentioned to treat the simple (non-tension) PTX thus created [12, 16].

Once the desired thoracostomy tube is placed, lung inflation should be confirmed by chest radiograph, preferably upright, and the amount of air leak, if any, should be noted. Failure of the lung to inflate with a large continuous air leak in the water seal chamber may indicate a tracheobronchial injury, which should be confirmed by bronchoscopy. If present, a second chest tube should be considered as the first maneuver. Thoracic specialty consultation should be obtained. The management of this injury is beyond the scope of this text. Failure of the lung to inflate without an air leak indicates mal-positioning of the tube, usually in the subcutaneous tissue or occlusion of the chest tube, drainage system, or bronchi. The system should be checked and bronchoscopy may be indicated. After placement of a thoracostomy tube, trauma patients treated for PTX should have a dynamic chest CT or CT angiogram contemplated to assess other latent thoracic injuries. It is well recognized that three thoracic injuries are identified on CT for every single injury noted on chest radiograph.

The increased sensitivity of CT scans will document occult PTX. Occult PTX is defined as a PTX noted only on CT scan but not evident on conventional chest radiograph [2, 17–20]. There is an increasing body of evidence and expert opinion that occult PTX are extremely unlikely to enlarge and can therefore be managed conservatively, as long as they remain stable in size and patients remain free of respiratory symptoms attributable to the PTX [13, 21]. Some have reported the successful deferral of thoracostomy even in the setting of positive pressure ventilation for surgical procedures [22]. However, the decision to defer thoracostomy should be approached cautiously in the multi-trauma patient. In this setting, an untreated PTX may create confusion when the patient suffers a hemodynamic or respiratory decompensation for unrelated reasons.

The spontaneous PTX due to congenital bleb in the young patient may be treated with a tube thoracostomy in the second interspace at the midclavicular line using a conventional tube or a pigtail catheter. The COPD patient with emphysematous bleb rupture may be treated similarly. However, in this situation a non-contrast chest CT should generally be obtained prior to tube placement (assuming that the patient is stable without evidence of tension physiology or respiratory compromise) to differentiate PTX from a giant emphysematous bleb [6–8, 23]. Placement of thoracostomy tubes into giant emphysematous blebs results in a bronchopleural fistula, which is very difficult to manage.

Small iatrogenic PTX due to attempted subclavian central venous catheter placement can generally be treated by

Table 15.1 Tube thoracostomy placement procedure

"Pearls" for tube thoracostomy placement
• Enter pleural space using a *blunt* Kelly clamp controlled by two hands
• Place index finger in pleural space prior to tube placement to assess for adhesions
• Place the tube attached to clamp. "Free hand" placement always fails with tube residing in subcutaneous tissue
• Fix the tube with "0" suture material, silk, braided polyester, or equivalent. Slightly indent tube with suture to assure firm hold
• Failure of lung to inflate without air leak means system obstruction or bronchial obstruction
• Failure of lung to inflate with large air leak may indicate central tracheobronchial injury. Second tube and/or bronchoscopy indicated

observation or by placement of an apical pigtail catheter with good results since the site of injury is known to be at the apex. Larger iatrogenic PTX should receive conventional thoracostomy tubes placed in the apical position [24]. Table 15.1 presents pearls for thoracostomy tube placement.

Once the chest tube is in place and inflation of the lung is confirmed on radiograph, numerous protocols and guidelines exist for tube management [25]. In general, once the lung is inflated and pleural surfaces are brought into apposition, the air leak should cease. The thoracostomy tube is then left to suction for 24–48 h to allow pleural symphysis or sealing to occur. Time to sealing will vary with the magnitude of the air leak and the patient's overall nutritional status. The removal of the tube from suction, known as placement on "water seal," is generally used to confirm healing of the pleural leak. The water seal chamber on the drainage system is monitored for recurrence of an air leak, and if none is noted a confirmatory radiograph is done, typically from 3 to 8 h later. However, there is very little evidence supporting the duration of time necessary on water seal before a radiograph is performed [26]. If a recurrent leak is noted in the drainage system leak chamber, the system is placed back on suction and a radiograph is done to confirm that the lung remains inflated. Suction is continued another 24–48 h before reattempting water seal.

Importantly, the lung may remain inflated on water seal even when small air leaks are present since a route of egress for the air is available. Removal of the tube in this setting will lead to a recurrent PTX. Therefore, it is important to identify even small leaks in the leak chamber of the drainage system. This can be done by checking for air leaks during forced expiration by asking the patient to take deep breaths in and out and to cough. If a forced expiratory air leak is identified the chest tube should remain in place until completely resolved.

As noted previously, failure of the lung to inflate after tube thoracostomy with a large air leak should raise concern for tracheobronchial injury. However, persistent failure of small air leaks to seal despite inflated lung or recurrent PTX on water seal may present both a diagnostic and therapeutic challenge. A CT scan with the thoracostomy tube on suction should be done to identify uninflated areas of lung that may be contributing to a persistent air leak. Additional thoracostomy tubes or radiologically guided drainage catheters may be required. Video-assisted thoracoscopic surgery (VATS) for pleurodesis may ultimately be needed [27–30]. Surgical pleurodesis involves the application of various irritants to the pleural surfaces to cause inflammatory adhesion of the visceral and parietal pleura and thereby seal air leaks. There is some literature advocating very early VATS intervention in persistent air leak in trauma patients at 48 h post injury [31, 32]. As of this writing, any benefit of such an approach for PTX alone has not been definitively demonstrated. Figure 15.3 shows a general composite algorithm for the management of traumatic PTX.

Importantly, with spontaneous PTX due to ruptured congenital or emphysematous blebs, the lungs are inherently abnormal and sealing of the air leak may take longer than 48 h or may even fail to occur. When tube thoracostomy fails to seal a pleural leak in this clinical setting, surgical intervention, typically VATS with pleurodesis, is required.

Complications

The most common complication of PTX is respiratory failure. In the trauma setting, this is usually due to the combined effect of the loss of lung volume, pain, and splinting from associated rib fractures, burden of associated injuries, and any preexisting pulmonary conditions. Consequently, in addition to reinflating the lung, a thorough approach must be taken in ameliorating the concomitant causes of respiratory failure in the trauma patient. Failure of lung inflation is a rare complication of conservative management without thoracostomy. This usually does not occur unless there is associated pleural blood (HTX) causing an inflammatory response and resultant trapped lung (further described in the next section).

The main iatrogenic complications of thoracostomy placement include injury to almost any intrathoracic structure. This can be avoided by carefully palpating and exploring with the operating finger through the thoracostomy incision prior to placing the tube. Adhesions are swept away and placement above the diaphragm is ensured. Often chest tube placement introduces some degree of additional pain and immobility to patients which is not desirable. Consequently, the decision to place a tube should be carefully considered in cases of smaller PTX. Reasonable respiratory benefit should be expected as a trade-off for the potential increase in splinting due to the presence of the tube.

Follow-Up

There is no evidence that patients who have had traumatic PTX inflated by a thoracostomy and show full inflation on "post-pull" radiograph several hours later need any further imaging as long as they remain clinically well. Nonetheless, it

Fig. 15.3 Algorithm for the management of acute traumatic pneumothorax

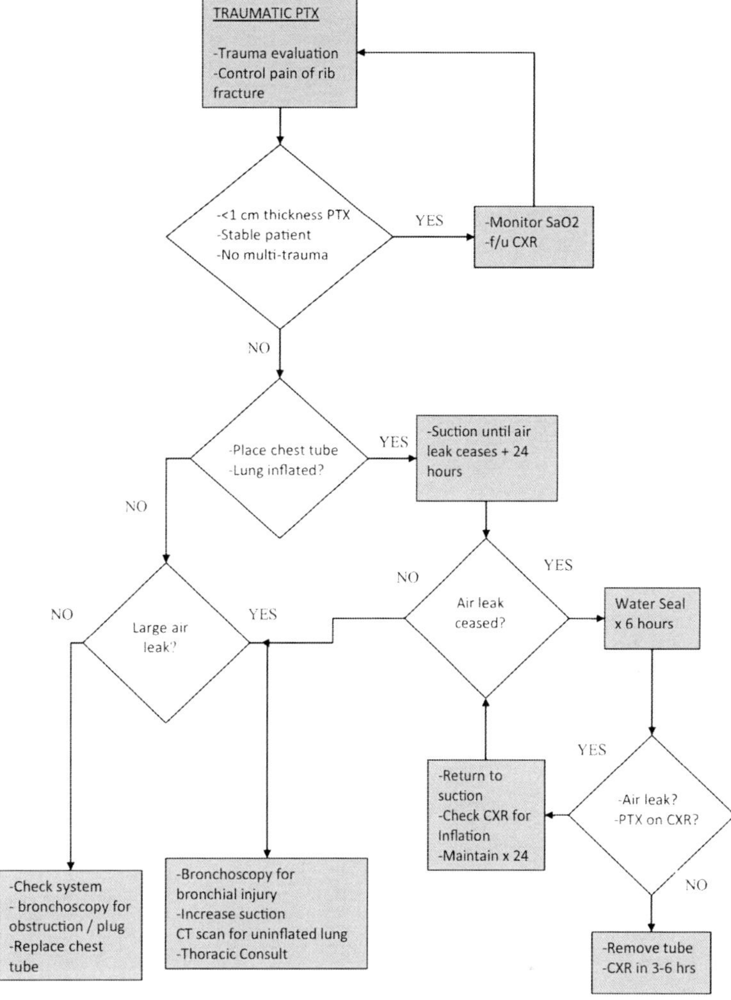

is the customary practice at many institutions to obtain a follow-up radiograph prior to discharge or at clinic visit. Patients who have been treated conservatively for small PTX generally receive a follow-up radiograph several weeks later to document full lung expansion, though the benefit of this also remains unclear. Recurrences are rare in otherwise healthy individuals in either situation. There is no standardized follow-up for patients with spontaneous PTX due to congenital bleb or emphysematous bleb rupture. These patients will generally become symptomatic if recurrences occur. They should maintain a close relationship with their pulmonologist or thoracic surgeon as recurrence rates may be as high as 50% [6–8].

Hemothorax

Epidemiology

The single major cause of HTX for all age groups is trauma, usually blunt [33]. Twenty-five percent of patients with chest trauma will be diagnosed with HTX [34]. Here the typical etiologic factor is intercostal vessel bleeding caused by fractured ribs, though other sources such as lung parenchyma laceration or hilar vascular injuries have been reported. Rare non-traumatic causes include pleural malignancy, iatrogenic injury, and spontaneous HTX due to pathologic coagulopathy [35]. For the purposes of this discussion we will be referring to traumatic HTX unless otherwise specified.

Clinical Presentation and Diagnosis

Three initial (acute) clinical presentations are common for HTX, each requiring its own approach to management. These include (1) immediate HTX with hemodynamic instability, (2) immediate HTX without hemodynamic instability, and (3) delayed HTX, which may appear up to 2 weeks after chest wall injury in up to 7% of all patients with rib fractures [33, 36, 37].

The unstable patient presenting to the trauma bay will have an appropriate history of mechanism, for example motor vehicle driver with side impact or stab wound to the thorax or upper abdomen. They may be hypotensive or merely tachycardic. Oxygen saturation may be low or normal depending upon loss of lung volume, other injuries, and pre-existing respiratory status. They may complain of dyspnea. Physical examination reveals absent breath sounds on the affected side. Here, diagnosis is often made by emergent placement of the thoracostomy tube and the expression of a large amount of blood.

The stable patient with HTX may have respiratory or pain-related complaints or both. Clinical examination may or may not identify decreased breath sounds but there will often be chest wall tenderness. Here diagnosis is made by chest radiograph, preferably in the semi-upright position. It should be remembered that on the supine radiograph, very significant fluid collections may yield only a barely detectable increased opacity on the injured side (Fig. 15.2). These HTX may not be suspected until incidentally noted on the lower thoracic cuts of an abdominal CT. Several centers have begun to utilize the FAST examination to identify HTX, but the efficacy of this has not yet been fully determined [38].

The patient presenting with a delayed HTX is often in-hospital or may even have been discharged to home, as this acute bleeding may occur up to 2 weeks after initial trauma [39, 40]. The mechanism here is hypothesized to improve pain control allowing for increased respiratory excursion that then results in a new tear of an intercostal vessel at a fracture site. The incidence of delayed HTX is increased with multiple and displaced rib fractures. Presentation is varied and may be predominantly one of blood loss with tachycardia, malaise, or overt hemorrhagic shock. Alternatively, it may manifest as respiratory symptoms ranging from mild exercise intolerance all the way to respiratory distress. Presentation may be very subtle and missed in the patient still incapacitated from distant injuries. For patients on mechanical ventilation, the HTX may be a surprising incidental finding on a routine chest radiograph.

Management

In severe or multi-trauma patients, the treatment of HTX, like that of any injury, should be prioritized based on the principles of ATLS [12]. If an HTX is suspected or documented on chest radiograph, a large thoracostomy tube, 36 or 40 French, is inserted in the fifth intercostal space at the posterior or mid-axillary line. If a massive HTX is expected based on radiograph or presentation, an autotransfusion attachment should be placed in line with the chest drainage system to scavenge and return shed blood. This may provide an immediate improvement in stability; however, it has not been shown to decrease transfusion requirements [36].

For the unstable patient whose immediate chest tube output is ≥1,500 ml, a massive HTX, and who remains unstable, immediate thoracotomy remains the treatment of choice along with autologous and banked blood resuscitation [12]. This has been based on the rationale that large shed blood volumes indicate injury to larger vessels, such as intercostal arteries, the internal mammary artery, or more central lung vasculature that are less likely to cease bleeding without operative control of the vessel in question. For patients with large initial thoracostomy outputs who are stable, or readily stabilized, VATS is being used successfully in the acute setting by several groups to avoid thoracotomy [31, 41]. It has been shown that this procedure can be safely performed by acute care surgeons with the appropriate experience with thoracic surgical backup as needed [42]. Electrocautery and clips can be applied thoracoscopically to control moderate hemorrhage. The lower morbidity of this procedure may make it applicable in the future to patients with lesser but still significant thoracostomy outputs for whom the risk/benefit ratio for full thoracotomy may be unfavorable.

Stable patients with lesser immediate chest tube output should have complete evacuation of the HTX with tube thoracostomy and subsequent lung inflation documented on an upright chest radiograph. The trauma workup should be completed as necessary. This should include chest CT to identify significant thoracic injuries related or unrelated to the HTX, especially in the setting of penetrating trauma. The chest tube output is monitored hourly and the patient monitored in at least an intermediate care setting. Numerous protocols exist to trigger surgery in such stable patients based on continuing chest tube output. Examples are 250 ml/h for 2 h or 125 ml/h for 4 h [12, 37]. These are not hard-and-fast rules, however, and there is no substitute for good surgical judgment. Factors to consider when deciding upon intervention, be it by thoracotomy or VATS, include trend in chest tube output, patient stability, associated injuries, and the patient's overall health. Sudden cessation of chest tube output during monitoring, particularly if the patient becomes unstable, should raise concern for occlusion of the thoracostomy tube and prompt an immediate chest radiograph to assess for re-accumulation.

Some success has been reported using angiographic embolization to control intercostal bleeding or internal mammary artery bleeding in stable patients for whom chest CT has shown contrast extravasation or a "blush" indicative of arterial bleeding [43]. More validation is required for use of this modality, but over time this may prove applicable to stable patients with moderate thoracostomy output. Figure 15.4 shows a patient successfully treated with angioembolization of the left internal mammary artery for HTX sustained due to a fall.

Patients with lesser initial chest tube drainage (<1,000 ml) and clearing of the chest radiograph who remain unstable should be investigated for extrathoracic injuries or non-traumatic causes of their shock. Figure 15.5 illustrates a composite of algorithms for the management of acute HTX.

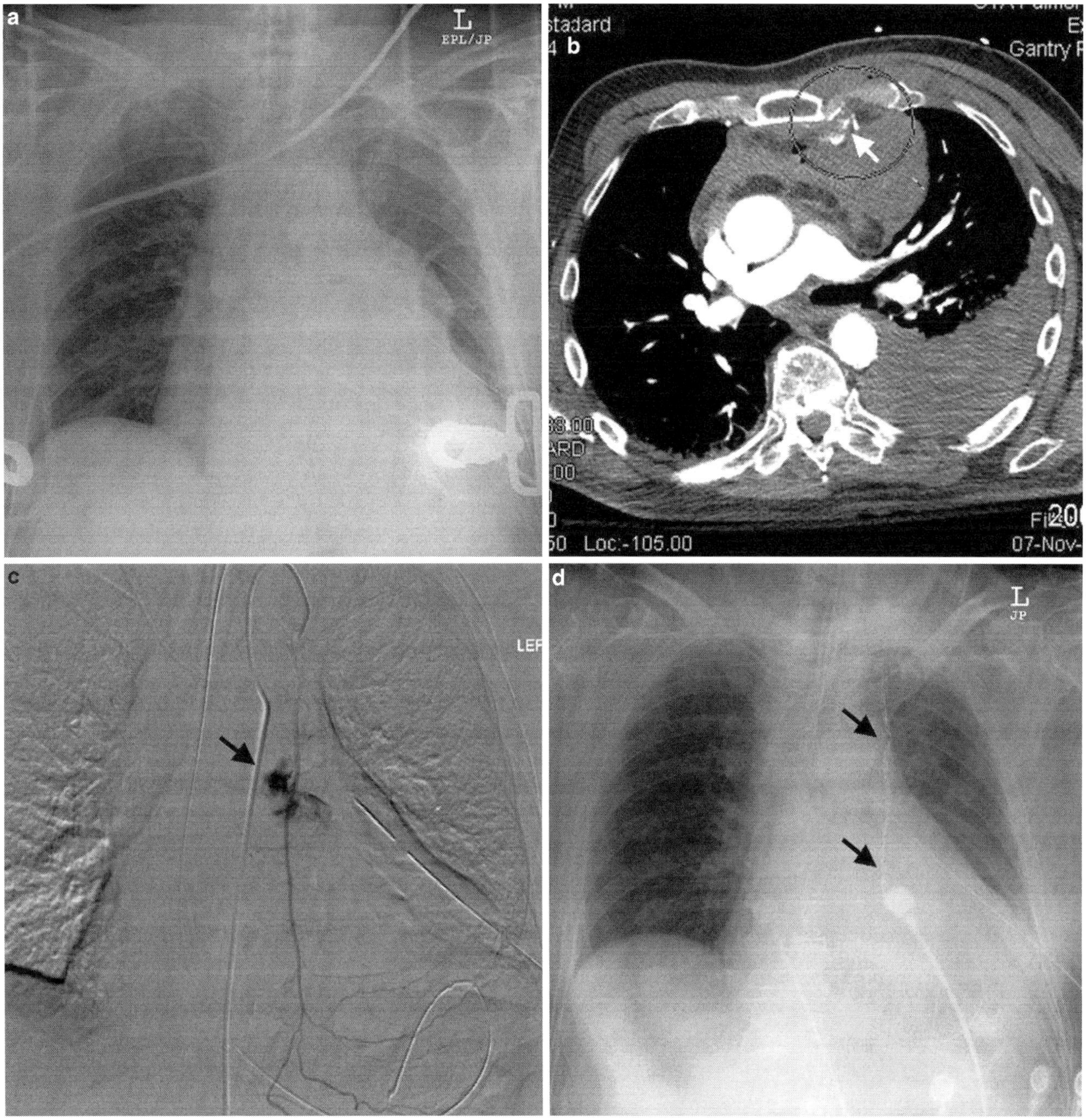

Fig. 15.4 An 88-year-old blunt trauma patient with sterna and rib fractures transferred to trauma center after left-sided chest tube placement for hemothorax. (**a**) Shows initial chest X-ray. *White arrow* in (**b**) shows contrast extravasation from the left internal mammary artery adjacent to bone fragments from the sterna fracture (*circled*). *Dark arrow* in (**c**) shows ongoing contrast extravasation at angiography. The patient was successfully treated with coil embolization as shown by the *dark arrows* in (**d**). Image courtesy of Dr. Suvaraju Ganguli and Ms. Stephanie Hanson, Massachusetts General Hospital

In stable patients with radiographic evidence of HTX, the question commonly arises as to how much volume of intrathoracic blood mandates drainage. Several studies have indicated that complications can occur with as little as 300–500 ml of intrathoracic blood [44]. In general, almost all traumatic HTX that completely opacify the costophrenic angle on plain radiographs should be evacuated as early as possible to prevent complications [37, 42]. In multi-planar CT imaging, this has been correlated to the thickness of the lateral pleural fluid stripe. Evidence suggests that a stripe >1.5 cm in thickness is an indication for a drainage intervention [45]. Table 15.2 illustrates pearls for the management of acute traumatic HTX.

Retained HTX after initial chest tube drainage is now recognized as a source of considerable morbidity, requiring late

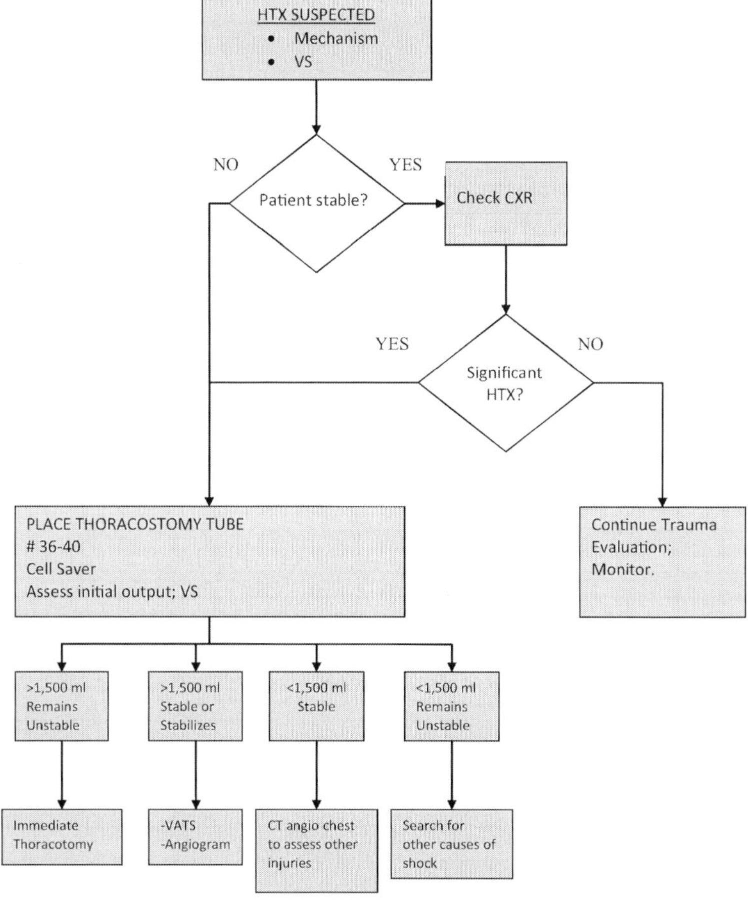

Fig. 15.5 Algorithm for the management of acute traumatic hemothorax

Table 15.2 Management of acute traumatic HTX

"Pearls" for management of acute traumatic hemothorax
• HTX greater than 300–500 ml (or those that opacify the costophrenic angle on upright CXR) should be evacuated as soon as possible
• Use a 36–40 Fr thoracostomy tube
• Use an in-line auto-transfuser for large HTX in unstable patients
• Confirm complete evacuation by CXR
• Monitor patients with multiple rib fractures for delayed HTX
• Early evacuation of retained HTX by VATS ideally within 2 days, but no later than 5 days

thoracotomy in up to 16.7% of patients with initial thoracostomy tube [42, 44–48]. Complications of retained HTX include prolonged or permanent loss of lung volume due to formation of a restrictive peel (fibrothorax) and pleural infection (empyema) in up to 15% of cases [49]. The volume of the retained intrathoracic blood has been shown to directly correlate with the risk of empyema [50]. Prompt and appropriate treatment of retained HTX is warranted because even mild to moderate loss of lung volume can lead to decreased exercise tolerance or to overt respiratory insufficiency in patients with pre-injury respiratory dysfunction.

An increasing number of groups now intervene early in retained HTX using VATS and pleural lavage to liquefy and aspirate the clot and early forming peel in the gelatinous phase prior to fibrous organization. High-pressure lavage has been shown to be very effective for this purpose [47]. The time frame appropriate for evacuation of retained HTX remains debated. Traditionally, a period of three to five days was felt to be appropriate as this was the minimum time for early solidification of the clot and good results have been shown with this algorithm. Others believe even earlier intervention should be performed for optimal results [48]. Consequently, a tube thoracostomy is placed at admission and clearing of the HTX monitored by chest radiograph. If there is failure of clearing after 48 h, VATS is performed. Figure 15.6 shows evacuation of an early clotted HTX via VATS.

Others have addressed the early retained HTX with repeated administration of thrombolytic agents such as streptokinase or more recently tissue plasminogen activator (TPA) via the thoracostomy tube. High rates of success without hemorrhagic complications have been reported in small studies [51]. The practical concern here relates to the administration of thrombolytics in such a close time frame to major trauma. Life-threatening hemorrhagic complications have been reported [52]. Administration of thrombolytics is contraindicated in patients with other injury sites where even modest bleeding would be catastrophic, such as the brain, spinal cord, or globe

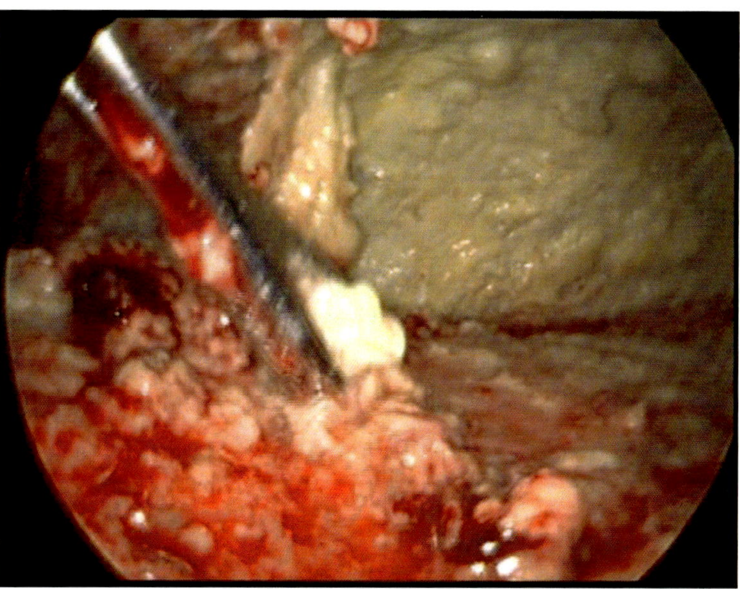

Fig. 15.6 Intra-operative photograph of evacuation of an early clotted hemothorax with video thoracoscopy (VATS). The *thick white surface at the top of the field* is the chest wall or parietal pleura with a fibrous inflammatory peel. The *area on the bottom of the field* represents residual hemorrhage adherent to the peel on the lung surface (visceral peel). The instrument pictured is a large-bore suction catheter

of the eye. It is also relatively contraindicated for patients with injuries for which surgical hemostasis has not been achieved such as pelvic fractures. The optimal dosing and number of treatments are yet to be determined. Figure 15.7 outlines an algorithm for the management of retained HTX.

Empyema

Epidemiology

Empyema is strictly defined as infection in the pleural space. This may range from grossly innocuous free pleural fluid in which an aspirate shows bacteria to a mature intrapleural abscess cavity formed when infection stimulates inflammatory fibrous in-growth on the pleural surfaces. This creates a "pseudocapsule" between the visceral and parietal pleura. The most common location for an empyema in the pleural space is dependant and posterior in the phrenic recess, as this is where the infected pleural fluid will accumulate.

A retained HTX is the greatest independent risk factor for the development of an empyema in the trauma population and the risk correlates directly with the volume of retained blood [50]. Other risk factors include prolonged duration of tube thoracostomy, length of intensive care unit (ICU) stay, presence of pulmonary contusion, overall injury severity, and need for laparotomy [53]. In the trauma patient, the infecting organism is usually *Staphylococcus* species acquired at the time of tube placement in blunt trauma or from the penetrating projectile, skin, or clothing fragments in penetrating trauma victims. On occasion, hematogenous spread may occur from other infectious sites or from primary bacteremias [54, 55]. The incidence of empyema after traumatic HTX is reported to be as high as 4% [56].

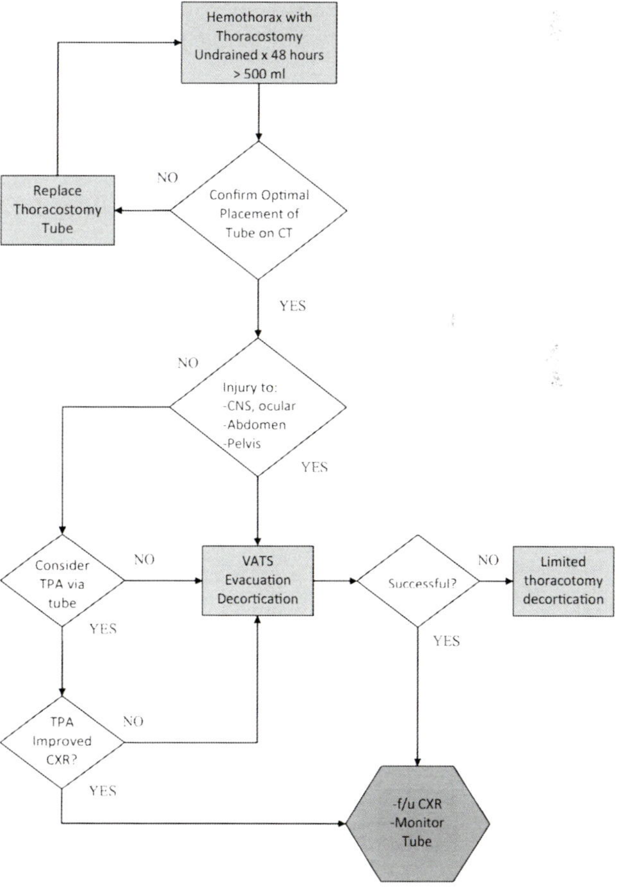

Fig. 15.7 Algorithm for the management of retained hemothorax

The most common cause of empyema in the non-trauma patient is consequent to a bacterial pneumonia that penetrates the visceral pleura spilling purulent material into the pleural space (parapneumonic empyema). Organisms here are again mostly *Staphylococcus* but may also be *Streptococcus*,

Pneumococus, and others. Gram-negative organisms are rarely reported. In patients with appropriate risk factors such as malnutrition, intravenous drug use, and immune compromise, *Mycobacterium tuberculosis* may also be causative [57]. The incidence of parapneumonic empyema is reportedly increasing and was as high as 6 per 100,000 in 2008 [58].

As far back as the 1960s, the natural history of empyema was recognized as having three pathologic stages: acute or exudative, transitional or fibrinopurulent, and chronic or fibrous [59]. The exudative phase is defined by outpouring of sterile fluid in response to inflammation. This inflammation can be due to a pleurisy associated with a pneumonia that has penetrated the pleura or to the inflammation of a degrading HTX. Classically, the fluid is thin, with a low cellular content, low lactate dehydrogenase (LDH) content, and a normal pH and glucose. Critical in this phase is the observation that the pleural surfaces are still mobile, which is critical to the treatment strategy.

The fibrinopurulent phase is characterized by thicker fluid due to increased neutrophil content and the beginning of fibrous in-growth into the pleura. This will begin the process of trapping the lung that still remains relatively mobile. Due to bacterial activity, the pH and glucose begin to fall and LDH begins to rise [14].

The fibrous phase is marked by development of the pleural peel with capillary in-growth and rigid fixation of the pleural cavity, known as the empyema space. The time to development of the fibrous phase has been noted to be anywhere from 7 days to 6 weeks after the start of the infectious process. Typically at this stage, pleural fluid glucose is less than 40 mg/dl and pH less than 7. However, the absence of these laboratory criteria does not rule out the presence of infection.

The pathologic stages of empyema may be less relevant when a retained HTX is the causative problem as opposed to a parapneumonic origin. The process of development of empyema here represents a continuum from organizing HTX with degrading clot, through contamination, to the development of gross pus [60]. A variable degree of inflammatory reaction and fibrous in-growth may occur from the HTX itself prior to bacterial contamination or multiplication of existing bacteria in the blood medium. Consequently the time course of development of empyema in retained HTX is variable.

Not uncommonly, purulent-appearing fluid evacuated from patients with clinical and radiographic manifestations of empyema is found to be sterile. Still, the patient improves after evacuation. This so-called sterile empyema likely represents a systemic inflammatory response to the degradation of the HTX.

Clinical Presentation and Diagnosis

Post-traumatic empyema may manifest in the ICU-confined patient on a ventilator, in the ambulatory patient on the surgical floor, or at home after discharge. The presentation in each case may differ significantly. In the ICU setting, the patient with a known thoracic injury will show a persistent chest opacity on radiograph or develop a new opacity, usually associated with signs of infection such as leukocytosis or fever. These parameters, however, may only be minimally elevated and are often attributed to a plethora of other infectious or noninfectious causes. Often there will be more subtle signs of infection in the ICU patient such as glucose intolerance, failure to wean from the ventilator, or failure to achieve an anabolic nutritional state. Fulminant septic shock with pressor dependence is not a common presentation of empyema [60]. Radiographic findings often lead to a CT scan of the chest, which may show the classical findings of a thickened pleural peel of the empyema space, high-density fluid, often heterogeneous, and possibly loculated air. These features combined with high clinical suspicion are felt to be most sufficient to prompt intervention without initial bacteriological confirmation [36, 57]. The classical findings may be absent, however, particularly if the injury course since HTX has been short. If empyema is still suspected, diagnostic thoracentesis under ultrasound or CT guidance should be undertaken. Figure 15.8 shows a right-sided empyema space with a well-formed fibrous pleural peel.

In the recovering patient on the surgical floor or already at home, an empyema often develops from a missed delayed HTX or underappreciated occult HTX. Here general malaise rather than respiratory symptoms is the predominant complaint. Hospital vital signs usually reveal low-grade temperature and/or mild tachycardia. The patient at home may note intermittent episodes of rigors or chills. In both cases, chest radiograph abnormalities will lead to CT scanning and diagnostic thoracentesis if CT findings are equivocal.

Patients with parapneumonic empyema may be sick inpatients with multiple medical problems who have recently had a health-care-associated pneumonia. In this case, the transition from pneumonia to empyema may be subtle and there may be only a brief period or no period with respiratory improvement and resolution of the signs of infection. Alternatively, the healthy ambulatory patient with an apparently mild community-acquired pneumonia may also develop empyema. In this case, an improvement in infectious and respiratory symptoms with pneumonia may be noted prior to apparent recurrence. Finally, in the otherwise healthy, ambulatory patient, the initial pneumonia may be missed by the patient, or noted as a "bad cold" and he or she may primarily present with the malaise and infectious symptoms of empyema.

Parapneumonic empyema may be as dependent as post-traumatic empyema or may be localized to the site of the pneumonia if the perforating process was effectively walled-off by the pleural surfaces. Because of this, changes in radiographic findings may be subtle and may be interpreted only as failure of clearance of the pneumonia.

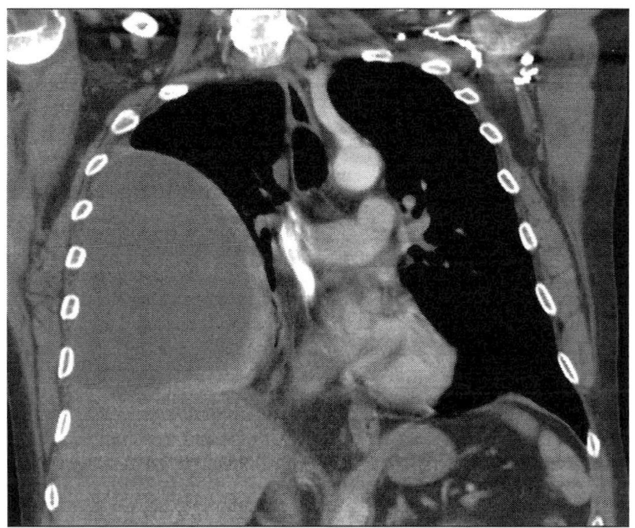

Fig. 15.8 CT scan showing a large empyema space with a well-formed, thick fibrous peel

Management

Once definitively diagnosed by microbiology, or highly suspected by clinical presentation, all empyemas should be evacuated. Concurrently, broad-spectrum antibiotics should be started for gram-positive and gram-negative organisms with the intent of narrowing spectrum once specific microbiology is obtained. The ultimate goal of treatment is to empty the empyema space and fully inflate the lung so that the pleural surfaces are in apposition and recurrence cannot occur. Antibiotics are ancillary and will be unsuccessful in curing the infection if residual empyema space persists.

The interventions required to evacuate empyema depend upon the pathologic stage at which the intervention occurs [36, 53, 61]. In the early or exudative phase, tube thoracostomy, either surgically or percutaneously placed, will usually evacuate the fluid and lead to lung inflation. A baseline CT scan should be obtained if not already done to assess for loculated collections and to prognosticate on the likelihood of success of nonoperative management. Visible peel indicates that pathologic stage II or III has been reached. Either way, thoracostomy drainage is the first mode of treatment; with the anticipation of thick fluid in the advanced stages a large surgical tube (32 to 36 French) is desirable.

Results are measured by tube output and clearing of the chest radiograph. If unsuccessful, thrombolytic dissolution may be attempted with TPA through the thoracostomy prior to surgical intervention as long as there are no contraindications such as those previously discussed. TPA is pushed through the thoracostomy tube with a syringe and the tube is then clamped for several hours as the patient assumes various positions to dwell the medication throughout the accessible pleural space. If partial improvement is obtained as measured by additional chest tube output and radiologic improvement, additional doses can be given, though the risk of hemorrhage may increase with additional doses [62, 63]. Several groups have reported that this method is highly successful in evacuating empyema spaces with rare nonlife-threatening hemorrhagic complications [62, 63]. Most patients studied were suffering from parapneumonic effusions. Thrombolytics are less likely to be successful in the chronic, fibrous phase of an empyema.

For patients who have failed thrombolytics or are felt to have a thickened chronic cavity unlikely to improve with TPA, surgical intervention will be required. Whether VATS decortication should be attempted prior to thoracotomy is based on the skill set and judgment of the surgeon, the duration and radiologic appearance of the empyema space, and the patient's overall condition. In general, chronic empyema spaces of long duration with thickened fibrous peels require open thoracotomy for drainage and decortication. It should also be noted that parapneumonic empyema in association with a badly destroyed lung may require concurrent pulmonary resection in order to achieve cure. Resection in the face of infection raises the risk of bronchial stump breakdown. These complex cases should be managed by a thoracic surgical specialist.

The critical principles of open decortication include full release of the peel on the visceral and parietal pleural surfaces. The major reason for recurrent empyema is failure to completely decorticate the diaphragmatic surface, thereby failing to enable full lung expansion. The hilar area should not be decorticated as little expansion normally occurs in this area and the danger of injury to hilar structures outweighs the benefits of the additional minor re-expansion. Optimal operative chest tube placement is critical to the outcome of decortication. Typically, three tubes are placed. In addition to the traditional anterior and posterior apical tubes, a tube, often curved, should be placed on the diaphragmatic surface to prevent re-accumulation in this location.

For patients who are judged to be too unstable or debilitated for open thoracotomy, open external drainage may be performed if CT indicates that the peel has fully excluded the empyema space from the rest of the pleural space. This is known as the Eloesser procedure and involves rib excision and "maturing" of the empyema space by suturing the thickened pleura to the skin. This creates permanent open drainage, which can then be treated by local wound care in a number of ways as the space gradually closes [64]. The modern Eloesser procedure can be assisted by CT or sonographic marking of the borders of the empyema so that optimal dependent drainage can be obtained. Figure 15.9 shows a typical guideline for empyema management. The reader is referred to any of a number of treatises on surgical procedures for empyema [65].

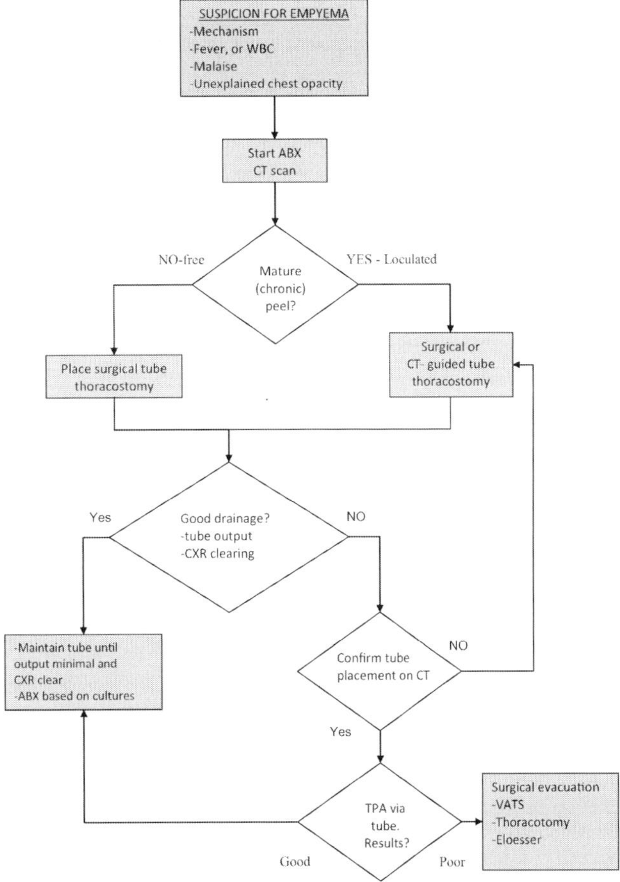

Fig. 15.9 Algorithm for the treatment of empyema

Complications and Follow-Up

The most concerning complication of inadequately treated empyema is that of persistent systemic symptoms with bacteremia and distant complications. The major surgical complication of concern is also persistent or recurrent infection. Signs of infection and persistence or worsening of chest opacity should prompt follow-up CT scanning. Small loculated residual empyema spaces are often drainable by a percutaneous radiologic approach.

The question often arises as to how long thoracostomy tubes draining empyema should remain in situ, whether the tubes were placed as the primary treatment or consequent to surgical decortication. The classic teaching has been that once the empyema space is presumed to be fully walled off from the pleural space, tubes should be cut off near the skin and opened to air as open drains or "empyema tubes." They are then slowly removed over a number of weeks while the empyema space presumably collapses down. Today, follow-up by modern CT scanning allows the surgeon to identify any residual spaces after thoracostomy. If the lung is fully inflated without residual space, many believe tubes can be removed after drainage effectively ceases.

Table 15.3 Management of empyema

"Pearls" in the treatment of empyema

- Presentation may be subtle in ICU or ambulatory patient
- Suspicion raised by persisting opacity after HTX or pneumonia with "soft" signs of infection
- May be culture positive or "complex effusion" with chemical criteria
- All effusions confirmed or highly suspicious for empyema should be evacuated
- Broad-spectrum antibiotics when empyema suspected and narrow based on microbiology. Duration of treatment is debated
- Tubes remain in until drainage ceases or longer if residual space

The question also arises as to the duration of antibiotic treatment for empyema. Infectious disease specialists will generally recommend many weeks of treatment for empyema [66]. In cases where the empyema has been surgically extirpated in its entirety and the lung fully inflated, many surgeons will treat until leukocytosis and temperature are normalized and the patient feels well. Other factors that may influence the duration of antibiotic treatment are the patient's overall health and immune status and the severity of the bacterial pleurisy noted at surgery. Table 15.3 lists pearls in the treatment of empyema.

References

1. Di Bartolomeo S, Sanson G, Nardi G, et al. A population-based study on pneumothorax in severely traumatized patients. J Trauma. 2001;51:677–82.
2. Ball CG, Dente CJ, Kirkpatrick AW, et al. Occult pneumothoraces in patients with penetrating trauma: does mechanism matter? Can J Surg. 2010;53:251–5.
3. Sahn SA, Heffner JE. Spontaneous pneumothorax. N Engl J Med. 2000;342:868–74.
4. Lu A, Aronowitz P. Pneumothorax in a patient with COPD after blunt trauma. J Hosp Med. 2010;5:E34–5.
5. Celik B, Sahin E, Nadir A, et al. Iatrogenic pneumothorax: etiology, incidence and risk factors. Thorac Cardiovasc Surg. 2009;57:286–90.
6. Haynes D, Baumann MH. Management of pneumothorax. Semin Respir Crit Care Med. 2010;31:769–80.
7. Noppen M. Spontaneous pneumothorax: epidemiology, pathophysiology and cause. Eur Respir Rev. 2010;19:217–9.
8. Murali R, Park K, Leslie KO. The pleura in health and disease. Semin Respir Crit Care Med. 2010;31:649–73.
9. Wilkerson RG, Stone MB. Sensitivity of bedside ultrasound and supine anteroposterior chest radiographs for the identification of pneumothorax after blunt trauma. Acad Emerg Med. 2010;17:11–7.
10. Dulchavsky SA, Schwarz KL, Kirkpatrick AW, et al. Prospective evaluation of thoracic ultrasound in the detection of pneumothorax. J Trauma. 2001;50:201–5.
11. Mariani PJ, Wittick L. Pneumothorax diagnosis by extended focused assessment with sonography for trauma. J Ultrasound Med. 2009;28:1601. author reply 2.
12. Surgeons ACo. ATLS—Advanced trauma life support course for doctors. 8th ed. Chicago, IL: American College of Surgeons; 2008.
13. Soldati G, Testa A, Sher S, et al. Occult traumatic pneumothorax: diagnostic accuracy of lung ultrasonography in the emergency department. Chest. 2008;133:204–11.

14. Blaivas M, Lyon M, Duggal S. A prospective comparison of supine chest radiography and bedside ultrasound for the diagnosis of traumatic pneumothorax. Acad Emerg Med. 2005;12:844–9.

15. Reddy VS. Minimally invasive techniqures in thoracic surgery. Semin Thorac Cardiovasc Surg. 2008;20:72–7.

16. Zengerink I, Brink PR, Laupland KB, et al. Needle thoracostomy in the treatment of a tension pneumothorax in trauma patients: what size needle? J Trauma. 2008;64:111–4.

17. Brar MS, Bains I, Brunet G, et al. Occult pneumothoraces truly occult or simply missed: redux. J Trauma. 2010;69:1335–7.

18. Kaiser M, Whealon M, Barrios C, et al. The clinical significance of occult thoracic injury in blunt trauma patients. Am Surg. 2010;76:1063–6.

19. Yadav K, Jalili M, Zehtabchi S. Management of traumatic occult pneumothorax. Resuscitation. 2010;81:1063–8.

20. Ball CG, Kirkpatrick AW, Feliciano DV. The occult pneumothorax: what have we learned? Can J Surg. 2009;52:E173–9.

21. de Moya MA, Seaver C, Spaniolas K, et al. Occult pneumothorax in trauma patients: development of an objective scoring system. J Trauma. 2007;63:13–7.

22. Wilson H, Ellsmere J, Tallon J, et al. Occult pneumothorax in the blunt trauma patient: tube thoracostomy or observation? Injury. 2009;40:928–31.

23. Noppen M. The utility of thoracoscopy in the diagnosis and management of pleural disease. Semin Respir Crit Care Med. 2010;31:751–9.

24. Huber-Wagner S, Korner M, Ehrt A, et al. Emergency chest tube placement in trauma care—which approach is preferable? Resuscitation. 2007;72:226–33.

25. Fitzgerald M, Mackenzie CF, Marasco S, et al. Pleural decompression and drainage during trauma reception and resuscitation. Injury. 2008;39:9–20.

26. Schulman CI, Cohn SM, Blackbourne L, et al. How long should you wait for a chest radiograph after placing a chest tube on water seal? A prospective study. J Trauma. 2005;59:92–5.

27. Casos SR, Richardson JD. Role of thoracoscopy in acute management of chest injury. Curr Opin Crit Care. 2006;12:584–9.

28. Carrillo EH, Kozloff M, Saridakis A, et al. Thoracoscopic application of a topical sealant for the management of persistent posttraumatic pneumothorax. J Trauma. 2006;60:111–4.

29. Ahmed N, Jones D. Video-assisted thoracic surgery: state of the art in trauma care. Injury. 2004;35:479–89.

30. Paci M, Annessi V, de Franco S, et al. Videothoracoscopic evaluation of thoracic injuries. Chir Ital. 2002;54:335–9.

31. Fabbrucci P, Nocentini L, Secci S, et al. Video-assisted thoracoscopy in the early diagnosis and management of post-traumatic pneumothorax and hemothorax. Surg Endosc. 2008;22:1227–31.

32. Divisi D, Battaglia C, De Berardis B, et al. Video-assisted thoracoscopy in thoracic injury: early or delayed indication? Acta Biomed Ateneo Parmense. 2004;75:158–63.

33. Meyer DM. Hemothorax related to trauma. Thorac Surg Clin. 2007;17:47–55.

34. LoCicero 3rd J, Mattox KL. Epidemiology of chest trauma. Surg Clin North Am. 1989;69:15–9.

35. Ng CS, Pang KK, Wong RH, et al. Spontaneous hemothorax: what is in a name? World J Surg. 2009;33:1780–1.

36. Molnar TF, Hasse J, Jeyasingham K, et al. Changing dogmas: history of development in treatment modalities of traumatic pneumothorax, hemothorax, and posttraumatic empyema thoracis. Ann Thorac Surg. 2004;77:372–8.

37. Livingston DH, Hauser CJ. Chest wall and lung. In: Feliciano DV, Mattox KL, Moore EE, editors. Trauma. 6th ed. New York: McGraw Hill Medical; 2008. p. 535–9.

38. Abboud PA, Kendall J. Emergency department ultrasound for hemothorax after blunt traumatic injury. J Emerg Med. 2003;25:181–4.

39. Sharma OP, Hagler S, Oswanski MF. Prevalence of delayed hemothorax in blunt thoracic trauma. Am Surg. 2005;71:481–6.

40. Misthos P, Kakaris S, Sepsas E, et al. A prospective analysis of occult pneumothorax, delayed pneumothorax and delayed hemothorax after minor blunt thoracic trauma. Eur J Cardiothorac Surg. 2004;25:859–64.

41. Crnjac A, Antonic J, Zorko A, et al. Video-assisted thoracic surgery–a new possibility for the management of traumatic hemothorax. Wien Klin Wochenschr. 2001;113 Suppl 3:18–20.

42. Morrison CA, Lee TC, Wall Jr MJ, et al. Use of a trauma service clinical pathway to improve patient outcomes for retained traumatic hemothorax. World J Surg. 2009;33:1851–6.

43. Hagiwara A, Yanagawa Y, Kaneko N, et al. Indications for transcatheter arterial embolization in persistent hemothorax caused by blunt trauma. J Trauma. 2008;65:589–94.

44. Vassiliu P, Velmahos GC, Toutouzas KG. Timing, safety, and efficacy of thoracoscopic evacuation of undrained post-traumatic hemothorax. Am Surg. 2001;67:1165–9.

45. Bilello JF, Davis JW, Lemaster DM. Occult traumatic hemothorax: when can sleeping dogs lie? Am J Surg. 2005;190:841–4.

46. Navsaria PH, Vogel RJ, Nicol AJ. Thoracoscopic evacuation of retained posttraumatic hemothorax. Ann Thorac Surg. 2004;78:282–5. discussion 5–6.

47. Tomaselli F, Maier A, Renner H, et al. Thoracoscopical water jet lavage in coagulated hemothorax. Eur J Cardiothorac Surg. 2003;23:424–5.

48. Villegas MI. Risk Factors associated with the development of posttraumatic retained hemothorax. Br J Trauma Emerg Surg 2010;

49. Macleod J, Ustin J, Kim J, et al. The epidemiology of traumatic hemothorax in a level 1 trauma center: case for early video-assisted thorascopic surgery. Eur J Trauma Emerg Surg. 2010;36:204–6.

50. Karmy-Jones R, Holevar M, Sullivan RJ, et al. Residual hemothorax after chest tube placement correlates with increased risk of empyema following traumatic injury. Can Resp J. 2008;15:255–8.

51. Kimbrell BJ, Yamzon J, Petrone P, et al. Intrapleural thrombolysis for the management of undrained traumatic hemothorax: a prospective observational study. J Trauma. 2007;62:1175–8. discussion 8–9.

52. Jerjes-Sanchez C, Ramirez-Rivera A, Elizalde JJ, et al. Intrapleural fibrinolysis with streptokinase as an adjunctive treatment in hemothorax and empyema: a multicenter trial. Chest. 1996;109:1514–9.

53. Eren S, Esme H, Sehitogullari A, et al. The risk factors and management of posttraumatic empyema in trauma patients. Injury. 2008;39:44–9.

54. Hoth JJ, Burch PT, Bullock TK, et al. Pathogenesis of posttraumatic empyema: the impact of pneumonia on pleural space infections. Surg Infect (Larchmt). 2003;4:29–35.

55. Stewart RM, Corneille MG. Common complications following thoracic trauma: their prevention and treatment. Semin Thorac Cardiovasc Surg. 2008;20:69–71.

56. Aguilar MM, Battistella FD, Owings JT, et al. Posttraumatic empyema. Risk factor analysis. Arch Surg. 1997;132:647–50.

57. Bailey KA, Bass J, Rubin S, et al. Empyema management: twelve years' experience since the introduction of video-assisted thoracoscopic surgery. J Laparoendosc Adv Surg Tech A. 2005;15:338–41.

58. Grijalva CG, Zhu Y, Nuorti JP, et al. Emergence of parapneumonic empyema in the USA. Thorax. 2011;66:663–8.

59. Society AT. Management of nontuberculous empyema. Am Rev Respir Dis. 1962;85:93.

60. Carrillo E, Williams M. Thoracic surgery. In: Civetta J, Taylor R, Kirby R, editors. Critical care. 3rd ed. Philadelphia: Lippincott—Raven; 1997. p. 1143.

61. Andrade-Alegre R, Garisto JD, Zebede S. Open thoracotomy and decortication for chronic empyema. Clinics. 2008;63:789–93.

62. Davies S, Richardson MC, Anthony FW, et al. Progesterone inhibits insulin-like growth factor binding protein-1 (IGFBP-1) production by explants of the Fallopian tube. Mol Hum Reprod. 2004;10:935–9.
63. Cameron R. Intraapleural fibrinolytic therapy versus conservative managementin the tratment of adult parapneumonic effusions and empyema. Cochrane Database Syst Rev. 2000;3:2312.
64. Ravitch MM, Steichen FM. Atlas of general thoracic surgery. Philadelphia: WB Saunders; 1988.
65. Pichlmaier H, Schildberg F. Thoracic surgery: surgical procedures on the chest and thoracic cavity. New York: Springer-Verlag; 1987.
66. Bryant RE, Salmon CJ. Pleural empyema. Clin Infect Dis. 1996;22:747–62.

Paul J. Schenarts, Mandy R. Maness,
and John R. Pender IV

Introduction

The terminology used to describe diaphragmatic hernias may be confusing. The first step is to differentiate hernias through the esophageal hiatus from hernias through the diaphragmatic musculature. These later type are more commonly congenital in nature such as Bochdalek or Morgagni hernias. They may also result from traumatic injuries, which may present immediately after the trauma or in a delayed fashion.

Hernias that occur through the esophageal hiatus are further classified into four distinct types based upon the location of the gastroesophageal (GE) junction and the contents of the hernia sac (Fig. 16.1). A type I hernia, also known as a sliding hernia, is characterized by an upward dislocation of the GE junction and the cardia of the stomach through the attenuated phrenoesophageal ligament into the posterior mediastinum. A type II hernia is a true paraesophageal hernia, which occurs when the fundus herniates through the hiatus alongside a normally located GE junction. A type III hernia has characteristics of both type I and type II, in that the GE junction, cardia, and fundus of the stomach are all intrathoracic. Because of the combination of these characteristics, another name for a type III is a mixed hernia. As the hiatus enlarges progressively more stomach herniates into the mediastinum. When more than one-third of the stomach is in the chest it is defined as a "giant paraesophageal hernia," whereas an "intrathoracic stomach" describes the situation when

greater than 75% of the stomach has herniated through the hiatus. When other organs such as the colon, small bowel, or spleen herniate into the chest along with the GE junction and stomach, the hernia is classified as a type IV hernia.

Although this anatomic classification system is accurate and easy to use, from a practical clinical standpoint, patients are divided into those with sliding hiatal hernias (type I) and paraesophageal hernias (types II, III, and IV). As type I hernias account for more than 95% of hiatal hernias, they typically present with symptoms of gastroesophageal reflux and are typically treated in an elective fashion, whereas symptomatic paraesophageal hernias represent an emergency that would more commonly require management by an acute care surgeon. Therefore the focus of the remainder of this chapter is on the pathophysiology, epidemiology, presentation, evaluation, and management of paraesophageal hernias.

Pathophysiology

The exact etiology causing the attenuation of the phrenoesophageal ligament remains unknown. There is a familial occurrence suggesting an autosomal-dominant pattern of inheritance and congenital (primary) paraesophageal hernias have been described in children. However, paraesophageal hernias typically present in old age, suggesting the fibromuscular degeneration of this ligament as the most common pathologic etiology [1–5]. This deterioration involves the thinning of the upper facial layer and loss of elasticity of the lower facial layer of this ligament. This results in the membrane stretching up into the posterior mediastinum with increased intra-abdominal pressure. Factors that are known to increase intra-abdominal pressure have also been associated with the development of hiatal hernias to include obesity, kyphosis in elderly women, and pregnancy [6–9]. Studies on the influence of gender have yielded contradictory results [9].

Once the stomach or other abdominal contents enter the hiatus, incarceration and strangulation with subsequent perforation into the mediastinum may occur. Abdominal contents

P.J. Schenarts, M.D., F.A.C.S. (✉)
Department of Surgery, College of Medicine, University of Nebraska, 983280 Nebraska Medical Center, Omaha, NE 68198, USA
e-mail: paul.schenarts@unmc.edu

M.R. Maness, M.D.
Department of General Surgery, Vidant Medical Center, Greenville, NC, USA

J.R. Pender IV, M.D., F.A.C.S.
Departments of General and Laparoscopic Surgery, Bariatric Surgery, Brody School of Medicine, Vidant Medical Center, Greenville, NC, USA

L.J. Moore et al. (eds.), *Common Problems in Acute Care Surgery*,
DOI 10.1007/978-1-4614-6123-4_16, © Springer Science+Business Media New York 2013

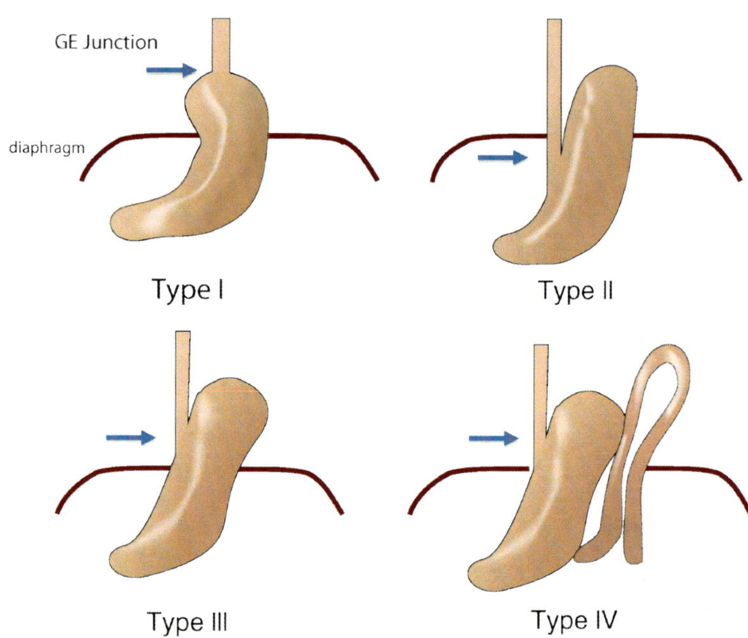

Fig. 16.1 Paraesophageal hernia types. A type I hernia is characterized by an upward dislocation of the gastroesophageal (GE) junction and the cardia of the stomach through the attenuated phrenoesophageal ligament into the posterior mediastinum. A type II hernia occurs when the fundus herniates through the hiatus alongside a normally located GE junction. In a type III hernia, the GE junction, cardia, and fundus of the stomach are all intrathoracic. In a type IV hernia, other organs such as the colon, small bowel, or spleen herniate into the chest along with the GE junction and stomach

may volumetrically displace contents in the inferior chest and mediastinum resulting in respiratory embarrassment [10]. Vascular engorgement of the gastric wall may also occur resulting in severe upper gastrointestinal hemorrhage. Gastric volvulus occurs when there is an abnormal rotation of the stomach of at least 180 degrees, thereby creating a closed loop obstruction. It is most common for the stomach to rotate around the longitudinal axis that connects the GE junction and the pylorus. When this occurs, the greater curvature of the stomach flips up into the chest, dragging the omentum with it. This situation is defined as an organoaxial volvulus. A less common variant is the mesenteroaxial volvulus, which occurs when the rotation is around the axis that runs from the greater curvature to the gastric angulus.

Epidemiology

Because the majority of patients are asymptomatic, the true incidence of hiatal hernias remains unknown. While type I hernias are thought to be relatively common, types II–IV account for only approximately 5% of all hiatal hernias [11]. Of those with paraesophageal hernias, the annual incidence of acute symptoms is 0.7–7%, with an annual probability of needing emergency surgery of approximately 1% [12]; however, the overall chance of developing acute symptoms and incarceration is approximately 30% [11, 12]. In a 15-year Finnish population-based study, the annual rate of hospital admission for patients with paraesophageal hernia was 8.2/1,000,000 with an annual mortality of only 0.6/1,000,000 [13]. Of those patients who underwent operative treatment the mortality was 2.7%, whereas it was 10% for those presenting

with a gangrenous stomach [13]. Given the pathophysiologic mechanisms described above, it is not surprising that patients presenting with paraesophageal hernias are typically older (60–90 years) and have multiple other co-morbidities.

Clinical Presentation

Acute incarceration of a paraesophageal hernia may occur suddenly against a background of nonspecific complaints such as postprandial discomfort or dyspepsia. Precipitating events are typically related to either the ingestion of a large meal or those which increased intra-abdominal pressure such as ileus, pregnancy, or parturition. On abdominal examination, patients have little epigastric tenderness and overall have no significant findings.

The classic constellation of symptoms of incarcerated paraesophageal hernia, referred to as Borchardt's triad, consists of chest pain, retching with an inability to vomit, and inability to pass a nasogastric tube. The chest pain is typically substernal and is caused by acute gastric obstruction, which if left untreated will progress to ischemia followed by perforation into the mediastinum leading to septic shock and ultimately death [14]. Acute presentations may also be atypical, leading to diagnostic confusion. Symptoms including the acute onset of respiratory collapse due to a grossly contaminated thoracic cavity, heart failure, perforation into adjacent organs, large-volume upper gastrointestinal hemorrhage, and tension gastrothorax have also been described [15–18].

While it is of paramount importance for an acute care surgeon to recognize the presentation of incarcerated paraesophageal hernias, these same surgeons are also frequently called upon to evaluate vague abdominal complaints. Although it is estimated that 50% of these hernias are asymptomatic, subtle findings may suggest either a chronic or subacute presentation [14]. Further complicating the subacute presentation of a paraesophageal hernia is the advanced age and associated co-morbidities of this patient population. For example, iron deficiency anemia in this population may have a multitude of other causes, of which chronic blood loss from Cameron ulcers, chronic linear lesions resulting from diaphragmatic shear forces in patients with paraesophageal hernias, would rank toward the bottom of the list [19–21]. After hernia repair, the anemia resolves in more than 90% of patients [21].

Symptoms may also be misattributed to the normal aging process. Increasing dyspnea developing over years is a common symptom in patients with paraesophageal hernias; however, in a population of elderly patients this cause may be overlooked. However, following hernia repair most patients note significant improvement in these symptoms, exercise capacity, as well as objective pulmonary function testing [22].

Chronic symptoms can be divided into two broad categories: obstructive and those related to gastroesophageal reflux disease (GERD). Gastroesophageal reflux-type symptoms are due to a dysfunctional lower esophageal sphincter and are manifest as heartburn, chronic cough, regurgitation of partially digested food, and aspiration. These symptoms predominate in patients with type 1 hiatal hernias. Those with type III hernias may also present with GERD symptoms by virtue of the fact that this type mixes the characteristics of both type I and type II [23]. Patients may also describe GERD symptoms that are supplanted by more obstructive symptoms.

Obstructive symptoms are most prominent in those patients with type II, III, and IV paraesophageal hernias. These hernias cause an outflow restriction at the hiatus when the cardia distends compressing the distal esophagus or by torsion of the GE junction as the stomach displaces into the chest [16]. Symptoms include epigastric pain, postprandial fullness or bloating, chest pain, dysphagia, and respiratory complaints. Of these, dysphagia and postprandial discomfort are most common, occurring in more than 50% of symptomatic patients [12].

Diagnosis

The evaluation of a patient with a suspected paraesophageal hernia depends on the acuity of the presentation. Because of the vague and variable presentation of these hernias, the goal of the diagnostic evaluation is to confirm or refute the diagnosis, define the anatomy, rule out associated pathologic processes, and determine the presence or the absence of GERD. Given that the acute care surgeon is most likely to encounter these patients when in crisis, it is important to simultaneously perform both diagnostic and resuscitative measures so that if surgery is required, the patient can tolerate induction and a general anesthetic without physiologic compromise [24].

Traditionally, paraesophageal hernias were diagnosed via an upright chest radiograph, revealing an air-fluid level behind the cardiac shadow. Radiographs may also reveal evidence of ischemia of the gastric wall or perforation manifested as pneumomediastinum or pneumoperitoneum. By enlarge, computed tomography (CT) scans have replaced plain radiographs as they provide greater detail and are now easily obtained in most hospitals. Computed tomography not only provides similar information as seen on radiographs, but it also provides additional anatomic information as to the type and location of the hernia. In a patient who presents in extremis, with the appropriate radiographic findings, no additional diagnostic studies are needed.

If clinically appropriate, the next most appropriate diagnostic test is an upper gastrointestinal series [24]. This contrast study provides important information as to the anatomic location of the esophagus, GE junction, and stomach, and may suggest the size of the diaphragmatic defect. Additionally, complete obstruction due to a gastric volvulus or occult perforation may be identified. Currently, this study is considered the gold standard for the diagnosis of paraesophageal hernias. Similarly a contrast CT scan may be used in a similar manner and provide the detail needed to plan an operative intervention.

Upper endoscopy provides useful information in diagnosing paraesophageal hernias, and most importantly, rules out concomitant pathology while defining the anatomy of the hernia. The most pertinent finding on endoscopy is the status of the gastric mucosa. If ischemia is present, the operative approach may change from laparoscopic to open. When evaluating anatomic relationships, type 1 hernias can be confirmed by finding the GE junction and gastric pouch above the impression made by the diaphragmatic crura, whereas with type II hernias, retroversion of the scope will demonstrate a second gastric orifice where the stomach has herniated alongside the GE junction and distal esophagus. Upper endoscopy in type III hernias may have difficulty in differentiating from type I hernias; however, it may be suspected if a large gastric pouch is seen above the diaphragm with the GE junction entering midway along the side of the gastric pouch [24]. When performing an upper endoscopy, care needs to be taken to avoid overinflation of the stomach to reduce the risk of cardiopulmonary compromise.

While not appropriate in patients with an urgent indication for surgery, in the more chronic setting, the use of manometry in the workup of paraesophageal hernias is controversial. Proponents of manometry argue that it provides additional information regarding the location of the lower esophageal sphincter and the possible need for an esophageal lengthening procedure. Those who argue against the routine use of manometry note that it adds little information to that provided by endoscopy and contrast upper GI series. Manometry is also technically difficult in patients with paraesophageal hernias and is unable to be completed in more than 50% of patients [24]. Due to the fact that most surgeons routinely perform a fundoplication procedure as part of the hernia repair, pH testing has been virtually eliminated from the preoperative examination of these patients, so obtaining this information does not alter the planned operation.

The goals in diagnostic evaluation of a patient for paraesophageal hernia are to first confirm the diagnosis, secondarily define the hernia's anatomy, and finally rule out associated or concurrent pathology. The acuity of the patient dictates if additional evaluation may be undertaken, or if an emergent operation must be pursued.

Management

The optimal management of paraesophageal hernias is less well defined. Controversial issues include:

1. When to operate on asymptomatic patients
2. Which operative approach to use (thoracic, versus abdominal; laproscopic versus open)
3. The need for the complete excision of the hernia sac
4. The closure of the crural defect
5. The use of mesh
6. An antireflux procedure
7. A gastropexy

While it is unlikely that an acute care surgeon would be required to manage a type I hernia, the mere presence of a paraesophageal hernia (types II, III, and IV) has traditionally been considered an indication for surgical repair. This view is based on the catastrophic complications of bleeding, infarction, and perforation that occur as the natural progression of these hernias. Clearly, patients with paraesophageal hernias who present with evidence of gastric volvulus, acute obstruction, ischemia, bleeding, or perforation require immediate surgical intervention [24, 25]. However the management of asymptomatic or minimally symptomatic patients with paraesophageal hernias is controversial. In their classic report, Belsey and Skinner found that nearly 30% (6 of 21) of patients with minimal symptoms whose paraesophageal hernias were managed non-operatively died and these deaths occurred without warning [12]. If surgery was delayed and was later required on an emergent basis, the operative mortality was 19% compared to 1% for elective repair [12]. While these findings are significant, advances in surgical critical care and the overall improved health of the elderly have altered this mandate. In a series of 23 patients who refused to undergo surgery and were followed for 78 months, there were no deaths and 83% of these patients had no change in their symptoms [25]. In another study with 15-year follow-up, elective hernia repair would have prevented only 12.5% of deaths [26]. Unfortunately, studies investigating the natural history of paraesophageal hernias consist of very small number of patients and are further limited by occurring over many years, during which other medical advances have occurred.

Further complicating this picture is the evolving experience with laparoscopy [27–30]. The general perception that laparoscopic repairs are associated with less pain and a more rapid recovery has provided additional impetus for those who favor an aggressive surgical approach [27]. However, laparoscopic repairs are often more difficult than open repairs, particularly for type III hernias. Additionally there is an evolving body of evidence that laparoscopic repairs are associated with a higher recurrence rate, up to 42% [28].

When patients present with clear evidence of gastric compromise or perforation, it is obviously prudent to proceed with open surgery [26]. For other patients with paraesophageal hernias, there are presently no concrete guidelines as to the timing of surgery, type of procedure to perform, or what should be done in the instance of a recurrence [24]. Given the limitations of the current literature, Fig. 16.2 provides a management algorithm, based on that described by Bawahab et al. [31]. If and when an operation is untaken, the fundamental steps remain the same, regardless of a laparoscopic or open approach.

Traditionally paraesophageal hernia repairs were performed through a thoracotomy or laparotomy. Advocates of the thoracic approach cited the ease of dissecting the contents of the hernia sac and the enhanced ability to fully mobilize the esophagus, thereby decreasing the need for an esophageal lengthening procedure. The major disadvantages of this approach were increased pain, the risk of pulmonary complications, and the need for a thoracostomy tube. There was also a potential risk of gastric volvulus occurring after the stomach was replaced into the abdomen.

The classic open abdominal repair includes excision of the hernia sac, reduction of the stomach into the abdomen, evaluation of the length of the esophagus, closure of the diaphragmatic crura, an antireflux procedure, and gastropexy [26]. Proponents of this approach emphasize the ease with which the stomach can be completely mobilized, improved reduction of the gastric volvulus, and recreation of normal anatomy. This approach also allows other abdominal procedures such as gastrostomy or anterior gastropexy. While mobilization of the esophagus may be more challenging, gastroplasty is still possible. To date, there are no randomized trials comparing abdominal to thoracic approaches.

As experience with advanced laparoscopic techniques increases, one would predict that a greater proportion of paraesophageal hernias will be approached laparoscopically. Overall the fundamental elements of the classic open procedure apply; however, laparoscopic repairs are technically more challenging and thus require significant experience with gastrointestinal laparoscopic surgery. In particular, the operative time is significantly longer, a wider dissection is required, anatomic restoration is more difficult, and the recurrence rate is higher. The specific steps of the laparoscopic approach follow, as we perform the procedure.

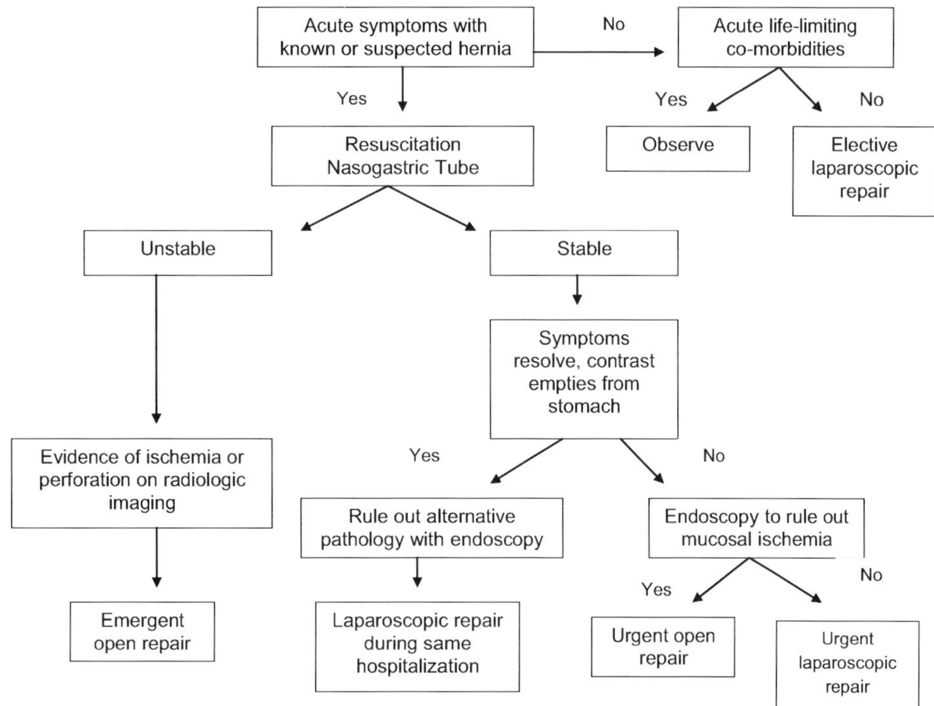

Fig. 16.2 Paraesophageal management algorithm

Sequence for Laparoscopic Paraesophageal Hernia Repair

The patient should be positioned in the supine position with the arms out and a footboard in place. After prepping and draping the abdomen, the patient is placed in steep reverse Trendelenberg position. The peritoneal cavity is accessed in the left mid-clavicular line, 2 cm off the costal boarder. After achieving a pressure of 15 mmHg CO_2 (20 mmHg CO_2 for obese patients) a 5 mm trocar is placed in the midline, 14 cm below the xyphoid process. A common error is to place this camera port in the supra umbilical skin fold as in preparation for a cholecystectomy. Placement of the camera port too low will make visualization and dissection of the crura posterior to the esophagus difficult if not impossible. A Nathanson liver retractor is inserted through a sub-xyphoid incision and used to hold up the left lobe of the liver. One or two 5 mm ports are placed to the left of the camera port. A 10 mm trocar is placed in the mid-clavicular line on the right and an additional 5 mm is placed lateral to this.

The case is begun by assessing the upper abdomen for signs of perforation or necrosis of any of the hernia contents. An attempt is then made to reduce the hernia. Occasionally this will occur with establishing pneumoperitoneum and placing the patient in steep reverse Trendelenburg. If the hernia must be reduced, one must be careful not to tear the tissues and cause perforation or bleeding. Dissection is begun through the gastrohepatic ligament extending up to the right crus using an ultrasonic dissector or cautery device. Dissection is then carried anteriorly. For large type III and IV paraesophageal hernias, this should be enough to reduce mostly everything except for the fundus of the stomach. Dissection is then started high on the greater curvature, taking the short gastric vessels with the ultrasonic dissector. Attempts are made to preserve as much of this blood supply as possible.

The dissection is carried up to the left crus of the diaphragm and then anteriorly. Utilization of the electrocautery hook can facilitate getting into the hernia sac as it curves along the diaphragmatic hiatus. Care is taken to identify the vagus nerves. This can be quite challenging in the face of a chronically thickened hernia sac with possible active inflammation. Maintaining hemostasis is of utmost importance. Blood in the operative field can make identification of the tissue planes even more challenging. Use of esophagogastroscopes, oral gastric tubes, and boogies can help to identify the anatomy and planes. Once the hernia sac is reduced, it is sometimes necessary to resect it using 3.5 mm staple loads. The sac can then be placed in an endoscopic bag to be removed at the end of the case.

If there is concern of gastric ischemia, now is a good time to perform an upper endoscopy to examine the mucosa. After reducing a large, incarcerated hernia, the stomach serosa can appear quite ecchymotic. Endoscopy can guide one's judgment as to if a gastric resection is required. The endoscopy will also aid in determining the location of the GE junction and its relationship to the crus of the diaphragm (critical to assessing esophageal length).

To achieve the 2–3 cm of intra-abdominal esophageal length required, the esophagus and stomach must be completely mobilized. Although the use of a 30 degree laparoscope can facilitate dissection in the area posterior to the GE junction, a 0 degree scope will provide a better view of the intrathoracic esophagus.

Unintended entrance into the plural space is rarely problematic and easily repaired. If left open, it rarely causes problems. Anesthesia may report a rise in the end tidal CO_2. If this becomes a problem, decrease the pneumoperitoneum pressure. Anesthesia should then increase the minute ventilation and place the patient on 100% oxygen. These same measures can be taken if the patient develops subcutaneous gas.

If adequate esophageal length is unobtainable, a decision must be made as to what direction the operation will go at this point. Assessment of the patient's overall condition, future quality of life, nutrition status, and age must guide the surgeon's decision as to whether efforts are made to obtain more length through extending the length of the operative time, performing a Collis gastroplasty, or converting to an open procedure.

In a damage control setting, a posterior crural repair can be performed using a zero braided permanent suture and a feeding gastrostomy inserted. The gastrostomy will act as both a gastropexy and as access for enteral nutrition. Closed suction drains can be left in place extending into the chest alongside the esophagus. If the patient is in good health and there is adequate esophageal length, a posterior crural repair should be undertaken. As there have been reports of complications such as erosion into the esophagus after using prosthetic mesh, we do not use prosthetic mesh to repair the crural defect. As for bioprosthetic meshes, long-term data does not demonstrate a reduced recurrence rate when compared to repairs without reinforcement.

A nissen fundoplication should be performed over a 60 French boogie. As these patients present emergently and no esophageal manomotery has been performed, it is better to perform a loose or "floppy" fundoplication so as to avoid postoperative dysphagia. This patient population can have higher rates of esophageal dysfunction than the rest of the population. Although there is some debate regarding the necessity of gastropexy, if a fundoplication and tension-free crural repair are able to be performed, it is our practice to routinely perform a gastropexy. This can easily be performed by placing a 2–0 permanent suture through the body of the stomach. The needle is then removed. Using a suture passer through a small stab wound, the two ends are brought up through two places on the anterior abdominal wall about 5 mm apart. The abdomen is deflated and the suture is tied. As there may be concern about gastric ischemia and gas bloat, a nasogastric tube should be placed under direct visualization before leaving the abdomen.

Controversies in Operative Management

Esophageal Shortening

Despite being a historically documented concern, the true incidence of esophageal shortening in patients with paraesophageal hernias is unknown and controversial [32, 33]. The most important factor associated with esophageal shortening is inflammation, often associated with chronic GERD and/or other inflammatory processes such as Crohn's disease or scleroderma. Esophageal shortening may limit the ability to reduce the stomach to its normal intra-abdominal position, predisposing to tension with an increased risk of recurrence. Preoperatively identifying the shortened esophagus is problematic, as there is no definitive test for this; therefore, the most accurate assessment is made in the operating room. When confirmed, options include further intrathoracic mobilization or a Collis gastroplasty. Those who do not believe in esophageal shortening, reason that it only appears shortened secondary to being pushed up into the chest by the stomach, which may explain why with the enhanced visualization during laparoscopy, esophageal shortening is less commonly identified.

Antireflux Procedure

Only limited data confirm the need to perform a fundoplication; however, this is commonly done as it is felt to help anchor the stomach within the abdomen [34, 35]. Additionally the amount of required dissection completely disrupts the hiatal mechanism, thereby rendering the GE junction incompetent and hence the need to recreate a barrier to reflux. Proponents of antireflux procedures favor a "floppy" fundoplication, to decrease the risk of dysphagia. On the contrary, some believe that avoiding the fundoplication eliminates the potential for postoperative dysphagia, as most patients with incarcerated hernias have not undergone manometry. This also decreases the operative time in elderly patients often with numerous co-morbidities. Others favor selective fundoplication in those patients with preexisting GERD. In particular, patients with a type III hernia may have reflux symptoms by virtue of the fact that the GE junction is above the diaphragm. In these patients, performance of an antireflux procedure would be reasonable.

Anterior Gastric Fixation

Another area of controversy is the necessity of fixing the stomach to the anterior gastric wall using either a gastropexy or placement of a gastrostomy tube [36, 37]. Anchoring the stomach to the abdominal wall is thought to prevent hernia recurrence. Those who oppose fixation claim that re-herniation is not prevented by fixation, as the stomach is pliable and merely stretches in response to increased intra-abdominal pressures. Unfortunately for those who favor fixation, there are no prospective randomized trials to guide them as to which fixation technique is superior. Proponents of the gastropexy note that it is a simple, fast procedure that adds little to the operative time; however, a high rate of recurrence has been reported using this technique. Those who favor gastrostomy argue that this technique not only provides a solid anchoring point but also effectively decompresses the stomach, thereby avoiding the need for a nasogastric tube.

Mesh Reinforcement of Crural Repair

The need to reinforce the crural repair with mesh remains an area of controversy. The failure of the crural closure is a common cause for re-herniation; therefore, some surgeons favor reinforcement of the crural closure with mesh [38, 39]. While this may decrease recurrence, it is important for the acute care surgeon to balance this potential benefit with the potential risk of mesh complications such as erosion or infection. Clear indications for placement of a mesh would be if the hiatus cannot be re-approximated or if there is concern that the crural closure is under tension. Unfortunately, there is no consensus in the literature as to the routine use of mesh as part of a paraesophageal hernia repair.

Postoperative Complications

The preceding section discussed controversies in the operative repair, mostly aimed at preventing recurrence. However, the clinical significance of such a recurrence is unknown. The risks and complications of nonoperative management have been outlined earlier in this chapter. In brief, the estimated mortality of a known yet untreated paraesophageal hernia has been estimated between 16 and 30%, while mortality from operative treatment has been demonstrated around 3% [24]. Although incarceration of these hernias is a relatively rare complication, it is preventable; therefore, elective repair of symptomatic patients continues to be recommended for patients without life-limiting co-morbidities.

By virtue of the fact that paraesophageal hernias occur most frequently in the elderly many of whom have other significant co-morbidities, acute exacerbation of these represents the most significant complication in the postoperative period. Because of this concern, the laparoscopic approach has been advocated. Unfortunately, recurrence rates for the laparoscopic approach range from 0 to 42% [27, 28, 30], hence the controversy surrounding the routine anterior gastropexy and the use of biologic mesh.

Conclusion

Overall follow-up after paraesophageal hernia repair is similar to other open or laparoscopic procedures. Because most patients with paraesophageal hernias are asymptomatic, in light of the contradictory data on need for operation versus watchful waiting after initial identification of the hernia, monitoring for the development of symptoms is a reasonable approach. On the other hand, if the surgeon is of the opinion that operative intervention is mandatory if identified, upper gastrointestinal contrast studies performed at routine intervals are also not unreasonable. Also given the reported higher recurrence rates with laparoscopic procedures, a lower threshold to actively seek out recurrence would be appropriate.

References

1. Schieman C, Grondin SC. Paraesophageal hernia: clinical presentation, evaluation, and management controversies. Thorac Surg Clin. 2009;19(4):473–84.
2. Luketich JD, Raja S, Fernando HC, Campbell W, Christie NA, Buenaventura PO, Weigel TL, Keenan RJ, Schauer PR. Laparoscopic repair of giant paraesophageal hernia: 100 consecutive cases. Ann Surg. 2000;232(4):608–18.
3. Mittal SK, Bikhchandani J, Gurney O, Yano F, Lee T. Outcomes after repair of the intrathoracic stomach: objective follow-up of up to 5 years. Surg Endosc. 2011;25(2):556–66.
4. Yano F, Stadlhuber RJ, Tsuboi K, Gerhardt J, Filipi CJ, Mittal SK. Outcomes of surgical treatment of intrathoracic stomach. Dis Esophagus. 2009;22(3):284–8.
5. Karpelowsky JS, Wieselthaler N, Rode H. Primary paraesophageal hernia in children. J Pediatr Surg. 2006;41(9):1588–93.
6. Eliska O. Phreno-oesophageal membrane and its role in the development of hiatal hernia. Acta Anat. 1973;86(1):137–50.
7. El Sherif A, Yano F, Mittal S, Filipi CJ. Collagen metabolism and recurrent hiatal hernia: cause and effect? Hernia. 2006;10(6):511–20.
8. Menon S, Trudgill N. Risk factors in the aetiology of hiatus hernia: a meta-analysis. Eur J Gastroenterol Hepatol. 2011;23(2):133–8.
9. Yamaguchi T, Sugimoto T, Yamada H, Kanzawa M, Yano S, Yamauchi M, Chihara K. The presence and severity of vertebral fractures is associated with the presence of esophageal hiatal hernia in postmenopausal women. Osteoporos Int. 2002;13(4):331–6.
10. Pandolfino JE, Kwiatek MA, Kahrilas PJ. The pathophysiologic basis for epidemiologic trends in gastroesophageal reflux disease. Gastroenterol Clin North Am. 2008;37(4):827–43.
11. Ellis Jr FH. Diaphragmatic hiatal hernias. Recognizing and treating the major types. Postgrad Med. 1990;88(1):113–4. 117–20, 123–4.
12. Skinner DB, Belsey RH. Surgical management of esophageal reflux and hiatus hernia. Long-term results with 1,030 patients. J Thorac Cardiovasc Surg. 1967;53(1):33–54.
13. Sihvo EI, Salo JA, Räsänen JV, Rantanen TK. Fatal complications of adult paraesophageal hernia: a population-based study. J Thorac Cardiovasc Surg. 2009;137(2):419–24.
14. Hill LD. Incarcerated paraesophageal hernia. A surgical emergency. Am J Surg. 1973;126(2):286–91.
15. Borchardt M. Zur pathogie und therapie des magenvolvulus [Pathology and therapy of gastric volulus]. Arch Klin Chir. 1904;74:243–60. in German.

16. Hunt GS, Gilchrist DM, Hirji MK. Cardiac compression and decompensation due to hiatus hernia. Can J Cardiol. 1996;12(3):295–6.

17. Tadler SC, Burton JH. Intrathoracic stomach presenting as acute tension gastrothorax. Am J Emerg Med. 1999;17(4):370–1.

18. Salling N, Falensteen AM, Larsen LG. Non-traumatic perforation of gastric ulcer in a hiatal hernia to the pericardium. Acta Med Scand. 1983;213(3):225–6.

19. Weston AP. Hiatal hernia with cameron ulcers and erosions. Gastrointest Endosc Clin North Am. 1996;6(4):671–9.

20. Pauwelyn KA, Verhamme M. Large hiatal hernia and iron deficiency anaemia: clinico-endoscopical findings. Acta Clin Belg. 2005;60(4):166–72.

21. Hayden JD, Jamieson GG. Effect on iron deficiency anemia of laparoscopic repair of large paraesophageal hernias. Dis Esophagus. 2005;18(5):329–31.

22. Low DE, Simchuk EJ. Effect of paraesophageal hernia repair on pulmonary function. Ann Thorac Surg. 2002;74(2):333–7.

23. Wo JM, Branum GD, Hunter JG, Trus TN, Mauren SJ, Waring JP. Clinical features of type III (mixed) paraesophageal hernia. Am J Gastroenterol. 1996;91(5):914–6.

24. Stylopoulos N, Gazelle GS, Rattner DW. Paraesophageal hernias: operation or observation? Ann Surg. 2002;236(4):492–500.

25. Allen MS, Trastek VF, Deschamps C, Pairolero PC. Intrathoracic stomach. Presentation and results of operation. J Thorac Cardiovasc Surg. 1993;105(2):253–8.

26. Low DE, Unger T. Open repair of paraesophageal hernia: reassessment of subjective and objective outcomes. Ann Thorac Surg. 2005;80(1):287–94.

27. Andujar JJ, Papasavas PK, Birdas T, Robke J, Raftopoulos Y, Gagné DJ, Caushaj PF, Landreneau RJ, Keenan RJ. Laparoscopic repair of large paraesophageal hernia is associated with a low incidence of recurrence and reoperation. Surg Endosc. 2004;18(3):444–7.

28. Targarona EM, Novell J, Vela S, Cerdán G, Bendahan G, Torrubia S, Kobus C, Rebasa P, Balague C, Garriga J, Trias M. Mid term analysis of safety and quality of life after the laparoscopic repair of paraesophageal hiatal hernia. Surg Endosc. 2004;18(7):1045–50.

29. Dahlberg PS, Deschamps C, Miller DL, Allen MS, Nichols FC, Pairolero PC. Laparoscopic repair of large paraesophageal hiatal hernia. Ann Thorac Surg. 2001;72(4):1125–9.

30. Draaisma WA, Gooszen HG, Consten EC, Broeders IA. Mid-term results of robot-assisted laparoscopic repair of large hiatal hernia: a symptomatic and radiological prospective cohort study. Surg Technol Int. 2008;17:165–70.

31. Bawahab M, Mitchell P, Church N, Debru E. Management of acute paraesophageal hernia. Surg Endosc. 2009;23(2):255–9.

32. Gastal OL, Hagen JA, Peters JH, Campos GM, Hashemi M, Theisen J, Bremner CG, DeMeester TR. Short esophagus: analysis of predictors and clinical implications. Arch Surg. 1999;134(6):633–6.

33. Horvath KD, Swanstrom LL, Jobe BA. The short esophagus: pathophysiology, incidence, presentation, and treatment in the era of laparoscopic antireflux surgery. Ann Surg. 2000;232(5):630–40.

34. Swanstrom LL, Jobe BA, Kinzie LR, Horvath KD. Esophageal motility and outcomes following laparoscopic paraesophageal hernia repair and fundoplication. Am J Surg. 1999;177(5):359–63.

35. Morris-Stiff G, Hassn A. Laparoscopic paraoesophageal hernia repair: fundoplication is not usually indicated. Hernia. 2008;12(3):299–302.

36. Ponsky J, Rosen M, Fanning A, Malm J. Anterior gastropexy may reduce the recurrence rate after laparoscopic paraesophageal hernia repair. Surg Endosc. 2003;17(7):1036–41.

37. Braslow L. Transverse gastropexy vs Stamm gastrostomy in hiatal hernia. Arch Surg. 1987;122(7):851.

38. Hui TT, Thoman DS, Spyrou M, Phillips EH. Mesh crural repair of large paraesophageal hiatal hernias. Am Surg. 2001;67(12):1170–4.

39. Frantzides CT, Madan AK, Carlson MA, Stavropoulos GP. A prospective, randomized trial of laparoscopic polytetrafluoroethylene (PTFE) patch repair vs. simple cruroplasty for large hiatal hernia. Arch Surg. 2002;137(6):649–52.

Sherry L. Sixta

Introduction

Peptic ulcer disease (PUD) was not well elucidated as a significant contributor to patient morbidity and mortality until the early 1900s. From that time up until the late twentieth century, PUD was felt to be caused by stress and dietary factors, with treatments focusing on dietary modification, bed rest, and later on, acid suppression and neutralization [1–3]. With the discovery of *Helicobacter pylori* in the 1980s and the subsequent development of improved medical regimens to treat the organism and suppress acid production, the incidence of PUD has decreased dramatically over the past 30 years [4]. Furthermore, data gathered from multiple countries within the same time period reveals a 40–50% global decline in incidence [5–7]. In accordance with the trend of successful medical management, surgeons have seen a steady decline in the rate of elective surgery for PUD over the past three decades. Procedures that were once common have become a rarity for today's surgical residents to encounter. However, though the rate of elective interventions has declined dramatically (80–97%), the rate of emergency surgery related to PUD has remained constant or increased [6, 8]. Wang et al. reported a 44% increase in emergent operative interventions related to PUD from 1993 to 2006, and in 2006, there were nearly 25,000 operations performed in the United States alone for perforated or bleeding peptic ulcers. With the evolution of therapeutic modalities for the treatment of PUD, including pharmaceutical advancements and endoscopic and therapies, surgical interventions have become more salvage in nature. The majority of surgical indications for PUD are now limited to complications from hemorrhage or perforation that have failed medical and minimally invasive interventions. Less frequently, surgical interventions are sought for rare causes of PUD such

S.L. Sixta, M.D. (✉)
Department of Surgery, Cooper University Hospital,
3 Cooper Plaza, Suite 411, Camden, NJ 08103, USA
e-mail: ssixta@yahoo.com

as gastrinoma or Zollinger–Ellison syndrome (ZES), antral G-cell hyperplasia, trauma, or burns. Elective operative gastric procedures, though rare, are primarily for lesions suspicious for malignancy or refractory PUD due to failed medical therapy, patient intolerance, or noncompliance [9]. Undoubtedly, the next generation of acute care surgeons will be called upon to manage the urgent and emergent complications of PUD, on a much more complicated population of patients, with significantly less experience than generations prior. The goal of this chapter is to provide a brief overview of the pathophysiology, epidemiology, and presentation of PUD with a more in-depth description of the management and operative techniques as they relate to the acute care surgeon in urgent and emergent situations.

Epidemiology

It is estimated that 1 in 10 Americans are plagued with symptoms related to PUD, with an overall 2% prevalence in the United States. The majority of patients who endure complications secondary to PUD are 70 years of age or older, and the rate of complications is estimated to be from 2 to 10% [10–12]. The prevalence of disease is 1.5 times greater in men than women. Yet in regard to the rate of perforation, the Data from the United States data reveals a rise in the female population and an overall decline in the male population [7, 13]. This is thought to be secondary to nonsteroidal anti-inflammatory drug (NSAID) use and smoking patterns [14]. Duodenal ulcers are more common than gastric ulcers, and are more likely to be the source of PUD in younger patients. However, there has also been an association established implicating increased risk of duodenal ulceration with chronic lung, liver, and pancreatic disease processes [13, 15]. Gastric ulcers account for only 5% of all PUD, yet more operative interventions are needed for gastric ulcers than for duodenal ulcers. Additionally, gastric ulcers are more frequently associated with the elderly, and are therefore associated with a higher mortality rate [16, 17]. Despite the overall

L.J. Moore et al. (eds.), *Common Problems in Acute Care Surgery*,
DOI 10.1007/978-1-4614-6123-4_17, © Springer Science+Business Media New York 2013

decline in PUD over the past 30 years, the rate of emergent operative intervention for bleeding, obstruction, or perforation has remained relatively unchanged in the United States. Moreover, there is data out of European countries that may reveal an actual increase in need for emergent operative interventions. There is an overall decrease in the prevalence of PUD in developed countries due to advances in pharmaceutical technology and sanitation that have significantly reduced the *H. pylori* infection rate [5, 6]. However, when considering the increased overall usage of NSAIDS in an increasingly older population, the explanation for the relative lack of improvement in the frequency of operative intervention becomes evident.

Anatomical Considerations

Peptic ulcers have characteristic anatomical occurrence patterns. Ninety-five percent of all duodenal ulcerations are located within 2 cm of the pylorus in the first portion, or the bulb, of the duodenum. These lesions are almost always non-malignant disease processes. There are five different classifications of gastric ulcers according to the most commonly used classification system, the Modified Johnson classification system. Type I ulcers occur along the lesser curvature of the stomach near the incisura angularis, and 60% of these are located within 6 cm of the pylorus [15]. Type II ulcers are pre-pyloric gastric ulcers. They occur in association with duodenal ulcers and are often referred to as "kissing ulcers." Type III gastric ulcers are located in the antrum or pre-pyloric region. Type IV ulcers are located near the gastroesophageal junction, on the proximal lesser curvature. Type V ulcers are the newest category: lesions that are secondary to NSAID or aspirin usage. They can be located anywhere throughout the stomach. Ninety-five percent of gastric ulcers are also benign in nature. Even giant ulcers, lesions greater than 2 cm, which were once thought to be malignant, are now known to be benign processes in 90% of patients. Ulcers located in the fundus of the stomach are very rare; however, these lesions should elicit concern as most are malignant [18].

Pathophysiology

Although there may be numerous factors that contribute to the development of gastroduodenal mucosal breakdown, we now recognize that the majority of gastroduodenal ulcerations are caused by *Helicobacter pylori (H. pylori)* infestation, NSAID use, or a combination of the two. 75% of patients with gastric ulcers and 90% of those with duodenal ulcers are infected with *H. pylori* yet only 15–20% of people colonized with the bacteria will develop PUD in their lifetime [14]. Greater than half of patients with PUD report recent NSAID use [18, 19]. Additionally, several studies have demonstrated a cumulative effect of cigarette smoking with H pylori that leads to an increased risk of complicated PUD [20, 21]. The overall mechanism of ulcerogenesis results from the inability of the mucosal barrier to protect the gastroduodenal mucosa from acidic gastric secretions [22]. There are multiple factors that have been associated with mucosal injury and excessive acid secretion including smoking, psychological stress, alcohol, drugs (including aspirin and cocaine), and various environmental associations [2].

The treatment philosophy for PUD was historically "no acid no ulcer." It remains a viable statement since acid suppression is the key management strategy to the promotion of healing. Prior to our understanding of the role of *H. pylori* and NSAIDs in ulcerogenesis, therapy was long-standing and consisted of avoidance of known ulcerogenic stimuli such as caffeine, smoking, and alcohol along with pharmaceutical management to relieve symptoms. Surgical intervention, such as antrectomy and vagotomy for acid suppression, was then used if relief was not obtained from conservative measures. Pharmaceutical therapy consisted of antacids, H2 blockers (introduced in the late 1960s), and various oral cytoprotective agents. Proton pump inhibitors (PPIs) were not introduced until the late 1980s. In 1984, Marshall and Warren published their discovery of "an unidentified curved bacilli in the stomach of patients with gastritis and peptic ulcerations," eventually known as *Helicobacter pylori* [23]. Multiple trials over the following several years established the etiology of *H. pylori* in PUD. Subsequently, evidence demonstrated that a short treatment course with antibiotics and antisecretory agents resulted in a cure for the majority of ulcers without recurrence [24–27]. In 1994, the National Institute of Health Consensus Conference officially recommended the medical eradication of *H. pylori* as the primary therapy for PUD [28].

It is now understood that *H. pylori* infection results in the alteration of gastric acid secretion that is observed in PUD. If the infection is localized primarily in the antrum, an impairment and alteration in the negative feedback loop results in increased acid productivity. The ultimate outcome is an increased prevalence of pre-pyloric and duodenal ulcers. Patients that have a global infection of the gastric mucosa consistently have decreased acid secretion in response to the chronic inflammation within the gastric body. This leads to impaired protective function of the gastric mucosa resulting in ulcer formation [2].

In regard to NSAIDs, as well as aspirin, the mechanism of insult is related to the inhibition of prostaglandins by both of these classes of drugs. Prostaglandins act to increase mucous secretion and bicarbonate production as well as to modulate the blood flow to the mucosal tissue [29]. The inhibition of the mucosal defense mechanisms along with decreased blood flow and impaired healing leads to the direct correlation of both

NSAIDs and aspirin with ulcer formation. In concordance, there is an additional synergistic effect that occurs in patients with underlying *H. pylori* infection that also take anti-inflammatory medications. The protective function of the mucosa is further weakened leading to increased ulcerogenesis [30]. The majority of gastric and duodenal ulcers are attributable to one or both of these two pathogens in combination. Taking this into account, it would be prudent to say that the majority of ulcerogenesis can be contributed to treatable or avoidable causes that can be managed medically [31]. Therefore, the current surgical approach in elective and emergent management of PUD has become reflective of this treatment philosophy.

Medical Management of Peptic Ulcer Disease

If PUD is in the differential diagnosis for a patient in accordance with symptoms or the chief complaint, a complete history and physical should focus on the cause or confounding factors associated with the disease process. Medical management can then focus on addressing these factors with the patient. Patients should be tested for *H. pylori* so that a treatment regimen can be initiated. An esophagogastroduodenoscopy (EGD) is not mandatory for diagnosis. Serology is the test of choice if endoscopy is not required. The urea breath test is also an option, but it is used more frequently as a test of cure after a treatment regimen has been completed. An EGD should be considered for all patients with symptomatology consistent with PUD for evaluation and diagnosis. Biopsies can be taken for *H. pylori* histology or culture, or a rapid urease assay can be performed. In addition, visualizing the location and overall presentation of the ulcerative disease helps to address the causative factors, especially if the patient uses NSAIDs chronically. Most physicians will presumptively treat for PUD with an H2 blocker or PPI in order to improve symptoms prior to attaining an EGD to verify the diagnosis. If symptoms persist and noninvasive testing is pending or inconclusive for *H. pylori*, an empiric therapeutic regimen is also a reasonable option. Although there are multiple ways to test or screen for *H. pylori,* the most accurate test is with a tissue sample for histology or culture.

All NSAIDs and aspirin should be discontinued if the patient has an upper GI bleed, a diagnosed ulceration, or if PUD is strongly suspected based upon the clinical presentation. For those who are on aspirin therapy for recent cardiac stent placement or other co-morbidities, there should be an expedited workup and thorough multidisciplinary evaluation of the risks and benefits associated with continued salicylate use. In addition, all practices that may be ulcerogenic such as smoking, caffeine intake, alcohol consumption, and cocaine abuse should be addressed and abandoned if PUD is suspected. It is essential that patients understand the importance of lifestyle modification on the progression and resolution of PUD.

Table 17.1 Treatment regimens for *Helicobacter pylori* (data from ref. (33))

Medications/dose/frequency	Duration
PPI + Clarithromycin 500 mg bid + Amoxicillin 1,000 mg bid	10–14 days
PPI + Clarithromycin 500 mg bid + Metronidazole 500 mg bid	10–14 days
PPI + Amoxicillin 1,000 mg bid then:	5 days
PPI + Clarithromycin 500 mg bid + Tinidazole 500 mg bid	5 days
Salvage regimens	
Bismuth subsalicylate 525 mg qid + Metronidazole 250 mg qid + Tetracycline 500 mg qid + PPI	10–14 days
PPI + Amoxicillin 1,000 mg bid + levofloxacin 500 mg daily	10 days

PPI = proton pump inhibitor

Acute presentations of PUD, such as pain, bleeding, or perforation, should be treated with continuous infusion of an intravenous PPI. Upon discharge, these patients should remain on an oral PPI or an H2 blocker for at least 3 months. A follow-up endoscopy should then be scheduled to monitor healing, especially if there is a chronic component to the presentation. Depending upon the initial pathology and the source of the lesion, healing has usually peaked by 4 weeks. Patients who are hospitalized for complications due to PUD, those with a repetitive history of PUD, and patients that require aspirin or NSAID therapy for other co-morbidities should be considered for lifelong maintenance with PPI or H2 receptor blocker therapy. Additionally, patients who are noncompliant with smoking cessation or alcohol abuse should remain on maintenance therapy as well if these behaviors were felt to be contributory to their PUD. Misoprostol as well as sucralfate are useful as adjuncts to antisecretory therapy. However, these drugs should be used only as preventative maintenance therapy, or in conjunction with H2 blockers or PPIs. They should not be used as sole therapy in patients who are acutely symptomatic. As previously mentioned, the majority of PUD can be attributed to an association with *H. pylori* infection. If *H. pylori* has been diagnosed via biopsy or serology, the patient should complete a treatment regimen for eradication [18, 32]. There are multiple acceptable regimens [33] (see Table 17.1).

Clinical Presentation of Peptic Ulcer Disease

The majority of patients who are diagnosed with PUD complain of pain in the epigastric region. The pain is often described as a localized burning, aching, or "gnawing" pain. Other symptoms include nausea, vomiting, bloating, anemia, and anorexia or weight loss due to decreased oral intake secondary to symptoms. An extensive and thorough history should be elicited from the patient. In particular, the questioning should focus on previous episodes or symptoms consistent with PUD, correlation with oral intake, and the patient's association with known ulcerogenic risk factors. An aggressive medication history should also be attained with a specific focus on NSAIDs, aspirin, antisecretory medications, consumption and correlation of antacid use, and a complete social history including alcohol, tobacco, and substance abuse as well as recent psychological stressors.

Duodenal ulcers characteristically have a cyclic type of associated pain. Patients often awake from sleep at night with epigastric pain; however it is usually resolved by the time they awake. Throughout the day, pain recurs 1–2 h after eating a meal and then temporarily dissipates with oral intake or antacids. Symptoms worsen and become more constant if the ulceration erodes posteriorly into the pancreas. Back pain may then also ensue. Pain with palpation during physical exam is an inconsistent and unreliable finding.

Gastric ulcers usually present with epigastric pain that is coupled with oral intake. Patients often complain of pain within 30 min of eating, and at times, symptoms can be aggravated by oral intake. In spite of this, many patients claim to have at least temporary relief of symptoms with oral intake or antacids. Symptoms from gastric ulcers can also be reliably vague and nonspecific in nature leading to a circuitous and extensive differential diagnosis and workup. PUD should be a differential diagnosis for any patient with abdominal symptomatology.

The most common indications for acute surgical intervention for PUD are bleeding and perforation [32]. Anemia may be the presenting symptom with chronic PUD; however, chronic bleeding is rarely managed surgically as most lesions will respond to medical management with compliance. Other reasons for surgical intervention due to PUD include intractable pain, refractory PUD, gastric outlet obstruction, known malignancy, and sequelae secondary to gastrinomas (ZES). Since the majority of emergent procedures for PUD involve perforation or bleeding, the remainder of the chapter addresses surgical management for this population of patients as it pertains to the acute care surgeon.

Bleeding Peptic Ulcer Disease

Sixty percent of all upper GI bleeds are secondary to PUD [34]. Of all deaths that are felt to be attributable to PUD, bleeding is the most common cause of mortality. This patient population is usually older than 65 years of age with concurrent chronic co-morbidities [15]. Although 80% of UGI bleeds are self-limited, there is an overall mortality of 8–10% in those that continue to bleed or have recurrent bleeds. Recurrent bleeds occur in 20–30% of patients and the mortality after a re-bleed ranges from 10 to 40%. Not surprisingly, the onset of a GI bleed during an unrelated hospital stay is associated with a higher mortality rate (33%) than an initial bleed outside of the hospital or before admission (7%) [14, 35]. The American Society of Gastrointestinal Endoscopy (ASGE) investigated the correlation of eight different disease co-morbidities with outcomes in patients with upper GI bleeding. These included central nervous system, cardiac, gastrointestinal, hepatic, pulmonary, neoplastic, renal, and psychological stress. The mortality rate for an upper GI bleed with no concurrent diagnoses was 2.5%. However, if the patient had three coexisting diagnoses, the mortality rate rose to 14.6%, and then to 66.7% with six diagnoses [36].

Due to the significant amount of blood supply to the stomach, 35–40% of gastric ulcers will bleed, but significant hemorrhage is more associated with type II and type III gastric ulcers [14]. Gastric ulcers are more commonly found in older patients. This explains the correlation with increased morbidity and mortality in patients with bleeding gastric ulcers in comparison to bleeding duodenal ulcers. The duodenum, however, also has a generous blood supply from the gastroduodenal artery (GDA), which lies just posterior to the duodenum. When a duodenal ulceration progressively erodes through the duodenal wall and into a branch of the GDA, or the artery itself, the resultant bleeding can be substantial. Fortunately, the majority of duodenal ulcers are superficial in nature, and most bleeds are self-limited or amenable to endoscopic interventions [35]. In reality, the majority of duodenal ulcers will present as minor bleeds with guaiac-positive stools or melana. However, approximately 25% of all upper GI bleeds that present for urgent treatment are due to duodenal ulcerations [14].

Acute upper gastrointestinal bleeding due to PUD presents as hematemesis, melana, or occasionally hematochezia with massive hemorrhage. Not uncommonly, patients will present after actively bleeding or possibly with syncope to the emergency department with a history of having been "found down" at home for some unknown amount of time. These patients are frequently hemodynamically unstable due to hemorrhagic shock. Aggressive resuscitation and transfusion may be required to stabilize the patient enough to even tolerate endoscopy for diagnostic or therapeutic measures.

As with any critically ill patient that is hemodynamically unstable, the standard airway, breathing, circulation (ABC) algorithm should be followed by verifying a patent or secure airway, ensuring adequate oxygenation and ventilation, and then focusing on the patient's circulation and hemodynamics. Two large-bore IVs should be attained for volume resuscitation with crystalloid or blood products if significant hemorrhage is suspected or known to have occurred. If peripheral access is not available, a central venous catheter, such as a large-diameter cordis catheter, should be placed to better facilitate resuscitation and transfusion. Blood products should be available and transfused as necessary, and coagulopathies should be addressed and corrected. A Foley catheter is usually placed so that accurate urine output can be monitored to reflect kidney perfusion. Central venous lines and arterial lines are often placed in order to accurately monitor hemodynamic parameters, volume status, and resuscitation efforts.

If the source of bleeding is unclear, an upper GI source versus a lower GI source, a nasogastric tube should be inserted and a gastric lavage should be performed looking for clots or bloody aspirate. Some would advocate irrigation with ice water or cold saline solution until the nasogastric tube irrigation is clear as the iced irrigation will usually stop or slow the bleeding. Although there is no evidence basis behind the practice, most practitioners will immediately start intravenous PPIs or H2 blockers while resuscitating. Once the patient is resuscitated and hemodynamically stable, the upper endoscopy can be facilitated. These patients are critically ill with the potential for instability, regardless of the endoscopy findings. The majority of these patients, and in particular the elderly, frail, or those patients with multiple co-morbidities, should be monitored in an ICU setting with serial hemoglobin monitoring for a minimum of 24–48 h after the initial event.

Endoscopy is first-line treatment for all upper GI bleeds, especially and including variceal bleeds. Many facilities will consult a gastroenterology service; however, many general surgeons also have privileges to perform interventional endoscopic procedures. A surgical endoscopist would also have the advantage of visualizing the anatomy and location of the bleed. This would be optimal should endoscopic measures be unsuccessful and operative intervention become necessary. Either way, the surgical team should be present to visualize the source of bleeding and the interventions attempted for hemorrhage control in order to formulate an operative plan. In the hands of a skilled endoscopist, surgical intervention is only required in 5–10% of bleeding ulcers, and many upper GI bleeds will actually stop spontaneously [31]. There are several different scoring systems that have been developed to predict the need for intervention for control of bleeding. The use of these prognostic scoring systems to identify patients at greater risk is one of the recommendations from the international consensus of recommendations for management of non-variceal upper GI bleeding that was published in 2010 in the *Annals of Internal Medicine* [37]. Gastroenterologists as well as surgeons should be comfortable and familiar with these scoring systems. Blatchford published a scoring system in *Lancet* in 2000 that is likely the most referenced. The system uses both clinical and laboratory data to help predict the likelihood of need for intervention to attain hemostasis. Patients with a score of less than or equal to 3 have a 6% chance of requiring intervention for hemostasis, whereas those with a score of 6 or higher have a greater than 50% chance of needing endoscopic or surgical intervention for control of hemorrhage [38] (see Table 17.2 and Fig. 17.1).

Table 17.2 Blatchford admission risk markers for peptic ulcer bleeding (adapted from ref. 39)

Admission risk marker	Score component value
Blood urea (mg/dl)	
6.5–8.0	2
8.0–10.0	3
10.0–25.0	4
>25.0	6
Hemoglobin (g/dl) for men	
12.0–13.0	1
10.0–12.0	2
<10.0	6
Hemoglobin (g/dl) for women	
10.0–12.0	1
<10.0	6
Systolic Blood Pressure (mmHg)	
100–109	1
90–99	2
<90	3
Other markers	
Pulse > 100 bpm	1
Presentation with melana	1
Presentation with syncope	2
Hepatic disease	2
Cardiac failure	2

Scores ≥6 have a greater than 50% chance of requiring intervention

The first goal of endoscopy is to locate and visualize the source of bleeding, and there are many endoscopic techniques used for control of upper GI hemorrhage. There is often excessive clot over the lesion, and irrigation is necessary to visualize the mucosa below the clots. This is done with caution as not to disturb the clot directly over the lesion and the hemostasis that may have already been achieved. Indications for endoscopic therapeutic intervention include active bleeding or oozing at an identified site, stigmata of a recent bleed such as a large blood clot, or the presence of a visible vessel at the base of the ulceration. If the lesion is no longer bleeding, or if it is merely oozing, epinephrine is often injected in or around the lesion and the surrounding mucosa in order to employ its vasoconstrictive properties for assistance with clot formation. Beyond injection, there are several other methods of direct vessel control depending upon the source and location of the bleed. Cautery may be used to provide hemostasis, or sclerosing agents may be directly injected into the bleeding vessel. Clips can be placed directly on a visualized vessel or circumferentially to address the rich vascularity of the region. Banding is more frequently used on variceal bleeds, but can also be successful depending upon the source. Most endoscopists will use epinephrine in association with another method of intervention such as clips or cautery. Dual intervention has been shown to improve the success of initial endoscopic hemorrhage control and also to decrease the incidence of recurrent bleeding [39, 40].

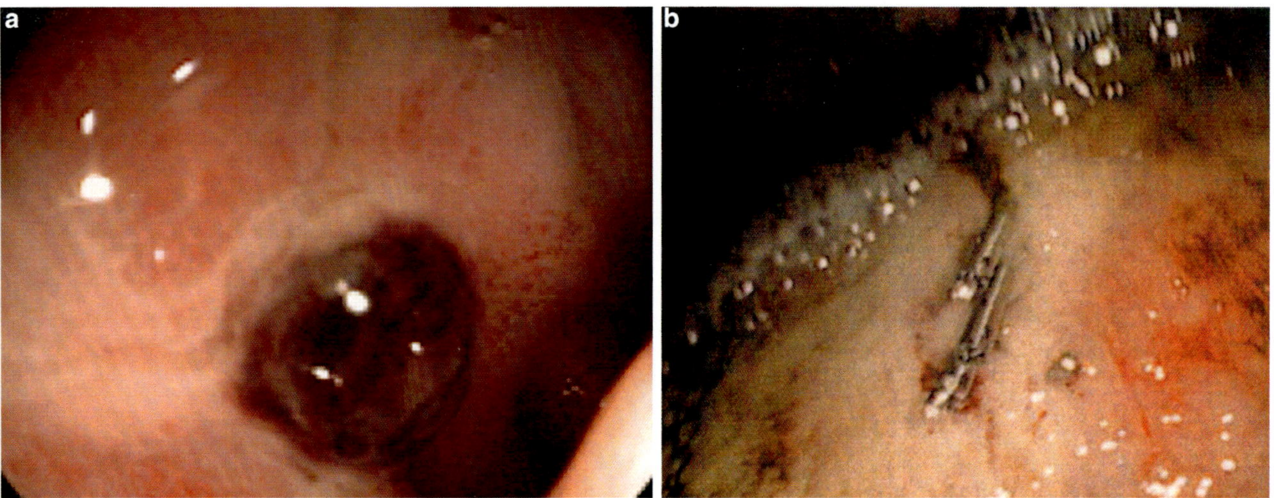

Fig. 17.1 (**a**) Ulcer in the bulb of the duodenum with overlying clot (**b**) Endoscopic clips used to control hemorrhage from a gastric ulcer

The majority of upper GI bleeds can be initially controlled via endoscopic interventions; however, 15–20% of patients will experience recurrence of bleeding from the site of ulceration [41]. It is the surgical team's responsibility to evaluate the patient and his or her co-morbidities, the cause of bleeding, and any other extenuating factors to decide if and when operative intervention is necessary. Historically, many surgeons have used a threshold of six transfused units of packed red blood cells as the deciding point to proceed with operative intervention. The number six certainly defines the need for excessive transfusion, but several other factors need to be considered along with the patient's transfusion requirements. The location of the ulcer should be influential in the decision of whether or not to intervene early. In particular, lesions in areas with grossly exposed vasculature, those with abundant blood supply such as posterior duodenal ulcers, or ulcers on the lesser gastric curvature with extensive inflow from the left gastric artery may benefit from early operative intervention.

Many endoscopists routinely perform a second-look procedure at 24 h after the initial endoscopic intervention. There is also frequently a trend to repeat therapies such as cautery or injection of epinephrine in order to prophylactically treat continued oozing or to reinforce previous interventions. If the re-bleed is significant, many practitioners will proceed with repeat endoscopic therapeutic interventions. However, if the source was visualized on previous endoscopy, operative intervention may be the more prudent decision. In a prospectively randomized study performed at a high-volume center, Lau and colleagues demonstrated a 75% success rate in control of re-bleeds via repeat endoscopic intervention. They also found similar mortality rates and decreased complication rates when compared to a similar group of patients who underwent surgical intervention. Additionally, their data recognized two factors that independently predicted failure of repeat endoscopic interventions for re-bleeding: hypotension and ulcers greater than 2 cm [42]. Elemunzer et al. did a meta-analysis of ten prospective studies to assess re-bleeding after endoscopic therapy for hemorrhage due to PUD. They found the rate of re-bleeding to be 16.4%. The following factors were found to be independently predictive of re-bleeding after endoscopic interventions: pre-endoscopic hemodynamic instability, comorbid illness, active bleeding at endoscopy, large ulcer size (>2 cm), posterior duodenal ulcerations, and ulcerations on the lesser gastric curvature [43]. Every patient must be individually evaluated and the transfusion requirements, hemodynamic status, and co-morbidities taken into consideration. However, it seems reasonable to proceed with early surgical intervention after the first endoscopy if the ulcer is greater than 2 cm, there is hemodynamic instability, there was extensive hemorrhage, the location of the ulcer is concerning (the posterior duodenum or the lesser gastric curvature), or the patient is greater than 60 years of age and/or has multiple co-morbidities (Fig. 17.2).

In complicated patients with intricate surgical or medical histories, localizing the source of the hemorrhage and identifying the best method to attain hemostasis may be challenging. A technetium-99 m tagged red blood cell scan is a nuclear study that can identify bleeding at 0.1 ml/min and therefore may be beneficial in identifying a slow GI bleed. The study may be difficult to facilitate as availability may be institution dependent, and although it may be somewhat sensitive, it lacks specificity in localization of hemorrhage [44]. However, this information can be instrumental at times in helping to guide the next stage of clinical intervention. Computed tomography angiograms (CTA) have recently been used more frequently with lower GI bleeding for source localization. Depending upon the patient and the clinical

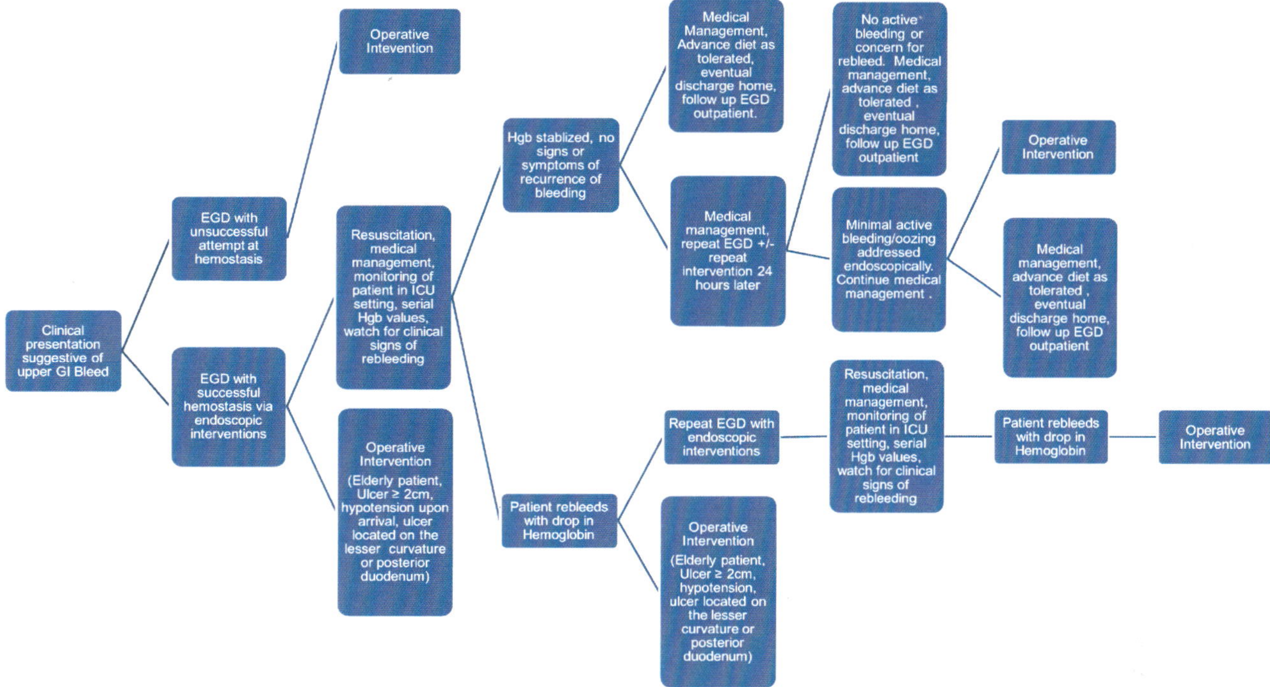

Fig. 17.2 Algorithm for contemporary management of upper GI bleed due to peptic ulcer disease

scenario, a CTA may be helpful in localizing bleeding in the upper GI tract as well. Modern-day multi-detector CT scans can detect bleeding at a rate of between 0.35 and 0.40 ml/min, which is improved sensitivity in comparison to angiography. CT scans may be useful for identification of an upper GI bleed; however rarely is there a practical need for the expense or the radiation exposure incurred without any means of truly effecting prognosis or outcomes.

A resource that has become increasingly more utilized in critically ill and complicated patients (those with re-bleeding, uncertain endoscopic findings, or those who are at high risk for general anesthesia) is angiography and interventional arterial embolization. Angiography can identify bleeding at a rate of 0.5 ml/min and is less sensitive than a tagged RBC scan. However, angiography can be used in conjunction with fluoroscopy to localize the region of bleeding and to then embolize the primary blood supply to that region. The most common vessel to be embolized in interventional procedures for bleeding PUD is the GDA followed by the left gastric artery. On average, active bleeding is demonstrated about 50% of the time leaving 50% of the interventions categorized as empiric therapy. Selective embolization is performed primarily using either coils or a gel foam material. Although the stomach and duodenum have a rich vascular supply, there is an associated risk of ischemia with any embolization procedure to not only the stomach and the duodenum but also the pancreas [45–47]. Therefore, interventional radiologic procedures should never be introduced as first-line therapy. All risks and benefits of embolization

should be thoroughly evaluated in relation to the patient and the clinical scenario. Post-procedurally, all patients should be monitored closely for any clinical signs of re-bleeding or ischemia with telemetry, serial abdominal exams, and serial laboratory values including base deficits, lactate levels, and complete blood counts to monitor for continued bleeding and leukocytosis.

Regardless of the decision to operate, to repeat endoscopy, to consult interventional radiology, or to observe closely with medical management, the surgical team should remain intimately involved in the care of this population of patients until they are hemodynamically stable and are tolerating oral intake without signs of continued bleeding.

Operative Intervention for Bleeding Peptic Ulcers

Once the decision has been made to operate on a patient with an upper GI bleed, a thorough evaluation of the intraoperative findings and the clinical scenario will help to guide which operation is most appropriate for the patient. With the advancements in endoscopic control of enteric bleeds, the patients that fail endoscopic management tend to be those with the highest risk factors for surgical intervention. Given the shift in the population now requiring these procedures, the historically indicated procedures for stable elective patients may not always be the safest and most appropriate intervention. The type of operation performed should initially be based on the patient's overall clinical picture and hemodynamic status. In unstable patients, the procedure should provide hemostasis within the least amount of time under general anesthesia. Additional procedures can be done at a later time, if necessary, once the patient has stabilized. Other factors that should be considered are the possibility of malignancy, coinciding perforation or obstruction, and the location of the ulcer.

The generalized surgical principles for the treatment of an acute bleed secondary to PUD are relatively straightforward. The most important goal is obviously hemostasis. The option of an antisecretory procedure with respective drainage as indicated may then be considered. Oversewing of the ulcer is the most common intervention for bleeding duodenal ulcers. Bleeding gastric ulcers, although rare, can also be oversewn, but they must additionally be biopsied to rule out malignancy. Dependent upon the patient's clinical presentation, the surgeon's experience, and the patient's history of PUD, medical compliance, and co-morbidities, a highly selective vagotomy (HSV) or a truncal vagotomy with drainage procedure may additionally be performed. The third category of treatment options includes resection or excision of the ulcer which may also involve a vagotomy and a drainage procedure dependent upon the location and indication.

Traditionally the decision of whether or not to do an antisecretory procedure was dependent upon the location of the ulcer. Type II and type III ulcers have classically been categorized as lesions that evolve secondary to acid hypersecretion. The historical recommendation has always been to perform a truncal vagotomy with a gastric emptying procedure. If the pylorus is not resected or bypassed, a pyloroplasty would be the necessary alternative. Some would advocate the use of a HSV to allow gastric emptying and avert the need for pyloroplasty or antrectomy. However, given the relative rarity of HSV in modern-day general surgery, the majority of younger surgeons do not have the exposure or experience to perform the procedure with dependably successful outcomes. In considering our advances regarding *H. pylori* treatment, the pathogenesis of ulcer formation, and the use of PPIs for acid suppression, the necessity for antisecretory procedures is ambiguous. Truncal vagotomies are associated with some level of dumping syndrome, whether it is clinically significant or not. HSV may be associated with lesser detrimental effects; however, the procedure is less common and certainly more time consuming. The patient's overall state of health, his or her hemodynamic status, and the location of the bleed must all be taken into consideration when the operative plan is established.

Most modern-day damage control surgery for acutely bleeding PUD involves either resection or oversewing of the ulceration. Patients are then treated postoperatively for assumed *H. pylori* with an appropriate regimen including PPIs or H2 blockers. In the era of the damage control laparotomy, resection alone also can be performed, leaving the patient in discontinuity with a properly placed nasogastric tube for decompression. A second-look laparotomy can then be utilized, after the patient is adequately resuscitated, for reconstruction or performance of definitive antisecretory and drainage procedures if they are indicated. Regardless of the choice of intervention, it should be understood that the majority of patients requiring surgical intervention for bleeding PUD in the current era have very little physiologic reserve. Operative interventions should focus on expediently addressing the source of the bleeding in order to return the patient back to the ICU for resuscitation and hemodynamic support.

Operative Approach for the Bleeding Gastric Ulcer

Gastric Resection

The procedure of choice for bleeding types I, II, and III ulcers (Fig. 17.3) is a distal gastric resection inclusive of the bleeding ulcer. A Billroth I or Billroth II reconstruction can then be performed depending upon the mobility of the duodenum. As always, the patient's hemodynamic status is the deciding factor as to whether or not it is appropriate to proceed forward with a definitive anastomotic procedure. If the patient is hypotensive, it would be prudent to do a wedge resection, an oversew procedure, or a damage control partial gastrectomy with nasogastric decompression and an eventual second laparotomy to establish continuity. A wedge resection can easily be performed if the ulcer is on the greater curvature, the antrum, or within the body of the stomach. However, resection may be difficult or inappropriate for type IV ulcerations, lesions on the lesser curvature, or those more proximal to the gastroesophageal junction. Multiple bleeding erosions may require total gastrectomy with eventual creation of a Roux-en-Y esophagojejunostomy or esophagogastrojejunostomy, depending upon the extent of gastric resection that is required to gain hemostasis.

Gastric resections, as well as ulcer excisions, are usually performed with a gastrointestinal anastomosis (GIA) stapler after the stomach is sufficiently mobilized and cleared of surrounding attachments. A Kocher maneuver is performed in order to mobilize the duodenum for the gastroduodenal anastamosis of a Billroth I procedure. The anastomosis is created by removing, or avoiding initial placement of, the staple line on the inferior portion of the gastrectomy. The anastomosis can then either be handsewn in a two-layer fashion using absorbable sutures or stapled with a GIA stapler placed through a gastrotomy.

If the duodenum is scarred or will not reach the distal stomach remnant, a Billroth II will need to be performed. There are several complications associated with this procedure including duodenal stump leaks and afferent or efferent

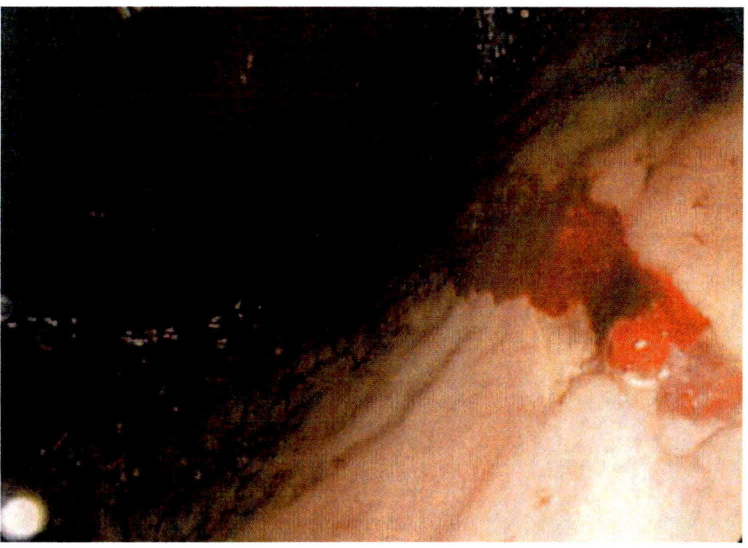

Fig. 17.3 Active arterial bleeding from a gastric ulcer on the lesser curvature of the stomach

limb syndromes. The Billroth I primary anastomosis has less incidence of complications, but if there is any tension on the anastomosis, a Billroth II is the procedure of choice. The proximal duodenum should be transected using either a TA stapler or a GIA stapler. Attention should be given to the anatomy in regard to the common bile duct, as it lies just posterior to this region. Additionally, the thickness and induration of the duodenal stump should be evaluated. It may be necessary to handsew the stump closed to avoid a stump leak. Many experienced surgeons would suggest placing an omental patch over the stump as well. In the case of a friable or extremely indurated stump, a lateral duodenostomy tube can be placed in a Stamm fashion to the lateral abdominal wall in order to decompress the duodenum, although this is recommended only in extreme conditions. There are several ways to perform the anastomosis for a Billroth II gastrojejunostomy. The jejunal afferent limb should reach the gastric remnant without any tension, but with no more than 20 cm of length from the ligament of Treitz. Placing the jejunum through a retrocolic window will decrease tension on the mesentery, but antecolic placement is functionally equivalent. There are several methods of constructing the gastrojejunostomy using staplers, 2′0 absorbable sutures, or a combination of both. If the anastomosis is handsewn, it should be a two-layered anastomosis with an outer layer of Lembert sutures and an inner layer of full-thickness absorbable sutures.

The Oversew Technique

Oversewing of a bleeding gastric ulcer is not the ideal procedure, but it may be the most appropriate procedure for a high-risk patient. Remember that all gastric ulcers must be biopsied if resection is not possible, and therefore, if the ulcer is oversewn, a biopsy must be procured. If the location of the ulcer is known, a gastrotomy is made to localize the lesion. The ulcer is then biopsied and oversewn with absorbable sutures to attain hemostasis. The gastrotomy should be closed in a two-layer fashion or via a TA stapler. In type IV ulcers, those lesions located near the gastroesophageal junction, oversewing the ulcer is the procedure of choice as this region is not readily amenable to wedge resection. The area also has a vast blood supply secondary to inflow from the left gastric artery. The appropriate procedure for a type IV lesion then includes oversewing the bleeding ulcer, ligation of the left gastric artery to prevent re-bleeding, and a vagotomy and drainage procedure (pyloroplasty) if the patient is hemodynamically stable.

Truncal Vagotomy and Pyloroplasty

In a stable patient, with straightforward anatomy, a truncal vagotomy should be considered for acid suppression as long as the procedure does not extensively prolong time spent in the operating room. In order to perform a vagotomy, the left lateral section of the liver as well as the triangular ligament must be mobilized. The esophagogastric junction must be retracted inferiorly using gentle tension in order to localize the proximal nerves. Once the nerves are localized, they are isolated using Penrose drains. Clips are placed proximally and distally on each nerve, and a 2 cm long portion of each proximal nerve is excised and sent off to pathology for verification. Exposure and extensive mobilization are often required for this procedure, and therefore should only be pursued in hemodynamically stable patients. If a truncal vagotomy is performed, the vagal intervention to the pylorus and distal stomach is disrupted. If a bypass procedure is not performed, pyloroplasty is necessary to allow for drainage of the gastric contents. The most commonly performed method of pyloroplasty is the Heineke–Mikulicz pyloroplasty. The pylorus is localized and bovie cautery is then used to create a longitudinal full-thickness pyloromyotomy extending from

1 cm proximal to 1–2 cm distal to the pylorus. Traction sutures are then placed superiorly and inferiorly and tension is applied superiorly and inferiorly to convert the longitudinal incision into a transverse incision. The defect is then closed transversely in a double-layer fashion with full-thickness bites using nonabsorbable suture. A Kocher maneuver and adequate duodenal mobilization may be necessary in order to close the incision without tension.

Operative Approach for Bleeding Duodenal Ulcer

As with the management of bleeding ulcers, the same principles of management apply in regard to an acutely bleeding duodenal ulcer. The ulcer can either be oversewn or resected in order to achieve hemostasis. The option to perform a vagotomy and drainage procedure then also needs to be contemplated. The most commonly used approach is by creation of the pyloromyotomy as previously described. The longitudinal duodenotomy incision is extended another 1 cm as needed in order to visualize the duodenal ulcer. As nearly all duodenal ulcerations are located on the posterior portion of the first part of the duodenum, this incision should give ample exposure. A Kocher maneuver can be performed if necessary for exposure and so that the left hand can be used to manually control bleeding. The source of bleeding is usually the gastroduodenal artery. Figure of eight sutures with a heavy suture material, such as 3′0 silk, should be placed superiorly and inferiorly at the base of the posterior duodenal ulcer for ligation of the vessel. Several sutures may need to be placed before hemostasis is attained. A U-stitch should also be placed at the base of the ulcer in order to control any possible hemorrhage from the transverse pancreatic arterial branches that enter the gastroduodenal artery from the posterior aspect. Once the bleeding has ceased, the ulcer should be manipulated in order to verify the stability of the arterial ligation. If true hemostasis has been achieved, the longitudinal incision can then be closed transversely in two layers as a Heineke–Mikulicz pyloroplasty. A Finney pyloroplasty can also be utilized if transverse reapproximation is not attainable. If the patient is stable, a truncal vagotomy would be the classic next step in management. However, the majority of surgeons, as evident by surveys performed in both the United Kingdom and the United States, no longer perform vagotomies on these patients [7, 48]. Although there is no level 1 evidence to support the change in practice patterns, the transition has come about since the availability of medical acid suppression with PPIs.

The other option for management of a bleeding duodenal ulcer is resection. An antrectomy is performed that extends distally to the first portion of the duodenum in order to encompass the bleeding ulcer. The surgeon must be acutely cognizant of the location of the common bile duct when performing the resection as it can easily be mistaken for thickened tissue within the stapler device. A vagotomy and accompanying reconstructive procedure will then also need to be performed. A Billroth II is usually the type of reconstruction used given the shortened length of the duodenal stump. However, if it can be attained without tension on the anastomosis, a Billroth I would be the procedure of choice. The GIA stapler is usually employed for the gastroduodenectomy procedure. The duodenal stump should be approached in the same fashion as previously described including the use of an omental patch. Complications from the procedure are similar to those previously described for gastric resection including duodenal stump leak, dumping syndrome, and anastomotic breakdown of the gastrojejunostomy. It is also imperative to insure that all of the antrum is resected as retained antrum can result in recurrent ulcerative disease.

As previously mentioned, the majority of surgeons opt to perform the less invasive of the two procedures, the duodenotomy and pyloroplasty. There is data from the early 1990s that supports similar mortality outcomes with either method. In 1991, Poxon published data comparing acid suppression with histamine blockers in combination with oversewing to vagotomy and pyloroplasty or antrectomy and found similar mortality rates [49]. However, the study was stopped early due to several re-bleeding episodes in the conservative group. In 1993, Millat published a randomized controlled study comparing vagotomy and pyloroplasty to excision of the ulcer that revealed increased incidence of re-bleeding (17% vs. 3%) with the less invasive procedure, though mortality outcomes were similar [50]. In analyzing these studies, it would seem that although the mortality outcomes are similar there is an increased incidence in re-bleeding with the less invasive method. The problem with all of these studies is that they are outdated, as all of these results were collected prior to the introduction of PPIs. Certainly we know that this class of drugs has completely changed the management of PUD. The majority of surgeons extrapolate the success of the PPIs in acid suppression to their choice in operative management. Many will perform the least invasive procedure with the caveat that these patients will remain on acid-suppressing medications. In saying that, there is no known literature to date that has analyzed either procedure in combination with PPIs. The literature in regard to reoperation for bleeding on patients after having received a pyloroplasty and vagotomy also comes from the early 1990s prior to the introduction of PPIs when the rate of re-bleed was somewhere between 6 and 17% [49, 50]. If a patient re-bleeds, endoscopic intervention is usually not an option, especially if the patient is in the acute postoperative period. Reoperation carries a much higher risk of morbidity and mortality; however if resection was not performed during the initial operation, this would be an option to achieve hemostasis. It has become increasingly more common to employ the expertise of interventional radiology for postoperative hemorrhage control with transarterial embolization under fluoroscopy. There are no studies to date that directly compare operative intervention with transarterial embolization; however, there is data from two large studies that indicate a 75% success rate in controlling recurrent bleeding after duodenostomy and oversewing of a bleeding ulcer [51, 52].

Perforated Peptic Ulcer Disease

Perforation is the second most common complication related to PUD. The majority of these ulcers tend to occur in the region of the pyloric channel or the first portion of the duodenum. Perforation is most common in the duodenal bulb (62%), followed by the pylorus (20%), and then the gastric body (18%) [53]. Duodenal ulcer perforations are classically located anteriorly or laterally. Although they can occasionally be associated with a concurrent UGI bleed, that is usually not the case. Most patients who present with perforated PUD do not have a history of PUD. The two strongest risk factors associated with perforation are a history of PUD and the use of NSAIDs [54].

Patients with perforated PUD present with an acute onset of pain. They may have been previously experiencing upper GI complaints consistent with PUD. Nonetheless, most patients can recall the exact time of perforation due to the acuteness of the symptoms. Peritonitis usually ensues over the next 2–12 h after perforation. At approximately twelve hours, patients will start mounting a systemic inflammatory response syndrome (SIRS) response with fever, abdominal distension, and changes in vital signs such as tachycardia and mild hypotension [31]. As with all surgical disease processes, elderly patients often have more complicated presentations. They may present with confusion, lethargy, falls, abdominal distension, or vague abdominal complaints. Elderly patients and those with concurrent co-morbidities often present in septic shock and may require aggressive resuscitation for stabilization before the workup for diagnosis can even be initiated.

In patients that are cooperative, the diagnosis of perforation can often be attained from a good history and physical exam with a correlative upright chest X-ray (CXR) revealing free air. Upright films will reveal pneumoperitoneum underneath the diaphragm in 80–90% of perforated patients [32]. If CXR is not confirmatory, a CT of the abdomen, preferentially with oral contrast, is diagnostic. Absolute intraoperative findings of duodenal perforation are not localized in 10–20% of patients, likely secondary to posterior and retroperitoneal perforations [55]. It is critical to expediently diagnose perforations given the extensive enteric spillage and resultant peritonitis that can occur. A delay in therapeutic

intervention beyond 12 h following perforation is associated with an increase in mortality and morbidity, and the prognosis is improved if addressed operatively within 6 h of perforation [56, 57]. All patients should be appropriately resuscitated and relatively stable prior to proceeding forward with operative intervention. In patients with multiple co-morbidities, medical optimization is preferential; however, often sepsis is the driving force behind the organ dysfunction and source control must be obtained prior to resolution. Patients should receive intravenous PPIs and broad-spectrum antibiotics and antifungals for coverage of gram-negative rods, anaerobes, oral flora, and fungus during the preoperative resuscitation, and all ulcerogenic agents should be discontinued [58, 59].

Surgical intervention is nearly always the management option of choice for perforation secondary to PUD. However, emergency surgery for the perforation is associated with a 6–30% risk of mortality [57]. The variables that have been associated with an increased mortality include age, American Society of Anesthesiologists (ASA) class, shock at the time of admission, hypoalbuminemia, elevated serum creatinine, and a preoperative metabolic acidosis [60]. Infrequently, nonoperative management can be used on a patient who is without hemodynamic compromise or peritonitis with CT findings of a contained perforation [61]. However, this encompasses no more than 5% of the disease population, and the decision to treat medically should be done cautiously with a dedicated plan for serial exams and hemodynamic monitoring. If the patient does not improve within the first 12–24 h of hospitalization, or if the patient exhibits any signs of clinical deterioration, operative intervention should be sought. In 1989, a randomized control study was published by Crofts et al. that randomized a total of 83 patients to either operative or nonoperative management for perforated PUD. Patients that did not improve within the first 12 h with nonoperative management went to the OR for surgical intervention. Morbidity and mortality rates were similar between both groups; however the length of stay for the conservative management group was longer, and failure of nonoperative management was more frequent in patients older than 70 [62]. Again, this study was performed prior to the introduction of PPIs, but the overall message is that older patients have worse outcomes. Considering that the majority of patients presenting with perforated ulcer disease are either elderly or have multiple co-morbidities, the decision to abstain from operative intervention will seldom be an option.

Operative Approach for Perforated Gastric Ulcers

Perforated gastric ulcers are much less common than duodenal perforations, but the mortality rates associated with the diagnosis are much greater. The difference is likely due to these patients being older with more chronic co-morbidities and typically larger ulcers. This population also tends to have delays in seeking medical attention which also leads to increased mortality [32].

Classically, the management options for a perforated gastric ulcer include resection, either via a wedge resection with vagotomy and pyloroplasty or by a partial gastrectomy. For types II and III gastric ulcers, an antrectomy and truncal vagotomy are performed with reconstruction by means of a Billroth I or Billroth II. The least invasive method of repair is via an omental patch. This may also then be paired with a vagotomy and pyloroplasty. Patch repair is a viable option for gastric perforations as long as the ulcer is appropriately biopsied. Considering that an antrectomy with vagotomy and reconstruction carries an associated 20% incidence of a post-gastrectomy or post-vagotomy syndrome, this may be the better option depending upon the overall clinical presentation of the patient [18]. All gastric ulcers must be biopsied, if not resected, as the rate of malignancy has been reported to be between 4 and 14% in gastric perforations [63]. Data from the late 1980s revealed a higher short-term complication rate (20% vs. 5%) and a higher recurrence rate (25% vs. 10%) in patch closure in comparison to distal gastrectomy [64]. This data was again published prior to our knowledge of the impact of *H. pylori* on ulcer formation as well as prior to the introduction of PPIs. It may be that the success of the gastrectomy was in part due to the control of *H. pylori* with the antrectomy procedure. Now that we can usually eradicate the bacteria quite easily, the resultant outcome is that vagotomies are being performed with increasingly less frequency.

As discussed previously with bleeding gastric ulcers, wedge resections are more feasible anatomically if the lesion is located in the antrum, the body, or along the greater curvature. The ulceration can easily be excised and the gastrotomy closed with a GIA or TA stapler. Depending upon the skill of the surgeon and the clinical presentation of the patient, these procedures can also be done laparoscopically with similar expected outcomes. However, the patient's clinical presentation should be used as a determining factor as patients in shock upon admission have poor tolerance for pneumoperitoneum. Wedge resections along the lesser curvature of the stomach are technically difficult due to the abundant arterial inflow from branches off of the left gastric artery. If the lesion is not amenable to closure via an omental patch, a distal gastrectomy will likely need to be performed. Proximal perforated gastric ulcers, similarly to proximal bleeding gastric ulcers, may definitively require subtotal gastrectomy or a Roux-en-Y esophagogastrojejunostomy. Please refer back to the section on approach to bleeding ulcers for further specifics regarding operative techniques.

Operative Approach for Perforated Duodenal Ulcers

The most commonly performed procedure for duodenal perforated PUD is an omental patch procedure (Graham Patch Repair). This repair has historically been performed with a truncal vagotomy and pyloroplasty or a HSV. The classic antrectomy and truncal vagotomy are usually reserved for those patients with some elicited history of chronic PUD, previous failed management, or need for chronic NSAID maintenance. Most recommend simple patch repair alone without vagotomy if the patient is in shock, has exudative peritonitis with greater than 24 h since perforation, or multiple medical co-morbidities.

Data published in the 1980s supports omental patching with an HSV as the procedure with the lowest risk of recurrence (4%). Truncal vagotomy was found to have a slightly greater risk (12%), and simple patch closure was shown to have the highest rate of recurrence at up to 63% [65]. Other literature from the same time era also validated the duodenal patch with accompanying HSV as the procedure with the least incidence of recurrence [66]. However, none of these studies included high-risk patients with hemodynamic instability, prolonged perforation, or at high risk due to advanced age or co-morbidities. Boey and colleagues demonstrated the mortality rate for perforated duodenal ulcer to be 100, 45, 10, or 0% based upon whether the patient has three, two, one, or zero of those respective risk factors [67]. Furthermore, this data was collected prior to the discovery of *H. pylori*'s influence on ulcerogenesis and the outcomes associated with eradication. Additionally, PPIs were not yet available. In 2000, Ng and colleagues published a randomized control trial of 99 patients who had an omental patch repair of a perforated duodenal ulcer. Successful treatment of *H. pylori* postoperatively decreased the recurrence rate from 38 to 5% [68]. It therefore seems reasonable that in the majority of patients that present with the need for emergent surgical intervention secondary to a perforated duodenal ulcer, a simple omental patch repair with copious peritoneal irrigation is sufficient treatment. The patient should also be treated empirically for *H. pylori* unless colonization is otherwise ruled out by negative serology, histology, or culture. Alternatively, if the patient is stable and there is a concern for recurrent PUD or postoperative noncompliance with completing the *H. pylori* regimen, a definitive operation is warranted. The type of operation should depend not only on the patient's presentation but also on the experience of the surgeon. Failure of HSV in novice hands can lead to a high incidence of recurrence, so the operative surgeon should be comfortable with the proposed interventions [69]. The complications involved in definitive procedures are similar to those discussed earlier and include duodenal stump leak, anastomotic breakdown, and post-gastrectomy and vagotomy syndromes.

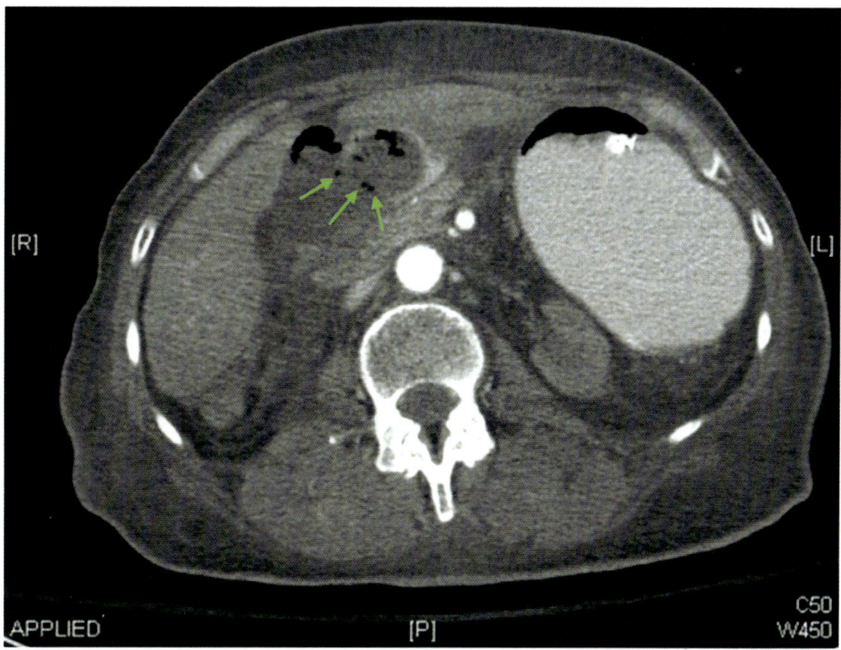

Fig. 17.4 Perforated giant duodenal ulcer on the lateral wall of the second portion of the duodenum. *Arrows* denote the perforation site

Omental Patch (Graham Patch) for Duodenal Perforation

Upon entering the peritoneal cavity, the perforation site must first be localized. The majority of ulcerations are located in the pyloric channel or in the first portion of the duodenum (Fig. 17.4). However, if the perforation is not visualized or accessible, the duodenum should be fully mobilized via a Kocher maneuver. Once the site of perforation is localized, the edges of the ulceration should be debrided back to healthy tissue. A modified Graham Patch is performed by placing several, usually 3 or 4, interrupted sutures with 2′0 absorbable suture. The tails of the tied sutures are then used to secure a pedicle of viable vascularized omentum over the now reapproximated edges of the defect. The sutures are then secure over the omentum with just enough tension to bolster the pedicle in place without compromising vascular flow. A true Graham Patch is used when the edges of the ulcer cannot be reapproximated either due to induration or because the narrowing would result in compromise of the duodenal lumen. A piece of omental pedicle is then used to plug the defect in a similar fashion without complete reapproximation of the duodenal tissue.

The omental patch procedure can also be approached laparoscopically in those patients who are hemodynamically stable. Patients with hypotension do not tolerate the cardiovascular effects of pneumoperitoneum. In the hands of a skilled surgeon, laparoscopic repair of a perforated duodenal ulcer can be more expedient than if performed by open technique. This was demonstrated by Siu and colleagues in a randomized controlled trial published in 2004 [70]. The technique has also been shown to have similar overall outcomes and postoperative complication rates in comparison to open procedures as long as patients are not in a state of shock upon admission. Additionally, as with many other laparoscopic procedures, the length of stay is shorter, patients report less postoperative pain and need for analgesia, and patients recover faster [70–72].

Giant Peptic Ulcers

Giant peptic ulcers are defined as having a diameter greater than 2 cm. These lesions have a higher risk of bleeding and perforation. In gastric lesions, although the risk of malignancy is less than historically predicted, the incidence is still around 10% [73, 74]. Classically, a giant peptic ulcer was an indication for surgical resection. However, the majority of these ulcers, greater than 80%, are now successfully treated conservatively with medical management for 6–8 weeks with follow-up endoscopy to evaluate the progression of healing [32]. There are no specific surgical treatment recommendations since the site of perforation and resultant effects on the surrounding anatomy must direct the necessary interventions. These patients are also frequently in septic shock upon presentation given the peritoneal spillage involved. This factor alone should significantly influence the choice of operative intervention. Giant gastric ulcers are most commonly located on the lesser curvature and will often require an antrectomy and reconstruction. For perforated giant duodenal ulcers, the defect is often much too large to secure patent reapproximation. Leak rates of up to 12% have been reported from attempted closure with an omental patch procedure [75]. The proximity of the defect and its relation to the common bile duct and ampulla of Vater must also be thoroughly investigated. Intraoperative cholangiogram may even be necessary to verify patent anatomy. There are several different procedures that have been described for duodenal defects such as a jejunal serosal patch, tube duodenostomy, and several variations of omental plugs and patches. Of course, an antrectomy with diversion is the classic and most commonly described intervention.

Given the relative rarity of exposure to bleeding and or perforated giant peptic ulcers, the operating surgeon should do the safest procedure in accordance with the level of experience. Affected patients are often in extremis at the time of presentation, and therefore a damage control procedure will likely be the safest and most appropriate operation for the patient. An antrectomy, with resection of the duodenal defect for duodenal ulcers, will allow for control of spillage. Depending upon the location of the duodenal defect, closure and diversion via antrectomy may be the safest method for damage control. The proximal gastric remnant should be decompressed with a nasogastric tube that was placed and verified intraoperatively. Anastomoses should be avoided in the setting of hypotension or hemodynamic instability, especially if the patient is requiring vasopressors. After copious abdominal irrigation, a temporary abdominal closure device can be placed. The patient can then be resuscitated appropriately in the ICU. The surgeon can return to the OR for re-exploration, restoration of continuity, possible vagotomy, and closure of the abdomen once the patient is hemodynamically stable.

Postoperative Management and Follow-Up

Since we now understand that the pathology behind the majority of PUD is infectious in nature, it is important that *H. pylori* is diagnosed either via biopsy or serology. A treatment regimen must then be prescribed and taken to completion. The patient should be tested for cure as the recurrence rate of ulceration with *H. pylori* eradication is 5% as compared to 38–70% without [13, 76]. Serology can be attained; however repeat endoscopy with biopsy for histology or culture is the most accurate method [18]. The urea breath test is another common test of cure, but it should not be attained until 4 weeks after treatment is completed. Patients should also be counseled and encouraged to avoid all ulcerogenic behaviors and medications. If the patient is unwilling to address long-standing behaviors such as smoking or alcohol intake, lifelong PPI therapy should be considered. Patients with medical conditions that require chronic NSAID use should also be started on maintenance PPI therapy. As with all surgical procedures, patients should have scheduled follow-up with the operating surgeon. Mandatory follow-up endoscopy is probably unnecessary, unless the patient is symptomatic or there were extenuating circumstances that need to me monitored or reevaluated.

Additionally, patients with truncal vagotomies or antrectomies should be monitored for post-gastrectomy and post-vagotomy syndromes. Recurrent symptoms after surgical intervention and appropriate *H. pylori* eradication should prompt a workup for less common causes of hyperacidity or hypergastrinemia such as ZES (gastrinoma), retained antrum, or incomplete vagotomy.

Conclusion

The discovery of *H. pylori* and its impact on our understanding and treatment of the PUD, pharmaceutical advances in acid suppression, and new and improved endoscopic and interventional therapies have dramatically changed our management of PUD over the past 30 years. The decision of how to proceed with the acute surgical management of PUD is no longer as straightforward as the classic surgical algorithms would suggest. The majority of PUD can be sufficiently and appropriately treated medically. This selects out a much more complicated and critically ill group of patients that require our surgical expertise. As described, there are a myriad of options and variations for the surgical treatment of perforated or bleeding PUD. It is important that the current generation of surgeons is familiar with not only the classic surgical interventions but also the interventions that will allow us to stabilize the patient. It is paramount that we understand the risks and potential benefits of each procedure and intervention as it translates historically as well as in collaboration with the use of modern medicinal regimens including PPIs and those that eradicate *H. pylori*. Evidence-based literature regarding acid-reducing surgical procedures in comparison to PPIs in relation to long-term outcomes are desperately needed. However, given that PPIs have become the standard of care, randomized controlled studies are difficult to perform, especially in such a critically ill population. We must use the data that we have to extrapolate those findings to our current patient population. Each specific patient and clinical scenario must be thoroughly evaluated before a definitive decision for management is implemented. The safest and likely the most prudent decision for the majority of these patients will be to control the source of bleeding or sepsis as expediently and safely as possible. Once the patient has been resuscitated and has stabilized postoperatively, further operative interventions can be performed to safely and definitively treat inciting event.

References

1. Friedenwald J. A clinical study of a thousand cases of ulcer of the stomach and duodenum. Am J Med Sci. 1912;144:157–70.
2. Malfertheiner P, Chan FK, McColl KE. Peptic ulcer disease. Lancet. 2009;374(9699):1449–61.

3. Harbison SP, Dempsey DT. Peptic ulcer disease. Curr Probl Surg. 2005;42:346–454.

4. Ramakrishnan K, Salinas RC. Peptic ulcer disease. Am Fam Physician. 2007;76(7):1005–12.

5. Groenen MJ, Kuipers EJ, Hansen BE, et al. Incidence of duodenal ulcers and gastric ulcers in a Western population: back to where it started. Can J Gastroenterol. 2009;23(9):604–8.

6. Paimela H, Paimela L, Myllykangas-Luosujarvi R, et al. Current features of peptic ulcer disease in Finland: incidence of surgery, hospital admissions and mortality for the disease during the past twenty-five years. Scand J Gastroenterol. 2002;37(4):399–403.

7. Wang YR, Richter JE, Dempsey DT. Trends and outcomes of hospitalizations for peptic ulcer disease in the United States, 1993 to 2006. Ann Surg. 2010;251(1):51–8.

8. Schwesinger WH, Page CP, Sirinek KR, et al. Operations for peptic ulcer disease: paradigm lost. J Gastrointest Surg. 2001;5(4):438–43.

9. Napolitano L. Refractory peptic ulcer disease. Gastroenterol Clin North Am. 2009;38:267–88.

10. Sonnenberg A, Everhart JE. The prevalence of self-reported peptic ulcer in the United States. Am J Public Health. 1996;86:200–5.

11. Brock J, Sauaia A, Ahnen D, et al. Process of care and outcomes for elderly patients hospitalized with peptic ulcer disease: results from a quality improvement project. JAMA. 2001;286(16):1985–93.

12. Behrman S. Management of complicated peptic ulcer disease. Arch Surg. 2005;140(2):201–8.

13. Ahsberg K, Ye W, Lu Y, et al. Hospitalisation of and mortality from bleeding peptic ulcer in Sweden: a nationwide time-trend analysis. Aliment Pharmacol Ther. 2011;33(5):578–84.

14. Mercer DW, Robinson EK. Chapter 47: Peptic ulcer disease. In: Townsend CM, editor. Sabiston textbook of surgery. 18th ed. Philadelphia: Elsevier Saunders; 2008.

15. Doherty GM, Way LW. Chapter 23. Stomach & duodenum. In: Doherty GM, editor. Current diagnosis & treatment: surgery. 13th ed. New York: McGraw-Hill; 2009.

16. Smith BR, Stabile BE. Emerging trends in peptic ulcer disease and damage control surgery in the *H. pylori* era. Am Surg. 2005;71(9):797–801.

17. Dempsey DT. Chapter 26: Stomach. In: Brunicardi FC, Andersen DK, Billiar TR, Dunn DL, Hunter JG, Matthews JB, Pollock RE, editors. Schwartz's principles of surgery. 9th ed. New York: McGraw-Hill; 2010.

18. Tinit MS, Trooskin SZ. Chapter 49: Perforated peptic ulcers. In: Rabinovici R, Frankel HL, Kirton OC, editors. Trauma, critical care and surgical emergencies: a case and evidence-based textbook. Informa, UK: Informa Healthcare; 2010.

19. Laine L. Approaches to nonsteroidal anti-inflammatory drug use in the high-risk patient. Gastroenterology. 2001;120:594–606.

20. Kurata JH, Nogawa AN. Meta-analysis of risk factors for peptic ulcer: nonsteroidal anti-inflammatory drugs, helicobacter pylori, and smoking. J Clin Gastroenterol. 1997;24:2–17.

21. Svanes C, Soreide JA, Skarstein A, et al. Smoking and ulcer perforation. Gut. 1997;41:177–80.

22. Mertz HR, Walsh JH. Peptic ulcer pathophysiology. Med Clin North Am. 1991;75:799–814.

23. Marshall BJ, Warren JR. Unidentified curved bacilli in the stomach of patients with gastritis and peptic ulceration. Lancet. 1984;1:1311–5.

24. Leodolter A, Kulig M, Brasch H, Meyer-Sabellek W, Willich SN, Malfertheiner P. A meta-analysis comparing eradication, healing and relapse rates in patients with *Helicobacter pylori*-associated gastric or duodenal ulcer. Aliment Pharmacol Ther. 2001;15:1949–58.

25. Van der Hulst RWM, Rauws EAJ, Koycu B, et al. Prevention of ulcer recurrence after eradication of *Helicobacter pylori*: a prospective long-term follow-up study. Gastroenterology. 1997;113:1082–6.

26. Graham DY, Lew GM, Klein PD, et al. Effect of treatment of *H. pylori* infection on the long-term recurrence of gastric or duodenal ulcer: a randomized, controlled study. Ann Intern Med. 1992;116:705–8.

27. Hentschel E, Brandstatter G, Dragosics B, et al. Effect of ranitidine and amoxicillin plus metronidazole on the eradication of *Helicobacter pylori* and the recurrence of duodenal ulcer. N Engl J Med. 1993;328:308–12.

28. NIH Consensus Conference. *Helicobacter pylori* in peptic ulcer disease. NIH Consensus Development Panel on *Helicobacter pylori* in peptic ulcer disease. JAMA. 1994;272(1):65–9.

29. Wallace JL. Prostaglandins, NSAIDs, and gastric mucosal protection: why doesn't the stomach digest itself? Physiol Rev. 2008;88(4):1547–65.

30. Huang JQ, Sridhar S, Hunt RH. Role of *Helicobacter pylori* infection and nonsteroidal anti-inflammatory drugs in peptic-ulcer disease: a meta-analysis. Lancet. 2002;359(9300):14–22.

31. Lee CW, Sarosi GA. Emergency ulcer surgery. Surg Clin North Am. 2011;91:1001–13.

32. Harbison SP, Dempsey DT. Peptic ulcer disease. Curr Probl Surg. 2005;42:346–454.

33. Chey WD, Wong BCY. Practice parameters committee of the American College of Gastroenterology: American College of Gastroenterology Guideline on the Management of *Helicobacter pylori* infection. Am J Gastroenterol. 1808;2007:102.

34. Loperfido S, Baldo V, Piovesana E, et al. Changing trends in acute upper-GI bleeding: a population-based study. Gastrointest Endosc. 2009;70(2):212–24.

35. Sandel MH, Kolkman JJ, Kuiper EJ, et al. Nonvariceal upper gastrointestinal bleeding: differences in outcome for patients admitted to internal medicine and gastroenterological services. Am J Gastroenterol. 2000;95:2357–62.

36. Silverstein FE, Gilbert DA, Tedesco FJ, et al. The national ASGE survey on upper gastrointestinal bleeding. Study design and baseline data. Gastrointest Endosc. 1981;27:73–9.

37. Barkun AN, Bardou M, Kuipers EJ, et al. International consensus recommendations on the management of patients with nonvariceal upper gastrointestinal bleeding. Ann Intern Med. 2010;152(2):101–13.

38. Blatchford O, Murray WR, Blatchford M. A risk score to predict need for treatment for upper-gastrointestinal haemorrhage. Lancet. 2000;356(9238):1318–21.

39. Laine L, McQuaid KR. Endoscopic therapy for bleeding ulcers: an evidence based approach based on meta-analyses of randomized controlled trials. Clin Gastroenterol Hepatol. 2009;7(1):33–47.

40. Lau JY, Leung JW. Injection therapy for bleeding peptic ulcers. Gastrointest Endosc Clin N Am. 1997;7:575–91.

41. Rockall TA, Logan RF, Devlin HB, et al. Risk assessment after acute upper gastrointestinal haemorrhage. Gut. 1996;38(3):316–21.

42. Lau JY, Sung JJ, Lam YH, et al. Endoscopic retreatment compared with surgery in patients with recurrent bleeding after initial endoscopic control of bleeding ulcers. N Engl J Med. 1999;340(10):751–6.

43. Elmunzer BJ, Young SD, Inadomi JM, et al. Systematic review of the predictors of recurrent hemorrhage after endoscopic hemostatic therapy for bleeding peptic ulcers. Am J Gastroenterol. 2008;103(10):2625–32.

44. Zink SI, Ohki SK, et al. Noninvasive evaluation of active lower gastrointestinal bleeding: comparison between contrast-enhanced MDCT and ^{99m}Tc-labeled RBC scintigraphy. Am J Roentgenol. 2008;191:1107–14.

45. Shapiro MJ. The role of the radiologist in the management of gastrointestinal bleeding. Gastroenterol Clin North Am. 1994;23:123–81.

46. Dempsey DT, Burke DR, Reilly RS, et al. Angiography in poor risk patients with massive nonvariceal upper gastrointestinal bleeding. Am J Surg. 1990;159:282–6.

47. Walsh RM, Anain P, Geisinger M, Vogt D, Mayes J, Grundfest-Broniatowski S, et al. Role of angiography and embolization for massive gastroduodenal hemorrhage. J Gastrointest Surg. 1999;3:61–5.

48. Gilliam AD, Speake WJ, Lobo DN, et al. Current practice of emergency vagotomy and *Helicobacter pylori* eradication for complicated peptic ulcer in the United Kingdom. Br J Surg. 2003;90(1):88–90.

49. Poxon VA, Keighley MRB, Dykes PW, et al. Comparison of minimal and conventional surgery in patients with bleeding peptic ulcer: a multicenter trial. Br J Surg. 1991;78:1344–5.

50. Millat B, Hay JM, Valleur P, Fingerhut A, Fagniez PL. Emergency surgical treatment for bleeding duodenal ulcer: oversewing plus vagotomy versus gastric resection, a controlled randomized trial French Associations for Surgical Research. World J Surg. 1993;17:568–74.

51. Holme JB, Nielsen DT, Funch-Jensen P, et al. Transcatheter arterial embolization in patients with bleeding duodenal ulcer: an alternative to surgery. Acta Radiol. 2006;47(3):244–7.

52. Eriksson LG, Ljungdahl M, Sundbom M, et al. Transcatheter arterial embolization versus surgery in the treatment of upper gastrointestinal bleeding after therapeutic endoscopy failure. J Vasc Interv Radiol. 2008;19(10):1413–8.

53. Bertleff MJ, Lange JF. Laparoscopic correction of perforated peptic ulcer: first choice? A review of literature. Surg Endosc. 2010;24(6):1231–9.

54. Lanas A, Serrano P, Bajador E, et al. Evidence of aspirin use in both upper and lower gastrointestinal perforation. Gastroenterology. 1997;112(3):683–9.

55. Grassi R, Romano S, Pinto A, et al. Gastro-duodenal perforations: conventional plain film, US and CT findings in 166 consecutive patients. Eur J Radiol. 2004;50(1):30–6.

56. Silen W. Cope's early diagnosis of the acute abdomen. 19th ed. New York: Oxford University Press; 1996.

57. Svanes C, Lie RT, Svanes K, et al. Adverse effects of delayed treatment for perforated peptic ulcer. Ann Surg. 1994;220(2):168–75.

58. Lee SC, Fung CP, Chen HY, et al. Candida peritonitis due to peptic ulcer perforation: incidence rate, risk factors, prognosis and susceptibility to fluconazole and amphotericin B. Diagn Microbiol Infect Dis. 2002;44(1):23–7.

59. Shan YS, Hsu HP, Hsieh YH, et al. Significance of intraoperative peritoneal culture of fungus in perforated peptic ulcer. Br J Surg. 2003;90(10):1215–9.

60. Moller MH, Shah K, Bendix J, et al. Risk factors in patients surgically treated for peptic ulcer perforation. Scand J Gastroenterol. 2009;44(2):145–52.

61. Donovan AJ, Berne TV, Donovan JA. Perforated duodenal ulcer: an alternative therapeutic plan. Arch Surg. 1998;133:1166–71.

62. Crofts TJ, Park KG, Steele RJ, Chung SS, Li AK. A randomized trial of nonoperative treatment for perforated peptic ulcer. N Engl J Med. 1989;320:970–3.

63. Lehnert T, Buhl K, Dueck M, et al. Two-stage radical gastrectomy for perforated gastric cancer. Eur J Surg Oncol. 2000;26(8):780–4.

64. Lanng C, Palnaes Hansen C, Christensen A, Thagaard CS, Lassen M, Klaerke A, et al. Perforated gastric ulcer. Br J Surg. 1988;75:758–9.

65. Boey J, Lee NW, Koo J, Lam PH, Wong J, Ong GB. Immediate definitive surgery for perforated duodenal ulcers: a prospective controlled trial. Ann Surg. 1982;196:338–44.

66. Tanphiphat C, Tanprayoon T, Na Thalang A. Surgical treatment of perforated duodenal ulcer: a prospective trial between simple closure and definitive surgery. Br J Surg. 1985;72:370–2.

67. Boey J, Wong J, Ong GB. A prospective study of operative risk factors in perforated duodenal ulcers. Ann Surg. 1982;195:265–9.

68. Ng EK, Lam YH, Sung JJ, et al. Eradication of *Helicobacter pylori* prevents recurrence of ulcer after simple closure of duodenal ulcer perforation: randomized controlled trial. Ann Surg. 2000;231(2):153–8.

69. Johnson AG. Proximal gastric vagotomy: does it have a place in the future management of peptic ulcer? World J Surg. 2000;24(3):259–63.

70. Siu WT, Leong HT, Law BK, Chau CH, Li AC, Fung KH, et al. Laparoscopic repair for perforated peptic ulcer: a randomized controlled trial. Ann Surg. 2002;235:313–9.

71. Siu WT, Chau CH, Law BK, Tang CN, Ha PY, Li MK. Routine use of laparoscopic repair for perforated peptic ulcer. Br J Surg. 2004;91:481–4.

72. Katkhouda N, Mavor E, Mason RJ, et al. Laparoscopic repair of perforated duodenal ulcers. Arch Surg. 1999;134:845–50.

73. Raju GS, Bardhan KD, Royston C, Beresford J. Giant gastric ulcer: its natural history and outcome in the H2RA era. Am J Gastroenterol. 1999;94:3478–86.

74. Barragry TP, Blatchford 3rd JW, Allen MO. Giant gastric ulcers: a review of 49 cases. Ann Surg. 1986;203:255–9.

75. Jani K, Saxena AK, Vaghasia R. Omental plugging for large-sized duodenal peptic perforations: a prospective randomized study of 100 patients. South Med J. 2006;99(5):467–71.

76. Bose A, Kate V, Ananthakrishnan N, et al. *Helicobacter pylori* eradication prevents recurrence after simple closure of perforated duodenal ulcer. J Gastroenterol Hepatol. 2007;22(3):345–8.

Gastric Outlet Obstruction

Randeep S. Jawa and David W. Mercer

Introduction

Gastric outlet obstruction (GOO) indicates obstruction of the distal stomach, pylorus, or proximal duodenum. The term is also used to encompass lesions in the second through fourth portion of the duodenum as the demarcation between gastric outlet obstruction and duodenal obstruction is inconsistent [1]. GOO can be the result of benign or malignant conditions. While classically GOO was ascribed to noncancerous pathology, a frequently cited review by Johnson et al. of 261 patients with GOO indicated that the epidemiology of GOO is changing [2]. They noted that between 1962 and 1975, malignancy accounted for 33% of GOO cases at their hospital in the United Kingdom. Between 1976 and 1985 malignancy accounted for 50% of cases. However, from 1987 to 1988 malignancy was responsible for 66% of cases of GOO. Current thinking is that GOO in adults is secondary to malignancy unless proven otherwise.

Benign Etiology in Adults

A variety of noncancerous lesions can cause GOO. By far, the most often etiology written about is peptic ulcer disease (PUD) and it is discussed first. In the symptomatic patient, GOO can be diagnosed radiographically, endoscopically, surgically, or through a combination of these modalities.

R.S. Jawa, M.D. (✉) • D.W. Mercer, M.D.
Department of Surgery, University of Nebraska Medical Center, 983280 Nebraska Medical Center, Omaha, NE 68198, USA
e-mail: rjawa@unmc.edu

Peptic Ulcer Disease

Epidemiology

The incidence of GOO has decreased in large part secondary to the introduction of H_2 blockers, proton pump inhibitors, and *Helicobacter pylori* treatment. In a population-based study in Finland from the 1970s to 1990s, the incidence of GOO secondary to gastric ulcers ranged from 0 to 0.7 per 10^5 inhabitants, and for duodenal ulcers from 0.3 to 2.8 per 10^5 inhabitants [3]. In the USA, GOO accounts for only 5–10% of all hospital admissions for PUD [4]. A range of frequencies for GOO in PUD have been reported, from a low of 5% to a high of 15% [5–8]. Less than 2% of patients with complicated gastric ulcer disease and less than 5% of patients with complicated duodenal ulcer disease will develop GOO [9].

GOO occurs less frequently than perforation or bleeding from PUD [5]. As of the late twentieth century, approximately 2,000 patients per year in the USA required operation for obstructive PUD [4, 10–12]. As compared to other complications of PUD, such as perforation and bleeding, GOO was the indication for surgery in only 8% of patients at one facility from 1993 to 1998 [4].

With regard to prevalence by type of gastric ulcer, GOO is more common with Type 3 ulcer (prepyloric ulcer), less common with Type 2 ulcer (combination of lesser curvature ulcer with duodenal ulcer), and uncommon with Type 1 ulcer (lesser curvature ulcer) [13]. With regard to the duodenum, greater than 95% of cases of GOO are secondary to obstruction in the duodenal bulb [9].

Clinical Presentation

The most common presentation of obstructing PUD is recurrent postprandial non-bilious vomiting [9, 10]. The vomiting is non-bilious because the obstruction is proximal to the sphincter of Oddi. The vomiting may be projectile, contain

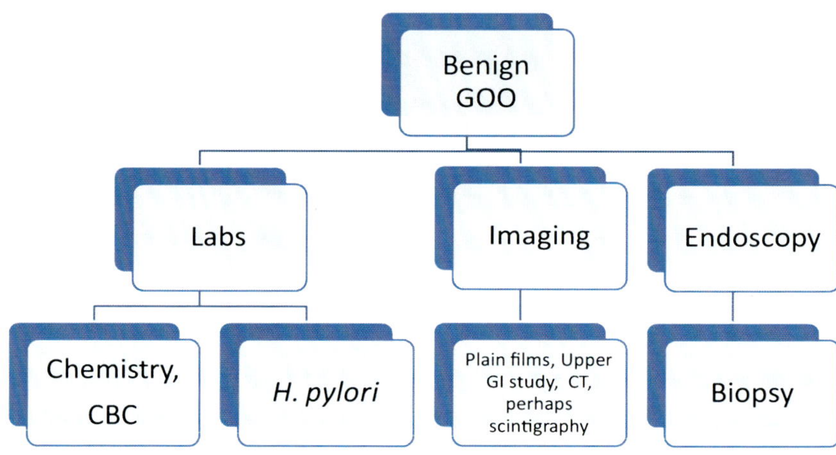

Fig. 18.1 Evaluation of peptic ulcer disease (PUD)-associated benign GOO

undigested food, and occur more than 24–48 h after oral intake [9, 10, 14–16]. Coffee-ground emesis occurs in less than 17% of patients [9]. These patients are at risk for aspiration pneumonia [15]. Patients also have nausea that improves with vomiting [9, 10, 14, 17]. Additional symptoms include chest/epigastric pain, heartburn, regurgitation, early satiety, and weight loss [9, 18–20]. With disease progression, patients decrease and then eliminate solid intake [10]. Patients can also present with severe dehydration that is accompanied by metabolic/acid–base abnormalities. With ongoing vomiting, lethargy, confusion, and rarely tetany secondary to severe alkalosis may occur [9]. Findings on examination may include abdominal tenderness, a distended stomach with visible peristalsis, and a succussion splash [16].

Diagnosis

GOO can present either acutely or chronically. While the acute form is believed to be secondary to edema and spasm of the gastric outlet, repeated episodes of healing and scarring with fibrosis can result in chronic GOO [13]. Diagnostic criteria for benign chronic GOO include a long (years) history of PUD, obstructive symptoms lasting several months, succussion splash, large gastric residual volume after an overnight fast, contrast radiography demonstrating gastric dilation and GOO, stenosis at endoscopy or surgery, and no evidence of malignancy (Fig. 18.1) [8, 21–23].

The classically described test for GOO (i.e., "gastric retention") is the saline load test described by Goldstein et al. in 1965 [24]. After evacuation of the stomach via a nasogastric tube (NGT), 750 mL of normal saline is instilled into the stomach over 3–5 min, and gastric contents aspirated 30 min later. In Goldstein's study of 92 subjects, of whom 69 were controls, they found that greater than 400 mL of saline remaining in the stomach at 30 min was highly suggestive of gastric retention [24]. They further noted that reversion of the test to normal with medical treatment indicated that surgery would not be required for that episode of GOO [24].

Imaging

Plain films of the abdomen may reveal massive gastric distention with an air-fluid level in the stomach and the absence of small bowel distention [5, 10]. Additional imaging studies that can aid in the diagnosis include upper gastrointestinal (UGI) contrast studies and computerized tomography (CT) scans [9]. Barium radiography typically reveals three layers in the stomach: air, retained gastric juice, and sediments at the bottom [5]. In normal individuals, the majority of the barium slurry will be emptied from the stomach within 2 h and all of it by 6 h on UGI study, whereas in GOO, more than 60% of liquid barium will be retained in the stomach for more than 4 h and some of it can be retained for more than 24 h [9, 10]. In interpreting these studies, it should be recalled that the $t_{1/2}$ of gastric emptying for water is around 10–20 min, depending on proximal gastric tone. Gastric emptying of solids is about 1–4 h and varies according to ease of liquefaction, contraction intensity, and composition of the meal [13]. Giant peristaltic waves may appear early during obstruction while a distended, atonic stomach during decompensated GOO may be noted on imaging studies [5]. Although the use of barium is commonly described, water-soluble contrast material is also used. Each contrast agent has advantages and disadvantages. CT scanning will further assist in the evaluation for malignant etiologies [9].

Gastric emptying scintigraphy was described by Griffith et al. in 1966 and has generally been regarded as the gold standard for evaluation of gastric emptying [25, 26]. Scintigraphy is generally performed for up to 2 h using 99mTc-sulfur colloid or 99mTc-DTPA [26]. A variety of test meal compositions (liquid, solid, or a combination thereof), as well as a variety of positions for testing, have been described [26]. Some reasons for the use of scintigraphy are its simplicity, reproducibility, and quantitative ability [27]. Of note, while several symptoms are often noted with GOO, a nuclear medicine study demonstrated that various commonly described symptoms of GOO such as epigastric discomfort, postprandial fullness, etc. are not reliable indicators of GOO or gastroparesis [27]. As such, objective testing for GOO is advisable.

Endoscopy

Endoscopy is the primary modality for localizing the site of obstruction and evaluating pathology [9]. GOO is generally diagnosed when a 9–11 mm endoscope cannot be passed through the stenosis [8, 9]. The degree of stenosis is assessed by comparing the size of the opening to the outer diameter of the endoscope and the ability to advance the endoscope into the duodenum, distal to the obstruction [28]. When performing endoscopy, biopsy is also advised to evaluate for malignancy and other, non-PUD-associated, causes of GOO [9]. Caution, however, must be exercised when solely using endoscopy to exclude malignancy in GOO, as a retrospective study of 40 patients with GOO found that endoscopic biopsy, including repeat biopsy and jumbo biopsy, had a sensitivity of only 37% for malignancy [29]. In a multivariate analysis, age and negative history of PUD were associated with increased risk for malignant GOO [29]. Given these findings, it was suggested that if the initial biopsy is negative then at least one more set of larger endoscopic biopsies should be performed in patients older than age 55 and without a history of PUD [29]. Even if the second set of biopsies is also negative for malignancy, a CT of the abdomen and pelvis for these high-risk individuals is still advisable [29].

Labs

Possible laboratory findings from persistent vomiting are a hypochloremic, hypokalemic metabolic alkalosis, secondary to loss of gastric contents that have high concentrations of sodium, chloride, and hydrogen [10, 13]. Additional chemistry findings include mild to moderate hyponatremia, increased serum bicarbonate, elevated BUN, and elevated creatinine [9]. A complete blood count may demonstrate hemoconcentration and normal or mildly elevated white blood cell count [9]. It may also demonstrate anemia; this may only become apparent with resuscitation [19]. A urinalysis may demonstrate high urine-specific gravity and paradoxically, aciduria [9]. The vomiting-induced loss of volume, sodium, and potassium forces the kidney to conserve sodium. To retain sodium, the kidney secretes hydrogen ions into the glomerular filtrate, resulting in paradoxical aciduria [9]. Potassium is also lost in the urine. The treatment is administration of isotonic saline to replace sodium and chloride deficits. Replacement of the sodium deficit in turn allows the kidney to excrete alkaline urine [5].

Because ionized calcium binds to plasma proteins that donated their hydrogen ions to compensate for the alkalosis, serum ionized calcium concentration is decreased, but total body calcium is initially unchanged [5]. Severe depletion of calcium, however, may rarely result in tetanus [9].

Management

GOO from PUD is usually secondary to a combination of edema, spasm, fibrotic stenosis, and gastric atony [3]. While acute GOO secondary to edema or spasm will usually resolve within 48–72 h, with the ability to resume a regular diet within 96 h, chronic GOO from PUD is unlikely to respond to nonoperative measures [9, 10]. Management of GOO secondary to PUD can be divided into three categories that are not mutually exclusive: medical, endoscopic/fluoroscopic, and surgical (Fig. 18.2).

Medical (Conservative) Management

Medical management includes *nil per os* (NPO) status, NG tube decompression, intravenous fluid rehydration, and antisecretory therapy via proton pump inhibitors (PPI) or histamine receptor type 2 (H_2) blockers infused intermittently or continuously [10, 13]. Normal saline is the preferred initial crystalloid for resuscitation [9, 10]. Lost potassium needs to be replaced. To this end, serial monitoring of electrolytes and acid–base status is advisable. Serum gastrin levels may be obtained if concern for gastrinoma is present; however, use of antisecretory agents may interfere with test results [9]. Parenteral nutrition may also be indicated after initial resuscitation [10]. Nonsteroidal anti-inflammatory drugs (NSAIDs) should be stopped. Once initial resuscitation is completed, consideration should be given to performing esophagogastroduodenoscopy (EGD). A complementary UGI study or CT scan may also be performed once resuscitation is well under way [10].

The role of *H. pylori* in GOO is unclear. Reported rates of *H. pylori* positivity are between 33 and 47% in small studies [4, 21]. Nevertheless, testing for *H. pylori* should be performed, as its presence may predict successful balloon dilation decreased ulcer complication rate [21]. It has been noted that patients without *H. pylori* infection have a more severe ulcer diathesis. [21] It is hypothesized that patients without *H. pylori* infection may have chronic scarring that is less amenable to balloon dilation [21]. *H. pylori* infection can be diagnosed with a rapid urease breath test or on pathologic examination of samples [21]. While readily available, stool antigen testing and serologic testing are considered less accurate indicators of active infection [30]. If testing is positive, then eradication therapy should be commenced; this can be intravenous until enteral access is achieved. A variety of treatment regimens for *H. pylori* are available, including omeprazole, amoxicillin, and clarithromycin [21]. Of note, there are several case reports demonstrating resolution of GOO with *H. pylori* treatment, without recurrent GOO [8, 31]. These studies concluded that GOO associated with PUD is primarily because of edema and spasm and not cicatrization of the pyloric canal, and hence recommend prolonging a trial of medical management to 2 weeks, before proceeding with interventional techniques [8, 31].

Medical management alone is generally favored in patients with first episodes of acute obstruction. Edema and gastritis are seen on endoscopy. This generally resolves quickly [9]. However, follow-up endoscopy is recommended to confirm *H. pylori* eradication and resolution of obstruction [9]. GOO unresponsive to medical therapy continues to be a

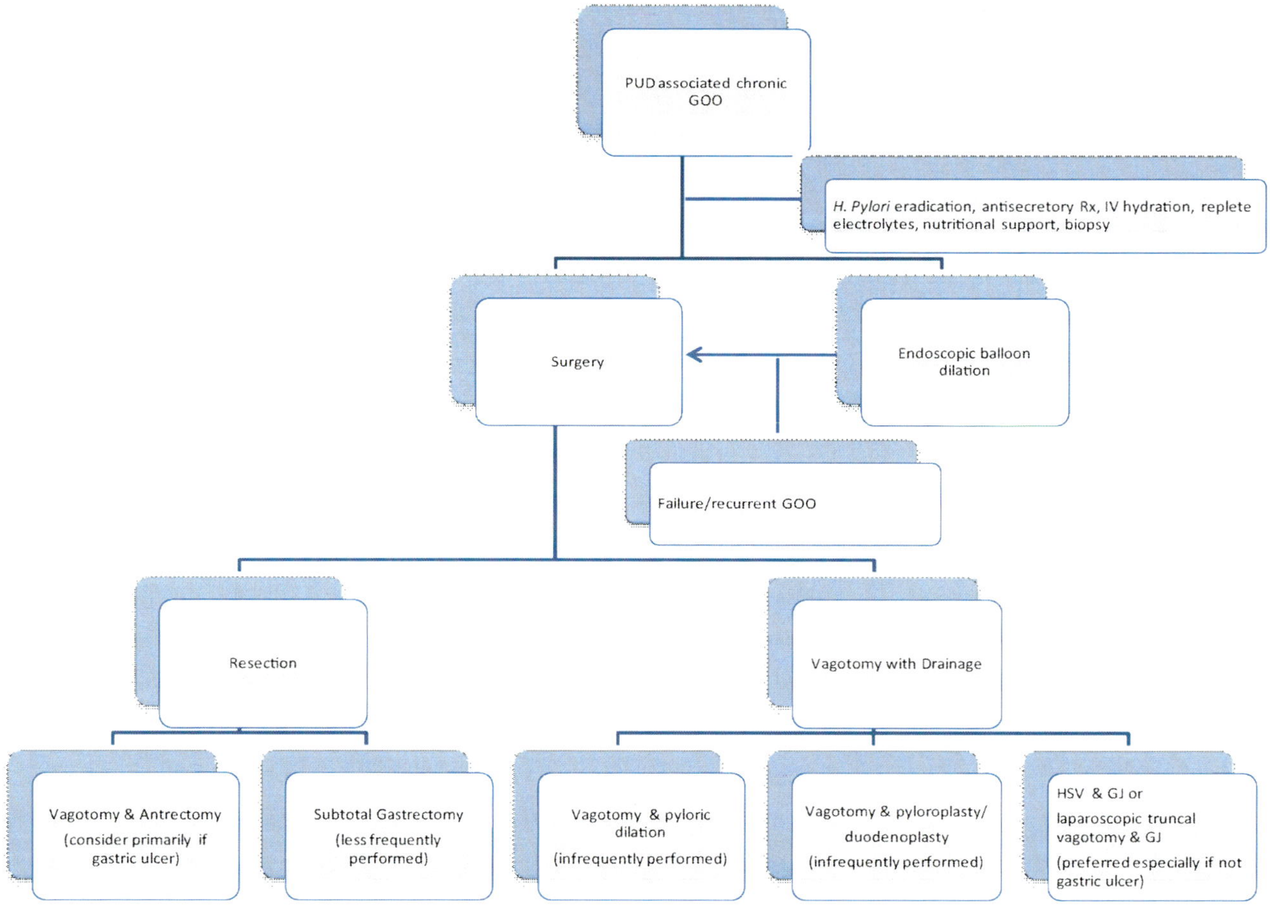

Fig. 18.2 Management of chronic PUD-associated GOO

problem in a small percentage of patients with PUD and is the main indication for surgery in a small percentage of patients requiring surgery for PUD [32]. Failure of medical management can be addressed via endoscopic/fluoroscopic balloon dilatation or surgery. The exact role of endoscopic balloon dilatation is still being defined. Surgery is recommended if there is concern for malignancy.

Endoscopic Management: Balloon Dilation

The primary therapeutic endoscopic modality for PUD-associated GOO is endoscopic balloon dilation (Table 18.1). It was first described by Benjamin et al., who used the principles of balloon catheter dilation in angiography to successfully perform through the scope (TTS) balloon dilation of a stenotic pylorus in a patient with GOO and acute myocardial infarction. Presently, balloon dilation is commonly done endoscopically; however the addition of fluoroscopy, with the use of contrast medium for balloon inflation, facilitates the procedure and may make it safer [21, 33]. Balloon dilation can also be performed under fluoroscopic guidance alone.

Several factors need to be considered prior to embarking on balloon dilation. First, malignancy needs to be excluded. This may be done via a combination of endoscopy with biopsy and CT scan. When endoscopy is done for PUD-associated GOO, multiple and perhaps repeat or jumbo biopsies should be taken to exclude malignancy [28, 29]. Second, in patients with *H. pylori* infection, both eradication therapy and balloon dilation appear necessary to decrease the risk of recurrent GOO [4]. Third, long-term antisecretory/antacid therapy will also be needed to decrease the recurrence rate [4, 5, 20]. Fourth, while generally effective initially, endoscopic balloon dilation has a high recurrence rate [10, 11]. Greater than 80% of patients treated with balloon dilation will eventually require surgical intervention [10].

Once the decision has been made to perform balloon dilation, the size of the balloon must be carefully considered, as smaller balloons are associated with higher recurrence rates, whereas larger balloons (greater than 15 mm diameter) are associated with an increased perforation risk [21, 33, 34]. In deciding upon balloon size, it should be recalled that the normal adult pyloric canal diameter is about 15 mm [35].

Endoscopic Balloon Dilation Results, Complications, and Follow-Up

Successful dilation has been defined as an expansion of the obstructed segment to 10–15 mm diameter and resolution of

Table 18.1 Selected studies comparing stenting and GJ in malignant GOO

Ref. number	Year	*n*	Type	Results
[103]	2004	18	Prospective, randomized Covered stent vs. open GJ	No statistically significant differences between the two groups in terms of morbidity, mortality, delayed gastric emptying, and clinical outcomes at 3-month follow-up
[104]	2004	36	Prospective SEMS vs. open GJ	100% of the patients that were alive in the stenting group could eat at 1 month 81% of the patients that were alive in the surgical group could eat at 1 month Shorter mean postoperative stay with stenting at 7.3 vs. 14.7 days Significantly less initial hospitalization cost with stenting, but the cost over the remaining lifetime was not significantly different between the stenting and surgery groups Advantage of stents in that they can be performed under conscious sedation
[70]	2005	47	Retrospective Stent vs. open GJ	Comparable technical success rates but lower clinical success rates in the surgery group Lower morbidity and 30-day mortality rate in the endoscopic group
[83]	2005	22	Retrospective review Stent vs. open GJ	100% technical success rate in both groups 77.3% clinical success rate in both groups Major reasons for clinical failure included peritoneal dissemination, dysmotility, anastomotic dysfunction in GJ patients 75% of stent patients and 72.2% of GJ patients became independent of parenteral support No significant difference in the incidence of post-op complications Chemotherapy following stent insertion did not increase the risk of complications
[105]	2006	41	Nonrandomized controlled Stent vs. open GJ	Stented patients achieved a significantly faster oral intake at an average of 2.4 days vs. 5 days for the surgical group Stenting group significantly shorter hospital length of stay at an average of 7.1 days vs. 11.5 days for the open group Significantly lower 30-day mortality rate of 16.6% in the stent group vs. 29.4% in the surgical group 68% of patients developed biliary obstruction
[82]	2008	50	Prospective, observational	Median overall survival 64 days, did not differ significantly between patients treated with stents, GJ, or PEG/PEJ Significantly shorter median hospital length of stay with stenting at 2.5 days than other therapies Similar re-intervention rates between surgical GJ and stented groups at 3 months Acceptable QOL scores in both surgical GJ and stent groups
[106]	2010	39	Multicentered, randomized Stent vs. open or laparoscopic GJ	No significant difference in survival between stent and surgery Hospital stay was significantly shorter in the stenting group at 7 days vs. 15 days in the surgical group Significantly shorter time to tolerance of oral intake in the stenting group, with a median of 5 days vs. 8 days By 2 months, food intake as measured by the GOOSS score was significantly better in the surgical group When including stent obstruction, there were significantly more major complications following stent placement Significantly more patients with stents required re-intervention for obstructive symptoms Hospital costs were significantly higher in the surgical group, primarily secondary to the longer hospital stay No significant differences in the health-related quality of life in follow-up between stenting and surgery

symptoms [21, 36]. Failed balloon dilation may be secondary to long, tortuous strictures and severe fibrosis with anatomic distortion [5]. Following endoscopic dilation, the diet is advanced as tolerated. Overall, endoscopic balloon dilation has a very favorable safety profile. However, post procedure, patients should be monitored for bleeding or perforation [28]. Perforation may occur in up to 6% of patients [11]. If perforation is suspected, diagnostic choices are an upper GI study with water-soluble contrast or CT scan with oral contrast [28]. To decrease perforation risk, some authors have suggested graded dilations at

1–2-week intervals as needed [21, 28]. A third complication is pain. It is not uncommon, but is generally self-limited.

In the majority of patients, symptoms tend to improve rapidly following balloon dilation and patients are able to resume oral intake shortly thereafter [19–21, 36]. Further evidence of the efficacy of balloon dilation is provided by scintigraphic scanning, which has demonstrated improved gastric emptying [36]. However, the long-term results tend to be less favorable [10]. Several small studies (40 patients or less) reported outcomes that varied from a 36% recurrence rate at 2 years, to 70% recurrence rate at 3.5 years, to an 84% recurrence at a median follow-up of a little less than 4 years [19–21]. In a study with 40 patients, 30% were relieved with a single dilation, and 30% were referred for surgery [34]. Another small study found that all patients were asymptomatic at a median follow-up of 43 months using a combination of antisecretory therapy, endoscopic balloon dilation, and removal of etiologic factors; however, 91% of patients required a median of two dilations [19].

Given the high likelihood of recurrent ulceration/GOO and concern for underlying malignancy, patients undergoing endoscopic dilation should have long-term follow-up. Also, in *H. pylori*-positive patients, *H. pylori* eradication should be confirmed. Patients with recurrent or intractable symptoms of GOO despite multiple attempts at endoscopic therapy should be considered for surgical intervention [28]. Underlying malignancy should be considered in patients who develop rapid restenosis after dilation [5]. Factors predictive of referral for surgery include younger age, technical failure, need for multiple dilations, need for endoscopic intervention after 1 year, and a long duration of treatment course [10, 34]. Given these considerations, some authors feel that balloon dilation should be reserved as a temporizing measure or used in patients who are otherwise too ill to undergo surgical intervention [10, 30].

Surgery

Given the remarkable efficacy of PPI, *H. pylori* eradication therapy, and NSAID avoidance, the role of a major surgical resection and/or vagal resection for complicated PUD has become less clear [17]. While this may be in part because endoscopic and interventional radiologic techniques are comparatively recent inventions, the need for salvage surgical intervention if other therapies fail or to treat complications of other interventions cannot be argued [4, 37]. Surgery appears to be the gold standard against which all others are judged. For patients with recurrent symptoms after two balloon dilations, and/or those who are *H. pylori* negative, surgical evaluation is suggested [4]. The goals of surgery are to eliminate long-term antiulcer medication use and cure the GOO with a single procedure [5]. Given gastric dysmotility with chronic GOO, consideration can be given to placement of a jejunal feeding tube and decompressive gastrostomy [38].

Preoperative Care

Surgery is usually delayed for 5–7 days while the patient is rehydrated and electrolyte imbalances are resolved [22]. Stomach lavage/decompression for at least the day prior to surgery is advisable [22]. NGT decompression is continued intra- and postoperatively. Deep venous thrombosis (DVT) prophylaxis and perioperative antibiotics are administered according to Surgical Care Improvement Project (SCIP) guidelines.

Resective Surgery

In selecting the operative intervention, factors that need to be considered are procedural morbidity, mortality, and ulcer/GOO recurrence rate. Some authors favor resective procedures, especially for gastric ulcer-associated GOO, while others do not [10]. Choices of surgical resection are procedural PUD-associated GOO include subtotal gastrectomy and antrectomy with vagotomy. Vagotomy is not necessary with subtotal gastrectomy. With antrectomy (also known as distal gastrectomy), whereby the distal 1/3 to 1/2 of the stomach are removed, a vagotomy is performed to further reduce acid secretion. Vagotomy may be truncal (at the esophageal hiatus, proximal to the hepatic and celiac branches of the vagus nerves) or selective (distal to the hepatic and celiac branches of the vagus nerves) (Fig. 18.3). Both subtotal gastrectomy and vagotomy with antrectomy (V&A) have higher perioperative morbidity rates but lower incidence of ulcer recurrence, as compared to non-resective procedures [39]. Specifically, V&A has a PUD recurrence rate of up to 1.5%, a 2% mortality, and significant morbidity [5]. The morbidity includes dumping syndrome in 25% of patients, although generally not severe and often resolving over time; alkaline reflux gastritis which affects 3–4% of patients and is persistent; diarrhea in up to 23% of patients; and nausea and bilious vomiting [5].

Following gastric resection, options for reconstruction include a Billroth I gastroduodenostomy, Billroth II gastrojejunostomy, or Roux-en-Y gastrojejunostomy. Data supporting Roux-en-Y reconstruction was provided by Csendes et al. in 2009 in a randomized study comparing Billroth II and Roux-en-Y anastomosis after partial gastrectomy with vagotomy [40]. They found significantly less symptoms, higher percentage of Visick I score (i.e asymptomatic) significantly more frequent normal distal esophageal endoscopic findings, significantly less frequent short segment Barrett's esophagitis, and significantly more frequent normal gastric endoscopic findings in patients undergoing Roux-en-Y reconstruction as opposed to Billroth II reconstruction [40].

Vagotomy and antrectomy are often reported as preferred management options for GOO secondary to gastric ulcer [10]. However, it is important to note that in some complicated cases of GOO, significant scarring between the stomach, pancreas, and duodenum can make performing a resection difficult. Resection may leave a difficult duodenal stump. It also carries much higher morbidity and mortality rates.

Non-resective Surgery (Vagotomy with Drainage)

If non-resective surgery is decided upon for duodenal or gastric ulcer, then biopsies, especially in the case of gastric ulcer, should be performed to exclude malignancy [10]. Therapeutic alternatives include vagotomy (truncal or highly selective vagotomy [HSV]) with drainage (pyloric

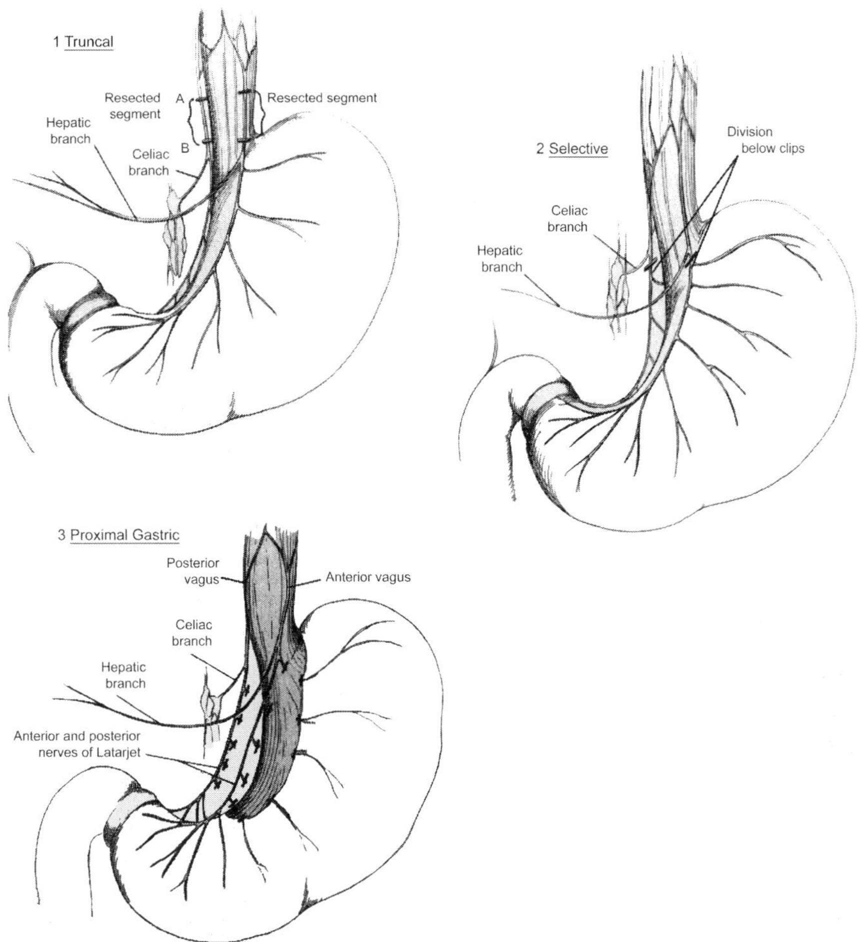

Fig. 18.3 Types of vagotomy. Figure reproduced by permission from Skandalakis L, Gray S, Skandalakis J. The history and surgical anatomy of the vagus nerve. Surgery, Gynecology & Obstetrics Journal, 1986;162:83 (ref. [108])

dilation, pyloroplasty, duodenoplasty, or gastroenterostomy). With HSV (also known as proximal gastric vagotomy or parietal cell vagotomy), the nerves of Latarjet (gastric divisions of the anterior and posterior vagus nerves) and Crow's feet innervation to the antropyloric area are preserved (Fig. 18.3). As classically described for PUD management, an HSV is not performed with a drainage procedure because innervation to the pylorus is preserved; however, in the setting of GOO, HSV must be performed with a drainage procedure [41]. There is little data available on selective vagotomy with drainage for GOO.

One drainage procedure is pyloric dilation. In performing pyloric dilation, Hegar or Bakes' dilators, a finger, or both can be used [5, 8]. A balloon-tipped catheter may also be used, especially if performing the procedure laparoscopically [38]. In a study of 30 patients with symptomatic PUD-associated GOO undergoing HSV with digital duodenal dilatation 90% of patients with initially symptomatic stenosis had no further problems with duodenal ulceration, with a follow-up time of up to 10 years [23]. Surgical dilatation

carries a perforation rate from 0% to 27% [5]. Dumping and diarrhea have been found in up to 7% of patients, and delayed gastric emptying has been reported in 3–47% of patients [5]. Restenosis rates of up to 16% have been reported in the literature [5]. It should be noted that this may also be performed in the duodenum. Because of the availability of endoscopic balloon dilation, antisecretory therapy, and *H. pylori* treatment, this approach is currently used infrequently [10].

A second option advocated by some for drainage following vagotomy is pyloroplasty, where choices include Heineke–Mikulicz, Finney, or Jaboulay pyloroplasty [5]. For a Heineke–Mikulicz pyloroplasty, the pylorus is longitudinally incised and then closed transversely. Alternatively, depending on stricture location, a duodenoplasty may be indicated. In this case, a longitudinal incision of the stricture is followed by subsequent transverse closure [5]. Some authors argue against pyloroplasty as a drainage procedure as dissection of the obstructing segment or pylorus and closure of the duodenal stump can be challenging

[10, 42]. Because of these reasons, and the availability of other techniques, vagotomy with pyloroplasty has fallen out of favor.

A third choice for drainage following vagotomy is gastroenteric anastomosis. The choice between pyloroplasty and gastrojejunostomy (GJ) is made in part by the appearance of the pyloric-duodenal area. A GJ is currently the favored approach. When a gastrojejunal anastomosis is chosen, decisions must be made as to whether the anastomosis will be retrocolic or antecolic, located on the posterior or anterior aspect of the stomach, and isoperistaltic or antiperistaltic. A retrocolic anastomosis will require the creation of a window in the gastrocolic omentum. In selecting the location of the gastroenteric anastomosis for benign disease, it is believed that an anastomosis with the posterior gastric wall facilitates drainage [43]. Furthermore, the anastomosis should be located on the most dependant part of the greater curve or antrum, as close to the pylorus as possible [22].

HSV with GJ is generally the preferred treatment for chronic GOO [13]. HSV maintains antral propulsive activity [41]. In comparing HSV with truncal V&A, complications such as delayed gastric emptying, gastric atony, dumping, alkaline reflux gastritis, diarrhea, cholelithiasis, and weight loss are less common with HSV because pyloric innervation is preserved [5, 10]. However, ulcer recurrence rates of 3–30% with HSV, depending on surgeon experience, are much higher than V&A, especially after greater than 10-year follow-up [5]. HSV is favored over V&A in poor-risk patients and/or those with problematic duodenums [10].

Two notable older trials compared open surgical management strategies in GOO. It should be noted that both trials included patients from the 1970s, around the time that H_2 blocker use was in its early stages and well before PPI were widely marketed. In 1993, Csendes et al. published the results of a prospective randomized study comparing open HSV with GJ, HSV with Jaboulay gastroduodenostomy, and selective vagotomy (SV) with antrectomy in 90 patients with GOO secondary to duodenal ulcer [41]. As compared to HSV with Jaboulay gastroduodenostomy, on late follow-up, there were a significantly higher number of patients with HSV with GJ with Visick I score. They concluded that HSV with gastrojejunostomy as compared to the other two operations was the procedure of choice in GOO secondary to duodenal ulcer. Meanwhile Makela et al. analyzed 99 patients with GOO secondary to PUD and noted a 5% post-operative mortality rate [3]. They found an 11% restenosis rate in patients undergoing Billroth I reconstruction, 0% incidence in Billroth II reconstruction, and 4% after Roux-en-Y reconstruction. They also noted a 5% incidence of restenosis in those undergoing selective vagotomy and antrectomy. Finally, they found a 42% rate of restenosis amongst those

undergoing HSV with pyloroduodenal dilatation, and consequently, they argued against its use.

Laparoscopic/Laparoscopically Assisted Surgery for GOO

While both laparoscopic and open surgical intervention is used, the trend has been towards a greater role for laparoscopic surgery in the management of GOO. Often cited reasons for favoring a laparoscopic over an open approach include less pain, less immobility, shorter hospital length of stay, smaller wounds, and a quicker return to activities of daily living [44]. While laparoscopic HSV with gastrojejunostomy may also be considered, the literature primarily promulgates truncal vagotomy with gastroenterostomy. Hence, this technique will be discussed. A retrospective study of 21 GOO patients comparing laparoscopic with open truncal vagotomy and gastrojejunostomy noted that laparoscopic surgery was associated with significantly reduced operating time, intraoperative blood loss, time to flatus, time to tolerance of semisolid diet, length of hospital stay [42]. While laparoscopic equipment costs more, these costs are generally believed to be offset by the shorter hospital stay [44]. In considering laparoscopic procedures, while intervention may be done purely laparoscopically, there are also a variety of laparoscopically assisted techniques which may offer some element of patient safety, especially for those who are not expert laparoscopic surgeons. In this regard, a 2005 study of 18 patients with GOO who underwent laparoscopic truncal vagotomy followed by an extracorporeal antecolic posterior gastrojejunostomy reported no mortality, no conversions, and a median hospital stay of 6 days [45]. This study noted a 16% incidence of postvagotomy diarrhea, which is slightly higher than that commonly reported. Similarly, extracorporeal antecolic anastomosis was performed in a study of 18 patients undergoing laparoscopic-assisted gastrojejunostomy with truncal vagotomy for cicatrizing duodenal ulcer with GOO [22]. This study also noted that no patient required conversion to a fully open procedure, no mortality, but one patient had an anastomotic leak requiring laparotomy. With a mean follow-up of 22.8 months, none of the patients developed recurrent obstruction.

Open Highly Selective Vagotomy with Gastrojejunostomy Technique: General Principles

The general principles of HSV, as described in a standard surgical text, is briefly discussed [46]. The dissection is started at a point approximately 7 cm proximal to the pylorus, on the lesser curvature. The vagal nerve fibers distal to this point are preserved. The nerves of Latarjet are identified and encircled with vessel loops. The nerves emanating from the nerves of Latarjet along the lesser curvature along with associated blood vessels are ligated and divided. Dissection proceeds proximally to the esophagus, first dividing the ante-

Fig. 18.4 Criminal nerve of Grassi. Reproduced by permission from Diesen D, Haney J, Pappas J. Laparoscopic management of peptic ulcer disease. In: Pappas T, Pryor A, Harnisch M, eds. *Atlas of laparoscopic surgery*. 3rd ed. New York: Current Medicine; 2008:65–79 (ref. [109])

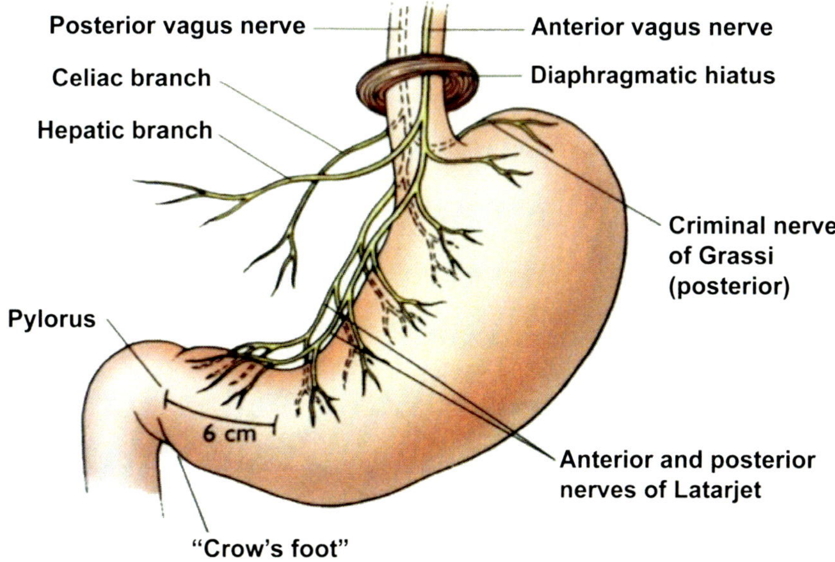

rior layer of nerves, followed by an irregular intermediate layer of nerves, and then the posterior layer of nerves. Finally, the esophagogastric junction is mobilized and branches to the stomach including the criminal nerve of Grassi, a branch of the posterior vagus nerve that supplies the cardia and can originate high in the mediastinum, are divided (Fig. 18.4). This generally involves clearing the distal 5 cm of the esophagus of vagal nerve fibers. A gastrojejunostomy is then performed near the antrum to the posterior wall of the stomach, along the greater curvature of the stomach using a gentle loop of jejunum [41].

Laparoscopic/Laparoscopic-Assisted Truncal Vagotomy with Gastrojejunostomy Technique

The technique, as described by several authors, follows [39, 43, 45]. The patient is placed in reverse Trendelenburg, in the Lloyd-Davis position, with the operating surgeon standing between the patient's legs. The peritoneal cavity is insufflated with carbon dioxide and several additional ports are inserted. The left lobe of the liver is retracted medially; subsequently the esophagus is identified by palpation of the previously placed nasogastric tube. The phrenosesophageal ligament is divided. The anterior vagus nerve is identified, clipped proximally and distally, transected, and the intervening segment is submitted for frozen section pathologic confirmation. Attention is then directed to the posterior vagus nerve; dissection in the peri-esophageal region between the right crus and esophagus facilitates exposure; again the main trunk is clipped and divided, and the intervening segment is submitted for frozen section pathologic analysis [39]. It is important not to carry the dissection too far towards the liver or too low over the gastric fundus [43]. A search is then made for additional branches of the vagus nerve, including the criminal nerve of Grassi [39, 43]. At least 5 cm of the distal esophagus is cleared of vagal fibers [39]. While the principles of laparoscopic vagal resection are the same as those in open surgery, with its magnified view, caution must be exercised to ensure that longitudinal esophageal muscles are not mistaken for the vagal nerves [43]. Gastrojejunostomy is performed using a loop of the jejunum that gives the shortest afferent loop, generally 30–40 cm from the ligament of Treitz [39, 43]. Ultrasonic dissection may be used to create the gastrostomy and jejunostomy [39]. The gastroenteric anastomosis can be completed intracorporeally or extracorporeally, using a gastrointestinal anastomosis stapling device or suture (Fig. 18.5). The opening at the anastomosis is then closed with suture or a stapler. All fascial incisions greater than 5 mm in diameter should be closed, unless a radially dilating type port is used. A radially dilating port may allow a slightly larger fascial incision to be left open.

Operative Pearls

In operating on the obstructed stomach, every effort should be made to evacuate fluid and gases from the stomach prior to entering the gastrointestinal tract [47]. Caution must be exercised in the use of electrocautery, as explosions have been reported secondary to retained gases [47]. When performing operations on the stomach for GOO, consideration should be given to performing hand-sewn anastomoses or using a greater tissue depth staple cartridge, to ensure adequate purchase on the hypertrophied stomach [10].

The appearance of the pylorus and proximal duodenum influences surgical intervention. Extensive inflammation may make a Billroth I procedure impossible; it may also yield a difficult duodenal stump with a Billroth II reconstruction [17, 30, 42]. In those patients with a difficult duodenal

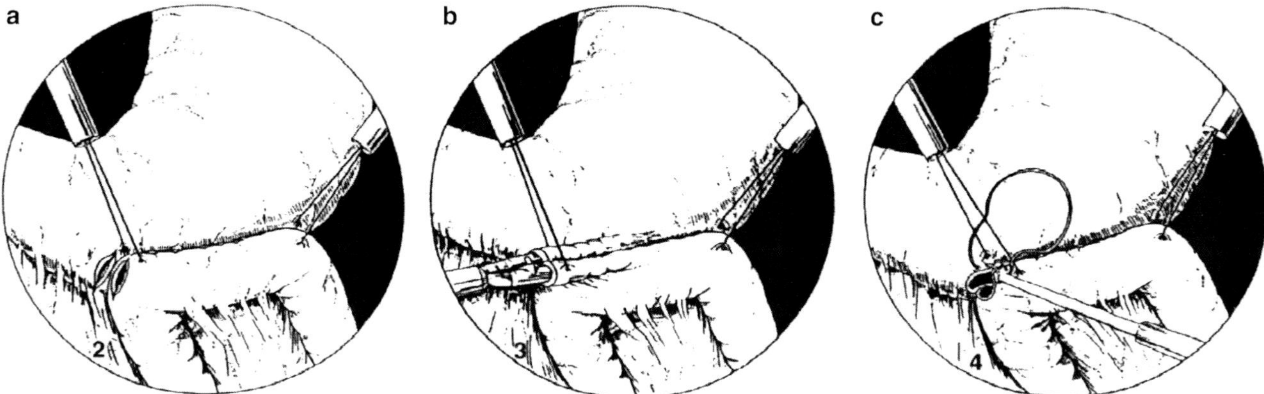

Fig. 18.5 Laparoscopic GJ diagram. (**a**) After placement of stay sutures, an opening is made in both the stomach and jejunum. (**b**) An endoscopic stapler is introduced into the adjacent stomach and jejunum. (**c**) The open end of the anastomosis is closed with sutures. Figure reproduced permission from Brune IB, Feussner H, Neuhaus H, Classen M, Siewert JR. Laparoscopic gastrojejunostomy and endoscopic biliary stent placement for palliation of incurable gastric outlet obstruction with cholestasis. *Surg Endosc.* 1997;11(8):834–837 (ref. [110])

closure, consideration can be given to performing a tube duodenostomy and perihepatic drainage [4]. However, it is better to avoid this situation altogether and perform a vagotomy with gastroenterostomy [4].

Postoperative Care, Complications, and Follow-Up After Surgery

Surgery is highly effective in the management of GOO. Postoperatively, the patient is admitted to a monitored floor. Fluid and electrolyte status need to be followed closely. Nutritional support should be continued. While the duration of NGT decompression is controversial, it should be recalled that patients with GOO may need NGT for a longer period of time secondary to delayed gastric emptying from chronic gastric atony as well as vagotomy. Follow-up with the surgeon is generally performed by about 2 weeks post discharge. A second follow-up visit may occur several weeks later, and then as needed to address any complications that may arise. Long-term follow-up is usually with the primary care physician and/or gastroenterologist.

Complications that may occur postoperatively include atelectasis, fever, arrhythmia, myocardial infarction, DVT, pulmonary embolism (PE), pneumonia, bleeding, wound infection, and in the case of an anastomosis, an anastomotic leak. Long-term complications of truncal vagotomy include gastric stasis, bilious vomiting, diarrhea, and dumping [42]. The literature suggests a 5–16% incidence of diarrhea following vagotomy [45]. Diarrhea from the dumping syndrome is secondary to massive outpouring of fluid from the vascular compartment into the bowel lumen, because early gastric emptying produces hyperosmolar intraluminal contents [45]. Additional complications of commonly performed PUD operations included anastomotic obstruction/stenosis, obstruction of the afferent or efferent loops, delayed gastric emptying, and marginal ulceration.

PUD Conclusions

In conclusion, while PUD-associated acute GOO often resolves with conservative measures, chronic GOO will generally require intervention. While the role of *H. pylori* in GOO is unclear, infection must be assessed and eradication therapy administered if it is found. Antisecretory medications are administered and malignancy must be excluded. Depending on patient preference and in poor-risk surgical candidates, it appears reasonable to offer a trial of endoscopic balloon dilation as it provides a rapid relief of symptoms and has a favorable safety profile, with the understanding that there is a high long-term recurrent GOO risk and long-term antisecretory therapy will be needed. In good-risk patients who are *H. pylori* negative, fail endoscopic treatment, wish to avoid long-term antisecretory medication treatment, or desire definitive treatment, surgical intervention should be performed. In deciding amongst the myriad of operations, one algorithm to consider is to perform vagotomy and antrectomy in the patient with a gastric ulcer with good performance status and simple anatomy. If the gastric ulcer patient has a limited performance status, then vagotomy with gastroenterostomy should be performed. If the patient has a duodenal ulcer, consider performing HSV with drainage or truncal vagotomy with drainage. While either technique can be performed laparoscopically, there is presently very little literature available on laparoscopic HSV with drainage for GOO. The decision between the two would depend on the surgeon's familiarity with the procedures; it has been reported that surgeons today may have limited operative experience with GOO [48]. Additional factors to guide decision-making are informed consent from the patient, regarding side effects from surgery and risk of recurrent ulceration. As previously discussed, HSV with drainage has fewer side effects but a higher risk of recurrent PUD than truncal vagotomy with drainage.

Other Benign Causes of Goo

Inflammatory Conditions

Several local and systemic inflammatory conditions can also cause GOO. Local conditions include acute and chronic pancreatitis, pancreatic pseudocyst, and obstruction secondary to cholecystoduodenal fistula with calculous cholecystitis (Bouveret's syndrome) [9, 49, 50]. Systemic inflammatory conditions include Crohn's disease. While gastroduodenal involvement in Crohn's disease is rare, with an incidence of about 5%, stenosis was noted in 78% of 54 patients in a small series of patients with gastroduodenal disease [51]. Other conditions include Behcet's disease and systemic lupus erythematosus [9]. Finally, eosinophilic gastroenteritis can result in intestinal obstruction due to muscular infiltration with eosinophils [15].

Postsurgical GOO Including Bariatric Surgery

Other causes of GOO include postsurgical complications. The obstruction can be secondary to adhesions or from to obstruction of a gastroenteric anastomosis. In turn, anastomotic obstruction may be secondary to stenosis, food impaction, or ulceration [52].

With regard to bariatric surgery, progressive stenosis of the gastroenteric anastomosis may result in GOO. Reported rates of this complication vary from a low 0.1% to a high 19%; however, rates may be lower with open surgery [52–54]. Fibrosis at the anastomosis typically occurs in the first 90 days [54]. These anastomotic strictures are frequently amenable to endoscopic balloon dilation. In a 2003 study of 562 patients, the mean time from bariatric surgery to initial endoscopic dilation was 7.7 weeks, with an average of 2.1 dilations performed per patient, and a 95% success rate [52]. Similarly, a study of 450 patients in 2003 found that the majority of the 14 patients with stenosis presented within approximately the first 3 months after surgery [55]. Thirteen patients had anastomotic stricture, while one had edema. With a mean follow-up of 18 months, nine patients had good long-term relief after initial dilation and five required a further dilation. There were no complications. Finally, a 2007 retrospective study of 801 patients found that 93% of the 43 patients with strictures were successfully managed by one or two dilations [54]. Another therapeutic option is fluoroscopic guided balloon dilation [53]. Advocates of fluoroscopy-guided dilation state that it has a lower risk of complications because the proximal bowel, stricture site, and distal bowel are radiographically visualized [53].

Infections

A variety of acquired immunodeficiency syndrome (AIDS)-related complications can also cause GOO. These include toxoplasmosis, cryptosporidiosis, tuberculosis, lymphoma, and Kaposi's sarcoma [9]. Additionally, cytomegalovirus (CMV) disease can result in GOO [15].

Etiologies less commonly seen in the USA include obstruction secondary to parasites and tuberculosis. GOO is the most common presentation of gastroduodenal tuberculosis [56]. In this case, GOO may be due to tissue hypertrophy or involvement of perigastric or peri-duodenal lymph nodes with subsequent fibrosis [56]. Biopsies of the bowel wall and lymph nodes are advised [56]. Gastrojejunostomy is preferred over pyloroplasty because intense fibrosis at the pylorus–duodenum will make pyloroplasty difficult [56]. Rao et al. recommend always performing a jejunojejunostomy with a gastrojejunostomy to address the problem of delayed gastric emptying [56]. Approximately 1 year of treatment with antitubercular drugs is recommended along with surgery [56].

Anatomic Variation/Pathologic Variations

Several anatomic/pathologic variations may also result in GOO in adults. These include annular and ectopic pancreas, congenital duodenal web, duodenal duplication, and superior mesenteric artery (SMA) syndrome [9, 10, 15]. Adult hypertrophic stenosis causing GOO is rare, but it can be due to PUD [9, 10, 15].

Acute gastric volvulus is a rare, but potentially fatal cause of GOO [57]. A triad of findings (Borchardt's) includes severe epigastric pain, abdominal distention, intractable retching without vomitus, and difficulty or inability to pass a nasogastric tube [57]. Dysphagia may also be the initial clinical symptom depending on the site of obstruction [57]. Surgical treatment is required; however the optimal surgical intervention remains to be clarified [57].

Rarely, an abdominal aortic aneurysm can cause duodenal obstruction by direct compression [58]. Patients will typically present with protracted emesis in association with a pulsatile abdominal mass. Treatment involves aneurysm repair.

Ingestions

While a majority of ingested foreign bodies will pass spontaneously, a small fraction will require therapeutic intervention [59]. There are three sites distal to the stomach where an ingested foreign body may cause obstruction: the pylorus, duodenal C-loop, and ileocecal valve [59]. Objects longer than 5 cm or more than 2.5 cm in diameter will have difficulty negotiating through the pylorus [59]. Bezoars may also be a source of GOO.

Caustic injury may result in GOO at a variety of time periods, as the injury evolves. Active ulceration and necrosis are present early [33]. The subacute phase is characterized by ongoing inflammation, ulceration, and sloughing of devitalized tissue [33]. In the chronic phase, cicatrix development starts at about 3 weeks, and is established by 8 weeks [33]. Small studies support endoscopic balloon dilation in the subacute and chronic phase of GOO [33, 60].

Trauma

Duodenal hematoma secondary to blunt trauma is more often found in children. Initially, it is generally initially managed conservatively with NPO status, nasogastric tube decompression, and intravenous fluids and perhaps parental nutrition. The obstruction generally resolves after a few weeks. However, if a duodenal hematoma is found during laparotomy for blunt trauma, then exploration of the hematoma is warranted.

Functional Disorders

A variety of disorders can induce functional GOO. One cause is diabetes-associated gastroparesis. Surgical vagotomy, unless antral innervation is preserved, and functional vagotomy from tumors, including those in the mediastinum, will induce delayed gastric emptying [10, 61]. Chronic bowel obstruction can also lead to GOO [9, 10].

The evaluation of functional disorders includes radiographic imaging studies and endoscopy to exclude an anatomic or mechanical etiology. Gastric emptying scintigraphy confirms the diagnosis [61]. The general management is supportive. A variety of drugs may help improve gastric emptying, including erythromycin, metoclopramide, and domperidone; they are generally used for a limited time period [62]. Domperidone is not presently available in the USA [62]. Off-label botulinum toxin A injection into the pylorus has been used with limited success in highly selected patients with pylorospasm [62]. A surgical procedure that is US Food and Drug Administration (FDA) approved at only a few centers is the use of gastric electrical stimulation [62]. The more commonly performed supportive surgical intervention is placement of a gastrostomy tube for gastric decompression and a jejunostomy tube for enteral nutrition [62].

Benign Neoplasms

As compared to PUD and malignancy, benign neoplasms are an infrequent cause of GOO. Benign tumors that can cause GOO include adenomatous polyp, lipoma, carcinoid, and gastrinoma.

Malignant Etiology in Adults

Epidemiology

The most common cause of GOO in Western countries today is malignancy [2, 10, 63, 64]. This also appears to be the case in developing countries [65]. Age greater than 55 and the absence of a history of PUD are independent predictors of malignancy in GOO [10]. The most frequent primary malignancies that are associated with GOO are adenocarcinoma of the pancreas or stomach and less frequently, duodenal adenocarcinoma [10]. While pancreatic cancer is listed as the most common cause of GOO by some, others suggest that adenocarcinoma of the stomach is more common. Specifically, GOO occurs in 10–33% of patients with advanced pancreatic/periampullary malignancy [9, 10, 66–69]. Additional causes include lymphoma, stromal tumors, cholangiocarcinoma, metastatic malignancy (e.g., from colorectal cancer), neuroendocrine carcinoma, advanced retroperitoneal/renal or ovarian cancer, and sarcoma [9, 70, 71].

Clinical Presentation

GOO can go undetected for a long period of time, because the stomach can distend significantly [14]. Characteristic features of GOO are nonbilious vomiting that contains undigested food particles [14]. This places patients at risk for aspiration pneumonia. Additional findings include nausea, bloating, abdominal pain, dehydration, and malnutrition. However, it should also be noted that nausea, vomiting, and inability to consume sufficient calories orally may be due to advancing malignancy and not GOO, and therefore these findings may not be an indication for gastroenteric bypass [72]. In this regard, 30–50% of patients with periampullary cancer will have nausea/vomiting, even though radiographs will demonstrate obstruction in only a small percentage of these cases [68, 73]. A variety of metabolic and electrolyte disturbances, as previously discussed, may also be present.

Management

Initial principles of management for malignant GOO are similar to those for benign GOO, namely, NPO status, nasogastric tube decompression, intravenous fluid hydration, and correction of electrolyte imbalance. Given the malnourished state, some form of nutritional support in the nonexpectant patient is usually indicated. Workup includes laboratory analyses, UGI study with small bowel follow-through contrast studies/CT scan, and endoscopy, as previously discussed in the PUD section. Once initial stabilization and workup are completed including tumor type identification, if possible, then interventional therapy can be planned. In choosing a therapy, it is vital that the diagnosis of malignancy is confirmed preoperatively. Usually, this is via endoscopic biopsy. GOO secondary to malignancy is unlikely to respond to medical management alone and will need interventional therapy, in the nonexpectant patient. There may also be a role for palliative chemotherapy as it may prolong oral intake [74].

Intervention in malignant GOO is most often performed for palliation as opposed to curative intent. There are many reasons for this, but principal among them are extent of local tumoral invasion that precludes curative resection and the increased likelihood of metastatic disease. These patients have a median survival of a few months [75]. Additional goals of management include amelioration of symptoms from tumor invasion of the biliary tree, duodenum, and splanchnic nerves [76]. The rationale for palliative intervention is to improve quality of life, as GOO leads to nausea/vomiting, abdominal distention, dehydration, electrolyte imbalance, malnutrition, and starvation [77]. While quality of life scores are not frequently obtained in GOO, various scoring systems of the ability to tolerate oral intake have been described. A commonly used scale is the GOO scoring system (GOOSS), where a score of 0 indicates no oral intake, 1 indicates liquids only, 2 indicates soft solids, and 3 indicates low residue or full diet [67]. This appears to be the most frequently used grading system. Several other systems have also been described [36, 78–80]. One commonly used gastrointestinal symptom score is the modified Visick score, where grade I indicates no symptoms, grade II indicates mild or moderate symptoms that do not interfere with habits and usual activities, grade III means moderate or severe symptoms that require medications and interfere with habits and usual activities, and grade IV is severe and incapacitating symptoms [36].

Interventional management focuses on two therapies: stenting (generally via endoscopy) and surgery. In choosing between these two therapies that can be used in a complementary manner, the first decision that has to be made is whether the patient can be cured of the malignancy by surgical resection (Fig. 18.6). While this is infrequent with malignant GOO, surgery with curative intent should be performed if possible. A study of 817 patients with antral gastric cancer found that while 78% of patients with pyloric stenosis could undergo resection, only 30% could have curative resection, as compared to 98 and 74%, respectively, for those without pyloric stenosis [81]. Patients with pyloric stenosis had a significantly higher incidence of serosal invasion, direct invasion of neighboring organs, liver metastases, lymph node metastases, and peritoneal dissemination [81]. If cure is not possible, then the alternatives are palliative resection, palliative gastroenteric bypass, endoscopic stenting, and less frequently decompressive gastrostomy with or without a feeding jejunostomy. In evaluating the choice of palliative intervention, factors that need to be considered are patient age, life expectancy, performance status, location of obstruction, length of obstruction, number of obstructions, extent of local tumoral invasion, distant metastases, presence of malignant ascites or carcinomatosis, and possibility of concomitant or future biliary obstruction [82, 83].

Stenting

The goals of stenting are relief of obstructive symptoms, resumption of normal diet, improvement of nutritional status, and improvement in quality of life [84]. As stenting for GOO is less commonly performed with only fluoroscopic guidance, the subsequent discussion will focus primarily on endoscopic stenting. Stenting is generally performed for a single stenosis, unequivocally unresectable disease on imaging, advanced disease at staging laparoscopy, malignant recurrent disease at surgical anastomosis, a short expected survival, and perhaps when incipient obstruction is found at the time of failed resection for malignant GOO [71, 84]. Contraindications to stenting include multiple gastric outlet or duodenal obstructions that cannot be bridged by one or two overlapping stents, distal obstruction, obstruction that prevents passage of a guidewire, suspected or impending perforation, acute or chronic infection, and free perforation with tension pneumoperitoneum or peritonitis [77, 84, 85].

Endoscopic stenting is performed with self-expandable metal stents that are composed of a variety of metal alloys that may produce artifact on CT [85]. While most stents appear to be magnetic resonance imaging (MRI) compatible, there may be some interference on signal intensity [85]. Stents appear to become incorporated into both tumor and native tissue via pressure necrosis. The degree of incorporation is dependent on whether it is a bare metal stent or a covered stent. The degree of incorporation is less with covered stents, thereby predisposing them to migration [85]. A prospective, single-center, randomized study of 80 patients with pyloric obstruction and inoperable gastric adenocarcinoma with metastatic disease found comparable (100%) technical success rate, clinical success rate as measured by the GOOSS score (90–95%), endoscopic patency at 8 weeks (61%), and median stent patency (13–14 weeks) between covered and uncovered stents [86]. While stent migration occurred significantly more frequently in the covered stent group (25.8% vs. 2.8%), restenosis occurred significantly less in the covered group (0% vs. 25%) on endoscopic follow-up at 8 weeks. These authors also published data on the use

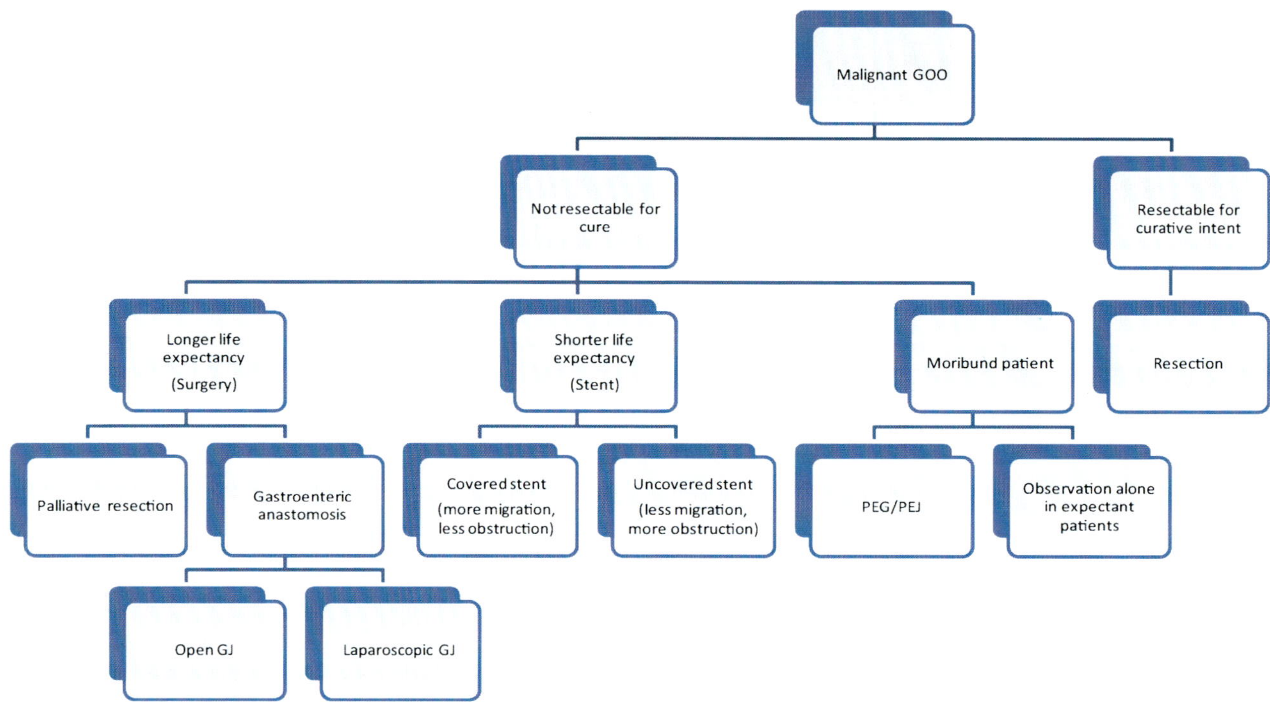

Fig. 18.6 Management of malignancy-associated GOO. Please note that stenting and surgery may also be used in a complementary manner. The algorithm is adapted from Adler et al. [67] and Schmidt et al. [82]

of endoscopic clips to secure a 3-layered (nitinol, PTFE, nitinol) stent to normal gastroduodenal mucosa [1]. Besides uncovered and covered, other considerations are braided versus woven stents. It should be noted that in the USA, as of 2011, the three FDA-approved stents for management of duodenal obstruction are all uncovered stents, two are braided, and one is a woven stent.

Prior to endoscopic stenting, a UGI with small bowel follow-through contrast study/CT scan is advisable to plan the procedure, i.e., determine stricture length and angulation and to exclude distal or multiple sites of obstruction [67]. Furthermore, evaluation of the biliary tree should be done preoperatively with possible placement of a biliary stent first as the ampulla can become inaccessible following stent placement [14, 67]. A meta-analysis indicated that between 24 and 51% of patients with malignant GOO require biliary bypass, pre-, post, or intra-operatively [87]. After gastroduodenal stenting, percutaneous transhepatic approaches will be needed to access the biliary system [67, 84]. In this regard, the deployment of a stent into the duodenum transhepatically, via a biliary access catheter, has been described [88]. Finally, as stenting is a palliative procedure, it is of paramount importance to have a diagnosis of incurable malignancy preoperatively. Nasogastric decompression prior to the procedure is advisable; it may be required preoperatively for days.

While endoscopic stenting is often performed under conscious sedation, an argument can be made for stent placement under general anesthesia with endotracheal intubation to protect the airway, given the likely voluminous gastric contents [14, 67]. Use of fluoroscopy during endoscopic stent placement is helpful because it delineates the length and geometry of the stricture, assists in stent positioning, documents successful stent placement, and can demonstrate early complications such as stent migration and perforation [14]. Stents are generally deployed in a TTS manner. Deployed stents should overlap the lesion by a few centimeters on each side; overlapping stents may be used to accomplish this. Fluoroscopy is used to confirm that the stent overlaps both sides of the lesion. This overlap is necessary in part because as certain stents expand radially over the ensuing days, they also shorten [88]. Post-procedurally, in large part depending on medical status, patients are nowadays often able to be discharged within a few days. Follow-up with the endoscopist is often done within about 1 week, where a follow-up radiograph to verify stent position can be obtained. Subsequent long-term follow-up may involve a multidisciplinary team including oncology, palliative care, primary care, and surgery.

Results of Stenting Trials

In examining various stenting trials, two commonly described parameters are technical success (i.e., satisfactory stent deployment) and clinical success [89]. Reported technical success rates are quite high, at greater than 90%.

However, clinical success rates vary from 79 to 91%, depending on the definition of clinical success, i.e., luminal patency versus resumption of oral intake versus resumption of normal oral intake [84, 89]. Most patients can take food orally within 24 h of stent placement; the diet is slowly advanced to a low-residue diet [14]. However, some patients with a functional stent will be unable to tolerate oral intake; this must be discussed with patients preoperatively [14]. In explaining the difference between technical and clinical success rate, it should be recalled that gastric emptying is a complex process involving grinding and emptying of the meal and it is unlikely that the reestablishment of a passage with stenting will be followed by a more rapid rate of gastric emptying [80]. To this end, a study of 14 patients following stenting found that although the patients had resumed oral intake within one week, gastric dysmotility/stasis on scintigraphy was still highly prevalent [26]. Specifically, while the time for gastric half-emptying was approximately 59 min for controls group, only 6/14 patients reached gastric half-emptying by 120 min. The presence of ongoing impaired emptying following stenting suggests that these patients have gastric dysmotility and that GOO is not simply due to mechanical obstruction [26]. Finally, it should be noted that weight loss may also continue to progress after stent insertion secondary to progression of disease [14].

In a 2002 study, 34 of 36 patients were able to tolerate an oral diet following stent placement, whereas only 17 could tolerate a diet preoperatively [67]. Of note, 44% had concomitant or subsequent development of biliary obstruction and 22% required re-intervention for recurrent symptoms. A prospective multicentered trial of palliative stenting in 43 inoperable patients demonstrated a technical success rate of 100% after the second attempt, with a median survival of 49 days post-procedurally [77]. While oral intake improved, the short form-36 (SF-36) quality of life score did not improve. Adverse events occurred in 23% of patients, and included stent occlusion or malfunction, perforation, sepsis, cholangitis, gastrointestinal hemorrhage, nausea, vomiting, and abdominal pain. By 7 days, 75% of patients had a GOOSS increase by 1 or more points; 80% were tolerating solid food by 28 days. Of those tolerating solid food, nearly 1/2 remained on solid food until last follow-up or death. In a 2010 study of 70 patients with malignant GOO, technical success rate was 93%, clinical success rate was 95%, median hospital stay was 2 days, median survival was 1.8 months, and 89% had improved GOOSS (0 before stenting to a median of 2 afterwards) [90]. Two patients required salvage gastrojejunostomy. A study in 2010 of 75 patients found that the use of covered stents with post-procedure chemotherapy significantly improved stent patency, without adversely affecting migration rate [91].

In a systematic review with 606 patients, Dormann et al. found that stent placement for malignant gastroduodenal obstruction was technically successful in 97% and clinically successful in 89% [92]. They found no procedure-related mortality. Major complications of bleeding or perforation occurred in 5%, stent migration in 18%, and stent obstruction, primarily due to tumor infiltration, occurred in 18% of patients. The mean survival was 12.1 weeks. They found that 87% of patients could take soft solids or a full diet postoperatively.

Complications

Stents are associated with a low complication rate and with little peri-procedural mortality [82]. Complications can occur early or late. A sudden decline in oral intake tolerance may indicate stent occlusion from tumor ingrowth/overgrowth, stent migration, or disease progression [14]. Immediate and early complications include complications of sedation or anesthesia, pain, stent obstruction from food or tumor intrusion, stent malposition, perforation, aspiration pneumonia, and bleeding [82, 84, 86]. Late complications include stent obstruction from food or tumor ingrowth or overgrowth, bleeding, perforation, stent migration, and fistula formation [84, 86]. Stent obstruction due to tumor intrusion may occur early or late. In early intrusion (a few days) after stent placement, the obstruction is felt to be secondary to wide mesh spacing which may have a "cheese-cutter"-type effect on friable tissue [77]. Obstruction secondary to tumor ingrowth may be treated by the placement of additional stents or even laser therapy [82]. While uncovered stents are less subject to migration, they are more subject to obstruction by tumor. The converse is true of covered stents. Stents may also kink [91]. Additional complications include pancreatitis, stent fracture, and ulceration [84, 88].

Conclusions: Stents

A literature review in 2009 concluded that endoscopic stenting is safe, minimally invasive, and cost-effective [84]. As indicated previously, consideration may be given to the administration of palliative chemotherapy to stented patients. In several clinical trials, stents have demonstrated at least non-inferiority to surgical intervention, if not superiority with regard to decreased hospital length of stay and cost [14]. Although stenting improves oral intake scores, the benefit to overall quality of life is not clear. A review of the literature in 2009 concluded that the available studies have not objectively evaluated quality of life using standardized questionnaires before and after stent treatment, nor were quantitative tests of gastric emptying performed [80]. Unfortunately, the one trial that used the SF-36 questionnaire was unable to demonstrate significant improvements in quality of life [77].

Surgery

In selecting surgical intervention, the decision first should be made as to whether the patient can undergo resection for curative intent. If this is possible, then it is the optimal choice, as a study found that operative curability in patients with gastric carcinoma with pyloric stenosis was associated with a 45.8% 5-year survival as compared to 7.4% 5-year survival in those that could not be operatively cured [81]. Furthermore, a 23.8% 5-year survival rate has been reported in patients with gastric cancer with pyloric stenosis undergoing resection as compared to a 0% 5-year survival in nonresected patients [81]. Besides the improved survival rate, additional arguments for resectional surgery as opposed to bypass surgery are the persistent impaired gastric motility and possibility of bleeding in the future from the tumor [93]. However, palliative gastrectomy carries significant morbidity and mortality rates [94]. Others argue that although comparisons of resective surgery with nonresective surgery generally favor palliative gastric resection, there are generally a variety of confounders, especially different disease stages, and therefore selection bias [93]. Given the high morbidity and mortality rates with palliative gastric resection, the primary focus for palliative surgery is currently gastrojejunostomy.

Gastrojejunostomy

In performing a GJ, as with stenting, the possibility of concomitant or future development of biliary obstruction must be considered. As such, palliative biliary bypass may be performed concomitantly. Alternatively, interventional radiology or endoscopic approaches to biliary bypass may be utilized pre-, intra-, or postoperatively in the event of development of biliary obstruction; arguably, the former may be preferable. In performing a GJ, both antecolic and retrocolic approaches are described. Whereas some favor the antecolic position due to concerns of placing an anastomosis close to the tumor, others believe that this concern is unfounded, and believe that a retrocolic, isoperistaltic GJ has a lower rate of delayed gastric emptying and recurrent obstruction [73, 95]. Antecolic versus retrocolic anastomosis is also determined by tumor location. GJ may be performed laparoscopically or open.

Laparoscopic Versus Open Surgery

While there are proponents of both open and laparoscopic approaches, the general trend is towards laparoscopic gastroenterostomy. Small, retrospective studies have noted a decreased length of hospital stay and fewer complications with the laparoscopic approach [66, 69]. One study also noted decreased postoperative analgesic requirements with laparoscopic surgery as compared with open surgery [66]. However, not all studies demonstrated a difference in outcomes between approaches, including median time

taken to tolerate a regular diet [96]. In comparing laparoscopic to open studies, it should be noted that some cases that start laparoscopically are converted to open. The reported laparoscopic to open conversion rate ranges from 0 to 20% [72, 75, 97, 98]. There is also a concern about port site recurrence with laparoscopic surgery. While some studies report no port site cancer recurrences with the laparoscopic approach, others have reported port site metastasis [69, 72].

Operative Pearls

Surgical intervention should generally be delayed until electrolyte abnormalities are corrected. Preoperative nasogastric tube decompression is performed. This is continued intra- and postoperatively. Informed consent detailing the possibility of delayed return of gastric emptying is obtained. DVT prophylaxis and perioperative antibiotics are provided according to SCIP guidelines.

It is important to note that unlike surgery for benign GOO, vagotomy is not generally performed with GJ. One reason for this is the limited patient life span which decreases, but does not eliminate, the likelihood of marginal ulcer development. A second reason is to reduce the likelihood of delayed gastric emptying [73].

Laparoscopic GJ Technique

The technique described by Kazanjian et al. and Gentileschi et al. follows [99, 100]. Following insufflation of the peritoneal cavity with carbon dioxide, the harmonic scalpel is used to expose the postero-inferior aspect of the stomach. An enterotomy is created in the first loop of jejunum distal to the ligament of Treitz that can easily reach the distended stomach. A gastrotomy is created on the posterior aspect of the most dependent part of the stomach, and is used for the creation of an antecolic gastrojejunostomy with two firings of the 45-mm endoscopic anastomosing stapler (Fig. 18.7). This stapler is also used to close the open end of the anastomosis. An "anti-obstruction" silk suture is also placed between the stomach and afferent jejunal limb.

Postoperative Care and Follow-Up After Gastrojejunostomy

Postoperatively, the patient is admitted to a monitored floor, and fluid and electrolyte levels are closely monitored. Ongoing nutritional support is provided. As previously noted, NGT decompression may be needed for a prolonged time period. Following surgical gastroenterostomy, some authors prefer to initiate oral feeding after clinical criteria are met and an upper GI study with Gastrografin demonstrates no anastomotic leak [69]. The reported median time to resumption of solid food orally following laparoscopic GJ was approximately 5 days in the study by Bergamaschi et al. [69].

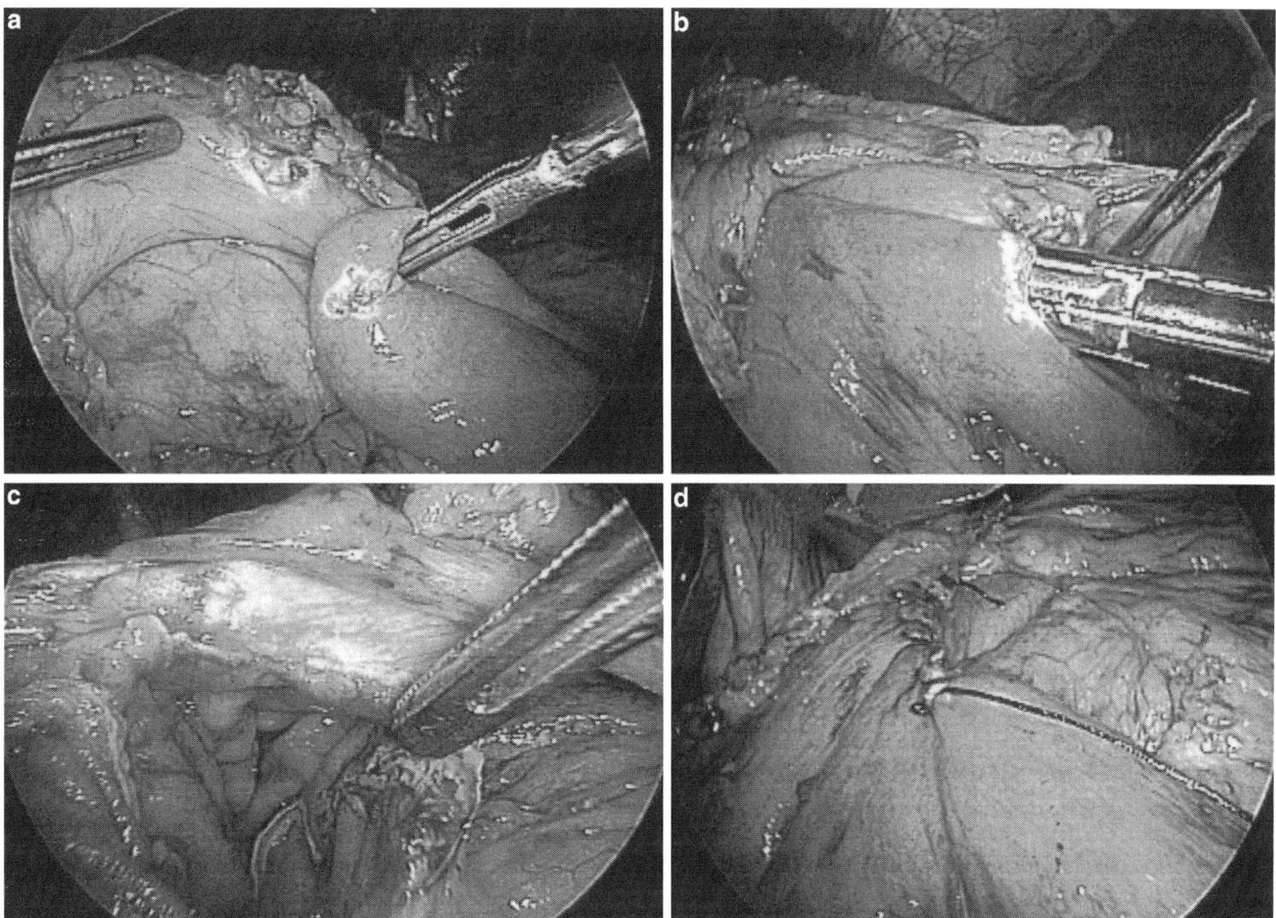

Fig. 18.7 Laparoscopic GJ operative photographs. (**a**) Opening made in posterior wall of stomach and also jejunum. (**b**) Endoscopic stapler is introduced to create an anastomosis. (**c**) The anastomosis is inspected for bleeding. (**d**) The anastomosis is sutured closed. Figure reprinted by permission from Dr. Michael Gagner, MD, Montreal, QC, Canada and *JSLS Journal of the Society of Laparendoscopic Surgeons*. Gentileschi P, Kini S, Gagner M. Palliative laparoscopic hepatico- and gastrojejunostomy for advanced pancreatic cancer. *JSLS*. 2002;6(4):331–338 (ref. [99])

Follow-up after discharge from the hospital with the surgeon is generally within about 2 weeks and a second visit after a few more weeks. Postoperative management is generally coordinated through the primary care physician, gastroenterologist, oncologist, surgeon, and/or palliative care team members as these patients generally have a limited life expectancy.

Results and Complications of Gastrojejunostomy for Malignant GOO

As indicated previously, surgical intervention achieves palliation in a majority of patients. Two small studies demonstrated successful palliation with laparoscopic GJ in 87–89% of patients [100, 101]. One of these studies also demonstrated the feasibility of salvage surgical GJ following stent placement as four patients had previous stent placement; another four were referred for surgery following unsuccessful stent placement attempts [100].

Surgery, however, carries relatively high mortality and morbidity rates. Complications can be divided into two groups: those that are specific to GJ and those that may occur after any surgical intervention. GJ has a perioperative/30-day mortality range of 2–32% [5, 71, 72]. Median survival in two studies was 4–6 months [5, 71, 72]. GJ has a perioperative/30-day morbidity rate of 20–39%, and up to 31% of patients do not experience sufficient symptom relief [5, 71, 72]. The most frequent minor complications after GJ are wound infections and delayed gastric emptying, which occurs in 14–29% of patients [26, 72, 87]. Delayed gastric emptying is defined as the inability to eat a regular diet by postoperative days 8–10 [26, 72]. Factors thought to be responsible for this include gastroparesis secondary to autonomic denervation and chronic gastric distention/atony [43, 69]. To decrease the adverse effects of this complication on nutrition, some authors recommend placing a feeding jejunostomy at the time of surgery. A variety of additional complications may occur postoperatively. These include GJ dysfunction, anastomotic leakage, marginal ulceration, and afferent or efferent limb obstruction [69, 76, 87]. Long-term administration of antisecretory medications to decrease the likelihood of marginal ulcer development is therefore advisable [73]. Anastomotic obstruction secondary to tumor progression may also occur; however, reported rates of recurrent GOO are less than 5% [72, 102]. In certain cases, recurrent GOO may be amenable to therapeutic endoscopic stent placement. In this regard, it should be noted that a number of patients undergoing GJ will require further intervention. Specifically, in one study, 17% of patients required re-intervention in the postoperative period [71]. The most common causes of early re-intervention were bleeding and anastomotic leakage; the most common causes of late surgical re-intervention were intestinal obstruction and anastomotic stenosis. Readmission after GJ in many cases is secondary to tumor progression rather than complications of surgery [72].

There can also be other complications including arrhythmia, myocardial infarction, fever, atelectasis, DVT and PE, urinary tract infection, wound infection, intra-abdominal bleeding, and intra-abdominal abscess to name a few. In general, patients with malignancy have a hypercoagulable state and are therefore prone to DVT and PE. They are also prone to aspiration pneumonia secondary to the distended, fluid-filled stomach.

Stents Versus Surgery

A basic difference between stenting and surgery is that surgery appears to provide longer lasting relief of obstruction; i.e., death after surgery is secondary to disease progression as opposed to complications of the palliation. Having said that, it seems that surgery and stenting for malignant GOO have complementary, as opposed to mutually exclusive, roles. Limited data suggests that "salvage" gastrojejunostomy is a feasible option for those with recurrent obstruction following endoscopic stenting. The converse is also true, whereby stents may be used to relieve gastroenteric anastomotic stenosis. Advantages of stenting over surgery include that it is a minimally invasive approach, carries a low morbidity rate, has high technical and clinical success rates, and is less expensive [84, 89]. The results of several studies comparing the two treatment modalities are detailed in Table 18.1; while some outcomes favor surgery, other favor stenting [70, 82, 83, 103–106].

Given the variable outcomes, several systematic reviews, decision analyses, and meta-analyses have been performed to help guide patient management. In interpreting the findings, it should be noted that the conclusions are largely based on smaller, non-randomized trials, with the possibility of selection bias being omnipresent. Furthermore, the same studies were included in more than one analysis. Even then, there is some discordance in the findings. However, it can be concluded that stenting has a favorable safety profile and does not preclude salvage gastrojejunostomy.

In a 2007 meta-analysis of 1,046 stented patients and 297 GJ patients who underwent palliation Jeurnink et al. found no significant difference in technical success rate, early or late major complication rate, and postoperative persistence of symptoms [87]. However, they found significantly more frequent recurrent obstructive symptoms (18% vs. 1%), shorter hospital stay (7 days vs. 13 days), and shorter mean survival (105 vs. 164 days) with stenting as compared with surgery. Of note, biliary drainage was required in 24% of patients who underwent stenting and in 51% of patients undergoing GJ, suggesting more advanced disease in the surgical patients [87].

Hosono et al., in a meta-analysis in 2007 of 9 studies with 153 patients undergoing 307 procedures, concluded that stenting had a significantly higher clinical success rate, shorter time to resumption of oral intake, lower incidence of delayed gastric emptying, and shorter hospital stay than gastroenterostomy [75]. However, there was no significant difference in 30-day mortality.

Ly et al. in a systematic review in 2009 of 514 patients echoed many of these findings, with the comment that there were few randomized controlled trials [107]. They found no significant difference in major complication rate, length of survival, or 30-day mortality following endoscopic stenting versus open GJ. However, patients undergoing open GJ had a significantly higher medical complication rate (e.g., respiratory infection, myocardial infarction, acute respiratory failure). They found that patients were more likely to tolerate oral intake following stenting than open GJ, and they were more likely to tolerate it earlier with stenting. Finally they also evaluated laparoscopic GJ and concluded that there was insufficient data to make an adequate comparison between stenting and laparoscopic GJ [107]. They also concluded that likely the differences in long-term benefits of stenting or GJ depend on the cause of the malignancy.

Siddiqui et al. in 2007 published the results of a decision analysis, based on 33 studies, comparing one-month outcomes of surgical bypass with endoscopic stenting in patients with malignant GOO [76]. They concluded that endoscopic stenting (ES) as compared to laparoscopic or open GJ had the highest rate of success, lowest mortality rate, leads to earlier resumption of oral intake, and was the most cost-effective. However they noted a higher 1-month complication rate with stenting primarily because of obstruction. These authors concluded that surgical bypass should be performed when expertise for ES is lacking or it fails to relieve the obstruction.

Other Interventional Procedures

A palliative modality that is used more often in patients with short life expectancy and poor performance status is the placement of a decompressive gastrostomy tube with or without a feeding jejunostomy tube [14, 85]. This may be performed open, laparoscopically, endoscopically, in interventional radiology, or via a combination of these modalities. Problems with these tubes include skin breakdown, tube dislodgement, and tube blockage [88]. The presence of ascites is considered a contraindication for percutaneous endoscopic gastrostomy/jejunostomy tube placement [88]. Therapies that have fallen out of favor include endoscopic balloon dilation and laser ablation because of low success rates [88].

Conclusion: Management of Malignant GOO

An algorithm adapted from Adler et al. [67] and Schmidt et al. [82] to guide therapeutic intervention is described in the following text and in Fig. 18.6. If a patient with malignant GOO has disease that can be resected with curative intent, then this should be performed. If the disease cannot be resected for curative intent and the patient is not moribund, then the options are palliative resection, gastroenteric bypass, or stenting. Open or laparoscopic surgery is favored in patients with good performance status, longer (at least 2 months) life expectancy, and slowly progressive disease. Meanwhile, those with poor performance status, single site of obstruction, widespread disease without carcinomatosis, and severe medical comorbidities are candidates for endoscopic stent placement. In patients with poor performance status, less than 30-day life expectancy, multiple obstructions, and peritoneal carcinomatosis and without malignant ascites, the placement of a jejunal feeding tube with a gastric decompressive tube can be considered. In the presence of malignant ascites, a nasojejunal feeding tube can be placed. A consideration in the expectant patient is observation alone with comfort care.

References

1. Kim ID, Kang DH, Choi CW, et al. Prevention of covered enteral stent migration in patients with malignant gastric outlet obstruction: a pilot study of anchoring with endoscopic clips. Scand J Gastroenterol. 2010;45(1):100–5.
2. Johnson CD, Ellis H. Gastric outlet obstruction now predicts malignancy. Br J Surg. 1990;77(9):1023–4.
3. Mäkelä JT, Kiviniemi H, Laitinen S. Gastric outlet obstruction caused by peptic ulcer disease analysis of 99 patients. Hepatogastroenterology. 1996;43(9):547–52.
4. Gibson JB, Behrman SW, Fabian TC, Britt LG. Gastric outlet obstruction resulting from peptic ulcer disease requiring surgical intervention is infrequently associated with *Helicobacter pylori* infection. J Am Coll Surg. 2000;191(1):32–7.
5. Barksdale AR, Schwartz RW. The evolving management of gastric outlet obstruction from peptic ulcer disease. Curr Surg. 2002;59(4):404–9.
6. Millat B, Fingerhut A, Borie F. Surgical treatment of complicated duodenal ulcers: controlled trials. World J Surg. 2000;24(3):299–306.
7. Piñero Madrona A, Robles R, López J, et al. Evolution of the need for operation for peptic pyloric stenosis over a period of 24 years (1976–1999). Eur J Surg. 2001;167(10):758–60.
8. Shabbir J, Durrani S, Ridgway PF, Mealy K. Proton pump inhibition is a feasible primary alternative to surgery and balloon dilation in adult peptic pyloric stenosis (APS): report of six consecutive cases. Ann R Coll Surg Engl. 2006;88(2):174–5.
9. Ferzoco S, Soybel D. Gastric outlet obstruction, peforation, and other complications of gastroduodenal ulcer. In: Wolfe M, editor. Therapy of digestive disorders. 2nd ed. Philadelphia, PA: Saunders; 2006. p. 357–72.
10. Berg D, Dempsey DT. Peptic ulcer disease: obstruction. In: Bland K, editor. General surgery principles and international practice. New York: Springer; 2009. p. 525–32.
11. Behrman SW. Management of complicated peptic ulcer disease. Arch Surg. 2005;140(2):201–8.
12. Richard K. Gastrointestinal dilation. In: Yamada T, Alpers D, Owyang C, editors. Textbook of gastroenterology. Philadelphia: Lippincott; 1990. p. 2039–54.
13. Helmer K, Mercer D. Gastric physiology and acid-peptic disorders. In: Miller T, editor. Modern surgical care. 3rd ed. New York: Informa; 2006. p. 333–67.
14. Adler DG. Enteral stents for malignant gastric outlet obstruction: testing our mettle. Gastrointest Endosc. 2007;66(2):361–3.
15. Mohammed AA, Benmousa A, Almeghaiseeb I, Alkarawi M. Gastric outlet obstruction. Hepatogastroenterology. 2007;54(80):2415–20.
16. Ellis H. Pyloric stenosis complicating duodenal ulceration. World J Surg. 1987;11(3):315–8.
17. Gaughan C, Dempsey DT. Management of duodenal ulcer. In: Cameron J, Cameron A, editors. Current surgical therapy. 10th ed. Philadelphia, PA: Elsevier Saunders; 2011. p. 68–73.
18. Mabogunje OA, Lawrie JH. Surgical management of duodenal ulcer in Zaria, Nigeria. J R Coll Surg Edinb. 1985;30(5):283–7.
19. Cherian PT, Cherian S, Singh P. Long-term follow-up of patients with gastric outlet obstruction related to peptic ulcer disease treated with endoscopic balloon dilatation and drug therapy. Gastrointest Endosc. 2007;66(3):491–7.
20. Kuwada SK, Alexander GL. Long-term outcome of endoscopic dilation of nonmalignant pyloric stenosis. Gastrointest Endosc. 1995;41(1):15–7.
21. Lam YH, Lau JY, Fung TM, et al. Endoscopic balloon dilation for benign gastric outlet obstruction with or without *Helicobacter pylori* infection. Gastrointest Endosc. 2004;60(2):229–33.
22. Abdel-Salam WN, Katri KM, Bessa SS, El-Kayal E-SA. Laparoscopic-assisted truncal vagotomy and gastro-jejunostomy: trial of simplification. J Laparoendosc Adv Surg Tech A. 2009;19(2):125–7.
23. Pollard SG, Friend PJ, Dunn DC, Hunter JO. Highly selective vagotomy with duodenal dilatation in patients with duodenal ulceration and gastric outlet obstruction. Br J Surg. 1990;77(12):1365–6.
24. Goldstein H, Boyle JD. The saline load test–a bedside evaluation of gastric retention. Gastroenterology. 1965;49(4):375–80.
25. Griffith GH, Owen GM, Kirkman S, Shields R. Measurement of rate of gastric emptying using chromium-51. Lancet. 1966;1(7449):1244–5.
26. Maetani I, Ukita T, Tada T, et al. Gastric emptying in patients with palliative stenting for malignant gastric outlet obstruction. Hepatogastroenterology. 2008;55(81):298–302.

27. Matolo NM, Stadalnik RC. Assessment of gastric motility using meal labeled with technetium-99m sulfur colloid. Am J Surg. 1983;146(6):823–6.

28. Yusuf TE, Brugge WR. Endoscopic therapy of benign pyloric stenosis and gastric outlet obstruction. Curr Opin Gastroenterol. 2006;22(5):570–3.

29. Awan A, Johnston DE, Jamal MM. Gastric outlet obstruction with benign endoscopic biopsy should be further explored for malignancy. Gastrointest Endosc. 1988;48(5):497–500.

30. Newman N, Mufeed S, Makary M. Benign gastric ulcer. In: Cameron J, Cameron A, editors. Current surgical therapy. 10th ed. Philadelphia, PA: Elsevier Saunders; 2011. p. 63–8.

31. Choudhary AM, Roberts I, Nagar A, Tabrez S, Gupta T. *Helicobacter pylori*-related gastric outlet obstruction: is there a role for medical treatment? J Clin Gastroenterol. 2001;32(3): 272–3.

32. Dempsey DT. Management of benign gastric outlet obstruction in the adult patient. Curr Surg. 2002;59(2):158–62.

33. Kochhar R, Poornachandra KS, Dutta U, Agrawal A, Singh K. Early endoscopic balloon dilation in caustic-induced gastric injury. Gastrointest Endosc. 2010;71(4):737–44.

34. Boylan JJ, Gradzka MI. Long-term results of endoscopic balloon dilatation for gastric outlet obstruction. Dig Dis Sci. 1999;44(9): 1883–6.

35. Kovacs T, Jensen D. Complications of peptic ulcer disease. In: DiMarino A, Benjamin SB, editors. Gastrointestinal disease: an endoscopic approach. 2nd ed. Thorofare, NJ: Slack; 2002. p. 411–38.

36. Artifon ELA, Sakai P, Hondo FY, et al. An evaluation of gastric scintigraphy pre- and postpyloroduodenal peptic stenosis dilation. Surg Endosc. 2006;20(2):243–8.

37. Harrell AG, Sing RF, Novitsky YW, et al. A re-evaluation of vagotomy and gastrojejunostomy for benign gastric outlet obstruction. J Laparoendosc Adv Surg Tech A. 2006;16(1):77–8. author reply 78.

38. Broderick T, Matthews J. Ulcer complications. In: Zinner M, Ashley S, editors. Maingot's abdominal operations. 11th ed. New York: McGraw-Hill Medical; 2007. p. 353–77.

39. Siu WT, Tang CN, Law BKB, et al. Vagotomy and gastrojejunostomy for benign gastric outlet obstruction. J Laparoendosc Adv Surg Tech A. 2004;14(5):266–9.

40. Csendes A, Burgos AM, Smok G, et al. Latest results (12–21 years) of a prospective randomized study comparing Billroth II and Roux-en-Y anastomosis after a partial gastrectomy plus vagotomy in patients with duodenal ulcers. Ann Surg. 2009;249(2): 189–94.

41. Csendes A, Maluenda F, Braghetto I, et al. Prospective randomized study comparing three surgical techniques for the treatment of gastric outlet obstruction secondary to duodenal ulcer. Am J Surg. 1993;166(1):45–9.

42. Kim S-M, Song J, Oh SJ, et al. Comparison of laparoscopic truncal vagotomy with gastrojejunostomy and open surgery in peptic pyloric stenosis. Surg Endosc. 2009;23(6):1326–30.

43. Wyman A, Stuart RC, Ng EK, Chung SC, Li AK. Laparoscopic truncal vagotomy and gastroenterostomy for pyloric stenosis. Am J Surg. 1996;171(6):600–3.

44. Saccomani GE, Percivale A, Stella M, Durante V, Pellicci R. Laparoscopic billroth II gastrectomy for completely stricturing duodenal ulcer: technical details. Scand J Surg. 2003;92(3):200–2.

45. Rangarajan M, Subramanian CS, Chandralathan TA. Laparoscopy-assisted truncal vagotomy with antecolic posterior gastrojejunostomy for benign gastric outlet obstruction. Surg Endosc. 2006;20(1):61–3.

46. Kelly K, Teotia S. Proximal gastric vagotomy. In: Fischer J, editor. Mastery of surgery. 5th ed. Philadelphia: Wolters Kluwer Health/ Lippincott Williams & Wilkins; 2007. p. 872–7.

47. Mills GH, Jones RB. Explosion during surgery for gastric outlet obstruction. Anaesthesia. 1993;48(6):544.

48. Søreide K, Sarr MG, Søreide JA. Pyloroplasty for benign gastric outlet obstruction–indications and techniques. Scand J Surg. 2006;95(1):11–6.

49. Maull KI, Price DC. Migratory gallstone causing duodenal obstruction. J Am Coll Surg. 2006;203(5):781.

50. Rodriguez Romano D, Moreno Gonzalez E, Jiménez Romero C, et al. Duodenal obstruction by gallstones (Bouveret's syndrome). Presentation of a new case and literature review. Hepatogastroenterology. 1997;44(17):1351–5.

51. Yamamoto T, Allan RN, Keighley MR. An audit of gastroduodenal Crohn disease: clinicopathologic features and management. Scand J Gastroenterol. 1999;34(10):1019–24.

52. Go MR, Muscarella 2nd P, Needleman BJ, Cook CH, Melvin WS. Endoscopic management of stomal stenosis after Roux-en-Y gastric bypass. Surg Endosc. 2004;18(1):56–9.

53. Vance PL, de Lange EE, Shaffer Jr HA, Schirmer B. Gastric outlet obstruction following surgery for morbid obesity: efficacy of fluoroscopically guided balloon dilation. Radiology. 2002; 222(1):70–2.

54. Peifer KJ, Shiels AJ, Azar R, et al. Successful endoscopic management of gastrojejunal anastomotic strictures after Roux-en-Y gastric bypass. Gastrointest Endosc. 2007;66(2):248–52.

55. Ahmad J, Martin J, Ikramuddin S, Schauer P, Slivka A. Endoscopic balloon dilation of gastroenteric anastomotic stricture after laparoscopic gastric bypass. Endoscopy. 2003;35(9):725–8.

56. Rao YG, Pande GK, Sahni P, Chattopadhyay TK. Gastroduodenal tuberculosis management guidelines, based on a large experience and a review of the literature. Can J Surg. 2004;47(5):364–8.

57. Yau KK, Siu WT, Cheung HYS, Yang GPC, Li MK. Acute gastric volvulus: an unusual cause of gastric outlet obstruction. Minim Invasive Ther Allied Technol. 2005;14(1):2–5.

58. Deitch JS, Heller JA, McGagh D, et al. Abdominal aortic aneurysm causing duodenal obstruction: two case reports and review of the literature. J Vasc Surg. 2004;40(3):543–7.

59. O'Carroll R, Kennedy R. Gastric outlet obstruction. Can J Surg. 2007;50(6):E29–30.

60. Kochhar R, Dutta U, Sethy PK, et al. Endoscopic balloon dilation in caustic-induced chronic gastric outlet obstruction. Gastrointest Endosc. 2009;69(4):800–5.

61. Savas J, Miller T, Mercer D. Derangements in gastrointestinal function secondary to previous surgery. In: Miller T, editor. Modern surgical care: physiologic foundations and clinical applications. 3rd ed. New York: Informa Healthcare; 2006.

62. Madriaga M, Soybel D. Motility disorders of the stomach and small bowel. In: Cameron J, Cameron A, editors. Current surgical therapy. 10th ed. Philadelphia, PA: Elsevier Saunders; 2011. p. 117–24.

63. Shone DN, Nikoomanesh P, Smith-Meek MM, Bender JS. Malignancy is the most common cause of gastric outlet obstruction in the era of H2 blockers. Am J Gastroenterol. 1995;90(10): 1769–70.

64. Khullar SK, DiSario JA. Gastric outlet obstruction. Gastrointest Endosc Clin N Am. 1996;6(3):585–603.

65. Misra SP, Dwivedi M, Misra V. Malignancy is the most common cause of gastric outlet obstruction even in a developing country. Endoscopy. 1998;30(5):484–6.

66. Al-Rashedy M, Dadibhai M, Shareif A, et al. Laparoscopic gastric bypass for gastric outlet obstruction is associated with smoother, faster recovery and shorter hospital stay compared with open surgery. J Hepatobiliary Pancreat Surg. 2005;12(6): 474–8.

67. Adler DG, Baron TH. Endoscopic palliation of malignant gastric outlet obstruction using self-expanding metal stents: experience in 36 patients. Am J Gastroenterol. 2002;97(1):72–8.

68. Lillemoe KD, Cameron JL, Hardacre JM, et al. Is prophylactic gastrojejunostomy indicated for unresectable periampullary cancer? A prospective randomized trial. Ann Surg. 1999;230(3):322–8. discussion 328–330.

69. Choi Y-B. Laparoscopic gatrojejunostomy for palliation of gastric outlet obstruction in unresectable gastric cancer. Surg Endosc. 2002;16(11):1620–6.

70. Del Piano M, Ballarè M, Montino F, et al. Endoscopy or surgery for malignant GI outlet obstruction? Gastrointest Endosc. 2005;61(3):421–6.

71. Medina-Franco H, Abarca-Pérez L, España-Gómez N, et al. Morbidity-associated factors after gastrojejunostomy for malignant gastric outlet obstruction. Am Surg. 2007;73(9):871–5.

72. Bergamaschi R, Arnaud JP, Mårvik R, Myrvold HE. Laparoscopic antiperistaltic versus isoperistaltic gastrojejunostomy for palliation of gastric outlet obstruction in advanced cancer. Surg Laparosc Endosc Percutan Tech. 2002;12(6):393–7.

73. House MG, Choti MA. Palliative therapy for pancreatic/biliary cancer. Surg Clin North Am. 2005;85(2):359–71.

74. Maetani I, Isayama H, Mizumoto Y. Palliation in patients with malignant gastric outlet obstruction with a newly designed enteral stent: a multicenter study. Gastrointest Endosc. 2007;66(2): 355–60.

75. Hosono S, Ohtani H, Arimoto Y, Kanamiya Y. Endoscopic stenting versus surgical gastroenterostomy for palliation of malignant gastroduodenal obstruction: a meta-analysis. J Gastroenterol. 2007;42(4):283–90.

76. Siddiqui A, Spechler SJ, Huerta S. Surgical bypass versus endoscopic stenting for malignant gastroduodenal obstruction: a decision analysis. Dig Dis Sci. 2007;52(1):276–81.

77. Piesman M, Kozarek RA, Brandabur JJ, et al. Improved oral intake after palliative duodenal stenting for malignant obstruction: a prospective multicenter clinical trial. Am J Gastroenterol. 2009;104(10):2404–11.

78. Song H-Y, Shin JH, Yoon CJ, et al. A dual expandable nitinol stent: experience in 102 patients with malignant gastroduodenal strictures. J Vasc Interv Radiol. 2004;15(12):1443–9.

79. Lowe AS, Beckett CG, Jowett S, et al. Self-expandable metal stent placement for the palliation of malignant gastroduodenal obstruction: experience in a large, single, UK centre. Clin Radiol. 2007;62(8):738–44.

80. Larssen L, Medhus AW, Hauge T. Treatment of malignant gastric outlet obstruction with stents: an evaluation of the reported variables for clinical outcome. BMC Gastroenterol. 2009;9:45.

81. Watanabe A, Maehara Y, Okuyama T, et al. Gastric carcinoma with pyloric stenosis. Surgery. 1998;123(3):330–4.

82. Schmidt C, Gerdes H, Hawkins W, et al. A prospective observational study examining quality of life in patients with malignant gastric outlet obstruction. Am J Surg. 2009;198(1):92–9.

83. Maetani I, Akatsuka S, Ikeda M, et al. Self-expandable metallic stent placement for palliation in gastric outlet obstructions caused by gastric cancer: a comparison with surgical gastrojejunostomy. J Gastroenterol. 2005;40(10):932–7.

84. Gaidos JKJ, Draganov PV. Treatment of malignant gastric outlet obstruction with endoscopically placed self-expandable metal stents. World J Gastroenterol. 2009;15(35):4365–71.

85. Baron TH, Harewood GC. Enteral self-expandable stents. Gastrointest Endosc. 2003;58(3):421–33.

86. Kim CG, Choi IJ, Lee JY, et al. Covered versus uncovered self-expandable metallic stents for palliation of malignant pyloric obstruction in gastric cancer patients: a randomized, prospective study. Gastrointest Endosc. 2010;72(1):25–32.

87. Jeurnink SM, van Eijck CHJ, Steyerberg EW, Kuipers EJ, Siersema PD. Stent versus gastrojejunostomy for the palliation of gastric outlet obstruction: a systematic review. BMC Gastroenterol. 2007; 7:18.

88. Singer SB, Asch M. Metallic stents in the treatment of duodenal obstruction: technical issues and results. Can Assoc Radiol J. 2000;51(2):121–9.

89. Aviv RI, Shyamalan G, Khan FH, et al. Use of stents in the palliative treatment of malignant gastric outlet and duodenal obstruction. Clin Radiol. 2002;57(7):587–92.

90. Shaw JM, Bornman PC, Krige JEJ, Stupart DA, Panieri E. Self-expanding metal stents as an alternative to surgical bypass for malignant gastric outlet obstruction. Br J Surg. 2010;97(6):872–6.

91. Cho YK, Kim SW, Hur WH, et al. Clinical outcomes of self-expandable metal stent and prognostic factors for stent patency in gastric outlet obstruction caused by gastric cancer. Dig Dis Sci. 2010;55(3):668–74.

92. Dormann A, Meisner S, Verin N, Wenk Lang A. Self-expanding metal stents for gastroduodenal malignancies: systematic review of their clinical effectiveness. Endoscopy. 2004;36(6):543–50.

93. Stupart DA, Panieri E, Dent DM. Gastrojejunostomy for gastric outlet obstruction in patients with gastric carcinoma. S Afr J Surg. 2006;44(2):52–4.

94. McFadden D, Schneider J. Gastric adenocarcinoma. In: Cameron J, Cameron A, editors. Current surgical therapy. 10th ed. Philadelphia, PA: Elsevier Saunders; 2011. p. 80–5.

95. Watanapa P, Williamson RC. Surgical palliation for pancreatic cancer: developments during the past two decades. Br J Surg. 1992;79(1):8–20.

96. Guzman EA, Dagis A, Bening L, Pigazzi A. Laparoscopic gastrojejunostomy in patients with obstruction of the gastric outlet secondary to advanced malignancies. Am Surg. 2009;75(2):129–32.

97. Nagy A, Brosseuk D, Hemming A, Scudamore C, Mamazza J. Laparoscopic gastroenterostomy for duodenal obstruction. Am J Surg. 1995;169(5):539–42.

98. Ghanem AM, Hamade AM, Sheen AJ, et al. Laparoscopic gastric and biliary bypass: a single-center cohort prospective study. J Laparoendosc Adv Surg Tech A. 2006;16(1):21–6.

99. Gentileschi P, Kini S, Gagner M. Palliative laparoscopic hepatico- and gastrojejunostomy for advanced pancreatic cancer. JSLS. 2002;6(4):331–8.

100. Kazanjian KK, Reber HA, Hines OJ. Laparoscopic gastrojejunostomy for gastric outlet obstruction in pancreatic cancer. Am Surg. 2004;70(10):910–3.

101. Alam TA, Baines M, Parker MC. The management of gastric outlet obstruction secondary to inoperable cancer. Surg Endosc. 2003;17(2):320–3.

102. Lillemoe KD, Sauter PK, Pitt HA, Yeo CJ, Cameron JL. Current status of surgical palliation of periampullary carcinoma. Surg Gynecol Obstet. 1993;176(1):1–10.

103. Fiori E, Lamazza A, Volpino P, et al. Palliative management of malignant antro-pyloric strictures. Gastroenterostomy versus endoscopic stenting. A randomized prospective trial. Anticancer Res. 2004;24(1):269–71.

104. Johnsson E, Thune A, Liedman B. Palliation of malignant gastroduodenal obstruction with open surgical bypass or endoscopic stenting: clinical outcome and health economic evaluation. World J Surg. 2004;28(8):812–7.

105. Espinel J, Sanz O, Vivas S, et al. Malignant gastrointestinal obstruction: endoscopic stenting versus surgical palliation. Surg Endosc. 2006;20(7):1083–7.

106. Jeurnink SM, Steyerberg EW, van Hooft JE, et al. Surgical gastrojejunostomy or endoscopic stent placement for the palliation of malignant gastric outlet obstruction (SUSTENT study): a multicenter randomized trial. Gastrointest Endosc. 2010;71(3): 490–9.

107. Ly J, O'Grady G, Mittal A, Plank L, Windsor JA. A systematic review of methods to palliate malignant gastric outlet obstruction. Surg Endosc. 2010;24(2):290–7.

108. Skandalakis L, Gray S, Skandalakis J. The history and surgical anatomy of the vagus nerve. Surg Gynecol Obstet. 1986;162:83.
109. Diesen D, Haney J, Pappas J. Laparoscopic management of peptic ulcer disease. In: Pappas T, Pryor A, Harnisch M, editors. Atlas of laparoscopic surgery. 3rd ed. New York: Current Medicine; 2008. p. 65–79.
110. Brune IB, Feussner H, Neuhaus H, Classen M, Siewert JR. Laparoscopic gastrojejunostomy and endoscopic biliary stent placement for palliation of incurable gastric outlet obstruction with cholestasis. Surg Endosc. 1997;11(8):834–7.

Lynn Gries and Peter Rhee

Introduction

Upper gastrointestinal bleeding (UGIB) is a common problem and frequently generates a consult for the acute care surgeon. Although very few patients with this complaint ultimately have any surgical intervention, surgeons have historically been intimately involved in the management of UGIB patients. With the discovery of *Helicobacter pylori*, effective *H. pylori* treatment and eradication regimens have greatly decreased the incidence of peptic ulcer disease as well as shifted the algorithm away from surgical treatment. Moreover, there appears to be a decreasing incidence and mortality of peptic ulcer disease as well as a decrease in acute UGIB related to peptic ulcer disease [1]. Recent data suggests that surgical intervention for any symptom or complication of peptic ulcer disease has declined more than 80% [2]. Moreover, the fields of diagnostic and therapeutic endoscopy as well as interventional radiology have expanded in directions that have had a huge impact on the treatment options available for the patient with an UGIB. The role of the surgeon will often be to assist their colleagues in guiding the patient into an informed and evidence based plan of action.

Epidemiology and Etiology of UGIB

An UGIB in the USA and other industrialized nations is a relatively common occurrence; it was the 30th most common principal diagnosis in a survey of US community hospital stays in 2009. There were 360,739 patients discharged with this diagnosis representing only 0.9% of all discharges. The average length of stay was 4.3 days and the mortality rate was 2.8% [3]. Around 70–80% of UGIBs will resolve spontaneously [4]. However, these statistics fail to portray a complete picture of UGIB in that they do not include noncommunity hospitals, patients whose primary diagnosis was not UGIB, or patients who sustained an UGIB during an admission for a different problem. Tertiary care centers and hospitals whose patient population is more elderly than most would likely have a higher mortality rate than a community hospital. Multiple studies done in the USA and Europe during the late 1990s through 2000 demonstrated a marked difference in mortality between emergency admissions (3.7–11% mortality) and in-hospital patients with UGIB (23–42% mortality) [5].

An UGIB is a diagnosis for which the etiology can range from a single, localized disorder such as a bleeding duodenal ulcer in a patient with an untreated *H. pylori* infection to several local and systemic conditions, all of which together create the conditions necessary for an UGIB, such as a hemorrhagic gastritis in a patient with an acute leukemia undergoing chemotherapy, immunosuppression, and systemic anticoagulation for a recent stroke. It is important to consider these possibilities when beginning the diagnostic evaluation. Table 19.1 lists the most common etiologies of UGIB.

Peptic Ulcer Disease

Peptic ulcer disease remains the most common etiology of UGIB. Duodenal ulcers are the most common cause of UGIB both historically and currently, accounting for 20–30% [2, 4, 5]. Unfortunately, most studies include all duodenal ulcers, gastric ulcers, and often gastritis under peptic ulcer disease, despite the evidence that several of these conditions have different etiologies and potentially different surgical management. The four major causes of gastric and duodenal inflammation, ulceration, and bleeding are overproduction of acid, *H. pylori* infection, nonsteroidal anti-inflammatory drug (NSAID)-induced loss of

L. Gries, M.D.
Department of Surgery, Division of Trauma, Critical Care and Acute Care Surgery, Arizona Health Science Center, University of Arizona Medical Center, Tucson, AZ, USA

P. Rhee, M.D., M.P.H., F.A.C.S., F.C.C.M., D.M.C.C. (✉)
Department of Surgery, Division of Trauma, Critical Care and Acute Care Surgery, University of Arizona Medical Center, 1501 N. Campbell Avenue, Room 5411, Tucson, AZ 85724, USA
e-mail: prhee@surgery.arizona.edu; lballesteros@surgery.arizona.edu

L.J. Moore et al. (eds.), *Common Problems in Acute Care Surgery*, DOI 10.1007/978-1-4614-6123-4_19, © Springer Science+Business Media New York 2013

Table 19.1 Etiology of upper gastrointestinal bleeding (UGIB)

Etiology	Frequency (%)
Duodenal ulcer	33.2
Gastric ulcer	16.9
Varices	11.5
Gastric erosions	10.4
Neoplasms	5.2
Esophagitis	4.3
Mallory–Weiss lesions	3.2
Anastomotic ulcer	3.0
Vascular malformations	2.8
Rare causes, including transpapillary bleeding	2.4
Undetermined	5.0

Source: Loperfido S, Baldo V, Piovesana E, Bellina L, Rossi K, Groppo M et al. Changing trends in acute upper-GI bleeding: a population based study. Gastrointestinal Endoscopy, 2009; 70(2): 212–224

mucosal defense, and stress-induced loss of mucosal defense. Gastric acid and pepsin produced in the stomach, both important for breakdown of food, are cytotoxic to the cells of the stomach and small intestine. The cells lining these organs are protected from these agents by a thick layer of mucus. When acid production and mucosal defense mechanisms are in balance, acid and pepsin can be safely secreted without harm to the tissue. If one of these components is altered, breakdown of the tissue with resultant inflammation, ulceration and bleeding may occur. The least common cause is true acid-overproduction, as seen in Zollinger–Ellison syndrome. The autoregulation of acid secretion is disrupted and overwhelms mucosal defense mechanisms.

All other causes of inflammation, ulceration, and bleeding are essentially caused by disruptions in mucosal defense. *H. pylori*, a motile bacterium which lives in the mucus layer of the stomach, secretes several different cytotoxins that weaken the mucus barrier protecting the underlying cells as well as damage the cells directly. Increased permeability of the mucus layer allows for direct damage by gastric acid and pepsin; underlying cell damage promotes an inflammatory response and decreases mucus production. It is estimated that 70% of gastric ulcers and 95% of duodenal ulcers are associated with *H. pylori* infection [6].

A second mechanism by which mucosal defenses are broken down is NSAID use. NSAIDs block cyclooxygenase (COX) activity. COX exists in two forms in the body, COX1 and COX2, and most NSAIDs on the market today inhibit both enzymes to some degree. COX1 is a constitutive enzyme in the gastric mucosa that converts arachidonic acid into prostaglandins. Prostaglandins play a cytoprotective role in the stomach by stimulating mucin, bicarbonate, and phospholipid secretion by epithelial cells. They stimulate local mucosal blood flow and promote epithelial cell division and migration, all important components of mucosal repair. NSAIDs also appear to interfere with several other mechanisms important to mucosal defense such as inducible nitric oxide activity but these remain less well defined at this time. Aspirin irrevers-

ibly binds to COX1 and the gastric mucosa requires 5–8 days after the last dose of aspirin to regain levels of COX1 adequate to perform its cytoprotective role. The transient inhibition of COX1 by other NSAIDs such as ibuprofen and naproxyn allows for a faster recovery of cytoprotection, but consistent use of these agents causes as much damage as aspirin [7]. The combination of *H. pylori* infection with NSAID use has a synergistic, additive effect on peptic ulcer disease. Both factors increase ulcer formation independently. *H. pylori* infection increases ulcer incidence fourfold, whereas NSAID use increases ulcer incidence threefold. The presence of both increases the risk of ulcers 17-fold over patients who were *H. pylori* negative and non-NSAID users. More importantly, NSAID use increases risk of UGIB by fivefold over nonusers. *H. pylori* infection and NSAID use together increased the risk of bleeding 20-fold over noninfected, nonusers [8].

Gastric ulcers have been categorized by their location in the stomach as well as by their association with acid secretion. The original classification scheme subdivided gastric ulcers by their location in the stomach. Type I ulcers are located on the lesser curvature of the stomach, while Type II ulcers are located on the lesser curvature and are accompanied by a duodenal ulcer. Type III ulcers are located in the prepyloric region. Type IV ulcers are located in the cardia near the GE junction. Type V ulcers are diffuse. Several studies done during the era prior to the discovery of *H. pylori* correlated gastric acid secretion levels with the locations of these ulcers [9, 10]. The evidence suggested Types II and III were associated with high gastric acid secretion and Types I, IV, and V were not. Unfortunately, this data has not been updated since the discovery of the role of *H. pylori* in the etiology of peptic ulcer disease. Infection with *H. pylori* can cause hypergastrinemia and increase gastric acid secretion [11]. Moreover, there is data demonstrating no correlation between the location of a gastric ulcer and basal acid output [12]. Duodenal ulcers seem to be most reliably associated with high acid secretion; they are also overwhelmingly associated with *H. pylori* infection. Further work needs to be done in this area and the historical surgical classification of ulcers based on high acid secretion status without consideration the *H. pylori* factor needs to be reevaluated.

Esophageal and Gastric Varices

Variceal bleeding accounts for 4–30% of all UGIBs depending upon the study population. More importantly, it accounts for 50–60% of UGIBs in cirrhotic patients. In a retrospective study of 403 cirrhotic patients with bleeding varices, 36% were diagnosed with cirrhosis during their first admission for an acute UGIB [13]. These data bring up two important points. First, it is important to assess any patient with an UGIB for signs and symptoms of cirrhosis and pursue this diagnosis with an ultrasound or computed tomography (CT) scan if necessary, as the patient may not have been diagnosed with the disease at the time of their first UGIB. Second, although the slight majority of cirrhotics with UGIBs will have variceal bleeding, a significant number will have a non-variceal source of hemorrhage. This distinction is important for the treatment options available to the patient and treating physician.

Portal Hypertensive Gastropathy

Portal hypertensive gastropathy (PHG) is a poorly understood phenomenon occurring in patients with portal hypertension, usually secondary to cirrhosis, in which alterations in the gastric mucosa results in macroscopic changes in the mucosa as well as mucosal and submucosal vascular ectasia without histological evidence of inflammation. This has been reported to cause acute and chronic UGIB in patients with cirrhosis or portal hypertension. The incidence of PHG as a cause of UGIB is difficult to estimate because the patients who present with this phenomenon may be misdiagnosed as having variceal bleeding, acute gastritis, or angiodysplastic lesions. These lesions appear to be caused by local changes in vascular tone, nitric oxide, and various cytokines. There is debate in the literature about the relationship between the degree of portal hypertension as measured by the hepatic venous pressure gradient and the presence or severity of PHG. The relationship between the severity of PHG and the severity of hepatic dysfunction, portal hypertension, and causes of hepatic dysfunction remain unclear [14].

Mallory–Weiss Tear

Historically known as Mallory–Weiss syndrome, this cause of UGIB was originally associated with a triad of signs and symptoms: vomiting, hematemesis, and alcohol abuse. The lesions found at endoscopy were acute linear mucosal tears at or around the gastroesophageal junction, often with brisk associated arterial bleeding. These tears are thought to be caused by rapid forceful dilation of the GE junction. It is now understood that this process can result from many different activities, including childbirth, esophageal intubation, seizures, blunt abdominal trauma, cardiopulmonary resuscitation (CPR), and many different causes of sustained retching or vomiting, including hyperemesis gravidarum, alcohol intoxication, and chemotherapeutic treatments. On endoscopy, the most common appearance is a single linear tear along the lesser curvature of the stomach at the GE junction. Less frequently, there is more than one tear and if present, the other sites are along the greater curvature, posteriorly, and very rarely anteriorly. Up to 90% of Mallory–Weiss lesions stop bleeding spontaneously with resuscitation, acid suppression, and antiemetics [15].

Neoplasm

Benign tumors of the esophagus, stomach, and duodenum will cause bleeding as their initial symptom in approximately 10% of patients. This is usually the result of ulceration of the mucosa overlying a submucosal mass. Malignant tumors of this area will also infrequently bleed although it is not a common presenting symptom. Malignancies in this area include esophageal cancer, gastric adenocarcinoma, gastrointestinal stromal tumors (GISTs), and duodenal adenocarcinomas. Massive UGIB secondary to neoplastic disease is uncommon.

Dieulafoy Lesions

Dieulafoy lesions, first accurately identified in 1898, are a rare cause of UGIB. They account for between 3 and 5% of UGIBs, although they are likely underreported and misidentified as arteriovenous malformations and angiodysplastic lesions. Pathologically, a Dieulafoy lesion results when an artery travelling through the wall of the gastrointestinal tract fails to narrow appropriately as it reaches the outer limits of its territory. This has also been described as a "caliber-persistent artery" in that it is a histologically normal vessel other than its constant diameter of 1–3 mm. Macroscopically these vessels run a tortuous course in the submucosa. Bleeding occurs when the mucosa overlying the vessel breaks down and the wall of the vessel is injured or eroded. These lesions are not evenly distributed throughout the gastrointestinal tract. 71% are found in the stomach, 15% in the duodenum, and 8% in the esophagus. The remaining 6% are relatively evenly distributed in the rest of the small bowel, colon and rectum. Bleeding Dieulafoy lesions are more common in elderly patients already hospitalized. 90% of patients with lesions will have comorbidities and 40–50% will be taking NSAIDs, aspirin, or warfarin. These data suggest stress or impairment of mucosal defense mechanisms leading to mucosal breakdown and vessel erosion may be the proximal cause of bleeding in these lesions but this link remains elusive. Bleeding from a Dieulafoy lesion can range from intermittent to massive and correspondingly, presentation can range from iron-deficiency anemia to combined hematemesis and melena [16, 17].

Aortoenteric Fistula

A primary fistulous connection between the upper GI tract and aorta is very rare. If present, it is associated with an atherosclerotic aortic aneurysm in 85% of patients. Much less likely causes include foreign body ingestion or an infectious, inflammatory or neoplastic process. On the other hand, aortoenteric fistulae after aortic reconstruction are far more common. The third portion of the duodenum often directly overlies the repair and is involved in 80% of all aortoenteric fistulae [18, 19]. Less common sites of secondary fistulization include the esophagus and stomach. The classic presentation of an aortoenteric fistula is abdominal pain, a pulsatile mass, and a spontaneously resolving "herald" GIB, followed eventually by massive bleeding, exsanguination, and death.

Transpapillary Hemorrhage

A less common but important group includes those pathologies that result in hemobilia, or transpapillary bleeding. The most common cause of transpapillary bleeding is iatrogenic injury from hepatic or biliary procedures done percutaneously or endoscopically. Others include trauma, malignancy, hepatic artery aneurysms, arteriovenous malformations, and hemosuccus pancreaticus [4, 20]. Hemosuccus pancreaticus occurs when a pancreatic pseudocyst or other pancreatic inflammatory process erodes the surrounding tissue and forms a communication between the pancreatic duct and a peripancreatic artery or the splenic artery. These patients usually present with abdominal or back pain and hematochezia. Although rare, it is most common in patients with chronic pancreatitis. On endoscopy, the bleeding will appear to be coming from the ampulla of Vater [4, 21].

Clinical Presentation and Initial Management

Patients with an UGIB may present with a range of symptoms depending upon the rapidity and severity of the bleeding. Symptoms include hematemesis, hematochezia, melena, occult fecal blood, anemia and fatigue. Hemodynamic instability may or may not accompany the symptoms.

Resuscitation

Management of an UGIB should begin before a diagnosis is made. Although many UGIBs will stop spontaneously, the clinicians treating a patient with an UGIB should assume it will not. All patients with an UGIB should be managed initially by following the fundamentals of resuscitation of shock. The patient's capacity to maintain a safe airway should be established and if in doubt, the patient should be intubated. The patient's cardiovascular status and the presence or absence of shock should be rapidly investigated and treated. If the patient has any signs of hemodynamic instability or visible evidence of large volume blood loss, the patient should have large-bore vascular access placed and the blood bank should be alerted for possible unmatched blood needs and a type and crossmatch for packed red blood cells. The physical exam is not as helpful in UGIB as it can be in other disease processes. Signs of shock,

stigmata of liver disease, presence of peripheral vascular disease, and evidence of previous surgery can usually be investigated. If gross blood or melena is not obvious, a digital rectal exam and fecal occult blood test should not be overlooked. Bloodwork should include a complete blood count, a coagulation panel, a comprehensive metabolic panel and a blood type and screen, at minimum. If there is any history that suggests the patient will have abnormal coagulation studies, dysfunctional, or absent platelets, fresh frozen plasma and platelets should be made available as well [21].

A complete blood count is useful for ruling out blood dyscrasias, and the presence or absence of thrombocytopenia. The hemoglobin level is useful; however, a trend in hemoglobin levels over time is usually more helpful depending on the clinical situation. The metabolic panel will be most helpful in assessing the patient's current level of renal or hepatic dysfunction, if any. Coagulation panels are useful in assessing the current level of coagulation impairment and should be correlated to medication history. If a patient is coagulopathic and not taking an anticoagulant, malnutrition, DIC, and underlying liver disease should be urgently considered and investigated. Consideration should be given to ordering platelet function assays in patients taking platelet-altering medications. There is some data to recommend platelet transfusions to normalize function assays in patients taking platelet inhibitors who are having a significant bleeding problem [22]. This has not been studied in the setting of UGIB but deserves consideration in the patient with a massive or hemodynamically significant bleed.

History

Concurrent to these events, as much history as possible should be elicited from the patient, the family, and any other physicians involved with the patient. In addition to the events surrounding the UGIB, attention should be paid to any previous history of peptic ulcer disease or other forms of GIBs. Also, any history of liver disease, renal disease, malignancy, and cardiovascular disorders will be important as each of these has an implication for the etiology and management of the UGIB. A medication history is vital and must include not only prescription medications, but also over-the-counter medications. Patients frequently have more difficulty identifying the type and quantity of over-the-counter drugs they are taking and often do not know the importance of their NSAID use, for example, in their diagnosis and management. The past surgical history is vital to obtain. The success of any possible intervention in these patients in particular relies on a clear understanding the pre-procedural anatomy. Any prior surgery of the foregut, hepatopancreaticobiliary system, aorta, peripheral vasculature, and other abdominal organs will alter the diagnostic and technical approach of the endoscopist, interventional radiologist, and acute care surgeon.

Nasogastric Intubation and Aspiration

The diagnostic pathway in an UGIB frequently overlaps with the treatment pathway but the first step is identifying the location of the blood loss as proximal or distal to the ligament of Trietz. Every step taken to localize and characterize the source of the bleed improves the chance of successful treatment. A common tool to differentiate an UGIB from lower gastrointestinal bleeding (LGIB) is placement of a nasogastric tube and evaluation of the aspirate. The conventional wisdom suggests a nasogastric aspirate which returns bilious, but not bloody, fluid should prompt a workup for a LGIB. The logic underlying this step is that an aspirate containing bile reflects the fluid composition in the duodenum as well as the stomach; thus, bilious non-bloody fluid should rule out a source proximal to the ligament of Trietz. Unfortunately, this intuitive step has little evidence to support its use. Palamidessi et al. reviewed the literature for studies correlating findings from a nasogastric aspirate with an esophagogastroduodenoscopy (EGD) in patients with melena or hematochezia without hematemesis. They found only three studies that fit their criteria. Among these the sensitivity and specificity of a positive NGT aspirate ranged from 42 to 84% and 54 to 91%, respectively, with the highest values in a cohort of inpatients being treated for a myocardial infarction when they began to have symptoms [23]. They conclude that a conversation with the consulting gastroenterologist concerning the value of an NGT may be worthwhile. If an endoscopist has assessed the patient and their plan to perform upper or lower endoscopy will not be affected by the results of an NGT aspirate, then foregoing this step may be reasonable. Otherwise, an NGT aspirate may still be considered helpful and warranted.

Diagnosis and Management

Diagnostic and Therapeutic Endoscopy

After the initial resuscitation is underway, the source and etiology of the UGIB must be localized. The best initial procedure is usually endoscopy. EGD has proven to be the most important initial procedure. This modality in skilled hands will also offer several therapeutic options. Localization of the source of the bleed is critical. The success of all endoscopic, angiographic, and surgical interventions depends upon localization of the bleeding source. At the minimum, and with the worst conditions, an EGD can differentiate an UGIB from a LGIB. Should the bleeding fail to stop spontaneously or be controlled endoscopically, narrowing down the source vessels or tissues as much as possible makes the possibility of a successful angiographic or surgical intervention with the least amount of morbidity much more likely.

Therapeutic options for the endoscopist have expanded considerably in the last two decades. The techniques used will depend upon the skill and comfort of the endoscopist and the site and etiology of the bleeding. Options include epinephrine or sclerosant injection, thermal coagulation, hemostatic clip application, banding, or a combination of these techniques. Multiple trials have demonstrated that all of these modalities have similar efficacy in arresting bleeding, preventing rebleeding, and reducing the need for urgent surgical intervention. Success after initial treatment can be as high as 98% [4, 24]. Additionally, biopsies can provide useful information and in some institutions, *H. pylori* testing from biopsied tissue can be done with results much faster than serology or other types of testing. Neoplastic causes of bleeding can also be established by biopsy and can play an important role in treatment strategies. Furthermore, in the case of transpapillary bleeding, endoscopic retrograde cholangiopancreatography (ERCP) can be helpful for both localization and treatment. Recurrent bleeding after endoscopic control is infrequent, occurring in <10% of patients in centers with strong endoscopy departments. Repeat endoscopy for bleeding after initial endoscopic control has been compared to surgical intervention and has been demonstrated to achieve long-term hemostasis in a majority of patients while avoiding the complications of surgery [24]. Repeat endoscopy is widely regarded as the appropriate response to evidence of rebleeding after initial endoscopic control [21].

CT Scan

Several studies have shown a role for high resolution multidetector CT (MDCT) scan with digital subtraction angiography in localizing GI bleeding, including UGIBs. The "pooled" sensitivity and specificity of MDCT for GIB are 86% and 95%, respectively [25]. In swine and in vitro models, high quality MDCT imaging has been shown to localize bleeding as slow as 0.35–0.5 ml/min [26]. MDCT is currently considered "usually appropriate" by the American College of Radiology as the next diagnostic step following a negative or inconclusive endoscopy [4]. MDCT may be the best next step in a patient in whom an aortoenteric fistula is suspected or in a postsurgical patient in whom the anatomy is unclear. Additionally, if complications of neoplastic disease are high on the differential diagnosis, a CT scan may be highly valuable in assessing the extent of disease and these data could dramatically change further diagnostic and therapeutic plans. Unfortunately, at this time MDCT offers few possible concurrent therapeutic maneuvers and remains a solely diagnostic modality.

Tagged Red Cell Scan

Technetium-99 m-labeled erythrocyte scans, commonly known as tagged red cell scans, are useful because they can detect bleeding as slow as 0.05–0.1 ml/min. The major drawback to this option is its limited value in localizing the bleeding site. In the case of a LGIB, the relatively immobility of the colon can offer adequate localization for the next therapeutic endeavor. If the source of bleeding is in freely mobile viscera such as the majority of the small bowel, this information is of limited value for any intervention. Surprisingly, given the relatively predictable placement of the stomach and duodenum, studies have shown that tagged red cell scan localization of bleeding lesions in these areas to be frequently inaccurate [27, 28]. Thus, for the UGIB, tagged red cell imaging is rarely appropriate.

Diagnostic and Interventional Angiography

With the exception of the discovery of the role of and treatment for *H. pylori* in peptic ulcer disease, nothing has revolutionized the treatment of GI bleeding as much as advances in interventional radiology in the last two decades. Initially, angiography was available as a purely diagnostic tool and still plays an important role in that respect. Diagnostic angiography can detect bleeding at rates as low as 0.5 ml/min. Although it is generally not as helpful as endoscopy in characterizing the cause of bleeding, angiography can provide anatomic or structural information about lesions which are bleeding at the time of angiography or those that appear to bleed intermittently. Selective visceral angiography is most helpful if the source is arterial; detection of venous bleeding during the venous phase of the imaging is less reliable. Transcatheter arterial embolization (TAE) of UGIB source vessels involves selective visceral angiography and localization of the bleed. This can be expedited by visualization of previously placed endoscopic clips. Thus, hemostatic clip placement at the time of endoscopy is ultimately useful even when the clip placement is not technically successful [29]. Once the site of hemorrhage has been identified, feeding arteries can be embolized with coils, polyvinyl alcohol particles, gelfoam, iso-butyl-2-cyanoacrylate, ethibloc, or a combination of these products. Most studies found no difference in outcomes based on the type of agent used, although no randomized trials have been done to confirm this observation [4, 30]. If the lesion has been at minimum localized to a region of the stomach or duodenum by endoscopy, but cannot be visualized by angiography, "blind" embolization of the vessels feeding this area can be done successfully.

Multiple studies have demonstrated the benefits of TAE in UGIB when endoscopic attempts are not successful. TAE procedural and early clinical success rates (absence of early rebleeding), for bleeding after failure of endoscopic control range from 75 to 100% and 72 to 78%, respectfully in studies published from 2000 onward [20, 31, 32]. This success is highlighted by the fact that many of these studies were done in patients considered too high risk for surgery. The rebleeding rate after TAE in recent studies ranges from 7 to 30%. The factors associated with the risk of rebleeding after TAE have been extensively studied and in multivariate analysis, the presence of coagulopathy or multiple organ failure are consistently associated with clinical failure or rebleeding [20]. The drawbacks of TAE as a treatment option include the requirement for a skilled interventionalist team with 24-h availability, possible inability to cannulate the access vessel secondary to narrow or tortuous vasculature, and inability to localize the bleeding lesion in areas where blind embolization is not an option. Procedural drawbacks include the need for contrast injection and its potential risk of contrast induced renal insufficiency, groin hematomas and pseudoaneurysms, transient hepatic or pancreatic ischemia after embolization, and late duodenal stenosis secondary to embolic ischemia.

There have been no randomized controlled trials comparing TAE to surgery for UGIBs that have failed endoscopic treatment. Several groups have retrospectively compared the two modalities. There are numerous methodological differences amongst these studies; however, most found that patients who underwent embolization rather than surgery were consistently older, had more comorbidities including coronary artery disease, and were more frequently on anticoagulation therapy at the time of the UGIB. Despite this, most showed no significant difference between surgery and TAE in terms of the incidence of recurrent bleeding (23–43%), nor the need for additional surgery [33–36]. This data strongly supports the argument to proceed with angiography and TAE if endoscopic management fails. In cases of transpapillary bleeding, TAE has had excellent results. In studies of TAE in transpapillary bleeding published since 1999, the technical and clinical success rates of TAE have been 88–100% and 75–100%, respectively. The rebleeding rates in these studies ranged from 0 to 21% with major complication rates of 0–3% [20].

The therapeutic options now available for interventional radiologists are various and are not confined to the angiographic approach. They include transjugular intrahepatic portosystemic shunts (TIPS) as well. TIPS insertion for variceal bleeding unresponsive to endoscopic management has excellent outcomes in cessation of bleeding. If combined with variceal embolization, the rate of rebleeding is reduced further. It is equally efficacious as surgical porto-systemic shunts in cirrhotics. Shunts of either type are associated with an increased risk or exacerbation of hepatic encephalopathy. The newer TIPS stents are associated with a secondary patency rate of 90% or higher; additionally, TIPS can be exchanged percutaneously for occlusion and downsized for medically refractory encephalopathy [4].

Surgery

Historically, surgical intervention was the definitive treatment of UGIBs. Fifty years ago, there were neither endoscopic nor angiographic options; medical treatment of *H. pylori* was unknown. The etiology of UGIB was different. Peptic ulcer disease was more common and occurred in younger patients. Fewer UGIB patients were elderly, on chronic immunosuppression or anticoagulation; none had freshly placed coronary artery stents. Critical care-related illnesses were infrequent as critical care was in its infancy. Transplants and TIPS procedures were not available for patients with end stage liver disease, nor was dialysis available for patients with end stage renal disease. The surgical therapy of UGIB evolved in a patient population and health care system very different from today. The procedures were developed with few goals in mind: cessation of bleeding and acid suppression for peptic ulcer disease and portosystemic shunts for complications of cirrhosis. The morbidity of these procedures was acceptable as there were seldom any alternatives to surgical therapy. Today, the patient population has changed, the etiologies of UGIBs have changed, and many nonsurgical therapies are available. However, surgery is still required in some cases and the procedures available to the surgeon need to be understood. Some acute care surgeons may work in austere environments in which other modalities are not available locally or regionally. Early surgical intervention is lifesaving if less invasive methods of hemostasis are not options. Once an operation has been selected, it needs to be performed well and efficiently. Fewer and fewer acute care surgeons have seen or done any of the procedures used for UGIB in training.

Duodenotomy and Ligation of the Bleeding Vessel

This approach is most frequently used for a bleeding duodenal ulcer on the posterior wall of the lumen. An upper midline incision is made. The duodenum is mobilized and palpated for the location of the ulcer. An anterior longitudinal duodenotomy is made at the level of the posterior ulcer. The bleeding source is usually an erosion into the lumen of the gastroduodenal artery. Nonabsorbable sutures are used to ligate the vessel proximal and distal to the bleeding lumen. A third "U-stitch" is placed medial to the bleeding area to control inflow from the tranverse pancreatic artery (see Fig. 19.1). All of these sutures must be placed with care and precision in order to avoid any injury to the adjacent common bile duct. Once hemostasis has been achieved, the duodenotomy is closed transversely, most often with the Heineke-Mikulicz pyloroplasty, to avoid any postoperative obstructive symptoms [37, 38].

Truncal Vagotomy and Pyloroplasty

At this point, a truncal vagotomy can be added to the procedure. The left lobe of the liver is retracted and the body of the stomach is retracted caudad. This facilitates exposure of the gastroesophageal junction. The peritoneum overlying the junction is divided with scissors. Blunt dissection with a finger is used to encircle the esophagus, which is then looped with a Penrose drain. The drain can be used to retract and maneuver the esophagus while the anterior and posterior trunks of the vagus are identified. A nerve hook can be used to elevate the

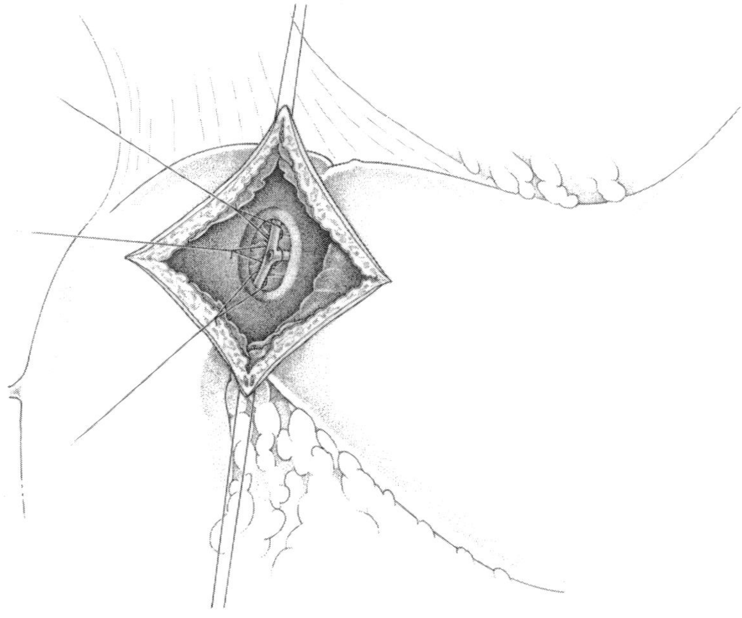

Fig. 19.1 Duodenotomy with appropriate suture placement on gastroduodenal and transverse pancreatic arteries. Reprinted with permission from Fischer JE, Jones DB. Chapter 77 In: *Mastery of Surgery*. 5th Edition. Fischer JE, Bland KI (eds). Philadelphia: Lippincott Williams & Wilkins; 2007

trunk up and away from the surrounding tissue. A 2 cm section of each nerve is resected, inspected to verify that it is neural tissue and then sent to pathology. At least 5 cm of space above the GE junction should be exposed to identify any accessory nerves not resected initially. The most common error here is missing the "criminal nerve of Grassi," a branch of the vagus originating from the posterior trunk which travels anteriorly and to the left of the esophagus. Once all accessory branches have been identified and ligated the area is inspected for hemostasis and the procedure is terminated [37].

Highly Selective Vagotomy

A highly selective vagotomy is intended to divide the vagal branches responsible for stimulation of the acid producing cells of the stomach while retaining smooth muscle innervation to the antrum of the stomach. The approach begins the same as the truncal vagotomy with exposure of the GE junction. The avascular plane along the lesser curvature of the stomach is divided. The anterior vagus is identified and the nerve of Latarjet is identified. This nerve gives off branches along the lesser curvature resembling "crow's feet." These branches are divided in a distal to proximal direction, leaving the branches 6 cm proximal to the pylorus intact. The rest can be ligated or divided using a harmonic scalpel all the way to the GE junction including any accessory branches 6–7 cm proximal to the GE junction. The posterior trunk is identified and the posterior nerve of Latarjet is identified and exposed down to the starting point, 6 cm proximal to the pylorus. Again, moving from distal to proximal, the "crow's feet" between the posterior nerve of Latarjet and the lesser curvature are divided all the way to the GE junction and any accessory branches found in the 6 cm cephalad to the GE junction. Lastly, the right gastroepiploic pedicle, found 10 cm proximal to the pylorus along the greater curvature of the stomach is identified and divided [37, 39].

Distal Partial Gastrectomy

The distal partial gastrectomy broadly describes any surgery removing the distal portion of the stomach, from antrectomy to subtotal gastrectomy. The more familiar eponymous names such as Bilroth I or Bilroth II refer to variations on how the remnant portion of the stomach is reconnected to the rest of the GI tract. The operations can be used for bleeding ulcer in the duodenum as well as bleeding ulcers in the stomach. These are usually done through an upper midline incision. Classically, the dissection begins by dividing the gastrocolic ligament and the gastroepiploic vessels midway along the length of the greater curvature. This area will eventually be the distal resection point of the stomach and form part of the gastroenteric anastomosis. This starting point can be modified depending upon the location of the bleeding ulcer in order to excise the inflamed tissue adequately and have healthy gastric tissue in this area to form the future anastomosis. Once the division point along the grater curvature has been selected, the gastrohepatic ligament is incised. Blunt dissection can be used to free the stomach from the underlying tissue of the lesser sac until a Penrose drain can be looped around the stomach. The duodenum is mobilized using a Kocher maneuver to loosen as much of the duodenum as possible for a tension free anastomosis if a gastroduodenal anastomosis is planned. Dissection along the stomach continues distally until the first portion of the duodenum is freed. The gastroduodenal artery is a good landmark for the transition between the free and the fixed portions of the duodenum. Once this is free, the dissection continues along the lesser curvature and includes ligation of the right gastric artery and preservation of the left gastric artery. When the distal stomach is free it is divided distally and proximally. The proximal division can be done prior to the dissection towards the duodenum as well. Both sutures and stapling devices have been used. The gastric remnant at the greater curvature is re-incised to form the gastric side of the gastroduodenal anastomosis. The duodenum and gastric remnant are brought together in an end-to-end fashion and closed using interrupted sutures. If a tension free anastomosis with healthy duodenal tissue cannot be achieved in an end to end fashion, there are several other options. The duodenal stump can be closed and the gastroduodenostomy formed between the stomach and the anterior wall of the duodenum, or an end-to-side anastomosis. Another technique that has been described for chronic bleeding ulcer of the posterior wall of the duodenal bulb in which the ulcer bed cannot be dissected away from the underlying tissue safely entails performing the distal gastrectomy as described, except for the resection of the posterior portion of the duodenum. The ulcer is oversewn and the ulcer bed left in place. The gastroduodenostomy is made with the posterior wall of the stomach sutured to the healthy duodenal mucosa just distal to the ulcer. The rest of the anastomosis proceeds in the same manner as the classical description. The difference is the ulcer bed remains in place but excluded from the GI tract. This method allows for suture placement in healthy tissue, an end-to-end reconstruction, and avoidance of the risks to the pancreas and portal vasculature that resection of the ulcer bed creates [40]. Lastly, if no gastroduodenal anastomosis is possible, the duodenal stump is closed either with a stapler or with suture, and the GI tract is reconstructed with an end-to-side gastrojejunal anastomosis [41].

Dieulafoy Lesions and Mallory–Weiss Lesions

These lesions share the distinction of being causes of UGIB related to neither acid production nor *H. pylori* infection. Thus, an acid-reducing procedure is not recommended for either of these lesions. Options range from a simple gastrotomy and oversew of the bleeding tissue to much larger gastric resections. Gastrotomy and oversew is most appropriate for a Mallory–Weiss lesion for two reasons. It is a benign, essentially traumatic, lesion without an underlying pathological process and is usually located in close proximity to the GE junction, an area well-known to be poorly tolerant of resections and anastomoses. As previously mentioned, Mallory–Weiss lesions rarely need surgical intervention and should it be necessary, the simplest approach to achieving hemostasis is recommended. Similarly, 90% of Dieulafoy lesions are successfully treated with one endoscopic therapy, most of the remainder are successfully treated with a second endoscopic approach. If both fail, and TAE is not an option; a simple gastrotomy and oversew or wedge resection would be appropriate [16, 17].

Gastric Wedge Resection

This has been used for bleeding from Type I ulcers located on the lesser curvature of the stomach and not associated with acid secretion. An upper midline incision is made, the lesser sac is entered as needed to palpate the lesion. If the preoperative localization and intraoperative palpation are excellent, the lesion can be resected in a wedge fashion using a stapling device. If the exact location cannot be determined, an anterior gastrotomy is made along a plane that can be incorporated into the future edge of the resection.

Gastric Ulcer Variations: Pauchet, Csendes, Kelling-Madlener

There are several surgical resection options described for Type IV gastric ulcers or other inflammatory processes that approach the GE junction. The Pauchet and Csendes procedures both involve resection of the ulcer and surrounding inflammatory tissue high along the lesser curvature of the stomach and bringing up a roux limb to prevent a prohibitive degree of narrowing of the gastric outlet. The Kelling-Madlener is described for giant gastric ulcers in which the ulcer bed or surrounding inflammation approaches the GE junction but given the size and appearance of the ulcer, an acid-related etiology is suspected. In this unusual case, multiple biopsies of the lesion are taken to rule out a neoplastic cause, the ulcer bed is rendered hemostatic, then a subtotal gastrectomy, truncal vagotomy, and roux-en-Y reconstruction is performed leaving the ulcer in place. The theory behind this procedure suggests that the acid-suppressive component of the procedure would allow the ulcerated tissue to heal [42].

Evidence-based Decision-making

As surgical management of UGIB becomes less and less common, it has become more difficult to make surgical decisions in an evidence-based manner. Surgical techniques for UGIB were designed in an era in which *H. pylori* was unknown and acid-suppressive medication was in its infancy. Medical management has evolved significantly while surgical management has not. When confronted with a patient who requires surgical intervention, the question of whether to perform a short hemostatic procedure or to perform a larger resection and various forms of vagotomy and reconstruction is difficult to answer.

There were two randomized controlled trials from the early 1990s which compared smaller interventions to conventional resections. Poxon et al. randomized patients with bleeding peptic ulcers to oversew or exclusion of the ulcer with postoperative ranitidine or a more conventional surgery of the surgeon's choice, ranging from oversew of the ulcer with pyloroplasty and vagotomy to partial gastrectomies without postoperative ranitidine. There was no significant difference in postoperative mortality. Both groups had rebleeding complications postoperatively. However, in the oversew and rantidine group, there was significantly higher mortality after rebleeding and the study was terminated [43].

The second study randomized patients with bleeding duodenal ulcers to either oversew of the ulcer with pyloroplasty and truncal vagotomy or distal gastric resection and Bilroth I or II reconstruction. Again there was no statistical difference in mortality. The oversew group had a higher rebleeding rate postoperatively. There was a trend towards higher duodenal leak rate in the Bilroth group and a significantly higher duodenal leak rate in patients who had a Bilroth II reconstruction. This study has been criticized for its very low accrual rate and significant dropout rate [44]. Both of these studies were completed before the advent of proton-pump inhibitors, *H. pylori* eradication, endoscopic therapy, or TAE. There has been no randomized controlled trial of surgical technique in UGIB for almost 20 years. The utility of these techniques is unclear. Certainly the skills to safely oversew an ulcer or resect a portion of the stomach or duodenum that would not tolerate a more minimal approach need to be maintained. However, the utility of adding the acid-suppressive components in the acute UGIB scenario is questionable. There is strong evidence that *H. pylori* infection or *H. pylori* infection with concomitant NSAID use are the causes of most peptic ulcer disease. In some areas, one of these two factors is involved in 98.4% of duodenal ulcers and 95.9% of gastric ulcers [45]. Two randomized controlled trials in 1995 demonstrated patients with bleeding duodenal ulcers who underwent *H. pylori* eradication had 0% recurrent bleeding at 1 year compared to 27–33% of controls [46, 47]. Patients taking

NSAIDs who are *H. pylori* positive have double the risk of an UGIB compared with NSAID users who are not [8].

There are a number of reports citing lower rates of *H. pylori* positivity in patients with bleeding ulcers, suggesting bleeding ulcers are less likely to be related to infection. However, further work has elucidated the weaknesses of *H. pylori* testing. Several tests such as the CLO test or urease breath test lack sensitivity even in ideal situations. False negativity is increased in situations which are fairly common for patients with an UGIB today. The best documented are the presence of fresh blood in the area and recent administration of antibiotics or proton pump inhibitors, all of which are very common in patients with an acute UGIB [48–50].

UGIB in Cirrhotic Patients

Variceal bleeding is a common, recurring problem in cirrhotic patients. It is the third most common cause of death in this group. Initial treatment is the same as for non-variceal bleeding: early resuscitation, correction of coagulopathy, and early endoscopy. Once endoscopic investigation has confirmed that the bleeding is secondary to varices, the management is different from that of non-variceal bleeding. Variceal bleeding is most frequently initially treated with endoscopic sclerotherapy, ligation, or a combination of both modalities and beta-blockade. If bleeding recurs, repeat endoscopy is a still an option. A second possibility is a surgical portosystemic shunt or a transjugular intrahepatic portosystemic shunting (TIPS). The purpose of either shunt is to decompress the portal system, lower the portal venous pressure and prevent rebleeding from varices. Both shunting procedures are associated with a risk of posttreatment encephalopathy. Multiple trials have investigated the benefits of TIPS versus endoscopic retreatment. A recent meta-analysis of 12 RCTs demonstrated TIPS was associated with a significant reduction in variceal rebleeding as well as death due to rebleeding. However, in the analysis of posttreatment encephalopathy and deaths due to all causes, endoscopic retreatment was associated with better outcomes [51].

Surgical Procedures for UGIB in Cirrhotics

TIPS procedures are modeled after earlier surgical portosystemic shunt procedures. These procedures are rarely done anymore because there are other modalities available for treatment and, in additional to the higher risks of surgical complications in cirrhotics, there has always been a risk of encephalopathy after shunting procedures. This belief has been challenged recently in an RCT of emergent portocaval shunt versus endoscopic sclerotherapy for acute bleeding esophageal varices. Orloff et al. found patients treated with a portocaval shunt had lower risks of variceal rebleeding, lower mean transfusions requirements, fewer readmissions and higher median, 5-year and 10-year survival rates. Moreover, the shunted group had a

lower incidence of posttreatment encephalopathy than those treated with sclerotherapy. Most episodes of encephalopathy in both groups appeared to be a result of dietary protein indiscretion, alcohol abuse, infection or uncontrolled diabetes. The major weakness of this approach was a significantly higher mortality rate in the first 14 days in the shunt group due to indeterminate causes. Despite these early deaths, it would appear the surgical shunting procedures were much more effective than has previously been reported. The authors note that the shunts were all done by two faculty surgeons who had extensive experience in shunting procedures; thus, the apparent success of these shunts may not be easily replicated by current acute care surgeons in practice who have little experience with shunting procedures [52].

The Modified Sagiura Procedure

For patients with variceal bleeding in whom a TIPS procedure is not feasible, usually secondary to anatomical issues, a second option which has been promoted in Southeast Asia is the Sagiura procedure. Initially described and modified by Sagiura in the 1960s and 1970s, the current method of this procedure involves an upper midline incision and devascularization of the distal 7 cm of the esophagus, the proximal 2/3rds of the stomach, and the short gastric vessels. For patients with bleeding esophageal varices, this is followed by esophageal transection and reanastomosis. Other surgeons have added other components including fundoplication, pyloroplasty, vagotomy, splenectomy, or oversewing of gastric varices [53]. Most early reports of the success of the Sagiura procedure were in patients with prehepatic portal hypertension, a condition infrequently seen in the acute care setting in the Western hemisphere [53]. However, later authors have found it useful in variceal bleeding in cirrhotic patients as well. Lee et al. reported on a case series of 41 cirrhotic patients with acute UGIB who had a modified Sagiura procedure: splenectomy, gastric and distal esophageal devascularization, fundectomy, pyloroplasty and occasionally esophageal transection. They had a 17.1% operative mortality rate and a 26.8% complication rate. For those who survived the operation, the five year survival rate was 62%. Survival was higher in those patients with lower Child Pugh classification and those without hepatocellular carcinoma. Although the operative mortality rate and complication rate are high, the procedure is worth considering for patients with few comorbidities, absence of hepatocellular carcinoma, and a potentially high postoperative quality of life [54].

Overall predictors of mortality in acute variceal bleeding include encephalopathy, presence of hepatocellular carcinoma, inpatient status prior to the UGIB, steroid usage, abnormal INR or prothrombin time, creatinine and bilirubin. Several prognostic indices such as the Child–Pugh score, the Garden score, and Gatta score have been compared and found to be similar in their predictive power of mortality [55].

Rebleeding and Mortality in Non-variceal UGIB

A European study of 2,660 patients with UGIB identified multiple predictors of poor outcomes which the authors defined as rebleeding, need for multiple procedures including surgery, in-hospital mortality and 30-day mortality. The characteristics identified were: advanced age, cardiac failure, ischemic heart disease, liver disease, renal insufficiency and renal failure, hematologic malignancy, disseminated malignancy, coagulopathy, inpatient status prior to the UGIB, and presentation with shock [55].

Rebleeding rates after UGIB range from 7 to 16%; however, the definition of rebleeding is highly variable and these estimates should be used with caution [2, 56]. Risk factors for rebleeding are consistent across multiple studies and include shock as well as multiple components of the initial presentation of the bleed: hematemesis, blood in the stomach, active bleeding or clot at the site, a visible vessel, and ulcer size. Two studies reported ulcer location at the posterior duodenal bulb or high lesser curvature as predictive as well although location has not been consistently predictive [55, 57–61]. Multiple models have been proposed to predict rebleeding and death: Forrest's classification, the Rockall scoring system, the Cedars-Sinai Predict Index, the Blatchford scoring system, and the Baylor college scoring system. Most are fairly sensitive predictors of rebleeding or death; however, the specificities and positive predictive values of each are very weak and consequently not great tools for surgical decision-making [62].

Mortality after an episode of UGIB has also been studied extensively. It is important to note that most mortality after an UGIB is not related to bleeding or rebleeding. With the exception of shock, the risk factors for rebleeding are different from the risk factors for mortality. In a prospective study of more than 10,000 patients with non-variceal UGIB, Sung and his colleagues found 80% of mortalities were not due to bleeding or rebleeding. Terminal malignancy was the most common cause of death at 33.7%. Pulmonary disease, multiple organ failure, and cardiac disease accounted for another 23.5%, 23.9%, and 13.5% respectively. Of those who died of bleeding related causes, 3% died of hemorrhage during surgery and 29% died of complications after surgical intervention for bleeding. In their analysis of factors associated with bleeding related mortality versus non-bleeding related mortality, use of NSAIDs, shock, and a clot or bleeding at the ulcer site increased a patient's risk of dying from bleeding related issues. Similar to other studies, predictors of death after an UGIB included advanced age, use of NSAIDs, inpatient status prior to the UGIB, rebleeding, and shock. Survivors were younger, more likely to have a prior history of peptic ulcer disease and *H. pylori* infection, and more likely to have been admitted for the UGIB itself [62, 63].

The Morbidity and Mortality of Surgical Therapy

The morbidity and mortality after surgical intervention for UGIB is difficult to measure. There have been very few studies designed to look specifically at the outcomes of surgical treatment of UGIB during the last 20 years. Many studies which compared other forms of treatment to surgery were designed to focus on the outcomes of the other intervention and detailed reports of the outcomes of surgical patients are lacking. As endoscopists and interventional radiologists gain expertise with treatment of UGIB, fewer patients need surgery; however, those who do tend to have failed other management strategies. The patients who present for surgery today are likely to be more acutely ill with more comorbidities than the patients who presented 50 years ago. The best recent data available concerning the morbidity and mortality of surgical treatment today can be extracted from the studies comparing TAE to surgery after failed endoscopic therapy. In a retrospective case–control study, Eriksson et al. reported the outcomes of 91 patients with UGIB who failed endoscopic therapy of whom 40 received TAE and 51 underwent surgery. The TAE group were largely selected by being poor surgical candidates; thus, the patients in the surgery group tended to be younger and have fewer comorbidities than the TAE group. Eighteen percent of the surgical group had continued bleeding or rebleeding postoperatively. There was a 37% complication rate with surgery and a 14% 30-day mortality rate. Ripoll et al. reported on a similar group of patients who had failed endoscopic management and were selected for surgery versus TAE on the basis of their surgical risk. Surgical patients had a rebleeding rate of 9%, and a mortality rate of 20.5%, most due to underlying disease. Eighteen percent had non-bleeding related complications which required a second procedure. Defreyne et al. retrospectively analyzed two groups of patients with endoscopically unmanageable UGIB. In this study the patients in the TAE group and the surgery group were not significantly different demographically, although patients with duodenal ulcers were more likely to have had surgical therapy than TAE. Lasting hemostasis was not achieved in 25.4% of the surgery group. Mortality was 27.5% for these patients, more than half died of multiple organ failure or underlying disease. Complications of surgery were not reported [30, 33, 34]. In Lau's study of the utility of repeat endoscopic treatment, one group of patients underwent surgery after the first endoscopic treatment failed. This group had a complication rate of 63%. The group allocated to repeat endoscopic treatment prior to salvage surgery had a complication rate of 46%. All the reported complications of respiratory failure, myocardial infarction, arrhythmia, stroke, wound dehiscence, wound infection, hepatic failure, renal failure, stump leak and bowel ischemia occurred in patients who had surgery. Lau's group found no significant difference in mortality. Only one retrospective analysis of surgical treatment of UGIB has been published in the last 20 years. Clarke et al. have published the only recent case series of surgical treatment of UGIBs. Over 12 years they had good documentation of only 41 surgical patients. Almost all had undergone endoscopy with and without therapeutic intervention; none had received TAE. Ninety percent of the procedures done on these patients were simple oversewing or excisions and 10% had partial gastrectomies. The authors reported a 56% postoperative complication rate and a 10% mortality rate. Only 15% of the complications were rebleeding; the rest were wound complications and cardiopulmonary complications. They do not report whether TAE was an option at their institution during the time period of the study [64].

All of these data suggest that patients in this era of endoscopic and interventional treatment who undergo ultimately undergo surgery for an UGIB do poorly. Rebleeding rates ranged from 9 to 18%. The mortality rates for these groups range from 14 to 27%; complication rates, when reported at all, range from 37 to 63%. Most deaths were from underlying disease or multiple organ failure; most complications were surgical infections or organ failure. None of these studies include information of the long-term outcomes of these patients. Specifically, it is unknown whether those who survived were able to return to independent living or whether they had any assessments of their quality of life. As the patients suffering from UGIBs refractory to initial medical and endoscopic management are consistently older and have more comorbities at presentation, these quality of life measures are important to consider. Surgeons consulted for these patients should consider the UGIB in the context of the of the patient's overall state of health. It is certainly valuable to discuss any end-of-life concerns or advance directives with the patient or the family prior to embarking on a surgical course.

Conclusion: Consultation, Cooperation, and Transfer

An UGIB associated with hemodynamic instability, large volume or ongoing blood loss, a transpapillary source of bleeding, or in a patient with significant comorbidities (such as cirrhosis, coronary artery disease, or renal insufficiency) or concurrent problems (such as malignancy, blood dyscrasias, recent cerebrovascular event, recent myocardial infarction, stent placement, or pulmonary embolus) will likely need a multidisciplinary approach. Diagnosis and treatment of these patients may require the services of a highly skilled endoscopist, interventional radiologist, intensivist, or surgeon. Their comorbid or concurrent conditions may require consultations from oncologists, cardiologists, neurologists, and nephrologists among others. They may require imaging, procedures,

and intensive care unit (ICU) care on a 24-h availability basis. The physicians caring for these patients need to remain in close contact with the specialists assisting with diagnosis and treatment in order to develop a treatment plan or algorithm for the patient. As information is collected and the complexity of the patient's problem is revealed, the resources available at the treating institution should be frequently reassessed. If it appears that complexity and possible needs of the patient are not appropriate to the institution, consideration should be made to transfer the patient to a facility that can provide these services. A consultation over the phone with a physician at a referral center can often help with a decision to keep or transfer a patient. Awareness of the strengths and weaknesses of the treating institution, close communication with other specialists involved in the patient's care, and a planned set of criteria for transfer are immensely helpful in providing quality patient care and resource management.

References

1. Lanas A. Editorial: upper GI bleeding-associated mortality: challenges to improving a resistant outcome. Am J Gastroenterol. 2010;105(1):90–2.
2. van Leerdam ME. Epidemiology of acute upper gastrointestinal bleeding. Best Pract Res Clin Gastroenterol. 2008;22(2):209–24.
3. Statistics for U.S. community hospital stays, prinicpal diagnosis based on CCS, 2009. 2011. Agency for Healthcare Research and Quality. 7-13-2001. Ref Type: Online Source
4. Schenker MP, Majdalany BS, Funaki BS, et al. ACR Appropriateness Criteria(R) on upper gastrointestinal bleeding. J Am Coll Radiol. 2010;7(11):845–53.
5. van Leerdam ME, Vreeburg EM, Rauws EA, et al. Acute upper GI bleeding: did anything change? Time trend analysis of incidence and outcome of acute upper GI bleeding between 1993/1994 and 2000. Am J Gastroenterol. 2003;98(7):1494–9.
6. Ford AC, Delaney BC, Forman D, Moayyedi P. Eradication therapy for peptic ulcer disease in *Helicobacter pylori* positive patients. Cochrane Database Syst Rev. 2006;(2):CD003840.
7. Feldman M, Shewmake K, Cryer B. Time course inhibition of gastric and platelet COX activity by acetylsalicylic acid in humans. Am J Physiol Gastrointest Liver Physiol. 2000;279(5):G1113–20.
8. Papatheodoridis GV, Papadelli D, Cholongitas E, Vassilopoulos D, Mentis A, Hadziyannis SJ. Effect of helicobacter pylori infection on the risk of upper gastrointestinal bleeding in users of nonsteroidal anti-inflammatory drugs. Am J Med. 2004;116(9):601–5.
9. Johnson HD. Gastric ulcer: classification, blood group characteristics, secretion patterns and pathogenesis. Ann Surg. 1965;162(6):996–1004.
10. Vesely KT, Kubickova Z, Dvorakova M. Clinical data and characteristics differentiating types of peptic ulcer. Gut. 1968;9(1):57–68.
11. Sachs G, Shin JM, Munson K, et al. Review article: the control of gastric acid and *Helicobacter pylori* eradication. Aliment Pharmacol Ther. 2000;14(11):1383–401.
12. Collen MJ, Sheridan MJ. Gastric ulcers differ from duodenal ulcers. Evaluation of basal acid output. Dig Dis Sci. 1993;38(12):2281–6.
13. Del Olmo JA, Pena A, Serra MA, Wassel AH, Benages A, Rodrigo JM. Predictors of morbidity and mortality after the first episode of upper gastrointestinal bleeding in liver cirrhosis. J Hepatol. 2000;32(1):19–24.

14. Curvelo LA, Brabosa W, Rhor R, et al. Underlying mechanism of portal hypertensive gastropathy in cirrhosis: a hemodynamic and morphological approach. J Gastroenterol Hepatol. 2009;24(9):1541–6.

15. Harbison SP, Dempsey DT. Mallory-Weiss syndrome. In: Cameron JL, editor. Current surgical therapy. 9th ed. Philadelphia, PA: Mosby Elselvier; 2008.

16. Baxter M, Aly EH. Dieulafoy's lesion: current trends in diagnosis and management. Ann R Coll Surg Engl. 2010;92(7):548–54.

17. Lara LF, Sreenarasimhaiah J, Tang SJ, Afonso BB, Rockey DC. Dieulafoy lesions of the GI tract: localization and therapeutic outcomes. Dig Dis Sci. 2010;55(12):3436–41.

18. Hollander JE, Quick G. Aortoesophageal fistula: a comprehensive review of the literature. Am J Med. 1991;91(3):279–87.

19. Pipinos II, Carr JA, Haithcock BE, Anagnostopoulos PV, Dossa CD, Reddy DJ. Secondary aortoenteric fistula. Ann Vasc Surg. 2000;14(6):688–96.

20. Mirsadraee S, Tirukonda P, Nicholson A, Everett SM, McPherson SJ. Embolization for non-variceal upper gastrointestinal tract haemorrhage: a systematic review. Clin Radiol. 2011;66(6):500–9.

21. Hungness ES. Gastrointestinal bleeding. In: Ashley S, Wilmore D, editors. ACS surgery: principles and practice. BC Decker: Hamilton, ON; 2011.

22. Rand ML, Leung R, Packham MA. Platelet function assays. Transfus Apher Sci. 2003;28(3):307–17.

23. Palamidessi N, Sinert R, Falzon L, Zehtabchi S. Nasogastric aspiration and lavage in emergency department patients with hematochezia or melena without hematemesis. Acad Emerg Med. 2010;17(2):126–32.

24. Lau JY, Sung JJ, Lam YH, et al. Endoscopic retreatment compared with surgery in patients with recurrent bleeding after initial endoscopic control of bleeding ulcers. N Engl J Med. 1999;340(10):751–6.

25. Chua AE, Ridley LJ. Diagnostic accuracy of CT angiography in acute gastrointestinal bleeding. J Med Imaging Radiat Oncol. 2008;52(4):333–8.

26. Kuhle WG, Sheiman RG. Detection of active colonic hemorrhage with use of helical CT: findings in a swine model. Radiology. 2003;228(3):743–52.

27. Bentley DE, Richardson JD. The role of tagged red blood cell imaging in the localization of gastrointestinal bleeding. Arch Surg. 1991;126(7):821–4.

28. Winzelberg GG, McKusick KA, Froelich JW, Callahan RJ, Strauss HW. Detection of gastrointestinal bleeding with 99mTc-labeled red blood cells. Semin Nucl Med. 1982;12(2):139–46.

29. Loffroy R, Guiu B. Role of transcatheter arterial embolization for massive bleeding from gastroduodenal ulcers. World J Gastroenterol. 2009;15(47):5889–97.

30. Defreyne L, De Schrijver I, Decruyenaere J, et al. Therapeutic decision-making in endoscopically unmanageable nonvariceal upper gastrointestinal hemorrhage. Cardiovasc Intervent Radiol. 2008;31(5):897–905.

31. Loffroy R, Guiu B, Cercueil JP, et al. Refractory bleeding from gastroduodenal ulcers: arterial embolization in high-operative-risk patients. J Clin Gastroenterol. 2008;42(4):361–7.

32. Loffroy R, Guiu B, Mezzetta L, et al. Short- and long-term results of transcatheter embolization for massive arterial hemorrhage from gastroduodenal ulcers not controlled by endoscopic hemostasis. Can J Gastroenterol. 2009;23(2):115–20.

33. Ripoll C, Banares R, Beceiro I, et al. Comparison of transcatheter arterial embolization and surgery for treatment of bleeding peptic ulcer after endoscopic treatment failure. J Vasc Interv Radiol. 2004;15(5):447–50.

34. Eriksson LG, Ljungdahl M, Sundbom M, Nyman R. Transcatheter arterial embolization versus surgery in the treatment of upper gastrointestinal bleeding after therapeutic endoscopy failure. J Vasc Interv Radiol. 2008;19(10):1413–8.

35. Defreyne L, Vanlangenhove P, De VM, et al. Embolization as a first approach with endoscopically unmanageable acute nonvariceal gastrointestinal hemorrhage. Radiology. 2001;218(3):739–48.

36. Larssen L, Moger T, Bjornbeth BA, Lygren I, Klow NE. Transcatheter arterial embolization in the management of bleeding duodenal ulcers: a 5.5-year retrospective study of treatment and outcome. Scand J Gastroenterol. 2008;43(2):217–22.

37. Schirmer BD. Bleeding duodenal ulcer. In: Fischer JE, Bland KI, editors. Mastery of surgery. 5th ed. Philadelphia: Lippincott Williams & Wilkins; 2007.

38. Winkleman BJ, Usatii A, Ellison EC. Duodenal ulcer. In: Cameron JL, editor. Current surgical therapy. 9th ed. Philadelphia, PA: Mosby Elselvier; 2008.

39. Donahue PE. Parietal cell vagotomy versus vagotomy-antrectomy: ulcer surgery in the modern era. World J Surg. 2000;24(3):264–9.

40. Guinier D, Destrumelle N, Denue PO, Mathieu P, Heyd B, Mantion GA. Technique of antroduodenectomy without ulcer excision as a safe alternative treatment for bleeding chronic duodenal ulcers. World J Surg. 2009;33(5):1010–4.

41. Siewert JR, Bumm R. Distal gastrectomy with Bilroth I, Bilroth II, or Roux-Y reconstruction. In: Fischer JE, Bland KI, editors. Mastery of surgery. 5th ed. Philadelphia: Lippincott Williams & Wilkins; 2007.

42. Fisher WE, Brunicardi FC. Benign gastric ulcer. In: Cameron JL, editor. Current surgical therapy. 9th ed. Philadelphia, PA: Mosby Elsevier; 2008.

43. Poxon VA, Keighley MR, Dykes PW, Heppinstall K, Jaderberg M. Comparison of minimal and conventional surgery in patients with bleeding peptic ulcer: a multicentre trial. Br J Surg. 1991;78(11):1344–5.

44. Millat B, Hay JM, Valleur P, Fingerhut A, Fagniez PL. Emergency surgical treatment for bleeding duodenal ulcer: oversewing plus vagotomy versus gastric resection, a controlled randomized trial. French Associations for Surgical Research. World J Surg. 1993;17(5):568–73.

45. Arroyo MT, Forne M, de Argila CM, et al. The prevalence of peptic ulcer not related to *Helicobacter pylori* or non-steroidal anti-inflammatory drug use is negligible in southern Europe. Helicobacter. 2004;9(3):249–54.

46. Miehlke S, Bayerdorffer E, Lehn N, et al. Two-year follow-up of duodenal ulcer patients treated with omeprazole and amoxicillin. Digestion. 1995;56(3):187–93.

47. Rokkas T, Karameris A, Mavrogeorgis A, Rallis E, Giannikos N. Eradication of *Helicobacter pylori* reduces the possibility of rebleeding in peptic ulcer disease. Gastrointest Endosc. 1995;41(1):1–4.

48. Leung WK, Sung JJ, Siu KL, Chan FK, Ling TK, Cheng AF. False-negative biopsy urease test in bleeding ulcers caused by the buffering effects of blood. Am J Gastroenterol. 1998;93(10):1914–8.

49. Grino P, Pascual S, Such J, et al. Comparison of diagnostic methods for *Helicobacter pylori* infection in patients with upper gastrointestinal bleeding. Scand J Gastroenterol. 2001;36(12):1254–8.

50. Gisbert JP, Calvet X. Review article: *Helicobacter pylori*-negative duodenal ulcer disease. Aliment Pharmacol Ther. 2009;30(8):791–815.

51. Zheng M, Chen Y, Bai J, et al. Transjugular intrahepatic portosystemic shunt versus endoscopic therapy in the secondary prophylaxis of variceal rebleeding in cirrhotic patients: meta-analysis update. J Clin Gastroenterol. 2008;42(5):507–16.

52. Orloff MJ, Isenberg JI, Wheeler HO, et al. Portal-systemic encephalopathy in a randomized controlled trial of endoscopic sclerotherapy versus emergency portacaval shunt treatment of acutely bleeding esophageal varices in cirrhosis. Ann Surg. 2009;250(4):598–610.

53. Mathur SK, Shah SR, Nagral SS, Soonawala ZF. Transabdominal extensive esophagogastric devascularization with gastroesophageal stapling for management of noncirrhotic portal hypertension: long-term results. World J Surg. 1999;23(11):1168–74.

54. Lee JH, Han HS, Kim HA, Koo MY. Long-term results of fundectomy and periesophagogastric devascularization in patients with gastric fundal variceal bleeding. World J Surg. 2009;33(10):2144–9.

55. Chiu PW, Ng EK. Predicting poor outcome from acute upper gastrointestinal hemorrhage. Gastroenterol Clin North Am. 2009;38(2):215–30.

56. Lanas A, Aabakken L, Fonseca J, et al. Clinical predictors of poor outcomes among patients with nonvariceal upper gastrointestinal bleeding in Europe. Aliment Pharmacol Ther. 2011;33(11):1225–33.

57. Villanueva C, Balanzo J, Espinos JC, et al. Prediction of therapeutic failure in patients with bleeding peptic ulcer treated with endoscopic injection. Dig Dis Sci. 1993;38(11):2062–70.

58. Brullet E, Calvet X, Campo R, Rue M, Catot L, Donoso L. Factors predicting failure of endoscopic injection therapy in bleeding duodenal ulcer. Gastrointest Endosc. 1996;43(2 Pt 1):111–6.

59. Brullet E, Campo R, Calvet X, Coroleu D, Rivero E, Simo DJ. Factors related to the failure of endoscopic injection therapy for bleeding gastric ulcer. Gut. 1996;39(2):155–8.

60. Guglielmi A, Ruzzenente A, Sandri M, et al. Risk assessment and prediction of rebleeding in bleeding gastroduodenal ulcer. Endoscopy. 2002;34(10):778–86.

61. Wong SK, Yu LM, Lau JY, et al. Prediction of therapeutic failure after adrenaline injection plus heater probe treatment in patients with bleeding peptic ulcer. Gut. 2002;50(3):322–5.

62. Kim BJ, Park MK, Kim SJ, et al. Comparison of scoring systems for the prediction of outcomes in patients with nonvariceal upper gastrointestinal bleeding: a prospective study. Dig Dis Sci. 2009;54(11):2523–9.

63. Sung JJ, Tsoi KK, Ma TK, Yung MY, Lau JY, Chiu PW. Causes of mortality in patients with peptic ulcer bleeding: a prospective cohort study of 10,428 cases. Am J Gastroenterol. 2010;105(1):84–9.

64. Clarke MG, Bunting D, Smart NJ, Lowes J, Mitchell SJ. The surgical management of acute upper gastrointestinal bleeding: a 12-year experience. Int J Surg. 2010;8(5):377–80.

Harry M. Richter III and Thomas M. Komar

Introduction

Biliary tract diseases requiring emergency or urgent surgical evaluation and treatment are among the most common acute conditions encountered by the general or acute care surgeon. The vast majority of these conditions represent complications of gallstones. Contained within the gallbladder, stones may lead to acute cholecystitis, followed by potential sequelae including gallbladder empyema, gangrene, perforation, liver abscess, or peritonitis. An impacted stone in the gallbladder infundibulum, together with the inflammation thus caused, may partially obstruct the hepatic duct, or even erode into the adjacent duct (Mirizzi syndrome). Similarly, the stone could erode into the adjacent adherent duodenum, ultimately obstructing the intestine. When smaller gallstones escape the gallbladder via the cystic duct into the common duct, the stones, howsoever small, may incite an attack of acute pancreatitis. Or they may obstruct the common duct, causing jaundice; if the bile happens to harbor bacteria, then the result could be acute cholangitis. Cholecystitis can occur without gallstones as a complication of trauma or other acute conditions. Finally, cholecystitis and cholangitis may complicate biliary stent treatment of malignant or benign bile duct stricture.

Acute Cholecystitis

Gallstones within the gallbladder are extremely common, and fortunately they may remain clinically silent for the lifetime of their host. Biliary colic is a syndrome of right upper quadrant or epigastric pain, lasting from several minutes to several hours,

usually accompanied by nausea and sometimes by vomiting. It is caused by the transient obstruction of the gallbladder outlet, being either the gallbladder infundibulum or the cystic duct, by a gallstone. Resolution of the pain follows dislodgement of the offending stone, which either slips back freely into the gallbladder or is propelled through the cystic into the common bile duct. But if the obstruction should persist long enough, local edema will further secure the errant stone in place. The gallbladder will become edematous and inflamed, and will distend with secreted fluid. This is acute calculus cholecystitis. In younger, nondiabetic patients with a short or no history of gallstones, the process will likely be sterile. The probability of infected gallbladder bile increases with age, presence of gallstones, diabetes, and prior elimination of the protection of the sphincter of Oddie, e.g., following endoscopic sphincterotomy or endobiliary stent placement.

Without treatment, acute calculus cholecystitis may evolve in one of several directions. If the bile is sterile, the obstructed gallbladder wall can remain intact, while the epithelium, having absorbed bile pigment, secretes a clear fluid to reach an equilibrium of distension with elevated pressure. This state of affairs is called hydrops of the gallbladder. While usually uncomfortable it may be tolerable for a surprisingly long duration before definitive resolution.

Regions of the gallbladder's wall are apt to become necrotic. Not always, but usually free perforation is prevented by the liver and by protective adhesions from the omentum, hepatic flexure of the colon and mesocolon, and the duodenum.

Gangrene is more common among diabetic patients [1] (as well as in those suffering acalculus cholecystitis) probably reflecting an ischemic mechanism compounding distension and infection (Fig. 20.1). A pericholecystic abscess may develop, contained either by surrounding omentum and viscera or within the adjacent liver substance. If the wall remains intact, infection can produce a pus-filled organ termed empyema of the gallbladder. Infection involving gas-producing organisms can generate gas within the lumen, or more especially gas within the wall of the gallbladder, called emphysematous cholecystitis [2].

H.M. Richter III, M.D., F.A.C.S. (✉)
Division of General Surgery, Department of Surgery, Stroger Hospital of Cook County, 1901 W. Harrison Street, Chicago, IL 60612, USA
e-mail: harry_richter@rush.edu

T.M. Komar, M.D.
Department of Surgery, Stroger Hospital of Cook County, Chicago, IL, USA

L.J. Moore et al. (eds.), *Common Problems in Acute Care Surgery*,
DOI 10.1007/978-1-4614-6123-4_20, © Springer Science+Business Media New York 2013

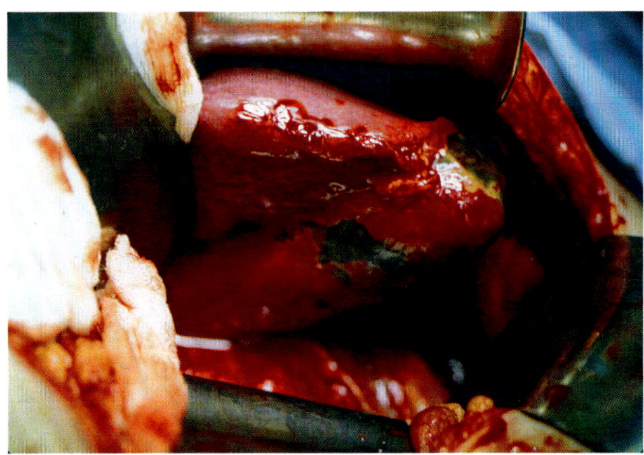

Fig. 20.1 Acute gangrenous cholecystitis (operative photograph)

On the other hand, even before the modern era of antibiotics and other interventions, acute cholecystitis did often enough certainly resolve spontaneously. In fact, with the judicious use of antibiotics and support with intravenous fluids and analgesics, recovery from acute calculus cholecystitis without definitive intervention is expected, despite the litany of dire complications enumerated above. What happens that permits the obstructed gallbladder to recover? In many patients the obstructing stone becomes dislodged. Perhaps progressive gallbladder distension, combined with sloughing of the mucosa surrounding the stone, frees the stone to slip back harmlessly into the body of the gallbladder. Restored patency of the gallbladder outlet can be documented in many patients who recover with the help of percutaneous gallbladder decompression (cholecystostomy), and these are typically patients selected for drainage because they did not quickly resolve on their own.

The anticipated successful outcome of medically treated acute cholecystitis engendered a traditional approach of "cooling off" the inflamed gallbladder, followed by an elective cholecystectomy not sooner than 6 weeks after resolution of symptoms. This delay typically permitted a nonhostile operative field for open cholecystectomy, where acute hyperemia of inflammation had subsided, and adhesions had resolved or softened.

Diagnosis of Acute Calculus Cholecystitis

The cardinal symptom of acute cholecystitis is abdominal pain of rapid but not sudden onset, developing generally in the right upper quadrant, or else in the epigastrium. Radiation of the pain toward the right scapula tip is common. Nausea and vomiting usually accompany the pain. The attack may follow prior episodes of biliary colic, the symptoms of which are similar but self-limited. Cholecystitis symptoms persist and worsen until finally emergency medical attention is sought. On exam the patient appears worried and uncomfortable. Fever is generally absent or low-grade. Visible jaundice is rare. Abdominal exam reveals marked right upper quadrant tenderness, typically with localized guarding. A distended gallbladder or inflammatory mass can often be palpated. On the other hand, the inflamed gallbladder may be protected by the right costal margin. In this case, a deep inspiratory breath will bring the gallbladder down to the palpating fingertips. "Murphy's sign," in common usage, is the abrupt cessation of inspiration due to pain caused by bringing the inflamed gallbladder into contact with the abdominal wall being depressed by the examiner's fingers. (A positive "ultrasonic Murphy's sign" is the analogous effect caused by the ultrasound probe.)

Basic laboratory investigation may disclose at most a modest leukocytosis unless gangrene or empyema has supervened. Similarly, liver function tests are often unremarkable. Bilirubin and alkaline phosphatase are sometimes mildly elevated, indicating either a concomitant common bile duct stone or compression of the common duct by the inflammatory reaction to an impacted gallbladder stone. Likewise, aminotransferase levels are normal unless secondary inflammation of the adjacent liver causes mild elevation. A reasonable differential diagnosis includes pyogenic or amoebic liver abscess, contained perforation of a duodenal or gastric ulcer, pancreatitis, or contained perforation of the hepatic flexure of the colon. Especially in older patients, concomitant gallbladder cancer has to be considered.

Ultrasound examination of the right upper quadrant is without doubt the single most appropriate test to evaluate presumed acute calculus cholecystitis [3]. In the hands of an experienced operator and interpreter, ultrasound reliably identifies the presence of gallbladder stones; discloses the presence of a nonmobile stone impacted in the infundibulum; suggests acute inflammation by recognizing gallbladder distension, wall thickness (edema), and pericholecystic fluid; discovers additional liver pathology; measures the caliber of the intra- and extrahepatic bile ducts; assesses the status of the right kidney; and may, absent overlying bowel gas, provide a useful view of the head of the pancreas (Fig. 20.2). If ultrasound confirms calculus cholecystitis in a non-jaundiced patient, then no other test is necessary before executing the therapeutic plan.

Unfortunately, quality ultrasound studies are not available in all emergency departments, and certainly not at all hours of the day or night. Computed tomography (CT) scan is often more readily obtainable, is far less operator dependent than ultrasound, and physicians and surgeons are generally more comfortable interpreting CT scans themselves, and acting upon their findings. As a consequence, CT scanning is often performed for all acute or potentially acute abdominal conditions, including likely cholecystitis. The disadvantages of CT scans are known: radiation exposure, potential nephrotoxicity

Fig. 20.2 Abdominal ultrasound examination demonstrating distended gallbladder with thickened gallbladder wall and impacted gallstone within infundibulum of gallbladder

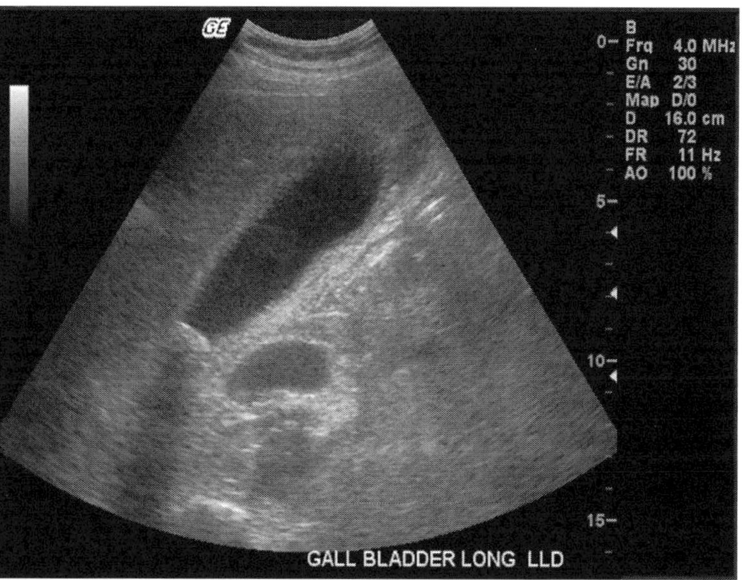

from IV contrast infusion; sequestration of the patient from caregivers for a potentially critical period of time; and expense. Additionally, CT scan is much less sensitive than ultrasound for confirming the presence of gallstones. CT scan does of course reliably confirm signs of acute cholecystitis: gallbladder distension, wall edema, pericholecystic edema, contained perforation (Fig. 20.3). Furthermore, alternative diagnoses are likely to be ruled out or in with certainty. What if CT scan confirms a strong clinical suspicion of acute cholecystitis but gallstones are not seen? While a simple ultrasound will settle the matter of stones, the therapeutic plan is nearly always unchanged by that added knowledge.

Treatment of Acute Calculus Cholecystitis

The medical treatment of acute cholecystitis is straightforward. The patient is admitted to the hospital and made NPO to minimize gallbladder stimulation and aggravation of nausea and vomiting. Nasogastric suction is not necessary. Intravenous hydration and parenteral pain medication are given. Antibiotics are withheld in the absence of signs of infection, but fever, leukocytosis, or other indications of sepsis are sufficient to initiate antibiotic treatment. The expected pathogens include mainly gram-negative bacilli (*E. coli*, *Klebsiella*, *Enterobacter*), for which the antibiotic regimen is chosen. Patients symptomatically improve because of this supportive treatment, regardless of the pathological condition of their gallbladder. They feel reassured by the attention received in the hospital, and claim to tolerate sips of clear liquids. True recovery, however, requires complete resolution of right upper quadrant tenderness, and the temptation of a flavorful fried meal should bring a guilty grin of anticipation.

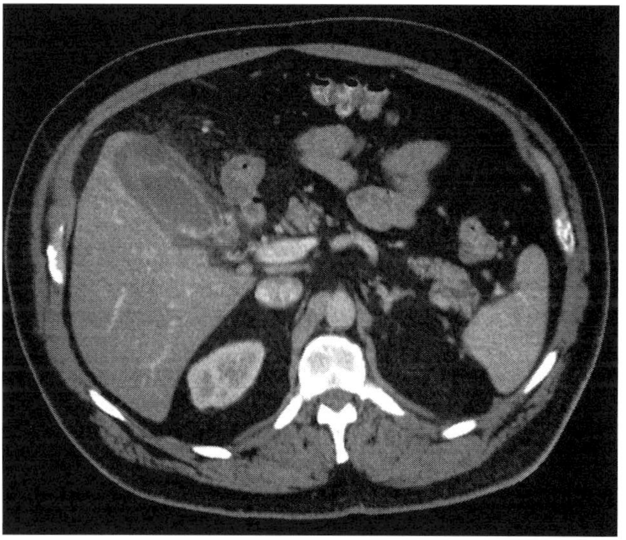

Fig. 20.3 Computed tomographic scan of abdomen showing signs of acute cholecystitis, including gallbladder wall thickening and pericholecystic edema

In the pre-laparoscopic era, medical resolution of acute cholecystitis followed by interval open cholecystectomy was generally effective, if admittedly inefficient. But failure of medical treatment required operation—either cholecystectomy or, when that was not safe, open cholecystostomy. After several days of failed treatment, even open cholecystectomy could be a tough and even treacherous operation. Cholecystectomy earlier in the acute attack, surgeons observed, was likely to be easier and safer. Adhesions were less dense and vascular, and edema between the gallbladder wall and the liver bed facilitated dissection of this plane. A policy of "early operation" for acute cholecystitis developed, in which "early operation" meant during the index hospitalization, at the first convenient opening in the surgeon's operating schedule. The early operation plan has been shown to be as safe as delayed cholecystectomy, while saving hospital days and preventing intercurrent biliary attacks.

Elective laparoscopic cholecystectomy rapidly replaced open elective cholecystectomy, in spite of the early frighteningly large risk of common bile duct injury. Acute cholecystitis was at first considered a contraindication to attempting laparoscopic operation. To preserve the advantages of minimally invasive cholecystectomy, many surgeons returned to the approach of medical treatment followed by delayed cholecystectomy. Fortunately the hazards and perceived difficulties of laparoscopic cholecystectomy in the face of acute inflammation have gradually been answered by experience, improved operative technique, and ongoing development of laparoscopic instrumentation. Once again, laparoscopic cholecystectomy early in the course of acute cholecystitis is demonstrably as safe as delayed operation, saves resources, and prevents further attacks [4–6]. The likelihood of needing to convert to an open operation is the same, whether done early or delayed.

The exact optimal timing of "early cholecystectomy" remains the subject of study and discussion. From the patient's point of view, the disease and its attendant misery and inconvenience should be resolved as soon as safely possible, i.e., as soon as resuscitation is complete and medical comorbid conditions have been optimized. From the gallbladder's perspective, so long as a stone is obstructing the infundibulum or cystic duct, the situation is getting worse. Distension, edema, hyperemia, lymphatic congestion, cystic duct lymph node enlargement are progressive. An intact gallbladder wall soon may face ischemia and necrosis. A few bacteria proliferate— will antibiotics arrive in time? and so on. A convenient window of 72 h after diagnosis and admission no longer qualifies as "early," because on a continuum of time, the earlier the operation is undertaken, the easier and safer the operation will be, the smaller the risk of having to convert to open cholecystectomy, and the sooner the patent is likely to leave the hospital and resume normal activities [7, 8].

However early the operation is conducted, whether laparoscopic or open, it must be given its due respect as a major, potentially challenging procedure. In other words, all possible support systems need to be in place or readily available. Are the anesthesiologists and recovery room nurses prepared for a potentially sick patient? Is the scrub and circulating operating room (OR) team intimately familiar with laparoscopic equipment? Is radiology rapidly available for intraoperative cholangiography? Are surgical assistants highly qualified? And for the neophyte attending surgeon, is senior backup easily at hand? In all but the busiest medical centers, these requirements argue against conducting the operation at night. With proper personnel and dedication, a weekend cholecystectomy seems reasonable. The surgeon should be relaxed and rested, not overly stressed or sleep deprived, in order to perform the operation with the requisite equanimity. An "acute care surgery" practice model can provide the apparent paradox of an earlier operation, still performed during regular daytime hours, with less disruption of the elective surgical schedule [9]. On the other hand, the patient will be ill-served by a surgeon who lacks an elective gallbladder practice and an interest in biliary disease. In other words, we agree with Strasburg that the operation for acute cholecystitis demands a surgeon who demonstrates expertise in complicated laparoscopic cholecystectomy [10].

Operative Technique in Detail

Laparoscopic Cholecystectomy

The operation for acute cholecystitis is merely an adaptation or modification as necessary of the standard laparoscopic cholecystectomy, with which the surgeon must be entirely familiar. What follows is a description of the technique as it has evolved in our clinic.

The patient is positioned supine on the operating table with arms extended or tucked according to surgeon and anesthesiologist agreement. The position must accommodate the possibility of maneuvering a C-arm into position for a cholangiogram, as well as attaching a self-retaining retractor (e.g., Bookwalter or Omni) in the event of an open operation. A Foley catheter is used, anticipating a lengthy operation. Antibiotic prophylaxis is used unless therapeutic antibiotic coverage is already ongoing. Deep venous thrombosis prophylaxis is instituted as well.

A standard four-port approach is used, beginning with an umbilical Hassan cannula placed using an open sharp technique. Insufflation to about 15 mmHg (adjusted higher or lower according to circumstance) allows inspection using a 10 mm 30 laparoscope. The lateral 5 mm port is placed near the anterior axillary line nearly opposite the umbilicus (higher if the patient is very tall). The patient is placed in reverse-Trendelenburg, left side down position, to allow omentum and colon to fall away from the gallbladder. Next an 11 mm epigastric port is inserted, entering the abdomen to the right of the falciform ligament (sometimes made easier by pulling the ligament to the left). The fourth port is not introduced until the need for gallbladder decompression has been determined. To do this, adhesions are separated from the gallbladder fundus. Omentum is pulled away with a blunt grasper. Then, exploiting the plane along the gallbladder wall, a Maryland-type dissector or, even better, the blunt-tipped suction-irrigator is insinuated and stroked upward and downward to gently separate tissues. Usually a turgid phlegmon of omentum, mesocolon, and colonic wall can be peeled off from the gallbladder in one piece, revealing the diseased organ. At least, a space must be cleared on the dome, to permit decompression as distension will otherwise preclude grasping the fundus. Once the need for decompression is determined, the fourth trocar is placed so as to provide a direct pathway through the dome along the long axis of the gallbladder, which can be partially stabilized using an instrument inserted through the epigastric port. The distended viscus may be aspirated using a long needle and syringe; a specimen is easily gotten for culture, but emptying the gallbladder is tedious and incomplete. Our preferred option is to reintroduce the stylette into the fourth port, and thrust this port directly into the gallbladder, carefully avoiding a through-and-through injury. Once the trocar is inside, the stylette is removed and suction applied to rapidly empty the fluid contents. A Lukens trap in the suction circuit may be used to secure a sample for culture. Some spillage of content is inevitable as the trocar is retracted. A grasper through the lateral port seizes the fundus, ideally closing the perforation as well, though closure is inessential, and regrasping elsewhere to provide optimal retraction and exposure of dissection is far more important. Upward retraction of the fundus now facilitates separation of the remaining adhesions and exposure of the infundibulum. The relationship of the pylorus and duodenum are assessed; a fistula to the duodenum may be encountered and must be recognized and repaired.

The next step is to grasp the infundibulum, where all too often an impacted stone renders this plan impossible. If the stone can be milked back into the gallbladder, the problem is solved. Otherwise, grasp the body of the organ above the stone; to attempt to grasp below it is unsafe until dissection confirms the safety of the common duct. Open the peritoneum over the leading edge of the gallbladder where its junction with the cystic duct is suspected. With the infundibulum pushed medially, continue in the subperitoneal plane posteriorly first, staying well up on the gallbladder wall, proceeding as far toward the fundus as possible. This opening is then deepened, gently spreading with the dissector and taking small bites of edematous connective tissue with the hook cautery. This is the first step in achieving a "critical view of safety" [11]. The dissection is carried anteriorly on the gallbladder, skirting above the enlarged cystic duct lymph node, and superficial to the hidden cystic artery. Again, peritoneum and subjacent connective tissue are divided as far toward the fundus as practical without frequent changes of grasping position.

The cystic duct and artery are commonly inapparent, concealed by edema and an enlarged cystic duct node. As gently as possible, peritoneum, fat and connective tissue is teased and swept away from the front and back of the gallbladder hilum; forceful grasping or cautery of tissue is avoided until duct and artery are brought into view. Often, the critical maneuver is the mobilization of the enlarged and inflamed cystic duct node. Having opened the peritoneum above the node, it is dissected from the gallbladder surface and gradually rolled downwards in the direction of the hepatoduodenal ligament. In this way, small bleeders can be cauterized with less risk, and dissection a plane too deep is more likely to open the gallbladder than the common duct. The field is hyperemic; some oozing is inevitable. The node can often be teased downward with the tip of the suction-irrigator, simultaneously maintaining adequate visualization with a combination of suction and hydro-dissection. Usually the discrete vascular pedicle of the node will be identified and, once dissected, can be cauterized and divided. The node may be excised and removed, or merely swept further downward.

This maneuver will generally expose portions of the cystic duct and artery, as well as the medial edge of the gallbladder infundibulum. While this identification of cystic duct will usually prove correct, the careful surgeon will now say aloud words to the effect of "This could well be the common duct" and assume that it is so until proven otherwise. The space between the cystic duct, artery, and gallbladder is now gently enlarged, both from the front and the back, by a combination of delicate spreading with the dissector, and a nuzzling action with the blunt tip of the suction-irrigator. Dissection in this space is always directed first toward the gallbladder. Often a frenulum of connective tissue binds anteriorly the proximal cystic duct to the gallbladder. When this tissue is isolated and divided with several fine applications of the hook cautery, the cystic duct straightens and further separates from the cystic artery.

As the surrounding connective tissue is swept away, the putative cystic duct and artery (which may branch into anterior and posterior branches) come into clearer view. Their identification is not final, however, until the gallbladder itself has been fully separated from the liver well up toward the fundus. The goal is to assure that the common or right hepatic duct or artery does not remain fused to the gallbladder, perhaps misidentified as the cystic duct or artery. Having achieved this "critical view of safety," the cystic duct and artery are controlled and divided. Cholangiography is performed selectively at this point to investigate the possibility of common duct stones, to resolve uncertain biliary anatomy, or to confirm the safety, or otherwise, of the common bile duct.

Dissection of the remaining portion of the gallbladder from the liver may proceed smoothly in the "cholecystectomy plane," which is superficial to the cystic plate of the gallbladder bed. The right hepatic duct or its tributaries, and the middle hepatic vein, or its tributaries, may lie immediately deep to the cystic plate. Aggressive attempts to remove the entire wall of the gallbladder will often penetrate deep to the cystic plate, especially if the operation is conducted after more than several days of acute inflammation, or if previous attacks have already fused the back wall of the viscus to the liver. At this point the operation becomes much easier and safer, and every bit as therapeutic, if a decision is made to leave the whole remaining back wall of the gallbladder in situ attached to the liver. The gallbladder usually has already been opened deliberately for the purpose of decompression. The remaining mucosa, if there is any still viable, may be cauterized, though the value of doing so is uncertain. The gallbladder is simply opened again near the liver, and its wall divided circumferentially using hook cautery or even a harmonic scalpel or other energy device. Gallstones that spilled are sought and extracted or placed along with the gallbladder in a retrieval bag inserted via the umbilical port. The operative field is generously irrigated and suctioned to remove debris and minimize residual contamination. A closed suction drain may be used if desired, exteriorized via one of the lateral port sites.

The indications to convert to an open operation are the same as for elective cholecystectomy, and arise somewhat more frequently. The patient should be well informed ahead of time that laparoscopic cholecystectomy may prove impossible, and that conversion to an open cholecystectomy is a very real possibility, executed solely for the protection of the patient's safety. The surgeon must never regard the decision to convert to an open operation as a complication or defeat, a failure of nerve, or an awkwardness of any other nature. Instead, it is a mature, conservative move that safeguards the patient's safety. Remember also that while the surgeon may feel a sense of exasperation for having spent time, material, and effort in the laparoscopic attempt, the remainder of the operating room team will feel only relief!

Technique of Open Cholecystectomy

The technique described applies equally to a deliberately open or a laparoscopic converted to open cholecystectomy. In either case, it is understood that the operation is inherently difficult (hence the open operation). Assistance must be adequate, and exposure optimal. An upper midline incision is used for a patient with a particularly narrow costal angle. Otherwise, a right upper quadrant oblique transverse incision provides both good exposure and a durable closure. A true subcostal "Kocher" incision is popular and adequate, but it invariably transects two intercostal nerves, weakening the muscle below the incision. A somewhat flatter, "sabre-slash" incision will require more forceful retraction but spares one of the two intercostal nerves. Either incision should divide the linea alba medially, and the round and falciform ligaments, to ensure adequate exposure. When converting a laparoscopic operation to open, the port sites are incorporated into the incision only if the exposure is not compromised by doing so.

After separating adhesions to the gallbladder, a mechanical retractor such as a Bookwalter retractor is attached to the table frame. Four retracting blades are used; moist lap pads beneath the retractor blades protect the underlying viscera and add a degree of friction, which minimizes slippage. A broad, deep blade retracts the hepatic flexure of the colon and its mesentery inferiorly. A narrower, flexible blade is adjusted to retract the duodenum inferomedially, putting the hepatoduodenal ligament on a slight stretch. A medium blade retracts segment four of the liver superiorly. The final blade elevates the costal margin superiorly, at least to begin. The value of good, stable exposure is so important that periodically during the operation, the retraction is adjusted, sometimes seemingly with obsessive concern. Occasionally, one or two moist packs are inserted over the liver to bring the gallbladder out from under the costal margin. The foramen of Winslow is explored with an index finger to prepare for a possible Pringle maneuver in case the cystic artery escapes control. A protective moist lap pad (all laps are moist) is placed in Morrison's pouch to absorb spilled gallbladder content. Then, through an untied purse-string suture in the fundus, the gallbladder is suctioned empty after a sample is taken for culture, and the suture tied (Fig. 20.4). The stones within the gallbladder are now palpable, including usually the troublemaker stuck in the infundibulum.

Open cholecystectomy is performed in a "fundus first" or top down sequence. The idea is similar to the concept of the "critical view of safety" applied to laparoscopic cholecystectomy. The cystic duct and artery are not divided until the gallbladder is attached only by those structures, and this performance ought to avoid inadvertent common duct injury. The theory is only as good as its execution. In a fundus-first cholecystectomy, the plane between gallbladder wall and liver (cystic plate) must be visualized and dissected with small gentle strokes, tissue not divided until it can be seen through. A clamp placed on the fundus aids retraction away from the liver. As the organ is separated, oozing of blood is inevitable. The tissue is hyperemic, and the cystic artery has not yet been tied. An assistant experienced with suctioning becomes truly invaluable. Once the gallbladder is about halfway detached from the liver, the retractor assigned to the costal margin is moved (replaced if necessary) to retract over a folded lap the bared gallbladder bed of the liver. This helps significantly with hemostasis; if possible, the retractor should elevate the liver, bringing the hilum of the gallbladder closer to the operator.

Now dissection continues to separate gallbladder from liver, and as the gallbladder becomes more mobile, anterior retraction permits separation of adhesive and developmental attachments between the infundibulum and duodenum. The top-down sequence brings the cystic artery into the field before the duct. The peritoneum overlying the artery is divided, permitting an adequate length to be freed. To ensure ultimate safety, the artery is ligated in continuity, using two ties on the proximal end, one tie on the gallbladder end, then dividing close to the gallbladder tie with a scalpel.

Now the cystic duct elongates and is cleared safely. A tie is secured on the gallbladder side of the duct and left long, not so much to prevent spillage from the gallbladder but to provide gentle traction for what follows. A decision will already have been made regarding the need for a cholangiogram.

Fig. 20.4 Aspiration of acutely distended and inflamed gallbladder (acute cholecystitis), an early step in open cholecystectomy

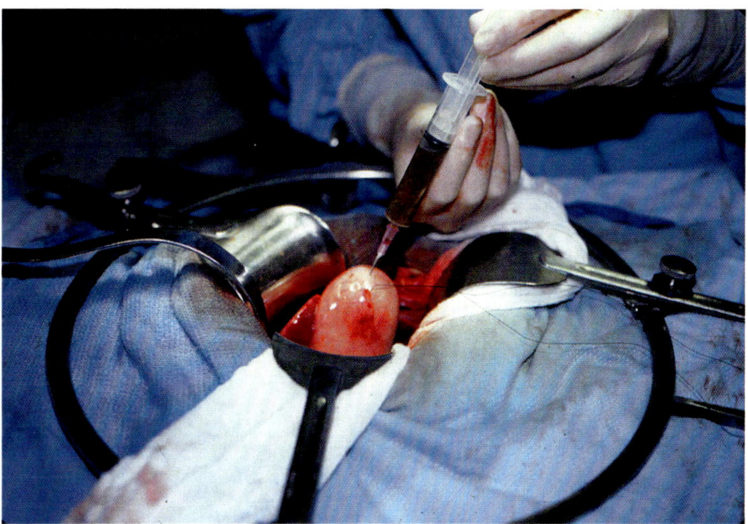

The cystic duct is partially opened (a knife carrying a number 11 blade does a good job of this). The duct is milked backward, as small stones may be lodged therein and these must be removed. If retrograde flow of bile emanates from the ductotomy, the duct is cannulated or secured. If no bile is seen, the cause is probably another small stone lodged more distally. The cystic duct is carefully mobilized in the direction of the common duct, stopping often to feel for the suspected stone. The duct can be opened longitudinally as the mobilization progresses, so long as enough intact duct is preserved for a safe closure. Once the duct has been cleared of stones, it may be closed with a tie or suture, or a cholangiogram may now be obtained.

Solid fusion of the gallbladder to the liver is discovered early in the operation and compels a strategic change to subtotal cholecystectomy. The gallbladder is opened widely and gallstones extracted. The wall is divided with cautery, or an energy device, close to the liver, downward toward the infundibulum, leaving the back wall safely attached. As the infundibulum is approached, the final stones are removed, including any distally impacted stone. Almost always, at this point, the cholecystectomy plane between gallbladder and cystic plate can be safely entered, and cautiously extended transversely behind the back wall, using a gently curved clamp. With the clamp as a guide, the back wall is transected, and the cut edge of the infundibular end grasped with one or two Allis forceps. Traction on these clamps permits cautious, safe dissection of the cystic duct and artery, allowing the operation to proceed as described previously.

Only very rarely is the final mobilization of the cystic duct and artery deemed too hazardous to proceed. Ideally, all stones can be removed, as suggested by the appearance of fresh bile within the infundibulum. Then, the gallbladder remnant may be simply sutured closed, or the duct orifice may be oversewn from within the open remnant. Another good option is to cannulate the cystic and thence the common duct with a 5–8 French sterile plastic tube provided with several side-holes (a sterile pediatric feeding tube serves this purpose). The tube is secured by one or two rapidly dissolved sutures (e.g., catgut) and the cystic duct or infundibulum closed as neatly as possible around the tube, which is then exteriorized across the abdominal wall and ultimately will be attached to a drainage bag, just like a T-tube. This intubation has several purposes. An intraoperative or postoperative cholangiogram can easily be obtained. An obstructed bile duct is decompressed, awaiting postoperative endoscopic clearance. And an insecure closure of the gallbladder or duct lumen is protected by temporary internal drainage of the bile duct. A closed suction drain is left in Morrison's pouch. The transcystic biliary tube is removed after about 3 weeks in the outpatient setting, following a satisfactory cholangiogram.

Percutaneous Cholecystostomy

Cholecystectomy may be the treatment of choice for acute calculus cholecystitis, but some patients are at least initially too sick to undergo a general anesthetic, pneumoperitoneum, or an operation of any sort. The reason may be an acute cardiac condition, pulmonary insufficiency, advanced malignancy, or any other constellation of comorbidities mitigating against operation. In addition, some otherwise healthy enough patients present with a 5- or 6-day history of unremitting pain, a tender right upper quadrant mass, and imaging confirming an advanced pericholecystic phlegmon. Here too, a direct operative assault may be unwise. Historically, operative tube cholecystostomy, performed through a small incision under local anesthesia, was required to salvage such patients. Now, fortunately, cholecystostomy is routinely accomplished using a percutaneous technique. The catheter usually traverses the liver substance to avoid risk of intraperitoneal bile spillage, but the transperitoneal route conversely avoids the rare complication of hemobilia, and works as well. A self-retaining pigtail catheter is left within the gallbladder lumen, a specimen of content collected for culture, and the catheter attached to a drainage bag.

Accompanied by antibiotics and resuscitative measures, percutaneous cholecystostomy is very effective at relieving the symptoms and the associated sepsis attributed to cholecystitis [12]. Output from the tube, after the initial drainage, is at first scant, since the cystic duct or infundibulum is obstructed. Over time, the obstruction may resolve, heralded by the onset of drainage containing bile. Contrast radiography via the tube can then be used to evaluate the gallbladder (not usually necessary) and the biliary tree if indicated.

One advantage of open tube cholecystostomy was the possibility that the gallbladder could sometimes be emptied of gallstones. In that case, the tube could be simply removed after a few weeks, without immediate recurrence of cholecystitis. Gallstones do eventually reform, and complications of stones might then develop, but patients enjoyed up to several years without renewed gallbladder distress. Percutaneous cholecystostomy, on the other hand, alleviates cholecystitis without eliminating the gallstones. Simply removing the drain after recovery is therefore not a good plan for the long term. Patients with a very short life expectancy, or prohibitive operative risk, may live indefinitely with the drain in place. Percutaneous gallbladder stone extraction, via the dilated matured drain tract, has been achieved, using techniques analogous to renal stone extraction. Most patients will be candidates for elective interval cholecystectomy. This is planned for at least 6 weeks after drainage, in analogy with the earlier protocol for delayed cholecystectomy for acute cholecystitis. There is no rush to operate, however, as the drain protects against recurrent cholecystitis, so patients can be medically optimized at a deliberate pace. Predictably, the cholecystectomy will not be easy. A laparoscopic start is reasonable, but conversion to open will be anticipated. Finally, it causes no harm to leave the percutaneous drain in place until the operation is clearly headed toward inevitable success. Removing the drain while prepping the abdomen constitutes "burning a bridge" that the surgeon may have cause to regret if the operation needs to be hastily concluded.

Mirizzi's Syndrome

When the pathology caused by one or more gallstones impacted in the gallbladder infundibulum or cystic duct extends to involve the adjacent common bile duct, the resulting clinical presentation is termed "Mirizzi's syndrome" in honor of the South American surgeon who characterized these specific coincident complications. In particular the impacted stone(s) and the edema caused thereby can cause bile duct obstruction by external compression. The dominant symptom may be cholecystitis, with concomitant jaundice, or the gallbladder disease may be comparatively quiescent, with jaundice being the principal symptom. The common duct is intrinsically intact, merely compressed. This is Type I Mirizzi's syndrome [13]. If the stone disease smolders long enough without earlier acute presentation, the infundibulum may fuse firmly to the hepatic duct; eventually pressure necrosis due to the impacted stone creates a fistula between these structures, and the true cystic duct is lost within the fistula and dense fibrotic reaction. Although stones may spill into the bile duct via the fistula, the originating impacted stone generally remains in situ in the infundibulum. This is now referred to as Type II Mirizzi's syndrome. Not rarely, a second gallbladder fistula, this one to the duodenum, is also present [14]. Patients with the Type II syndrome may present either acutely, as cholecystitis or cholangitis, or more chronically with biliary type pain and abnormal liver function tests.

A preoperative diagnosis of Mirizzi's syndrome is useful enough to warrant an extended workup when possible [15]. A standard evaluation beginning with ultrasound will confirm the presence of stones with inflammation and should identify biliary ductal obstruction. Because gallbladder cancer or cholangiocarcinoma will be considered in all but the youngest patient, a CT scan has appeal. The bile ducts require visualization, the choice lying between magnetic resonance imaging/magnetic resonance cholangiopancreatography (MRI-MRCP) or endoscopic retrograde cholangiopancreatography (ERCP). The former can substitute for a CT scan while simultaneously ruling in or out luminal filling defects (i.e., stones) in the bile ducts. On the other hand, ERCP can not only diagnose but, with sphincterotomy can generally clear common duct stones. Furthermore, a preoperatively placed endobiliary stent confirms several benefits. Jaundice and associated cholangitis improve. The bile duct is more easily identified within an inflammatory phlegmon if the stent is palpable. Finally, if definitive operative relief of the biliary obstruction for some reason cannot be accomplished, the preexisting endobiliary drain allows for a more graceful retreat.

Traditional open operation is still preferred, though patients with a presumed Type I Mirizzi syndrome may be operated laparoscopically [16]. All of the methods and caveats embraced for acute cholecystitis apply. Early opening of the gallbladder, and removal of the stone(s) not only facilitates the dissection, but an unexpected fistula to the duct must be found early on. At some point after the infundibulum has been mobilized a cholangiogram should be performed, even if preoperative duct imaging suggested simple extrinsic compression.

All but the hardiest laparoscopists will approach a known Type II Mirizzi patient via an open approach. Likewise, if a fistula is discovered laparoscopically, conversion to an open operation is warranted. The strategy is to open the gallbladder and remove all accessible stones. The cholecystocholedochal fistula is seen from within the gallbladder lumen.

An endobiliary stent, if present, is seen and retained. The gallbladder is excised, leaving a cuff of wall around the orifice of the fistula. The common duct may be explored, at least in a limited fashion using a flexible choledochoscope to search for extra stones, and to identify a true stricture (the compression effect will have been relieved by extracting the gallbladder stones). The simplest conclusion of this operation is to insert a T-tube into the duct (through the fistulous opening) and close the cuff of residual gallbladder wall around the exiting limb of the tube with fine absorbable suture [17]. The closure may not be air-tight, but the decompression provided by the T-tube (and stent if present) will limit the bile leak. Closed suction drainage is of course used. If the residual gallbladder cuff defies any semblance of passable closure around the T-tube, the defect is managed by anastomosis to a roux-en-y limb of jejunum. After preparation of the limb in the conventional manner, it is brought, preferably through an opening in the right side of the transverse mesocolon, anterior to the duodenum, to lie on top of the bile duct/gallbladder cuff. Near the closed end of the roux limb, on the antimesenteric side, an opening is made to correspond to the size of the gallbladder cuff. Using fine absorbable interrupted suture, the opened roux limb is anastomosed to the gallbladder cuff. External drainage is provided. The anastomosis, as it heals, will not narrow the lumen of the bile duct. A bile leak will heal, especially with the aid of the endobiliary stent likely already in place.

Gallstone Ileus

The term "gallstone ileus" refers to a mechanical small bowel obstruction of the obturation type, caused by a gallstone within the bowel lumen. The stone usually obstructs near the terminal ileum, where the bowel lumen is narrowest. The stone entered the bowel via a cholecystoduodenal fistula, this caused by chronic pressure necrosis of the stone in the gallbladder, gradually burrowing its way into the duodenum. The gallbladder itself is chronically diseased, scarred and adhered, but not acutely inflamed. Indeed, the spontaneous internal drainage of the gallbladder all but completely prevents acute cholecystitis.[1]

The affected patient is usually elderly, presenting with signs and symptoms of a complete mechanical intestinal obstruction. Plain abdominal films confirm the obstruction, may demonstrate the offending gallstone in the right lower quadrant, and may also subtly display air within the gallbladder and biliary tree. A CT scan is by no means out of order, and will illustrate the plain X-ray findings with greater clarity. Complete resuscitation is accomplished without undue

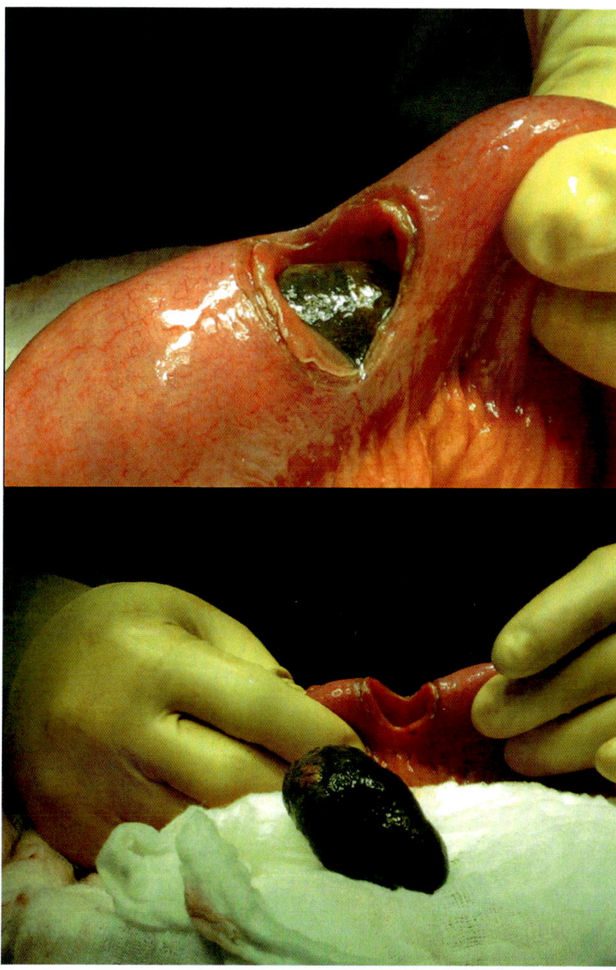

Fig. 20.5 Gallstone ileus (operative photographs). *Top*: Gallstone revealed within distal ileum. *Bottom*: Gallstone extracted via transverse enterotomy

haste. The obstruction is complete and requires operation, but by the same token this mechanism of obstruction poses no risk of strangulation.

The goals of operation are twofold. First, relieve the obstruction by removing the responsible gallstone. Second, search for other stones lurking silently within the lumen of the bowel, and remove them also. The stone(s) are delivered through a short enterotomy (Fig. 20.5). Whether created transversely or lengthwise, the opening is closed in a transverse direction to prevent narrowing of the ileal lumen. Patency of the lumen through to the cecum is confirmed. This operation is so satisfying that the surgeon is now tempted to address the pathology in the right upper quadrant. STOP! The patient is old, maybe frail, and suffering the pathophysiological consequences of a bowel obstruction. The exposure is imperfect. And above all, the next step is no simple cholecystectomy! In other words, immediate corrective biliary surgery is virtually never indicated. Recurrent gallstone ileus occurs, but is rare. The cholecystoduodenal fistula may spontaneously close. In any event, the patient will be in much better condition to tolerate definitive cholecystectomy

---

[1] J.B. Murphy of Chicago developed his mechanical aid to intestinal anastomosis, the "Murphy button," in part to facilitate the operation cholecystoenterostomy for complications of calculus gallbladder disease.

and reconstruction after full recovery from the bowel obstruction and the urgent laparotomy required to correct it.

References

1. Landau O, Watemberg S, Kott I, et al. Gangrenous cholecystitis: seventeen years of experience. Dig Surg. 1995;12:318–20.
2. Shrestha Y, Trottier S. Emphysematous cholecystitis. N Engl J Med. 2007;357(12):1238.
3. Benarroch-Gampel J, Boyd C, Sheffield K, et al. Overuse of CT in patients with complicated gallstone disease. J Am Coll Surg. 2011;213:524–30.
4. Teoh AYB, Chong CN, Wong J, et al. Routine early laparoscopic cholecystectomy for acute cholecystitis after conclusion of a randomized controlled trial. Br J Surg. 2007;94:1128–32.
5. Casillas RA, Yegiyants S, Collins C. Early laparoscopic cholecystectomy is the preferred management of acute cholecystitis. Arch Surg. 2008;143:533–7.
6. Gurusamy K, Samraj K, Gluud C, et al. Meta-analysis of randomized controlled trials on the safety and effectiveness of early versus delayed laparoscopic cholecystectomy for acute cholecystitis. Br J Surg. 2010;97:141–50.
7. Madan AK, Aliabadi-Wahle S, Tesi D, et al. How early is early laparoscopic treatment of acute cholecystitis? Am J Surg. 2003;183:232–6.
8. Banz V, Gsponer T, Candinas D, et al. Population-based analysis of 4113 patients with acute cholecystitis. Ann Surg. 2011;254:964–70.
9. Britt RC, Bouchard C, Weireter LJ, et al. Impact of acute care surgery on biliary disease. J Am Coll Surg. 2010;210:595–601.
10. Strasberg SM. Acute calculous cholecystitis. N Engl J Med. 2008;358:2804–11.
11. Strasberg SM, Brunt LM. Rationale and use of the critical view of safety in laparoscopic cholecystectomy. J Am Coll Surg. 2010;211:132–8.
12. Byrne MF, Suhocki P, Mitchell RM, et al. Percutaneous cholecystostomy in patients with acute cholecystitis: experience of 45 patients at a US referral center. J Am Coll Surg. 2003;197:206–11.
13. McSherry CK, Ferstenberg H, Virshup M. The Mirizzi syndrome: suggested classification and surgical therapy. Surg Gastroenterol. 1982;1:219–25.
14. Beltran MA, Csendes A, Cruces KS. The relationship of Mirizzi syndrome and cholecystoenteric fistula: validation of a modified classification. World J Surg. 2008;32:2237–43.
15. Mithani R, Schwesinger WH, Bingener J, et al. The Mirizzi syndrome: multidiscipliary management promotes optimal outcomes. J Gastrointest Surg. 2008;12:1022–8.
16. Erben Y, Benavente-Chenhalls LA, Donohue JM, et al. Diagnosis and treatment of Mirizzi syndrome: 23-year mayo clinic experience. J Am Coll Surg. 2011;213:114–21.
17. Dewar G, Chung SC, Li AKC. Operative strategy in Mirizzi syndrome. Surg Gynecol Obstet. 1990;171:157–9.

Bile Duct Injury

21

Adnan Alseidi, Abigail Wiebusch, Ryan K. Smith, and W. Scott Helton

Introduction

Among the most challenging patients for surgeons are those with bile duct injuries (BDIs). BDI is associated with substantial morbidity, impaired quality of life, and mortality [1–4]. Morbidity following BDI is reported to be as high as 47% and mortality anywhere from 1.7 to 9% [1, 5, 6]. Morbidity and mortality is related not only to the severity of the BDI and associated bowel injury, but also to delays in management, inadequate management, or complications directly related to failed repair. Failed repairs can result in postoperative peritonitis, biliary sepsis, anastomotic stricture that can result in long-term recurrent cholangitis, biliary cirrhosis, and death. Numerous studies have noted that the level of BDI correlates with surgical outcome, with worse outcomes occurring more frequently in patients with higher levels of BDI [7–9].

Swift recognition of BDIs will decrease the chances of significant early complications such as organ failure, sepsis or death. Preventative measures should always be employed where BDI is a risk. Sound judgment, knowledge and management are necessary to avoid BDI in patients at risk. However, BDI can occur to any surgeon, at any time, in any environment. If and when BDI occurs, successful outcomes require swift recognition and the knowledge of appropriate management pathways.

The acute care surgeon may encounter a patient with BDI through a variety of avenues. They may create a BDI themselves, they may be called to the operating room by a colleague who has made an injury, or they may inherit a patient transferred to their care from an outside facility or through their hospital's emergency room. This chapter provides a guide for the acute care surgeon on how to avoid a BDI, the workup of patients suspected of having a BDI (both intraoperatively and postoperatively), and the management of patients with BDIs (Fig. 21.1a–c). The guiding principles discussed herein are provided while keeping in mind the complexity of the problem as it tends to merge variable patient, surgeon, and setting-specific factors.

Epidemiology and Background

Definitions

BDI is a broad term used to describe a transection of, an excision of, a leak from, or a stricture of the biliary tree. Transection is the division of any duct in the extrahepatic or intrahepatic tree that results in loss of communication between segments of biliary branches. Excisions are identical to transections with the exception of a loss of an indeterminate amount of the bile duct. Both injuries could result, but not necessarily so, in drainage of bile into the peritoneal cavity, i.e., bile leak. Stricture is another problematic injury and does not include bile drainage into the peritoneal cavity; however, biliary communication with ducts downstream of the stricture is prevented or hindered by the narrowing of the afflicted ducts and consequent dilation of the upstream ducts.

The Strasberg Classification System

There are a number of systems that have been used to classify BDIs. Such systems are important for understanding how the injury occurred, for management decisions, and for long-term reporting of outcomes. Of the various methods used to classify BDI, we recommend the Strasberg classification because it provides a reasonable approach to treatment based upon the type of injury [10]. The Strasberg classification organizes BDIs using key features and is used in this chapter to help direct the physician in a predetermined care pathway.

The Strasberg classification categorizes BDI from A through E (see Fig. 21.2, Table 21.1). Type A through D

A. Alseidi, M.D., Ed.M. • A. Wiebusch, M.D. • R.K. Smith, B.A.
Department of Surgery, Virginia Mason Medical Center,
Seattle, WA, USA

W.S. Helton, M.D. (✉)
Department of Surgery, Liver, Pancreas and Bile Duct Surgical Center of Excellence, Virginia Mason Medical Center,
1100 Ninth Avenue, Mail Stop C6-GS, Seattle, WA 98101, USA
e-mail: scott.helton@vmmc.org

L.J. Moore et al. (eds.), *Common Problems in Acute Care Surgery*,
DOI 10.1007/978-1-4614-6123-4_21, © Springer Science+Business Media New York 2013

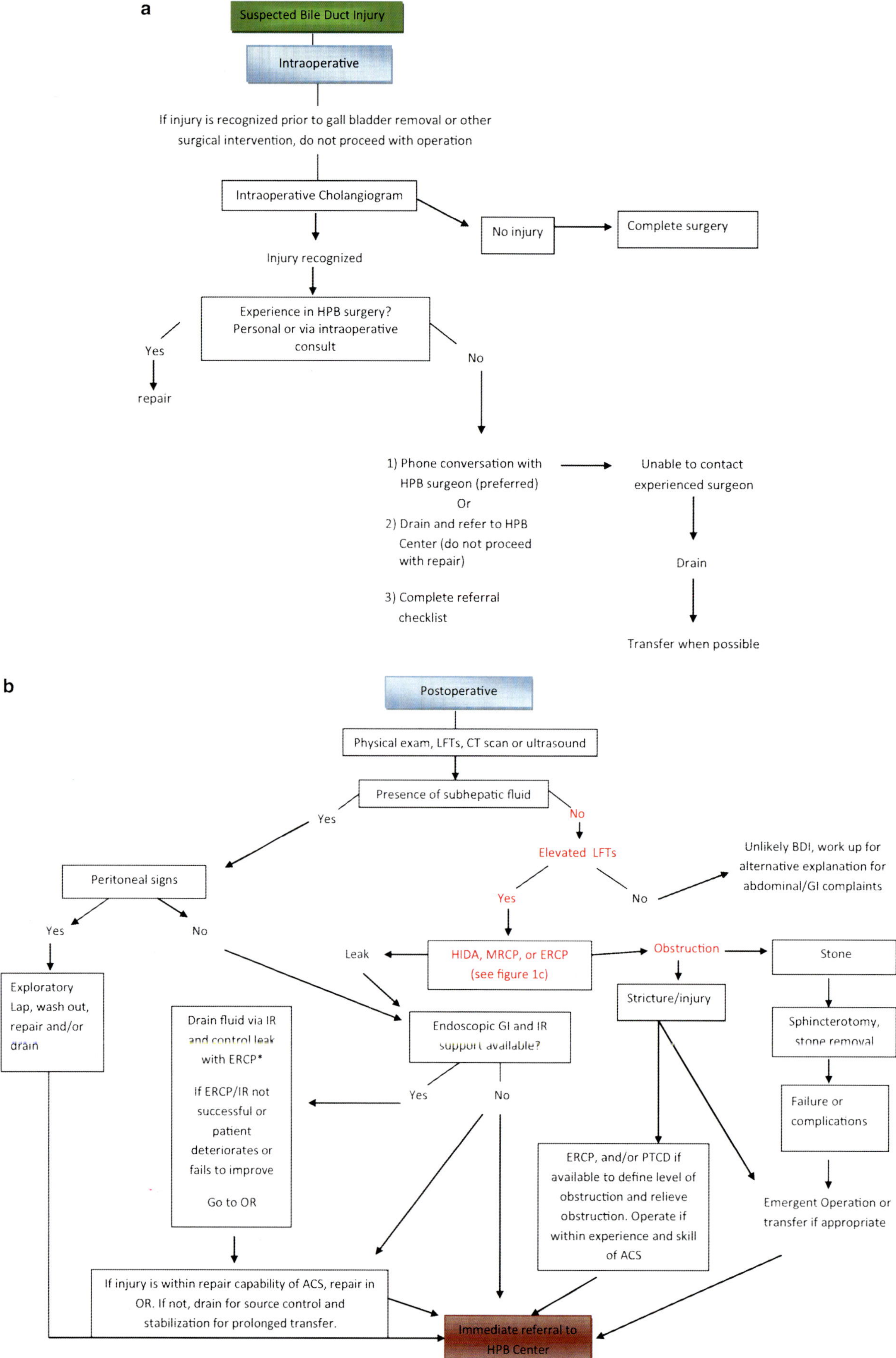

Fig. 21.1 (a–c) Algorithm for management of suspicion of BDI

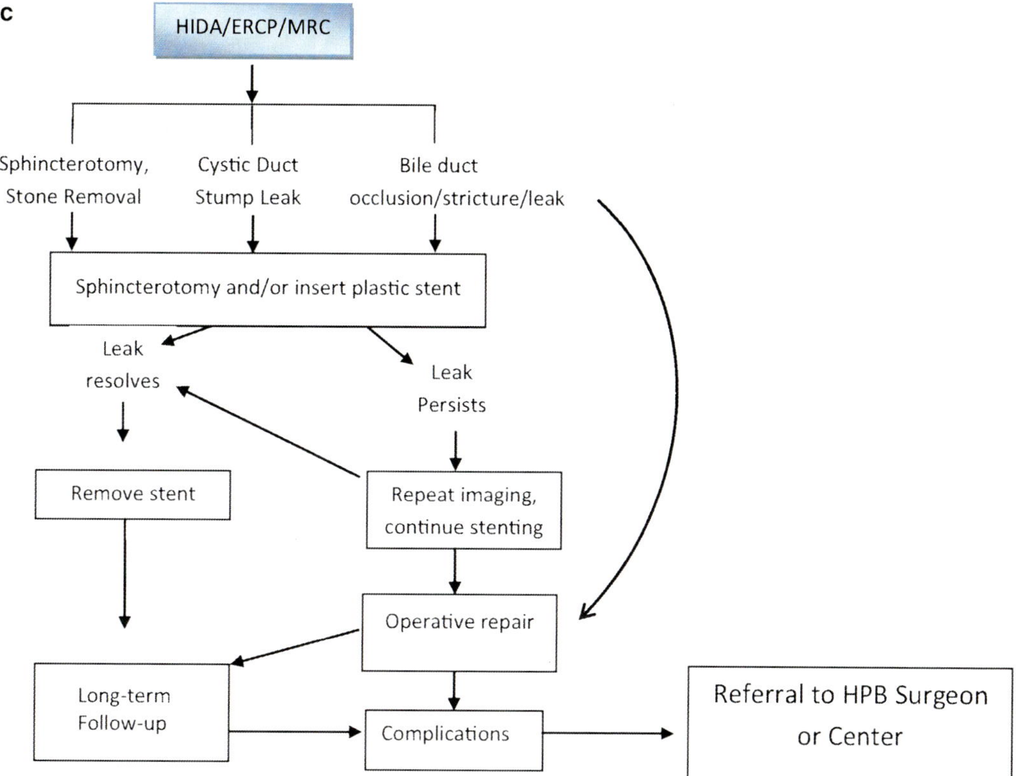

Fig. 21.1 (continued)

injuries categorize leaks, lateral injuries, occlusions and transected minor ducts. The defining characteristic of these injuries is the intact communication between the intrahepatic ducts and the duodenum. However, this communication is lost in type E injuries, which are further subclassified into E_1–E_5. Each of these subcategories is indicative of a loss of direct communication between the intrahepatic ducts and the duodenum. This separation of the liver from the duodenum can be because of duct stenosis, complete occlusion of the duct or because of loss of ductal tissue as a consequence of duct resection. E_2, E_3, and E_4 injuries are the most common type of BDIs that occur during laparoscopic cholecystectomy [10, 11].

Etiology, Incidence, and Pathogenesis

Iatrogenic injury, through operative trauma, is the main cause of BDI, accounting for 96% of all BDIs. Injuries arise through mechanical causes or anatomical misidentification. Mechanical causes of BDI vary from direct injury via inadvertent transection, excision, or clip application, to indirect injury caused by excessive traction or cautery. Anatomical misidentification is commonly associated with mistaking the common bile duct for the cystic duct or an aberrant duct, which has been termed the "classic injury" [12]. Any operation

performed in the right upper quadrant of the abdomen poses a risk for BDI. Operative procedures such as gastrectomy, pancreatectomy, hepatic resection, or exploration of the common bile duct (be it via endoscopic, laparoscopic, interventional transhepatic, or open approach) have been implicated in BDIs. However, the highest risk procedure for operative biliary injury is cholecystectomy, with the laparoscopic approach being the leading cause [13].

Laparoscopic cholecystectomy is known to provide many benefits, namely, less pain postoperatively, earlier return of bowel function, fewer cosmetic defects, shorter length of hospital stay, earlier return to full activity, and decreased overall cost in comparison to open cholecystectomy [14–16]. However, the incidence of BDI has dramatically increased with the adoption of laparoscopy as the method of choice for gallbladder removal. The traditional open approach to cholecystectomy demonstrated a stable 0.16–0.2% rate of BDI [10, 17]. This is in stark contrast to more recent data suggesting the incidence of BDIs resulting from laparoscopic cholecystectomy to be between 0.3 and 0.7% [18]. These injuries, according to two recent studies, are more often complex, Strasberg class E (Table 21.1) [11, 19].

The relative low incidence of BDI during cholecystectomy is magnified by the volume of cholecystectomies performed nationally. In the United States, there are approximately 750,000 cholecystectomies performed every year, making it

Table 21.1 Strasberg classification of bile duct injury

Type of injury	Description	Examples	Presentation	Treatment	
A	Bile leak from a transected minor duct or cystic duct that does not disturb the continuity with the common bile duct	Transected small duct of Luschka from gallbladder fossa or cystic duct leak	1. Pain 2. Fever 3. Sepsis 4. Mild hyperbilirubinemia 5. Biloma or biliary ascites 6. Possible peritonitis	Clip or ligate if operated upon or endoscopic stenting	Maintains continuity between the central biliary tree and duodenum
B	Ligation of aberrant right posterior sector duct or aberrant segment duct VI or VII	Occlusion of aberrant right hepatic duct using a clip	1. Asymptomatic elevation in AST, ALT, and alkaline phosphatase with normal bilirubin 2. Late presentation as pain or segmental cholangitis in obstructed liver segment 3. Liver atrophy of proximal liver segment or right posterior sector 4. Compensatory hypertrophy of left lobe or right anterior	Observation initially	
C	Bile leak from a duct not in communication with the common bile duct	Transection of an aberrant right posterior sector or segment duct	Same as A injury	Ligation, drainage only, or RY hepaticojejunostomy	
D	Lateral injury to major ducts of the extrahepatic biliary tree	Laceration or tear of the CHD, necrosis of lateral bile duct wall from cautery	Same as A injury	Primary repair, T-tube, or RY hepaticojejunostomy	
E1	CHD stricture or occlusion >2 cm below the biliary bifurcation	Resection/ablation with cautery; stenosis above the cystic duct junction with at least 2 cm of CHD before the bifurcation	Obstructive jaundice if total occlusion and no leak. Signs and symptoms similar to Classes A, C, D if leak present from proximal duct(s)	RY hepaticojejunostomy, bilateral hepaticojejunostomy, or right hemihepatectomy with left hepaticojejunostomy if serious vascular injury to R lobe	Disruption between major biliary tree and duodenum
E2	CHD stricture or occlusion within 2 cm of the biliary bifurcation	Resection/ablation with cautery; stenosis above the cystic duct junction with less than 2 cm of CHD before the bifurcation			
E3	Injury to common hepatic duct and biliary confluence with preservation of the back wall	Resection/ablation with cautery; stenosis at the bifurcation of the right and left hepatic ducts resulting in no CHD			
E4	Injury to the confluence including the back wall resulting in the loss of communication between right and left hepatic ducts	Resection/ablation with cautery of the CHD including the bifurcation			
E5	Common hepatic duct and right duct injury	Resection/ablation with cautery of the hepatic duct along with injury to aberrant right duct			

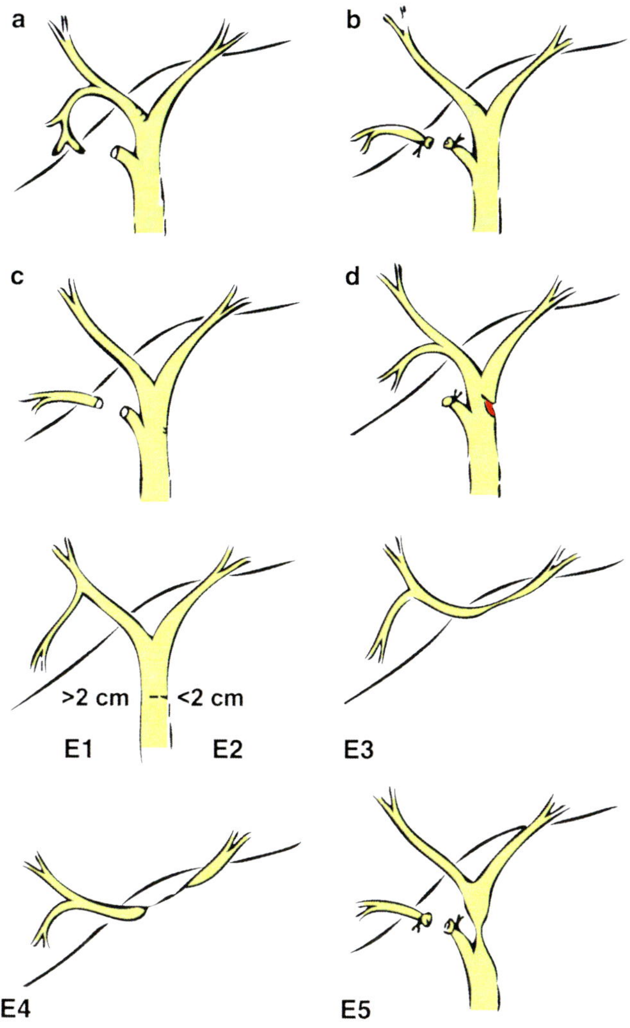

Fig. 21.2 The Strasberg classification system for biliary injury

the most common abdominal operation [18]. This number reflects not only the burden of gallstone disease on the US population, but also the onus on surgeons to recreate a procedure with exceptional high standards and to practice preventive methods to avoid BDIs. Given the high volume of cholecystectomy and incidence of biliary injury, it is estimated that between 2,250 and 5,250 BDIs occur each year.

Prevention and Avoidance

Avoidance of BDIs requires a change in the way a surgeon manages cholecystitis, prior to operating, and how he/she manages a suspicion of BDI, once in the operating room. The latter is discussed later in this chapter. Dr. Steven Strasberg has stressed the importance of "changing the culture of cholecystectomy" as a means to teach surgeons how to reduce BDIs during cholecystectomy [20, 21]. In his article, he encourages surgeons to constantly assess ways to

prevent entering into situations that increase the chance of causing a BDI. An example of such a circumstance is when operating on a severely inflamed gall bladder. In such settings, cholecystostomy tube and antibiotics may be a safer option [22–24]. While retrospective studies have concluded that operating on a severely inflamed gallbladder may be safe, these were uniformly underpowered to assess BDIs and it is the experts' opinion that in such setting BDI is more likely and a surgeon should consider drainage procedures as part of the treatment pathway [20, 21, 25].

Once in the operating room, achieving the critical view of safety, prior to duct or artery transaction, is universally recognized as the safest and most appropriate manner of avoiding BDI during cholecystectomy [10, 26–28]. Unfortunately, the critical view of safety cannot be safely obtained in a large percentage of patients because inflammation, bleeding, or anatomic variations preclude safe dissection at the neck of the gallbladder. When this situation occurs, the ACS should adopt alternative techniques for addressing the gallbladder disease. Such techniques include early cholangiography through the gallbladder, cholecystostomy tube, conversion to open cholecystectomy, fundus first approach, partial cholecystectomy, and asking for assistance from another experienced surgeon [29]. Failure to employ these techniques, and proceed with dissection when there is unclear anatomy or inability to achieve a clear critical view of safety is ill advised and increases the risk of causing a BDI.

Clinical Presentation

Approximately 20–30% of BDIs are appreciated during the index operation [10, 30, 31]. The type of injury and the surgical approach used are factors in predicting early or late recognition. Major injuries to the main bile duct, those classified as types D and E, are identified intraoperatively one quarter to one half of the time [10, 32]. Type A and B injuries, however, being more subtle in nature, are rarely identified during the index operation [10]. The timing of recognition also differs in open versus laparoscopic cases. As may be expected, open cases that result in biliary injury are more likely to be appreciated during the index operation that those than occur during laparoscopic procedures [32].

A BDI should be suspected or placed high on the differential diagnosis of any patient following a recent operation in the right upper quadrant who presents in one of two ways. The first is with elevation of liver function tests. More specifically, total bilirubin and alkaline phosphatase levels will incrementally elevate beyond the patient's normal levels. The second presentation is due to symptoms caused by bilious drainage within the peritoneal cavity. This can result in a biloma or become diffuse in the peritoneal cavity resulting in biliary ascites or bile peritonitis.

Patient Characteristics

Patient demographics tend to mirror that of those that require procedures on or around the biliary tree. A 2005 report compiled patient, institutional, and outcome characteristics from 1991 to 2000 on patients who required reconstruction after sustaining a BDI resulting from laparoscopic cholecystectomy [3]. This series found that about 2/3 of injuries occur in female patients with an age range of 40–75 years old. A common misconception is that most patient with BDI present via the emergency department. The fact is that only about 35% of patients with BDI present through the ER while 61% present in other medical settings (clinics, offices) and a small proportion (2.5%) are transferred from other institutions [3]. Emergency cholecystectomy is associated with a higher rate of BDI (57%) compared to elective surgeries (31.8%). Upon discharge, the majority of patients with BDI (74.9%) are routed home, while 19.6% are transferred to short-term hospitals or skilled nursing facilities [3].

Bile Duct Injury Diagnosis and Patient Management

It is important to note that proper management of BDI starts prior to definitive diagnosis of an injury. Ignoring the suspicion of BDI is in fact often the main cause in patient deterioration, and often, cause for medicolegal complications (see section on "Litigation"). The ACS is advised to treat any deviation in a patient's expected postoperative recovery as a potential BDI until proven otherwise.

Suspicion of BDI can occur intraoperatively (surgeon's intuition, presence of bile, unexpected anatomy of structures) or postoperatively (deviation from normal postoperative recovery pathways). The exact management pathway an ACS follows when such suspicion arises is influenced heavily by several factors: surgeon factors (his/her experience level), setting factors (resources at hand included IR and GI support), and patient factors (patient stability and comorbidity and patient and family wishes). This section and the algorithm presented in Fig. 21.1a–c should help the ACS navigate these variables to achieve a favorable outcome. Any surgeon that is in the position of having to manage BDIs is encouraged to understand these factors and assess their personal ability, their operating room's equipment, their local and regional resources, and their comfort level with managing BDI repair. The surgeon should develop a management plan for addressing BDI that is specific to their situation and ensures the best possible recovery of the patient.

Intraoperative BDI Suspicion

BDI avoidance extends into the operating room before and after suspicion that such an injury had occurred (Fig. 21.1a). Intraoperatively, the avoidance of BDI starts by halting further progression in the operation once a suspicion of BDI exists. Often progression would result in a worst BDI due to the surgeon being in the wrong plane and, in the attempt to reenter into the correct plan, cause biliary or vascular structural injuries. Thus, as soon as a BDI is suspected intraoperatively, the procedure stops and the management of the possible injury begins.

In such a setting, the surgeon is advised to employ methods to better define the anatomy, such as intraoperative cholangiography (IOC) or asking for a second surgeon to scrub in and assist in the assessment and management of the injury. A properly performed IOC that clearly shows all parts of the biliary tree (duodenum, CBD, CHD, CD, right anterior section, right posterior section, and left liver) should reassure the surgeon to proceed with the procedure. An IOC that is not complete, i.e., does not show all parts listed, can easily be misinterpreted and the ACS is advised not to ignore his/her suspicion and utilize techniques to complete the IOC (see section on "Cholangiography") or ask for a second opinion. The ACS may also request radiology to formally read an IOC if there is any doubt in biliary or hepatic anatomy.

If a BDI is demonstrated, then the surgical expertise of the operating surgeon for managing BDI or that of an in house surgeon, dictates the next step in management. It is important to note that BDIs occur across a spectrum and while expertise and skill may exist to manage low BDIs (Strasberg A, D, E_1), high injuries (Strasberg E_2–E_4), posterior sector duct injuries (Strasberg B, C, E_5) [33–35] and/or vasculobiliary injuries [36, 37] require a different set of expertise and hepatobiliary capability that typical does not exist except in specialized hepatobiliary units.

In the event that repair of a particular BDI is beyond the surgeons' or hospital's ability, immediate phone contact with a HPB referral surgeon or center is advised to ensure the best patient outcome. This is best accomplished immediately from the operating room. Again, these referral patterns are best established in advance. If immediate phone conversation is not possible, the surgeon is advised not to proceed and to establish good drainage of the injury, talk to the family and patient, and refer the patient with all documentations, images, and ensure surgeon–surgeon phone conversation in a timely manner. The use of a referral checklist (Table 21.2) is recommended to avoid errors of omission and affect a safe transfer to a higher level of care hospital and HPB surgeon.

Table 21.2 Transfer checklist

- ☐ Communicate with patient and key family members rational and need for transfer
- ☐ Name of receiving physicians and hospital
- ☐ Medical records/chart
- ☐ Key laboratory tests
- ☐ Current medications
- ☐ Brief note on physical/physiologic status
  - ☐ Patient cognition, awareness of situation
  - ☐ Urine output
  - ☐ IV access
  - ☐ Drains—clearly label, secure
  - ☐ Pain control plan
- ☐ All pertinent imaging studies on a disk
- ☐ Operative note
- ☐ Define the biliary injury as understood
  - ☐ Hand drawn figure portraying injury/anatomy and position of drains
  - ☐ Cholangiograms
  - ☐ Send intraoperative digital picture if possible
- ☐ Surgeon to surgeon communication
  - ☐ Before transfer
  - ☐ Follow-up communication plan

If the type of BDI lends itself to immediate intraoperative repair, i.e., absence of a vascular injury and the presence of sufficient surgical expertise, such repair should proceed based on best standards for such injury. In this situation, the surgeon is advised to leave the operating room, if safe, in order to inform the patient's family or whomever has accompanied them to the hospital that an injury has occurred and additional surgery is going to occur in an effort to repair the injury. Immediate disclosure to the patient about the nature of the injury and repair should occur as soon as the patient is awake and alert. Caution is advised in ignoring an injury to the right hepatic artery or an accessory right hepatic artery or in underestimating the level of injury because immediate repair in such setting may result in poor long-term outcomes [5, 38, 39].

Postoperative Suspicion of BDI

The ACS may be confronted with a patient with complications of BDI in the immediate postoperative period or months to years after a previous right upper quadrant operation (Fig. 21.1b). Patients presenting in the immediate postoperative period (e.g., less than 30 days) will usually give a history of never having felt well in the postoperative period and usually show signs of acute illness. The evaluation and management of these patients is discussed in detail below. In contrast, patients who present with a bile duct problem months to years later usually have an insidious onset of symptoms that is related to an underlying bile duct stricture, which manifests itself in the form of abdominal pain, jaundice, and/or

cholangitis. These strictures may be secondary to an unrecognized injury made at the time of operation related to a clip or cautery damage to the bile duct. Alternatively, a bile duct stricture may have evolved following BDI that was addressed in the immediate postoperative period from reoperation, endoscopic or percutaneous management. These patients should be referred to a surgeon and/or endoscopist experienced in the management of biliary strictures. Discussion of these patients is beyond the scope of this chapter and the interested reader can read about the approach [40–42].

As stated previously, suspicion of BDI should occur when any patient undergoing RUQ surgery complains of abdominal problems in the early postoperative period or has an unexpected postoperative course. A prompt and thorough evaluation of these patients to exclude BDI is indicated. This evaluation should include physical examination, laboratory studies (to include liver function tests), and abdominal imaging. While this evaluation is being initiated, the patient should be resuscitated and broad-spectrum antibiotics initiated. An important early step in the evaluation process of a presumed BDI is for the surgeon to determine if the patient has an active bile leak as part of their biliary injury or if they have a ligated or clipped duct without a leak. This is important because if a bile leak exists, surgical site control of the leak becomes the next priority (see later section on "Source control of bile leak"). If a leak does not exist, the management follows a different pathway (Fig. 21.1b).

Abdominal imaging is best achieved by either ultrasound or CT scan. If ultrasound is performed, the sonographer should be asked to interrogate the arterial and portal flow to the right lobe of the liver as well. In many patients ileus, obesity or intestinal gas may prevent clear views of the subhepatic or subdiaphragmatic spaces by ultrasound. For this reason, an abdominal/pelvic CT scan with iv and oral contrast provides the most information because it can identify fluid collections anywhere in the abdomen as well as provide anatomical detailed information about the critical structures in the porta hepatis as well as integrity of arterial and portal blood supply to the liver. However, I.V. contrast should not be given to a patient if they are dehydrated or have an elevated creatinine.

A bile leak will usually lead to diffuse ascites or loculated fluid collections. It is important to note that patients with an active leak with large amounts of bile in their peritoneal cavity may have little to no tenderness while others with a small amount of bile in the peritoneal cavity may have peritoneal irritation. So the absence of peritoneal signs on examination does not exclude a major bile leak and the acute care surgeon should not be lulled into complacency regarding the potential dire consequences of an active bile leak, when a patient does not yet have systemic illness or peritoneal irritation. An active bile leak that is walled off from the peritoneal cavity (usually in the subhepatic or subdiaphragmatic spaces

Table 21.3 Typical presentation scenarios of bile duct injury and the suggested management

Scenario 1

Marked elevation in bilirubin, alkaline phosphatase, AST, ALT

No peritoneal fluid seen on imaging

No peritoneal irritation or abdominal guarding

Additional clips are seen in midline than cannot be explained if just the cystic duct and cystic artery were ligated. Clips positioned along the same vertical axis should be suspected to be on the common bile duct and hepatic ducts

Possibilities: (1) obstruction from stone; (2) clip completely across bile duct (E1, E2) or right and left ducts (E4) with no bile duct transection; (3) complete transection of duct with complete occlusion of proximal biliary system (any E)

Scenario 2

Mild elevation in liver function tests (bilirubin <3, and near normal alkaline phosphatase) with abdominal fluid present

Abdominal tenderness may or may not be present

Possibilities: Strasberg A, D, C or any E if one side of liver is not occluded

Scenario 3

Mild elevation in AST, ALT, bili (<3). Moderate elevation in alkaline phosphatase. No fluid observed on CT. No leak demonstrated by HIDA with intact flow into small bowel. ERCP shows no obstruction or bile leak and is commonly interpreted as normal by endoscopist and radiologist. However, failure to fill a right posterior sector or segment VI or VII ducts is a partially clipped or unclipped transected right posterior sector duct (see Fig. 21.3)

Probable: Strasberg B. Diagnosis confirmed by absence of right posterior sector or segmental ducts on ERCP, differential perfusion of right posterior segments VI or VII or right posterior section on a four phase CT scan, cholangiography filling right posterior sector ducts without filling of common bile duct

Scenario 4

High bile duct injury suspected or observed

Decreased perfusion to the right hemi-liver during the arterial phase of CT, or enhanced perfusion to the right hemi liver during the portal venous phase of CT scan is indirect evidence of right hepatic arterial ligation

Marked elevation in AST, ALT without elevation in bilirubin shortly after operation

Possibility: vasculobiliary injury

(biloma)) often is not accompanied by abdominal tenderness. It is important to also understand that many patients with a biliary leak from BDI can also have partial or complete obstruction of other parts of their biliary tree.

If no fluid collections or ascites is found on CT or ultrasound, and the patient has normal liver function tests, BDI is probably not the cause of the patient's symptoms and physical findings. In such circumstances, alternative causes of the patient's complaints need to be further investigated.

Alternatively, if no fluid collections or ascites are found on CT or ultrasound and the patient is jaundiced, or has elevated liver function tests, then it is presumed that the patient has biliary obstruction (follow red text in Fig. 21.1b). The most common cause of obstruction in the postoperative period would be a retained common bile duct stone, or an inadvertent clipped common or hepatic bile duct. A HIDA scan or ERCP can confirm the presence of obstruction and also exclude with confidence a bile leak. ERCP, if available, is the diagnostic test of choice as it cannot only identify the point of obstruction, but also because it can be therapeutic by relieving obstruction through removal of a stone or placement of a stent across a partially clipped but intact duct.

With an understanding of how BDIs occur, experienced HPB surgeons can usually predict the type of BDI a patient has after reviewing only the operative report, the CT or ultrasound and lab studies, and noting the presence, number and position of clips on abdominal radiographs or CT scan. This knowledge and understanding is also important for the ACS evaluating and managing patients with BDIs because it can alert them to specific types of BDI that they may elect not to explore in favor of early referral. A number of typical scenarios are provided to serve as examples of how various BDIs present in Table 21.3.

Understanding some important physiologic facts can help the ACS properly interpret liver function tests in the setting of BDI. A mild elevation in bilirubin (<3 mg/dl) with otherwise normal LFTs or minimally elevated LFTs can result from bile in the peritoneal cavity. Marked elevation in serum bilirubin and clinical jaundice usually occurs only with complete bile duct obstruction. If one half of the liver is not obstructed, marked jaundice usually does not develop. However, serum alkaline phosphatase will become elevated with obstruction of just a single liver segment.

Once the presence or absence of a fluid collection and biliary obstruction is determined, the ACS needs to use his/her judgment as to the next best course of action depending upon a number of factors: his experience and comfort level of dealing with a BDI, the physiologic condition of the patient, availability of resources, and availability and time necessary for transfer to a tertiary center that can provide multidisciplinary HPB care.

We recommend that patients with diffuse intra-abdominal fluid collections accompanied with physical signs of peritonitis, or systemic toxicity be explored urgently once they are reasonably resuscitated. This is important, even if the ACS is not experienced in surgically correcting BDI for two reasons. First, the goal of exploration is drainage of bile collections, peritoneal toilet and surgical site control of the leaking bile duct(s). This is thoroughly and rapidly accomplished with exploration of the abdomen. Second, abdominal exploration is the best way to identify and treat a hollow viscous injury, which frequently accompanies biliary injury [43] and can be difficult to distinguish from BDI. In fact, a duodenal or small bowel perforation can be misinterpreted as a BDI and these injuries are not effectively managed with percutaneous drainage. In addition, failure to recognize, drain and control a hollow viscus injury in a timely manner (e.g., <24 h) is associated with substantially increased risk for death. Abdominal exploration can be initiated safely via a laparoscopic approach and in fact, is preferred in patients who were initially operated upon laparoscopically. The rational for starting abdominal exploration laparoscopically is in case the patient is found to have a simple cystic duct leak or type D injury that lend themselves to management without laparotomy.

An additional reason for exploring patients laparoscopically is when the ACS chooses to not repair the BDI and only drain it externally. Drainage is easily and rapidly accomplished and spares the patient the morbidity of a laparotomy incision just prior to hospital transfer. If for any reason, effective irrigation and drainage of the peritoneal cavity and a leaking bile duct cannot be accomplished laparoscopically, or if hollow viscus injury not confidently ruled out, the ACS should proceed to general laparotomy. By following this approach, the surgeon eliminates the devastating consequences of a missed bowel injury, rapidly stabilizes the patient by eliminating bile peritonitis and reduces the probability of the patient developing SIRS or organ failure as they are being prepared for transfer to a tertiary care center. If the hospital and acute care surgeon lack the ability to safely perform emergent laparoscopy or laparotomy, immediate contact and transfer to a higher level of care is advised.

While uncommon, a small bile leak can exist without a large fluid collection being detected by imaging. Therefore, if BDI is suspected for any reason, even in the absence of intra-abdominal fluid collections, a HIDA scan, MRCP, or ERCP can be obtained preferably in that order (from least invasive to most invasive) (see Fig. 21.1c). When the preliminary evaluation is normal, the patient should be resuscitated and monitored for at least a day with close follow-up once discharged from hospital.

In the setting of previous cholecystectomy, bile duct obstruction is presumed to be either a common bile duct stone or a ligated or clipped bile duct. If the patient had a non biliary right upper quadrant operation, and presents postoperatively with jaundice and/or subhepatic fluid collections, BDI should be considered as part of the differential diagnosis (Fig. 21.1c).

Source Control of Bile Leak

Once a bile leak is identified or heavily suspected, source control should be attempted emergently, even in stable patients in order to avoid the development of organ failure, SIRS and abdominal sepsis, through percutaneous, endoscopic or even operative drainage. If a patient is systemically ill, shows any signs of peritonitis, presents shortly after surgery (<48 h), or has diffuse ascites, we recommend emergent laparoscopy or laparotomy as opposed to percutaneous drainage. Alternatively, patients who present in a more delayed manner, are hemodynamically stable, have no peritoneal signs, and localized fluid collections, percutaneous drainage is appropriate and usually sufficient for source control of a bile leak.

The inexperienced surgeon should not endeavor to repair any BDI laparoscopically unless it is an easily identified cystic duct leak nor should they dissect in the porta hepatis in an effort to identify an injured bile duct for they could cause further damage and/or bleeding. The principle goal of the acute care surgeon at the time of laparoscopic exploration is to achieve source control of the leak as a means to stabilize the patient. Secondary goals of exploration are to identify the source and nature of the bile leak. If laparoscopy is not possible, or unsuccessful at evacuating blood clots and bile, then a small laparotomy through a right upper quadrant incision should be used to achieve source control and effective drainage.

Once a patient is resuscitated and stable, an effort to classify the type and level of BDI should be performed via ERCP, MRCP, or PTC. This is a critical step in the management of any BDI because bile leakage from a Strasberg class A, B, or C injury may be easily and appropriately managed by the acute care surgeon whereas a higher injury at or above the bifurcation may be beyond the capabilities of the surgeon and/or hospital. Even an experienced HPB surgeon must try to understand the level and complexity of a BDI prior to operation so that an appropriate and safe reconstructive operation can be planned and carried out. If ERCP, MRCP, and/or PTCD are not available and hence the nature and location of the injury cannot be determined preoperatively, the acute care surgeon must decide if the patient is stable for transport to a higher level of care or if emergent damage control laparotomy is warranted as a means of stabilization prior to transport. Source control can almost always be easily achieved no matter what type of injury via good external drainage. The type of BDI encountered coupled with the surgeon's experience and judgment will dictate if the injury can be definitively managed at the time of exploration (e.g., simple cystic duct leak or small laceration of common bile duct) or if definitive repair should be deferred such as Strasberg class E or vasculobiliary injury. Based on the type of injury identified, the center specific pathways should define the best method of management. This may be endoscopic management (i.e., stent), percutaneous or surgical management if expertise and resources allow. Again, patients with a BDI at or above the biliary bifurcation, vasculobiliary injury, or who fail to respond to resuscitation should be immediately transferred to a center where multidisciplinary expertise exists in HPB disease.

Cholangiography

Intraoperative cholangiography is an essential tool in the ACS arsenal, and he/she are advised to know the exact ability of their operating room in advance [18, 44]. The ability to have live fluoroscopy is essential. Further, the ability to replay the fluoroscopy run is very helpful and essential for accurate determination of the presence BDI and level of injury [45]. The surgeon needs to also be comfortable in utilizing techniques that allow for better visualization of proximal ducts. These techniques are often necessary in patients with a history of sphincterotomy where obtaining enough intrabiliary contrast pressure to view intrahepatic ducts can be challenging.

The surgeon should not accept an incomplete cholangiogram as sufficient to alleviate suspicion of BDI. An improperly read cholangiogram, read as normal, in the presence of a BDI is a common phenomenon primarily because the cholangiogram is incomplete. A complete IOC must include visualization of the CBD, CHD, CD, left liver ducts, right anterior and posterior section ducts. It must also show passage of contrast into duodenum. Adjunct techniques to achieve a complete cholangiogram may be needed. These include placing the patient in Trendelenburg position, rotating the patient left or right, clamping the distal bile duct to facilitate proximal filling and using a smaller syringe to obtain higher injection pressure, using a balloon occlusion in the duct (with the ability to inject proximal and distal to the balloon), needle cholangiography via the common bile duct, duct irrigation with saline, and use of sphincter relaxants such as glucagon. Cholangiographic pictures and cine loops obtained intraoperatively are critically important information to transfer to the surgeon who ultimately manages the repair.

If immediate surgical repair is not performed at the time of the index operation, subsequent cholangiography can be performed via the subhepatic drains once they are well walled off from the abdominal cavity or via percutaneous transhepatic drainage catheters (see Fig. 21.3).

Repair Goals

The goals of biliary reconstruction are to provide definitive internal biliary drainage, to ensure long-term anastomotic patency with low chance of stricture and the avoidance of major postoperative complications such as bile leak, sepsis, organ failure and death. To achieve these goals, surgeons repairing BDIs should possess appropriate knowledge about

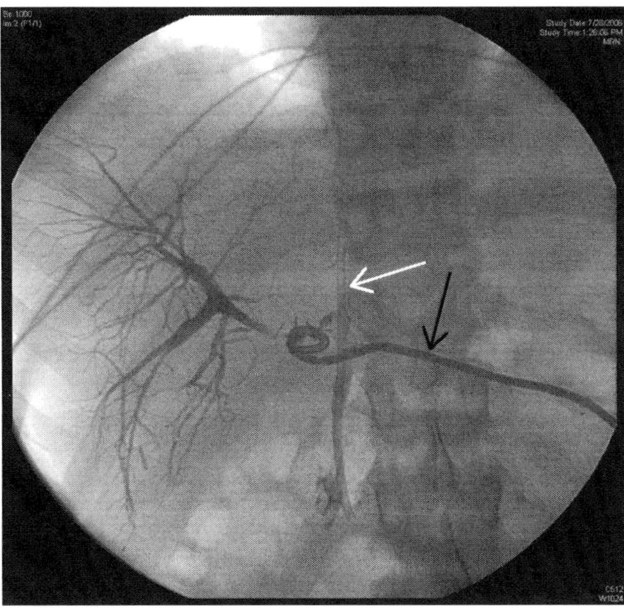

Fig. 21.3 Fluoroscopic image of right posterior section injury demonstrated via percutaneous drainage pigtail catheter (black arrow) cholangiogram. Note: straight endoprosthesis (white arrow) is in common bile duct with no communication with the right posterior sector duct injury

Table 21.4 Conditions for going ahead with bile duct repair

- Physiologically stable
- No systemic or localized infection
- No significant edema of the bile duct or intestine
- Absence of concomitant major vascular injury
- Minimal or well controlled medical comorbidities
- Complete cholangiography of all liver segments obtained

biliary anatomy and injury, exercise solid judgment with respect to the timing of repair, the choice of repair and possess sufficient experience and technical skill in biliary surgery [9, 11, 19, 31, 46, 47]. An ACS who elects not to repair a BDI still plays a pivotal role in achieving the best possible outcome for the patient by timely diagnosis, stabilization through surgical site control, and early referral.

Basic Principles of Bile Duct Injury Repair

There are no set rules in BDI repair. However, there are general principles that a surgeon should follow as a means to achieve the best possible outcomes for the patient with BDI (see Tables 21.4 and 21.5). Optimal clinical outcomes of BDI repair begins with appropriate timing of the repair. The timing of surgical repair must always be individualized and will vary from patient to patient [9, 19, 46, 48]. As discussed earlier, the best possible outcome is achieved if a BDI is recognized at the time it occurs and repaired during the same operation [46, 49]. Unfortunately, for most patients, the BDI is not recognized at the time it occurs and the patient subsequently presents in the postoperative period. When an

Table 21.5 Surgical checklist for considering emergent repair

The following guidelines can serve as a surgical checklist for the surgeon who is faced with the challenge of repairing a bile duct. A yes answer to any of these questions is grounds for not performing repair, delaying repair, or transferring the patient to an experienced surgeon in biliary repair

- Is there systemic or intra-abdominal sepsis?
- Is the patient hemodynamically unstable?
- Is there significant inflammation in the porta hepatis or bowel wall edema?
- Is the level of injury at or above the bifurcation (Strasberg E2 or higher)?
- Is there a right posterior sector duct injury?
- Is there significant thermal injury to the bile duct close to the bifurcation or to any of the sector ducts?
- Are the orifices of the hepatic duct or sector ducts <3 mm?
- Is there evidence of concomitant vascular injury, such as ligation of the right or an accessory right hepatic artery?
- Is the surgeon unable to delineate all liver segments with cholangiography?
- Is the surgeon not able to identify healthy proximal hepatic duct below the bifurcation with good blood supply that is at least 5 mm in diameter?

experienced HPB surgeon is confronted with a patient several days after BDI has occurred, he/she has to evaluate and use their judgment if an early versus a late repair should be performed. There is no high level medical evidence to support one approach over the other though many reports have shown that delayed repair results in excellent outcomes [48]. In fact, it is not realistic to perform a prospective, controlled, randomized trial to solve this question because of the variations in patients' anatomy, inflammatory response, and type of injury. However, some basic criteria for proceeding with immediate repair are offered in Table 21.4 while other criteria for delaying repair are listed in Table 21.5.

Patients satisfying the criteria for early repair (e.g., within 2–4 days of injury) can have excellent long-term outcomes when repaired by experienced HPB surgeons [50, 51]. However, when a patient satisfying these criteria is explored early and found to have significant inflammation of the porta hepatis and/or of their intestines or an unexpected vasculo-biliary injury, long-term results of repair are less satisfactory and postoperative complications are high [36, 39, 52]. Under such circumstances the surgeon must decide to risk repair and accept a high rate of early and late failure or to delay repair, typically for 6 weeks to 3 months. This is a critically important decision that requires keen judgment and experience [2, 8, 31, 41, 47, 48, 51].

If the surgeon decides not to repair a BDI at initial laparotomy, then the right upper quadrant should be adequately drained via transabdominal drains placed in the subhepatic space. Also, when a patient has high biliary transection (e.g., Strasberg E_2–E_4), or very small ducts in whom percutaneous transhepatic catheters have not yet been placed, the orifices

of the transected ducts can be cannulated with small pediatric feeding catheters (usually 5 French) which are secured to the edge of the transected duct and then exteriorized. These catheters can subsequently be used to obtain cholangiograms to help delineate the patient's biliary anatomy and to serve as guides for future biliary reconstruction. Additional subhepatic drainage is always indicated in these patients because even with ductal cannulation and drainage, bile will leak around these catheters into the subhepatic space.

Patients with localized intra-abdominal or systemic sepsis or hemodynamic instability within the first few days of a BDI should not undergo early repair. Management should be centered around and limited to achieving source control thorough external drainage of all collections, as well as controlling sepsis and correcting organ dysfunction. Effective trans abdominal drainage via two large (at least #15 French) soft silastic round closed suction drains is perhaps the most important thing that an ACS can and should ensure as a means of stabilizing the patient should he/she decide to transfer them to a higher level of care. Round drains are preferred over flat drains because they are more easily exchanged over a guide wire and replaced with pigtail catheters should the need arise down the road. One drain is placed in the sub-diaphragmatic space and right colonic gutter and the other in the subhepatic space; both exit posterior laterally through the abdominal wall. Patients rarely become systemically ill when external biliary diversion is managed by transabdominal drains and usually promptly improve. Subhepatic drains, while providing early safe and effective drainage of intra-abdominal biliary leaks should ideally not be kept in place long term because of the risk for eroding into bowel loops and causing biliary-enteric cutaneous fistulae [43]. This however is not something that the acute care surgeon will usually have to deal with but rather rests with the surgeon managing delayed repair.

When complete biliary intestinal disconnection exists as occurs with complete transection or ligation of the hepatic or common bile duct (Strasberg E), external biliary drainage is ultimately best managed via a percutaneous transhepatic biliary drainage (PTCD) tube. Such drains can traverse the opening of the transected biliary tree and even drain the subhepatic space. Complete biliary diversion creates a special physiologic situation that the ACS can play an important role in managing through placing a GJ or feeding jejunostomy tube at the time of initial exploration. This is important for patients who must be repaired in a delayed manner so that bile collected through their PTCD catheters can be fed through a feeding tube into their proximal small bowel. Bile should not be fed through a G tube or placed down a NG tube because it can cause bile gastritis; it must be placed into the duodenum or farther downstream. (See later section on "Postoperative complications for the importance of bile refeeding").

General Operative Principles and Practices

Long-term studies have demonstrated that superior outcomes are obtained when BDIs are repaired by surgeons experienced in HPB surgery [6, 13, 19, 31, 46, 49]. This is particularly true for high biliary injuries (Strasberg E), vasculobiliary injury, or posterior sector duct injuries. These outcomes may be related not only to proper surgical technique but overall better management in a center with experienced interventional radiologists and interventional endoscopists. Timing of repair, quality of repair, and follow-up are all important factors in determining the best long-term outcome. The fact that the majority of BDIs are of the complex variety provides a strong argument that the inexperienced surgeon should defer definitive repair of these injuries in favor of good drainage and early referral to a tertiary care facility. The following principles are considered essential elements of managing BDIs.

- All biloma and intra-abdominal infected collections should be drained and the patient free from recent infection and cholangitis prior to any consideration of elective operative repair of BDI.

- A road map of the biliary tree is very important in surgical planning and should be obtained prior to definitive repair when possible. This may require some combination of imaging and direct cholangiography (e.g., MRCP or injection cholangiography). Cholangiography may also require more than one route to show all bile ducts (via PTCD catheter, subhepatic drain, and/or ERCP). At the time of surgery, all bile duct orifices should be cannulated and cholangiograms obtained. All segmental intrahepatic bile ducts should be demonstrated by cholangiography. Failure to delineate all segments in the liver via cholangiography suggests that an aberrant duct injury is missed.

- Percutaneous transhepatic biliary drainage should be achieved if at all possible prior to operative repair. This not only facilitates cholangiography but can also help guide the surgeon in identifying the common hepatic duct in the setting of significant inflammation and scarring of the biliary tree as well as serve as a stent across the anastomosis should the surgeon desire this.

- High BDIs, Strasberg E_2–E_4 and some Ds, are best managed by creating a side to side anastomosis to the biliary bifurcation carried out onto the left hepatic duct using the approach described by Hepp–Couinaud [40, 41]. This approach always requires elevating the hilar plate at the base of segment IV and sometimes requires a partial resection of segment IV and V in order to expose the anterior aspect of the right and left main hepatic ducts [53]. One must avoid dissection on the cephalad or caudal aspect of the biliary bifurcation as well as preserve its back wall in order to preserve the transverse hilar marginal artery and hilar epicholedochal plexus that provide collateral arterial blood flow from the left hepatic duct across to the right hepatic duct [54]. The Hepp–Couinaud anastomosis or variations of this approach are preferred to anastomoses below the bifurcation because it is made to healthy bile duct without edema with excellent blood supply remote from injury and the size of the anastomosis is large and less likely to become stenotic over time [11, 55]. Surgeons not experienced with this approach should not endeavor to employ this technique in emergent repairs of the bile duct.

- Devitalized bile duct tissue from cautery or crush injury as well as dense scar should be excised to bleeding edges of healthy appearing bile duct [46]. This may lead to a much more proximal site of anastomosis than the actual site of biliary transection or ligation. In so doing, the surgeon must be cognizant of the location of the biliary bifurcation and the take off of all sector ducts as they may have an aberrant point of joining the common hepatic duct below the bifurcation.

- Electrocautery should not be used to control bleeding from the cut edges of the bile duct. Instead, hemostasis from the marginal vessels on the bile duct at the 3 and 9 o'clock anatomical positions should be achieved by using 6-O absorbable sutures.

- Permanent sutures should never be used in the bile duct because they are lithogenic and provide a nidus for chronic inflammation which, in turn, can lead to stricture and biliary stone formation [56]. 4-O to 6-O caliber sutures on fine taper needles (RB1 or RB2) are preferred.

- A tension free anastomosis is most easily accomplished by use of a Roux-en Y jejunal limb that is delivered through a right sided retrocolic window into the subhepatic space. Hepaticoduodenostomy, while possible without tension, is not recommended for high BDIs.

- The use of biliary stents in biliary reconstruction is highly individualized but are not necessary to obtain a high quality anastomosis and do not prevent biliary stricture [11, 57].

- Many groups have shown excellent results in complex injuries by delaying the surgery using temporary stents for percutaneous drainage [48] (see also reference [8]).

- Subhepatic drains should not be left for a long period of time because of the risk of intestinal fistulization. When the condition of the patient requires substantial delay in repair, subhepatic drains should be changed to percutaneous transhepatic drains in order to avoid this complication [43].

Type of Repair

The type of BDI repair that should be performed in any given patient will depend more than anything else upon the nature and extent of the injury [17]. In the section that follows, a general discussion about repair using the Strasberg classification is provided.

Class A Injuries

These injuries are repaired by simple suture ligation or a clip placed on the bile duct side or at the base of the liver side when a small transected duct is identified. Prior to ligating a small bile duct draining from the gall bladder fossa, it is important to identify whether or not it is a small end duct that drains only a small section of segment V deep to the gallbladder bed (these are ducts of Luschka) or if it may represent the orifice of a segment VI, VII or right posterior sector duct [33]. This is accomplished by cannulating the duct with a small pediatric or cholangiocatheter and obtaining a cholangiogram through the duct as well as cholangiography through the hepatic duct. Ducts of Luschka will only penetrate into the liver by a centimeter or so. These can be ligated safely without adverse sequelae.

Class B and C Injuries

These injuries are similarly assessed as class A injuries. If ligation or division of a right posterior sector duct or segment VI or VII segment duct is found in the immediate postoperative period and the patient is not contaminated and the duct is small (<3 mm), it can usually be safely ligated. If on the other hand, a small transected aberrant duct occurs in a patient with obvious abdominal infection, it should not be ligated for fear of causing segmental cholangitis and intrahepatic abscess [47]. These small ducts should also not be treated via construction of a biliary enteric anastomosis because of a high probability of stricture and future cholangitis and abscess in the liver section or sector being drained [33]. Instead, these contaminated small ducts are best initially managed with external drainage because more than 50% of such ducts will stricture down over time (average 56 days) and not cause any problems [34]. For those ducts that fail to close over time, reconstructive surgery or right posterior sectionectomy can be considered. Two recent publications report that nonoperative management of right posterior sector duct injuries provides equivalent long-term outcomes as surgical reconstruction [34, 35]. Hence, a conservative approach should be strongly considered as the first option in patients with type B and C injuries.

Larger right posterior sector ducts (see Fig. 21.3) can be drained into a RY jejunal limb successfully by an experienced HPB surgeon. However, if this anastomosis becomes stenotic over time, it can be difficult to access endoscopically or transhepatically as a means to dilate or drain. Should these efforts fail and the patient develops recurrent infection in the obstructed hepatic segment, segmentectomy or right posterior sectionectomy may be required.

Class D Injuries

If less than 30% of the circumference of the common bile duct or hepatic duct is damaged by sharp laceration or traumatic tear, primary closure alone is safe. Primary closure of lateral injuries is similar to closure of a choledochotomy and should be done with interrupted fine monofilament absorbable sutures using surgical loops. In contrast, a type D injury involving the lateral wall of the right or left hepatic ducts or to a small aberrant right posterior sector duct can be very difficult to repair primarily because of their small size and are subject to early and late complications. The ACS is advised not to attempt to repair these ducts primarily but rather to refer the patient emergently to an expert HPB surgeon. Instead, such lateral injuries should be well drained externally.

Primary repairs of type D injuries of the common and main hepatic duct should be decompressed by some means. This can be through a T-tube placed below the suture closure, by deploying an endobiliary stent that traverses the ampulla or by a transcystic duct catheter that is exteriorized and placed to gravity drainage. We recommend the latter technique so that the advantages of a primary closure without a T-tube can be achieved which are decreased operating time, decreased postoperative and biliary complications, shorter time until return to work, and decreased hospital costs [58–61]. This can be achieved with a 5 or 8 French pediatric feeding catheter whose tip is cut off. The catheter is threaded downstream into the common bile duct and secured to the cystic duct with a double absorbable ligature. It is advisable to leave a subhepatic closed suction drain in these patients in the event there is any additional biliary leakage. After 2 weeks, the pediatric transcystic catheter can be used to obtain cholangiography to ascertain the integrity of the bile duct repair and emptying into the duodenum. If all looks well, then the pediatric and closed suction drains can be discontinued. If the repair is stenotic and/or there is impeded contrast flow into the duodenum, the pediatric catheter is left in place to facilitate ERCP. At that time, a glide wire can be inserted through the pediatric catheter to guarantee that the endoscopist can cannulate the biliary tree, a technique commonly referred to as modified rendezvous. An internal endoscopic stent can then be deployed to bridge the stricture. The advantage of transcystic duct decompression is avoidance of T-tube specific problems such as dislodgment, biliary leak and stricture.

When a type D injury involves more than 30% of the bile duct circumference, primary repair is not advised as it usually will result in a stricture; this is particularly true in small ducts <1 cm. An end to end repair, while easy, is also inadvisable, because blood supply is usually insufficient and results in long-term biliary stricture [46, 50, 62]. In the report by Stewart, every primary end to end repair over a T-tube was unsuccessful in every case in which the duct had been divided [46]. Therefore, RY hepaticojejunostomy is the preferred approach for repairing Class D injuries when there is substantial division of the bile duct wall so long as the bile duct diameter is of sufficient size (>3 mm) [47]. Should the patient's condition not allow for RY hepaticojejunostomy or the surgeon is uncomfortable in performing RY hepaticojejunostomy due to a small size duct, then repair over a T-tube or a pediatric feeding catheter placed into the lumen of the bile duct along with subhepatic drainage and immediate transfer is advisable.

Type E Injuries

E injuries that are below or at the biliary bifurcation without compromise to the left or right hepatic ducts in a patient with good size bile duct (>8 mm) with good blood supply can be safely managed with RY hepaticojejunostomy. This is easily performed by an end of bile duct to side of jejunum. However, as stated previously, the Hepp–Couinaud approach with a side to side anastomosis is preferred and associated with the best long-term results [11, 41, 55, 63]. E_3, E_4, and E_5 injuries may require bilateral hepaticojejunostomy. It is important for the ACS to know that higher BDIs, are frequently associated with right hepatic artery injury or ligation [5, 36, 52]. For this reason, it is strongly recommended that the hepatic arterial anatomy be assessed as part of any major BDI. While this can be accomplished by visceral angiography it is preferably done by thin-collimation CT angiography when available [64]. If an E injury is accompanied by vascular injury, right hemihepatectomy with left hepaticojejunostomy may be necessary [5, 52, 65–67]. This latter operation should not be performed emergently or in the immediate post-injury phase unless absolutely necessary as a life saving maneuver in a patient with hepatic ischemic necrosis and sepsis.

Bile Duct Injury Due to Nonoperative Trauma

Non-iatrogenic Trauma

It is estimated that BDIs resulting from non-iatrogenic trauma account for approximately 4% of overall biliary injuries. Isolated biliary injury without trauma to associated intra-abdominal structures is extremely rare. The vast majority of these injuries are associated with external penetrative trauma to the abdomen and very few from blunt trauma. The management of penetrating or blunt trauma BDI will usually be quite different from the management of operative iatrogenic injury because they are associated with major torso trauma and multiple organ injury. Management of a BDI in the trauma patient will be determined by the nature and extent of the injury, the presence or absence of associated injuries, the physiologic condition of the patient, and experience of the operating surgeon. In critically injured and hemodynamically unstable patients or in those with major blood loss, the principles of damage control laparotomy take precedent over diagnosis and management of the BDI. Control of hemostasis, hollow viscous injury and general resuscitation

are the first priorities in these patients. External drainage via close suction drains in combination with abdominal packing is sufficient for short term management of BDI in unstable patients, whether it is intrahepatic or extrahepatic. More definitive diagnosis and management can be obtained when the patient returns to the operating room for secondary laparotomy. Conversely, in a hemodynamically stable trauma patient without significant other major organ injuries or penetrating injury, in whom non operative management principles are being followed, BDI may not be evident and present late. Abdominal CT scan showing a hematoma in the porta hepatis or fractured liver and obstructive pattern on the liver function tests may suggest a BDI. Peritoneal lavage may also show the presence of bile.

Management principles of external traumatic injury to the bile duct can be grouped according to location of the injury into one of three zones: intrahepatic, extrahepatic, and intrapancreatic.

Intrahepatic Bile Duct Injury

These injuries can be associated with major high grade liver injuries, occurring in response to blunt trauma or high velocity gunshot wounds, in which case, packing and drainage is the principal first line management [68, 69]. While liver resection is necessary in only 2–4% of all patients with major traumatic liver injury, ongoing intrahepatic bile leak is a major reason why liver resection is required in some patients [69]. BDI in patients managed nonoperatively occurs in less than 1% of patients and may present with delayed biliary peritonitis or biloma [70]. T-tubes should not be placed into the extrahepatic bile duct in patients with suspected or proven intrahepatic BDI. The subhepatic and perihepatic space should be drained widely with close suction drains. Postoperative ERCP with transpapillary stenting may help resolve subsequent biliary fistula. Many such injuries may scar down and leave an intrahepatic stricture. Such strictures can be addressed electively in a tertiary center with a multidisciplinary team experienced in hepatopancreaticobiliary disease. Liver resection for acute intrahepatic BDI from trauma is rarely if ever indicated or appropriate. On the other hand, liver resection may be necessary to manage delayed problems or recurrent hepatic abscesses [68].

Extrahepatic Injury

BDIs that occur caudal to the biliary bifurcation and superior to the pancreatic head usually show contusion, edema, fresh clot formation, or active bleeding in the porta hepatis. Management of active bleeding is the first priority and requires exploration of the portal structures after obtaining proximal and distal control. If BDI is found, it can be managed with primary repair, T-tube drainage or RY reconstruction. Primary repair is not recommended for complete transection of the bile duct or if more than 40% of the circumference of the bile duct is divided [71]. T-tube drainage is a conservative, safe repair option if there is only partial disruption of the bile duct wall. But the surgeon must be cautious using a T-tube if the diameter of the bile duct is less than 8 mm. If primary repair with common duct decompression is used by the surgeon as a means of quick surgical source control, they must appreciate that in the long term this type of repair may increase the likelihood of biliary stricture. We recommend that T-tubes be avoided and that transcystic common duct decompression or endobiliary stent decompression be employed when primary repair is performed as it will avoid problems related to T-tubes (see prior section under repair of Strasberg "Class D injuries"). Complete transection of the bile duct or when there is more than 40% disruption of bile duct wall is best managed by RY hepaticojejunostomy or choledochoduodenostomy if the injury is low on the bile duct and the duodenum is non-injured. However, biliary enteric anastomosis is not recommended in any unstable patient or someone with associated other organ injury or if the surgeon is not experienced in biliary reconstruction techniques. This is particularly true if the diameter of the bile duct is less than 8 mm. Definitive repair of these injuries can be accomplished upon return to the operating room when the physiologic state of the patient is improved and inflammation and edema to the proximal biliary tree and bowel is reduced. Since the latter is often unlikely in a critically injured patient with other intra-abdominal organ injury, delayed biliary reconstruction, if possible, will result in a more satisfactory long-term repair, especially when it is performed by an experienced HPB surgeon. This is particularly the case when the level of BDI is high in the porta (type E). Under such circumstances, intubation of the bile duct with a soft silastic tube and/or ample external drainage with closed suction drains followed by percutaneous transhepatic biliary drainage is usually sufficient to tide the patient over for delayed definitive repair.

Intrapancreatic Injury

The most serious BDIs from external trauma are those that occur within the pancreatic head. The retroduodenal region of the superior portion of the pancreas is the most common site of biliary transection following blunt trauma though this is extremely rare. Because injury may be contained within the retroperitoneum, delay in diagnosis is common. If there is hematoma or bile staining around the pancreatic head, the duodenum should be kocherized to facilitate retroperitoneal exploration. Cholecystectomy or cholecystostomy can be rapidly performed and cholangiography performed via the cystic duct or gallbladder to evaluate the distal bile duct. If stricture, occlusion or leakage of the bile duct within the pancreatic head is found, biliary decompression through the gallbladder, cystic duct, or T-tube in that order is recommended unless pancreaticoduodenectomy is performed. When there is active hemorrhage or an expanding hematoma within the pancreatic head, associated with severe duodenal and/or pancreatic parenchymal injury, pancreatoduodenectomy may be necessary [72, 73]. BDI in these patients is addressed as part of the biliary reconstruction that accompanies pancreaticoduodenectomy.

Austere Environments

Surgeons in a remote or isolated setting may find themselves in a circumstance where the patient has a suspected BDI, no interventional radiology support, no gastroenterology support, and the inability to transfer the patient due to lack of immediate resources. In such a setting, appropriate source control and drainage, operatively, is the primary goal. The secondary goal, when safe and feasible is operative repair using the principles discussed earlier. Definitive repair in the presence of wide contamination, severe inflammation, sepsis, or patient instability has rather poor outcomes and should not be contemplated. If the patient is found to have a complete biliary disconnection with total biliary diversion, and is subject for prolonged external drainage (e.g., months) then the ACS should give consideration to bile refeeding. This can be accomplished by placing a feeding jejunostomy tube at the time of laparotomy or via a nasoduodenal feeding tube postoperatively. Once the patient is stable, they can be transferred to a higher level of care.

Potential Complications

Short and long-term complications associated with the treatment of BDIs are not uncommon. Considerable morbidity is experienced in the form of intra-abdominal abscesses, bilomas, biliary fistulae, cholangitis, hemorrhage, and hepatic insufficiency, both pre- and post-reconstruction [1, 5, 6, 74, 75]. Late complications are usually the result of anastomotic strictures and can present many years after biliary-enteric reconstruction [10, 13, 74, 76]. It is important to note that surgically related complications are less frequently encountered in patients whose injury is repaired in a tertiary care hospital or by an experienced HPB surgeon [13, 76]. In fact, several series have reported excellent long-term results in the majority of patients undergoing definitive operative repair at tertiary referral centers [13, 48, 75–77]. Again, this highlights the importance of early recognition of BDI and expeditious referral to a specialized center with hepatobiliary expertise in order to decrease the incidence and impact of further complications.

In order to maintain a heightened awareness of patients at risk for complications, one should recognize those factors which are associated with greater morbidity and mortality. Overall morbidity ranges from 38 to 47% in the literature [2, 78]. Several studies have identified late referral to tertiary medical center as a one of the greatest risk factors for early perioperative complications, including intra-abdominal abscess and prolonged ICU stay, as well as delayed complications, such as anastomotic stricture [76, 79]. Many of these complications are potentially avoidable if earlier surgical site control was achieved prior to transfer to higher levels of care. Hence, the importance of early drainage as discussed under management.

Conditions that influence long-term outcome after hepaticojejunostomy include presence of active peritonitis at the time of repair, concomitant biliary and vascular injury, and the level of injury at or above the biliary bifurcation [2, 46, 49, 74, 76]. Also of significant importance, is whether the operation was performed by the primary injuring surgeon or by an expert at a specialized center, as overall success rates vary from 35% in the former to over 90% in the latter [74]. While morbidity is fairly high, the operative mortality after definitive repair of a BDI is generally very low, with a reported range of 0–9% in several large series [1, 2, 5, 6, 13, 74–77, 79]. Factors affecting mortality include the number of previous operations, a history of severe infection, a high BDI (Strasberg E), low preoperative serum albumin concentration, and the presence of liver disease with portal hypertension [74]. All of these issues should be taken into account in order to minimize the perioperative risks when treating patients with BDIs.

Patients undergoing delayed repair are subject to complications not seen in patients operated upon immediately. These include the development of recurrent fluid collections, the occlusion or dislodgment of temporizing drains or stents [10, 80, 81], cholangitis, organ space or superficial wound infection, biliary-enteric or bilio-cutaneous fistulae, metabolic derangement, and progressive malnutrition. However, these complications rarely require reoperation [80]. Patients need to be followed closely and advised to contact their physician should any fever or new onset abdominal pain or wound problems occur. Rapid assessment by physical examination, lab investigation (CBC and LFTs), CT scan and tube sinograms or cholangiograms usually will identify the problem and guide management. Percutaneous measures by a skilled and experienced interventional radiologists or endoscopists in collaboration with the surgeon usually are successful in managing recurrent abscess, biloma, or cholangitis. The important point to be made is that these patients must be managed very meticulously and promptly in order to get them successfully to reconstructive surgery [10, 80].

Bile Refeeding and Nutritional Support

Patients with complete biliary enteric disconnection are at risk for metabolic derangement and malnutrition because excessive losses of bile can lead to dehydration, metabolic acidosis, progressive loss of protein, and malabsorption. Collection of bile and refeeding it into the small bowel helps prevent dehydration, metabolic derangement, improves the digestion and absorption of fat, and reduces the volume of hepatic bile output through the enterohepatic recirculation of bile salts. Most patients can tolerate bolus infusion of bile into their small bowel of 150 cc or less every 4 h and they can be taught to do this on their own at home. But, if a patient has a feeding jejunostomy or a GJ tube, it is preferable to provide bile refeeding in a continuous manner. Our recipe for doing this is as follows. Bile should be collected over 4 h increments from the PTCD or subhepatic drain (if the latter is clear and not turbid). It is then strained and put into a sterile bag where it is then reinfused with the aid of an infusion roller pump through a separate line that is Y connected to their feeding tube. Bile should not be put into a feeding tube bag, allowed to sit stagnant in a drainage bag for longer than 4 h nor sit in a bag for infusion at room temperature for longer than 4 h in order to avoid significant bacterial overgrowth. This approach minimizes intestinal intolerance to bile infusions and minimizes bacterial overgrowth.

Malnourished patients with complete biliary disconnection and external biliary fistula may require specialized semi elemental diets to avoid fat malabsorption. Diets rich in medium chain triglycerides which do not require bile salt micelles for absorption are preferred over diets containing long chain triglycerides. These patients are also at risk for fat soluble vitamin deficiency and should be offered water soluble forms of vitamin E, A, D and K either orally or through a feeding tube.

The overall success rate of biliary reconstruction after BDI, when carried out in a specialized center, is greater than 90% [13, 74, 75, 77, 78]. In cases when a primary repair has failed early, it is not always necessary to perform a surgical revision [10]. Occasionally, the problem is simply a bile leak from an adequate anastomosis, or a slightly stenotic anastomosis [10]. Most significant leaks are evidenced by bilious drainage from intra-operatively placed drains or visualized as extravasation during postoperative cholangiography [78]. These are often successfully managed by the placement of percutaneous transhepatic stents, reserving reoperation for failure of these procedures [10, 13, 77, 78]. In fact, the same nonoperative interventions are predominantly utilized in late failures as well. These failures typically present months to years after the initial operation as recurrent cholangitis, jaundice, or pruritus, or on laboratory evaluation by rising alkaline phosphatase or liver transaminases [78, 82]. All of these findings should raise suspicion of an anastomotic stricture [78]. Often times, patients have been on repeated courses of antibiotics for recurrent cholangitis before the diagnosis is made and the stricture is identified [78]. Advanced biliary cirrhosis may result from delayed diagnosis and management of a biliary stricture [2, 78]. Two-thirds of restenoses are diagnosed in the first 2 years after repair but restenosis has been described after 10 years time [10, 74, 76]. The restenosis rate varies from 5 to 28% both in choledochoduodenostomy and hepaticojejunostomy, with the majority of strictures amenable to percutaneous or endoscopic balloon dilation [31, 76]. Only a small percentage of patients with stenotic biliary enteric anastomotic strictures require reoperation for resolution [76].

Follow-up

Pre-repair

Patients in the pre-repair phase of BDI require vigilant observation with prompt intervention to control bile leakage and peritoneal contamination while they await definitive repair. Obviously, unstable or septic patients need aggressive resuscitation with broad-spectrum antimicrobial therapy and urgent radiologic investigations for any un-drained biloma or abscess. Properly placed transhepatic biliary drains should be able to control bile leakage; however, supplemental percutaneous drains may be necessary to control large abdominal bile collections [48]. Laparotomy may be required when hemorrhage is suspected, when adequate bile drainage cannot be obtained percutaneously, in the setting of peritonitis or when radiologic support is unavailable [48]. Once patients are stabilized and adequate drainage achieved, biliary ductal anatomy should be elucidated, as this is a critical component of the workup and allows operative planning to commence [47, 48, 74]. This can be accomplished by reconciling the anatomy through a combination of CT scans and cholangiograms, often via the percutaneous transhepatic approach, or even retrograde through subhepatic drains [48]. During the period between presentation and delayed repair, patients should be seen at regular intervals [48]. Subhepatic drains are often removed in the interim, so as to avoid intestinal fistulae [48]. At any sign of infection, cholangitis, or sudden change in bile drainage, manifesting as fever, leukocytosis, abdominal pain, or elevated liver enzymes, rapid workup for abscess, biloma, or occluded biliary drains should be undertaken. Bile should be cultured to target appropriate antimicrobials to specific organisms. Clinical and laboratory exams should be routine to maximize therapy while the acute inflammation resolves so that successful reconstruction can occur in an elective fashion.

Post-repair

Long-term follow-up is necessary to fully evaluate the results of biliary reconstruction for BDIs [75]. Restenosis of a biliary enteric anastomosis can manifest many years following operative repair. In fact, up to 10 years has been described, although the majority of patients are symptomatic within 2 years [75]. All patients who have had a repair of a BDI should have regular and frequent follow-up (q 3 months), particularly in the early postoperative period. This includes clinical evaluation, inquiring about symptoms of fever, jaundice, or pruritus, laboratory values, including monitoring of liver function tests, and radiologic studies [77, 80]. Before operatively placed drains and stents are removed, a cholangiogram should be performed to evaluate the anastomosis [10, 80]. Over the long term, once the stents have been removed, MRC, PTC, or ERC may have to be obtained if anastomotic stricture is suspected by features of biliary obstruction [77]. However, on routine laboratory monitoring, stricture is most commonly heralded by a rising alkaline phosphatase [80, 82]. As many patients have a low level elevation at baseline, the more concerning feature is a consistent upward trend [80]. However, it is not uncommon for the alkaline phosphatase to remain mildly elevated for the first year after biliary reconstruction [82]. Recurrent anastomotic stricture on MRC is best managed by proceeding to PTC and ERC which can define the anatomy further as well as allow for interventions in the form of balloon dilation and or stenting [77, 80]. If the patient was reconstructed with a hepaticojejunostomy then all interventions are likely achieved by percutaneous transhepatic route, though double balloon enteroscopy with ERCP is also possible in expert hands [83]. Endoscopic retrograde access is safely utilized in patients with hepaticoduodenostomies [78, 80]. Surgical revision and hepatic resection are reserved for refractory cases, although in most large series, this is a rare necessity [2, 10, 13, 74–76, 78, 80, 81, 84]. Progression to biliary cirrhosis leading to liver failure, intrahepatic abscesses and need for liver transplantation while rare, occurs in patients who have recurrent or inadequately treated biliary stricture as well as those who had vasculobiliary injury [85].

Litigation

Litigation is common after BDI during cholecystectomy and the majority of such cases that go to trial are decided in favor of the patient [30, 86–88]. Factors identified that were more likely to lead to litigation include treatment failures by nonspecialists in immediately recognized injuries, complications as a result of delay in diagnosis, misinterpretation of cholangiogram, and vasculobiliary injury [30, 86]. The acute care surgeon can play a pivotal role in preventing undesirable litigation by the patient against the operating surgeon by following some basic practices. The three most important factors in preventing litigation are the following: prevention of serious injury, timely recognition of injury, and prompt and appropriate care once injury is recognized. Severity of injury can be

Table 21.6 Intraoperative checklist

- Explore all quadrants of abdomen and run entire small bowel and colon
- Evacuate all clots, biloma
- Irrigate, wash out
- Define hepatic arterial anatomy by palpation and Doppler
- Identify any non ligated major end blood vessels
- Doppler liver to listen for intrahepatic portal and arterial signals
- Is there evidence of liver disease? If so, perform core needle biopsy
- Culture bile
- Identify and tag all bile duct orifices
- Perform cholangiography and define all liver segments under fluoroscopy
- Record size of common bile duct, hepatic duct, any segmental ducts
- Record level of bile duct injury and define using Strasberg Class
- Record presence and location of clips
- If transected common bile duct, identify and ligate distal duct in suprapancreatic location
- Observe and record if evidence of cautery injury
- Take digital picture of injury if possible using videoscope or cell phone and include in record and send to receiving surgeon

minimized by performing routine cholangiography and correct interpretation of cholangiograms [18, 44, 45, 89]. Intraoperative identification of injury is important because immediate repair by an experienced surgeon is the best management strategy, and hence the importance of intraoperative consultation or immediate referral to an expert center (Table 21.6). In the absence of such expertise, the acute care surgeon can often avoid or minimize the risk for future litigation by doing the right thing in the OR. This includes calling another colleague to the OR, consulting with a surgeon experienced in BDI, and then either appropriately repairing the injury or preparing the patient for safe transfer. Postoperative timely recognition of injury is another important practice that can avoid litigation. The basic concept here is to have an extremely low threshold for suspecting injury. Any patient who calls the office with unexpected complaints or returns to the emergency department in the immediate postoperative period with abdominal complaints, or abnormal LFTs should be considered to have a BDI until proven otherwise. Such patients should be seen by the surgeon or their covering physician and followed up closely; admission to hospital and/or quick workup to rule out injury is indicated.

Timely, honest and clear communication with the patient and their family about all aspects of a biliary injury is another important practice to reduce the risk of litigation [21]. If the acute care surgeon performed the operation in which biliary injury occurred, preoperative clear and detailed communication about risks and nature of BDIs is a critically important preventive step. If the acute care surgeon is the recipient of a

transfer from another facility then communication with the referring physician(s) about all aspects of the patient's condition and injury is critically important. Clear and accurate documentation in the medical record that is timed and dated of all notes as well as discussions with referring physicians, patients and their family will help in the successful defense of a litigated case. The surgeon needs to be honest and forthright about the nature of the injury and its severity and what this portends with respect to management; the situation should not be "sugar coated." The surgeon should discuss what he or she learned from the referring surgeon about what was done in the operating room to either repair the injury or to stabilize the patient in the event the injury was not repaired (e.g., placement of a drain) in preparation for safer more experienced repair by transfer to a higher level of care. If the ACS is of the opinion that the patient should be transferred to another facility for any number of reasons (e.g., ERCP, PTC, and/or surgical expertise), those reasons should be explained to the patient and their family. In the event a transfer is going to occur, the name of the accepting surgeon should be given to the patient and all of their medical records should be forwarded. The need for additional workup, diagnostic testing, and consultation should be carefully discussed and documented. The surgeon should demonstrate remorse and apologize for the injury and express concern for the patient's safety and recovery. Finally, the surgeon should manifest an extra effort to make him or herself available for all questions and concerns that the patient or their designated family members have.

In contrast to the practices and behaviors discussed previously, a surgeon creating a BDI will invite litigation by "washing their hands of the patient's care after the injury" by referring them to a gastroenterologist or other physician without first clearly communicating the nature of the injury, by being an ineffective communicator, by acting aloof and not admitting that they made a mistake and lack of concern for the patient's well-being. Failure of the original surgeon to offer his or her care to the patient long term when they return to their community can be perceived by the patient and their family as an act of abandonment and also invite litigation. Poor medical record documentation, poor patient communication, lack of timely attention to patient complaints and failure to refer patients in a timely manner or reoperate in a timely manner to gain source control resulting in adverse outcomes are practices that weaken defense in court.

References

1. Flum DR, Cheadle A, Prela C, Dellinger EP, Chan L. Bile duct injury during cholecystectomy and survival in medicare beneficiaries. JAMA. 2003;290(16):2168–73.
2. Walsh RM, Henderson JM, Vogt DP, Brown N. Long-term outcome of biliary reconstruction for bile duct injuries from laparoscopic cholecystectomies. Surgery. 2007;142(4):450–6.

3. Dolan JP, Diggs BS, Sheppard BC, Hunter JG. Ten-year trend in the national volume of bile duct injuries requiring operative repair. Surg Endosc. 2005;19(7):967–73.

4. Melton GB, Lillemoe KD, Cameron JL, Sauter PA, Coleman J, Yeo CJ. Major bile duct injuries associated with laparoscopic cholecystectomy: effect of surgical repair on quality of life. Ann Surg. 2002;235(6):888–95.

5. Buell JF, Cronin DC, Funaki B, et al. Devastating and fatal complications associated with combined vascular and bile duct injuries during cholecystectomy. Arch Surg. 2002;137(6):703–8.

6. Sicklick JK, Camp MS, Lillemoe KD, et al. Surgical management of bile duct injuries sustained during laparoscopic cholecystectomy: perioperative results in 200 patients. Ann Surg. 2005;241(5):786–92.

7. Johnson SR, Koehler A, Pennington LK, Hanto DW. Long-term results of surgical repair of bile duct injuries following laparoscopic cholecystectomy. Surgery. 2000;128(4):668–77.

8. Mercado MA, Chan C, Orozco H, et al. Prognostic implications of preserved bile duct confluence after iatrogenic injury. Hepatogastroenterology. 2005;52(61):40–4.

9. Mercado MA. Early versus late repair of bile duct injuries. Surg Endosc. 2006;20(11):1644–7.

10. Strasberg SM, Hertl M, Soper NJ. An analysis of the problem of biliary injury during laparoscopic cholecystectomy. J Am Coll Surg. 1995;180(1):101–25.

11. Winslow ER, Fialkowski EA, Linehan DC, Hawkins WG, Picus DD, Strasberg SM. "Sideways": results of repair of biliary injuries using a policy of side-to-side hepatico-jejunostomy. Ann Surg. 2009;249(3):426–34.

12. Davidoff AM, Pappas TN, Murray EA, et al. Mechanisms of major biliary injury during laparoscopic cholecystectomy. Ann Surg. 1992;215(3):196–202.

13. Lillemoe KD, Melton GB, Cameron JL, et al. Postoperative bile duct strictures: management and outcome in the 1990s. Ann Surg. 2000;232(3):430–41.

14. Barkun JS, Barkun AN, Sampalis JS, et al. Randomised controlled trial of laparoscopic versus mini cholecystectomy. The McGill Gallstone Treatment Group. Lancet. 1992;340(8828):1116–9.

15. Bass EB, Pitt HA, Lillemoe KD. Cost-effectiveness of laparoscopic cholecystectomy versus open cholecystectomy. Am J Surg. 1993;165(4):466–71.

16. Soper NJ, Barteau JA, Clayman RV, Ashley SW, Dunnegan DL. Comparison of early postoperative results for laparoscopic versus standard open cholecystectomy. Surg Gynecol Obstet. 1992;174(2):114–8.

17. Adamsen S, Hansen OH, Funch-Jensen P, Schulze S, Stage JG, Wara P. Bile duct injury during laparoscopic cholecystectomy: a prospective nationwide series. J Am Coll Surg. 1997;184(6):571–8.

18. Flum DR, Dellinger EP, Cheadle A, Chan L, Koepsell T. Intraoperative cholangiography and risk of common bile duct injury during cholecystectomy. JAMA. 2003;289(13):1639–44.

19. Perera MT, Silva MA, Hegab B, et al. Specialist early and immediate repair of post-laparoscopic cholecystectomy bile duct injuries is associated with an improved long-term outcome. Ann Surg. 2011;253(3):553–60.

20. Strasberg SM. Biliary injury in laparoscopic surgery: part 1. Processes used in determination of standard of care in misidentification injuries. J Am Coll Surg. 2005;201(4):598–603.

21. Strasberg SM. Biliary injury in laparoscopic surgery: part 2. Changing the culture of cholecystectomy. J Am Coll Surg. 2005;201(4):604–11.

22. Berber E, Engle KL, String A, et al. Selective use of tube cholecystostomy with interval laparoscopic cholecystectomy in acute cholecystitis. Arch Surg. 2000;135(3):341–6.

23. Borzellino G, de Manzoni G, Ricci F, Castaldini G, Guglielmi A, Cordiano C. Emergency cholecystostomy and subsequent cholecystectomy for acute gallstone cholecystitis in the elderly. Br J Surg. 1999;86(12):1521–5.

24. Byrne MF, Suhocki P, Mitchell RM, et al. Percutaneous cholecystostomy in patients with acute cholecystitis: experience of 45 patients at a US referral center. J Am Coll Surg. 2003;197(2):206–11.

25. Halpin V, Gupta A. Acute cholecystitis. Clin Evid (Online) 2011;pii:0411.

26. SAGES Guidelines for the Clinical Application of Laparoscopic Biliiary Tract Surgery. 2012. http://www.sages.org/publication/id/06/

27. Yegiyants S, Collins JC. Operative strategy can reduce the incidence of major bile duct injury in laparoscopic cholecystectomy. Am Surg. 2008;74(10):985–7.

28. Avgerinos C, Kelgiorgi D, Touloumis Z, Baltatzi L, Dervenis C. One thousand laparoscopic cholecystectomies in a single surgical unit using the "critical view of safety" technique. J Gastrointest Surg. 2009;13(3):498–503.

29. Strasberg SM. Biliary injury in laparoscopic surgery: part 2. Changing the culture of cholecystectomy. J Am Coll Surg. 2005;201(4):604–11.

30. Carroll BJ, Birth M, Phillips EH. Common bile duct injuries during laparoscopic cholecystectomy that result in litigation. Surg Endosc. 1998;12(4):310–3.

31. Lillemoe KD. Current management of bile duct injury. Br J Surg. 2008;95(4):403–5.

32. Russell JC, Walsh SJ, Mattie AS, Lynch JT. Bile duct injuries, 1989–1993. A statewide experience. Connecticut Laparoscopic Cholecystectomy Registry. Arch Surg. 1996;131(4):382–8.

33. Lillemoe KD, Petrofski JA, Choti MA, Venbrux AC, Cameron JL. Isolated right segmental hepatic duct injury: a diagnostic and therapeutic challenge. J Gastrointest Surg. 2000;4(2):168–77.

34. Perera MT, Monaco A, Silva MA, et al. Laparoscopic posterior sectoral bile duct injury: the emerging role of nonoperative management with improved long-term results after delayed diagnosis. Surg Endosc. 2011;25(8):2684–91.

35. Mazer LM, Tapper EB, Sarmiento JM. Non-operative management of right posterior sectoral duct injury following laparoscopic cholecystectomy. J Gastrointest Surg. 2011;15(7):1237–42.

36. Strasberg SM, Helton WS. An analytical review of vasculobiliary injury in laparoscopic and open cholecystectomy. HPB (Oxford). 2011;13(1):1–14.

37. Pulitano C, Parks RW, Ireland H, Wigmore SJ, Garden OJ. Impact of concomitant arterial injury on the outcome of laparoscopic bile duct injury. Am J Surg. 2011;201(2):238–44.

38. Strasberg SM. Error traps and vasculo-biliary injury in laparoscopic and open cholecystectomy. J Hepatobiliary Pancreat Surg. 2008;15(3):284–92.

39. Koffron A, Ferrario M, Parsons W, Nemcek A, Saker M, Abecassis M. Failed primary management of iatrogenic biliary injury: incidence and significance of concomitant hepatic arterial disruption. Surgery. 2001;130(4):722–8.

40. Hepp J. Hepaticojejunostomy using the left biliary trunk for iatrogenic biliary lesions: the French connection. World J Surg. 1985;9(3):507–11.

41. Mercado MA, Chan C, Orozco H, Tielve M, Hinojosa CA. Acute bile duct injury. The need for a high repair. Surg Endosc. 2003;17(9):1351–5.

42. Jarnagin W, Blumgart LH. Blumgart's surgery of the liver, pancreas and biliary tract. 5th ed. Philadelphia, PA: Elsevier Saunders; 2012.

43. Mercado MA, Chan C, Orozco H, et al. Iatrogenic intestinal injury concomitant to iatrogenic bile duct injury: the second component. Curr Surg. 2004;61(4):380–5.

44. Fletcher DR, Hobbs MS, Tan P, et al. Complications of cholecystectomy: risks of the laparoscopic approach and protective effects of operative cholangiography: a population-based study. Ann Surg. 1999;229(4):449–57.

45. Carroll BJ, Friedman RL, Liberman MA, Phillips EH. Routine cholangiography reduces sequelae of common bile duct injuries. Surg Endosc. 1996;10(12):1194–7.

46. Stewart L, Way LW. Bile duct injuries during laparoscopic cholecystectomy. Factors that influence the results of treatment. Arch Surg. 1995;130(10):1123–8.

47. Chapman WC, Abecassis M, Jarnagin W, Mulvihill S, Strasberg SM. Bile duct injuries 12 years after the introduction of laparoscopic cholecystectomy. J Gastrointest Surg. 2003;7(3):412–6.

48. Strasberg SM, Picus DD, Drebin JA. Results of a new strategy for reconstruction of biliary injuries having an isolated right-sided component. J Gastrointest Surg. 2001;5(3):266–74.

49. Stewart L, Way LW. Laparoscopic bile duct injuries: timing of surgical repair does not influence success rate. A multivariate analysis of factors influencing surgical outcomes. HPB (Oxford). 2009;11(6):516–22.

50. Wudel Jr LJ, Wright JK, Pinson CW, et al. Bile duct injury following laparoscopic cholecystectomy: a cause for continued concern. Am Surg. 2001;67(6):557–63.

51. Mercado MA, Franssen B, Dominguez I, et al. Transition from a low: to a high-volume centre for bile duct repair: changes in technique and improved outcome. HPB (Oxford). 2011;13(11):767–73.

52. Stewart L, Robinson TN, Lee CM, Liu K, Whang K, Way LW. Right hepatic artery injury associated with laparoscopic bile duct injury: incidence, mechanism, and consequences. J Gastrointest Surg. 2004;8(5):523–30.

53. Blumgart LH. Hilar and intrahepatic biliary enteric anastomosis. Surg Clin North Am. 1994;74(4):845–63.

54. Gunji H, Cho A, Tohma T, et al. The blood supply of the hilar bile duct and its relationship to the communicating arcade located between the right and left hepatic arteries. Am J Surg. 2006;192(3):276–80.

55. Jarnagin WR, Blumgart LH. Operative repair of bile duct injuries involving the hepatic duct confluence. Arch Surg. 1999;134(7):769–75.

56. Verbesey JE, Birkett DH. Common bile duct exploration for choledocholithiasis. Surg Clin North Am. 2008;88(6):1315–28. ix.

57. Mercado MA, Chan C, Orozco H, et al. To stent or not to stent bilioenteric anastomosis after iatrogenic injury: a dilemma not answered? Arch Surg. 2002;137(1):60–3.

58. Gurusamy KS, Samraj K. Primary closure versus T-tube drainage after laparoscopic common bile duct stone exploration. Cochrane Database Syst Rev 2007;(1):CD005641.

59. Leida Z, Ping B, Shuguang W, Yu H. A randomized comparison of primary closure and T-tube drainage of the common bile duct after laparoscopic choledochotomy. Surg Endosc. 2008;22(7):1595–600.

60. Zhu QD, Tao CL, Zhou MT, Yu ZP, Shi HQ, Zhang QY. Primary closure versus T-tube drainage after common bile duct exploration for choledocholithiasis. Langenbecks Arch Surg. 2011;396(1):53–62.

61. Jameel M, Darmas B, Baker AL. Trend towards primary closure following laparoscopic exploration of the common bile duct. Ann R Coll Surg Engl. 2008;90(1):29–35.

62. Csendes A, Diaz JC, Burdiles P, Maluenda F. Late results of immediate primary end to end repair in accidental section of the common bile duct. Surg Gynecol Obstet. 1989;168(2):125–30.

63. Mercado MA, Orozco H, de la Garza L, Lopez-Martinez LM, Contreras A, Guillen-Navarro E. Biliary duct injury: partial segment IV resection for intrahepatic reconstruction of biliary lesions. Arch Surg. 1999;134(9):1008–10.

64. Keleman AM, Imagawa DK, Findeiss L, et al. Associated vascular injury in patients with bile duct injury during cholecystectomy. Am Surg. 2011;77(10):1330–3.

65. Heinrich S, Seifert H, Krahenbuhl L, Fellbaum C, Lorenz M. Right hemihepatectomy for bile duct injury following laparoscopic cholecystectomy. Surg Endosc. 2003;17(9):1494–5.

66. Thomson BN, Parks RW, Madhavan KK, Garden OJ. Liver resection and transplantation in the management of iatrogenic biliary injury. World J Surg. 2007;31(12):2363–9.

67. Mercado MA, Sanchez N, Urencio M. Major hepatectomy for the treatment of complex bile duct injury. Ann Surg. 2009;249(3):542–3.

68. Parks RW, Chrysos E, Diamond T. Management of liver trauma. Br J Surg. 1999;86(9):1121–35.

69. Polanco P, Leon S, Pineda J, et al. Hepatic resection in the management of complex injury to the liver. J Trauma. 2008;65(6):1264–9.

70. Parks NA, Davis JW, Forman D, Lemaster D. Observation for nonoperative management of blunt liver injuries: how long is long enough? J Trauma. 2011;70(3):626–9.

71. Rodriguez-Montes JA, Rojo E, Martin LG. Complications following repair of extrahepatic bile duct injuries after blunt abdominal trauma. World J Surg. 2001;25(10):1313–6.

72. Krige JE, Beningfield SJ, Nicol AJ, Navsaria P. The management of complex pancreatic injuries. S Afr J Surg. 2005;43(3):92–102.

73. Asensio JA, Petrone P, Roldan G, Kuncir E, Demetriades D. Pancreaticoduodenectomy: a rare procedure for the management of complex pancreaticoduodenal injuries. J Am Coll Surg. 2003;197(6):937–42.

74. Machado NO. Biliary complications postlaparoscopic cholecystectomy: mechanism, preventive measures, and approach to management: a review. Diagn Ther Endosc. 2011;2011:967017.

75. Ahrendt SA, Pitt HA. Surgical therapy of iatrogenic lesions of biliary tract. World J Surg. 2001;25(10):1360–5.

76. de Reuver PR, Grossmann I, Busch OR, Obertop H, van Gulik TM, Gouma DJ. Referral pattern and timing of repair are risk factors for complications after reconstructive surgery for bile duct injury. Ann Surg. 2007;245(5):763–70.

77. Pottakkat B, Vijayahari R, Prakash A, et al. Incidence, pattern and management of bile duct injuries during cholecystectomy: experience from a single center. Dig Surg. 2010;27(5):375–9.

78. Hall JG, Pappas TN. Current management of biliary strictures. J Gastrointest Surg. 2004;8(8):1098–110.

79. Fischer CP, Fahy BN, Aloia TA, Bass BL, Gaber AO, Ghobrial RM. Timing of referral impacts surgical outcomes in patients undergoing repair of bile duct injuries. HPB (Oxford). 2009;11(1):32–7.

80. Haney JC, Pappas TM. Management of common bile duct injuries. Oper Tech Gen Surg. 2008;9:175–84.

81. Woods MS, Traverso LW, Kozarek RA, et al. Characteristics of biliary tract complications during laparoscopic cholecystectomy: a multi-institutional study. Am J Surg. 1994;167(1):27–33.

82. Fialkowski EA, Winslow ER, Scott MG, Hawkins WG, Linehan DC, Strasberg SM. Establishing "normal" values for liver function tests after reconstruction of biliary injuries. J Am Coll Surg. 2008;207(5):705–9.

83. Raithel M, Naegel A, Dormann H, et al. Modern enteroscopic interventions and characterization of nonmalignant postsurgical biliary anastomosis by double-balloon endoscopy. Surg Endosc. 2011;25(8):2526–35.

84. Nuzzo G, Giuliante F, Giovannini I, et al. Advantages of multidisciplinary management of bile duct injuries occurring during cholecystectomy. Am J Surg. 2008;195(6):763–9.

85. de Santibañes E, Ardiles V, Gadano A, Palavecino M, Pekolj J, Ciardullo M. Liver transplantation: the last measure in the treatment of bile duct injuries. World J Surg. 2008;32(8):1714–21.

86. Perera MT, Silva MA, Shah AJ, et al. Risk factors for litigation following major transectional bile duct injury sustained at laparoscopic cholecystectomy. World J Surg. 2010;34(11):2635–41.

87. Kern KA. Malpractice litigation involving laparoscopic cholecystectomy. Cost, cause, and consequences. Arch Surg. 1997;132(4):392–7.

88. Kern KA. Medicolegal analysis of bile duct injury during open cholecystectomy and abdominal surgery. Am J Surg. 1994;168(3):217–22.

89. Fletcher DR. Biliary injury at laparoscopic cholecystectomy: recognition and prevention. Aust N Z J Surg. 1993;63(9):673–7.

Edie Chan and Marc Mesleh

Introduction

There are two types of liver abscesses that may necessitate surgical intervention: pyogenic and amoebic. This chapter reviews the epidemiology, clinical presentation, diagnosis, and management of these diseases and gives a brief overview of echinococcal cysts.

Pyogenic

Epidemiology

Pyogenic abscesses are bacterial in origin and are caused by either direct extension into the liver from the abdominal cavity, via the bile ducts, via the portal vein, hematogenously via the hepatic artery, or direct trauma. In the early twentieth century, appendicitis was the most frequent cause of hepatic abscess [1]. However, with the advent of antibiotics, biliary disease, whether benign or malignant, became the most common source of pyogenic abscesses. A recent case review by Huang et al. spanning 42 years at a single institution identified biliary malignancy to be the most common cause in the latter period of the study [2].

The incidence of pyogenic liver abscesses appears to vary depending on the geographic region. In the United States, a recent population based study calculated an annual incidence of 3.6 cases per 100,000 people, whereas population based reports in other countries have varied from 1 to 17.6 per 100,000 people [3]. More recent studies have also shown an increasing slight male preponderance for the disease that was not seen in earlier published studies and it is more often seen in patients older than 50 years of age [1, 3–5]. The incidence of hepatic abscesses appears to be increasing and this may be attributable to the use of newer immunosuppressive drugs, the increase in immunocompromised patients, the more frequent use of indwelling biliary stents, and the use of hepatic artery embolization. Other risk factors include diabetes, immunocompromised state (human immunodeficiency virus [HIV], liver transplantation), intravenous drug abuse, and biliary malignancies [6].

Clinical Presentation

The majority of patients (~90%) present with fever as their first clinical sign. Approximately half of the patients will also present with chills. Other symptoms include jaundice, right upper quadrant pain, anorexia, weight loss, hepatomegaly, and weakness. The most common laboratory abnormalities include an elevated WBC (white blood cell count), hypoalbuminemia, anemia, and prolonged prothrombin time. Many patients will also demonstrate abnormal liver function tests including total bilirubin, alkaline phosphatase, aspartate aminotransferase, and alanine aminotransferase. However, these changes may not be present if the patient has an indwelling biliary stent.

Abscess cultures are positive approximately 2/3 of the time, whereas blood cultures are positive approximately only 60% of the time. The most common organisms isolated are gram-negative aerobes with *Klebsiella pneumoniae*, *Escherichia coli*, and *Pseudomonas aeruginosa* being the most commonly isolated organisms. *Streptococcus* is the most common gram-positive aerobe isolated and usually indicates a biliary source. Anaerobes are isolated 10–30% of the time and include *Bacteroides* and *Clostridium*. Approximately half of the patients will demonstrate a single isolate; however, multiple organisms are cultured approximately 33% of the time. Patients who are blood culture positive have concordant cultures with the abscess only 50–60% of the time [2, 5].

E. Chan, M.D. (✉) • M. Mesleh, M.D.
Department of Surgery, Rush University Medical Center,
1725 W. Harrison Street, Suite 161, Chicago, IL 60612, USA
e-mail: ediechan@hotmail.com

L.J. Moore et al. (eds.), *Common Problems in Acute Care Surgery*,
DOI 10.1007/978-1-4614-6123-4_22, © Springer Science+Business Media New York 2013

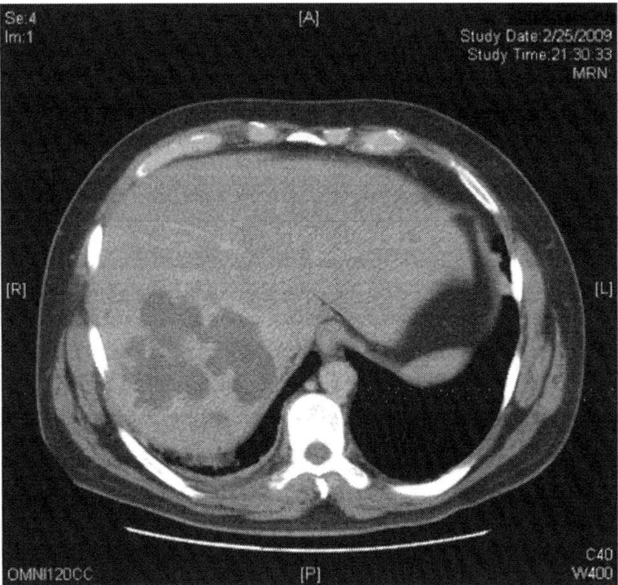

Fig. 22.1 A 52-year-old Mexican male who presented with RUQ pain and jaundice with pyogenic abscess

Diagnosis

Approximately half of the patients will have an abnormal chest X-ray (CXR). Typical findings include an elevated right hemidiaphragm, a right pleural effusion, or gas or fluid collection below the diaphragm. An ultrasound of the liver is often obtained. Although it is less expensive, faster, and no radiation side effects, it is often operator-dependent and not able to determine the location of smaller lesions especially near the diaphragm. The diagnostic test of choice is a computed tomography (CT) scan. It can differentiate small abscesses from small cysts, determine the presence of air within the abscess, and clearly delineate multiple loculations as well as multiple separate abscesses. On CT, hepatic abscesses have a lower attenuation than normal liver parenchyma and the abscess wall demonstrates enhancement on a contrast enhanced CT (Fig. 22.1). Hepatic abscesses more commonly occur in the right lobe, followed by the left lobe, and less frequently bilateral. Most recent reports have noted that liver abscesses also tend to be solitary now compared to multiple abscesses. This may reflect the changes associated with indwelling biliary stents, hepatic artery embolizations, and malignancies [2, 5].

Treatment

The initial treatment of any patient suspected of having a possible liver abscess is initiation of broad spectrum antibiotics. The development of broad spectrum single agents (imipenim, piperacillen/tazobactam) has replaced the traditional treatment of the combination of ampicillin, aminoglycoside, and an anaerobic drug such as metronidazole [7]. The duration of antibiotic use remains debatable, and is usually based on treatment response and the abscess characteristics.

Percutaneous drainage was first reported in 1953 but did not become accepted as standard therapy until the 1980s. It has now become the treatment of choice for pyogenic hepatic abscesses. It is usually performed either with ultrasound or CT guidance, and success rates range from approximately 60–90%. There is still some debate, however, as to percutaneous aspiration alone versus catheter drainage. Several studies have demonstrated the efficacy of percutaneous aspiration alone. Giorgio et al. reviewed 39 patients with hepatic abscesses who were treated with aspiration alone; 36 of the 39 (92.3%) were successfully treated with a single aspiration, and the other three patients only required one more aspiration. There were no deaths or complications in his study [8]. Yu et al. demonstrated a 96.8% success rate in 64 patients with aspiration alone; approximately half (49.5%) required a single aspiration and the rest of the patients required multiple aspirations. In his study, two patients died of overwhelming sepsis and another required surgical intervention for a liver laceration. However, other studies have demonstrated superiority of catheter drainage [9]. Rajak et al. randomly assigned 50 patients to aspiration or catheter drainage. Residual abscess after two aspirations was considered failure in the aspiration group, and residual abscess after catheter drainage was considered failure in the catheter group. Only 60% responded to the needle aspiration, whereas 100% responded in the catheter drainage group [10]. Zerem et al. prospectively randomized patients to percutaneous aspiration versus catheter drainage. Similar to the last study, percutaneous aspiration was successful in 67% of patients, whereas catheter drainage was successful 100% of the time [11].

Catheter drainage appears to also be successful in patients with multiloculated or multiple abscesses. A series by Liu et al. found no difference between single and multiple abscesses and had very high clinical success rates of treatment of 87% for a single abscess and 92% for multiple abscesses with catheter drainage. That study also found an 88% success rate for treatment of a single multiloculated abscess as well as a 90% success rate for multiple multiloculated abscesses [12]. Failure of catheter drainage appears to be decreasing but still exists in approximately 10% of patients. A recent case series by Mezhir et al. demonstrated only a 66% success with catheter drainage; however, in this study, 88% of patients had a history of gastrointestinal malignancy. Nine percent of these patients required surgical intervention, whereas the rest of the patients who failed percutaneous drainage died with indwelling catheters. Independent predictors of failure of catheter drainage included positive yeast cultures and communication with the biliary tree [7].

Surgical therapy is rarely necessary as the first line of intervention. If necessary, it is usually in patients with an obstructed biliary system than is not amenable to nonsurgical decompression or a ruptured abscess with sepsis. More commonly, surgical intervention is now reserved only when percutaneous drainage has failed, the abscess is not amenable to percutaneous drainage (multiloculated or large), or when there is a complication from percutaneous drainage [6].

Surgical Therapy

If the cause of the hepatic abscess is unknown, a careful exploration of the abdomen should be performed to rule out any other abdominal pathology. Surgical drainage of the abscess is then performed by localization of the abscess via ultrasound or needle localization with ultrasound guidance. The abscess is then bluntly opened and the pus evacuated. Blunt finger manipulation can be used to break up loculations and adhesions. Careful hemostasis should be obtained to prevent residual fluid collections or recurrent abscess. Large bore drains are then left in place for irrigation and suction of the abscess cavity. Tan et al. retrospectively reviewed 80 patients with pyogenic abscesses >5 cm who were treated either with surgical drainage (44 patients) or percutaneous drainage (36 patients). Eighty percent of these patients had multiloculated abscesses. In this study, the surgical drainage group had less treatment failure, less secondary procedures, and a shorter length of stay. The mortality for the surgical drainage group was 4.5% and 2.8% for the percutaneous group, which was not statistically significant [13].

Some case reports have advocated primary liver resection for hepatic abscess. Hope et al. retrospectively reviewed patients with >3 cm multiloculated pyogenic abscess who were treated with percutaneous drainage along with antibiotics versus treatment with partial liver resections. The resection group had a 100% success rate of treatment and 7.4% mortality in this group, whereas the drainage group only had a 33% success rate for treatment and 4.7% mortality. Eight patients in the latter group required repeat drainage and five required surgical resection. The mortality rates between the two groups also did not reach statistical significance. The authors concluded that for large multiloculated abscesses, surgical treatment may be the primary mode of treatment of the disease [14]. Strong et al. reviewed 49 patients who underwent resection for hepatic abscesses after either failed conservative treatment or underlying hepatobiliary pathology. All of the patients had resolution of their abscesses and no patients required reoperation. The authors did report 4% mortality in their group after abscess rupture in two patients [15].

Conclusion

Pyogenic abscesses are bacterial in origin and more likely to be associated with a hepatobiliary pathology. Primary treatment is broad spectrum antibiotics along with percutaneous treatment via aspiration or catheter drainage. Rarely, a patient may need surgical therapy for failed percutaneous treatment. Mortality for this disease is approximately 10% and appears to be improving from previous early reports. However, appropriate management with antibiotics and consideration of appropriate drainage are still required for best outcomes (Fig. 22.2).

Amoebic

Pathogenesis

Amoebic liver abscesses are caused by the protozoan *Entamoeba histolytica*, which is endemic in tropical or developing countries. Humans are both the principal hosts and the infective carriers and the disease is usually transmitted fecal-orally. Infected cysts may be passed through water or produce contaminated with feces, foods contaminated by food handlers or by direct transmission. Most infected patients are asymptomatic but some patients will develop invasive disease of the colon. The liver is the most common extra-intestinal site for infection [16].

Once ingested, the cysts are capable of resisting acid degradation in the stomach. They are then released in the trophozoite from the cysts triggered by the neutral intestinal juice in the small intestine. Passing into the large intestine and they adhere to the colonic mucosa and invade into the tissue. These infections may manifest as mucosal thickening or more classically, as ulcerations through the mucosa and into the submucosa [17]. It is believed they cause hepatic disease by ascending through the portal system or via direct extension into the liver. Amoebic abscesses consist of three stages: acute inflammation, granuloma formation, and advancing necrosis with subsequent abscess formation. The abscess itself contains necrotic proteinaceous debris with a rim of trophozoites invading the surrounding tissue.

Since the abscess is essentially composed of blood and necrotic hepatic tissue, its appearance is typically described as *anchovy sauce*. It is usually odorless and sterile, unless there is secondary bacterial infection. The abscess will continue to progress and grow until it reaches Glisson's capsule since the capsule is resistant to hydrolysis by the trophozoites. This lends to the classic imaging appearance of the lesion abutting the liver capsule (Fig. 22.3).

Fig. 22.2 Algorithm for treatment of pyogenic liver abscesses

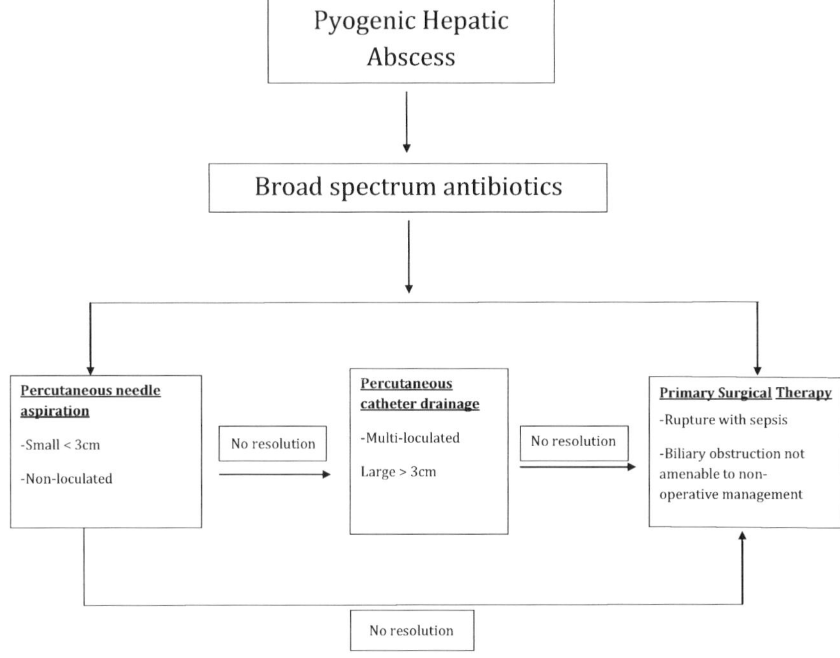

Fig. 22.3 A 49-year-old Chinese female who presented with RUQ pain caused by an amoebic abscess

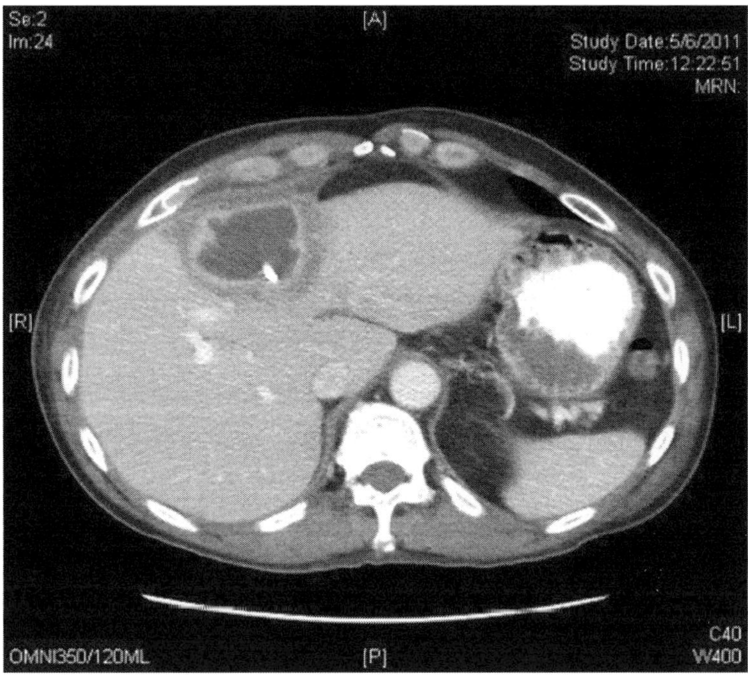

Epidemiology

Amoebic liver abscesses usually occur in developing or tropical countries with poor sanitation systems. Areas of the world with endemic disease include Central and South America, Mexico, India, and East and South Africa. The best estimate of the prevalence of amebiasis was by the World Health Organization (WHO) in 1995 that estimated approximately 40–50 million people become symptomatic per year with intestinal colitis or hepatic abscess, resulting in 40,000–100,000 deaths from the disease. A more recent population-based study in the United States identified the incidence to be 1.38 per million population with a 2.4% average decline during the course of the study (1993–2007) [16]. The mortality in that study was also lower than what has been previously reported and was approximately 1%.

Hispanic males between the ages of 20 and 40 with a history of travel to endemic regions of the world are most commonly affected by amoebic liver abscess, which is in contrast to pyogenic abscesses, which tend to occur in older patients [16]. There is also a heavier preponderance in the male gender although this is not well understood. One theory is alcohol use in men may lead to impaired Kupffer cell function or impaired immune response. Immunosuppressed patient are also at greater risk for amoebic liver abscess and predisposing conditions include HIV, steroid use, malnourished patients with severe hypoalbuminemia, and post-splenectomy patients.

Clinical Presentation

The most common clinical features of amoebic liver abscesses include fever and abdominal pain. Hepatomegaly with pain on palpation over the liver or below the ribs is one of the most important clinical signs that may help distinguish this disease from pyogenic abscesses. Other symptoms include chills, nausea, weight loss, and diarrhea. Jaundice is seen less commonly with amoebic abscesses.

Common laboratory findings include an elevated white blood cell (WBC) count and anemia. Patients with acute amoebic abscess tend to have an elevated AST and a normal alkaline phosphatase, whereas patients with chronic amoebic abscess will have a normal AST and almost always an abnormal alkaline phosphatase. In contrast, patients with pyogenic abscesses tend to have an elevated bilirubin and abnormal liver transaminases [17].

Diagnosis

Amoebic abscesses need to be distinguished from pyogenic abscesses. Like pyogenic abscesses, the majority of patient with amoebic abscesses will have an abnormal CXR, which may demonstrate an elevated hemidiaphragm, pleural effusion, or atelectasis. An abdominal ultrasound can help make the diagnosis of amoebic abscess and has an accuracy of 95%; however, it is operator dependent. Typical ultrasound findings include a round or oval lesion that is hypoechoic and homogenous in appearance without wall echoes and abutting the liver capsule. In addition the majority of lesions (>80%) are found in the right lobe of the liver.

Abdominal CT is another imaging modality that is extremely sensitive for detecting liver abscesses. Its advantage is the ability to distinguish an abscess from benign or malignant tumors; however, it does not always distinguish between pyogenic and amoebic abscess. The lesion is typically peripheral in the liver without an enhanced rim. Magnetic resonance imaging (MRI) is another imaging modality, but like CT, cannot distinguish between amoebic and pyogenic abscesses. It is also more expensive and is relatively inaccessible from an emergent standpoint.

Serologic testing is a useful adjunct to making a diagnosis of amoebic liver abscess. The majority of patients will not have any detectable parasites in their stools; however, >90% of patients will have antibodies to *E. histolytica* [18]. The enzyme linked immunoassay test has largely replaced all tests for *E. histolytica* as it is fast, highly sensitive, and widely available. Its sensitivity is ~99% with a specificity of 90%. Although the test cannot distinguish between acute and chronic infections, it is helpful in a patient with a typical story for amoebic hepatic abscess and a mass on imaging studies for making a determination of amoebic abscess.

Treatment

Metronidazole is the treatment of choice for amoebic abscesses. The drug enters the parasite by diffusion and is converted by reduced ferredoxin or flavodoxin into reactive cytotoxic nitro radicals. A 10-day treatment of 750 mg orally three times per day has a >95% efficacy in most patients [17]. Symptomatic improvements are usually seen by 3 days of treatment and there is little, if any, resistance to the drug. If the patient is unable to tolerate metronidazole, emetine hydrochloride or chloroquine phosphate can be substituted. Emetine hydrochloride is limited in its usefulness since it is administered intramuscularly and has significant cardiac side effects. Chloroquine phosphate can be used in pregnancy and has some associated side effects such as gastrointestinal upset, headaches, and pruritis. The majority of its use is limited to recurrent or resistant hepatic amebiasis.

After the patient has been treated for the amoebic abscess, they should be treated for the intestinal colonization with an agent such as iodoquinol, paromomycin, or diloxanide furoate. The risk of hepatic relapse is approximately 10% in patients not treated for their colonization.

Percutaneous drainage or aspiration of the abscess has been debated in the literature. A recent Cochrane review of image guided percutaneous drainage plus metronidazole versus metronidazole alone did not demonstrate any benefit to drainage [19]. The authors did note that the majority of studies were of low quality and that further confirmation with larger trials would be necessary to confirm their results. In a recent population-based study on amoebic abscess in the United States, percutaneous drainage was performed in 48% of cases and surgical drainage was performed in another 7% [16]. The indications for drainage were not noted in the study. There was no mortality associated with percutaneous drainage but the authors did note a 0.09% mortality when treated conservatively without drainage (either percutaneous or surgical). Other studies have reached mixed conclusions and there is currently no consensus on the placement of drains or aspiration.

Complications

Approximately 3–17% of the time, the abscess can rupture into the peritoneum, pleural cavity, hollow viscera, or pericardium. The majority of these ruptures are contained by the diaphragm, omentum, or abdominal wall. Free rupture into the abdominal cavity is rare as is rupture into a hollow viscus; however, there are reports of ruptures into the stomach and the colon. Most authors now advocate free ruptures into the peritoneum to be managed by percutaneous drainage of the pus. Aggressive surgical management in early published reports led to very high mortality rates, whereas patients who are conservatively managed tended to fare better.

Exploratory laparotomy is indicated when the diagnosis is uncertain, when there is life-threatening hemorrhage, or failure of conservative management. However, published mortality rates are high with surgical management. The abscess is usually seen to be on the surface of the liver. The portal triads will be traversing within the abscess since they are covered by Glisson's capsule and are not degraded by the amoeba. Care must be taken to not disrupt these triads or significant hemorrhage can occur. Since the bile ducts also are found here, disruption can lead to postoperative bile leaks. The abscess cavities can be irrigated gently with saline and then instilled with emetine hydrochloride. Drains should be left in place to widely drain the residual cavity.

Amoebic abscesses can also spontaneously rupture into the pleural cavity or pericardium. Patients will develop an acute shortness of breath with opacification of their lung on CXR. An ultrasound or CT imaging will reveal the hepatic abscess near the dome of the liver with a large opacified fluid collection in the lung. The treatment of choice for the pleural cavity is adequate drainage of the fluid. Left untreated or poorly drained, the patient will develop a secondary infection requiring decortications. If a patient develops a rupture into their pericardium, it can be difficult to diagnose unless there has been abdominal imaging. A high index of suspicion is often necessary to make the diagnosis. Treatment of the pericardial effusion either with percutaneous drainage or subxiphoid window is necessary in cases of tamponade or impending tamponade.

Conclusion

Amoebic abscesses are caused by the protozoan *Entamoeba histolytica*. The typical patient is a young Hispanic male with recent travel to endemic areas of the world. Primary treatment is with metronidazole. The majority of patients will respond within 3 days of treatment. Uncomplicated amoebic abscesses are easily treated with a low mortality; however, complications can arise which can significantly increase mortality (Fig. 22.4).

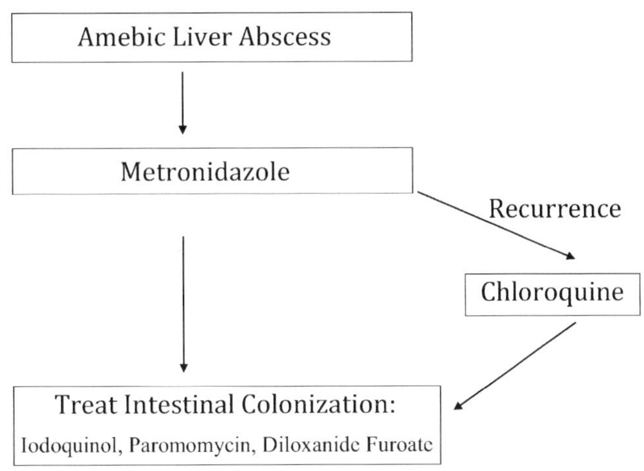

Fig. 22.4 Algorithm for treatment of amoebic liver abscesses

Echinococcal Cysts

Echinococcal cysts (hydatid cysts) of the liver are caused by the adult or larval stages of the tapeworm *Echinococcus granulosus*. This zoonotic disease occurs mostly in areas of the world associated with sheep grazing, but is common worldwide because dogs are the definitive host.

Pathogenesis

The adult tapeworm (*Echinococcus granulosus*) inhabits the small intestine of the definitive host (usually dogs). Eggs from the tapeworm are released into the feces, which are then ingested by an intermediate host. This can include sheep, cattle, goats, horses, or humans. Within the intestine, the egg hatches and releases an oncosphere larva. This oncosphere larva contains hooks that allow it to penetrate the bowel mucosa and enter the bloodstream where it then migrates to the liver or other solid organs, such as the lungs. There, the oncosphere larva develops into a 2-layer cyst surrounded by a host-derived fibrous capsule, referred to as the pericyst. The 2 layers consist of an inner germinal layer and an outer gelatinous membrane. This cyst continues to enlarge as protoscolices bud from the germinal layer and fill the interior of the cyst. With enough time, the cysts will form internal septations and other daughter cysts. In the intermediate host, such as humans, the protoscolices can only develop into more daughter cysts and cannot further differentiate into tapeworms. After the cyst containing organs of the infected intermediate host are ingested by the definitive host, such as a dog or sheep, the protoscolices then evaginate and attach to the intestinal mucosa. Within the intestine, they develop into the adult tapeworm, ready to be transmitted to its next host (Fig. 22.5).

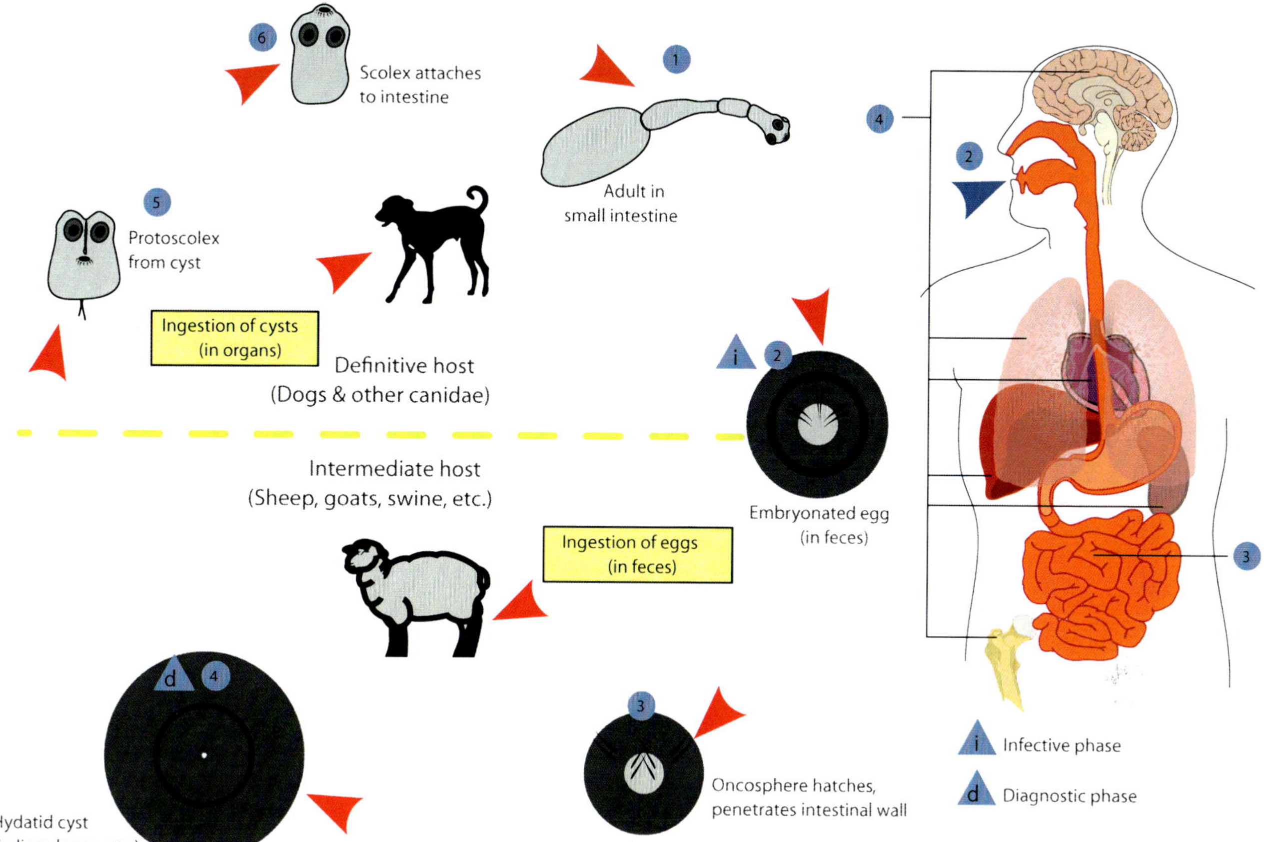

Fig. 22.5 Life cycle of *Echinococcus granulosus*. Reproduced via Wikimedia Commons from User:Slashme (Redrawn from file:CDC Echinococcus Life Cycle.jpg) [GFDL (http://www.gnu.org/copyleft/ fdl.html) or CC-BY-SA-3.0-2.5-2.0-1.0 (http://creativecommons.org/ licenses/by-sa/3.0)]

Epidemiology

Echinococcal disease is found worldwide especially in areas involved with sheep farming, but is most common in temperate regions such as the Mediterranean areas, South America, China, the Soviet Union, Central Asia, and Africa. In the United States, the majority of cases are found in immigrants from countries where echinococcosis is prevalent. The actual incidence and prevalence of echinococcosis is variable depending on the area of the world, but most estimates are thought to be misleading from the lack of actual data collecting. In most countries where the disease is prevalent, echinococcosis is not considered to be a reportable disease and rural settings present a challenge to acquiring epidemiologic data. The estimates may also be false as this disease is difficult to detect early on, and it is prevalent in areas with a weak healthcare systems, with a high population of stray dogs, and illegal slaughtering. However, several retrospective reviews demonstrate the incidence to be similar in many countries despite geographical difference. Reported data on the annual surgical incidence in Turkey was estimated to be 6.4 per 100,000 inhabitants, the incidence in Sardinia from 2001 to 2005 was 6.2 per 100,000 inhabitants, and the incidence in Tanzania was 10 per 100,000 [20, 21].

Clinical Presentation

Most hydatid cysts are asymptomatic and slow growing, and therefore are present for years before being detected. Most primary infections in humans consist of a single cyst, and the liver is the most common location, accounting for over 70% of cases, with the lung being the second most likely, seen in 25% of cases [22]. Signs and symptoms are vague and typically due to the mass effect of the large cyst on the involved and surrounding organs; these include hepatomegaly, abdominal pain, nausea, vomiting, and jaundice. Often, patients will present with a complication of the cyst as their initial presentation, which can include cyst rupture or secondary infection appearing similar to a pyogenic abscess [23].

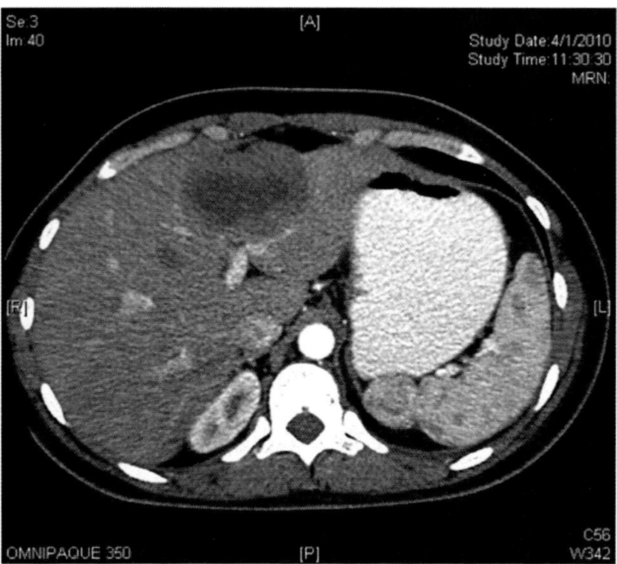

Fig. 22.6 A 34-year-old female who presented with RUQ pain due to large echinococcal cyst

Diagnosis

Abdominal ultrasound has become the diagnostic method of choice for imaging of hydatid cysts. It is easily available and can determine the number of cysts, the size, and the viability of the cyst based on the morphology of the cyst wall. It has been used worldwide because its availability, portability and accuracy. Typical findings include a well-circumscribed cyst with budding lesions on the cyst membrane. The cyst fluid may be simple or heterogeneous with classic hyperechoic contents creating a "snowflake sign." When the cyst is degenerating, it may be filled with an amorphous mass, which is composed of the degenerating membrane. CT or MRI is also often used, and these reveal large cystic lesions and when present, calcifications in the wall are nearly diagnostic for hydatid disease (Fig. 22.6). In addition, immunologic serum assays to detect antibodies to *E granulosus* are used to confirm the diagnosis. The sensitivity of these tests are limited to the fact that antigens are sequestered within the cyst cavity and therefore do not illicit an immune response from the host [22]. But, this modality is also helpful in the follow-up surveillance of patients after surgical or pharmacological treatment.

Treatment

Surgical treatment for hydatid cysts within the liver is the most successful method of treatment with the lowest incidence of recurrence [22]. The goal of surgery is complete removal of the cyst wall and contents with a surrounding rim of hepatic parenchyma, referred to as pericystectomy. In addition, larger or more complicated cysts may be best resected via partial hepatectomy or hepatic lobectomy. Other more conservative operative techniques include simple drainage, marsupialization of the cyst wall, or placing omentum within the cyst. Reported recurrence rates vary from 2% to 25%, while more radical interventions have the lowest rate of recurrence at the cost of higher operative risk [23]. Any communication with the biliary system must be recognized and treated in the operating room, and it is often repaired with a simple suture-ligature of the exposed ducts. Failing to recognize and repair this will lead to biliary leak and likely infected biloma.

The most severe consequence of surgery for hydatid cysts is the incidence of anaphylactic reaction due to spillage of the cyst contents. One important step is preoperative preparation and communication, as the anesthesia team should have epinephrine and steroids prepared to treat any anaphylactic reaction [1]. Other methods employed to minimize this risk include aspirating the cyst at the start of the operation and instilling ethanol or hypertonic saline within the cavity. The intra-abdominal surgical field should be isolated with laps so that any spillage is contained and interaction of the cyst contents and other tissues are minimal. In addition, soaking the laps in hypertonic saline has been described. Due to the pathogenesis of liver cyst formation, surgeons must be aware that the cyst contains 2 layers that must be removed en masse. Pericystectomy involves creating a dissection plane through healthy liver parenchyma, thus ensuring complete resection of both layers, and decreasing the risk of entering the cyst cavity.

In addition, there are an increasing number of reports of minimally invasive laparoscopic approaches to resection or drainage of hydatid cysts [24]. The same principles of surgery apply, including packing the liver to control drainage and complete removal pericyst tissue with normal hepatic parenchyma and detecting and treating any biliary communications.

Contraindications to surgery include pregnancy, patient refusal, or medical comorbidities. In these cases, medications used in the treatment of hydatid disease include albendazole and mebendazole. Medical therapy is effective in 60–80% of patients, and most often in those with small (<7 mm), isolated cysts, surrounded by minimal adventitial reaction [22]. Treatment typically lasts a minimum of 3 months, and patients must be monitored for adverse reactions such as neutropenia and hepatic toxicity.

"PAIR" (Puncture–Aspiration–Injection–Reaspiration) is gaining popularity as a third method of treatment of hydatid cyst disease. The procedure begins with image-guided puncture of the cyst, and can be done with either sonography or CT. Following aspiration of the entire cyst contents, the cavity is injected with a protoscolicidal agent such as 95% ethanol or hypertonic saline for 15–30 min, completed by reaspiration of this fluid. Reports indicate that the incidence of anaphylaxis is only 8%, compared to 25% during surgical resection [25]. When used as a part of a multimodality approach, the technique has been shown in a large meta-analysis to be slightly more effective than surgery with decreased rates of morbidity, mortality, hospital stay, and recurrence [25]. This approach includes a 7-day pretreatment course of albendazole or mebendazole, followed by at least 1 month of these medications post-procedure. Importantly, PAIR must not be used in patients whose cysts communicate with the biliary system as injection of the sclerosing agents can induce a severe sclerosing cholangitis. The presence of biliary communication must be detected with pre-procedural ERCP, cholangiography during the procedure, or testing the cyst fluid for bilirubin.

Complications

Initial symptoms of hydatid cysts are often vague; therefore often the first presentation is due to a complication. Most commonly cysts rupture freely into the peritoneal cavity, causing disseminating echinococcosis creating cysts in multiple intra-abdominal organs. In addition, the sudden release of cyst contents can precipitate allergic reactions that vary from mild to fatal anaphylaxis. It is reported that there is a 10% rate of severe anaphylactic reactions [23]. When recognized early, patients are treated with epinephrine or steroids to support them through this reaction. Within the liver, the cyst can rupture into the biliary tree and cause secondary cholangitis. Other complications include biliary obstruction by daughter cysts or simple extrinsic compression. In addition, the cyst cavity is a potential site of secondary bacterial infection. These are diagnosed and treated as pyogenic liver abscesses.

Conclusion

Echinococcal cysts (hydatid cysts) of the liver are caused by the tapeworm *Echinococcus granulosus*. While detected worldwide, they are more prevalent in temperate climates where humans are in contact with the definitive hosts, sheep and dogs. They most often cause cysts within the liver, detected by imaging and immunoassays. Symptoms are often due to mass effect; however, rupture and spillage of contents are associated with severe anaphylaxis. Primary treatment involves complete surgical resection of the cyst either via laparotomy or laparoscopic approach. Newer methods such as Percutaneous Aspiration–Injection–Reaspiration (PAIR) are growing in popularity as an effective and safe treatment option (Fig. 22.7).

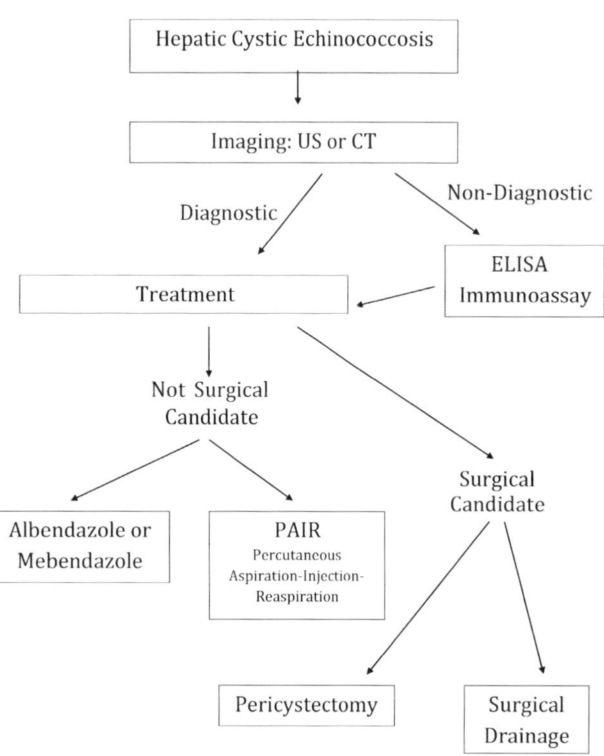

Fig. 22.7 Algorithm for treatment of echinococcal cysts (hydatid cysts) of the liver. *US* ultrasound, *CT* computed tomography, *ELISA* enzyme-linked immunosorbent assay

References

1. D'Angleica M, Fong Y. The Liver. In: Townsend CM, Beauchamp RD, editors. Sabiston textbook of surgery. 18th ed. Philadelphia, PA: Saunders Elsevier; 2008. p. 1463–523.
2. Huang C, Pitt HA, Lipsett PA, et al. Pyogenic hepatic abscess: changing trends over 42 years. Ann Surg. 1996;223:600–9.
3. Meddings L, Myers RP, Hubbard J, et al. A population-based study of pyogenic liver abscesses in the United States: incidence, mortality, and temporal trends. Am J Gastroenterol. 2010;105:117–24.
4. Kaplan GG, Gregson DB, Laupland KB. Population-based study of the epidemiology of and risk factors for pyogenic liver abscess. Clin Gastroenterol Hepatol. 2004;2:1032–8.
5. Rahimian J, Wilson T, Oram V, Holzman RS. Pyogenic liver abscess: recent trends in etiology and mortality. Clin Infect Dis. 2004;39:1654–9.
6. Strong RW. Pyogenic liver abscess. In: Blumgart LH, editor. Surgery of the liver, biliary tract, and pancreas. 4th ed. Philadelphia, PA: Saunders Elsevier; 2007. p. 927–34.
7. Mezhir JJ, Fong Y, Jacks LM, et al. Current management of pyogenic liver abscess: surgery is now second-line treatment. J Am Coll Surg. 2010;210:975–83.
8. Giorgio A, Stefano G, DiSarno A, et al. Percutaneous needle aspiration of multiple pyogenic abscesses of the liver: 13-year single-center experience. Am J Roentgenol. 2006;187:1585–90.
9. Ch Yu S, Hg Lo R, Kan PS, et al. Pyogenic liver abscess: treatment with needle aspiration. Clin Radiol. 1997;52:912–6.
10. Rajak CL, Gupta S, Jain S, et al. Percutaneous treatment of liver abscesses: needle aspiration versus catheter drainage. Am J Roentgenol. 1998;170:1035–9.

11. Zerem E, Hadzic A. Sonographically guided percutaneous catheter drainage versus needle aspiration in the management of pyogenic liver abscess. Am J Roentgenol. 2007;189:138–42.

12. Liu CH, Gervais DA, Hahn PF, et al. Percutaneous hepatic abscess drainage: do multiple abscesses or multiloculated abscesses preclude drainage or affect outcome? J Vasc Interv Radiol. 2009;20:1059–65.

13. Tan Y, Chung AY, Chow PK, et al. An appraisal of surgical and percutaneous drainage for pyogenic liver abscesses larger than 5 cm. Ann Surg. 2005;241:485–90.

14. Hope WW, Vrochides DV, Newcomb WL, et al. Optimal treatment of hepatic abscess. Am Surg. 2008;74:178–82.

15. Strong RW, Fawcett J, Lynch SV, Wall DR. Hepatectomy for pyogenic liver abscess. HPB. 2003;5:86–90.

16. Congly SE, Aziz AA, Meddings L, et al. Amoebic liver abscess in USA: a populations-based study of incidence, temporal trends and mortality. Liver Int. 2011;31:1191–8.

17. Hughes MA, Petri WA. Amebic liver abscess. Infect Dis Clin North Am. 2000;14:565–82.

18. Lodhi S, Sarwari AR, Muzammil M, et al. Features distinguishing amoebic from pyogenic liver abscess: a review of 577 adult cases. Trop Med Int Health. 2004;9:718–23.

19. Chavez-Tapia NC, Hernandez-Calleros J, Tellez-Avila FL et al. Image-guided percutaneous procedure plus metronidazole vs. metronidazole alone for uncomplicated amoebic liver abscess. Cochrane Database Syst Rev. 2009;1. Art. No:CD004886.

20. Concheda M, Antonelli A, Caddori A, et al. A retrospective analysis of human cystic echinococcosis in Sardinia, an endemic mediterranean region, from 2001 to 2005. Parasitol Int. 2010;59: 454–9.

21. Gonlugur U, Ozcelik S, Gonlugur TE, et al. The retrospective annual surgical incidence of cystic echinococcosis in Sivas, Turkey. Zoonoses Public Health. 2009;56:209–14.

22. Moro P, Schantz PM. Echinococcosis: a review. Int J Infect Dis. 2009;13:125–33.

23. McManus DP, Zhang W, Li J, et al. Echinococcosis. Lancet. 2003;362:1295–304.

24. Foster EN, Hertz G. Echinococcus of the liver treated with laparoscopic hepatectomy. Permanente J. 2010;14:45–6.

25. Smego RA, Bhatti S, Khaliq A, et al. Percutaneous aspiration-injection-reaspiration drainage plus albendazole or mebendazole for hepatic cystic echinococcosis: a meta-analysis. Clin Infect Dis. 2003;37:1073–83.

Steven M. Cohen, Andrew H. Nguyen,
and H. Leon Pachter

Introduction

Acute pancreatitis is characterized by localized pancreatic inflammation, but may progress to disease with systemic effects, such as distant organ dysfunction. Alcohol and gallstones are the most common causes of pancreatitis, although other etiologies such as metabolic disturbances, obstruction, or medications may less frequently cause pancreatitis. The inflammatory process of acute pancreatitis is thought to begin in the pancreatic acinar cells with co-localization of pancreatic zymogens and lysozymes in the cytoplasm, resulting in inappropriate activation. This process leads to acinar cell damage, followed by a robust infiltrate of leukocytes, further propagating this inflammatory process. Patients typically present with severe epigastric pain, radiating to the back, associated with nausea and vomiting. While most cases of acute pancreatitis are self-limiting, the disease can progress to severe acute pancreatitis and be complicated by a systemic inflammatory response syndrome, organ failure, shock, and death.

Epidemiology

The overall occurrence of pancreatitis may be as low as 4.9 persons per 100,000 person population [1]; however, there has been a recent trend in increasing incidence of acute pancreatitis in epidemiological studies in the United States.

S.M. Cohen, D.O. FACS (✉)
Department of Surgery, New York University Medical Center,
530 First Avenue, HCC 6C, New York, NY 10016, USA
e-mail: Steven.Cohen@med.nyu.edu

A.H. Nguyen, M.D.
Department of Surgery, David Geffen School of Medicine
at UCLA, 757 Westwood Plaza, Los Angeles, CA 90095, USA
e-mail: ahnguyen@mednet.ucla.edu

H.L. Pachter, M.D.
Department of Surgery, New York University Medical Center,
530 First Avenue, HCC 6C, New York, NY 10016, USA
e-mail: Leon.Pachter@nyumc.org

In a recent review of hospital discharges in the United States, more than 235,000 cases of pancreatitis were found to be admitted to hospitals with a calculated population incidence of 78 persons per 100,000 person population [2]. The increasing incidence over the past 20 years may be attributed to improvements in imaging technologies and laboratory tests that aid in the diagnostic assessment of nonspecific abdominal pathology. However, the more recent increases in incidence over the past 10 years may be attributed to the greater prevalence of obesity and an accompanying increase in incidence of gallstone pancreatitis [3]. Acute pancreatitis may have even greater incidence as many mild cases are under reported and a proportion of patients with severe acute pancreatitis go undiagnosed only until autopsy [4].

In the United States, the total cost of admissions for acute pancreatitis reaches approximately $2.2 billion per year. The average cost per hospitalization is just under $10,000 with a mean cost per hospital day of $1,670 during a 6.1 day average length of stay [5]. In subgroups such as elderly patients, average hospitalization tends to cost more, primarily due to a more complicated hospital course and extended lengths of stay.

Historically, acute pancreatitis has been a disease associated with a high mortality rate. Early studies in the 1940s reported a mortality rate of 25% in patients managed conservatively, with a mortality rate of 54% for those managed operatively [6]. By the early 1970s, Ranson et al. reported an overall mortality rate of 15% in acute pancreatitis [7]. In these early studies, patients often succumbed to death as clinicians had difficulty predicting and identifying those patients that would progress to severe acute pancreatitis. In addition, many more patients with severe disease were operated upon and thus, were exposed to the significant operative risks.

Currently, high rates of mortality in acute pancreatitis are still frequently cited, although some of these rates refer to specific sub-populations of patients. The overall mortality of all hospitalized patients with acute pancreatitis ranges from 2% to 5% (17% in severe acute pancreatitis, 1.5% in mild acute pancreatitis) [8]. Of patients admitted to the intensive care unit with acute pancreatitis, mortality was found to be

L.J. Moore et al. (eds.), *Common Problems in Acute Care Surgery*,
DOI 10.1007/978-1-4614-6123-4_23, © Springer Science+Business Media New York 2013

31.5% and later 10.3% for those patients transferred out of the intensive care unit [9]. The patients with highest risk of mortality in pancreatitis are those admitted to the intensive care unit or those with disease characterized as severe acute pancreatitis, when there are local complications of the pancreas or distant organ failure. Approximately 15–20% of patients with acute pancreatitis experience this severe form of disease. In severe acute pancreatitis, much of the morbidity and mortality is associated with organ failure, with organ failure occurring in approximately 50% of patients with severe acute pancreatitis [10]. The mortality in severe acute pancreatitis has been reported to range from as low as 17 to up to 69% [11–13]. However, in studies conducted at medical centers with specialized medical and surgical expertise in the management of pancreatic disease, the mortality in severe acute pancreatitis may be under 10% and as low as 6%, even when considering only the patients with necrotizing pancreatitis [14, 15].

There is a broad variety of etiologies of acute pancreatitis, although gallstone or biliary pancreatitis remains the most common cause. The mechanism is thought to be due to small gallstones that develop and pass via the cystic duct to be retained in the distal common bile duct. By blocking drainage of the common bile duct near the ampulla of Vater, it is thought that biliary fluids containing bile salts may reflux up into Wirsung's duct, causing damage to pancreatic acinar cells. Gallstone pancreatitis accounts for approximately 35–40% of all cases of acute pancreatitis [16, 17]. In the general population, however, there is a high prevalence of asymptomatic gallstones and less than 10% of patients with symptomatic gallstones actually develop pancreatitis [18]. Of ethnic groups, Caucasians, Hispanics, and Native Americans tend to have the highest rates of gallstone pancreatitis when compared to people of other ethnic backgrounds [19–21]. Well-defined risk factors associated with gallstone pancreatitis include female sex, pregnancy, and obesity.

The second most common cause of acute pancreatitis is due to chronic and excessive alcohol consumption. Alcoholic pancreatitis accounts for approximately 30% of cases of pancreatitis in the United States. The mechanism by which alcohol causes acute pancreatitis is presently unknown, although it is hypothesized to occur in the context of increased pancreatic duct secretions with sphincter of Oddi spasm, causing pancreatic ductal hypertension. Interestingly, pancreatitis associated with alcohol use rarely occurs with "binge drinking," but more typically occurs in patients with chronic alcohol intake, who already have either changes of chronic pancreatitis. Patients with alcoholic cirrhosis rarely also have pancreatitis and vice versa. Alcoholic pancreatitis occurrence peaks during the 4th and 5th decades of life [19]. The incidence of alcoholic pancreatitis is 2–3% per year in chronic alcoholics [22]. Alcoholic pancreatitis has been associated with greater mortality compared to gallstone pancreatitis, although this may be due to lower baseline nutrition and health status that occurs with chronic alcohol abuse.

In the absence of a history chronic alcohol abuse and gall-stones in the biliary system, other causes of pancreatitis may be investigated, which account for 30% of cases. These other causes may include tumor, infection, anatomic anomaly, trauma, iatrogenic injury, medication, metabolic dysfunction, autoimmune disease, or genetics. With resolution of symptoms in mild acute pancreatitis, it is permissible to defer an extensive investigation in the absence of clear etiology. However, with severe acute pancreatitis, repeated bouts of acute pancreatitis, or other more worrisome signs, a more thorough investigation is appropriate.

Tumor obstructing the main pancreatic duct is a rare, but serious cause of acute pancreatitis. Most frequently, ampullary tumors may cause pancreatitis, although masses anywhere along the pancreatic ducts may be a source for disease. Mucous from intraductal papillary mucinous neoplasm can also cause obstruction. Pancreatitis associated with weight loss, jaundice, steatorrhea, and pale-colored stools is concerning for a mass obstructing the pancreatic duct.

An even less prevalent cause of obstruction in the United States, helminth infestation, has been known to cause pancreatitis. These parasitic worms migrate via the small intestines into the pancreaticobiliary duct system and can induce pancreatitis by obstructing pancreatic fluid outflow. The most common culprits are *Ascaris lumbricoides* and *Clonorchis sinensis*, although both are rare in the United States. In the United States, helminth infestation is most common in immigrants from endemic countries.

Pancreas divisum, an anatomic anomaly where the majority of the pancreas drains by the duct of Santorini, has been associated with recurrent bouts of acute pancreatitis. Autopsy series have found that the prevalence of pancreas divisum ranges from 5% to 7% in the general population [23]. However, only a subpopulation of patients with pancreas divisum ever experiences symptomatic disease associated with this anomaly. It has been postulated that pancreatitis occurs because of a "relative obstruction" of the minor papilla, which drains the majority of pancreatic glandular tissue [24, 25].

Blunt trauma to the epigastrium can cause a severe pancreatic duct injury, where the main duct is compressed against the spine, or mild pancreatic inflammation and edema, due to contusion. Traumatic injury to the pancreas most commonly occurs in the context of motor vehicle and bicycle accidents with a forceful strike to the abdomen by the steering wheel or handlebars. Severe injury to the pancreatic duct can cause severe inflammation, pancreatic duct leak, pseudocyst formation, and a complicated hospital course.

Pancreatitis following endoscopic retrograde cholangiopancreatography (ERCP) is a well recognized cause. Although 75% of patients who have an ERCP will have elevations in post-procedure serum amylase [26], the incidence of abdominal pain and pancreatitis is only 4–5%, based on recent large clinical trials [27, 28]. At this time, there are no medications to prevent post-ERCP pancreatitis, although numerous agents have been studied [29–31]. Multiple studies have shown benefit of short-term prophylactic pancreatic stent placement for the prevention of post-ERCP pancreatitis [32].

Medications are another infrequent cause of pancreatitis, accounting for less than 1% of cases of acute pancreatitis [33]. It is often difficult to deduce a causative relation between medications and disease, as pancreatitis tends to be self-limiting and resolution may occur spontaneously, coincidentally at the same time of medication cessation. However, there are a number of medications that have consistently been associated with pancreatitis such as those for acquired immunodeficiency syndrome (AIDS) (didanosine, pentamidine), antibiotics (metronidazole, tetracycline), diuretics (furosemide, thiazides), inflammatory bowel disease drugs (sulfasalazine, 5-ASA), immunosuppressives (L-asparaginase, azathioprine), valproic acid, and steroids.

Metabolic disturbances such as hypertriglyceridemia and hypercalcemia can cause pancreatitis. Elevated triglycerides causing acute pancreatitis can be as low as 500 mg/dL, but are more typically found at levels greater than 1,000 mg/dL. Hypercalcemia causing pancreatitis often occurs in the context of hyperparathyroidism, but also can occur secondary to malignancy, total parenteral nutrition, or sarcoidosis.

Autoimmune pancreatitis is an etiology that typical occurs as sub-acute or chronic pancreatitis and can present later as a pancreatic head mass that could mimic pancreatic malignancies in initial presentation. It was first identified by Yoshida et al. in 1995 and had accounted for 5–6% of cases of idiopathic pancreatitis in Japan [34, 35]. Autoimmune pancreatitis is associated with elevated serum levels of IgG4 and other self-antigens and is highly responsive to corticosteroid therapy.

In younger patients, pancreatitis may occur from genetic causes, together categorized as "hereditary pancreatitis." In 1996, Whitcomb et al. reported a single-gene missense mutation affecting cationic trypsinogen, leading to clusterings of pancreatitis in an autosomal dominant pattern of inheritance [36]. Mutations in the cystic fibrosis transmembrane conductance regulator (CFTR) gene, causing defects in chloride ion channel and the disease cystic fibrosis is another genetic cause of pancreatitis. Serine protease inhibitor Kazal type I (SPINK-1) has also been found to be a hereditary cause of pancreatitis.

Infectious causes of acute pancreatitis include viruses, bacteria, and fungi. Viruses causing pancreatitis include mumps, Coxsackie virus, hepatitis B, cytomegalovirus, and varicella-zoster virus. Bacterial causes of pancreatitis tend to be exceedingly rare, but cases caused by Mycoplasma, Legionella, and Salmonella have been reported. Of fungi, aspergillus has been reported to rarely cause acute pancreati-

tis. Additionally, bites from various vectors, including the brown recluse spider, a scorpion found in the region surrounding Trinidad (*Tityus trinitatis*), and the Gila monster have been known to induce pancreatitis in their victims, via hyperstimulating cholinergic innervations to the pancreas, resulting in hypersecretion and sphincter spasm.

Clinical Presentation

The classic presentation of acute pancreatitis is acute onset of mild to severe epigastric pain, radiating to the back with associated nausea and vomiting. Up to 70% of patients with acute pancreatitis will have this classic pattern of symptoms. At onset, the pain typically develops over an hour and may be characterized as a pressure-like, dull and constant, or even throbbing epigastric abdominal discomfort. Patients may notice that the pain is better appreciated in the supine position and may be mildly alleviated in a sitting position and leaning forward. Variations in pain severity with exertion or the respiratory cycle would be atypical. In mild cases of acute pancreatitis, pain may resolve within 1 or 2 days, or can potentially persist for weeks. Interestingly, it is also not uncommon for patients to have pancreatitis, but have minimal or no pain symptoms.

On physical exam, patients with acute pancreatitis may be found to be febrile, tachycardic, and occasionally jaundiced. In cases of severe acute pancreatitis, the patient may appear pale, in respiratory distress, and hypotensive. On exam of the abdomen, in mild pancreatitis, epigastric tenderness on deep palpitation may be elicited. However, in more severe disease, abdominal exam may be significant for abdominal rigidity, guarding, and rebound tenderness. While rarely present on exam, signs of severe pancreatitis and retroperitoneal hemorrhage may include bruising around the umbilicus (Cullen's sign), along the flanks (Grey-Turner's sign), or along the inguinal ligaments (Fox's sign).

Diagnosis of acute pancreatitis relies on the patient's presentation—typically epigastric pain accompanied by nausea and vomiting, followed by clinical suspicion for pursuing such a diagnosis. Further evaluation of acute pancreatitis to confirm diagnosis would begin with laboratory tests of serum pancreatic enzymes, such as amylase and lipase. The elevation of these pancreatic enzymes is thought to occur when there is a physical blockade in secretion via the ducts, followed by leakage of pancreatic enzymes from acinar cells via the basolateral membrane and into the systemic circulation.

Amylase is the most commonly used biochemical marker to assist in the diagnosis of acute pancreatitis. Mild elevations in serum amylase concentration tend to be nonspecific. In addition to the pancreas, amylase also originates from salivary glands, fallopian tubes and small bowel and elevations can occur in a number of other intra-abdominal pathologies. Measurement of serum amylase can be more specific for pancreatitis by using a laboratory test that measures the isoform of amylase specific to the pancreas, P-isoamylase, rather than the standard serum amylase assay [37]. A level of three times the upper limit of normal is typically used as the cutoff for raising the likelihood of a diagnosis of pancreatitis. Elevations of serum amylase in acute pancreatitis occur rapidly within 12 h of onset of symptoms and similarly fall rapidly within 3 days. In patients with renal insufficiency, elevations in amylase may last longer or may be falsely elevated as well. Alternatively, in mild acute pancreatitis in the context of chronic pancreatitis or hypertriglyceridemia, amylase may remain within the normal limits during the duration of disease.

Measurement of serum lipase is both more sensitive and specific for acute pancreatitis. Elevations in serum lipase originate from the pancreas, making this study more specific compared to the standard serum amylase assay. Additionally, elevations in lipase tend to remain elevated for as long as a week after onset of disease. Sensitivity has been found to be as high as 100% with 96% specificity [38]. Similar to amylase, lipase is cleared by the kidneys and may remain abnormally elevated in patients with renal insufficiency.

Initial measurements of serum pancreatic enzymes is useful in making a diagnosis of pancreatitis, but repeat studies or further use in the assessment of severity is of limited value. After having a positive study at admission, repeating measurements of the biochemical markers is unnecessary, although some clinicians choose to trend pancreatic enzymes with the thought that decreasing levels may suggest resolution of disease. However, studies have found that levels of pancreatic enzymes are unable to predict either severity of disease or the course [39].

While physical exam findings are generally nonspecific and laboratory studies take time to return, simple imaging studies, such as with plain film X-ray, can be completed quickly, although less commonly used in the era of computed tomography and magnetic resonance imaging. Nonspecific findings such as diffuse ileus and a left upper abdominal "sentinel loop" of bowel may be observed. In chronic pancreatitis, calcifications may also be observed on abdominal X-ray. Chest X-ray may demonstrate pleural effusions in more severe disease.

Abdominal ultrasound can be a good early study in evaluating a patient with acute pancreatitis. On ultrasound, identification of an enlarged, hypoechoic pancreas is consistent with pancreatitis, although more focal disease may also be identified. Peripancreatic fluid collections identified by ultrasound can also indicate severity of inflammation. During the same imaging study, evaluation of etiology with imaging of the gallbladder and biliary tree can also be completed with about 70% sensitivity [40]. Ultrasound is insufficient in identifying pancreatic necrosis and is unable to view all potential locations where fluid may collect. Thus, while ideal for assessing biliary etiologies of pancreatitis, technical limitations in altrasound studies reduce the overall value for diagnosis and severity assessment.

Computed tomography (CT) is the most valuable imaging modality for determining the diagnosis and severity of acute pancreatitis. All patients scanned for pancreatitis should receive oral and intravenous contrast when safe and follow a CT protocol for optimal visualization of the pancreas [41]. Intravenous contrast is particularly helpful because of the dense vascular network of the pancreas, allowing the identification of pancreatic edema and/or necrosis in areas of abnormal contrast enhancement. CT scan is also accurate in the identification of peripancreatic fluid collections. While imaging studies may aid in early diagnosis, CT scan of the pancreas should be delayed to 48–72 h after onset of symptoms. Earlier scans can miss developing complications such as pancreatic necrosis that takes up to 4 days to develop, so an early normal scan may be falsely reassuring. After a week of hospitalization with persistent organ failure or worsening clinical condition, repeat CT scan may be appropriate to reassess severity of disease. CT scans can also be completed without the use of intravenous contrast in patients with renal insufficiency; however, such a study would be severely limited in the evaluation of pancreatic edema or necrosis.

While not yet a standard imaging modality in the evaluation of pancreatitis, magnetic resonance imaging (MRI) of the pancreas is becoming more available. Magnetic resonance cholangiopancreatography (MRCP) is the most commonly used of magnetic resonance technology in the evaluation of pancreatic disease. MRI with gadolinium can identify pancreatic necrosis with similar accuracy to CT images [42]. Gadolinium contrast used with MRI is a less nephrotoxic agent compared with the iodinated contrasts used with CT imaging and MRI does not expose patients to the high levels of radiation from the CT scanner. Additionally, some studies have found that MRI may be better than CT at assessing peripancreatic fluid collections [43]. Diffusion-weighted imaging (DWI) is a newer MRI protocol that can be applied to patients with pancreatitis. DWI of the abdomen has been found to be equivalent to contrast-enhanced CT imaging in the ability to detect acute pancreatitis [44]. Limitations of MRI include resource availability, time required for the study and patient participation. Thus, CT remains the primary imaging modality for the evaluation of pancreatitis, although as technological advances in MRI continue, magnetic resonance techniques may become more widely utilized.

Prognostication

Even prior to the confirmation of diagnosis, the early management of suspected acute pancreatitis should include prognostication of severity. As the disease course of pancreatitis can be unpredictable, the prognostication of the severity of disease is paramount. For patients with pancreatitis accompanied with significant gastrointestinal bleeding, hypoxia, alteration of mental status, hypotension, tachycardia, or other signs of multiple organ failure, immediate triage to an intensive care unit is appropriate.

In acute pancreatitis, patients are stratified into one of two groups: mild acute pancreatitis and severe acute pancreatitis, as defined by the 1992 Atlanta classification (Table 23.1) [45]. The majority of patients experience mild acute pancreatitis, which tends to follow a benign course of disease over a few days with mortality in less than 3% of patients. In mild pancreatitis, there is interstitial inflammation of the pancreas without necrosis and patients are without distant organ failure. In the 15–20% of patients who experience severe acute pancreatitis, their disease is characterized by severe local inflammation as well as systemic effects, frequently leading to a more complicated and prolonged disease course. By Atlanta classification, those with severe acute pancreatitis have a Ranson score of 3 or more or an Acute Physiology and Chronic Health Evaluation II (APACHE II) score of 8 or more and have signs of organ failure and/or local pancreatic complications. Organ failure is defined as shock (systolic blood pressure <90 mmHg), pulmonary insufficiency (PaO$_2$ <60 mmHg), renal failure (serum creatinine >2 mg/dL), or gastrointestinal bleeding (>500 mL blood loss within 24 h). Local pancreatic complications are defined as having the presence of pseudocyst, abscess, or >30% or more than 3 cm of pancreatic necrosis. While the Atlanta classification uses specific terms to differentiate severe versus mild disease, there still is disagreement in defining severe acute pancreatitis due to terms that are frequently used to describe pancreatic disease that had not been included in the classification. Studies conducted prior to 1992 did not utilize this classification and thus, patients in these studies who were categorized as having severe disease may not have the same disease considered severe in more modern times. Confusion also exists over the utilization of terms not defined by Atlanta classification, such as pancreatic phlegmon, which typically is a description of a complication due to more severe disease. Atlanta classification also does not differentiate between sterile versus infected necrosis. Finally, since 1992, there is greater understanding in organ dysfunction in pancreatitis and some groups recommend that transient organ failure that resolves within 48 h should not be considered an indicator of severe acute pancreatitis [46].

Table 23.1 1992 Atlanta classification

Severe acute pancreatitis as defined by presence of one or more of the following:

1. Ranson score: ≥3
2. APACHE II score: ≥8
3. Presence of one or more organ failures
4. Presence of one or more local complications

Organ failure, defined as:

A. Shock: systolic blood pressure <90 mmHg
B. Pulmonary insufficiency: PaO$_2$ <60 mmHg on room air
C. Renal failure: serum creatinine >2 mg/dL after fluid resuscitation
D. Gastrointestinal bleeding: blood loss >500 mL over 24 h
E. Coagulopathy: thrombocytopenia, hypofibrinogenemia, presence of fibrin split products in plasma
F. Severe hypocalcemia: serum calcium ≤7.5 mg/dL

Local complications, defined as:

A. Pancreatic necrosis
B. Pancreatic abscess
C. Pancreatic pseudocyst

Table 23.2 Ranson's criteria

At admission
Age: >55 years old
WBC: >16,000/µL
Glucose: >200 mg/dL
LDH: >350 U/L
SGOT (AST): >250 U/L
At 48 h
Calcium: <8 mg/dL
BUN change: >1.8 mmol/L (5 mg/dL)
Hct fall: >10%
Base deficit: >4 mEq/L
PaO$_2$: <60 mmHg
Fluid seq: >6 L

While Atlanta classifications sets the ground work for categorizing patients within the two categories of severity in acute pancreatitis, there is still the task of predicting patients into one of the two disease courses. Ranson's criteria is the most well-known strategy for predicting the severity of acute pancreatitis (Table 23.2). John H. Ranson's original study was conducted between 1971 and 1972 and included 100 consecutive patients with acute pancreatitis at New York University Medical Center and Bellevue Hospital [7]. Forty-three objective findings were measured and recorded during the first 48 h of admission. These 100 patients were stratified into three groups: those who died, those who were "seriously ill" (≥7 days in the intensive care unit), and those who were without significant serious illness. From these data, Ranson identified 11 prognostic factors that predicted severe disease with 5 measured at admission and 6 measured within 48 h of admission. In the study, the presence of 3 or more positive signs was more consistent with severe disease, which included those patients that either died or were "seriously ill." At the time of the study, the sensitivity of predicting severe disease was 65% with a specificity of 99%. Although Ranson's criteria is more than 35 years old, it still is frequently used in discussion of severity of acute pancreatitis. Following Ranson's criteria, a number of similar scoring systems were developed with similar criteria and organization. These scores are easily applied to patients based on common clinical and biochemical parameters. However, there are a number of limitations to Ranson's criteria. Since it depends on parameters measured at admission and at 48 h, it is unable to evaluate severity of disease immediately at admission or later in a patient's hospital course. With the use of Ranson's criteria in present day, there is a high false positive rate with Ranson's parameter cutoffs. A recent meta-analysis found that Ranson's criteria has a sensitivity closer to 75%, a specificity of 77%, a low positive predictive value of 49%, and a high negative predictive value of 91% [47]. With such a high negative predictive value, it may be more appropriate to utilize a low Ranson's score in the predication of a benign hospital course in acute pancreatitis. Recently, preliminary data for a revision of the Ranson's criteria was presented at the 2012 American College of Surgeons Clinical Congress by our group.

As Ranson's criteria can only be applied within the first 48 h of admission, other severity scores, such as the APACHE II score, are used to follow changes in severity later in the hospital course. The APACHE II score was originally developed to stratify a broad range of critically ill patients [48]. Severe disease in pancreatitis presents similarly to severe disease by other mechanisms such as sepsis, being accompanied with multi-organ dysfunction. Thus, the APACHE II score has become a powerful tool in the assessment of severity in acute pancreatitis. The APACHE II score consists of 12 physiologic and biochemical measures, including temperature, mean arterial pressure, heart rate, respiratory rate, alveolar-to-arterial oxygen gradient, pH, sodium concentration, potassium concentration, creatinine, hematocrit, white blood cell count, and Glasgow coma score. While different cutoffs may be used to assess severity, typically, APACHE II scores greater than 7 indicate more severe disease with sensitivities ranging from 65% to 76% and specificities ranging from 76% to 84% [47]. The greatest utility in using the APACHE II score is being able to regularly reevaluate clinically ill pancreatitis patients to assess improvement or worsening of a patient's condition.

Newer prognosis scores have included parameters such as presence of obesity, lung findings, and hemoconcentration. Obesity, defined as a body mass index (BMI) >30 kg/m², has been found to be associated with higher risk of severe acute pancreatitis [49]. It is thought that obesity affects the immune response to injury as these patients tend to have elevated levels of several pro-inflammatory cytokines [50–52]. Severity

scores such as the modified APACHE II (APACHE-O) and Panc 3 have included obesity as a prognostic factor. Chest X-ray findings of pleural effusions have been strongly linked to severe acute pancreatitis. A study in 1997 found that 84% of patients with severe acute pancreatitis had pleural effusions by chest X-ray, compared to 9% of patients with mild acute pancreatitis [53]. Further, a study of 143 patients with acute pancreatitis evaluated the use of identification of pleural effusion by ultrasound, reporting greater accuracy in predicting severe disease with the determination of pleural effusion alone, compared to Ranson's criteria or APACHE II [54]. Hemoconcentration is another marker of more severe disease. Hemoconcentration is the increased concentration of blood cells, which may be due to decreased fluid volume in the veins and arteries. This may occur due to extravasation of fluid out of the vasculature and into the interstitial space, secondary to systemic inflammation. While hemoconcentration at admission has low sensitivity, ranging from 34% to 74%, persistent hemoconcentration after fluid resuscitation at 24 h after admission can predict severe acute pancreatitis with sensitivities of 91–94% [55, 56].

In the last few years, a number of simpler approaches to prognostic scoring have been developed that do not require complicated calculations or the measurement of 11 or 12 clinical parameters. The Panc 3 score, published in 2007, uses only 3 widely available clinical variables for the prediction of severe acute pancreatitis [57]. This scoring system evaluates the presence of a hematocrit >44%, BMI >30 kg/m², and pleural effusions on chest X-ray at initial presentation. While signs of hemoconcentration was found to be the most predictive of severe disease in this study, having all three prognostic factors was associated with a >90% likelihood of developing severe acute pancreatitis. In 2008, the Bedside Index for Severity in Acute Pancreatitis (BISAP) score was published, which included 5 clinical parameters that are measured within the first 24 h of admission [58]. The BISAP score was derived from 17,992 cases of acute pancreatitis from 212 hospitals between the years 2000 and 2001. The scoring system was then validated on data from 18,256 cases of acute pancreatitis from 177 hospitals between 2004 and 2005. Conveniently, the name BISAP stands for the five parameters that were found to predict in-hospital mortality, which include BUN >25 mg/dL, impaired mental status, presence of systemic inflammatory response syndrome (SIRS) (>2 criteria), age >60 years, and the presence of a pleural effusion. With the presence of all 5 parameters, the likelihood of mortality was found to be approximately 20%, while 4 parameters was approximately 10%, 3 parameters was approximately 5%, 2 parameters 2%, and 0 or 1 parameters was less than 1% [58].

In 2009, another simple scoring system was published, but taking an alternative approach to how severity assessment in acute pancreatitis is typically thought about. Rather than predicting patients who will have a severe disease course, the Harmless Acute Pancreatitis Score (HAPS) predicts those patients who will have a benign course of pancreatitis [59]. Similar to the Panc 3 score, HAPS limits the number of prognostic parameters to predict a non-severe course: no rebound tenderness and/or guarding, normal hematocrit level, and normal serum creatinine level. With the presence of all three parameters for mild disease, the investigators found a 98% accuracy in identifying patients who would not require management at an intensive care unit level of care.

A number of individual laboratory tests have been evaluated to assess severity of disease due to inflammation of the pancreas. C-reactive protein (CRP) is widely available and should be part of the standard laboratory tests in the evaluation of acute pancreatitis. CRP is an acute phase reactant produced in the liver in response to elevations in the plasma concentration of interleukin-6 (IL-6). While serum CRP measured at admission does not predict severity well with a sensitivity of only 38%, serum CRP is best at 48 h with a sensitivity of 86% and a specificity of 61% [60]. Currently, CRP is the best individual biochemical marker as a predictor of severity in pancreatitis. Trypsinogen activation peptide (TAP) is another such biochemical marker that may be measured in serum or urine with commercially available enzyme-linked immunosorbent assay (ELISA) tests for the prediction of severe acute pancreatitis. TAP is produced as a side product during the activation of the pancreatic pre-enzyme trypsinogen to the enzyme trypsin. Urine TAP tests tend to have lower sensitivity in the 50–60% range, but specificity in the 70–80% range. Serum TAP tests tend to have higher sensitivities in the 70–90% range with specificities in the 60–70% range, varying based on different cutoffs [60]. Procalcitonin is a marker of inflammation which has been found to be useful in evaluating the likelihood of progression to severe acute pancreatitis [61]. Within the first 24 h of admission, measurement of procalcitonin has a sensitivity of 92% and a specificity of 84%. A rapid dipstick test is available that can measure levels greater than 0.5 ng/mL. This test for procalcitonin has great potential in the future for the prediction of severe acute pancreatitis given its high sensitivity and specificity and ability to produce rapid results. Measurements of serum cytokines, produced by inflammatory cells in acute pancreatitis, are another group of laboratory tests that may be used to assess severity of disease. The most studied serum cytokine in the prognostication of acute pancreatitis is IL-6 with sensitivities ranging from 70% to 100% and specificities ranging from 67% to 92% [60]. Other cytokines, such as interleukin-8 (IL-8) and interleukin-1 (IL-1), have also been evaluated, although the variability in study designs make it difficult to compare the use of one cytokine measurement from another. Measurement of serum IL-6 has the greatest potential in

becoming a more frequently used biochemical test in the assessment of severity of acute pancreatitis.

Contrast-enhanced CT scans with pancreatic protocol have become a standard tool in the evaluation of severe acute pancreatitis. The relatively quick completion of studies, wide availability, and ease of interpretation make CT scans of the pancreas an ideal study in the assessment of severify. Patients should be evaluated by CT scan at least 48 h after admission as radiographic signs of severe acute pancreatitis, such as with pancreatic necrosis, may not develop until a few days after initial admission. CT scan of the pancreas should be scored by the CT severity index, which was developed by Emil Balthazar et al. at New York University Medical Center in the late 1980s [62]. Over the past 20 years, this scoring system has held as a reliable means of assessing severity. The CT severity index is a combination of Balthazar grade, which evaluates the presence of pancreatic edema and peripancreatic fluid collections, and necrosis points, which classifies the degree of pancreatic necrosis. While a CT severity index of 0–3 points is associated with low mortality of 0–3%, with a CT severity index of 7–10 points, mortality ranges from 13% to 17% [62, 63]. Notably, the presence of significant necrosis is a poor prognostic sign in acute pancreatitis and tends to be associated with organ failure and worse outcomes. While most clinical and biochemical measures in evaluating severity of acute pancreatitis only give prognostic information, CT scan can not only help predict hospital course, but can also direct immediate management if significant pancreatic necrosis is present.

While not yet standard practice, MRI can be used to characterize pancreatic inflammation, peripancreatic fluid collections, and degree of pancreatic necrosis, much like CT [43]. Studies have found close correlation between CT severity index and MR severity index in acute pancreatitis, even when the two scans are conducted on an individual patient one day apart [64]. The benefits of MRI include less nephrotoxicity with gadolinium contrast when compared to iodinated contrast, no exposure to radiation, and better characterization of pancreatic ductal anatomy. MRI technology may be particularly useful in children, as most clinicians defer CT scans due to concerns of radiation exposure. However, MRI in the pediatric population often requires sedation for adequate quality images. MRI, is also limited by a number of other factors, such as lengthy process in acquiring a scan, limited hospital resources, and local expertise in performing and interpreting less commonly utilized MRI protocols.

Management

Accompanying severity assessment and triage (Fig. 23.1a, b), fluid resuscitation should be started immediately for any patient with pancreatitis to prevent hypovolemia and associated complications. In acute pancreatitis, an array of inflammatory mediators are released into the circulation, leading to increased vascular permeability, resulting in fluid collecting outside in the interstitial space as well as peritoneal and pleural cavities. Fluid resuscitation may help prevent cardiovascular collapse, pre-renal azotemia, as well as improve blood flow to the pancreatic microcirculation. Crystalloid fluids, such as normal saline or Lactated Ringer's solution, are typically delivered at rates ranging from 250 to 1,000 mL per hour, depending on the clinical scenario. While the optimal volume of intravenous fluids to be delivered has yet to be determined, the importance of aggressive fluid resuscitation, evaluated by timely resolution of hemoconcentration, has been well studied. Urine output of at least 0.5 mL/kg body weight per hour and resolution of hemoconcentration can be monitored as measures of adequate fluid resuscitation. During aggressive fluid delivery, patients should be closely monitored with regular lung exams, especially in more vulnerable patients with preexisting cardiac or pulmonary dysfunction. Patients with persistent hemoconcentration as identified on the complete blood count after 24 h of fluid delivery may require closer monitoring as these patients may be at greater risk of developing severe acute pancreatitis [65].

Pain management should be implemented along with fluid resuscitation in acute pancreatitis. Severe pain is often one of the primary complaints, due to the rich afferent sensory network surrounding the pancreas, primarily in the celiac plexus. With severe nausea, oral pain medications are often not well tolerated. Parenteral analgesia with morphine, hydromorphone, or other narcotics is most commonly used in acute pancreatitis for controlling pain. Morphine had been avoided in the past due to concerns of sphincter of Oddi spasm, which is thought to exacerbate pancreatitis, but these concerns are unfounded. With severe pain requiring frequent dosing of parenteral medications, patient-controlled analgesia may be appropriate. Increasing dosages and more frequent administration may be required for adequate relief. In cases of very severe pain, resistant to parenteral analgesia, epidural analgesia can considered [66].

In acute pancreatitis, mild hypoxia may occur and require supplemental oxygen. The disease course can be complicated by severe diffuse respiratory disease such as acute lung injury and acute respiratory distress syndrome, complications associated with mortality rates as high as 30%. These processes are largely mediated by inflammatory leukocytes and the production of cytokines like tumor necrosis factor-alpha (TNF-α) and chemokines like monocyte chemoattractant protein-1 (MCP-1). Severe inflammation in the lung parenchyma results in microvascular injury and alveolar damage. Clinically, the nearby inflammation of the pancreas and the local cellular driven inflammatory response within the lungs may result in pleural effusions and acute respiratory distress syndrome. In cases of severe acute pancreatitis, arterial blood gas measurement as well as continuous pulse oximetry may aid management. With persistent hypoxia and respiratory compromise, intubation and mechanical ventilation may be necessary. Elderly patents and those with preexisting respiratory disease should have respiratory status monitored closely as these patients are at greatest risk of more significant respiratory complications.

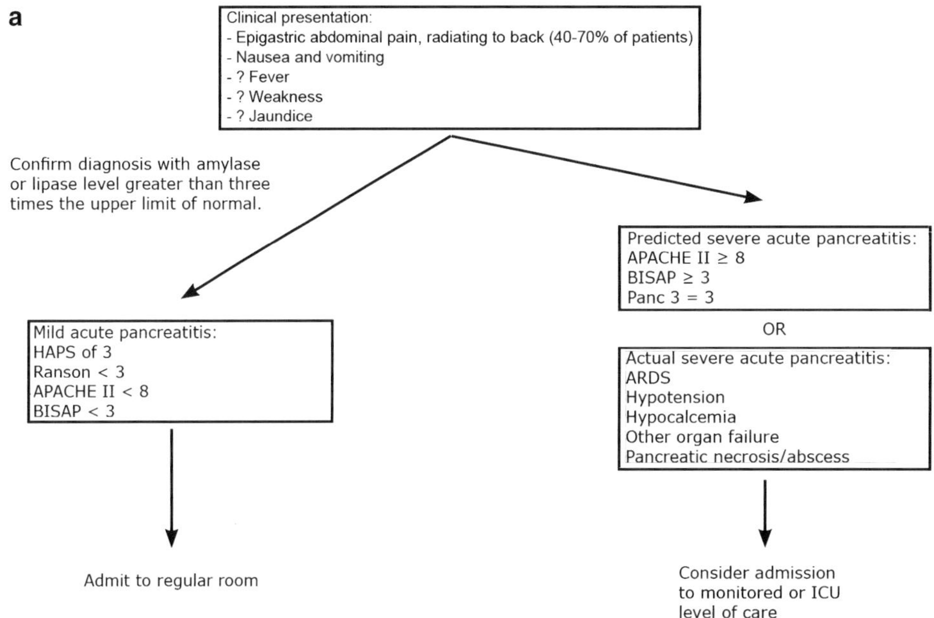

Fig. 23.1 Pancreatitis protocol. (**a**) Triage strategy for patients with acute pancreatitis. (**b**) Full algorithm for treatment of pancreatitis

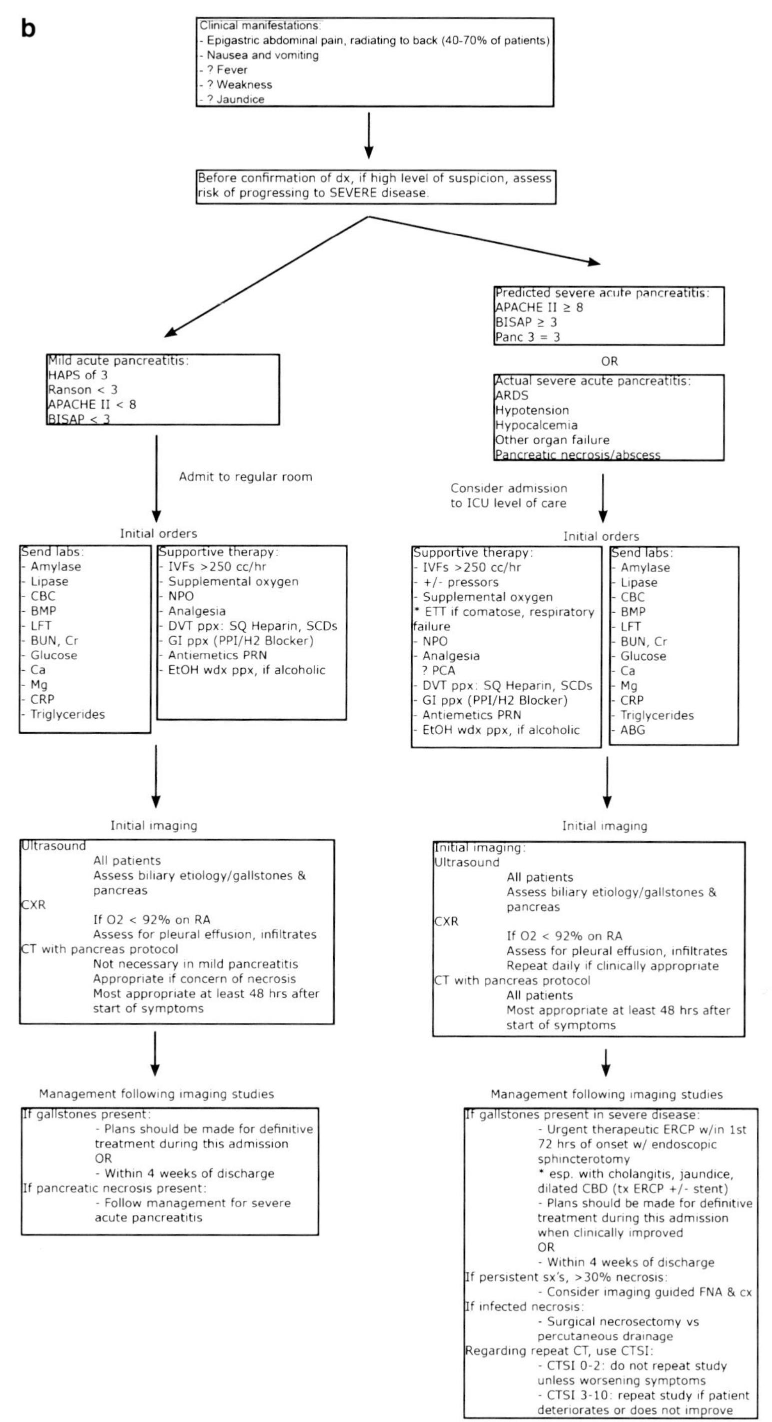

Fig. 23.1 (continued)

With the immense fluid requirements and considerable fluid shifts occurring during resuscitation in acute pancreatitis, electrolyte and metabolic disturbances may be commonly identified on the blood chemistry tests. Alterations in potassium, phosphate, and magnesium should be corrected with oral or parenteral supplementation. Hypocalcemia may occur and usually does not require correction, unless calculated free calcium levels are low or clinical signs of hypocalcemia are observed. Hyperglycemia in acute pancreatitis is common, and may require temporary administration of an insulin sliding-scale while the patient is admitted with the goal of maintaining blood glucose within the 100–200 mg/dL range.

Hypertriglyceridemia (<500 mg/dL) is also common in acute pancreatitis, occurring in approximately 20% of patients. In cases of severe hypertriglyceridemia (>1,000 mg/dL), plasmapheresis can quickly reduce serum levels.

Nutrition is important in acute pancreatitis, especially when patients have not been eating for a few days. Most patients at admission are ordered for nothing by mouth, due to nausea, vomiting, and poor oral tolerance. In mild acute pancreatitis with a short hospital course, patients may resume a normal diet once nausea resolves. For patients who are unable to tolerate oral nutrition for over 7 days, artificial feeding should be considered. Recently, there has been a trend away from total parenteral nutrition (TPN) to enteral feeding by naso-jejunal tube. TPN had been originally standard care as it was thought to reduce stimulation of the pancreas. However, there is no good evidence that such strategies of pancreatic rest reduce organ failure or other complications. Additionally, nutrition by TPN has the additionally risks of catheter-related infections and severe hyperglycemia. In cases of persistent ileus, TPN may be a practical solution to delivering nutrition, when any enteral nutrition would be poorly tolerated. Recent studies have shown benefit in enteral feeding over TPN, in reducing complications and lowering costs [67]. Enteral feeding has the additional benefit of maintaining gastrointestinal immunity. A naso-jejunal tube should be placed to feed distal to the ligament of Treitz. Some studies have found nasogastric feeding to be safe [68], although there may be increased pulmonary complications when compared to more distal feeding [69]. Currently, there is limited data regarding the type of enteral diet that should be delivered in acute pancreatitis, although elemental diets are often used with the thought of minimizing pancreatic stimulation.

In severe acute pancreatitis, there is often concern of infected pancreatic necrosis versus sterile pancreatic necrosis, with the former being associated with high mortality as high as 40% (Fig. 23.2). With infected pancreatic necrosis, broad antibiotic coverage should cover the endogenous gastrointestinal flora, which would be the most likely source of bacterial infection. A related topic that is frequently discussed is the role of prophylactic antibiotics in acute pancreatitis. Consideration of prophylactic antibiotics should be reserved only for acute pancreatitis with evidence of extensive pancreatic necrosis. The risk of infected necrosis tends to be low when pancreatic necrosis is limited to less than a third of the pancreas. Most studies show no significant benefit with the use of prophylactic antibiotics [70]. Thus, it is not recommended to prophylactically start patients on antibiotics for acute pancreatitis.

Acute need for operative management in pancreatitis is infrequently required, but can be life saving in carefully selected cases. Patients with mild acute pancreatitis typically only need to be managed conservatively. Selected cases

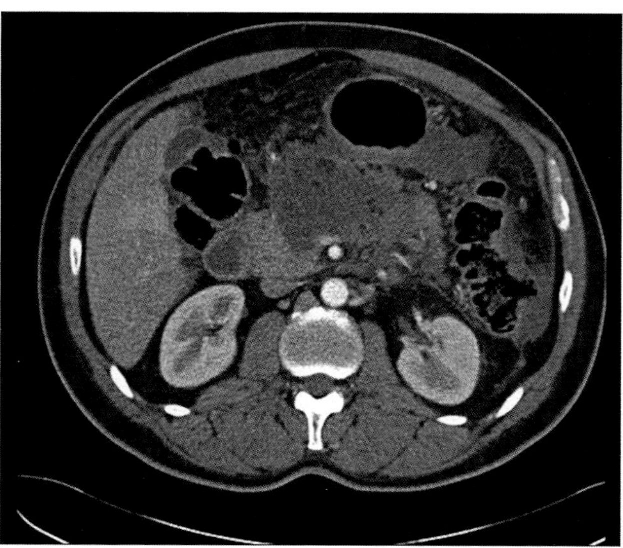

Fig. 23.2 Pancreatic necrosis with areas of poor enhancement and heterogeneity. Notably, the pancreatic head appears intact

requiring operative management tend to be limited to gallstone pancreatitis or severe acute pancreatitis complicated by infected necrosis.

In gallstone pancreatitis, operative management is reserved for cases where the causative gallstone is found to remain in the biliary tract during active disease or following a bout of acute gallstone pancreatitis with an elective cholecystectomy. In most cases of gallstone or biliary pancreatitis, the causative gallstone has usually passed through the common bile duct and into the duodenum. Some patients, however, may still have one or more gallstones in the common bile duct. In these circumstances, removal of the gallstone is appropriate, especially if disease is complicated by cholangitis. Therapy may be completed with ERCP, followed by sphincterotomy, although surgical management may be necessary if these less invasive endoscopic approaches fail. In cases of mild, uncomplicated pancreatitis associated with gallstones, (less than Balthazar Grade C) laparoscopic cholecystectomy is appropriate once symptoms resolve or within 2 weeks of discharge. Failure to complete cholecystectomy puts the patient at risk of recurrent pancreatitis.

In severe acute pancreatitis complicated by infected pancreatic necrosis, intervention to remove necrotic tissue, which serves as a nidus for further infection, is usually necessary. Diagnosis of infected necrosis can be made by radiology with the identification of air or gas within the pancreatic necrotic collections or by a fine needle aspiration with evaluation of necrotic tissue. CT or ultrasound-guided fine needle aspiration should be performed in patients with greater than 30% pancreatic necrosis with clinical suspicion of sepsis and aspirate samples should be sent for gram stain and culture. In cases of severe acute pancreatitis complicated by sterile

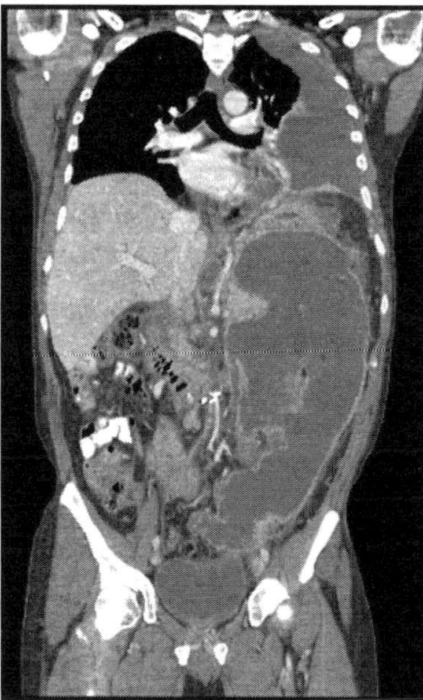

Fig. 23.3 Complicated pancreatic pseudocyst with extension to the pelvis and *left*-sided pleural effusion

pancreatic necrosis, surgical debridement and drainage is typically not required. However, patients with infected necrosis do require debridement or drainage, which can be approached endoscopically, radiologically, or surgically. Endoscopic drainage has become more common, involving placement of stents, frequently transgastrically, to drain of necrotic fluid into the gastrointestinal tract. Radiological drainage may also be appropriate with softened or liquefied pancreatic abscess, although, like with endoscopic drainage, there is a high rate of failure due to obstruction of drainage by solid necrotic debris. Success of radiological drainage ranges from 30% to 50% [71, 72]. Surgical debridement may be preferred, in addition to drainage, thorough debridement of necrotic tissue while leaving viable pancreatic tissue can be performed. The abdomen can be closed over drains, packed and left open, or closed over drains with pancreatic irrigation. These decisions depend largely on clinically derived experience, local expertise, and considerations regarding the patient anatomy and condition.

Over time, sterile pancreatic necrosis may evolve into a collection of pancreatic debris. Pancreatic necrosis can become walled off with the formation of a fibrotic capsule, much like a pseudocyst. If this walled-off necrosis contains purely liquid contents, endoscopic drainage may be possible; however, with any solid debris, surgical drainage by laparotomy or a laparoscopic approach may be taken.

Pseudocysts are collections of pancreatic fluid over time that can form a non-epithelial fibrous lining (Fig. 23.3). These typically develop following disruption of the pancreatic duct in pancreatitis. While many of these fluid col-

lections resolve spontaneously, others may persist and cause symptoms. Small pseudocysts, typically less than 6 cm in diameter, can be managed conservatively, especially if asymptomatic. Larger pseudocysts should be evaluated with CT, MRI, or endoscopic ultrasound to assess pseudocyst contents and potentially evaluate for a means of drainage. Persistent pseudocyst causing pain or obstructive symptoms should be drained. Drainage procedures should be performed after the pseudocyst has a well-developed lining or after 6 weeks following formation of the pseudocyst. If pseudocysts are without pancreatic debris, transgastric endoscopic stenting may relieve symptoms, although drainage may fail if debris occludes the stents. Open and laparoscopic procedures may be preferred, but specific technique and approach depends on patient-specific anatomy and disease. During operative drainage procedures, biopsy of pancreatic pseudocyst wall should be completed and sent to pathology for exclusion of cystic neoplasm of the pancreas.

Potential Complications

The major complications in acute pancreatitis are classically described by a bimodal distribution with separate peaks during the first and second weeks of the disease course. This distribution in pancreatitis has changed over the past 30 years with improvements in critical care madicine and monitoring. Within the first week, severe pancreatitis may be characterized by a significant rise in serum cytokines, which clinically results in systemic inflammatory response syndrome (SIRS) and distant organ dysfunction. Organ dysfunction often resolves within 48 h, although for other patients with persistent organ failure, they may continue along a poor clinical course.

Pancreatic necrosis and associated complications occur at the end of the first week or later in the second week. In some instances, pancreatic necrosis may be infected, which is thought to be due to translocation of gut bacteria to the pancreas. These patients continue to have severe SIRS, but necrotic pancreatic tissue also serves as a more significant inflammatory nidus.

With the intense inflammation of the pancreas, other acute complications local to the pancreas and the lesser sac occur. Acute fluid collections located in the pancreas or in peripancreatic regions are not uncommon. These often resolve spontaneously or persist and become pseudocysts. Also secondary to nearby inflammation, the splenic vein may develop a thrombus, which rarely can contribute to the development gastric variceal bleeding. Splenic vein thrombosis is relatively common, occurring in up to 19% of patients with acute pancreatitis [73]. However, in most situations no intervention is required. Only patients with history of gastric varices may need further evaluation and treatment.

Later complications following a bout of acute pancreatitis may include pseudocyst, fistula, recurrent pancreatitis, and chronic pain.

Pseudocyst formation, as discussed earlier, occurs by leakage of pancreatic fluid that persists and becomes walled off by non-epithelial layers of fibrous tissue. While some may spontaneously resolve, those that cause nausea, obstructive symptoms, or abdominal pain need to be drained. Pseudocysts may also become further complicated by infection, which require external drainage.

Pancreatic fistulas are abnormal communications between the pancreas and other organs. Fistula often occurs following surgery, such as following necrosectomy or pseudocyst drainage. However, fistula may also occur following pancreatic duct trauma or chronic pancreatitis. Pancreatic fistula often present in the context of abnormally high abdominal drain outputs in the postoperative period. The drain fluid can be sent for amylase or lipase studies to confirm suspicions. Treatment may include dietary restriction, octreotide to reduce secretions, and possibly surgical intervention. With a stable pancreatic fistula, conservative management can result in spontaneous resolution in approximately three-quarters of patients. In patients who have a persistent pancreatic fistula, operation to reroute pancreatic duct drainage with a Roux-en-Y operation or partial pancreatectomy can be performed.

In some patients after a first bout of acute pancreatitis, pancreatitis may recur. In the absence of gallstones or history of alcohol abuse, a more extensive workup is appropriate. Untreated recurrent pancreatitis can lead to chronic pancreatitis, characterized by parenchymal fibrosis and damage to the pancreatic duct. These patients frequently experience chronic pain that may require definitive treatment by pancreatic resection.

Conclusion

In the majority of cases, acute pancreatitis occurs as a single isolated event, not requiring extensive follow-up. For those with mild gallstone pancreatitis (less than Balthazar Grade C), patients should undergo cholecystectomy during the same admission or within 2 weeks of discharge. Patients with alcohol-induced pancreatitis should seriously consider abstinence, which can be aided with joining a substance abuse support group or other formal program. Patients with pancreatitis of unknown etiology may not require follow-up unless symptoms recur. For patients who progress to chronic pancreatitis, regular follow-up may be required for management of chronic pain symptoms and for discussion of potential operative management. Patients with pancreatic fistula may be followed with regular clinic visits in the hopeful anticipation of spontaneous resolution.

References

1. Vege SS, Yadav D, Chari ST. Pancreatitis. In: Talley NJ, Locke GR, Saito YA, editors. GI epidemiology. 1st ed. Malden, MA: Wiley-Blackwell; 2007.
2. Hall MJ, DeFrances CJ, Williams SN, Golosinskiy A, Schwartzman A. National Hospital Discharge Survey: 2007 summary. Natl Health Stat Rep. 2010;29:1–20, 24.
3. Hall MJ, Owings MF. 2000 National Hospital Discharge Survey. Adv Data. 2002;329:1–18.
4. Lankisch PG, Schirren CA, Kunze E. Undetected fatal acute pancreatitis: why is the disease so frequently overlooked? Am J Gastroenterol. 1991;86(3):322–6.
5. Fagenholz PJ, Fernandez-del Castillo C, Harris NS, Pelletier AJ, Camargo Jr CA. Direct medical costs of acute pancreatitis hospitalizations in the United States. Pancreas. 2007;35(4):302–7.
6. Taylor RA. The aetiology, pathology, diagnosis and treatment of acute pancreatitis; a review of 110 cases. Ann R Coll Surg Engl. 1949;5(4):213–39.
7. Ranson JH, Rifkind KM, Roses DF, Fink SD, Eng K, Spencer FC. Prognostic signs and the role of operative management in acute pancreatitis. Surg Gynecol Obstet. 1974;139(1):69–81.
8. Cavallini G, Frulloni L, Bassi C, et al. Prospective multicentre survey on acute pancreatitis in Italy (ProInf-AISP): results on 1005 patients. Dig Liver Dis. 2004;36(3):205–11.
9. Harrison DA, D'Amico G, Singer M. The Pancreatitis Outcome Prediction (POP) Score: a new prognostic index for patients with severe acute pancreatitis. Crit Care Med. 2007;35(7):1703–8.
10. Li X-Y, Wang X-B, Liu X-F, Li S-G. Prevalence and risk factors of organ failure in patients with severe acute pancreatitis. World J Emerg Med. 2010;1(3):201–4.
11. Shaheen MA, Akhtar AJ. Organ failure associated with acute pancreatitis in African-American and Hispanic patients. J Natl Med Assoc. 2007;99(12):1402–6.
12. Halonen KI, Pettila V, Leppaniemi AK, Kemppainen EA, Puolakkainen PA, Haapiainen RK. Multiple organ dysfunction associated with severe acute pancreatitis. Crit Care Med. 2002;30(6):1274–9.
13. Lytras D, Manes K, Triantopoulou C, et al. Persistent early organ failure: defining the high-risk group of patients with severe acute pancreatitis? Pancreas. 2008;36(3):249–54.
14. Gloor B, Muller CA, Worni M, Martignoni ME, Uhl W, Buchler MW. Late mortality in patients with severe acute pancreatitis. Br J Surg. 2001;88(7):975–9.
15. Warshaw AL. Pancreatic necrosis: to debride or not to debride-that is the question. Ann Surg. 2000;232(5):627–9.
16. Kingsnorth A, O'Reilly D. Acute pancreatitis. BMJ. 2006;332(7549):1072–6.
17. Whitcomb DC. Clinical practice. Acute pancreatitis. N Engl J Med. 2006;354(20):2142–50.
18. Moreau JA, Zinsmeister AR, Melton 3rd LJ, DiMagno EP. Gallstone pancreatitis and the effect of cholecystectomy: a population-based cohort study. Mayo Clin Proc. 1988;63(5):466–73.
19. Frey CF, Zhou H, Harvey DJ, White RH. The incidence and case-fatality rates of acute biliary, alcoholic, and idiopathic pancreatitis in California, 1994–2001. Pancreas. 2006;33(4):336–44.
20. Chwistek M, Roberts I, Amoateng-Adjepong Y. Gallstone pancreatitis: a community teaching hospital experience. J Clin Gastroenterol. 2001;33(1):41–4.
21. Shaffer EA. Gallstone disease: epidemiology of gallbladder stone disease. Best Pract Res Clin Gastroenterol. 2006;20(6):981–96.
22. Lankisch PG, Lowenfels AB, Maisonneuve P. What is the risk of alcoholic pancreatitis in heavy drinkers? Pancreas. 2002;25(4):411–2.
23. Cotton PB. Congenital anomaly of pancreas divisum as cause of obstructive pain and pancreatitis. Gut. 1980;21(2):105–14.

24. Gregg JA. Pancreas divisum: its association with pancreatitis. Am J Surg. 1977;134(5):539–43.
25. Yedlin ST, Dubois RS, Philippart AI. Pancreas divisum: a cause of pancreatitis in childhood. J Pediatr Surg. 1984;19(6):793–4.
26. Pieper-Bigelow C, Strocchi A, Levitt MD. Where does serum amylase come from and where does it go? Gastroenterol Clin North Am. 1990;19(4):793–810.
27. Wang P, Li ZS, Liu F, et al. Risk factors for ERCP-related complications: a prospective multicenter study. Am J Gastroenterol. 2009;104(1):31–40.
28. Cheon YK, Cho KB, Watkins JL, et al. Frequency and severity of post-ERCP pancreatitis correlated with extent of pancreatic ductal opacification. Gastrointest Endosc. 2007;65(3):385–93.
29. Chan HH, Lai KH, Lin CK, et al. Effect of somatostatin in the prevention of pancreatic complications after endoscopic retrograde cholangiopancreatography. J Chin Med Assoc. 2008;71(12):605–9.
30. Woods KE, Willingham FF. Endoscopic retrograde cholangiopancreatography associated pancreatitis: a 15-year review. World J Gastrointest Endosc. 2010;2(5):165–78.
31. Barkay O, Niv E, Santo E, Bruck R, Hallak A, Konikoff FM. Low-dose heparin for the prevention of post-ERCP pancreatitis: a randomized placebo-controlled trial. Surg Endosc. 2008;22(9):1971–6.
32. Singh P, Das A, Isenberg G, et al. Does prophylactic pancreatic stent placement reduce the risk of post-ERCP acute pancreatitis? A meta-analysis of controlled trials. Gastrointest Endosc. 2004;60(4):544–50.
33. Werth B, Kuhn M, Hartmann K, Reinhart WH. Drug-induced pancreatitis: experience of the Swiss Drug Adverse Effects Center (SANZ) 1981–1993. Schweiz Med Wochenschr. 1995;125(15):731–4.
34. Yoshida K, Toki F, Takeuchi T, Watanabe S, Shiratori K, Hayashi N. Chronic pancreatitis caused by an autoimmune abnormality. Proposal of the concept of autoimmune pancreatitis. Dig Dis Sci. 1995;40(7):1561–8.
35. Nishimori I, Tamakoshi A, Otsuki M. Prevalence of autoimmune pancreatitis in Japan from a nationwide survey in 2002. J Gastroenterol. 2007;42 Suppl 18:6–8.
36. Whitcomb DC, Gorry MC, Preston RA, et al. Hereditary pancreatitis is caused by a mutation in the cationic trypsinogen gene. Nat Genet. 1996;14(2):141–5.
37. Ventrucci M, Pezzilli R, Gullo L, Plate L, Sprovieri G, Barbara L. Role of serum pancreatic enzyme assays in diagnosis of pancreatic disease. Dig Dis Sci. 1989;34(1):39–45.
38. Gumaste VV, Roditis N, Mehta D, Dave PB. Serum lipase levels in nonpancreatic abdominal pain versus acute pancreatitis. Am J Gastroenterol. 1993;88(12):2051–5.
39. Yadav D, Agarwal N, Pitchumoni CS. A critical evaluation of laboratory tests in acute pancreatitis. Am J Gastroenterol. 2002;97(6):1309–18.
40. Wang SS, Lin XZ, Tsai YT, et al. Clinical significance of ultrasonography, computed tomography, and biochemical tests in the rapid diagnosis of gallstone-related pancreatitis: a prospective study. Pancreas. 1988;3(2):153–8.
41. Megibow AJ. CTA solidifies role in the evaluation of pancreatic disease. *Applied Radiology*. Dec 2004; Suppl:21–9.
42. Pamuklar E, Semelka RC. MR imaging of the pancreas. Magn Reson Imaging Clin N Am. 2005;13(2):313–30.
43. Morgan DE, Baron TH, Smith JK, Robbin ML, Kenney PJ. Pancreatic fluid collections prior to intervention: evaluation with MR imaging compared with CT and US. Radiology. 1997;203(3):773–8.
44. Shinya S, Sasaki T, Nakagawa Y, Guiquing Z, Yamamoto F, Yamashita Y. The efficacy of diffusion-weighted imaging for the detection and evaluation of acute pancreatitis. Hepatogastroenterology. 2009;56(94–95):1407–10.
45. Bradley 3rd EL. A clinically based classification system for acute pancreatitis. Summary of the International Symposium on Acute Pancreatitis, Atlanta, Ga, September 11 through 13, 1992. Arch Surg. 1993;128(5):586–90.
46. Johnson CD, Charnley R, Pancr, Rowlands B, et al. UK Working Party for Acute Pancreatitis. Gut. 2005;54(Suppl 3):iii1–9.
47. Larvin M. Assessment of clinical severity and prognosis. In: Beger H, Warshaw A, Buchler M et al., editors. The pancreas. Oxford: Blackwell Science; 1998. p. 489–502.
48. Knaus WA, Draper EA, Wagner DP, Zimmerman JE. APACHE II: a severity of disease classification system. Crit Care Med. 1985;13(10):818–29.
49. Funnell IC, Bornman PC, Weakley SP, Terblanche J, Marks IN. Obesity: an important prognostic factor in acute pancreatitis. Br J Surg. 1993;80(4):484–6.
50. Lyon CJ, Law RE, Hsueh WA. Minireview: adiposity, inflammation, and atherogenesis. Endocrinology. 2003;144(6):2195–200.
51. Dandona P, Weinstock R, Thusu K, Abdel-Rahman E, Aljada A, Wadden T. Tumor necrosis factor-alpha in sera of obese patients: fall with weight loss. J Clin Endocrinol Metab. 1998;83(8):2907–10.
52. Visser M, Bouter LM, McQuillan GM, Wener MH, Harris TB. Elevated C-reactive protein levels in overweight and obese adults. JAMA. 1999;282(22):2131–5.
53. Heller SJ, Noordhoek E, Tenner SM, et al. Pleural effusion as a predictor of severity in acute pancreatitis. Pancreas. 1997;15(3):222–5.
54. Ocampo C, Silva W, Zandalazini H, Kohan G, Sanchez N, Oria A. Pleural effusion is superior to multiple factor scoring system in predicting acute pancreatitis outcome. Acta Gastroenterol Latinoam. 2008;38(1):34–42.
55. Brown A, Orav J, Banks PA. Hemoconcentration is an early marker for organ failure and necrotizing pancreatitis. Pancreas. 2000;20(4):367–72.
56. Baillargeon JD, Orav J, Ramagopal V, Tenner SM, Banks PA. Hemoconcentration as an early risk factor for necrotizing pancreatitis. Am J Gastroenterol. 1998;93(11):2130–4.
57. Brown A, James-Stevenson T, Dyson T, Grunkenmeier D. The panc 3 score: a rapid and accurate test for predicting severity on presentation in acute pancreatitis. J Clin Gastroenterol. 2007;41(9):855–8.
58. Wu BU, Johannes RS, Sun X, Tabak Y, Conwell DL, Banks PA. The early prediction of mortality in acute pancreatitis: a large population-based study. Gut. 2008;57(12):1698–703.
59. Lankisch PG, Weber-Dany B, Hebel K, Maisonneuve P, Lowenfels AB. The harmless acute pancreatitis score: a clinical algorithm for rapid initial stratification of nonsevere disease. Clin Gastroenterol Hepatol. 2009;7(6):702–5. quiz 607.
60. Rettally CA, Skarda S, Garza MA, Schenker S. The usefulness of laboratory tests in the early assessment of severity of acute pancreatitis. Crit Rev Clin Lab Sci. 2003;40(2):117–49.
61. Rau B, Steinbach G, Gansauge F, Mayer JM, Grunert A, Beger HG. The potential role of procalcitonin and interleukin 8 in the prediction of infected necrosis in acute pancreatitis. Gut. 1997;41(6):832–40.
62. Balthazar EJ, Robinson DL, Megibow AJ, Ranson JH. Acute pancreatitis: value of CT in establishing prognosis. Radiology. 1990;174(2):331–6.
63. Simchuk E, Travers L. Computed tomography severity index is a predictor of outcomes for severe pancreatitis. 86th Annual Meeting of the North Pacific Surgical Association. Vancouver, British Columbia, Canada 1999.
64. Arvanitakis M, Delhaye M, De Maertelaere V, et al. Computed tomography and magnetic resonance imaging in the assessment of acute pancreatitis. Gastroenterology. 2004;126(3):715–23.
65. Brown A, Baillargeon JD, Hughes MD, Banks PA. Can fluid resuscitation prevent pancreatic necrosis in severe acute pancreatitis? Pancreatology. 2002;2(2):104–7.
66. Bernhardt A, Kortgen A, Niesel H, Goertz A. Using epidural anesthesia in patients with acute pancreatitis—prospective study of 121 patients. Anaesthesiol Reanim. 2002;27(1):16–22.

67. Marik PE, Zaloga GP. Meta-analysis of parenteral nutrition versus enteral nutrition in patients with acute pancreatitis. BMJ. 2004;328(7453):1407.

68. Eatock FC, Chong P, Menezes N, et al. A randomized study of early nasogastric versus nasojejunal feeding in severe acute pancreatitis. Am J Gastroenterol. 2005;100(2):432–9.

69. Eckerwall GE, Axelsson JB, Andersson RG. Early nasogastric feeding in predicted severe acute pancreatitis: a clinical, randomized study. Ann Surg. 2006;244(6):959–65. discussion 965–957.

70. Isenmann R, Runzi M, Kron M, et al. Prophylactic antibiotic treatment in patients with predicted severe acute pancreatitis: a placebo-controlled, double-blind trial. Gastroenterology. 2004;126(4): 997–1004.

71. Mithofer K, Mueller PR, Warshaw AL. Interventional and surgical treatment of pancreatic abscess. World J Surg. 1997;21(2):162–8.

72. Freeny PC, Hauptmann E, Althaus SJ, Traverso LW, Sinanan M. Percutaneous CT-guided catheter drainage of infected acute necrotizing pancreatitis: techniques and results. AJR Am J Roentgenol. 1998;170(4):969–75.

73. Mortele KJ, Mergo PJ, Taylor HM, Ernst MD, Ros PR. Splenic and perisplenic involvement in acute pancreatitis: determination of prevalence and morphologic helical CT features. J Comput Assist Tomogr. 2001;25(1):50–4.

Alicia J. Mangram, Alexzandra Hollingworth,
and James K. Dzandu

Introduction

Small bowel obstruction is a common clinical condition that accounts for 20% of all surgical admissions for acute abdomens [1]. Late, misdiagnosis, or even appropriate management of small bowel obstruction has likely been a source of frustration for many practicing general surgeons at some time during their surgical careers. Because of the acute onset of small bowel obstruction the majority of these patients present in the emergency room (ER). Therefore patient evaluation, subsequent operations and management are often performed by the "surgeon on call." With the new paradigm shift regarding the management of surgical emergencies, the majority of patients with small bowel obstruction are now being managed by the Acute Care Surgeon (ACS). The ACS is accustomed to dealing with difficult cases, and operating on a patient with small bowel obstruction is often a complicated procedure. There are multiple issues to address when operating on patients with small bowel obstruction including entering hostile abdomens, enterostomies, fistulas, wound infections, short bowel issues, and recurrent obstructions, just to name a few of the problems. The traditional surgical dictum "the sun should never rise and set on a complete small bowel obstruction" is no longer considered an entirely valid statement. This caveat may be attributed in part to the surgeon's diagnostic ability to differentiate complete obstruction, which could compromise intestine viability, from a partial obstruction, which could be amenable to nonoperative management. Thus in the absence of signs suggesting strangulation, a patient with partial obstruction

can be treated and managed effectively using nonoperative modalities.

Complex patients with multiple medical problems with indeterminate small bowel obstruction are initially observed until deteriorating patient clinical conditions force the hand of the surgeon. The availability of sixty-four-plus slice computed tomography (CT) scans now allows accurate determination of the site and cause of complete obstructions. In addition, there are now national guidelines for the management of small bowel obstruction [2] and each individual surgeon's experience adds needed refinements to this knowledge base.

Epidemiology

Small bowel obstruction is a clinical condition defined as a blockage of the small bowel loops resulting in an impairment, stoppage or reversal of the normal flow of intestinal contents towards the anus. Small bowel obstruction accounts for 20% of all acute surgical admissions [1]. Among acute surgical obstruction admissions, 80% are due to small bowel obstruction and large bowel obstruction accounts for the remaining 20% [3].

The etiology of small bowel obstruction is multifactorial (Table 24.1) and includes three major causes: extraluminal, intrinsic, and intraluminal [4]. Extraluminal obstructions are caused by adhesions, neoplasms, hernias, constricted bands malrotations, and intra-abdominal abscesses.

Adhesions

The most common cause of small bowel obstruction is adhesions, accounting for 60% of all cases. The risk of developing small bowel obstruction secondary to adhesions postoperatively has been estimated to be 9% in the first postoperative year and then increases to 19% by 4 years postoperatively and 35% by 10 years postoperatively [5].

A.J. Mangram, M.D., F.A.C.S. (✉) • A. Hollingworth, M.D.
J.K. Dzandu, Ph.D.
Trauma/Acute Care and Critical Care Services, John C. Lincoln Health Network, 250 East Dunlap Avenue, Phoenix, AZ 85020, USA
e-mail: alicia.mangram@jcl.com; aliworth@yahoo.com;
james.dzandu@jd.com

L.J. Moore et al. (eds.), *Common Problems in Acute Care Surgery*,
DOI 10.1007/978-1-4614-6123-4_24, © Springer Science+Business Media New York 2013

Table 24.1 Causes of small bowel obstruction

Extrinsic lesion	Intrinsic lesion	Obstruction of normal bowel
Adhesions	Intussusception	Gallstones
Hernia	Congenital malformation	Feces or meconium
Volvulus	Neoplasms	Bezoar
Extrinsic neoplasms	Intussuception	Gallstones
Intra-abdominal abscesses	Congenital malformation	Feces or meconium
Aneurism	Neoplasms	Bezoar
Hematomas	Inflammatory strictures	Ascaris infection
Endometriosis	Crohn's disease	Barium

Adapted from [4]

Table 24.2 Association between surgical type or surgical procedure and the incidence of adhesion-induced small bowel obstruction

Procedure type/group	Incidence of SBO
Ileal pouch-anal anastomosis	19.3% (1,018/5,268)
Open colectomy	9.5% (11,491/121,085)
Gynecological procedures	11.1% (4,297/38,752)
• Open anexal surgery	• 23.9%
• After cesarean section	• 0.1%
Cholecystectomy	
• Open	• 7.1%
• Laparoscopy	• 0.2%
Hysterectomy	
• Total hysterectomy	• 15.5%
• Laparoscopy	• 0.0%
Adnexal operations	
• Open	• 23.9%
• Laparoscopy	• 0.0%
Appendectomy	
• Open	• 1.4%
• Laparoscopy	• 1.3%

Adapted from [6]

Thus, informed consent for any abdominal operation should include the risk of developing adhesions and the potential need for further surgery in the future. It is difficult to predict when the patient will develop small bowel obstruction. In a study of 446,331 abdominal operations Barmparas et al. showed a strong and independent association between surgical procedure type utilized and the proportion of patients with adhesion-induced small bowel obstruction (Table 24.2) [6]. The identification of surgical procedure type as an independent risk factor for small bowel obstruction may have a predictive value for stratifying patients. A recent report by Angenete et al. suggests that factors such as age, previous abdominal surgery and comorbidity are important predictors of risks of hospitalization for small bowel obstruction or surgery for small bowel obstruction [7]. The incidence of small bowel obstruction among patients who have had bariatric surgery, including gastric bypass, was 3.2%. The estimated overall incidence of small bowel obstruction among patients who underwent abdominal trauma surgery operations was 4.6% [6].

Neoplasm

Neoplasms are the second most common cause of small bowel obstruction, comprising 20% of the cases [8]. If an adult patient presents with a small bowel obstruction and has a virgin abdomen (meaning the patient has not had any previous abdominal procedures) the etiology of a neoplasm as the source of obstruction must be entertained. Other causes could include inflammatory bowel disease, gallstones, ileus, or intussusceptions. More common origins of neoplasms include colorectal carcinoma, and ovarian carcinoma in women. Extrinsic compression, adhesions, and carcinomatosis are often seen as the etiology of small bowel obstruction in these cases.

Hernias

Hernias are the third leading cause of small bowel obstruction, comprising 10% of cases [8]. When examining a patient with a small bowel obstruction, the surgeon must be cognizant of the potential hernia etiologies. A meticulous examination of the groin, femoral region, parastomal region, and old surgical scar sites is warranted. In thin females an obturator hernia can be the cause of small bowel obstruction. One must have a high index of suspicion and this type of hernia can be identified with abdominal CT.

Other Extrinsic Causes

Malrotation and congenital or acquired hernias are less common causes of small bowel obstruction. Malrotation can present in both the pediatric and adult populations. Congenital hernias include transmesenteric, transomental, and paraduodenal hernias [9]. Acquired hernias develop after a resection of bowel where there exists a mesenteric defect. Bowel can herniate through this defect and cause a small bowel obstruction. The idea has been proposed that with the increase in laparoscopic procedures, defects are not closed as often, and the incidence of internal hernia increases. Experience with laparoscopic Roux-en-Y-gastric bypass (LRYGB) has attempted to answer these questions about small bowel obstruction and internal hernia incidence. However, the literature is mixed. What is important for the acute care surgeon to realize is that you will be seeing these patients come into the emergency department with small bowel obstruction secondary to internal hernias. There are three potential

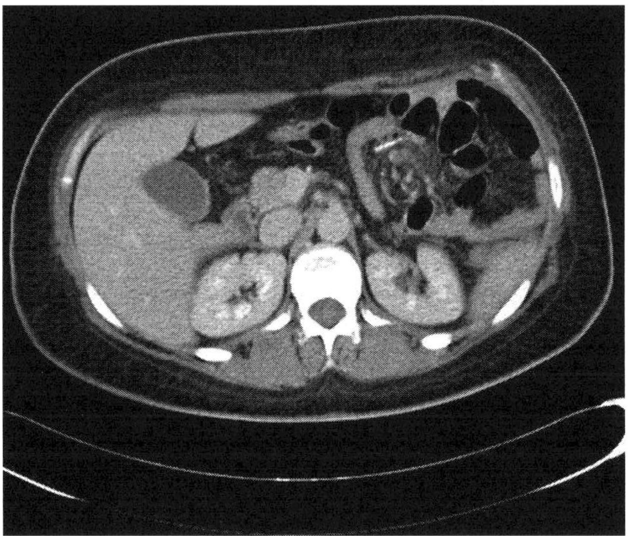

Fig. 24.1 Axial CT demonstrating Petersen's hernia with swirling of the mesentery evident in this image. Small bowel is seen herniating above the level of the stomach. There is a potential space posterior to the gastrojejunostomy where this herniation occurs. Radiopaedia.org (http://radipaedia.org/cases/peterserns-hernia), case ID: 14053

spaces: Petersen's space, the mesocolic space, and the mesomesenteric space. The Petersen's hernia occurs in a potential space posterior to the gastrojejunostomy (for example: See Fig. 24.1). Laparoscopic Roux-en-Y gastric bypass is done with an antecolic or retrocolic anastomosis. If a retrocolic anastomosis is performed, a defect in the mesocolon is necessary and there exists a potential space. The mesomesenteric potential space at the jejunojejunostomy is another area where an internal hernia can develop. Intra-abdominal abscesses may cause bowel obstruction via extrinsic causes by kinking the bowel as it adheres to the abscess cavity or even within it.

Intrinsic Causes

Intrinsic obstructions are due to such causes as aganglionic megacolon, primary tumors, Crohn's disease, tuberculosis, and intussusceptions. Crohn's disease causes strictures responsible for small bowel obstruction. Multiple resections of small bowel in patients with Crohn's can eventually lead to an endpoint of short bowel syndrome. Strictures can also be caused by radiation and ischemia. Irradiated bowel is very friable and the risks of enterotomies and subsequent fistula development are high. Intussusception is commonly identified with CT scans; however, the clinical significance can be questionable. However, when the intussusception is the lead point for small bowel obstruction in an adult, malignancy should be ruled out. In trauma, small bowel hematomas can cause bowel obstruction. The duodenum is particularly susceptible because a portion is fixed in the retroperitoneum.

Most duodenal hematomas resolve without the need for operative interventions.

Intraluminal obstructions are caused by impacted feces, gallstones, enterolith, bezoar, tumors, large polyps, and ingested foreign bodies. Small bowel tumors are rare but an important etiology of small bowel obstruction. They present with vague abdominal symptoms and ultimately cause small bowel obstrution. These include small bowel adenocarcinoma, carcinoid tumors, and lymphoma.

There is clinically significant morbidity associated with small bowel obstruction, although the mortality rate for patients with mechanical obstruction has been dramatically reduced in recent years. The observed improvements in mortality rate have been attributed to early diagnosis, appropriate strategic use of isotonic fluid resuscitation, gastric tube decompression, antibiotics, and surgery.

Clinical Presentation and Diagnosis

A well-conducted patient history is essential for formulating an initial working diagnosis for small bowel obstruction. Informative patient symptoms include the following: abdominal pain, nausea, vomiting, abdominal distension, obstipation, fever, tachycardia, or diarrhea secondary to increased peristalsis. Pain paroxysms at 4–5 min intervals are associated more frequently with distal obstructions whereas nausea and vomiting are sometimes more common in patients with more proximal obstructions. The past surgical history should be detailed. As shown in Table 24.2, there is strong association between surgical procedure type/group and the risk of developing a small bowel obstruction. On physical examination, a patient with a small bowel obstruction can present with tachycardia, fever, distended abdomen, and evidence of previous surgical scars. The time course of development of a small bowel obstruction is often reflected in an early rise in hyperactive bowel sounds (e.g., borborygmi) followed by significant reduction or complete cessation of bowel sounds. In refining the diagnosis for small bowel obstruction, it is important to exclude specific explanatory etiologies such as incarcerated hernias in the groin, the femoral triangle, and the obturator triangle. Extraluminal masses need to be excluded and distal colon obstruction can sometimes be excluded by rectal examination. Patients with positive rectal exam results should prompt a test for occult blood to assess for the possibility of a malignancy, intussusception, or infarction. The abdominal exam is extremely important in the diagnosis of a small bowel obstruction. Patients with suspect small bowel obstruction often have abdominal distension and tenderness. The tenderness may be localized but more often is diffuse. The reason the physical exam is so important is because patients with small bowel obstruction either resolve or progress and the intestines can become ischemic if not taken to the operating room in a timely manner. A worsening physical exam may be a signal of bowel necrosis. Consequently, the patient may begin to exhibit signs of peritonitis, diffuse tenderness, rebound, and guarding. Laboratory data should be obtained to include complete blood count (CBC) and basic metabolic panel at a minimum. Other tests such as liver function tests, arterial blood gas (for base deficit) and lactate may be helpful but are not absolutely essential. An increasing white blood cell (WBC) count, increasing base deficit or lactate, intravascular volume depletion, and low urine output are measures of a patient that is getting worse clinically (for treatment algorithm see Fig. 24.2).

Patients who present with partial small bowel obstruction or low-grade obstruction are treated with nasogastric decompression, nothing by mouth (NPO), and intravenous fluids. If no resolution occurs with this treatment, then repeat CT with water soluble contrast, CT enteroclysis, CT enterography, or small bowel series with oral contrast is indicated to further delineate the area of obstruction. The small bowel series should be done with water soluble contrast in case the patient needs to go to the operating room for a bowel resection. Computed tomography enteroclysis is valuable in low-grade and partial small bowel obstruction where the etiology is not clear on regular CT. The CT enteroclysis has the advantage of active luminal distension whereby the lumen can be evaluated. Thus, cross-sectional analysis of the bowel is feasible. It involves the insertion of a nasojejunal tube that lies at the duodenojejunal junction. Barium is directly injected into the bowel. Computed tomography enterography with large volume contrast compares in accuracy to enteroclysis without the need for a nosojejunal tube. The sensitivity of CT enteroclysis is 93.1% and specificity 96.9% as reported by Dixon and coworkers [10].

There is some controversy over the use of plain films in patients with small bowel obstruction. Based on the authors' personal exposure and experience, plain films are not necessary if one is going to obtain a CT scan. However, in the absence of CT scans, plain films can be extremely useful (see Fig. 24.3). The Eastern Association for the Surgery of Trauma (EAST) practice management guidelines recommend plain films on all patients who are being evaluated to rule out small bowel obstruction [2]. The plain films should consist of flat and upright abdominal films along with a chest X-ray (CXR) also known as an abdominal series. Serial plain films may be necessary to add to the physical exam during the hospital course. Computed tomography scans of the abdomen and pelvis are commonly obtained during the initial evaluation in the ER. The use of CT scans has largely replaced plain films in many hospitals and has proven to be very sensitive for the diagnosis of small bowel obstruction [2]. The sensitivity increases when the CT is performed with oral and intravenous contrast. As with plain films, the CT

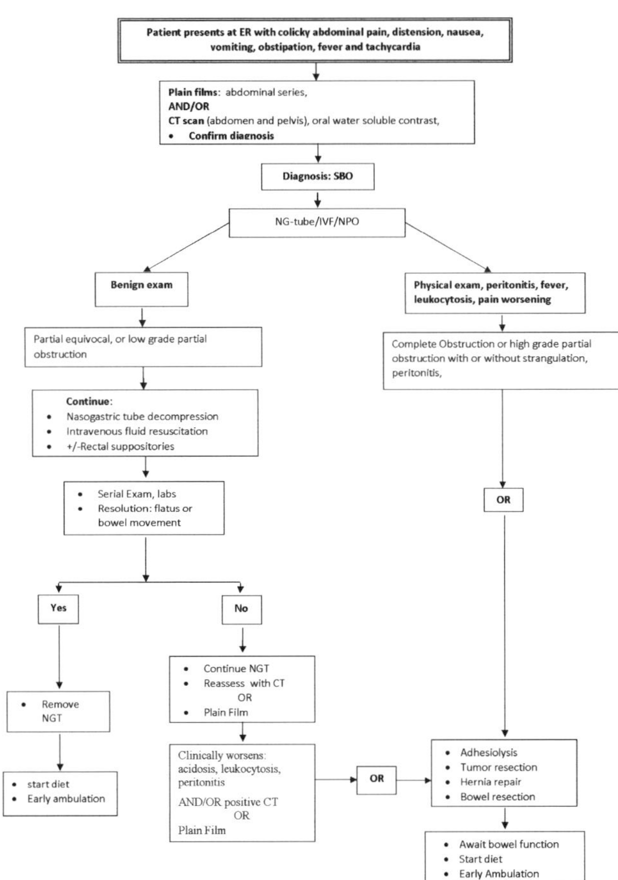

Fig. 24.2 An algorithm for the diagnosis and management of small bowel obstruction

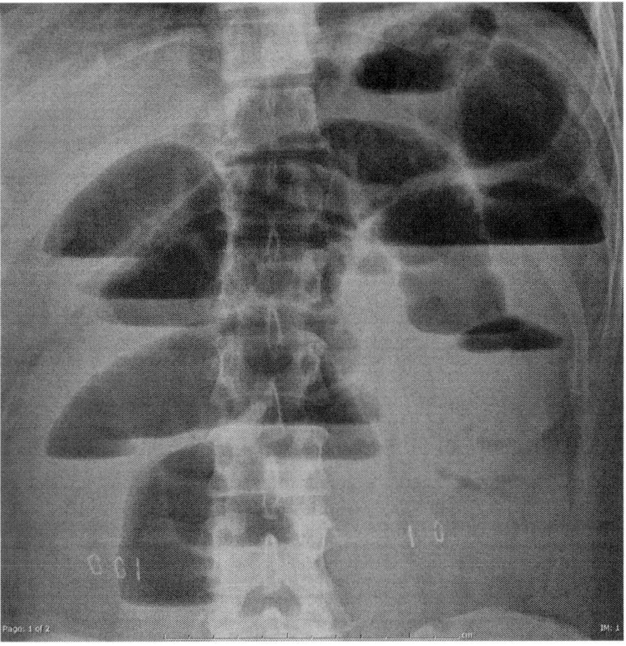

Fig. 24.3 Plain abdominal X-ray demonstrates air fluid levels in small bowel obstruction

scan may need to be repeated during the hospital course to assess small bowel obstruction progression or resolution. There are certain characteristics on CT scans that are helpful in planning the management of a patient with a small bowel obstruction. Identification of a transition zone between normal and abnormal intestinal diameter may localize the area of the obstruction and the probable cause of the obstruction. Similarly, proximal dilation of the small bowel (diameter >2.5 cm) and the presence of multiple free air-fluid levels are highly suggestive. Thus specific CT findings include the following: (1) dilated small bowel loops usually greater than 2.5 cm, (2) small bowel feces, (3) extrinsic causes such as hernias, (4) gas-filled loops, (5) intussuception, and (6) mesenteric vessel abnormalities such as haziness, obliteration congestion, or hemorrhage. The CT findings are best in determining the site, cause as well as complications of small bowel obstruction (Figs. 24.4–24.9).

Jones et al. performed a retrospective study to attempt to answer the question regarding the usefulness of a CT scoring system in predicting need for surgery in patients with small bowel obstruction [11]. The results demonstrated that CT can successfully predict the necessity for surgery 75% of the time. The CT scoring system when used in combination with specific criteria increased the ability to predict the need for surgery from 75 to 79%. Other modalities that have been used to aid in the diagnosis of small bowel obstruction include ultrasound and magnetic resonance imaging (MRI), but these are not commonly used and have not proved to be as sensitive as the previously mentioned studies. The presence of pneumatosis intestinalis on CT scan is a late finding and an ominous sign of bowel ischemia. Air in the portal system also may indicate gangrenous bowel in the face of small bowel obstruction.

The diagnosis of small bowel obstruction is not a difficult diagnosis to make. A patient presents with a history consistent with bowel obstruction and confirmed with a CT scan or plain films and the diagnosis is made. The challenge is management of this patient.

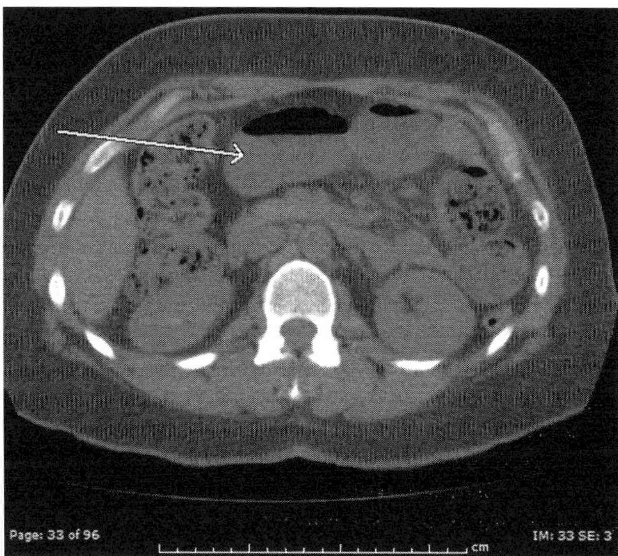

Fig. 24.4 Axial CT demonstrating dilated small bowel in a patient with SBO

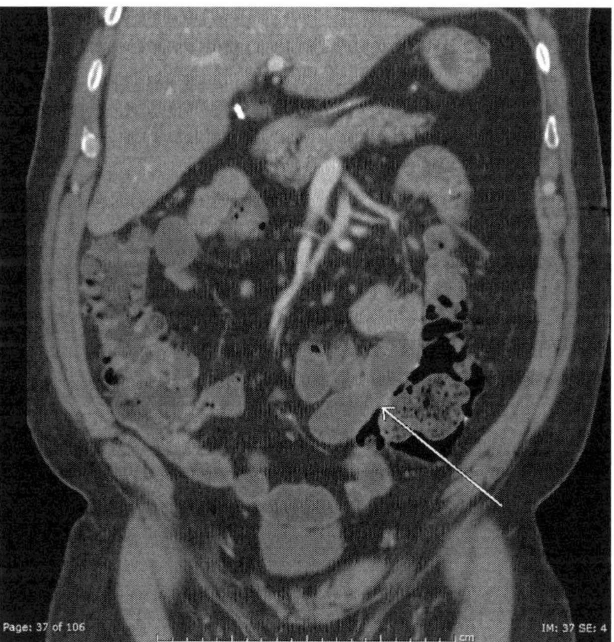

Fig. 24.5 Coronal CT showing dilated and fluid filled small bowel in partial small bowel obstruction

Management

A patient with a CT scan showing complete obstruction in the presence of peritoneal signs on physical exam will need operative intervention, particularly in the presence of fever, leukocytosis, and tachycardia. A well-timed decision to manage small bowel obstruction surgically is crucial to minimize the morbidity and mortality associated with intestinal strangulation. Thus surgery before onset of irreversible ischemia is a priority. This is prudent because the distinction between a patient with simple obstruction and a patient with strangulation cannot always be made reliably based on laboratory, clinical and imaging findings. Standardized and appropriate surgical procedures are performed based on the cause of the small bowel obstruction. These include lysis of adhesions, resection of tumors or reduction and repair of hernias. Invariably, viability of the intestine must be assessed by visual inspection and when necessary Doppler probe studies and arterial perfusion evaluations, including the use of Woods lamp.

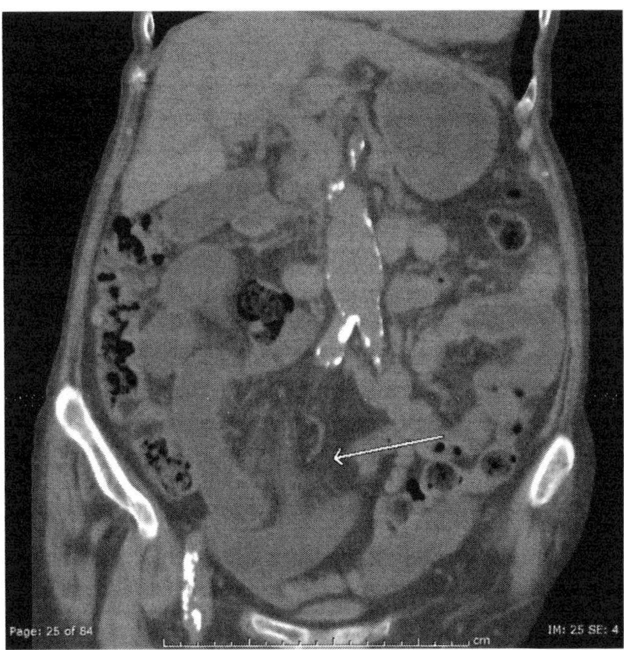

Fig. 24.6 Coronal CT showing closed loop obstruction with twisting of the mesentery

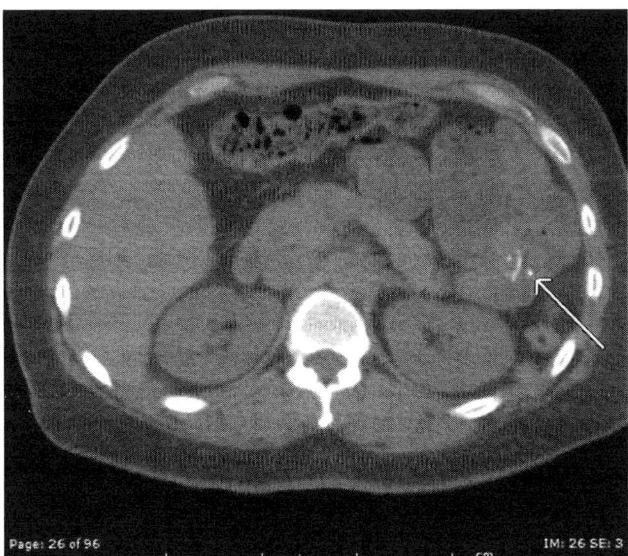

Fig. 24.8 Axial CT showing jejunojejunal anastomosis as site of obstruction

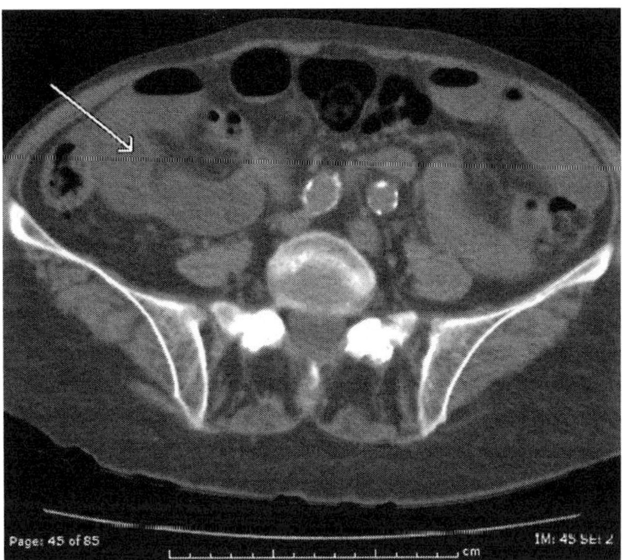

Fig. 24.7 Axial CT view showing the closed loop obstruction

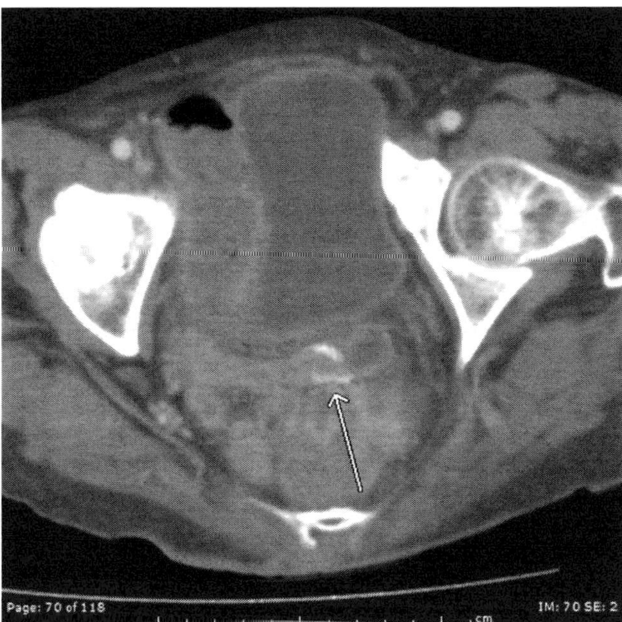

Fig. 24.9 Axial CT revealing transition zone at the anastomosis

The majority of patients with small bowel obstruction can initially be managed safely by conservative nonsurgical treatment. Conservative treatment involves the administration of intravenous (IV) fluids, nothing by mouth (NPO), placement of a nasogastric tube if the patient has significant emesis or if the patient has abdominal distension, and performance of serial abdominal exams to evaluate for worsening abdominal pain or the presence of peritonitis. The exact definition of serial abdominal exams is controversial. Should serial exams be performed every 4 h, every 6 h, every 8 h, or longer? This is a complicated question because how often the serial exam is performed should be based on the patient's clinical presentation at the time of the exam. If the exam continues to improve, the time interval between serial exams may increase. If the patient's abdominal exam is not improving or worsening, then the frequency of examination should increase. During this time, daily monitoring with laboratory testing including a CBC and electrolyte panel is a useful adjunct to track response to conservative treatments. Repeat CT scan and or plain films are usually done in the first 48 h to monitor progression or resolution.

The use of enemas, suppositories, and cathartics is controversial. Patients with bowel obstruction are contraindicated for enemas including those containing sodium phosphate [12]. However, in the case of partial small bowel obstruction, there have been reports of success with all the above interventions.

Prior to the evolution of laparoscopic surgery, the surgical management of small bowel obstruction was accomplished through an exploratory laparotomy. A midline incision is made when feaseable, the peritoneum is entered, and dissection is performed until the point of obstruction is identified. The etiology of the obstruction will dictate the procedure. If the obstruction is due to adhesion then adhesiolysis is performed. Small bowel obstruction can present at the previous suture line or anastomotic site (Figs. 24.8 and 24.9). If the obstruction is due to tumor then resection should be performed if possible. In the event that resection is not possible, then diversion is an option. In those patients with malignancy affecting large segments of the small bowel performance an enteroenterostomy (bypass) may be the only option available at the time of laparotomy. Indeed, cancers of the colon, stomach or metastasis from the lung or breast are often common causes of bowel obstruction. If a hernia is present then perform the appropriate hernia procedure; reduce the hernia, examine the bowel for viability, and perform hernia repair. In the case of internal hernias, the defect must be closed and bowel resection is often necessary. When taking a patient to the operating room for a small bowel obstruction that has previously undergone a Roux-en-Y gastric bypass, remember the mesomesenteric potential space at the jejunojejunostomy is often the site of the internal hernia. Closed loop obstructions pose a special problem. In this situation the surgeon must obtain control of the mesentery prior to untwisting the mesentery. The mesentery of the ischemic bowel must be clamped off proximally and distally in order to prevent the release of toxic substances within the closed loop. If the loop is released prior to obtaining control then bacteria and toxins can be released into the systemic circulation.

In the case of foreign body ingestion, usually operative management is warranted if the foreign body causes overt obstruction or perforation. Intra-abdominal abscesses causing an abdominal obstruction can often be managed nonoperatively with a drain placed by interventional radiology, nasogastric tube, and antibiotics.

Practical Operative Considerations

There are a few key issues to take into consideration when entering the abdomen for a small bowel obstruction:

1. Enter the abdomen in an area away from the prior scar or known hernia defect. Entering the abdomen above or below previous incisions can help avoid inadvertent enterotomies.
2. When the bowel is adherent to the undersurface of the abdominal wall use scissors (Metzenbaum or Cooley scissors) or a knife to take sharply down the adhesions. Avoid the use of electrocautery in these areas, as it may result in inadvertent thermal injury to the bowel that may be unrecognized at the time of operation.
3. When it is difficult to take down an area you have worked in without making much progress, it is prudent to leave the area, dissect somewhere else and then return later to complete your dissection.
4. Take your time with the dissection and get a second pair of hands if possible to facilitate exposure.
5. Resect bowel that has been "beat up" too much to avoid postoperative complications (strictures, adhesions, leaks).
6. If bowel viability is in question "damage control" is an option. Place a temporary abdominal closure and plan to come back after 12–24 h for a second look laparotomy.

Laparoscopic surgery for patients who need operative intervention for small bowel obstruction is becoming much more common place for those surgeons who are facile with the laparoscope. Proposed advantages of laparoscopy compared to open surgery include quicker postoperative recovery and reduced hospital length of stay. The increasing popularity of laparoscopy contrasts with experience in the past when small bowel obstruction was considered a contraindication for laparoscopy. While there is good agreement on feasibility, safety and efficacy of laparoscopy in the management of small bowel obstruction, there is some debate about its appropriateness for patients with an acute obstruction. It had been reported that only 50% of cases of small bowel obstruction could be managed successfully with laparoscopy [13]. Nevertheless, there is excellent prospect for increased utilization of laparoscopy for small bowel obstruction since open surgery increases the risk of the development of postoperative small bowel obstruction due to adhesion formation by at least fourfold compared to laparoscopy [7].

Since postsurgical adhesions often result in small bowel obstruction, there have been concerted efforts to prevent adhesions through the use of adhesion barriers during laparotomy. Currently, there are three US Food and Drug Administration (FDA)-approved adhesion barriers including Seprafilm (Genzyme), Adept (Baxter), and Interceed (Gynecare). Seprafilm has been reported to decrease the severity but not the incidence of postsurgical adhesions [14]. Interceed has a black box warning and is contraindicated as a haemostatic agent in laparoscopic surgery. The product labeling for Adept carries more contraindications than Seprafilm and Interceed. These include infections, laparotomy incision, bowel resection, appendectomy, and allergy to cornstarch.

Potential Complications

Potential complications of surgery for small bowel obstruction include sepsis, intra-abdominal abscess, wound dehiscence, aspiration, fistula formation, colostomy, short bowel syndrome, and death. It is important for the operating surgeon to have a detailed discussion with the patient and family prior to proceeding to the operating room. The estimated overall mortality rate after surgical treatment for small bowel obstruction has been reported to be as high as 5% [15]. Some of the factors that influence postsurgical mortality in patients with small bowel obstruction include: old age, the presence of a comorbid condition, the presence of bowel gangrene at laparotomy, and delay in diagnosis. Although comorbidity is strongly associated with older patients, it seems that comorbidity, especially cardiovascular and pulmonary comorbidities are independent predictors of death after surgery for small bowel obstruction. In addition to increased mortality rates, complication rates are also higher in patients older than 60 years compared to younger patients. Treatment delays of more than 24 h, nonviable or strangulated bowel and recurrent surgeries are also factors that increase complications risk.

Follow-up

Prognosis for the majority of cases of non-strangulated small bowel obstruction is very good, as bowel obstruction may resolve spontaneously. Patients with partial small bowel obstructions who are managed nonoperatively may spend 2–5 days for recovery and recurrence is low. However, patients who were managed surgically through resection or adhesiolysis generally spend more time in the hospital. The incidence of recurrence of small bowel obstruction in patients managed surgically was 5.8% and risk factors for recurrence were age <40 years, adhesions, and postsurgical complications [16].

Conclusion

The diagnosis and management of small bowel obstruction has always been accomplished quite successfully by general surgeons. Acute care surgeons are increasingly being relied upon to treat patients with small bowel obstruction. Undoubtedly, thorough physical examination, appropriate imaging studies, close monitoring, and timely laparotomy or laparoscopy will lead to a reduction in the morbidity and mortality of patients presenting with small bowel obstruction.

References

1. Foster NM, McGory ML, Zingmond DS, Ko CY. Small bowel obstruction: a population-based appraisal. J Am Coll Surg. 2006;203:170–6.
2. Diaz Jr JJ, Bokhari F, Mowery NT, Acosta JA, Block EF, Bromberg WJ, et al. Guidelines for management of small bowel obstruction. J Trauma. 2008;64(6):1651–64. East Practice Parameter Workgroup.
3. McLean A. Investigation of small bowel obstruction. J HK Coll Radiol. 2004;7:3–7.
4. Schwartz SI. Manifestations of gastrointestinal disease. In: Schwartz SI, editor. Principles of surgery. 7th ed. New York: McGraw-Hill; 1999. p. 1033–79.
5. Parker MC, Ellis H, Moran BJ, Thompson JN, Wilson MS, Menzies D, McGuire A, et al. Postoperative adhesions: ten-year follow-up of 12,584 patients undergoing lower abdominal surgery. Dis Colon Rectum. 2001;44:822.
6. Barmparas G, Branco BC, Schnuriger B, Lam L, Inaba K, Demetriades D. The incidence and risk factors of post-laparotomy adhesive small bowel obstruction. J Gastrointest Surg. 2010;14:1619–28.
7. Angenete E, Jacobsson A, Gellerstedt M, Haglind E. Effect of laparoscopy on the risk of small-bowel obstruction: a population-based register study. Arch Surg. 2012;147:359–65.
8. Kendrick ML. Partial small bowel obstruction: clinical issues and recent advances. Abdom Imaging. 2009;34:329.
9. Newsom BD, Kukora JS. Congenital and acquired internal hernias, unusual cause of small bowel obstruction. Am J Surg. 1986;152: 279–85.
10. Dixon PM, Roulston ME, Nolan DJ. The small bowel enema: a ten year review. Clin Radiol. 1993;47:46–8.
11. Jones K, Mangram AJ, Lebron RA, Nadalo L, Dunn E. Can a computed tomography scoring system predict the need for surgery in small-bowel obstruction? Am J Surg. 2007;194:780–4.
12. Hsu HJ, Wu MS. Extreme hyperphosphatemia and hypocalcemia coma associated with phosphate enema. Intern Med. 2008;47:643–6.
13. Zermatten MS, Halkic N, Martinet O, Bettschart V. Laparoscopic management of mechanical small bowel obstruction. Surg Endosc. 2000;14:478–83.
14. Fazio VW, Cohen Z, Fleshman JW, et al. Reduction in adhesive small-bowel obstruction by Seprafilm adhesion barrier after intestinal resection. Dis Colon Rectum. 2006;49:1–11.
15. Fevang BT, Fevang J, Strangeland L, et al. Complications and death after surgical treatment of small bowel obstruction a 35-Year Institutional Experience. Ann Surg. 2000;231:529–37.
16. Duron JJ, Jourdan-Da Silva N, Tezenas du Montcel S, et al. Adhesive postoperative small bowel obstruction: incidence and risk factors of recurrence after surgical treatment. Ann Surg. 2006;244:759–75.

Acute Appendicitis

Krista L. Turner

K.L. Turner, M.D., F.A.C.S. (✉)
Department of Surgery, The Methodist Hospital, Weill Cornell
Medical College, 6550 Fannin St, SM 1661A,
77030 Houston, TX, USA
e-mail: kristaturnermd@hotmail.com

Introduction

Acute appendicitis (AA) can be considered the signature disease encountered by the acute care surgeon. It is the most frequent abdominal diagnosis treated by surgeons with more than 500,000 appendectomies performed yearly in the USA [1]. Its classic presentation, commonality, and relative ease of cure can lull the surgeon into underestimating the morbidity that can arise from complicated cases. Generally considered a purely surgical disease with a singular treatment pathway, advances in surgical and medical treatment have pushed the branches of the decision tree. Recently, large national databases of surgical disease have provided data that can help the surgeon decide which pathway best serves a particular patient population. Current controversies exist over laparoscopic versus open technique, appropriate timing of intervention, and the appropriateness of nonoperative management.

Epidemiology and Pathology

Inflammation of the appendix was initially described more than 120 years ago by Fitz who recommended operative intervention. McBurney subsequently described a series of eight patients who presented with acute appendicitis who underwent operative management by appendectomy, thus dictating the preferred management for the disease that went unchanged for over a century [2]. Appendectomy remains one of the most commonly performed emergency general surgery procedures, and is classically one of the first procedures learned as a surgical trainee. The epidemiology of the disease reflects a younger male demographic. A minority of patients may have a complicated course, primarily occurring in the elderly population.

The pathophysiology of AA is typically described as obstruction of the appendiceal lumen, either by edema, bacteria, stool (appendicolith), or tumor. Hyperplasia of the submucosal lymphoid follicles in response to systemic inflammation is often present in the pediatric population and is termed catarrhal appendicitis. The clinicopathologic presentation ranges in spectrum from early acute appendicitis, suppurative appendicitis, gangrenous appendicitis, perforated appendicitis, to perforated appendicitis with phlegmon or abscess. Stump appendicitis, in which inflammation of a remaining portion of appendix occurs after appendectomy, has also been described.

The stepwise temporal progression of appendiceal inflammation to gangrene to perforation has been questioned, with emerging consideration that perforated and non-perforated appendicitis are actually two different disease processes [3]. Cytokine data suggest that the pathophysiology of perforated appendicitis follows a more virulent pathway from the onset of the disease. Polymorphisms of the promotor for the proinflammatory cytokine IL-6 have been compared to clinical pathology of appendicitis, with decreased IL-6 production correlating with a lowered incidence of complicated appendicitis [4, 5]. Epidemiologic data comparing AA and acute diverticulitis have likewise suggested that perforation is a separate disease process [6]. Both diseases are considered a function of intraluminal pressure and bacterial overgrowth. Both are rare in geographic regions where hygiene is poor and diets are high in fiber. The incidence of non-perforated diverticulitis follows the same pattern as non-perforated AA in these regions [7]. This evidence seeks to refute the idea that perforated AA is ultimately the result of untreated appendicitis.

L.J. Moore et al. (eds.), *Common Problems in Acute Care Surgery*,
DOI 10.1007/978-1-4614-6123-4_25, © Springer Science+Business Media New York 2013

Presentation

The history and physical presentation in the healthy, young adult as classically described generally does not waver: the onset of peri-umbilical pain, with migration to the right lower quadrant, nausea following the onset of pain, tenderness at McBurney's point, and mild leukocytosis. Despite the consistency of this presentation, the ease of obtaining a computed tomography (CT) scan means these patients often undergo unnecessary radiation exposure and time wasted verifying AA before a surgeon is even consulted. Occasionally, images from the scan may help guide trocar placement for a laparoscopic approach in the case of a retrocecal appendix, for example. Often this same information can be obtained simply from a more dedicated physical exam, specifically the presence of a psoas or obturator sign. Variation in the clinical history may indicate a ruptured appendix, as indicated by the patient with increasing pain in the right lower quadrant over several days, which then suddenly improves but never fully resolves. Palpation of an inflammatory mass in the right lower quadrant may indicate rupture with phlegmon formation.

Acute appendicitis outside of the young, healthy demographic, however, may have an extremely varied presentation, earning the moniker of "the great imitator." Older patients often have more vague symptoms, with mild to moderate nonspecific abdominal pain, which is often tolerated for longer periods of time before presentation. Associated symptoms of diarrhea, nausea, and urinary symptoms may be more frequently encountered. The differential diagnosis of right-sided abdominal pain is broader in a population with comorbidities, previous surgeries, complicating medications, immunocompromise, and in the woman of childbearing age. Table 25.1 lists the more common differential diagnoses to consider. Various scores have been developed in an effort to more accurately diagnose AA based on signs and symptoms, such as the modified Alvarado Score depicted in Table 25.2. Although these types of scoring systems are helpful, a high index of suspicion for AA should be entertained for any older patient with abdominal pain.

Table 25.1 Differential diagnosis of right lower quadrant abdominal pain

Gastrointestinal origin
Appendicitis
Mesenteric adenitis
Intussusception
Terminal ileitis
Cecal diverticulitis
Epiploic appendagitis
Typhlitis
Inflammatory bowel disease
Constipation

Urogenital
Ureteral stone
Urinary tract infection

Gynecologic
Tubo-ovarian abscess
Ovarian torsion
Ectopic pregnancy
Hemorrhagic ovarian cyst of corpus luteum remnants
Ruptured ovarian cyst
Pelvic inflammatory disease
Perforated duodenal ulcer with retroperitoneal extension
("Valentino's Appendix")
Pancreatic abscess with retroperitoneal extension

Table 25.2 Modified Alvarado's score [71]

Symptom	Points
Migratory right iliac fossa pain	2
Nausea/vomiting	1
Sign	
Right lower quadrant pain	2
Rebound tenderness	1
Fever	1
Rovsign's sign	1
Laboratory value	
Leukocytosis	2

Based on patient presentation, a combination of signs, symptoms, and laboratory data are totaled to predict likelihood of acute appendicitis
1–4 Points: acute appendicitis unlikely
5–6 Points: probable appendicitis
6–7 Points: definite appendicitis

Imaging

As described previously, a careful history and physical exam in combination with isolated leukocytosis will often provide the diagnosis of AA. Prior to the omnipresence of the CT scanner, a 20% negative appendectomy rate was considered an acceptable variance. A higher number indicated hasty procession to the operating room, while a lower number led to the concern that cases were being missed. By 1997, the frequent use of CT scanning had reduced the negative appendectomy rate to 15%, with numbers continuing to decrease to 10% with the use helical or multidetector CT scanners [8, 9]. Since the potential postoperative complications for a negative appendectomy are the same as for appendicitis, the benefits of obtaining a CT scan should be weighed against the risks. While a scan increases cost, radiation exposure, and potential time prior to proceeding to the operating room, it can also provide valuable information for plan of care. The presence of a phlegmon, predominant inflammation of the terminal ileum or cecum, identification of other pathology, or nonspecific findings in a high-risk patient can all save a patient from an unnecessary or dangerous operation and guide alternate therapy.

Acute appendicitis can often be readily identified on the different variations of abdomen/pelvis CTs performed with a sensitivity and specificity of approximately 94% [10]. Non-contrast (both intravenous and oral) CTs, those with both types of contrast or with oral and rectal contrast may all be helpful in making the diagnosis. Findings include an enlarged appendix, fat stranding around the tip or in the right lower

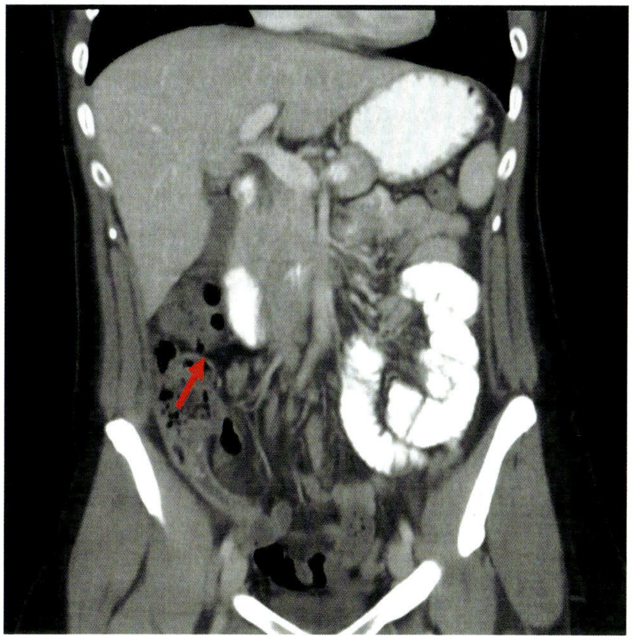

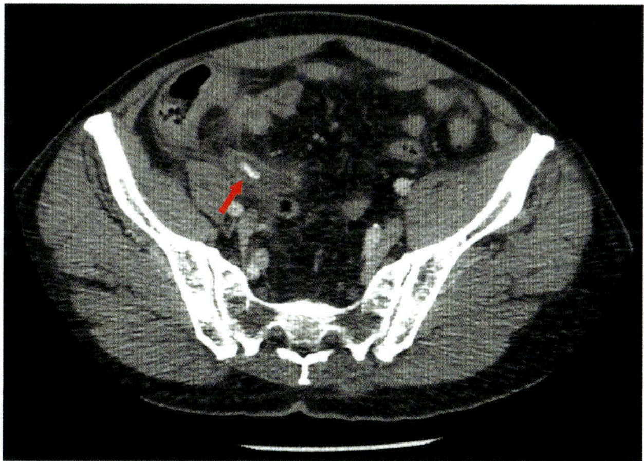

Fig. 25.1 Coronal CT image of acute non-perforated appendicitis. A dilated tubular structure (*arrow*) in the right lower quadrant is demonstrated. Inflamed periappendiceal fat can also be appreciated by darkening of the fat plane around the structure

Fig. 25.2 Axial CT image of acute appendicitis with appendicolith. The appendicolith (*arrow*) is noted as a white structure within the lumen of the mid-portion of the appendix

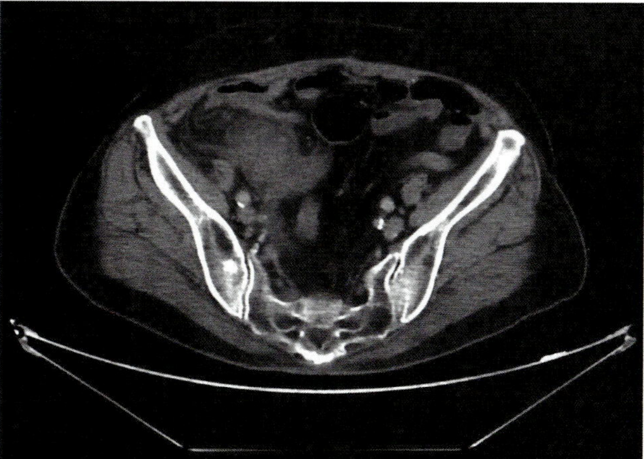

Fig. 25.3 Axial CT image of perforated appendicitis with phlegmon. Dense mass is noted with no definite separation of cecum from appendix. Generalized inflammation is noted in the right lower quadrant

should be limited. Ultrasound (US) is often used for the pediatric population, as it can be an extension of the exam and does not require sedation or travel out of the emergency room. The inflamed appendix on US appears as an incompressible, blind-ended, tubular structure with diameter greater than 6–7 mm. With graded compression, differentiation between normal loops of bowel and the appendix can be achieved [11]. Sensitivity and specificity of US for AA is approximately 83 and 93% [10]. MRI is often utilized for the pregnancy patient, as excellent imaging can be obtained with no radiation exposure. Contrast agents should not be administered. Although MRI is costly and may not be widely available, the risk of unnecessary laparoscopy or missed appendicitis in the pregnant patient can increase preterm contractions and fetal mortality. The sensitivity and specificity of MRI for AA in this patient population is approximately 100% and 93%, respectively [12].

Plain abdominal films are often obtained initially when in the emergency room, but these provide little information indicative of appendicitis unless an appendicolith is present, and are primarily used to rule-out more acute disease processes such as a perforated viscus or complete bowel obstruction.

quadrant, the presence of an appendicolith, non-filling of the appendix with oral or rectal contrast, or a phlegmon with or without abscess (see Figs. 25.1–25.3). Patients with little visceral adiposity make the diagnosis slightly more difficult, as there are reduced fat planes to highlight inflammation. Enlarged fallopian tubes or adnexal pathology in the female patient may also be difficult to distinguish from appendiceal inflammation on CT scan.

Ultrasonography or magnetic resonance imaging (MRI) may be obtained for patients in whom radiation exposure

Surgical Management

Most cases of AA will present in an uncomplicated manner and often proceed to the operating room with little deliberation regarding management. This holds true for the patient with little comorbidity and with suspected non-perforated appendicitis. Although a prompt operation is considered standard procedure, cases in select patient populations can often be delayed up to 12 h with no increase in morbidity [13]. In a large retrospective observational dataset, the risk of rupture for appendicitis was not increased with a delay of up to 24 h from hospital admission to operation[14]. A 6% increase in rupture rate was encountered if a delay over 36 h was noted. Again, the pathology of ruptured versus non-ruptured appendicitis has been debated, with less emphasis given to early operation for the prevention of rupture. A significant delay in surgery should still be avoided, however, as an expedited operation can reduce the suffering of the patient, in addition to reducing hospital cost by an extended length of stay. Preoperative preparation should be straightforward, with initiation of intravenous fluids, and demonstration of a negative pregnancy test for women of child-bearing age. Deep venous thrombosis prophylaxis and antibiotic prophylaxis should be initiated prior to surgery as indicated by standard guidelines [15].

Postoperative morbidity associated with appendectomy ranges from 10 to 20% for non-perforated appendicitis versus 30% for those with perforation. Most of these complications are infectious in nature [16]. Mortality for appendectomy is low, with a rate of 0.07–0.7% without perforation, and 0.5–2.4% with perforation [3, 17]. The mortality rate increases with comorbidities including cardiac risk factors, pulmonary disease, and morbid obesity. Age also increases mortality, with rates of 2.5% for patients in their 70s, 6.8% in their 80s, and 16.4% for those 90 years of age and older [18].

Laparoscopic Versus Open Technique

Standard open surgical technique for appendectomy includes an approximately 5 cm incision in the right lower quadrant through which the peritoneum is reached via a muscle slitting technique. The appendix and mesoappendix can then be suture ligated and divided, and the wound closed in layers after irrigation. With the availability and mastery of laparoscopic techniques, as well as the advancing rate of obesity of the population, this open technique is often considered a secondary approach. The laparoscopic approach is usually performed using three ports placed on the left side of the patient, with left arm tucked for better movement of the surgeon and assistant on the same side (see Fig. 25.4). A Foley catheter is placed to decompress the bladder as suprapubic ports are often placed. The appendix can be divided with an endovascular stapling device or with suture ligation. The mesoappendix may also be divided using a stapler, or various cautery devices. In theory, the laparoscopic approach provides better visualization of the abdomen when other pathology may be suspected. There is also the bias towards laparoscopy due to potential reduction of pain, infection, or resumption of diet.

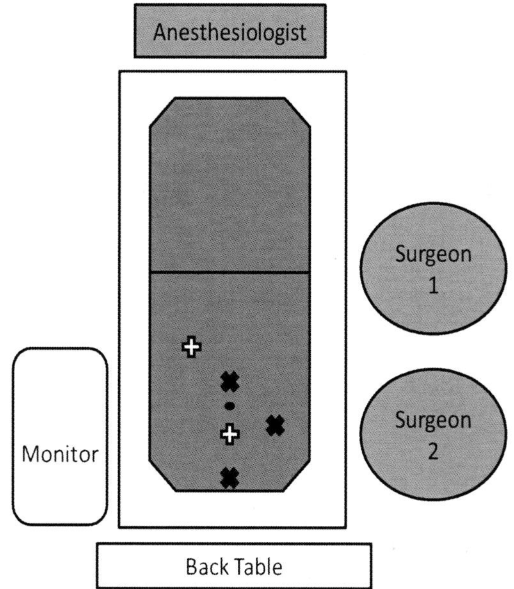

Fig. 25.4 Operative configuration for laparoscopic appendectomy. Possible operating room configuration for laparoscopic appendectomy is illustrated. Both surgeon and assistant stand on the patient's left for better ergonomic approach to the right lower quadrant of the abdomen. The patient's left arm should therefore be tucked to prevent excessive extension at patient's shoulder. *Black X shapes* demonstrate common port site placement for appendectomy, although additional or replaced ports may be placed as illustrated by the *white plus shapes*

The specific merits of a laparoscopic appendectomy (LA) over open appendectomy (OA) have been debated, however, particularly for obese patients or those with complicated AA. Initial series of comparative studies demonstrated possible faster recovery, earlier resumption of diet, and improved wound healing with LA versus OA. Other studies during the same time demonstrated no benefit. Most of these publications were small, and were thus underpowered. A meta-analysis performed in 2010 included 44 studies, pooling the results of appendectomy on 5,292 patients [19]. The only significant differences in outcome between the two techniques included slightly (8.67 min) longer operative time and slightly shorter length of hospital stay (0.6 days) for laparoscopic cases. Further, a Cochrane review in 2010 reviewed 56 studies [20]. This likewise demonstrated longer operative time (10 min) and shorter length of stay (1 day) with LA. These patients also had a lower subjective pain scale on postoperative day 1. While operative costs were significantly higher for laparoscopic cases, the out-of-hospital costs were lower.

The National Surgical Quality Improvement Program (NSQIP) provides a large standardized dataset of sampled surgical outcomes that can be accessed on a continuous basis. Based on a 2008 query that included 32,683 patients, 76.4% of appendectomies were performed laparoscopically [21]. Patients who underwent an open technique were statistically older, with increased comorbidities. On multivariate analysis, patients with LA had a decreased likelihood of developing any morbidity postoperatively, none of which were considered serious. Caution must be taken when interpreting this data, however, as causality cannot be ascertained. Those patients with comorbidities may have had an open procedure performed due to perceived decrease in operative time, inability to tolerate pneumoperitoneum due to cardiopulmonary disease, or other concerns by the surgeon.

Further query of the NSQIP dataset delineates more specific outcomes for appendectomy, particularly infection risk [22]. When adjusted for body mass index (BMI), sepsis, and operative time, wound infection had a risk reduction of 63% with LA. When adjusted for confounders, however, a 44% higher risk of organ space infection was noted for LA. Patients with wound class II, III, and IV had higher risk of organ space infection with a laparoscopic approach. In summary, the overall risk of complications was lower for LA, mostly due to a lower rate of wound infections; however, those patients with a greater degree of contamination had a higher risk of deep space infection postoperatively when LA was performed. This opposes the conventional wisdom that the laparoscopic approach affords a more thorough ability to washout the abdomen. The suction/irrigator may simply spread bacteria throughout the pelvis to a greater degree than with the limited view and dissection of the open technique.

Often surgeons advocate for the laparoscopic approach when operating on the obese patient. Less soft tissue dissection and greater visibility are often cited. Obese patients may also present a problem for the laparoscopic approach, however, due to diminished ability to ventilate during pneumoperitoneum and difficulty placing trocars or achieving appropriate angles for dissection due to soft tissue thickness. While reports of diminished wound infections in obese patients are noted in smaller reports, larger series comparing open to laparoscopic appendectomy demonstrate no difference in postoperative complications for these patients [23].

In summary, in a setting where basic laparoscopic expertise and equipment are available, LA has various slight advantages over OA, though some effects are small and of limited clinical significance. Women should be considered for a laparoscopic approach, as other adnexal pathology can be determined at operation. Young, employed, and more ambulatory patients also demonstrate added benefit from LA over OA, particularly in terms of resumption of activity and work.

Appendiceal Phlegmon or Abscess

Patients outside of the young, healthy demographic or who complain of prolonged periods of pain, may in fact present with an appendiceal phlegmon or abscess instead of simply suppurative appendicitis. A phlegmon consists of a mass of dense inflammatory tissue, often consisting of periappendiceal fat, but which may also include the cecum and/or terminal ileum. When encountered in the operating room, a phlegmon can significantly increase the difficulty of dissection, resulting in injury to adjacent tissues, or necessitating cecectomy or right hemicolectomy in order to achieve margins of resection that are not inflamed. An appendiceal abscess likewise represents a process which has walled itself off and clinically may result in less peritonism or systemic sequelae. In these cases, the acute process has already run its course, and secondary stages of inflammation with fibrosis have begun. Once inflammation has progressed to this stage, operative intervention becomes more dangerous, with risks of complications threefold higher in surgical versus nonsurgical management of cases of appendiceal phlegmon [24].

Overall, 2–6% of patients with AA will have some sort of inflammatory mass, and of those with an abscess, 20% will require drainage [25]. Of those requiring drainage, 2–6% will need to be approached in the operating room, due to inability to either access or adequately drain the collection percutaneously [26]. The early case series of patients treated in this manner were primarily pediatric, as the clinical presentation of symptoms was often late and surgical intervention less desirable. These patients often underwent treatment with antibiotics, with or without drainage, with planned interval appendectomy often 6–12 weeks later. Delayed operation was favored as the majority of the inflammation had subsided by this point, making operative intervention safer with reduced risk to adjacent organs [27, 28]. With success of this approach in the pediatric population, the adult population was treated similarly. Overall, conservative management of an appendiceal phlegmon was successful (i.e., did not require operative intervention) 76–97% of the time [29–32]. One of the larger studies comparing patients who underwent immediate surgery versus percutaneous drainage and interval appendectomy for AA with periappendiceal abscess included 104 patients. Patients who underwent immediate operation had a significantly higher rate of complications at initial hospitalization (58% versus 15%, $p < 0.001$). This group likewise had longer length of hospital stay [33].

Interval Appendectomy

The necessity of interval appendectomy after successful treatment with percutaneous drainage and antibiotics has been recently debated. Although expeditious surgical treatment has been considered the treatment of choice, the concept of delaying operation until inflammation has subsided has been proposed since the early 1900s [34]. Interval appendectomy is often recommended based on risk of subsequent AA or of risk of missing an incidental malignancy. A large retrospective study demonstrated a total recurrence rate of 14.6% in patients treated with antibiotics alone for phlegmon [35]. The majority of these recurrences occur within 3–6 months [31, 36, 37]. At this rate, interval appendectomy at 12 weeks would only prevent half of the potential recurrences. The recurrences that do occur have a relatively mild clinical course [24, 38]. There are likewise risks to operating in this setting, with complication rates for interval appendectomy ranging from 4 to 17% [29, 30]. This information has led some practitioners to approach an interval appendectomy with more expectant management depending on patient preference and perceived risk of malignancy [39].

Acute appendicitis associated with a phlegmon represents complicated inflammatory disease, and as such, should carry a higher index of suspicion for aberrant pathology. As an acute care surgeon, malignancy should be considered for any common inflammatory condition that has a variant presentation. A growing body of literature advocates for interval appendectomy for this reason. In a meta-analysis examining immediate versus interval appendectomy for AA, malignant disease was detected on follow-up in 1.2% of those who underwent interval appendectomy, approximately twice that reported for immediate appendectomy [24]. Patients at higher risk are those over 40 years of age, with type of tumor stratified per age group. Younger patients (mean 38 years old) present with carcinoid more commonly, while mucinous adenocarcinoma and intestinal-type adenocarcinoma are found in an older population (mean 60 years old) [40]. Colonic malignancy is strongly associated in those diagnosed with AA as age increases. The odds ratio for having concurrent colonic malignant disease was 38.5 for those over 40 years of age in a large population-based study [41]. For these reasons, patients who are over age 40 years or who are unreliable for dedicated follow-up should have interval appendectomy and/or follow-up colonoscopy performed.

Incidental Appendiceal Malignancy

Any neoplasm of the colon can also occur in the appendix, due to embryologic development of the appendix off of the cecum. Tumors of the appendix can obstruct the lumen and present as appendicitis. The acute care surgeon will therefore encounter appendiceal neoplasms either as detected on preoperative imaging or during operation. The majority are discovered only on the pathologic specimen, however. Approximately 0.7–1.7% of specimens will contain either benign or malignant appendiceal neoplasm [42, 43].

Carcinoid is the most common primary neoplasm of the appendix [44]. These appear as small round, well-demarcated tumors, usually at the tip of the appendix. Due to their small size and low metastatic potential, these are typically only discovered at time of follow-up. Metastatic potential is increased in tumors larger than 2 cm and with mesoappendiceal extension [45]. Based on this metastatic risk, patients with carcinoid larger than 2 cm, with any mesoappendiceal invasion, or any involvement of the base of the appendix should undergo right hemicolectomy. If these criteria are not met, then simple appendectomy is adequate resection [46].

Appendiceal adenocarcinomas are discovered on 0.08–0.1% of specimens [40]. Several histologic subtypes exist, including mucinous, intestinal type, signet ring, neuroendocrine, mixed, or undifferentiated. Subtype alone is not a significant prognostic factor, however. These tumors require treatment with a right hemicolectomy [47, 48]. In cases of perforated mucinous type (pseudomyxoma peritonei or "jelly belly"), a right hemicolectomy should only be performed in the setting of cytoreductive surgery and intraperitoneal chemotherapy (Sugarbaker procedure) [49, 50]. Handling of the tumor can result in further dissemination of peritoneal disease at time of the original procedure.

Specific information regarding rare neoplasms, as well as oncologic principles and follow-up are beyond the scope of this chapter. However, the acute care surgeon should be able to appropriately direct initial management when neoplasm is encountered in the setting of AA. If a suspicious mass or peritoneal mucin is noted on preoperative imaging, serum markers CEA, CA-125, and CA 19-9 should be sent and consideration given to biopsy prior to operative intervention. If diagnostic laparoscopy is performed, ports should be placed in the midline as these can be resected later if further definitive surgical therapy is needed. Colonoscopy may also help guide diagnosis and therapy prior to operative intervention.

If neoplasm is encountered incidentally at the time of operation, additional steps are needed to work up the disease process. The surgeon should search for extra-appendiceal disease, paying particular attention to the colon, liver, and omentum. If mucin, local lymph node spread, or other peritoneal seeding is noted, biopsies of these specimens should be sent to pathology. Unless the patient is at a center in which cytoreductive therapy is performed, the safest plan is to obtain good specimen for pathology, perform appendectomy, and refer the patient based on final pathology. If there is no evidence of additional peritoneal disease, and the tumor is less than 2 cm in size, an appendectomy should be performed [51]. Care should be taken to remove all of the mesoappendix and to do extensive washout of the peritoneal cavity and wounds. The specimen should be removed intact when able. If the mass is larger than 2 cm and there is no mucin or extraperitoneal spread is present, the case should be converted to open and a right hemicolectomy performed [52].

Most often the case exists in which no obvious tumor is noted either on preoperative imaging or during surgery, but neoplasm is reported on the final pathology report. If the histology is benign or carcinoid less than 2 cm and confined to the appendix, then no further therapy is needed. If the tumor has periappendiceal spread or it is larger than 2 cm, then right hemicolectomy needs to be performed. For any mucinous tumor or perforated epithelial tumor, obtaining tumor markers, staging CT scan, colonoscopy, and possible referral to a specialist are indicated [53].

Nonoperative Management of Acute Non-perforated Appendicitis

With the relative ease and satisfaction of performing an appendectomy, the concept of nonoperative management of non-perforated appendicitis is almost equivalent to heresy for the general surgeon. Pathophysiologic comparison to diverticulitis, as well as recognition of success with nonoperative management of perforated appendicitis has brought this concept back into consideration, however. While operative morbidity is low, there are still risks to surgery, with complication rates reported from 8 to 23% [54, 55].

Series of nonoperative cases of AA were initially reported from regions in which operative intervention is either unavailable or not practical. In 1956, Coldrey first reported on 471 patients with AA who were treated with antibiotics alone with documented low morbidity and mortality [56]. A 1977 report from the Chinese Medical Journal documented the successful nonoperative treatment of 425 patients with appendicitis [57]. Likewise, reports of Russian and US sailors on submarines treated with antibiotics alone for AA have been more recently published with favorable outcomes [58].

Subsequently, randomized trials have been conducted examining appendectomy versus antibiotic therapy for acute non-perforated appendicitis. The first of these was conducted in 1995 and included approximately 80 patients [59]. Of those treated with antibiotics alone, the success rate (no subsequent operative intervention required) was 97%. The recurrence rate at 1 year was 18% in the antibiotic group. An additional study of approximately the same size demonstrated 10% recurrence rate at 1 year [60].

Two larger randomized trials demonstrate feasibility of nonoperative management for non-perforated appendicitis, while providing valuable data regarding long term outcome after this approach. In a Swedish multicenter trial, 252 patients were randomized to appendectomy versus antibiotics [61]. Antibiotics consisted of IV infusion for 48 h, followed by oral antibiotics for 10 days. Of the antibiotic group, 86% improved without surgery. Recurrence rate of this group was 14% at 1 year. Of those who underwent appendectomy, a 14% complication rate was described. Reported pain by the antibiotic group was less and of shorter duration. The authors' conclusion was that AA could be successfully treated with antibiotics, with a recurrence rate similar to that of operative complication rate. These conclusions are not widely applicable to current practice, however. All patients included in the study were men younger than 50 years of age, and only 6% of patients underwent laparoscopic procedures. Also, patients who required operation within the first 24 h were not included in the number of those considered to have failed nonoperative management.

In a second larger trial, 369 patients were randomized to appendectomy or antibiotic therapy [62]. There was a high degree of cross-over, however, with half of the patients randomized to antibiotic therapy receiving appendectomy. Reasons for cross-over included patient preference and surgeon choice. This introduced bias toward operative intervention demonstrated by the fact that patients who underwent operation had higher white blood cell counts, pyrexia and peritonism compared to the antibiotic group. The authors concluded that antibiotic treatment was successful in 90.8% of patients. Patient receiving antibiotic therapy had a 13.9% recurrence rate at 16 months follow-up. Complications were three times higher in the appendectomy group, consisting of wound infections, small bowel obstruction, and intra-abdominal infection. Potentially due to this increase in complications, as well as operative costs, the antibiotic group had 20–25% less cost induced over the study period [63].

In summary, nonoperative treatment for AA has regained attention as a viable option. Antibiotics are effective in treating selected patient populations (including pediatrics) 68–95% of the time [64, 65]. Antibiotic strategy includes intravenous antibiotics for 48 h, then oral antibiotics for 7–10 days, with coverage aimed at gram-negative and anaerobic organisms [66]. Recurrence appendicitis occurs in 10–15% of patients at 1 year, is typically mild in presentation, and has no increased risk of perforation with time [67]. Nonoperative failure occurs most commonly when appendicolith is noted on imaging, or when the patient has a complicated or accelerated clinical course [68–70]. Overall indications for nonoperative management for AA includes: complicated appendicitis (phlegmon), a nonsurgical setting (boat), high operative risk, early appendicitis without appendicolith, and a compliant patient with access to follow-up. Due to risk of malignancy, any patient over age 40 years who elects for nonoperative management should undergo colonoscopy at 6 weeks.

Conclusion

Acute appendicitis is commonly encountered by the acute care surgeon. While most cases are straightforward, complicated appendicitis may still present some management challenges. Laparoscopic and open techniques of appendectomy are both appropriate options, with some minor advantages to laparoscopy. Perforated appendicitis with phlegmon should be approached nonoperatively initially, with percutaneous drainage of an abscess if present. The necessity of interval appendectomy is debated, although patients over 40 years of age should have appendectomy due to increased risk of incidental malignancy. Tumors of the appendix may often present as acute appendicitis, and the acute care surgeon should be adept at appropriate initial management of these neoplasms when encountered. Finally, nonoperative management with antibiotics for acute appendicitis has been described. This may be a viable option for patients at low risk of malignancy, in remote areas, or with prohibitive operative risk.

References

1. Addiss DG, Shaffer N, Fowler BS, Tauxe RV. The epidemiology of appendicitis and appendectomy in the United States. Am J Epidemiol. 1990;132(5):910–25.
2. McBurney II C. The indications for early laparotomy in appendicitis. Ann Surg. 1891;13(4):233–54.
3. Luckmann R. Incidence and case fatality rates for acute appendicitis in California. A population-based study of the effects of age. Am J Epidemiol. 1989;129(5):905–18.
4. Rivera-Chavez FA, Peters-Hybki DL, Barber RC, et al. Innate immunity genes influence the severity of acute appendicitis. Ann Surg. 2004;240(2):269–77.
5. Rivera-Chavez FA, Wheeler H, Lindberg G, Munford RS, O'Keefe GE. Regional and systemic cytokine responses to acute inflammation of the vermiform appendix. Ann Surg. 2003;237(3):408–16.
6. Livingston EH, Fomby TB, Woodward WA, Haley RW. Epidemiological similarities between appendicitis and diverticulitis suggesting a common underlying pathogenesis. Arch Surg. 2011;146(3):308–14.
7. Barker DJ, Osmond C, Golding J, Wadsworth ME. Acute appendicitis and bathrooms in three samples of British children. Br Med J (Clin Res Ed). 1988;296(6627):956–8.
8. Birnbaum BA, Wilson SR. Appendicitis at the millennium. Radiology. 2000;215(2):337–48.
9. Flum DR, Koepsell T. The clinical and economic correlates of misdiagnosed appendicitis: nationwide analysis. Arch Surg. 2002;137(7):799–804. discussion 804.
10. Doria AS, Moineddin R, Kellenberger CJ, et al. US or CT for diagnosis of appendicitis in children and adults? A meta-analysis. Radiology. 2006;241(1):83–94.
11. Puylaert JB. Acute appendicitis: US evaluation using graded compression. Radiology. 1986;158(2):355–60.
12. Pedrosa I, Lafornara M, Pandharipande PV, Goldsmith JD, Rofsky NM. Pregnant patients suspected of having acute appendicitis: effect of MR imaging on negative laparotomy rate and appendiceal perforation rate. Radiology. 2009;250(3):749–57.
13. Shindoh J, Niwa H, Kawai K, et al. Predictive factors for negative outcomes in initial non-operative management of suspected appendicitis. J Gastrointest Surg. 2010;14(2):309–14.
14. Bickell NA, Aufses Jr AH, Rojas M, Bodian C. How time affects the risk of rupture in appendicitis. J Am Coll Surg. 2006;202(3):401–6.
15. Berenguer CM, Ochsner Jr MG, Lord SA, Senkowski CK. Improving surgical site infections: using National Surgical Quality Improvement Program data to institute Surgical Care Improvement Project protocols in improving surgical outcomes. J Am Coll Surg. 2010;210(5):737–41. 741–3.
16. Hale DA, Molloy M, Pearl RH, Schutt DC, Jaques DP. Appendectomy: a contemporary appraisal. Ann Surg. 1997;225(3):252–61.
17. Blomqvist PG, Andersson RE, Granath F, Lambe MP, Ekbom AR. Mortality after appendectomy in Sweden, 1987–1996. Ann Surg. 2001;233(4):455–60.
18. Blomqvist P, Ljung H, Nyrén O, Ekbom A. Appendectomy in Sweden 1989–1993 assessed by the Inpatient Registry. J Clin Epidemiol. 1998;51(10):859–65.
19. Li X, Zhang J, Sang L, et al. Laparoscopic versus conventional appendectomy—a meta-analysis of randomized controlled trials. BMC Gastroenterol. 2010;10:129.
20. Sauerland S, Jaschinski T, Neugebauer EA. Laparoscopic versus open surgery for suspected appendicitis. Cochrane Database Syst Rev. 2010;(10):CD001546.
21. Ingraham AM, Cohen ME, Bilimoria KY, et al. Comparison of outcomes after laparoscopic versus open appendectomy for acute appendicitis at 222 ACS NSQIP hospitals. Surgery. 2010;148(4):625–35. discussion 635–7.
22. Fleming FJ, Kim MJ, Messing S, et al. Balancing the risk of postoperative surgical infections: a multivariate analysis of factors associated with laparoscopic appendectomy from the NSQIP database. Ann Surg. 2010;252(6):895–900.
23. Clarke T, Katkhouda N, Mason RJ, et al. Laparoscopic versus open appendectomy for the obese patient: a subset analysis from a prospective, randomized, double-blind study. Surg Endosc. 2011;25(4):1276–80.
24. Andersson RE, Petzold MG. Nonsurgical treatment of appendiceal abscess or phlegmon: a systematic review and meta-analysis. Ann Surg. 2007;246(5):741–8.
25. Arnbjörnsson E. Management of appendiceal abscess. Curr Surg. 1984;41(1):4–9.
26. Gillick J, Velayudham M, Puri P. Conservative management of appendix mass in children. Br J Surg. 2001;88(11):1539–42.
27. Thomas DR. Conservative management of the appendix mass. Surgery. 1973;73(5):677–80.
28. Marya SK, Garg P, Singh M, Gupta AK, Singh Y. Is a long delay necessary before appendectomy after appendiceal mass formation? A preliminary report. Can J Surg. 1993;36(3):268–70.
29. Skoubo-Kristensen E, Hvid I. The appendiceal mass: results of conservative management. Ann Surg. 1982;196(5):584–7.
30. Willemsen PJ, Hoorntje LE, Eddes E-HH, Ploeg RJ. The need for interval appendectomy after resolution of an appendiceal mass questioned. Dig Surg. 2002;19(3):216–20. discussion 221.
31. Lai H-W, Loong C-C, Chiu J-H, et al. Interval appendectomy after conservative treatment of an appendiceal mass. World J Surg. 2006;30(3):352–7.
32. Jordan JS, Kovalcik PJ, Schwab CW. Appendicitis with a palpable mass. Ann Surg. 1981;193(2):227–9.
33. Brown CVR, Abrishami M, Muller M, Velmahos GC. Appendiceal abscess: immediate operation or percutaneous drainage? Am Surg. 2003;69(10):829–32.
34. Ochsner AJ. VI. Ileus caused by neoplasms. Ann Surg. 1901;33(4):457–65.
35. Tekin A, Kurtoğlu HC, Can I, Oztan S. Routine interval appendectomy is unnecessary after conservative treatment of appendiceal mass. Colorectal Dis. 2008;10(5):465–8.

36. Kaminski A, Liu I-LA, Applebaum H, Lee SL, Haigh PI. Routine interval appendectomy is not justified after initial nonoperative treatment of acute appendicitis. Arch Surg. 2005;140(9):897–901.

37. Hoffmann J, Lindhard A, Jensen HE. Appendix mass: conservative management without interval appendectomy. Am J Surg. 1984;148(3):379–82.

38. Dixon MR, Haukoos JS, Park IU, et al. An assessment of the severity of recurrent appendicitis. Am J Surg. 2003;186(6):718–22. discussion 722.

39. Eriksson S, Styrud J. Interval appendicectomy: a retrospective study. Eur J Surg. 1998;164(10):771–4. discussion 775.

40. McCusker ME, Coté TR, Clegg LX, Sobin LH. Primary malignant neoplasms of the appendix: a population-based study from the surveillance, epidemiology and end-results program, 1973–1998. Cancer. 2002;94(12):3307–12.

41. Lai H-W, Loong C-C, Tai L-C, Wu C-W, Lui W-Y. Incidence and odds ratio of appendicitis as first manifestation of colon cancer: a retrospective analysis of 1873 patients. J Gastroenterol Hepatol. 2006;21(11):1693–6.

42. Bucher P, Mathe Z, Demirag A, Morel P. Appendix tumors in the era of laparoscopic appendectomy. Surg Endosc. 2004;18(7):1063–6.

43. Connor SJ, Hanna GB, Frizelle FA. Appendiceal tumors: retrospective clinicopathologic analysis of appendiceal tumors from 7,970 appendectomies. Dis Colon Rectum. 1998;41(1):75–80.

44. Carr NJ, Sobin LH. Neuroendocrine tumors of the appendix. Semin Diagn Pathol. 2004;21(2):108–19.

45. Goede AC, Caplin ME, Winslet MC. Carcinoid tumour of the appendix. Br J Surg. 2003;90(11):1317–22.

46. Gouzi JL, Laigneau P, Delalande JP, et al. Indications for right hemicolectomy in carcinoid tumors of the appendix. The French Associations for Surgical Research. Surg Gynecol Obstet. 1993;176(6):543–7.

47. Nitecki SS, Wolff BG, Schlinkert R, Sarr MG. The natural history of surgically treated primary adenocarcinoma of the appendix. Ann Surg. 1994;219(1):51–7.

48. Lo NSF, Sarr MG. Mucinous cystadenocarcinoma of the appendix. The controversy persists: a review. Hepatogastroenterology. 2003;50(50):432–7.

49. Sugarbaker PH, Chang D. Results of treatment of 385 patients with peritoneal surface spread of appendiceal malignancy. Ann Surg Oncol. 1999;6(8):727–31.

50. González-Moreno S, Sugarbaker PH. Right hemicolectomy does not confer a survival advantage in patients with mucinous carcinoma of the appendix and peritoneal seeding. Br J Surg. 2004;91(3):304–11.

51. Stocchi L, Wolff BG, Larson DR, Harrington JR. Surgical treatment of appendiceal mucocele. Arch Surg. 2003;138(6):585–9. discussion 589–90.

52. Navarra G, Asopa V, Basaglia E, et al. Mucous cystadenoma of the appendix: is it safe to remove it by a laparoscopic approach? Surg Endosc. 2003;17(5):833–4.

53. Murphy EMA, Farquharson SM, Moran BJ. Management of an unexpected appendiceal neoplasm. Br J Surg. 2006;93(7):783–92.

54. Liu K, Ahanchi S, Pisaneschi M, Lin I, Walter R. Can acute appendicitis be treated by antibiotics alone? Am Surg. 2007;73(11):1161–5.

55. Tingstedt B, Johansson J, Nehez L, Andersson R. Late abdominal complaints after appendectomy—readmissions during long-term follow-up. Dig Surg. 2004;21(1):23–7.

56. Coldrey E. Treatment of acute appendicitis. Br Med J. 1956;2(5007):1458–61.

57. Anon. Combined traditional Chinese and western medicine in acute appendicitis. Chin Med J. 1997;3(4):266–9.

58. Adams ML. The medical management of acute appendicitis in a nonsurgical environment: a retrospective case review. Mil Med. 1990;155(8):345–7.

59. Eriksson S, Granström L. Randomized controlled trial of appendicectomy versus antibiotic therapy for acute appendicitis. Br J Surg. 1995;82(2):166–9.

60. Malik AA, Bari S. Conservative management of acute appendicitis. J Gastrointest Surg. 2009;13(5):966–70.

61. Styrud J, Eriksson S, Nilsson I, et al. Appendectomy versus antibiotic treatment in acute appendicitis: a prospective multicenter randomized controlled trial. World J Surg. 2006;30(6):1033–7.

62. Hansson J, Körner U, Khorram-Manesh A, Solberg A, Lundholm K. Randomized clinical trial of antibiotic therapy versus appendicectomy as primary treatment of acute appendicitis in unselected patients. Br J Surg. 2009;96(5):473–81.

63. Davies GM, Dasbach EJ, Teutsch S. The burden of appendicitis-related hospitalizations in the United States in 1997. Surg Infect (Larchmt). 2004;5(2):160–5.

64. Nadler EP, Reblock KK, Vaughan KG, et al. Predictors of outcome for children with perforated appendicitis initially treated with nonoperative management. Surg Infect (Larchmt). 2004;5(4):349–56.

65. Oliak D, Yamini D, Udani VM, et al. Nonoperative management of perforated appendicitis without periappendiceal mass. Am J Surg. 2000;179(3):177–81.

66. Sakorafas GH, Mastoraki A, Lappas C, et al. Conservative treatment of acute appendicitis: heresy or an effective and acceptable alternative to surgery? Eur J Gastroenterol Hepatol. 2011;23(2):121–7.

67. Varadhan KK, Humes DJ, Neal KR, Lobo DN. Antibiotic therapy versus appendectomy for acute appendicitis: a meta-analysis. World J Surg. 2010;34(2):199–209.

68. Bufo AJ, Shah RS, Li MH, et al. Interval appendectomy for perforated appendicitis in children. J Laparoendosc Adv Surg Tech A. 1998;8(4):209–14.

69. Akbar F, Yousuf M, Morgan RJ, Maw A. Changing management of suspected appendicitis in the laparoscopic era. Ann R Coll Surg Engl. 2010;92(1):65–8.

70. Tsai H-M, Shan Y-S, Lin P-W, Lin X-Z, Chen C-Y. Clinical analysis of the predictive factors for recurrent appendicitis after initial nonoperative treatment of perforated appendicitis. Am J Surg. 2006;192(3):311–6.

71. Malik AA, Wani NA. Continuing diagnostic challenge of acute appendicitis: evaluation through modified Alvarado score. Aust N Z J Surg. 1998;68(7):504–5.

Diverticulitis

Michael S. Truitt and Anand Lodha

Introduction

Epidemiology

Diverticular disease is one of the most common causes of abdominal pain in the Western world. In addition, it appears to be increasing in incidence and demonstrates an age-dependent distribution. For example, diverticulosis affects only 5% of people age 40, but can be found in two-thirds of adults by age 85 [1]. Approximately 20% of patients with diverticulosis will suffer from at least one episode of diverticulitis. In fact, the prevalence of diverticulitis across all age groups in the United States is 60 per 100,000 [2]. Over a 7-year period from 1998 to 2005, Etzioni et al. demonstrated a 26% increase in hospital admissions secondary to diverticulitis. In this study, the largest increase (82%) was in the youngest cohort of patients age 18–44 [3]. The etiology for this increase is unknown, but may be related to dietary considerations. A gender predilection for diverticulitis has been demonstrated in some studies, but not duplicated in others [1, 4]. Obesity has been implicated but these findings have been inconsistent as well. In contrast, geographic patterns have been firmly established. While diverticular disease is predominately left sided (98.5%) in Western societies, it is much more common on the right (70%) in Asia [5].

M.S. Truitt, M.D., F.A.C.S. (✉)
Methodist Hospital of Dallas, 221 W. Colorado Blvd, Pav 2,
Suite 425, Dallas, TX 75208, USA
e-mail: mike_truitt@hotmail.com

A. Lodha, M.D.
Department of Surgery, Methodist Hospital of Dallas,
Dallas, TX, USA

Clinical Presentation

Colonic diverticula are classified as "false" or pulsion diverticula since they do not contain all layers of the bowel wall. The colon is predisposed to develop diverticulosis at four well-described points secondary to a weakness of the bowel wall where the vasa recta penetrate the circular muscle layer (Fig. 26.1) [6]. Although the vast majority of patients with diverticulosis will remain asymptomatic throughout their lives (70%), others will suffer severe and sometimes repeated bouts of diverticulitis (20%) and diverticular bleeding (10%).

Diverticulitis refers to inflammation or infection of a diverticulum. The patient with diverticulitis will commonly present with fever, leukocytosis, and left lower quadrant pain; however, the absence of these does not preclude a diagnosis of diverticulitis as about half of patients will not have a fever or leukocytosis [7]. The presence or absence of symptoms can be attributed to the severity of the underlying inflammatory process. Therefore, the diagnosis of diverticulitis is further characterized into uncomplicated and complicated to reflect the severity of the episode. Uncomplicated diverticulitis may be clinically silent with the exception of a mild variance in bowel habits. It accounts for the majority (75%) of cases and is usually amenable to medical therapy. Complicated diverticulitis refers to inflammation of the diverticula in concert with perforation, abscess, obstruction, or fistula. The majority of patients with complicated diverticulitis will require intervention.

Bleeding is the other major complication of diverticular disease. The etiology of a lower gastrointestinal bleed in this setting is secondary to progressive weakening of the vasa recta as the diverticulum forms. The vessels are placed under tension and the protective layers are progressively thinned, ultimately leaving them exposed to injury and rupture [8]. Diverticular disease accounts for approximately 40% of all lower gastrointestinal (GI) bleeding and is self-limiting 90% of the time. Massive bleeding occurs in 5–7% of cases and risk

L.J. Moore et al. (eds.), *Common Problems in Acute Care Surgery*,
DOI 10.1007/978-1-4614-6123-4_26, © Springer Science+Business Media New York 2013

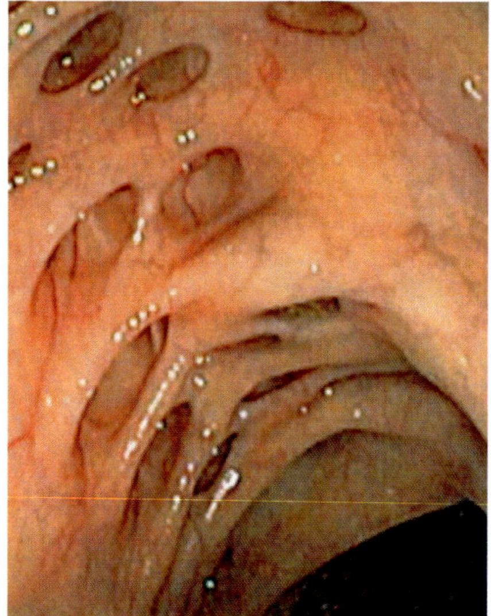
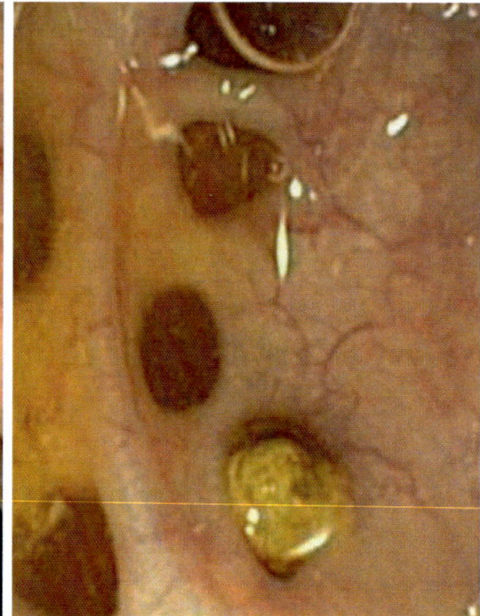

Fig. 26.1 Diverticular disease: (*left*) diverticulosis, (*right*) diverticulitis

factors are anticoagulation, ischemic heart disease, and the use of nonsteroidal anti-inflammatory drugs. Despite accounting for only 10% of diverticula, the right side of the colon is the bleeding source in 50% of cases. Diverticulitis does not increase the risk of diverticular bleeding and inflammation is not classically present during a bleeding episode [9].

Diagnosis

The initial evaluation of a patient with suspected acute diverticulitis includes a history and physical examination, a complete blood count (CBC), urinalysis, and plain abdominal radiographs in selected clinical scenarios. A diagnosis of acute diverticulitis can often be made based on history and physical exam findings, especially in patients with a history of diverticulitis. However, in many cases of abdominal pain, it may be unclear whether diverticulitis is the causative etiology and adjunctive studies may be helpful and warranted. Alternative diagnoses include irritable bowel syndrome, gastroenteritis, bowel obstruction, inflammatory bowel disease, appendicitis, ischemic colitis, colorectal cancer, urinary tract infection, kidney stone, and gynecologic disorders. An elevated white blood cell count often is helpful in confirming the presence of an inflammatory process. Pyuria may reveal a urinary tract infection, and hematuria may suggest a kidney stone. Plain abdominal films may show pneumoperitoneum from a perforated viscus, or signs of bowel obstruction.

In the modern era, computerized tomography (CT) scan of the abdomen and pelvis is usually the most appropriate imaging modality in the assessment of suspected diverticulitis (Fig. 26.2). Accuracy is enhanced if oral, intravenous, and rectal contrast is used. In this setting, CT is highly sensitive and specific, with a low false-positive rate [10]. Features typical of diverticulitis on CT are: presence of diverticula in

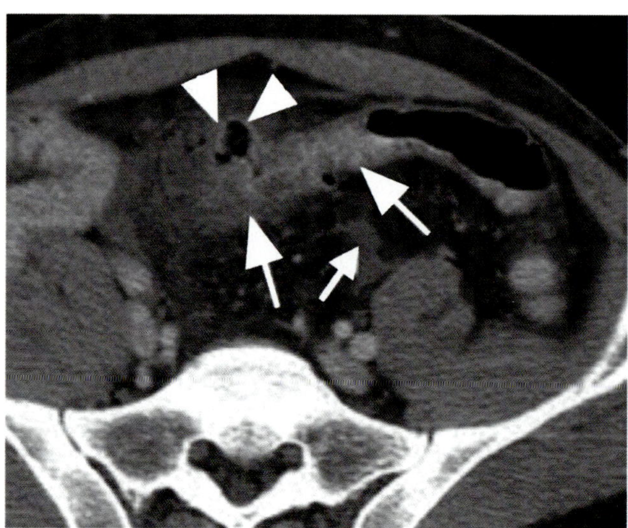

Fig. 26.2 CT findings of diverticulitis

descending or sigmoid colon, surrounding fat stranding, and bowel wall thickening. Complications, such as phlegmon, abscess, adjacent organ involvement and fistula, can also be identified and may alter the treatment regimen. A large abscess found on initial CT scan may prompt early percutaneous drainage and delay operative intervention. Severity staging, most commonly utilizing the Hinchey classification system, aids in the selection of patients who are most likely to respond to conservative therapy (Table 26.1) [11]. The severity of diverticulitis at the time of the first CT scan not only predicts an increased risk of failure of medical therapy on index admission but also a high risk of secondary complications after initial nonoperative management [12]. The incidence of a subsequent complication is highest in patients with severe disease on the initial CT scan [13].

Table 26.1 Hinchey classification system

Hinchey stage	
I	Pericolic abscess
II	Retroperitoneal or pelvic abscess
III	Purulent peritonitis
IV	Fecal peritonitis

Contrast enema and endoscopy are also occasionally useful in the initial evaluation of a patient with suspected acute diverticulitis. A gently administered single contrast enema may show stenosis/spasm with intact mucosa and associated surrounding diverticulosis. Diverticular strictures may also be apparent as they are usually longer and more regular than in carcinoma [14]. This diagnostic modality has largely been abandoned given the risk of perforation and subsequent complications. Endoscopy has limited use in the acute setting and may exacerbate inflammation or cause perforation [15]. As a follow-up modality, however, endoscopy should be utilized to exclude an oncologic component to the inflammatory disease process. An Australian study conducted by Lau et al. examined the incidence of malignancy after an acute attack of left-sided diverticulitis [16]. Almost 3% of patients received a diagnosis of colorectal cancer, while 26% of patients were diagnosed with polyps >1 cm. The odds of a diagnosis of colorectal cancer were 4 times higher in patients with local perforation, 6.7 times higher in patients with an abscess, and 18 times higher in patients with a fistula when compared to patients with uncomplicated diverticulitis. Once the acute attack has resolved, colonoscopy should be performed to exclude malignancy prior to elective operative intervention.

Management of Diverticular Disease

Uncomplicated Diverticulitis

The treatment of patients with diverticulitis has changed significantly in recent years. Patients may be treated on an outpatient basis in the absence of systemic signs. If they demonstrate mild abdominal tenderness, low-grade fever, and the ability to tolerate oral intake, reliable patients can be treated with oral antibiotics, low residue diet, and close follow-up. Antibiotics should be directed toward typical lower gastrointestinal flora. Oral antibiotic regimens, based on consensus rather than randomized trials, include gram-negative coverage typically with a fluoroquinolone or sulfa-based drug. Anaerobic coverage should be provided with metronidazole or clindamycin. Patients not meeting outpatient criteria will need to be hospitalized for intravenous fluids and antibiotics. Immunocompromized patients will also benefit from inpatient treatment. Intravenous antibiotic regimens such as ampicillin-sulbactam, timentin-clavulanate, or piperacillin/tazobactam are appropriate in this setting. For patients who require intravenous antibiotics but have a demonstrated beta-lactam intolerance, alternative regimens consist of a fluoroquinolone and metronidazole or monotherapy with a carbapenem. Subsequent to successful treatment of acute diverticulitis with conservative therapy, approximately 1/3 of patients will experience another episode. After a second episode, another 1/3 of patients will be subjected to a third attack. Of all patients with diverticulitis, about 1/5 will ultimately require operative intervention [17].

Elective resection can be safely performed 4–6 weeks after the most recent episode has resolved. Guidelines from the American Society of Colorectal Surgeons (ASCRS) taskforce in 2000 recommended segmental resection after two uncomplicated attacks of diverticulitis or after a single episode of complicated diverticulitis. This traditional surgical dictum has been called into question since that time. In a study from the Lahey Clinic, Hall et al. demonstrated that although diverticulitis recurrence was common (36%) following an initial attack that was managed medically, complicated recurrence was uncommon (3.9%) over a follow-up period of 5 years. Right-sided diverticulitis also had a low rate of recurrence [18]. Family history of diverticulitis, length of involved colon >5 cm, and a retroperitoneal abscess were independent risk factors associated with recurrence. In light of these and other data [19] we have become more liberal in our application of expectant management, but still generally endorse the guidelines from the ASCRS while also taking into consideration:

1. Physiologic reserve
2. Frequency of attacks
3. Severity of attacks
4. Impact on quality of life

Overall, morbidity after open colectomy for diverticulitis ranges from 9 to 54%, while mortality ranges from 0 to 1.2%. Risk factors for morbidity after elective left colectomy for diverticular disease are [20]:

1. Greater than 10% weight loss
2. Body mass index (BMI) >30
3. Left hemicolectomy (versus left segmental colectomy)

Traditionally, patients afflicted with an episode of diverticulitis are initially treated with bowel rest. Once the clinical picture begins to improve they are instructed to consume a clear liquid diet. The diet is then advanced as tolerated. A more aggressive approach limits the concept of bowel rest, with immediate resumption of a low-residue diet instead. Once an acute flare has subsided, a high fiber maintenance diet has been advocated. This may decrease both the formation of diverticula and the chance of a symptomatic recurrence. This recommendation is based on the idea that long-term fiber supplementation produces a bulky stool that results in a larger diameter colon, thereby decreasing segmentation and subsequent pressure, which may be protective in the formation of diverticula. The data in support of this and other dietary measures is not conclusive. Other anecdotal recommendations are to avoid caffeine, alcohol, and tobacco but the data do not indicate that these are risk factors [21]. Additional dietary restrictions frequently given to patients are to avoid seeds, corn, and nuts. While this advice makes intuitive sense, these small difficult to digest particles could become lodged in a diverticulum and predispose a patient to diverticulitis or perforation, a large observational study did not reveal an association with diverticular disease [22].

Complicated Diverticulitis

Small localized and intramural abscesses may resolve without intervention. Larger abscesses (>3 cm) are best managed with percutaneous drainage. After source control has been achieved, clinical improvement should occur within 48 h. In the absence of clinical improvement or if the condition of the patient worsens, repeat imaging may identify a previously undetected abscess, or worsening of an existing abscess, which would prompt a change of therapy. Conservative management of diverticulitis has grown more aggressive, recognizing the benefits of converting an emergency surgical intervention into an elective one. Advances in imaging, critical care, parenteral nutrition, and interventional techniques have lent themselves towards this goal. Mutch et al. examined the efficacy of nonoperative management in acute complicated diverticulitis [23]. Complicated diverticulitis was defined as having an associated abscess or free air diagnosed by CT scan. Out of 136 patients, 28% required percutaneous drainage, and 27% required parenteral nutrition. In total, only 5% (seven patients) failed medical management and required urgent surgery. Forty-eight percent then went on to have elective resections of their diverticular disease. Contraindications to a nonoperative approach include hemodynamic instability, generalized peritonitis, CT scan with significant free air and fluid, or immunosuppression. Operative intervention is also required for clinical deterioration after a period of expectant management.

Operative Approaches

The principles surrounding operative intervention focus on control of sepsis and determination of proper intestinal continuity. Preoperative considerations consist of aggressive intravenous fluid resuscitation and correction of electrolyte abnormalities. Bowel preparation is not indicated in the emergent setting. Historically there have been four basic approaches:

1. Staged procedure of (a) proximal diversion and drainage, (b) subsequent resection, and (c) final restoration of bowel continuity at a third procedure.
2. Resection and colostomy (modified Hartmann procedure)
3. Resection with primary anastomosis and diversion
4. Resection with primary anastomosis

The first has largely been abandoned secondary to high infectious complications resulting in substantial morbidity and mortality [24]. Rarely, it can be utilized as a temporizing procedure in a patient with severe diverticulitis and a frozen operative field. By diverting the fecal stream, diverticulitis that has been recalcitrant to antibiotic therapy may respond, rendering the subsequent operation less hostile.

Indications for a modified Hartmann's procedure include: fecal peritonitis, immunosuppression, malnutrition, significant intraoperative fluid or vasopressor requirements, and uncertain viability of the bowel. Preoperative placement of ureteral stents may prove useful during dissection. A dense inflammatory reaction precludes the usual lateral-to-medial dissection. A more appropriate conduct of operation is to go from proximal-to-distal, beginning the dissection along the lateral peritoneal reflection of the descending colon and distally in the rectum. Careful dissection is often necessary to separate the attached viscera, often a "pinching" or finger fracture maneuver aids in this endeavor. The proximal resection margin should incorporate the entire thickened segment. The distal margin should always extend to the recto-sigmoid junction, as the extension of the tenia coli around the rectum prevents diverticula from occurring at this level. The rectal stump should be labeled with a long, nonabsorbable suture and pelvic drains may be considered. In a study from the Mayo Clinic recurrent diverticulitis as it relates to the level of distal resection was investigated. Recurrent diverticulitis was noted in 12.5% of patients with use of the distal sigmoid in the anastomosis versus 6.7% where the rectum was used. Reoperation was required in 3.4% in the former, and 2.2% in the latter [25].

Recent papers have compared resection and primary anastomosis (PRA) with and without diversion to Hartmann's procedure and concluded that PRA may be superior except in high-risk patients [26]. In 1982, Farkouh et al. reported on 15 patients with perforated diverticulitis and diffuse peritonitis on whom an immediate anastomosis was constructed. Their criteria for anastomosis required: the bowel must not be distended; the bowel must be empty of feces; there should be minimal edema of the bowel wall at the resection edge; the distal segment of colon should be above the peritoneal reflection; there should be no fecal contamination and the patient's general medical condition should be reasonably good [27]. Under these rigid and uncommon circumstances, they recommended resection and primary anastomosis.

More recently other authors have shown that one-stage operations can be safely performed in Hinchey III/IV patients in the absence of immunosuppression or chronic kidney disease [28].

There is a growing body of evidence regarding the use of laparoscopic lavage and drainage in the face of sealed, purulent peritonitis with low morbidity and mortality rates [29]. This was born out of documentation in the literature that a discreet perforation site was rarely identified in patients that underwent urgent operation for diverticulitis with free air. Dissection of the phlegmon to identify the perforation should be avoided as this may create more spillage and bleeding. Franklin et al. reported on 40 patients who underwent intraoperative peritoneal lavage with excellent results. None required more invasive operative intervention during the index admission, 50% underwent elective laparoscopic colectomy after resolution of the acute attack, and none of the remaining 50% required surgical intervention at a follow-up of 8 years [30]. Given these recent reports of success, this may be another effective tool in the hands of an appropriately trained surgeon to mitigate the morbidity of an urgent operation and diminish the need for colostomy.

Recently, the management of peritonitis has been stratified into one concerning purulent peritonitis (peritonitis with abscess) versus fecal peritonitis (peritonitis with fecal soilage). Feculent peritonitis appears to carry with it an increased morbidity and mortality (35% vs. 6%) when compared directly to purulent peritonitis [31]. This may indicate the need for a more conservative operative approach in the setting of feculent peritonitis. Despite these differences, the management of generalized peritonitis warrants several key points, as offered by Fazio:

1. Resect the perforated segment.
2. Do not do more than is required.
3. Do not open further avenues of sepsis by performing extensive peritoneal dissection (i.e., entering the presacral space).
4. Do not create a mucous fistula.
5. Examine the open specimen for malignancy.

Other Considerations

Emergent colorectal resections carry with them high risk of morbidity and mortality, especially in the rapidly growing elderly population. A retrospective review of 292 patients 65 years and older undergoing emergency colorectal procedures revealed a 35% overall complication rate. Pneumonia (25%), persistent or recurrent respiratory failure (15%), and myocardial infarction (12%) were the most frequent complications. Operative time, shock, renal insufficiency and significant intra-abdominal contamination were independent risk factors associated with morbidity. Age, septic shock at presentation, large estimated intraoperative blood loss, delay to operation, and development of a complication were associated with in-hospital mortality [32].

The management of diverticulitis in young patients is more controversial. Small and older studies have pointed towards diverticulitis being more aggressive in younger patients, and hence, these patients were more likely considered for early resection. Recently, however, studies have called into question the natural history and severity of diverticulitis in younger patients. A study from Switzerland compared older and younger patients (<50 years) regarding clinical and radiologic parameters of acute left colonic diverticulitis to determine whether differences existed in its presentation and treatment. Younger patients needed fewer emergency surgical procedures and fewer colostomies. In addition, conservative treatment was more successful in younger patients [33]. Other studies have shown no significant differences in outcomes for younger patients [34, 35]. The most recent ASCRS practice parameters on sigmoid diverticulitis state: "There is no clear consensus regarding whether younger patients (less than 50 years) treated for diverticulitis are at increased risk of complications or recurrent attacks. Nevertheless, because of their longer life span, younger patients will have a higher cumulative risk of recurrent diverticulitis, even if the virulence of their disease is no different than that of older patients." Authors from Oxford performed an analysis of the literature for the management of diverticulitis in younger patients. They concluded that the risk of recurrence after conservative treatment is related to the severity of the attack at presentation rather than the age of the patient [36].

Complications of diverticulitis can present acutely, in the form of strictures, fistulas, or persistent inflammation. Strictures often do not present as complete bowel obstruction, rather with recurrent partial obstructive symptoms. Patients should be evaluated endoscopically and radiographically to exclude a malignant process and undergo resection when appropriate. Colocutaneous fistulas usually present as a complication of percutaneous drainage tracts. In men, fistulas are often associated with the genitourinary tract and symptoms such as pneumaturia or recurrent urinary tract infections may be present on history and physical exam. Computed tomography is the diagnostic procedure of choice with the finding of air in the non-instrumented bladder being pathognomonic. Women can also have colovesicular fistulas, but if a prior hysterectomy has been performed, they are also at risk for a colovaginal fistula. Symptoms include passage of flatus or stool per vagina, vaginitis, or recurrent urinary tract infections. Workup with a water-soluble contrast enema or a methylene blue enema with a vaginal tampon can aid in the diagnosis.

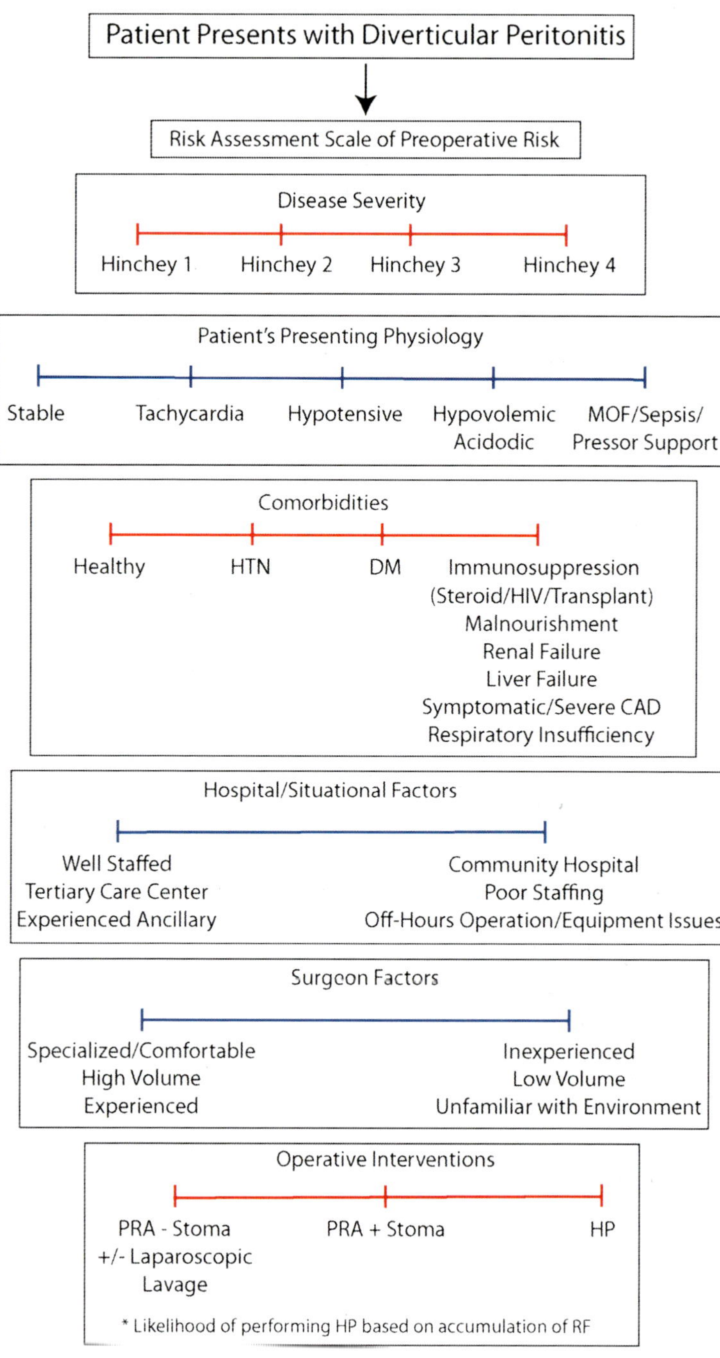

Fig. 26.3 Proposed treatment algorithm. Adapted from Bauer VP. Emergency management of diverticulitis. Clin Colon Rectal Surg. 2009 August;22(3):161–8

Conclusion

The treatment of diverticulitis is more "complicated" than ever before. What was once straightforward and amenable to a simple algorithm now requires thoughtful consideration of individual patient comorbidities, physiology at the time of presentation, and the treating surgeon's experience with an ever-expanding number of treatment options (Fig. 26.3).

References

1. Parks TG. Natural history of diverticular disease of the colon. Clin Gastroenterol. 1975;4:53.
2. Fry RD, Mahmoud N. Segmental resection for diverticulitis. Cameron current surgical therapy. 9th ed. Philadelphia, PA: Mosby Elsevier; 1516.
3. Etzioni DA, Mack TM, Beart RW, Kaiser AM. Diverticulitis in the United States: 1998–2005: changing patterns of disease and treatment. Ann Surg. 2009;249:210.

4. Rodkey GV, Welch CE. Changing patterns in the surgical treatment of diverticular disease. Ann Surg. 1984;200:466.

5. Fischer MG, Farkas AM. Diverticulitis of the cecum and ascending colon. Dis Colon Rectum. 1984;27:454.

6. Meyers MA, Alonso DR, Gray GF, Baer JW. Pathogenesis of bleeding colonic diverticulosis. Gastroenterology. 1976;71:577.

7. Ambrosetti P, Robert JH, Witzig JA, et al. Acute left colonic diverticulitis: a prospective analysis of 226 consecutive cases. Surgery. 1994;115:546.

8. Buttenschoen K, Buttenschoen DC, Odermath R, et al. Diverticular disease-associated hemorrhage in the elderly. Arch Surg. 2001;386(1):8–16.

9. Lewis M. Bleeding colonic diverticula. J Clin Gastroenterol. 2008;42(10):1156–8.

10. Doringer E. Computed tomography of colonic diverticulitis. Crit Rev Diagn Imaging. 1992;33:421–35.

11. Detry R, James J, Kartheuser A, et al. Acute localized diverticulitis: optimum management requires accurate staging. Int J Colorectal Dis. 1992;7:38–42.

12. Ambrosetti P, Grossholz M, Becker C, Terrier F, Morel P. Computed tomography in acute left colonic diverticulitis. Br J Surg. 1997;84:532–4.

13. Chautems RC, Ambrosetti P, Ludwig A, Mermillod B, Morel P, Soravia C. Long-term follow-up after first acute episode of sigmoid diverticulitis: is surgery mandatory? a prospective study of 118 patients. Dis Colon Rectum. 2002;45:962–6.

14. Hiltunen KM, Kolehmainen H, Vuorinen T, et al. Early water-soluble contrast enema in the diagnosis of acute colonic diverticulitis. Int J Colorectal Dis. 1991;6:190–2.

15. Chappuis CW, Cohn Jr I. Acute colonic diverticulitis. Surg Clin North Am. 1988;68:301–13.

16. Lau KC, Spilsbury K, Farooque Y, et al. Is colonoscopy still mandatory after a CT diagnosis of left-sided diverticulitis: can colorectal cancer be confidently excluded? Dis Colon Rectum. 2011;54:1265–70.

17. Wong WD, Wexner SD, Lowry A, et al. Practice parameters for the treatment of sigmoid diverticulitis-supporting documentation. The Standards Task Force. The American Society of Colon and Rectal Surgeons. Dis Colon Rectum. 2000;43:290.

18. Hall JF, Roberts PL, Ricciardi R, et al. Long-term follow-up after an initial episode of diverticulitis: what are the predictors of recurrence? Dis Colon Rectum. 2011;54(3):283–8.

19. Anaya DA, Flum DR. Risk of emergency colectomy and colostomy in patients with diverticular disease. Arch Surg. 2005;140:681–5.

20. Piessen G, Muscari F, Rivkine E, et al. Prevalence of and risk factors for morbidity after elective left colectomy: cancer vs noncomplicated diverticular disease. Arch Surg. 2011;146:1149.

21. Aldori WH, Giovanucci EL, Rimm EB, et al. A prospective study of physical activity and the risk of symptomatic diverticular disease in men. Ann Epidemiol. 1995;5:221.

22. Strate LL, Liu YL, Syngal S, et al. Nut, corn, and popcorn consumption and the incidence of diverticular disease. JAMA. 2008;300:907.

23. Dharmarajan SM, Hunt SR, Mutch MG, et al. The efficacy of nonoperative management of acute complicated diverticulitis. Dis Colon Rectum. 2011;54:663–71.

24. Adson MA, Pemberton JH, Nagorney DM. Sigmoid diverticulitis with perforation and generalized peritonitis. Dis Colon Rectum. 1985;28:71–5.

25. Benn PL, Wolff BG, Ilstrup DM. Level of anastomosis and recurrent colonic diverticulitis. Am J Surg. 1986;151:269–71.

26. Constantinides VA, Heriot A, Remzi F, et al. Operative strategies for diverticular peritonitis: a decision analysis between primary resection and anastomosis and Hartmann's procedure. Ann Surg. 2007;245:94–107.

27. Farkouh E, Hellou G, Allard N, et al. Resection and primary anastomosis for diverticulitis with perforation and peritonitis. Can J Surg. 1982;25(3):314–6.

28. Richter S, Lindemann W, Kollmar O, et al. One-stage sigmoid colon resection for perforated sigmoid diverticulitis. World J Surg. 2006;30(6):1027–32.

29. Myers E, Winter DC. Adieu to Henri Hartmann? Colorectal Dis. 2010;12(9):849–50.

30. Franklin ME, Portillo G, Trevino JM, et al. Long-term experience with the laparoscopic approach to perforated diverticulitis plus generalized peritonitis. World J Surg. 2008;32(7):1507–11.

31. Nagorney DM, Adson MA, Pemberton JH. Sigmoid diverticulitis with perforation and generalized peritonitis. Dis Colon Rectum. 1985;28:71.

32. McGillicuddy EA, Schuster KM, Davis KA, et al. Factors predicting morbidity and mortality in emergency colorectal procedures in elderly patients. Arch Surg. 2009;144(12):1157–62.

33. Kotzampassakis N, Pittet O, Schmidt S, et al. Presentation and treatment outcome of diverticulitis in younger adults: a different disease than in older patients? Dis Colon Rectum. 2010;53(3):333–8.

34. Biondo S, Pares D, Marti Rague J, et al. Acute colonic diverticulitis in patients under 50 years of age. Br J Surg. 2002;89:1137–41.

35. Nelson RS, Velasco A, Mukesh BN. Management of diverticulitis in younger patients. Dis Colon Rectum. 2006;49:1341–5.

36. Janes S, Meagher A, Faragher IG. The place of elective surgery following acute diverticulitis in young patients: when is surgery indicated? An analysis of the literature. Dis Colon Rectum. 2009;52:1008–16.

Laura E. White and Heitham T. Hassoun

Introduction

Acute mesenteric ischemia (AMI) is an uncommon yet life-threatening syndrome with a grave prognosis. Despite advancements in readily available diagnostics and improvements in the ability to care for critically ill patients, patients presenting with AMI face a mortality rate approaching 65% [1–3]. This high predicted mortality has remained relatively unchanged over the past several decades even in the era of evolving endovascular approaches to management of AMI. While the reasons for this stubborn trend are likely multifactorial, failure of physicians to quickly recognize symptoms of AMI on presentation most likely drives these devastating outcomes. Once the diagnosis of AMI is entertained, prompt diagnostic studies and swift therapeutic interventions are essential to successful treatment. With any delay in intervention, AMI leads to bowel necrosis, inciting a cascade of both local organ injury and remote organ system dysfunction, which is most often irreversible and fatal.

AMI can result from a number of pathophysiologic conditions; however, the clinical syndrome can be divided into four clinical presentations:

1. *Embolic* occlusion of the superior mesenteric and/or celiac arteries.
2. Acute *thrombosis* of one of these mesenteric arterial vessels.
3. *Non-occlusive* mesenteric ischemia (NOMI).
4. Mesenteric *venous thrombosis* (MVT).

L.E. White, M.D.
Department of Surgery, The Methodist DeBakey Heart and Vascular Center, The Methodist Hospital, Houston, TX, USA
e-mail: LHollinger@tmhs.org

H.T. Hassoun, M.D. (✉)
Departments of Surgery and Cardiovascular Surgery, The Methodist Hospital Physician Organization, 6550 Fannin Street, SM 1401, Houston, TX 77030, USA
e-mail: hhassoul@jhmi.edu

This chapter will first describe the clinical presentation and diagnostic evaluation of AMI. Subsequently, we will provide algorithms for surgical and nonsurgical management, guidelines for perioperative and long-term patient care, and review current clinical outcomes data for this challenging surgical emergency.

Epidemiology

AMI is a devastating but rare disease, occurring slightly more frequently than ruptured abdominal aortic aneurysms. In a review spanning 12 years, the overall incidence of AMI diagnosed at either autopsy or operation was estimated to be 12.9/100,000 person-years[4]. The prevalence of AMI is increasing in the United States, in part as a consequence of the aging populations and the high prevalence of associated and etiological comorbidities [2]. Roughly two-thirds of cases are caused by acute superior mesenteric artery (SMA) occlusion, whereas MVT and NOMI compromise the remaining third [4]. The incidence was found to increase with age, and is distributed equally between genders. Many patients (up to 73%) have a history of symptoms consistent with prior chronic mesenteric ischemia [4]. Despite advancements in diagnostic technology and therapeutic modalities, including endovascular management of AMI, the risk of death in AMI remains 60–70%, emphasizing the importance of early diagnosis and prompt intervention in this devastating disease [5, 6].

Clinical Presentation

The classic presentation of AMI is pain out of proportion to that produced upon physical exam. This clinical scenario in which the patient complains of excruciating abdominal pain prior to the onset of peritonitis, especially in patients at risk, is a well-established paradigm that should incite quick diagnostic pursuits and a high index of suspicion for AMI. Signs

L.J. Moore et al. (eds.), *Common Problems in Acute Care Surgery*,
DOI 10.1007/978-1-4614-6123-4_27, © Springer Science+Business Media New York 2013

of peritonitis typically develop after the onset of irreversible intestinal ischemia and bowel infarction, and waiting for peritonitis prior to intervention results in unacceptably high patient morbidity and mortality. In a study of all causes for AMI, 95% of patients presented with abdominal pain, 44% with nausea, 35% with vomiting, 35% with diarrhea, and 16% with blood per rectum [7]. Approximately one-third of patients present with the triad of abdominal pain, fever, and heme-positive stools. In most patients, severe abdominal pain progressively worsens while bowel infarction causes the initially lagging physical exam findings to catch up with the onset of peritonitis.

Different etiologies of AMI may be associated with slightly different clinical presentations; for example, patients with thrombotic mesenteric occlusion have the typical sudden onset of out-of-proportion abdominal pain, but may report a chronic history of postprandial abdominal pain and significant weight loss. Patients with NOMI have pain that is generally more diffuse and may wax and wane. Patients with MVT present a challenging diagnosis, as abdominal complaints may be nonspecific and include nausea, vomiting, diarrhea, abdominal cramping, and non-localized abdominal pain. Most symptoms in patients with MVT are non-acute, and a study of MVT patients found that 84% presented with abdominal pain, and of these only 16% presented with peritoneal signs; other presenting symptoms included diarrhea (42%), nausea and vomiting (32%), malaise (16%), and upper gastrointestinal (GI) bleeding (10%) [8].

Several risk factors for AMI have been identified and may facilitate prompt diagnosis for this scenario. In one study of patients with AMI, 78% had a history of hypertension, 71% had a history of tobacco use, 62% presented with a history of peripheral vascular disease, and 50% had a history of coronary artery disease [7]. Independent predictors of perioperative mortality for AMI include the presence of cardiac illness, elevated plasma urea levels, and the presence of both large and small bowel involvement [9]. Specific etiologies of AMI also garner certain risk factors; embolic occlusion of the mesenteric circulation is typically associated with recent cardiovascular events (myocardial infarction, atrial fibrillation, mural thrombosis, mitral valve disease, or left ventricular aneurysm) or previous embolic disease. In fact, nearly 50% of patients presenting with embolic AMI have atrial fibrillation [7] and approximately one-third of patients have a prior history of arterial embolus. Additionally, a "paradoxical" SMA embolism may occur in patients who have cardiac defects with a right-to-left shunt such as atrial septal defect (ASD) or patent foramen ovale (PFO). Patients with thrombotic occlusion typically have other manifestations of diffuse atherosclerotic disease such as coronary artery disease, carotid stenosis, and peripheral artery disease. Risk factors for NOMI differ in that NOMI is typically associated with low-flow states and severe mesenteric vasoconstriction.

Patients at risk for NOMI include ambulatory patients taking ergot alkaloids or digitalis, the critically ill with vasopressor requirements, and those undergoing dialysis with large volume fluid removal. Finally, patients with a history of previous venous thrombosis or pulmonary embolism, a known hypercoagulable state, and those taking oral contraceptives or estrogen supplementation are at an increased risk for MVT.

Diagnosis

Given the often nonspecific presentation of patients with AMI, the diagnosis is often delayed. The importance of prompt surgical evaluation cannot be overemphasized. After onset of symptoms, a delay in surgical consultation of greater than 24 h or a delay in operation of more than 6 h results in an increase in mortality [10]. Surprisingly, patients who presented with abdominal distention, elevated lactate, acute renal failure, shock, and lack of abdominal pain were more likely to have a delay in surgical consultation. Therefore a heightened awareness of AMI may lead to swift surgical evaluation, diagnosis, and treatment and allow for improved outcomes.

Laboratory Tests

The diagnosis of AMI generally relies heavily on a thorough history and physical examination combined with a high index of suspicion. Laboratory tests can alert the physician of the diagnosis, although none are specific to AMI. Indicators of systemic inflammation such as an elevated white blood cell (WBC) count (>20,000/mm^3) and signs of metabolic acidosis such as an increased base deficit and elevated serum lactate levels are frequently found. In a Mayo clinic study, 98% of patients with AMI had an elevated WBC count and 50% had counts higher than 20,000 mm^3 [7]. Additionally, 91% had elevated lactate levels (61% higher than 3 mmol/L), 71% had an elevated AST, and 52% had an abnormal base deficit. Other studies have identified D-dimer as a potential diagnostic marker for AMI; however, while the sensitivity was 94.7%, the specificity only approached 78.6% due to many other pathologies that may cause increased D-dimer levels [11]. Therefore, this diagnostic tool must be used with caution.

Abdominal X-Rays

Abdominal radiographs can neither establish nor exclude the diagnosis of AMI; however, they may reveal signs consistent with bowel ischemia if obtained late in presentation of this disease. Thumb printing along with a generalized pattern of ileus, and in severe cases, gas in the bowel and/or portal venous system may be identified. Patients who have abnormalities by the time abdominal radiography is obtained have a 78% mortality rate compared to 38% in patients with normal films, indicating the severity of disease progression required to produce abnormal plain radiography [12]. Most commonly, abdominal plain films reveal an ileus or are completely unremarkable, but can be helpful for excluding other causes of abdominal pain such as bowel obstruction, perforation of a hollow viscus, or kidney stones.

Duplex Ultrasonography

The role of duplex ultrasonography (US) in diagnosing chronic mesenteric ischemia is well established, however, in the acute setting, US has a limited application. Given the nature of disease in patients with AMI, bowel ileus with excessive bowel gas and bowel edema hinders visualization of the mesenteric vessels. Additionally, after-hours presentation of AMI often precludes availability of the vascular laboratory. Furthermore, while duplex US provides accurate imaging of stenotic and occlusive lesions at the origin of the mesenteric vessels, it fails to adequately image beyond the proximal portion of the vessel. Accordingly, duplex US is of little value in the presence of NOMI.

Computed Tomography

Traditional computed tomographic (CT) scanning has provided successful identification of arterial patency and anatomy, and additionally, has been able to evaluate bowel health and identify other causes of abdominal pain such as bowel perforation, bowel obstruction, and pancreatitis. For example, if identified along with signs of necrotic bowel, the presence of hepatic venous portal gas portends a >50% mortality rate in AMI [13]. With advancements in helical (spiral) CT scanning and multi-slice, multi-array helical CT scanning, the visceral arterial anatomy can now be visualized with three-dimensional special resolution. Consequently, CT angiography (CTA) has surpassed angiography as the diagnostic evaluation of choice due to its combined ability to accurately define mesenteric arterial anatomy and identify secondary signs of ischemia [14]. Spiral CTA has a reported 75% sensitivity and 100% specificity for detecting >75% stenosis of the celiac artery and a sensitivity of 100% and a specificity of 91% for detection of SMA stenosis [15]. Recent studies with multi-detector 16 row CTA reveal a sensitivity and specificity of 96.4% and 97.9%, respectively, in diagnosing AMI with an overall accuracy of 95.6% [16, 17].

While sophisticated CT technology provides excellent image clarity and definition, limitations persist. The origins of the celiac artery and the SMA are well visualized with CT, but secondary and tertiary branches are less apparent, and contrast angiography remains the gold standard for these small mesenteric vessels. CTA also tends to overestimate the degree of critical stenosis compared to conventional angiography; however, this limitation appears to be diminishing with refinements in multi-array or multi-detector technology. Additionally, significant calcification at vessel origins can interfere with CTA and make it difficult to determine the true degree of stenosis.

Computed tomography retains a valuable role in diagnosing MVT and is the preferred diagnostic imaging modality in patients presenting with abdominal pain who have a history of deep vein thrombosis (DVT) or a known hypercoagulable disorder [18]. It readily identifies superior mesenteric vein (SMV) thrombosis, with or without bowel abnormalities, and in fact, the identification of SMV thrombosis in asymptomatic patients has expanded our understanding of the pathophysiology and broad spectrum of this disease. Computed tomographic scanning correctly identifies 100% of patients with acute MVT and 93% of those with chronic MVT, whereas conventional angiography correctly diagnoses MVT in only five of nine patients [8, 19].

Progress in contrast-enhanced, three-dimensional magnetic resonance angiogram (MRA) technology has decreased the time requirement for this exam and made vast improvements in practicality and its applicability to the diagnosis of AMI. MRA also contains the advantage of employing a less nephrotoxic contrast agent, gadolinium, than the contrast agents for CT scans. This exam must be avoided, however, in patients with end stage renal disease due to the risk of nephrogenic fibrosing dermopathy. Like computed tomography angiography (CTA), MRA does not accurately image the distal mesenteric branch vessels. Studies comparing CTA and MRA demonstrate excellent agreement for proximal celiac and SMA disease; however, identification of intrahepatic arterial branches are much more variable [20].

Contrast Angiography

Contrast angiography has long been the gold standard for imaging the visceral vessels. This modality can visualize the aorta and the main trunks of the mesenteric vessels and can adequately asses several orders of distal branches. The images obtained with contrast angiography are superior to those obtained with CTA or MRA. The procedure can be performed from a transfemoral or a transbrachial approach using a modified Seldinger technique, and should be performed in both anterior–posterior (AP) and lateral views to identify proximal segments of the celiac, superior mesenteric, and inferior mesenteric arteries. The origins of the celiac artery and the SMA are best seen on the lateral view,

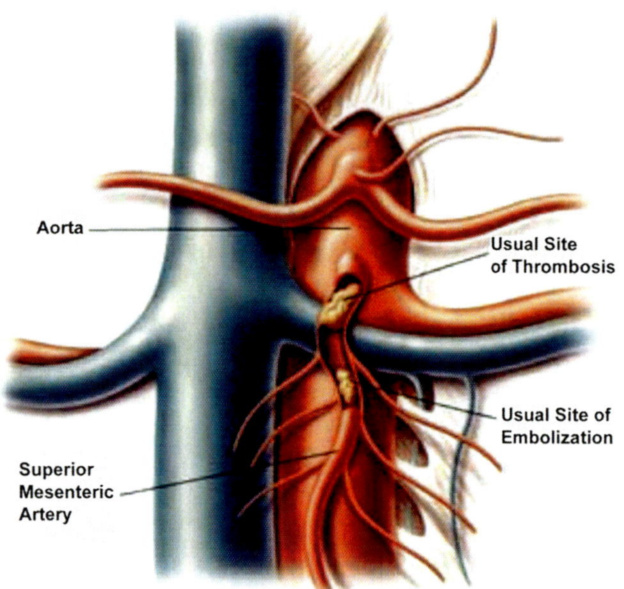

Fig. 27.1 Depiction of usual sites of SMA embolus versus thrombosis. Note sparing of proximal jejunal branches with more distal lodgment of an embolus. Reprinted with permission from Hassoun HT: Acute mesenteric ischemia. Chapter in: Current surgical therapy, 9th ed. Cameron JL (ed.), Mosby, Inc., pp. 884–889

whereas the middle and distal SMA and IMA are best seen on the AP view.

Classic angiographic patterns can distinguish AMI due to SMA embolism versus thrombosis. The SMA is by far the most likely visceral vessel for an embolism because its take-off angle from the aorta is much less acute than that of the celiac or inferior mesenteric arteries. SMA emboli usually lodge distal to the middle colic and proximal jejunal branches, while SMA thrombosis usually occurs at the SMA origin where there is formation of an atherosclerotic plaque (Figs. 27.1 and 27.2a, b). Angiographic findings in patients with AMI secondary to NOMI include narrowing of the origins of SMA branches, alternate narrowing/dilation of branch vessels, generalized spasm of distal arteries, and absent filling of distal intramural branches. These patterns are often best seen in the AP projection, and delayed views are often useful in evaluating a patient for NOMI.

Angiography is less useful for the diagnosis of MVT. Typically, MVT is diagnosed on the venous phase of selective arterial contrast injection; however, conventional angiography is less sensitive and specific for MVT than CTA: the diagnostic imaging modality of choice.

In addition to providing superior imaging quality, contrast angiography enables the surgeon to perform selective injection of any of the mesenteric vessels and to perform therapeutic intervention. In patients with NOMI, for example, the SMA may be selectively catheterized and a vasodilator such as nitroglycerine or papaverine infused directly into the vessel (Fig. 27.3). In a stable patient with AMI

from a partially occluding embolus but no peritoneal signs, selective catheterization of the SMA allows the institution of catheter-directed thrombectomy or intra-arterial thrombolytic therapy. Thus, contrast angiography not only represents the gold standard for diagnostic imaging but also provides important therapeutic options.

Given the current state of imaging technology, either CTA or MRA can confirm the diagnosis of AMI. Once the cause of ischemia is confirmed, and, in the case of SMA thrombosis, if distal targets are identified for revascularization, it is conceivable that the patient could be explored in the operating room without prior conventional contrast angiography. However, if institutions lack access to a hybrid endovascular suite, formal contrast angiography remains the best imaging modality for evaluation of the mesenteric vasculature.

Management

Embolic Occlusion of Mesenteric Vessels

The goals in surgical treatment of AMI are (1) to restore normal pulsatile flow to the SMA, (2) to resect any nonviable intestine, and (3) to perform second-look laparotomy when viability of the intestine is questionable. In general, revascularization precedes resection. The therapeutic approach varies, depending on the specific underlying cause. For embolic disease of the SMA, the standard treatment is surgical embolectomy.

After initial resuscitation with intravenous (IV) fluids, systemic heparinization, and antibiotics, the patient is taken to the operating room where a midline incision is performed for abdominal exploration. The transverse colon is reflected superiorly and the small bowel is reflected laterally to the patient's right. The ligament of Treitz is fully incised and the root of the mesentery is fully mobilized. The SMA is easily palpated by placing four fingers of the surgeon's hand behind the root of the mesentery with the thumb opposite and anterior to the root. The SMA is identified as the firm tubular structure, which may or may not have a palpable pulse. Alternatively, the SMA can also be identified by following the middle colic artery through the transverse colon until it enters the SMA at the root of the mesentery. Proximal and distal control is then obtained by sharp dissection, exposing the artery from its surrounding mesenteric tissue. Patients with SMA embolus will typically have an identifiable pulse proximally in the root of the mesentery with absent pulse distally. Once proximal control is obtained, an arteriotomy (either transverse or longitudinal) is them performed and a Fogarty balloon embolectomy is performed both proximally and distally. The embolus is usually removed with restoration of both back-bleeding as well as return of inflow. The arteriotomy is then closed either primarily or with a patch

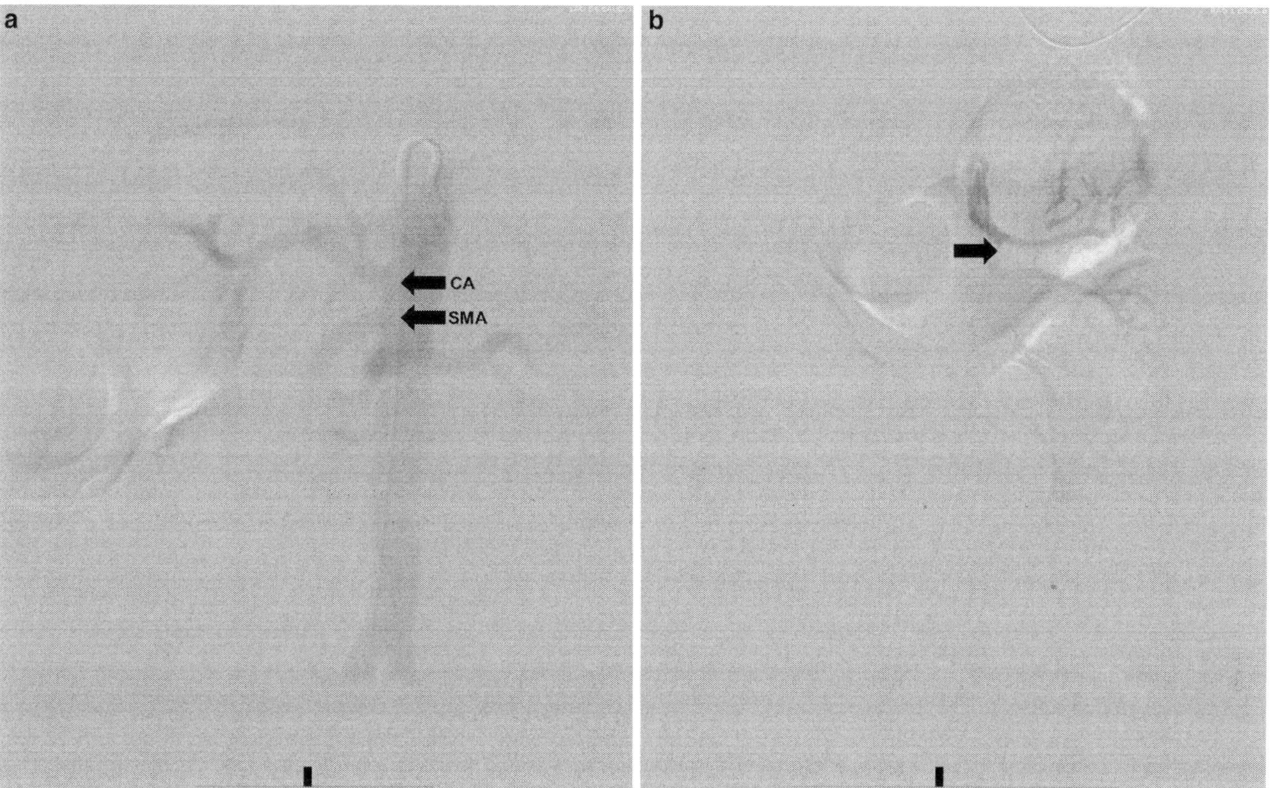

Fig. 27.2 (**a**) Aortogram demonstrating patent origins of the celiac artery (CA) and SMA. (**b**) Selective SMA angiogram demonstrating embolic occlusion of the SMA (*arrow*)

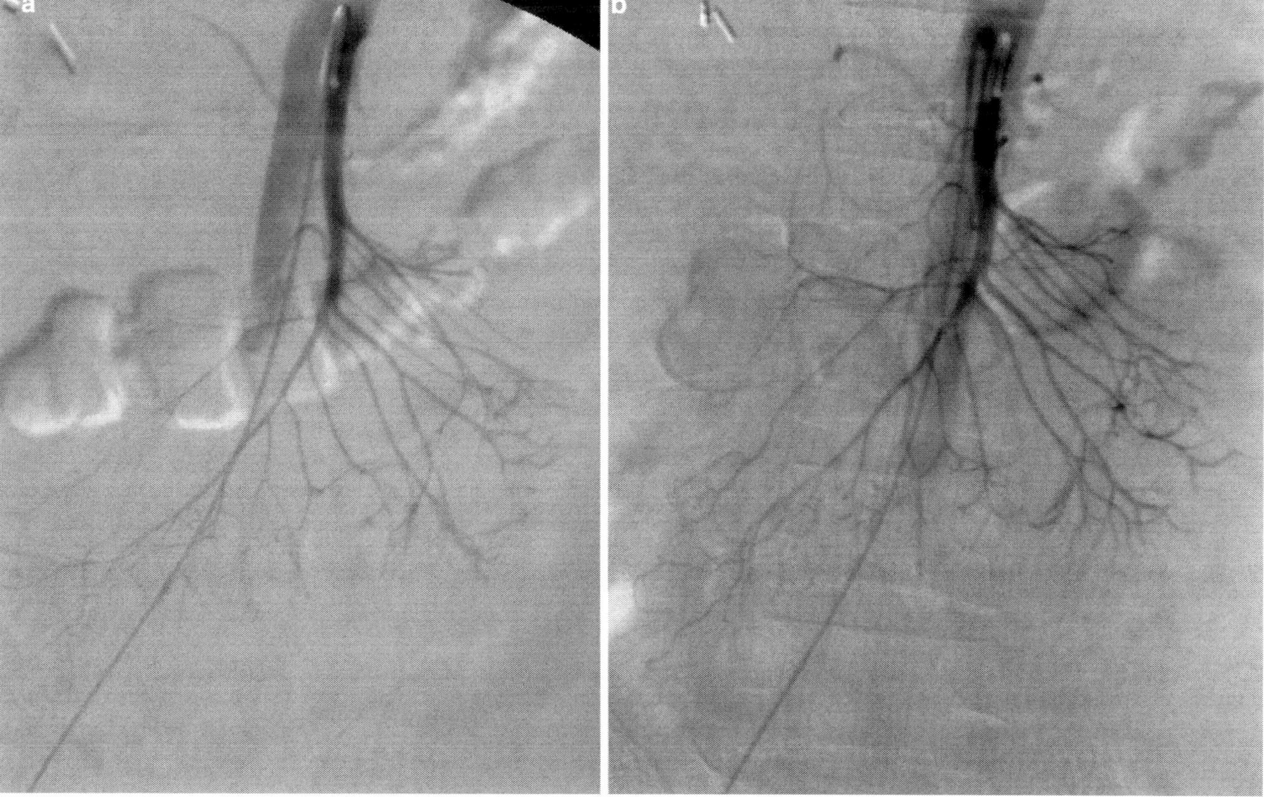

Fig. 27.3 Selective SMA angiogram in a patient with NOMI before (**a**) and after (**b**) treatment with catheter-directed papaverine infusion. Note improved filling of more distal SMA branches after treatment

angioplasty. After restoration of flow, a hand-held continuous wave Doppler can be used to detect the adequacy of intestinal blood flow.

Next, an assessment of bowel viability is performed followed by resection of clearly necrotic or nonviable intestine at this initial exploration. For cases of SMA embolism, the distal small bowel and proximal colon are typically affected with sparing of the proximal jejunum and transverse colon. Determination of bowel viability of marginally perfused intestine can be difficult even in the most experienced hands. Continuous wave Doppler ultrasound of the anti-mesenteric border, intraoperative IV administration of fluorescein and transcutaneous oxygen measurements have all been described, but none of these modalities are sensitive or specific for predicting ultimate bowel viability. Therefore, if any sections of intestine demonstrate questionable viability, the patient should be scheduled for a second-look laparotomy within 24–48 h for resection of nonviable tissue. The decision to perform second-look laparotomy should be made at the initial operation and adhered to strictly; often patients will improve clinically with resuscitation yet will still harbor necrotic bowel that must be removed to prevent systemic sepsis.

Percutaneous interventional treatment of the SMA occlusion has been described in the literature. At present, however, the applicability of this approach is limited, since most patients present with symptoms that warrant an exploratory laparotomy for evaluation of intestinal viability. In patients who present with abdominal pain and have no peritoneal signs that would necessitate immediate laparotomy, catheter-directed intra-arterial thrombolytic therapy of partially occlusive SMA emboli can be considered. Case reports have documented successful thrombolytic therapy, angioplasty and stenting in patients with AMI [21]; however, this route should be used cautiously and in the correct patient population (i.e., those without peritoneal signs or radiographic suggestion of bowel infarction). These patients will require close monitoring in the intensive care unit (ICU) setting with frequent abdominal examinations, and even if catheter-directed therapy does restore flow to affected bowel, the patient may still experience pain sufficient to warrant exploration. For these reasons, our use of thrombolytic therapy is highly selective.

SMA Thrombosis

AMI secondary to acute SMA thrombosis occurs in patients with long-standing atherosclerotic disease of the mesenteric vessels, and the entire midgut is usually involved. Surgical treatment consists of a bypass procedure, which may be done in either an anterograde or retrograde manner. The decision regarding the optimal method is often made intraoperatively based on the quality of the inflow vessels and patient condition. The conduit of choice is a reversed autologous greater saphenous vein graft. If possible, synthetic graft material should be avoided in the setting of acute bowel ischemia, given the risk of transmural infarction and bowel perforation. There are several inflow options for revascularization of the SMA including the supraceliac aorta, the infra-renal aorta, and the iliac arteries. While antegrade bypass graft of the supraceliac aorta to the SMA tunneled behind the pancreas is the optimal configuration because of less susceptibility to kinking, retrograde bypass from either the infra-renal aorta or iliac artery may be easier to perform in the acute setting when rapid revascularization is the ultimate goal. Additionally, retrograde bypass results in less hemodynamic compromise by avoiding supraceliac clamping and associated mesenteric and renal ischemia. Many of these patients, however, will have severe atherosclerotic disease precluding retrograde bypass and therefore the surgeon should be ready to perform revascularization from either approach.

Recently, a combined open and endovascular approach has been described [22]. With this technique, the infracolic SMA is exposed as usual and following thrombectomy and patch angioplasty, a sheath is placed in the infracolic SMA through the distal end of the patch for retrograde cannulation and stenting of the lesion. This hybrid technique offers both the advantages of open laparotomy for assessment of bowel viability and endovascular management for rapid revascularization, thus limiting ischemic time.

Patients with severe comorbidities without signs of peritonitis who present with acute SMA thrombosis may occasionally be treated with catheter-directed thrombolysis followed by percutaneous angioplasty and stenting; however, this treatment modality should be performed selectively and patients should be monitored closely for the need to undergo surgical exploration.

Non-occlusive Mesenteric Ischemia

Management of NOMI is largely nonoperative, and once the diagnosis has been established with angiography, treatment of the underlying precipitating cause is the key therapeutic intervention. Fluid resuscitation, optimization of cardiac output, and elimination of vasopressors are primary measures that greatly impact outcome. Selective SMA catheterization and papaverine infusion (30–60 mg/h) offers adjunctive therapy, and the infusion is continued for 24–48 h with repeat angiography at regular intervals to gauge efficacy. This algorithm is reserved for patients with hemodynamic stability and no signs of peritonitis on physical examination. Alternative therapy has been described using intra-arterial tolazoline and glycerol trinitrite as local dilators with good success [23].

If a patient presents with peritoneal signs, an exploratory laparotomy will be required for resection of frankly necrotic or gangrenous bowel. Intra-arterial papaverine infusion started prior to operation can be continued throughout surgical exploration. Additionally, given the propensity of NOMI to wax and wane in severity, a second-look laparotomy becomes imperative (see later section: Second-Look Laparotomy).

Mesenteric Venous Thrombosis

The mainstay of therapy for MVT is anticoagulation; however, if the patient's condition does not improve or worsens or if signs or symptoms of bowel ischemia develop, abdominal exploration is warranted. Most patients with MVT can be successfully managed with anticoagulation alone [8]; however, many will still require small bowel resection. Thrombolytic therapy can also treat MVT, with the catheter being placed into either the SMA for lysis of portal vein thrombus [8] or into the SMV or portal vein intraoperatively [24].

Additionally, once the diagnosis of MVT has been established, a hypercoagulable workup should be initiated to identify the underlying cause. If the patient has a hematologic hypercoagulable state, lifelong anticoagulation is recommended; however, if the cause is reversible, anticoagulation can be discontinued after 3–6 months.

Second-Look Laparotomy

Second-look laparotomy is an essential part of AMI management. Regardless of which adjunctive measure is employed intraoperatively to assess bowel perfusion and viability, second-look laparotomy is the most reliable means of determining the viability of marginally perfused bowel after revascularization. Indications for a second look include presentation with a low-flow state, requirement for small bowel resection and anastomosis, or requirement of a mesenteric thromboembolectomy [25]. Prior to a second look, appropriate fluid resuscitation and correction of any metabolic imbalances should be undertaken. Furthermore, the decision to return to the operating room for a second look should be made upon initial exploration, and should not be foregone regardless of the patient's condition 24–48 h later. Often, patients may retain necrotic bowel even after correction of metabolic derangements and volume status.

Some authors have advocated the use of second-look laparoscopy as an alternative to repeat laparotomy, citing lower operative times, shortened anesthesia requirements, and fewer postoperative complications such as wound complications [26]. The role of laparoscopic second-look operations remains unknown; however, an increasing number of recent publications reflect the widening experience with this modality [25, 27].

Anatomic Considerations

The splanchnic vasculature follows a well-described pattern with commonly identified variations that are crucial to understanding the presentation and pathogenesis of AMI. Important variations from classic splanchnic arterial anatomy include a common celiacomesenteric trunk, "replaced" hepatic arterial branches from the superior mesenteric artery (SMA) supply as opposed to their usual celiac origin, and the "Arch of Buhler": persistent ventral anastomosis between the proper hepatic and the replaced right hepatic from the SMA [28].

The SMA arises from the abdominal aorta 1–2 cm below the origin of the celiac trunk. Classically, the hepatic arteries arise from the celiac axis via the common and proper hepatic arteries; however, the right hepatic artery obtains its origin from the SMA in 15–20% of patients and the left hepatic artery branches from the left gastric artery in 25% of patients [29]. Should the celiac or superior mesenteric arteries experience an acute occlusion, the gastroduodenal artery becomes an important source for collateral flow. Additional SMA vascular anastomotic arcades occur with varying degrees of development among patients, with important implications during AMI. Large-vessel anastomoses arise along the 10–20 jejunal and ileal branches from the SMA. An anastomosis between the SMA and inferior mesenteric artery (IMA) occurs between the middle and left colic branches of the SMA and the IMA at the splenic flexure of the colon, termed "Griffith's point," a watershed area. The IMA arises from the abdominal aorta 5–6 cm below the origin of the SMA, supplying the left half of the transverse colon and the descending colon via the left colic artery. The marginal artery of Drummond and the arc of Riolan are important SMA and IMA collaterals that are capable of enlarging upon occlusion of the proximal splanchnic arteries.

The venous anatomy of the splanchnic system parallels the arterial anatomy, and the confluence of the superior mesenteric and splenic veins forms the portal vein, supplying vital perfusion to the liver. Hepatic blood then drains into the systemic circulation via the right, left, and middle hepatic veins into the superior vena cava. Specific sites of porto-systemic collateral circulation are of great importance during portal hypertension, which is beyond the scope of this chapter. However, in the event of MVT, these collaterals may become enlarged similar to the pattern seen in patients with portal hypertension.

Intestinal blood flow comprises 10–20% of the cardiac output, with significant increases in SMA, but not celiac, flow occurring 20–30 min after meal ingestion and sustain for 90 min. The intestinal mucosa comprises 1/2 of intestinal mass; however, it receives 75% of resting intestinal blood flow, with the remainder supplying the muscular and serosal layers. The sympathetic nervous system serves as the primary regulator of splanchnic blood flow, with influences from metabolic, myogenic, and extrinsic factors. Sympathetic stimulation increases splanchnic vascular tone, decreasing blood flow. Numerous hormonal and molecular substances contribute to the regulation of splanchnic blood flow in addition to many pharmaceuticals, some which may contribute to AMI in states of low systemic blood pressure.

Potential Complications

Mesenteric Ischemia and Reperfusion

Although AMI is initially managed surgically, patients face a significant risk of morbidity and mortality after treatment from systemic inflammation and subsequent multiple organ dysfunction syndrome (MODS). Mesenteric ischemia–reperfusion injury (IRI) promotes local synthesis of inflammatory mediators that exacerbate gut injury, priming circulating neutrophils for enhanced superoxide anion production and subsequent remote (i.e., pulmonary, hepatic) injury [30]. At the cellular level, mesenteric IRI activates a cascade of oxidative stress-sensitive protein kinases that converge on specific transcriptional factors to regulate expression of pro-inflammatory genes. These gene targets include enzymes (inducible nitric oxide synthase [iNOS] cyclooxygenase, and phospholipase A2), cytokines (tumor necrosis factor-α [TNF-α] and interleukin [IL]-1), chemokines (IL-8), and adhesion molecules (intercellular adhesion molecule-1 [ICAM-1]) [31–36]. Excessive gene activation leads to a maladaptive systemic inflammatory response syndrome (SIRS) that can trigger early MODS. Locally, this hyperinflammatory state can cause gut dysfunction characterized by histologic evidence of mucosal injury, increased intestinal epithelial and microvascular permeability, and impaired motility. Patients then become more susceptible to bacteremia, endotoxemia, and eventually, late MODS.

Experimental therapies directed at attenuating these pathways have been successful in laboratory models of mesenteric IRI, and may eventually translate into patient care. However, clinical trials investigating the efficacy of pharmacologic blockade of individual mediators (TNF-α, IL-1, and iNOS) have been largely unsuccessful and even deleterious in treating patients with sepsis and MODS [37]. The reasons for failure are probably multifactorial, but it appears that both the redundancy and breadth of the inflammatory cascade and poor timing of therapy are major contributing factors. The application of more broadly based therapeutic modalities like regional hypothermia for organ protection during ischemia may overcome these limitations

and prove to be efficacious in the clinical setting [38, 39]. Nevertheless, it is likely that to achieve any meaningful improvements in the care of patients with AMI, we must expand our knowledge of the early molecular pathways involved in the activation and proliferation of both local and systemic inflammation.

Surgical Outcomes

Most large studies examining outcomes of patients with AMI report perioperative mortalities ranging from 32 to 69% with 5-year survival rates ranging from 18 to 50% [40–42]. The morbidity and mortality associated with this condition largely depends on the underlying etiology. In general, in-hospital mortality is highest for NOMI, lower for acute SMA occlusion (with mortality rates for thrombotic occlusion exceeding those for embolic occlusion), and lowest (~20%) for MVT [4, 43, 44]. The difference in mortality between embolic and thrombotic disease may be accounted for by the tendency for thrombosis to occur more proximally and thus to be associated with a greater degree of bowel infarction than that of embolic disease, and that patients with thrombotic disease have a greater burden of underlying cardiovascular comorbidity. Multiple organ failure is the most frequent cause of death [7]. Peritonitis and bowel necrosis were found to be independent predictors of death or survival dependent upon total parenteral nutrition [43, 44]. In another institutional review, independent predictors of survival include age less than 60 years, bowel resection, and the absence of a major cardiovascular procedure [7]. A recent review of the National Surgical Quality Improvement Program (NSQIP) database revealed that among patients undergoing bowel resection for AMI, preoperative and intra-operative variables associated with mortality included do not resuscitate orders, open wound, low albumin, dirty versus clean-contaminated case, and poor functional status [42]. The authors developed a preoperative risk variable calculator to assist with identifying high risk patients and aiding the informed consent process.

A recent paper has highlighted a trend in the United States towards use of endovascular techniques for revascularization during AMI and its potential impact on improved outcomes [43]. The study investigated outcomes of 1,857 patients who underwent SMA percutaneous transluminal angioplasty with or without stenting versus 3,380 patients who underwent open surgical exploration from the Nationwide Inpatient Sample during 1988–2006. In-hospital mortality was significantly less for patients treated with percutaneous angioplasty (15.6%) versus surgical exploration (38.6%). While this large retrospective study has inherent limitations with regards to comparative effectiveness analysis, novel less-invasive therapies may prove to be effective in reducing the tremendous morbidity and mortality associated with this disease. In another prospective review of 257 patients treated for AMI before and after the development of endovascular techniques, there were no differences in operative morbidity, mortality, or length of stay between patients treated with open repair versus endovascular techniques, and at 5-year follow-up, there continued to be no differences between the groups for primary and secondary patency rates and recurrence-free survival [45].

Follow-Up

Patients treated with open or endovascular techniques for revascularization during AMI are evaluated by combined history and physical examination and duplex ultrasonography after hospital discharge. While there is no standard algorithm for graft patency surveillance, most surgeons recommend a clinical examination and duplex ultrasound study prior to discharge from the hospital, every 6 months during the first year, and annually thereafter. Rates of restenosis are high in patients with both acute and chronic mesenteric ischemia, varying from 20 to 66%, and of those nearly half will require reintervention because of symptom recurrence or progression of the lesion to a preocclusive state [46]. Interventions to correct recurrent stenosis vary depending on surgeon's preference as no guidelines exist for therapeutic reinterventions, and many surgeons employ percutaneous angioplasty techniques to correct visceral artery restenosis.

Conclusion

AMI is a rare but devastating disease with severe implications for the surviving patient. Therapeutic modalities range from open operative repair to endovascular revascularization, with overall morbidity and mortality largely equal across treatment modalities. Timely diagnosis, prompt surgical intervention, adequate support measures and appropriate second-look interventions are mainstays of therapy and improve outcomes in all causes of AMI. Future endeavors towards early and accurate diagnosis along with prevention of mesenteric ischemia–reperfusion injury and multiple organ failure may potentially improve outcomes in this deadly disease.

References

1. Lock G. Acute intestinal ischaemia. Best Pract Res Clin Gastroenterol. 2001;15(1):83–98.
2. Oldenburg WA, Lau LL, Rodenberg TJ, Edmonds HJ, Burger CD. Acute mesenteric ischemia: a clinical review. Arch Intern Med. 2004;164(10):1054–62.
3. Cho JS, Carr JA, Jacobsen G, Shepard AD, Nypaver TJ, Reddy DJ. Long-term outcome after mesenteric artery reconstruction: a 37-year experience. J Vasc Surg. 2002;35(3):453–60.
4. Acosta S. Epidemiology of mesenteric vascular disease: clinical implications. Semin Vasc Surg. 2010;23(1):4–8.
5. Mamode N, Pickford I, Leiberman P. Failure to improve outcome in acute mesenteric ischaemia: seven-year review. Eur J Surg. 1999;165(3):203–8.
6. Sachs SM, Morton JH, Schwartz SI. Acute mesenteric ischemia. Surgery. 1982;92(4):646–53.
7. Park WM, Gloviczki P, Cherry Jr KJ, Hallett Jr JW, Bower TC, Panneton JM, et al. Contemporary management of acute mesenteric ischemia: factors associated with survival. J Vasc Surg. 2002;35(3):445–52.
8. Morasch MD, Ebaugh JL, Chiou AC, Matsumura JS, Pearce WH, Yao JS. Mesenteric venous thrombosis: a changing clinical entity. J Vasc Surg. 2001;34(4):680–4.
9. Acosta-Merida MA, Marchena-Gomez J, Hemmersbach-Miller M, Roque-Castellano C, Hernandez-Romero JM. Identification of risk factors for perioperative mortality in acute mesenteric ischemia. World J Surg. 2006;30(8):1579–85.
10. Eltarawy IG, Etman YM, Zenati M, Simmons RL, Rosengart MR. Acute mesenteric ischemia: the importance of early surgical consultation. Am Surg. 2009;75(3):212–9.
11. Akyildiz H, Akcan A, Ozturk A, Sozuer E, Kucuk C, Karahan I. The correlation of the D-dimer test and biphasic computed tomography with mesenteric computed tomography angiography in the diagnosis of acute mesenteric ischemia. Am J Surg. 2009;197(4):429–33.
12. Ritz JP, Runkel N, Berger G, Buhr HJ. Prognostic factors in mesenteric infarct. Zentralbl Chir. 1997;122(5):332–8.
13. Nelson AL, Millington TM, Sahani D, Chung RT, Bauer C, Hertl M, et al. Hepatic portal venous gas: the ABCs of management. Arch Surg. 2009;144(6):575–81. discussion 81.
14. Wyers MC. Acute mesenteric ischemia: diagnostic approach and surgical treatment. Semin Vasc Surg. 2010;23(1):9–20.
15. Cikrit DF, Harris VJ, Hemmer CG, Kopecky KK, Dalsing MC, Hyre CE, et al. Comparison of spiral CT scan and arteriography for evaluation of renal and visceral arteries. Ann Vasc Surg. 1996;10(2):109–16.
16. Ofer A, Abadi S, Nitecki S, Karram T, Kogan I, Leiderman M, et al. Multidetector CT angiography in the evaluation of acute mesenteric ischemia. Eur Radiol. 2009;19(1):24–30.
17. Aschoff AJ, Stuber G, Becker BW, Hoffmann MH, Schmitz BL, Schelzig H, et al. Evaluation of acute mesenteric ischemia: accuracy of biphasic mesenteric multi-detector CT angiography. Abdom Imaging. 2009;34(3):345–57.
18. Kaleya RN, Sammartano RJ, Boley SJ. Aggressive approach to acute mesenteric ischemia. Surg Clin North Am. 1992;72(1):157–82.
19. Rhee RY, Gloviczki P, Mendonca CT, Petterson TM, Serry RD, Sarr MG, et al. Mesenteric venous thrombosis: still a lethal disease in the 1990s. J Vasc Surg. 1994;20(5):688–97.
20. Ernst O, Asnar V, Sergent G, Lederman E, Nicol L, Paris JC, et al. Comparing contrast-enhanced breath-hold MR angiography and conventional angiography in the evaluation of mesenteric circulation. AJR Am J Roentgenol. 2000;174(2):433–9.
21. Demirpolat G, Oran I, Tamsel S, Parildar M, Memis A. Acute mesenteric ischemia: endovascular therapy. Abdom Imaging. 2007;32(3):299–303.
22. Wyers MC, Powell RJ, Nolan BW, Cronenwett JL. Retrograde mesenteric stenting during laparotomy for acute occlusive mesenteric ischemia. J Vasc Surg. 2007;45(2):269–75.
23. Sommer CM, Radeleff BA. A novel approach for percutaneous treatment of massive nonocclusive mesenteric ischemia: tolazoline and glycerol trinitrate as effective local vasodilators. Catheter Cardiovasc Interv. 2009;73(2):152–5.

24. Kaplan JL, Weintraub SL, Hunt JP, Gonzalez A, Lopera J, Brazzini A. Treatment of superior mesenteric and portal vein thrombosis with direct thrombolytic infusion via an operatively placed mesenteric catheter. Am Surg. 2004;70(7):600–4.

25. Yanar H, Taviloglu K, Ertekin C, Ozcinar B, Yanar F, Guloglu R, et al. Planned second-look laparoscopy in the management of acute mesenteric ischemia. World J Gastroenterol. 2007;13(24):3350–3.

26. Meng X, Liu L, Jiang H. Indications and procedures for second-look surgery in acute mesenteric ischemia. Surg Today. 2010;40(8):700–5.

27. Anadol AZ, Ersoy E, Taneri F, Tekin EH. Laparoscopic "second-look" in the management of mesenteric ischemia. Surg Laparosc Endosc Percutan Tech. 2004;14(4):191–3.

28. Ibukuro K, Tsukiyama T, Mori K, Inoue Y. The congenital anastomoses between hepatic arteries: angiographic appearance. Surg Radiol Anat. 2000;22(1):41–5.

29. Reuter SR, Redman HC. Gastrointestinal angiography. 2nd ed. Philadelphia, PA: WB Saunders; 1971.

30. Hassoun HT, Kone BC, Mercer DW, Moody FG, Weisbrodt NW, Moore FA. Post-injury multiple organ failure: the role of the gut. Shock. 2001;15(1):1–10.

31. Hassoun HT, Weisbrodt NW, Mercer DW, Kozar RA, Moody FG, Moore FA. Inducible nitric oxide synthase mediates gut ischemia/reperfusion-induced ileus only after severe insults. J Surg Res. 2001;97(2):150–4.

32. Panes J, Granger DN. Leukocyte-endothelial cell interactions: molecular mechanisms and implications in gastrointestinal disease. Gastroenterology. 1998;114(5):1066–90.

33. Sonnino RE, Pigatt L, Schrama A, Burchett S, Franson R. Phospholipase A2 secretion during intestinal graft ischemia. Dig Dis Sci. 1997;42(5):972–81.

34. Tamion F, Richard V, Lyoumi S, Daveau M, Bonmarchand G, Leroy J, et al. Gut ischemia and mesenteric synthesis of inflammatory cytokines after hemorrhagic or endotoxic shock. Am J Physiol. 1997;273(2 Pt 1):G314–G21.

35. Turnage RH, Kadesky KM, Bartula L, Guice KS, Oldham KT, Myers SI. Splanchnic PGI2 release and "no reflow" following intestinal reperfusion. J Surg Res. 1995;58(6):558–64.

36. Welborn 3rd MB, Douglas WG, Abouhamze Z, Auffenburg T, Abouhamze AS, Baumhofer J, et al. Visceral ischemia-reperfusion injury promotes tumor necrosis factor (TNF) and interleukin-1 (IL-1) dependent organ injury in the mouse. Shock. 1996;6(3):171–6.

37. Huber TS, Gaines GC, Welborn 3rd MB, Rosenberg JJ, Seeger JM, Moldawer LL. Anticytokine therapies for acute inflammation and the systemic inflammatory response syndrome: IL-10 and ischemia/reperfusion injury as a new paradigm. Shock. 2000;13(6):425–34.

38. Hassoun HT, Miller 3rd CC, Huynh TT, Estrera AL, Smith JJ, Safi HJ. Cold visceral perfusion improves early survival in patients with acute renal failure after thoracoabdominal aortic aneurysm repair. J Vasc Surg. 2004;39(3):506–12.

39. Santora RJ, Lie ML, Grigoryev DN, Nasir O, Moore FA, Hassoun HT. Therapeutic distant organ effects of regional hypothermia during mesenteric ischemia-reperfusion injury. J Vasc Surg. 2010;52(4):1003–14.

40. Edwards MS, Cherr GS, Craven TE, Olsen AW, Plonk GW, Geary RL, et al. Acute occlusive mesenteric ischemia: surgical management and outcomes. Ann Vasc Surg. 2003;17(1):72–9.

41. Klempnauer J, Grothues F, Bektas H, Pichlmayr R. Long-term results after surgery for acute mesenteric ischemia. Surgery. 1997;121(3):239–43.

42. Gupta PK, Natarajan B, Gupta H, Fang X, Fitzgibbons Jr RJ. Morbidity and mortality after bowel resection for acute mesenteric ischemia. Surgery. 2011;150(4):779–87.

43. Schermerhorn ML, Giles KA, Hamdan AD, Wyers MC, Pomposelli FB. Mesenteric revascularization: management and outcomes in the United States, 1988–2006. J Vasc Surg. 2009;50(2):341.el–8.

44. Schoots IG, Koffeman GI, Legemate DA, Levi M, van Gulik TM. Systematic review of survival after acute mesenteric ischaemia according to disease aetiology. Br J Surg. 2004;91(1):17–27.

45. Ryer EJ, Oderich GS, Bower TC, Macedo TA, Vrtiska TJ, Duncan AA, et al. Differences in anatomy and outcomes in patients treated with open mesenteric revascularization before and after the endovascular era. J Vasc Surg. 2011;53(6):1611.e2–8.

46. Tallarita T, Oderich GS, Macedo TA, Gloviczki P, Misra S, Duncan AA, et al. Reinterventions for stent restenosis in patients treated for atherosclerotic mesenteric artery disease. J Vasc Surg. 2011;54(5):1422.e1–9.

Quan P. Ly and James A. Edney

Introduction

There are many causes of colonic obstruction ranging from anatomic to physiologic etiologies (Table 28.1). The type of obstructions also differ depend on region. In the United States, the most common cause of adult colonic obstruction is colorectal cancer, whereas in Russia and Africa, colonic volvulus is much more common. Clinical presentation, diagnosis, and management differ depending on the etiology; however, the initial assessment of the patient is similar regardless.

Clinical Presentation

As with any assessment, a thorough history and physical examination will help in delineating the problem. Most patients with colonic obstruction will present with abdominal distention, nausea, and vomiting. The duration of these symptoms can define the acuteness the process. Any associated pain implies urgency of the situation. Weight loss and melena would be concerning for a malignant process, as would a strong family history of cancer. Passing of flatus and stool differentiate between complete and partial obstruction. A history of previous cancer or current cancer would raise the concern for recurrence or disease progression. A previous history of abdominal surgery increases the likelihood of obstruction (adhesions) or incisional hernia. A complete assessment of the patient's comorbidities and medications is essential to the overall care of the patient.

Q.P. Ly, M.D., F.A.C.S
Department of Surgery, University of Nebraska Medical Center, Omaha, NE, USA

J.A. Edney, M.D., F.A.C.S. (✉)
Department of Surgical Oncology, 984030 Nebraska Medical Center, University of Nebraska Medical Center, Omaha, NE 68198, USA
e-mail: jedney@unmc.edu

On physical examination, it is important to assess the patient's vital signs for hemodynamic stability (instability witnessed in cases of dehydration, sepsis…). Patients with colonic obstruction often have abdominal distention and tympany. Dullness to percussion implies ascites as the cause of distention. Examine the abdomen for incisional scars and hernias. Be mindful of both internal hernias and adhesions as a cause of obstruction. The transverse and sigmoid colon have been reported to be incarcerated in hernias leading to obstruction. As always, a digital rectal examination is a key component of the physical examination.

Diagnosis

Laboratory tests that are usually obtained include a complete blood count (CBC), basic metabolic panel, lactate level, and coagulation panel. Additional laboratory studies should be ordered as indicated. The CBC may point to an infectious process with a leukocytosis or a malignancy with anemia. The metabolic panel evaluates the patient's electrolyte balance and renal function as well as the hydration status. A lactate level is frequently ordered in patients with abdominal pain to rule out an ischemic process. Coagulation studies and a type and screen are usually indicated if surgical intervention is entertained.

The first radiologic study commonly ordered is an acute abdominal series comprised of an upright chest radiograph, and an upright and flat abdominal radiograph. If free air is seen under the diaphragm (pneumoperitoneum), emergent surgical exploration is usually indicated. The presence of stool and/or air throughout the colon and rectum often (yet not always) points to a nonsurgical etiology. Occasionally, foreign bodies are seen on the radiographs. The classic radiographic presentation of sigmoid volvulus is described as a coffee bean, omega loop, or bent inner tube appearance (two dilated colonic limbs with the round loop in the right upper quadrant and the tip pointed to the left lower quadrant). A cecal volvulus appears as a dilated loop in the mid-abdomen, sometimes described as

Table 28.1 Causes of adult colonic obstruction

Neoplasms (polyps, adenoma, and carcinoma)
Volvulus (cecal, transverse, and sigmoid)
Diverticulitis
Incarcerated hernia
Inflammatory bowel disease
Intussusception
Ischemic colitis
Pseudo-obstruction (Ogilvie's syndrome)
Fecal impaction
Benign stricture
Foreign body

a "comma," and often seen with dilated small bowel on the right of the abdomen on radiographic imaging. It is important to measure the cecal diameter in all cases of colonic obstruction as a diameter of 10–12 cm poses an increased risk of perforation and may require emergent decompression either endoscopically or surgically. Computed tomography of the abdomen and pelvis is often performed as a subsequent study. It provides significantly more data as to the underlying pathology. It has been reported to be highly accurate in diagnosing volvulus demonstrating a "swirl sign" of the twisted mesenteric pedicle.

Contrast enemas can be both diagnostic and therapeutic. Water-soluble contrast, such as gastrografin, can help evacuate the colon in patients with stool impaction. A double contrast enema with barium is helpful in cases when the colonoscopy in incomplete and localization of the stricture site is necessary for surgical planning. However, barium should be avoided in cases of high-grade or complete obstruction and in patients with perforation or potential perforation.

Endoscopy is also both diagnostic and therapeutic in certain types of colonic obstruction. It is invaluable in the diagnosis of malignant colonic obstructions. With self-expanding metallic stents, it can change an acute colonic obstruction with possible two-stage surgery to an elective one-stage resection. It has also been recommended to be the first decompressing therapy for volvulus. Colonoscopy is also helpful in diagnosing ischemic colitis as well as pseudomembranous colitis.

Treatment

Fluid resuscitation and electrolyte correction are the first line of treatment for patients with colonic obstruction. Nasogastric tube is indicated only in those with nausea and vomiting. A Foley catheter is required for close monitoring of the urine output, an indication of the patient's volume status. The definitive management for differing pathologies will follow.

Neoplasms

Despite the fact that neoplasms are the most common cause of colonic obstruction in the United States, the majority of the patients with colorectal cancer do not present with acute obstruction. According to Phang et al. 10% of patients with rectal cancer presented with a bowel obstruction and needed emergent intervention [1].

Several studies have documented endoscopy with self-expanding metallic stents as a useful bridge to surgical therapy or as definitive palliative treatment [2–4]. Self-expanding metallic stents are successful greater than 90% of the time and have been associated with decreased lower overall morbidity, mortality, and hospital length of stay. However, they are not without risks. Complications include stent occlusion from tumor growth, stent migration, severe pelvic pain, incontinence, bleeding, and perforation. Currently, contraindications to self-expanding metallic stents are low rectal cancer, a long stricture segment, and severe angulation.

Indications for emergent surgical intervention in malignant colonic obstruction include impending perforation, failure of stenting, and early stage cancer. The surgical approach in most cases of complete malignant colonic obstruction is diverting ostomy, either open or laparoscopic. Curative resection with primary anastomosis can be done in patients with early cancer, whom are hemodynamically stable, and have minimal comorbidities. If a malignant process is suspected, especially when a resection is planned, tumor markers should be obtained preoperatively so as to aid with long-term follow-up. In resecting a primary tumor, oncologic principles should be maintained: negative margins and adequate nodal sampling with high ligation of the mesenteric vessels. Fig 28.1 depicts an algorithm for the management of malignant colonic obstructions.

Cecal Volvulus

Cecal volvulus was first described in 1837 by Rokitansky. It accounts for 1% of all adult intestinal obstructions and 30% of colonic volvulus [5–7]. It occurs when an abnormally mobile cecum twists axially or when the ascending colon hyperflexes upon itself (a bascule). The patient may present with chronic intermittent abdominal pain with spontaneous resolution, acute obstruction with increasing abdominal cramping pain and vomiting, or toxic with evidence of peritonitis. Laboratory studies are neither sensitive nor specific, but are helpful to assess fluid status and electrolyte balance. Classic signs on abdominal radiography include cecal dilation, cecal apices in the left upper quadrant, and absence of gas in the remainder of the colon. Computed tomography findings including the "whirl" sign, transition points, and

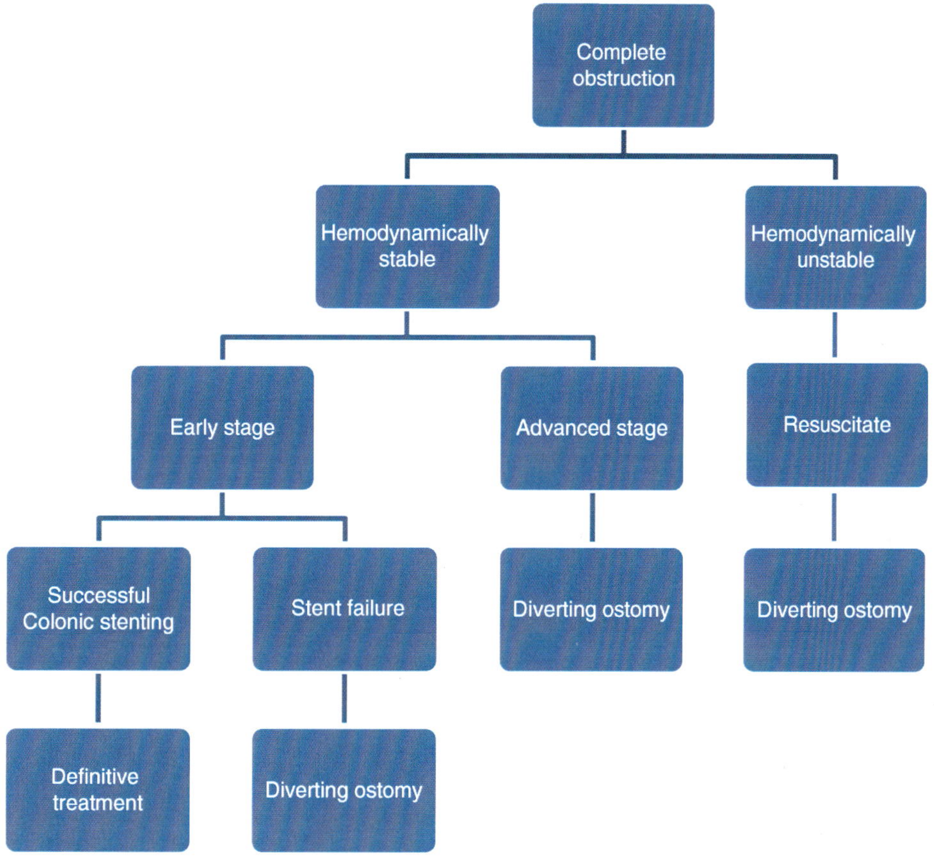

Fig. 28.1 Algorithm for the management of malignant colonic obstructions

distal colon decompression are highly sensitive and specific [8]. Barium enema and colonoscopy have been proposed in the past as both diagnostic and therapeutic, but is not recommended now as their diagnostic value has been supplanted by CT scans and as therapies have been shown to have a high recurrence rate.

Definitive surgical therapy for cecal volvulus is a right hemicolectomy with primary ileocolic anastomosis. Detorsion with suture pexy and tube cecostomy is recommended only in debilitated and malnourished patients, or those with multiple comorbidities or a hostile abdomen.

Sigmoid Volvulus

In the Western world, the incidence of sigmoid volvulus ranges from 1 to 3% of all intestinal obstruction, but increases to 42% in Iran and 55% in Russia [5, 9]. It is more likely to occur in the elderly, those who are institutionalized, and/or those who are taking neuropsychiatric medications. Sigmoid volvulus also occurs in children, mostly from Hirschprung disease (in the United States) and Chagas or other parasitic diseases (in less industrialized countries). Like cecal volvu-

lus, sigmoid volvulus is resultant from a redundant, mobile sigmoid colon that twists on its short mesenteric axis. Most patients present with a history of chronic constipation and abdominal distention long before their volvulus occurs. Abdominal examination can range from mild localized tenderness to diffuse peritonitis. As documented above, the plain abdominal radiograph can be diagnostic in 80% of cases. A barium enema is more helpful in the pediatric population than in the adult, with the "twisted tape" sign. Computed tomography has a greater sensitivity and specificity with its "swirl" sign and gives more details of bowel wall thickening and pneumatosis coli (air in the bowel wall).

Endoscopic decompression with either rigid or flexible sigmoidoscopy is the management of choice for noncomplicated sigmoid volvulus and is found to be successful 70–90% of the time [5, 9]. However, recurrent volvulus has been reported in 18–90% of cases with a mortality of 5–35% [5, 9]. Thus, endoscopic decompression is a mean of converting an emergent situation to that of an elective one. Definitive surgical intervention should be done within the same admission due to a high recurrence rate after endoscopic reduction. The recommended definitive surgery is a sigmoid resection with primary anastomosis. This procedure does have a mortality of approximately 8%, morbidity of 13–26%, and recurrence of 1.2% [5, 9]. In instances where elective resection is not possible like when there is sign of ischemic bowel present, an emergent resection is indicated. Whether to perform a primary anastomosis or an end colostomy depends on bowel viability and the patient's hemodynamic stability and comorbidities.

It has been believed that chronic constipation, colonic redundancy, and colonic atony or dysmotility may contribute to the recurrent volvulus or symptoms of volvulus. Some authors recommend a subtotal colectomy to prevent recurrence of volvulus [10–13]. This recommendation seems drastic to many who feel that a simple sigmoidectomy is sufficient. It would seem that in cases where there is megacolon present, a subtotal colectomy would be wise.

Pseudo-Obstruction (Ogilvie's Syndrome)

Acute colonic pseudo-obstruction accounts for at least 20% of large bowel obstruction. Because of the multiple comorbidities of these patients, delays in diagnosis, and inappropriate treatment, the overall mortality ranges from 25 to 31% with 40–50% of the patients having ischemia or perforation [14]. Predisposing factors includes post-orthopedic or spinal procedures, severe burns, myocardial infarction, infection, and neuropsychiatric medications. Water-soluble contrast enemas or CT scans can be done to rule out the presence of a mechanical obstruction; of note, the CT scan gives a more accurate measurement of the cecal diameter, better detail of the bowel wall (edema and intramural air), and mesenteric inflammation. Colonoscopy can be both diagnostic and therapeutic in ruling out mechanical obstruction, assessing mucosal ischemia, and decompressing the bowel distention.

Supportive therapy such as fluid resuscitation and electrolyte replacement (specifically hypokalemia and hypomagnesemia) is the first line of therapy. Remove narcotics, anticholinergics, and calcium channel blockers from the patient's medication list. Lactulose is contraindicated in this disease as it may promote bacterial fermentation and increase gas production in the colon. Although a 12 cm cecal diameter has been the teaching of an "at risk" cecum, perforation has occurred in cecal diameters less than 10 cm and resolution has occurred in one greater than 16 cm. In a retrospective review, patients with cecal diameters greater than 14 cm have a twofold increase in mortality.

Neostigmine (0.4–0.8 mg/h IV over 24 h) has been shown to be effective in three trials [15–17]. It is effective approximately 80% of the time. Although no major side-effects were reported in most studies, its use is not without potential complications. During infusion, vital signs and electrocardiogram should be continuously monitored for bradycardia, bronchospasm, and hypotension. Bradycardia is a significant concern. As such, patients should be in a monitored setting,

and Atropine should be readily available. Care should be taken in patients with history of myocardial infarction, asthma, renal failure, or in those taking beta-blockers.

If neostigmine fails, endoscopic decompression should be attempted with an 80% success rate; however, 20% of patients require a second colonoscopy for recurrence. The risk of perforation is approximately 2%. Surgical intervention is also associated with high morbidity and mortality. In patients with signs of ischemia or perforation, partial or subtotal resections are recommended. In patients too ill for surgery, a radiologically placed percutaneous tube cecostomy has been shown to be effective with few complications.

Obstruction Due to a Foreign Body

Another cause of colonic obstruction is foreign body insertion. Patients are often not forthcoming about the presence of the object, reason, or duration. In a systematic review, it has been found that the characteristic of the patient tends to be male (37:1) with a mean age of 44 years [18]. The majority of the removals (76.8%) can be removed with manual manipulation with or without endoscopy. Twenty-three percent of the time, a laparotomy with or without colectomy is required to remove the object. General anesthesia or spinal anesthesia is required in many of the cases (89%). Perforation and peritonitis occurs in 6.6% of reported cases either from the inserted object or from failed attempts at extraction [18]. Although most objects can be removed without complication or invasive surgery, it is important to diagnose and intervene in a timely manner to prevent complication.

Summary

Colonic obstruction has many possible etiologies that can lead to high morbidity and mortality. Accurate diagnosis, adequate resuscitation and appropriate treatment are keys to a successful outcome. Depending on the cause of the colonic obstruction and the hemodynamic stability of the patient, diagnostic and therapeutic options may involve radiologist, endoscopists and/or surgeon.

References

1. Phang PT, MacFarlane JK, Taylor RH, Cheifetz R, Davis N, Hay J, McGregor G, Speers C, Coldman A. Effect of emergent presentation on outcome from rectal cancer management. Am J Surg. 2003;185:450–4.
2. Hunerbein M, Krause M, Moesta KT, Rau B, Schlag PM. Palliation of malignant rectal obstruction with self-expanding metal stents. Surgery. 2005;137:42–7.

3. Watt AM, Faragher IG, Griffin TT, Rieger NA, Maddern GJ. Self-expanding metallic stents for relieving malignant colorectal obstruction: a systematic review. Ann Surg. 2007;246:24–30.

4. Ronnekleiv-Kelly SM, Kennedy GD. Management of stage IV rectal cancer: palliative options. World J Gastroenterol. 2011;17(7): 835–47.

5. Ballantyne GH, Brandner MD, Beart RW, Ilstrup DM. Volvulus of the colon, incidence and mortality. Ann Surg. 1985;202(1):83–92.

6. Habre J, Sautot-Vial N, Marcotte C, Benchimol D. Clinical image caecal volvulus. Am J Surg. 2008;196:e48–e9.

7. Martin MJ, Steele SR. Twists and turns: a practical approach to volvulus and intussusception. Scand J Surg. 2010;99:93–102.

8. Rosenblat JM, Rozenblit AM, Wolf EL, DuBrow RA, Den EI, Levsky JM. Findings of cecal volvulus at CT. Radiology. 2010; 256:169–75.

9. Raveenthiran V, Madiba TE, Atamanalp SS, De U. Volvulus of the sigmoid colon. Colorectal Dis. 2010;12:e1–e17.

10. Lau KCN, Miller BJ, Schache DJ, Cohen JR. A study of large-bowel volvulus in urban Australia. Can J Surg. 2006;49(3):203–7.

11. Chung YF, Eu KW, Nyam DC, Leong AF, Ho YH, Seow-Choen F. Minimizing recurrence after sigmoid volvulus. Br J Surg. 1999; 86(2):231–3.

12. Morrissey TB, Deitch EA. Recurrence of sigmoid volvulus after surgical intervention. Am Surg. 1994;60(5):329–31.

13. Katsikogiannis N, Machairiotis N, Zarogoulidis P, Sarika E, Stylianaki A, Zisoglou M, et al. Management of sigmoid volvulus avoiding sigmoid resection. Case Rep Gastroenterol. 2012;6(2): 293–9.

14. De Giorgio R, Knowles CH. Acute colonic pseudo-obstruction. Br J Surg. 2009;96:229–39.

15. Amaro R, Rogers AI. Neostigmine infusion: new standard of care for acute colonic pseudo-obstruction? Am J Gastroenterol. 2000;95:304–5.

16. Ponec RJ, Saunders MD, Kimmey MB. Neostigmine for the treatment of the acute colonic pseudo-obstruction. N Engl J Med. 1999;341:137–41.

17. Van der Spoel JI, van Oudemans-Straaten HM, Stoutenbeek CP, Bosman RJ, Zandstra DF. Neostigmine resolves critical illness-related colonic ileus in intensive care patients with multiple organ failure: a prospective, double-blind, placebo-controlled trial. Intensive Care Med. 2001;27:822–7.

18. Kurer MA, Davey C, Khan S, Chintapatla S. Colorectal foreign bodies: a systemic review. Colorectal Dis. 2010;12:851–61.

Lower Gastrointestinal Bleeding

Tricia Hauschild and Daniel Vargo

Introduction

The lower gastrointestinal tract consists of all gastrointestinal elements distal to the ligament of Treitz, including the jejunum, ileum, cecum, appendix, colon, rectum, and anus. Lower gastrointestinal bleeding can originate from any of these locations and thus represents a broad range of clinical entities. Most studies of lower gastrointestinal hemorrhage specifically reference lesions of the colon, rectum, and anus, and the majority of studies cited herein adhere to this convention.

Within the acute care surgical setting, these patients may present anywhere along the spectrum extending from occult bleeding demonstrated on fecal testing to frank, even massive, gastrointestinal hemorrhage. Although upper gastrointestinal bleeding is found to account for approximately five times the number of annual hospital admissions due to hemorrhage from lower gastrointestinal sources [1], lower gastrointestinal bleeding remains a frequently encountered clinical entity and can represent a diagnostic and therapeutic challenge for the acute care surgeon.

Epidemiology

Lower gastrointestinal bleeding accounts for a significant number of hospital admissions; the reported incidence in the US adult population is about 20–22 cases per 100,000 admissions, representing 0.5–0.7% of all annual hospital admissions in the acute care setting [2, 3]. The incidence of lower gastrointestinal bleeding is directly correlated with increasing patient age, with patients in the ninth decade of life experiencing an annual lower gastrointestinal bleeding rate

approximately two hundred times greater than comparable patients in the third decade of life [2, 3]. As the US demographic shift toward an older population continues, lower gastrointestinal bleeding can be expected to increase in overall incidence in coming years.

Hospitalization for acute lower gastrointestinal bleeding is also somewhat more common in males than females, with a reported annual incidence of about 24 per 100,000 in males versus 17 per 100,000 in females [2].

It should be intuitively obvious that certain etiologies of lower gastrointestinal bleeding are more common in particular age groups, and patient age is certainly a factor to be taken into account when developing a reasonable differential diagnosis for lower gastrointestinal bleeding. For example, bleeding due to angiodysplasia, diverticular disease, and colorectal malignancy are all markedly more common in older individuals, a reflection of the increasing incidence of these diagnoses in older populations.

Patients with lower gastrointestinal bleeding are more likely to require surgical intervention in comparison to those with upper gastrointestinal bleeds [3]. The severity of lower gastrointestinal bleeding varies widely, and a number of predictive models have been developed to identify which of these patients are at greatest risk for massive bleeding. Strate and colleagues identified seven factors which, taken together, predict the severity of lower gastrointestinal bleeding, including tachycardia, hypotension, syncope, benign abdominal examination, rectal bleeding, aspirin usage, and the presence of greater than two significant comorbidities [4]. According to this model, patients with four or more risk factors were classified as high risk (approximately 80% were expected to experience severe bleeding), patients with one, two, or three risk factors were classified as moderate risk (approximately 43% were expected to experience severe bleeding), and patients with no risk factors were classified as low risk, with an expected rate of severe bleeding less than 10% [5]. Severe bleeding was defined generally as a requirement for 2 U of packed red blood cells and/or a decrease in hematocrit of 20% or greater within the first 24 h after presentation in this

T. Hauschild, M.D. • D. Vargo, M.D., F.A.C.S (✉)
Department of Surgery, University of Utah School of Medicine, 3B-202 SOM, 30 North 1900 East, Salt Lake City, UT 84132, USA
e-mail: daniel.vargo@hsc.utah.edu

L.J. Moore et al. (eds.), *Common Problems in Acute Care Surgery*, DOI 10.1007/978-1-4614-6123-4_29, © Springer Science+Business Media New York 2013

study. Velayos and colleagues studied patients admitted with lower gastrointestinal hemorrhage in an acute care setting and found three factors noted within the first hour after initial presentation that were associated with the severity of bleeding and adverse outcomes: abnormal vital signs (hypotension or tachycardia) 1 h after initial evaluation, an initial hematocrit at or below 35%, and gross blood on initial rectal examination [6].

Fortunately most patients who present with lower gastrointestinal hemorrhage will stop bleeding spontaneously without any procedural or surgical intervention; in some series estimates range as high as 80% [7–10]. Estimates of mortality from major lower gastrointestinal bleeding in the acute setting vary widely, with reported rates from 2.1 to 21% in various case series [6, 11–13]. Higher mortality is seen in patients who initially present with lower gastrointestinal bleeding while already hospitalized for treatment of another condition; in this circumstance, the reported mortality rises to about one in four [2].

Clinical Presentation

The clinical presentation of a patient with lower gastrointestinal bleeding can run the gamut from occult bleeding identified on a stool guaiac assay to frank, even profuse, bleeding per rectum. Alternative presentations include fatigue, syncope, anemia, abdominal pain, and hemodynamic instability [3]. In many cases a patient may report a history of bright red blood per rectum that occurs intermittently and may not be present to any degree at the time of the actual clinical examination. The majority of patients presenting with a complaint of hematochezia or melena will be clinically stable at the time of presentation, and a thorough and complete diagnostic workup can be performed.

In some cases, however, particularly in a patient presenting with significant hematochezia, there may be significant vital sign abnormalities and other evidence of physiologic derangement, such as electrolyte imbalances and/or altered mental status, evident at the time of presentation. In these patients, as with all patients presenting with instability in the acute care setting, the detailed, comprehensive workup is briefly and appropriately deferred while initial stabilization and resuscitation measures are instituted.

Diagnosis

The diagnostic algorithm pertaining to a patient with lower gastrointestinal bleeding will to some extent be dependent on the severity and acuity of the clinical presentation; a patient experiencing torrential lower gastrointestinal hemorrhage would of course represent a differing set of initial

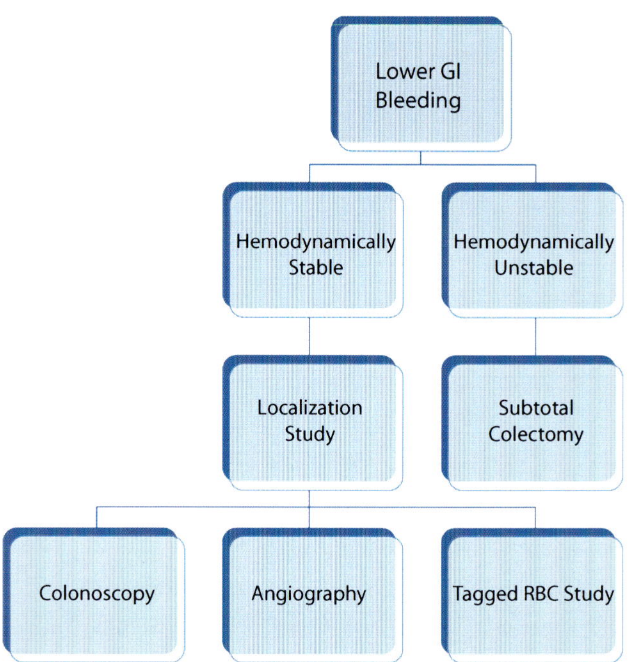

Fig. 29.1 Initial assessment of lower gastrointestinal bleeding

management priorities compared with a patient who reported intermittent bright red droplets of blood with defecation (Fig. 29.1). However, in the acute care setting, the initial management priorities for all patients would always prioritize ensuring hemodynamic stability and adequate resuscitation prior to a more detailed evaluation. If there is any concern that a patient presenting with a stable clinical picture is at risk of significant deterioration, the prudent clinician will establish intravenous access and have crystalloid and, possibly, blood products available to support resuscitation. If resuscitation is begun, a urinary catheter should be placed to monitor urine output as a marker for the adequacy of resuscitation. It should also be kept in mind that up to 15% of cases of significant lower gastrointestinal bleeding can be traced to an upper gastrointestinal source [7]. Unless there is a specific contraindication, patients presenting with lower gastrointestinal bleeding should have a nasogastric tube placed to help rule out the possibility of an upper gastrointestinal source. The presence of bilious nasogastric aspirate is an important indicator that upper gastrointestinal bleeding is unlikely; conversely, clear aspirate is not useful in eliminating upper gastrointestinal sources from the differential [14].

An important diagnostic caveat must be kept in mind in the evaluation of lower gastrointestinal bleeding, specifically that multiple sources of bleeding are not infrequently identified in this patient population. Among patients admitted in the acute care setting for lower gastrointestinal bleeding, the number of patients with multiple sources of hemorrhage is estimated at 4.4% [13]. In a prospective study of patients presenting with a chief complaint of intermittent bright red blood per rectum, Graham and colleagues documented additional abnormal findings on colonoscopy in 27% of patients with identifiable abnormalities on rectal examination [15]. The workup is therefore not complete once a single likely source of bleeding is identified; rather, optimal patient care dictates that a comprehensive evaluation be completed and other reasonably likely etiologies ruled out clinically.

As with any clinical situation, a thorough evaluation must begin with a detailed history and physical examination. A relevant history for the evaluation of lower gastrointestinal bleeding should, at a minimum, address the following areas:

- Acute bleeding symptoms: What is the nature of the bleeding? Is the patient experiencing hematochezia or melena? While traditional clinical dogma holds that hematochezia signifies a lower gastrointestinal bleed while melena is indicative of an upper gastrointestinal source of hemorrhage, the clinical reality is frequently less clear-cut, and it is widely acknowledged that particularly brisk upper gastrointestinal bleeding can present with hematochezia. Is the bleeding continuous or intermittent? Lower gastrointestinal bleeds are, in fact, intermittent in nature, making localization a true diagnostic challenge. How long has the bleeding been occurring? Has the patient experienced previous episodes of upper or lower gastrointestinal bleeding? Is there any pain associated with the bleeding?
- Possibly related systemic symptoms: Is the patient experiencing angina, palpitations, syncope, of unusual fatigue? Does the patient report any fevers or chills? Is nausea or vomiting present? Is there associated diarrhea or constipation? Does the patient report a history of gastroesophageal reflux or antacid use? Has there been any recent unintentional weight loss?
- Relevant medical history: Has the patient previously experienced any type of upper or lower gastrointestinal bleeding? Any history of inflammatory bowel disease, diverticulosis, hemorrhoids, gastrointestinal neoplasm, liver disease? Does the patient report any history of gastric or duodenal ulcer? Is there a known history of atrial fibrillation or other cardiac dysrhythmia? Does the patient report a history of peripheral vascular disease or ischemia? Any history of hematologic disorders, including thrombocytopenia or clotting cascade abnormalities? Has the patient ever experienced a transient ischemia attack or cerebrovascular accident? Has the patient recently been treated with radiation therapy?
- Medication history, including both prescription and non-prescription agents as well as herbal preparations. Specific inquiry regarding warfarin, aspirin, nonsteroidal anti-inflammatory agents, or other anticoagulant agents is of obvious importance.

- Health maintenance: Has the patient undergone any health screening that might reveal gastrointestinal disease, such as fecal occult blood testing, flexible sigmoidoscopy, or colonoscopy? When were these studies done, and what were the results? Has the patient recently had a polypectomy performed?
- Family history: Any relatives with any form of cancer, particularly cancers of the gastrointestinal tract? Any relatives with a history of inflammatory bowel disease? Any record of hereditary coagulopathies or other hematologic abnormalities?
- Social history: Is there any history of alcohol and/or tobacco usage? Recent travel, particularly to less-developed countries or regions? Recent sick contacts?

A focused yet thorough physical examination is also indicated as a key element of the initial workup. Vital signs will often be within normal limits in the setting of a lower gastrointestinal bleed unless the rate of bleeding is so substantial as to cause a significant volume depletion effect; in that case, tachycardia would be observed somewhat earlier, while hypotension and/or altered mental status would represent later findings associated with the acute loss of greater than 30% of the circulating blood volume (class III or higher hemorrhagic shock) [16]. Any evidence of vital sign alteration due to blood loss should prompt immediate placement of large-bore peripheral access and the institution of aggressive resuscitation with crystalloid and/or, in especially severe cases, blood products. In this circumstance, restoration and stabilization of volume status is the clinician's priority, and the further detailed physical examination is accordingly deferred until physiologic stability has been achieved.

A generalized visual inspection of the patient should reveal any anemic pallor, jaundice, or cachexia which might be present and associated with particular underlying conditions that could be associated with lower gastrointestinal bleeding. The abdominal examination should evaluate for generalized or focal tenderness, firmness or rigidity, any peritoneal signs such as guarding or rebound, organomegaly, and the presence of palpable masses. Presence of pain on abdominal examination generally argues in favor of an inflammatory process, while lower gastrointestinal bleeding due to diverticular disease or angiodysplasia in more commonly associated with a benign abdominal examination. Importantly, in the setting of a lower gastrointestinal bleed of unclear etiology, the examining clinician should perform a cardiac and peripheral pulse examination with particular attention to evidence of atrial fibrillation.

The rectal examination is among the most critical components of the physical examination in the patient with an acute lower gastrointestinal bleeding. A thorough and complete rectal exam should establish the presence or absence of gross blood, the existence of internal or external hemorrhoids or other perianal lesions including fistulae or fissures, and the presence and position of any palpable rectal masses. If no gross blood is apparent upon rectal examination, a stool guaiac test can be quickly performed in either the clinic or emergency department setting to establish the presence of occult gastrointestinal bleeding. Be aware, however, that the sensitivity of this assay is relatively low [17], and is further reduced in patients who take iron supplements or who have recently consumed red meat or peroxidase-rich fruits and vegetables, and specificity is reportedly diminished if a patient's diet is rich in citrus fruits or other concentrated sources of vitamin C [18, 19].

Initial laboratory studies should be sent to aid in the immediate evaluation of both the etiology and magnitude of a lower gastrointestinal bleed. A complete blood count (CBC) might be expected to reveal a decreased hematocrit in a patient with an active gastrointestinal hemorrhage; however, if the hemorrhage is of particularly acute onset, the intravascular volume may not yet be fully re-equilibrated and thus the hematocrit may be artificially elevated relative to true oxygen-carrying capacity. The CBC would also be expected to reveal evidence of thrombocytopenia, albeit with the same caveat that a hyperacute process might not permit an adequate intravascular re-equilibration interval before the laboratory study is drawn. Presence of a significant leukocytosis on CBC should prompt further consideration of an infectious process as the inciting etiology versus an inflammatory or ischemic mechanism.

Basic laboratory studies of electrolyte status as well as hepatic and renal function may serve the dual purposes of elucidating underlying comorbidities which may contribute to a gastrointestinal bleed while also identifying physiologic imbalances which could potentially be corrected prior to surgical or other procedural interventions. Likewise, coagulation parameters in this patient population may uncover underlying coagulopathies contributing to the presenting problem and permit the practitioner to order blood products where appropriate. It should be noted that the routine administration of vitamin K to correct patients on chronic warfarin therapy should be avoided in the setting of a lower gastrointestinal hemorrhage due to the difficulty and delay this presents when attempting to reestablish therapeutic anticoagulation once the acute hemorrhagic episode has been resolved [8].

Radiographic imaging may play an important role in establishing a definitive diagnosis in patients with lower gastrointestinal bleeding. Most patients with lower gastrointestinal bleeding who report concurrent abdominal pain acutely will undergo plain abdominal radiographs prior to the surgical consult. The information gleaned from these studies is somewhat limited; however, findings such as pneumoperitoneum or closed-loop obstruction may narrow the differential diagnosis That being said, the utility of plain abdominal radiographs is of limited utility in the evaluation of lower gastrointestinal bleeding.

Most patients in the acute setting of lower gastrointestinal bleeding with concurrent abdominal pain will, if hemodynamically stable, be appropriate candidates for computed tomography (CT) scanning of the abdomen and pelvis. A CT with oral and intravenous contrast may help identify mass lesions, such as colorectal adenocarcinomas, as well as sites of inflammation or potential perforation, as is seen with acute diverticulitis or inflammatory bowel disease. Bowel wall thickening or pneumatosis may also be noted in the case of ischemia or hypoperfusion-mediated bowel injury; an acute thromboembolic process would be expected to demonstrate these types of pathologic changes within a discrete vascular territory, while a more global low-flow mechanism would be expected to generate corresponding diffuse bowel involvement. Optimally, a CT scan in this setting would be performed with the administration of both oral and intravenous contrast. The patient's history should be reviewed for mention of impaired renal function or radiographic contrast allergy; initial laboratory studies including blood urea nitrogen and serum creatinine should likewise be reviewed prior to contrast administration.

Ultimately, the majority of patients undergoing an evaluation for lower gastrointestinal bleeding will undergo a colonoscopy. In addition to its utility as a diagnostic study, colonoscopic evaluation offers the advantage of potential therapeutic interventions. In acute lower gastrointestinal bleeding, the reported diagnostic utility of colonoscopy ranges between 45 and 89% [7, 20–23]. Complications of colonoscopy in the acute care setting, most significantly perforation, occur in up to 3% of cases [24].

The utility of colonoscopy in the acute setting is influenced by a number of factors including the quality of bowel preparation prior to the procedure, the rate of active bleeding (very slow bleeds may be below the diagnostic threshold of the procedure, while very brisk bleeding may impair adequate visualization and source localization), whether or not the bleeding is continuous or intermittent, and the skill/experience of the endoscopist. Additionally, not all facilities have 24-h availability of this procedure.

The quality of bowel preparation that can be achieved prior to colonoscopy has a clear influence on the success of the procedure from both a diagnostic and therapeutic perspective. That being said, a lack of bowel preparation does not preclude the successful use of endoscopic techniques in the diagnosis and treatment of lower gastrointestinal bleeding. In fact, some clinicians report that lower gastrointestinal bleeding actually acts to help purge the colon, and any impaired visualization on colonoscopy can be addressed via flushing the scope during the procedure, although diagnostic yield in this circumstance is only about 35% [23]. If a routine oral electrolyte-polyethylene glycol prep solution is administered prior to colonoscopy in the setting of an acute lower gastrointestinal bleed, improved diagnostic yields, approaching 80% are reported [25].

If colonoscopy is performed for acute lower gastrointestinal bleeding, and a definitive source is identified, therapeutic options include the following: sclerotherapy via direct epinephrine injection in a 1:10,000 concentration, bipolar or monopolar coagulation, and endoscopic clip application. Jensen and colleagues directly compared urgent colonoscopic intervention versus surgical treatment in a prospective study of patients with severe diverticular bleeding and demonstrated comparable efficacy [26].

In cases where resource issues or other patient factors make colonoscopy an unsuitable clinical option, flexible sigmoidoscopy may be utilized for visualization of the distal gastrointestinal tract. In cases in which a hemorrhagic lesion is identified within this segment of the colon, sigmoidoscopy can prove to be a valuable clinical adjunct for both diagnostic and treatment purposes. One must keep in mind that a significant portion of patients with distal lesions are also found to have more proximal sources of hemorrhage [15]; therefore, the performance of flexible sigmoidoscopy does not obviate the requirement for a more thorough examination via a complete colonoscopy at a later point in time.

If an anorectal source of bleeding is evident on examination or is suspected based on the clinical history and patient presentation, anoscopy is another tool which may be utilized to facilitate direct visualization and examination. Again, the identification of a distal lesion as a source of lower gastrointestinal hemorrhage does not in any way preclude the existence of a more proximal lesion. Therefore, it is advisable that these patients also be scheduled for a complete colonoscopy at a later date.

While colonoscopy is the preferred initial investigation for lower gastrointestinal bleeding [7, 27], angiography is another modality that offers the advantage of both diagnostic and therapeutic capabilities if colonoscopy is unavailable. The sensitivity for visceral angiography in the detection of active gastrointestinal bleeding is approximately 0.5 cm^3/min [10, 28]. Angiography is similarly poor in detecting venous bleeding, intermittent bleeding, and bleeding from small vessels. Finally, angiography is not without complications to include: hemorrhage at the catheter insertion site, arterial dissection, microembolization, pseudoaneurysm formation, puncture site infection, allergic reaction to contrast, and contrast-induced nephropathy [20, 29].

The reported success rates for angiography in the localization of lower gastrointestinal bleeding vary widely, with recent studies citing rates between 30.5 and 86% [7, 12, 30]. If angiography is able to detect a discrete bleeding source, several therapeutic interventions are possible including: embolization therapy and direct injection of vasopressin or sclerosing agents at the bleeding site. Unfortunately, angiographic capabilities are not available on a 24-h basis universally. If a significant delay in angiography is anticipated, other diagnostic and therapeutic modalities should be considered.

Radionuclide scintigraphy is yet another diagnostic modality for identification of the site of hemorrhage in a patient presenting with lower gastrointestinal bleeding. This technique can utilize either technetium-99m sulfur colloid or technetium-99m-labeled red blood cells. The latter technique, commonly referred to as a tagged red blood cell scan, is utilized more frequently. Sulfur colloid scanning has the advantage of relative ease of preparation in comparison with preparation of tagged red blood cells. However, it clears quickly, thus decreasing the likelihood of repeat scanning following a single infusion (an option with tagged red blood cell scans). All that being said, the detection rates are similar between the two techniques [31].

Radionuclide scintigraphy is able to identify bleeding at rates as low as 0.1 cm^3/min [32]. Thus, the tagged red blood cell scan is of greatest utility in identifying slow bleeds that are not localizable via other diagnostic techniques. Ng and colleagues evaluated the question of whether time to positive radionuclide scan ("blush") correlates with, and can be used to predict, the yield on angiographic intervention. In their series, 60% of patients with an immediate appearance of blush on radionuclide scan subsequently underwent a positive angiogram. Among patients in whom no blush had appeared after 2 min, only 7% had a positive angiogram [33]. While sensitivity of the tagged red blood cell scan can surpass either colonoscopy or angiography in the setting of active bleeding and can be used to predict which patients will benefit from angiogram, radionuclide scanning does have the significant disadvantage of representing a diagnostic modality only, with no capability for direct therapeutic intervention. Furthermore, 27% of patients who undergo a negative radionuclide study will experience recurrent lower gastrointestinal bleeding at a later date [34].

Despite these many modalities, bleeding will cease spontaneously and no definitive source of lower gastrointestinal bleeding will occur in 10.7–22.8% of patients [2, 22, 35–37]. However, it must be emphasized that a thorough workup which fails to identify a definitive source of bleeding is not without benefit to the patient, in that a number of potentially serious causes of lower gastrointestinal bleeding, such as colorectal adenocarcinoma, can be effectively eliminated from the differential diagnosis following the workup.

Management

In the majority of cases (70–85%), the lower gastrointestinal bleeding will cease without any therapeutic intervention (Table 29.1) [8, 9]. Re-bleeding is not uncommon, occurring in up to 25% of cases [38]. Thus, the absence of active bleeding at a particular point in time should not preclude definitive evaluation and treatment of the underlying condition.

Severe, persistent hemorrhage is the clinical presentation of lower gastrointestinal bleeding which most frequently

Table 29.1 Treatment options in lower gastrointestinal bleeding

Etiology	Treatment options
Diverticular disease	1. Resection ± anastomosis
	2. Angiography with embolization
Angiodysplasia	1. Colonoscopy with hemostatic maneuvers
	2. Angiography with embolization
	3. Resection ± anastomosis
Ischemic colitis	1. Resuscitation and antibiotics
	2. Resection with diversion
Infectious colitis	1. Resuscitation with antibiotics
	2. Resection ± anastomosis
Hemorrhoids	1. Anoscopy with resection
Neoplasm	1. Resection ± anastomosis
Radiation proctitis	1. Intraluminal steroids
	2. Colonoscopy with hemostatic maneuvers

requires surgical management. General indications for surgery include continued hemodynamic instability despite adequate resuscitation, requirement for transfusion of four or more units of packed red blood cells over 24 h, or severe recurrent bleeding [10]. Among patients who require a blood transfusion for the management of lower gastrointestinal bleeding, approximately one in four will ultimately require surgery [39]. The operative procedure of choice is a segmental resection for those patients in whom a hemorrhage source can be localized [40]. This approach is associated with greater control of bleeding and lower morbidity in comparison with the primary surgical alternative, a subtotal colectomy [7].

If efforts of localization are unsuccessful, as is the case in 8–12% of cases of acute lower gastrointestinal hemorrhage [25, 41], a subtotal colectomy is required to establish definitive control of bleeding [10]. Patients who undergo a total colectomy for control of lower gastrointestinal hemorrhage are at risk for considerable morbidity and mortality; overall mortality in this circumstance is between 10 and 20%, and those individuals with a transfusion requirement of ten or more units are subject to a mortality rate approaching 50%, likely mirroring the severity of underlying illness [42].

Given that a lower gastrointestinal bleed may result from a broad range of clinical conditions, the management of this patient population is dependent on the underlying diagnosis; however, there are general principles applicable to the management of all patients presenting with this clinical complaint.

Diverticular disease (Fig. 29.2) is the most frequently cited etiology for lower gastrointestinal bleeding in which a definitive source is identified, accounting for approximately 40–55% of all cases of acute lower gastrointestinal bleeding [2, 20]. The pathophysiology of bleeding due to diverticular disease is related to stretching and weakening of the vasa recta at the site of a colonic diverticulum. Diverticula are

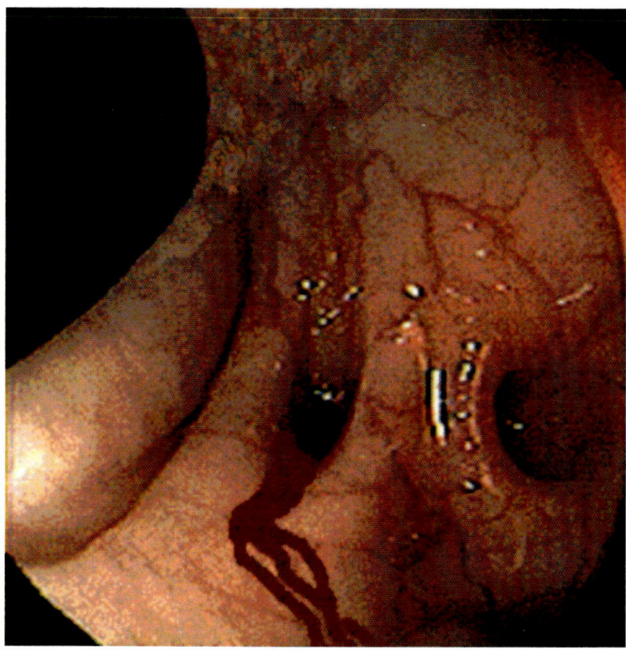

Fig. 29.2 Bleeding diverticulum

typically multiple. Diverticulosis is more commonly found in the left colon, in particular the sigmoid colon [10], but, curiously, diverticular bleeds are more commonly localized to the ascending colon [9]. Approximately one in six patients with diverticular disease will experience some degree of bleeding [10].

It is worth noting that lower gastrointestinal bleeding related to diverticular disease can occur within the setting of acute diverticulitis, but an acute episode of diverticulitis is by no means a prerequisite to bleeding. Although it might seem intuitive that the inflammatory changes associated with an episode of acute diverticulitis would increase the risk of acute hemorrhage, most diverticular bleeding occurs outside of acute diverticulitis. For unclear reasons, the hemorrhage is almost exclusively into the bowel lumen rather than into the extraluminal tissues [43].

Patients with acute diverticular hemorrhage present with painless, often brisk hematochezia, and in many cases, physiologic evidence of significant blood loss. Diverticular bleeding is highly unusual in patients under the age of 40, but the incidence rises with advancing age. The regular use of nonsteroidal anti-inflammatory drugs (NSAIDs) is also correlated with an increased likelihood of diverticular bleeding [44]. Ultimately, only a minority of patients with diverticular disease will experience bleeding, and of those patients who do, spontaneously resolution of bleeding occurs in approximately 75–80% [11, 45]. Re-bleeding is common, the rate of first re-bleed is estimated at 25–30%, and once this has occurred, the risk of subsequent re-bleeding is upwards to 50% [9].

The management of diverticular bleeding is dependent on several factors, including the severity of bleeding, whether or not the patient is experiencing a concurrent episode of acute diverticulitis, and the patient's history of previous episodes of diverticular bleeding and/or diverticulitis [46]. A diverticular bleed in the absence of acute diverticulitis is generally well-suited to an initial attempt at evaluation and treatment via colonoscopy. If bleeding is ongoing and of sufficient rate, colonoscopy can localize the bleeding site and endoscopic treatments can be undertaken with a goal of achieving hemostasis. In patients with a history of recent diverticular bleeding who do not appear to be actively bleeding at the time of examination, colonoscopic evaluation is nonetheless worthwhile, because in many instances, the stigmata of recent bleeding, including adherent clots and visible vessels [10], are readily identified.

In the setting of acute diverticulitis, colonoscopy is generally contraindicated due to the acute inflammation and perforation associated with this diagnosis. For hemodynamically stable patients experiencing lower gastrointestinal bleeding concomitant with acute diverticulitis, the diverticulitis is the clinical priority in accordance with evidence-based standards of care. Milder cases are generally managed with a regimen of bowel rest, appropriate antibiotics, and serial abdominal examinations. More severe cases, especially those characterized by evidence of purulent or feculent peritonitis (i.e., Hinchey grade III or IV disease), are managed operatively. Surgical resection is also indicated for patients experiencing recurrent lower gastrointestinal hemorrhage due to diverticular disease. This represents a significant portion of patients with diverticulosis, with the incidence ranging from 10% at 2 years to 25% at 4 years [2].

If bleeding is severe in a patient with acute diverticulitis, angiography is a reasonable option for localization of the hemorrhagic site and establishment of hemostasis. In the event angiography is unsuccessful, surgical exploration is often required. Approximately 5% of patients admitted for diverticular bleeding ultimately require surgical intervention [47]. Such exploration may be performed via either laparoscopic or open approach based on surgeon preference and experience. Surgical resection is also the standard of care following a second significant diverticular bleed given the high (approximately 50%) risk of subsequent re-bleeding [48].

The question of primary anastomosis at the time of initial bowel resection depends in part on whether or not the patient is experiencing active and extensive diverticulitis-mediated inflammation; if such is not present, as is true in the majority of cases, primary anastomosis of the remaining viable bowel is generally deemed safe and appropriate. If active inflammation is present to a considerable extent, the surgeon may reasonably elect to perform a diverting ostomy with a plan for delayed anastomosis to take place once the acute inflammatory changes have resolved.

Angiodysplasia encompasses a broad range of lesions including arteriovenous malformations, vascular ectasias, and angiomas [9]. It is commonly considered in cases of lower gastrointestinal bleeding; however, its incidence is only 2.7% (hospital admissions for acute lower gastrointestinal bleeding, with age-specific bleeding rates showing a strong, positive correlation) [2, 49]. The pathophysiology is thought to relate to normal age-related degeneration of smaller venous structures located within the gastrointestinal submucosa. It is therefore seen predominantly in older patient populations. Boley and colleagues hypothesized that the lesions arise largely due to chronic, low-grade obstruction of the submucosal venous system [50]. The cecum is the most common site of angiodysplastic lesions [10]. There appears to be a possible correlation between angiodysplastic lesions and aortic stenosis and/or renal failure; however, there is no strong evidence to suggest a causative relationship [49, 51].

The bleeding associated with angiodysplastic lesions often presents as a history of intermittent, painless, bright red blood per rectum. In most circumstances, angiodysplasia-associated bleeding is subtle and may not be noted overtly by the patient. In these cases, the signs and symptoms of anemia may be the only evidence pointing to a gastrointestinal bleed, and angiodysplasia may be discovered as part of a broader workup. In approximately 15% of cases, however, angiodysplasia presents with significant hemorrhage [9]. Abdominal pain is infrequently associated with bleeding due to angiodysplasia, and a complaint of significant abdominal pain in a patient with known angiodysplasia should prompt a thorough workup for other diagnoses.

While angiodysplastic bleeding ceases spontaneously in roughly 90% of cases [41, 52], the majority of patients who present with one angiodysplastic bleed will bleed again, ultimately requiring a comprehensive evaluation [9]. Colonoscopy is the diagnostic and therapeutic modality of choice in the treatment of acute lower gastrointestinal bleeding due to angiodysplasia. The lesions have a characteristic stellate, bright red appearance on colonoscopic examination which facilitates identification. The right colon, in particular the cecum, is the most frequent site of bleeding angiodysplastic lesions [9, 50].

Angiography is sometimes used in the identification and treatment of bleeding angiodysplastic lesions. While angiography enjoys an overall greater diagnostic sensitivity in comparison with colonoscopy, it is thought by some authors to be less sensitive in identifying and treating the small venous lesions which are characteristic of angiodysplasia, while others cite increased sensitivity for angiography versus colonoscopy in this setting [53]. Overall, most patients with angiodysplastic bleeding are diagnosed and treated via colonoscopy. Endoscopic treatments include electrocautery, laser, and heater probe as well as the increasingly well-studied argon plasma coagulation (APC) technique. The APC technique appears to be well tolerated and is associated with fewer complications and lower risk of re-bleeding [8, 54]. Because of the documented explosive risk associated with APC in this setting, a complete bowel preparation is strongly recommended prior to utilization [55, 56].

In some instances, a patient with a history compatible with angiodysplasia-mediated lower gastrointestinal bleeding may present for evaluation between active bleeds, this may prove to be quite difficult or impossible. Patients should be warned that angiodysplastic lesions are likely to re-bleed in the majority of cases (up to 80% in some series) [52] and that timely evaluation in the event of a re-bleed may greatly increase the likelihood of successful identification and treatment of the lesion in question. Colon resection is generally employed as a last resort when recurrent angiodysplastic bleeding is unable to be controlled through colonoscopic treatment or angiography [7].

Bleeding secondary to colonic ischemia or hypoperfusion, termed ischemic colitis, is not infrequently encountered and should be entertained in the differential diagnosis for any patient presenting with acute lower gastrointestinal bleeding, particularly in those with abdominal pain and bloody diarrhea. "Pain out of proportion to the physical examination" is commonly associated with intestinal ischemia. In a large series of patients admitted for acute lower gastrointestinal bleeding, 8.7–11.8% of cases were ultimately attributed to ischemic colitis [2, 57]. Typically hemorrhage is a relatively minor component of the clinical presentation and blood loss is not of sufficient magnitude to independently affect hemodynamic stability [7]. Although acute mesenteric ischemia may present with a similar clinical picture, colonic ischemia is in fact considerably more common secondary to the relatively poorly collateralized vascular supply to the colon in comparison to the small intestine. Those areas with poorly collateralized vascular supply are at highest risk for colonic ischemia, namely, the ascending colon, splenic flexure, and rectosigmoid junction. Conventional wisdom has held that Griffith's point is the single most common site of ischemic colitis, but rigorous investigation has failed to support this contention [58]. The diagnosis of ischemic colitis can be confirmed via colonoscopy with the characteristic findings including mucosal edema, erythema, mucosal necrosis, and hemorrhage with a clearly demarcated boundary between involved and uninvolved regions of bowel, reflective of the underlying vascular distribution [20, 59].

The pathophysiology of ischemic colitis is hypoperfusion of the involved segments secondary to cardiovascular issues, the administration of vasopressors, thromboembolic disease or known hypercoagulability, and generalized hypovolemia. Fernandez and colleagues identified diabetes mellitus, dyslipidemia, heart failure, peripheral arterial disease, and treatment with digoxin or aspirin as variables independently

associated with the development of ischemic colitis [60]. Another large series found that a majority of ischemic colitis patients were receiving vasoactive agents prior to the development of the condition [59]. All that being said, in many cases of ischemic colitis, no specific underlying cause is identified.

Most cases of ischemic colitis resolve with conservative management alone [20]. If such measures fail and there is evidence of bowel compromise (increasing abdominal pain and distention, peritoneal signs, rising lactate, and pronounced leukocytosis), surgical resection of the involved segment is indicated [10]. This is reported to occur in approximately 15–22% of all cases of ischemic colitis, and is associated with significant mortality [59, 61]. O'Neill and colleagues identified four factors—ischemia localized to the right colon, guarding on physical examination, lack of bleeding per rectum, and a history of chronic constipation—as being associated with severe ischemic colitis, defined as patients who either required surgical intervention and/or died from the disease process [62].

Ischemic colitis is diffuse rather than focal, and as such, endoscopic and angiographic treatment modalities are not well suited to the management of this condition. In cases where compromise is uncertain, a colonoscopy should be performed to assess bowel viability. If a bowel resection is required, it should encompass the vascular territory involved. A second-look laparotomy may be useful in further delineating overall bowel viability. Patients who undergo surgery for ischemic colitis have increased mortality rates versus those managed medically, which is reflective of a more severe disease process in these individuals as evidenced by variables including serum lactate, acute renal failure, duration of vasoactive drug administration, and the requirement for mechanical ventilation [61, 63].

Another etiology of lower gastrointestinal bleeding which can present similarly to ischemic colitis is hemorrhagic colitis of infectious origin. There are several commonly recognized infectious agents which can present with bloody diarrhea and associated abdominal pain, including *Campylobacter*, *Clostridium difficile*, *Escherichia coli* O157:H7, *Histoplasma*, *Salmonella*, *Shigella*, and *Yersinia*. Recent research has investigated strains of *Klebsiella oxytoca* linked to antibiotic-associated hemorrhagic colitis [64]. Cytomegalovirus is also recognized as a relatively common cause of bloody diarrhea in immunocompromised individuals. An evaluation for an infectious etiology should be largely dictated by the patient's history, with a focus on possible foodborne or waterborne exposures, development of diarrhea antecedent to lower gastrointestinal bleeding, recent antibiotics administration in the case of *C. difficile* or *K. oxytoca*, and any history of immune system compromise. Colonoscopy is infrequently utilized as the primary diagnostic modality in cases of infectious colitis; however, if it is, characteristic pseudomembranes are seen in cases of *C. difficile* colitis. Laboratory assays are available to identify the presence of each of these pathogens, and as such, serve as the primary diagnostic modality. Timely administration of the appropriate pathogen-specific antimicrobial or antiviral agents constitutes the cornerstone of treatment. Adjunctive treatment is largely supportive in nature, and surgical intervention is not generally required for colitis of infectious origin. A notable exception is the development of toxic megacolon in the setting of *C. difficile* colitis; this fulminant colitis frequently necessitates emergent colectomy.

Hemorrhoids represent another significant source of lower gastrointestinal bleeding, about 5% of all lower gastrointestinal bleeds evaluated in the acute inpatient setting [2] and the majority of cases in the outpatient setting [10]. Among younger adult patients, hemorrhoids represent by far the most common etiology of bright red blood per rectum. While many patients with hemorrhoids will report only intermittent rectal bleeding in small amounts, in some cases hemorrhoidal bleeding can be profuse and result in clinically significant blood loss. While many patients may report typical hemorrhoidal symptomatology such as anorectal pruritus, pain, a sensation of rectal fullness, and/or a history of constipation and pain with defecation, some patients with hemorrhoids are entirely asymptomatic except for bleeding. Therefore, hemorrhoids need to be ruled out on physical examination in any patient with lower gastrointestinal bleeding, regardless of the presence of typical hemorrhoidal symptoms.

Anoscopy is the diagnostic modality of choice in the detection and evaluation of hemorrhoids, with detection rates superior to flexible sigmoidoscopy [65]. This examination may be performed in the clinic or emergency department, but in some cases patient discomfort precludes effective examination. If hemorrhoidal disease is highly suspected, some surgeons prefer to perform examination under general anesthesia in the operating room. An advantage of this approach is that a full range of therapeutic interventions may be undertaken during the course of the same operation. However, it should be noted that surgical intervention is not, as a rule, required for the management of most hemorrhoidal bleeding, and most patients with this complaint will respond well to conservative measures such as Sitz baths, stool softeners, and increased dietary fiber [66]. Where conservative medical management fails, the most common treatment modalities include band ligation, sclerosant injection, cryotherapy, electrocautery, and laser photocoagulation [67]; among these options, band ligation appears to offer the greatest efficacy [68].

Absolute indications for endoscopic or surgical therapy in patients with hemorrhoidal bleeding include hemodynamically significant hemorrhage as well as persistent lower-volume bleeding that is unable to be controlled through conservative measures. It should also be noted that, as with all patients presenting with a lower gastrointestinal bleed, multiple concurrent sources of bleeding may be present. In particular in patients with hemorrhoidal bleeding over age 40 or with any evidence of elevated risk for colorectal adenocarcinoma, a colonoscopy should be performed to rule out concurrent malignancy. It is not mandatory that this study be carried out in the acute care or emergency setting, but rather the patient can be scheduled for colonoscopy on an outpatient basis several weeks after the acute lower gastrointestinal bleeding issue has been addressed.

Other anorectal lesions may also present with bleeding, including anal fissure and fistula-in-ano. Patients with anorectal fissure often present with complaints of anal pain, particularly with defecation, and small amounts of bright red blood per rectum. It is unusual for there to be profuse bleeding due to anal fissure, and large volume blood loss in a patient with anal fissure should prompt a thorough search for an alternate, concurrent etiology. Anal fissure is frequently readily detectable on basic physical examination. Anoscopy can also prove to be an important diagnostic adjunct in this circumstance [7]. In almost all cases, anal fissure will respond well to conservative management and surgical intervention will not be required to control bleeding.

Stercoral rectal ulcerations may also cause significant rectal bleeding if the ulcerative lesion erodes into a major blood vessel. In some cases the blood loss from this etiology can be of sufficient magnitude to affect hemodynamic stability. The most common pathophysiology of stercoral ulceration relates to severe constipation and fecal impaction; patients will typically report a significant prior history of constipation. Plain radiography and CT imaging in this case will often reveal a considerable stool burden, and these patients are obviously at risk for stercoral perforation elsewhere in the lower gastrointestinal tract.

If stercoral ulceration has not yet progressed to bowel perforation, endoscopic therapy can be employed for both diagnostic and therapeutic purposes. The ulcers have a sharp, nodular border with associated edema and erythema. Treatment consists primarily of thermal probe application, often with concomitant injection of epinephrine [69]. In cases of profuse hemorrhage due to stercoral perforation, most patients will typically require surgical correction as well as aggressive peritoneal irrigation to reduce the burden of contamination.

There are a number of less common causes of lower gastrointestinal bleeding which may be seen in the acute setting. Rectal and/or anal trauma may, depending on mechanism, result in hemodynamically significant hemorrhage. Trauma to adjacent structures (i.e., pelvic fractures) may also result in lower gastrointestinal bleeding if bone fragments disrupt the bowel wall. The digital rectal examination performed on as part of advanced trauma life support provides an initial screen for gross blood and obvious deformities which could indicate penetration or disruption of the bowel wall. This examination is typically performed quickly as part of the initial trauma patient assessment and may well overlook more subtle injuries. Practitioners caring for trauma patients who identify significant damage to adjacent structures, particularly pelvic fractures, should maintain a high index of suspicion for involvement of adjacent bowel, particularly if laboratory studies demonstrate evidence of ongoing blood loss and no other obvious source of hemorrhage is identified. These types of bleeds may be amenable to angiographic intervention if they fail to stop spontaneously.

Inflammatory bowel disease, including both Crohn's disease and ulcerative colitis, occasionally present with acute lower gastrointestinal bleeding, most commonly seen as bloody diarrhea [7]. However, more commonly these disease entities present with a history of abdominal and/or anorectal pain, recurrent diarrhea, and unintentional weight loss. Massive hemorrhage is unusual in the setting of inflammatory bowel disease, occurring in only 6% of patients with inflammatory bowel disease [70, 71], while occult blood loss is considerably more common. In most cases gastrointestinal blood losses in patients with Crohn's disease or ulcerative colitis are managed via treatment aimed at controlling the underlying inflammatory pathology. In such cases, lower gastrointestinal bleeding stops spontaneously in about half of patients [70], but roughly one third of these patients will experience recurrent bleeding [10]. For this reason, most surgeons will recommend resection after one episode of significant lower gastrointestinal bleeding in this clinical setting. Total abdominal colectomy is the standard operation in this setting unless the rectum is the source of major bleeding, in which case coloproctectomy should be performed [7].

Colonic neoplasms infrequently cause overt lower gastrointestinal hemorrhage. Often, the only indication of bleeding is the development of an otherwise-unexplained anemia. This type of bleed may also be detected on a routine screening fecal occult blood test. Although most cases of lower gastrointestinal bleeding are not associated with a neoplastic process, it is critically important to rule this out in the evaluation of these patients. Hence, the importance of a full colonoscopic examination in patients presenting with lower gastrointestinal bleeding, even those in whom an "obvious" source is identified.

Radiation proctitis/colitis is another unusual cause of lower gastrointestinal bleeding. This diagnosis will be either included or excluded from the differential on the basis of a thorough and accurate patient history, with special attention given to any history of prostate, rectal, bladder, cervical, or uterine cancer for which the patient was treated with radiation therapy. Confirmation is obtained via endoscopic examination which demonstrates friable mucosa with telangiectatic lesions [10, 20]. Bleeding due to this etiology is typically lower-grade and chronic [8], and massive hemorrhage

secondary to radiation proctitis/colitis is rare [20]. Nevertheless, this diagnosis must be kept in mind for that portion of the patient population who possess the appropriate history. Conservative therapy, including rectal steroids, rectal sucralfate, and short-chain fatty acid enemas [72], is successful in controlling bleeding due to radiation. If conservative therapies fail, endoscopic applications including argon laser [73], argon plasma coagulation [74], and electrocautery are frequently successful.

Clinically significant bleeding can also occur after a recent polypectomy, and estimates of the frequency of this complication range from 2.2 to 6.1% [75, 76]. Post-polypectomy bleeding can be either immediate or delayed. If immediate, the bleed is usually noted by the endoscopist and appropriate treatment, via either direct pressure on the residual polyp stalk, epinephrine injection, electrocautery, or clip application, is provided at that time. In other cases, bleeding after polypectomy may be delayed for up to 1 month [7, 8, 77]. The use of aspirin and NSAIDs prior to the procedure does not appear to increase the bleeding risk [75, 77], although warfarin therapy, even with a non-supratherapeutic international normalized ratio (INR), is correlated with an increased risk [75]. Bleeding will typically cease spontaneously. If bleeding is persistent, standard endoscopic interventions (epinephrine, cautery, or clipping) are first line therapy [78]. If the hemorrhage proves difficult or impossible to control, or the patient demonstrates signs of hemodynamic instability, urgent surgical intervention is necessary.

Complications

A number of diverse complications can occur in the management of patients with lower gastrointestinal bleeding, reflective of the diverse etiologies attributable to this condition. Each treatment modality carries distinct risks. While conservative management is often the least "risky" clinical strategy, it can only be considered as such for the appropriately selected patient population. In the acute setting, patients with significant lower gastrointestinal bleeding may require considerably more aggressive interventions to avoid significant morbidity and mortality.

Patients undergoing colonoscopy for either diagnostic or therapeutic purposes in the setting of lower gastrointestinal bleeding are at risk for bowel perforation during the procedure, in some series up to 3% [24]. This risk is likely elevated in the setting of significant inflammation. It also seems logical that perforation risk would increase in the setting of brisk bleeding which might compromise effective visualization during the procedure.

Angiography carries its own set of unique risks, including the development of a hematoma, pseudoaneurysm, or uncontrolled bleeding at the puncture site. There is also a nontrivial risk of damage to vascular structures along the path of the angiographic catheter. Additionally, there is an increased risk of thromboembolic events associated with angiographic intervention. Patients are also subject to the standard risks of contrast dye administration and the associated contrast-induced nephropathy. Targeted vasopressin therapy must be closely monitored due to the risks of systemic cardiovascular effects, and this therapy confers a significantly increased risk to patients with severe cardiovascular disease [32]. Embolization of larger-caliber bleeding vessels can result in bowel ischemia, in some cases progressing to bowel necrosis. These risks will, of course, vary based on the underlying risk profile of the patient as well as the skill and experience of the angiographer.

Surgical intervention for the management of lower gastrointestinal bleeding carries all of the risks of major abdominal surgery. As with all surgical procedures; the risk profile for the procedure must be adjusted based on the patient's underlying comorbidities, as well as the physiologic state at the time of operation. A patient with lower gastrointestinal bleeding of significant magnitude to warrant acute or emergent surgical intervention is, by definition, not physiologically stable to the same degree as a patient undergoing a planned, elective procedure; therefore, the risk profile is elevated as with any patient undergoing an urgent or emergent procedure. In all but the most emergent of circumstances, the patient going to the operating room for the management of lower gastrointestinal bleeding will benefit from appropriate preoperative fluid resuscitation and correction of electrolyte abnormalities. Similarly, patients with any evidence of coagulopathy should also be aggressively corrected prior to operative intervention if possible.

Conclusion

The appropriate follow-up for patients presenting with acute lower gastrointestinal hemorrhage is determined in large part by the underlying etiology of the bleeding, the severity of the presentation, and any operative or procedural interventions that were undertaken to address the bleeding. Patients who present with an initial lower gastrointestinal bleed are at elevated risk of a subsequent bleed, and should be counseled as such. For patients who present with recurrent bleeding, the recurrent nature of the problem should be weighed when considering whether surgical intervention is appropriate.

For patients who presented with chronic low-grade bleeding and anemia, it may be worthwhile to follow serial hematocrits on an outpatient basis as a noninvasive preliminary screen for recurrent bleeding. Fecal occult blood testing can also be performed intermittently, although the yield from a single test is relatively low. If this method of surveillance is selected, testing should occur at least annually. With regard to longer term surveillance, all patients over 50 with a non-elevated risk profile should be receiving colon cancer screening per the US Preventive Services Task Force recommendations [79] via either annual fecal occult blood testing, flexible sigmoidoscopy every 3 years, or colonoscopy every 10 years. A history of lower gastrointestinal bleeding does not, per se, alter these screening recommendations; however, if the etiology of the lower gastrointestinal bleed represents a factor associated with elevated risk for colorectal adenocarcinoma (i.e., lower gastrointestinal bleeding in the setting of ulcerative colitis), the screening intervals should be shortened accordingly.

References

1. Longstreth GF. Epidemiology of hospitalization for acute upper gastrointestinal hemorrhage: a population-based study. Am J Gastroenterol. 1995;90:206–10.
2. Longstreth GF. Epidemiology and outcome of patients hospitalized with acute lower gastrointestinal hemorrhage: a population-based study. Am J Gastroenterol. 1997;92(3):419–24. Research Support, Non-U.S. Gov't.
3. Peura DA, Lanza FL, Gostout CJ, Foutch PG. The American College of Gastroenterology Bleeding Registry: preliminary findings. Am J Gastroenterol. 1997;92(6):924–8. Research Support, Non-U.S. Gov't.
4. Strate LL, Saltzman JR, Ookubo R, Mutinga ML, Syngal S. Validation of a clinical prediction rule for severe acute lower intestinal bleeding. Am J Gastroenterol. 2005;100(8):1821–7. Research Support, Non-U.S. Gov't Validation Studies.
5. Strate LL, Orav EJ, Syngal S. Early predictors of severity in acute lower intestinal tract bleeding. Arch Intern Med. 2003;163(7):838–43. Research Support, U.S. Gov't, P.H.S.
6. Velayos FS, Williamson A, Sousa KH, Lung E, Bostrom A, Weber EJ, et al. Early predictors of severe lower gastrointestinal bleeding and adverse outcomes: a prospective study. Clin Gastroenterol Hepatol. 2004;2(6):485–90. Research Support, Non-U.S. Gov't.
7. Vernava 3rd AM, Moore BA, Longo WE, Johnson FE. Lower gastrointestinal bleeding. Dis Colon Rectum. 1997;40(7):846–58. Review.
8. Whitlow CB. Endoscopic treatment for lower gastrointestinal bleeding. Clin Colon Rectal Surg. 2010;23(1):31–6.
9. Hoedema RE, Luchtefeld MA. The management of lower gastrointestinal hemorrhage. Dis Colon Rectum. 2005;48(11):2010–24. Review.
10. Edelman DA, Sugawa C. Lower gastrointestinal bleeding: a review. Surg Endosc. 2007;21(4):514–20. Review.
11. Bloomfeld RS, Rockey DC, Shetzline MA. Endoscopic therapy of acute diverticular hemorrhage. Am J Gastroenterol. 2001;96(8):2367–72.
12. Browder W, Cerise EJ, Litwin MS. Impact of emergency angiography in massive lower gastrointestinal bleeding. Ann Surg. 1986;204:530–6.
13. Leitman IM, Paull DE, Shires 3rd GT. Evaluation and management of massive lower gastrointestinal hemorrhage. Ann Surg. 1989;209(2):175–80.
14. Cuellar RE, Gavaler JS, Alexander JA, Brouillette DE, Chien MC, Yoo YK, et al. Gastrointestinal tract hemorrhage. The value of a nasogastric aspirate. Arch Intern Med. 1990;150(7):1381–4. Research Support, U.S. Gov't, P.H.S.

15. Graham DJ, Pritchard TJ, Bloom AD. Colonoscopy for intermittent rectal bleeding: impact on patient management. J Surg Res. 1993;54(2):136–9.

16. Gutierrez G, Reines HD, Wulf-Gutierrez ME. Clinical review: hemorrhagic shock. Crit Care. 2004;8(5):373–81. Review.

17. Allison JE, Tekawa IS, Ransom LJ, Adrain AL. A comparison of fecal occult-blood tests for colorectal-cancer screening. N Engl J Med. 1996;334(3):155–9. Comparative Study Research Support, Non-U.S. Gov't.

18. Friedman A, Chan A, Chin LC, Deen A, Hammerschlag G, Lee M, et al. Use and abuse of faecal occult blood tests in an acute hospital inpatient setting. Intern Med J. 2010;40(2):107–11. Comparative Study Multicenter Study.

19. Sinatra MA, St John DJ, Young GP. Interference of plant peroxidases with guaiac-based fecal occult blood tests is avoidable. Clin Chem. 1999;45(1):123–6. Comparative Study Research Support, Non-U.S. Gov't.

20. Strate LL. Lower GI, bleeding: epidemiology and diagnosis. Gastroenterol Clin North Am. 2005;34(4):643–64. Research Support, N.I.H., Extramural Review.

21. Al Qahtani AR, Satin R, Stern J, Gordon PH. Investigative modalities for massive lower gastrointestinal bleeding. World J Surg. 2002;26(5):620–5. Evaluation Studies.

22. Tada M, Shimizu S, Kawai K. Emergency colonoscopy for the diagnosis of lower intestinal bleeding. Gastroenterol Jpn. 1991;26 Suppl 3:121–4.

23. Vellacott KD. Early endoscopy for acute lower gastrointestinal haemorrhage. Ann R Coll Surg Engl. 1986;68(5):243–4.

24. Damore 2nd LJ, Rantis PC, Vernava 3rd AM, Longo WE. Colonoscopic perforations. Etiology, diagnosis, and management. Dis Colon Rectum. 1996;39(11):1308–14. Review.

25. Caos A, Benner KG, Manier J, McCarthy DM, Blessing LD, Katon RM, et al. Colonoscopy after Golytely preparation in acute rectal bleeding. J Clin Gastroenterol. 1986;8(1):46–9. Research Support, U.S. Gov't, Non-P.H.S.

26. Jensen DM, Machicado GA, Jutabha R, Kovacs TO. Urgent colonoscopy for the diagnosis and treatment of severe diverticular hemorrhage. N Engl J Med. 2000;342(2):78–82. Clinical Trial Research Support, U.S. Gov't, P.H.S.

27. Bounds BC, Friedman LS. Lower gastrointestinal bleeding. Gastroenterol Clin North Am. 2003;32(4):1107–25. Review.

28. Steer ML, Silen W. Diagnostic procedures in gastrointestinal hemorrhage. N Engl J Med. 1983;309(11):646–50.

29. Chaudhry V, Hyser MJ, Gracias VH, Gau FC. Colonoscopy: the initial test for acute lower gastrointestinal bleeding. Am Surg. 1998;64(8):723–8.

30. Pennoyer WP, Vignati PV, Cohen JL. Mesenteric angiography for lower gastrointestinal hemorrhage: are there predictors for a positive study? Dis Colon Rectum. 1997;40(9):1014–8.

31. Ponzo F, Zhuang H, Liu FM, Lacorte LB, Moussavian B, Wang S, et al. Tc-99m sulfur colloid and Tc-99m tagged red blood cell methods are comparable for detecting lower gastrointestinal bleeding in clinical practice. Clin Nucl Med. 2002;27(6):405–9. Comparative Study.

32. Beck DE, Margolin DA, Whitlow CB, Hammond KL. Evaluation and management of gastrointestinal bleeding. Ochsner J. 2007;7(3):107–13.

33. Ng DA, Opelka FG, Beck DE, Milburn JM, Witherspoon LR, Hicks TC, et al. Predictive value of technetium Tc 99m-labeled red blood cell scintigraphy for positive angiogram in massive lower gastrointestinal hemorrhage. Dis Colon Rectum. 1997;40(4):471–7.

34. Hammond KL, Beck DE, Hicks TC, Timmcke AE, Whitlow CW, Margolin DA. Implications of negative technetium 99m-labeled red blood cell scintigraphy in patients presenting with lower gastrointestinal bleeding. Am J Surg. 2007;193(3):404–7. Discussion 7–8.

35. Schmulewitz N, Fisher DA, Rockey DC. Early colonoscopy for acute lower GI bleeding predicts shorter hospital stay: a retrospective study of experience in a single center. Gastrointest Endosc. 2003;58(6):841–6.

36. Ohyama T, Sakurai Y, Ito M, Daito K, Sezai S, Sato Y. Analysis of urgent colonoscopy for lower gastrointestinal tract bleeding. Digestion. 2000;61(3):189–92.

37. Strate LL, Syngal S. Timing of colonoscopy: impact on length of hospital stay in patients with acute lower intestinal bleeding. Am J Gastroenterol. 2003;98(2):317–22. Research Support, U.S. Gov't, P.H.S.

38. Imdahl A. Genesis and pathophysiology of lower gastrointestinal bleeding. Langenbecks Arch Surg. 2001;386(1):1–7. Review.

39. McGuire Jr HH. Bleeding colonic diverticula. A reappraisal of natural history and management. Ann Surg. 1994;220(5):653–6.

40. Wright HK, Pelliccia O, Higgins Jr EF, Sreenivas V, Gupta A. Controlled, semielective, segmental resection for massive colonic hemorrhage. Am J Surg. 1980;139(4):535–8.

41. Boley SJ, DiBiase A, Brandt LJ, Sammartano RJ. Lower intestinal bleeding in the elderly. Am J Surg. 1979;137(1):57–64.

42. Bender JS, Wiencek RG, Bouwman DL. Morbidity and mortality following total abdominal colectomy for massive lower gastrointestinal bleeding. Am Surg. 1991;57(8):536–40. Discussion 40–1.

43. Almy TP, Howell DA. Medical progress. Diverticular disease of the colon. N Engl J Med. 1980;302(6):324–31. Review.

44. Laine L, Connors LG, Reicin A, Hawkey CJ, Burgos-Vargas R, Schnitzer TJ, et al. Serious lower gastrointestinal clinical events with nonselective NSAID or coxib use. Gastroenterology. 2003;124(2):288–92. Clinical Trial Randomized Controlled Trial Research Support, Non-U.S. Gov't.

45. McGuire Jr HH, Haynes Jr BW. Massive hemorrhage for diverticulosis of the colon: guidelines for therapy based on bleeding patterns observed in fifty cases. Ann Surg. 1972;175(6):847–55.

46. Lopez DE, Brown CV. Diverticulitis: the most common colon emergency for the acute care surgeon. Scand J Surg. 2010;99(2):86–9. Review.

47. Klein RR, Gallagher DM. Massive colonic bleeding from diverticular disease. Am J Surg. 1969;118(4):553–7.

48. Wolff BG, Devine RM. Surgical management of diverticulitis. Am Surg. 2000;66(2):153–6. Review.

49. Richter JM, Hedberg SE, Athanasoulis CA, Schapiro RH. Angiodysplasia. Clinical presentation and colonoscopic diagnosis. Dig Dis Sci. 1984;29(6):481–5. Comparative Study.

50. Boley SJ, Sammartano R, Adams A, DiBiase A, Kleinhaus S, Sprayregen S. On the nature and etiology of vascular ectasias of the colon. Degenerative lesions of aging. Gastroenterology. 1977;72(4 Pt 1):650–60.

51. Bhutani MS, Gupta SC, Markert RJ, Barde CJ, Donese R, Gopalswamy N. A prospective controlled evaluation of endoscopic detection of angiodysplasia and its association with aortic valve disease. Gastrointest Endosc. 1995;42(5):398–402. Comparative Study.

52. Helmrich GA, Stallworth JR, Brown JJ. Angiodysplasia: characterization, diagnosis, and advances in treatment. South Med J. 1990;83(12):1450–3. Review.

53. Baum S, Athanasoulis CA, Waltman AC, Galdabini J, Schapiro RH, Warshaw AL, et al. Angiodysplasia of the right colon: a cause of gastrointestinal bleeding. AJR Am J Roentgenol. 1977;129(5):789–94. Research Support, U.S. Gov't, P.H.S.

54. Olmos JA, Marcolongo M, Pogorelsky V, Herrera L, Tobal F, Davolos JR. Long-term outcome of argon plasma ablation therapy for bleeding in 100 consecutive patients with colonic angiodysplasia. Dis Colon Rectum. 2006;49(10):1507–16.

55. Nurnberg D, Pannwitz H, Burkhardt KD, Peters M. Gas explosion caused by argon plasma coagulation of colonic angiodysplasias. Endoscopy. 2007;39 Suppl 1:E182. Case Reports.

56. Manner H, Plum N, Pech O, Ell C, Enderle MD. Colon explosion during argon plasma coagulation. Gastrointest Endosc. 2008;67(7):1123–7. Review.

57. Chavalitdhamrong D, Jensen DM, Kovacs TO, Jutabha R, Dulai G, Ohning G, et al. Ischemic colitis as a cause of severe hematochezia: risk factors and outcomes compared with other colon diagnoses. Gastrointest Endosc. 2011;74(4):852–7.

58. Glauser PM, Wermuth P, Cathomas G, Kuhnt E, Kaser SA, Maurer CA. Ischemic colitis: clinical presentation, localization in relation to risk factors, and long-term results. World J Surg. 2011;35(11):2549–54.

59. Scharff JR, Longo WE, Vartanian SM, Jacobs DL, Bahadursingh AN, Kaminski DL. Ischemic colitis: spectrum of disease and outcome. Surgery. 2003;134(4):624–9. Discussion 9–30.

60. Cubiella Fernandez J, Nunez Calvo L, Gonzalez Vazquez E, Garcia Garcia MJ, Alves Perez MT, Martinez Silva I, et al. Risk factors associated with the development of ischemic colitis. World J Gastroenterol. 2010;16(36):4564–9.

61. Paterno F, McGillicuddy EA, Schuster KM, Longo WE. Ischemic colitis: risk factors for eventual surgery. Am J Surg. 2010;200(5):646–50. Comparative Study.

62. O'Neill S, Elder K, Harrison SJ, Yalamarthi S. Predictors of severity in ischaemic colitis. Int J Colorectal Dis. 2012;27(2):187–91.

63. Reissfelder C, Sweiti H, Antolovic D, Rahbari NN, Hofer S, Buchler MW, et al. Ischemic colitis: who will survive? Surgery. 2011;149(4):585–92.

64. Joainig MM, Gorkiewicz G, Leitner E, Weberhofer P, Zollner-Schwetz I, Lippe I, et al. Cytotoxic effects of Klebsiella oxytoca strains isolated from patients with antibiotic-associated hemorrhagic colitis or other diseases caused by infections and from healthy subjects. J Clin Microbiol. 2010;48(3):817–24. Comparative Study Research Support, Non-U.S. Gov't.

65. Korkis AM, McDougall CJ. Rectal bleeding in patients less than 50 years of age. Dig Dis Sci. 1995;40(7):1520–3.

66. Alonso-Coello P, Mills E, Heels-Ansdell D, Lopez-Yarto M, Zhou Q, Johanson JF, et al. Fiber for the treatment of hemorrhoids complications: a systematic review and meta-analysis. Am J Gastroenterol. 2006;101(1):181–8. Comparative Study Meta-Analysis Research Support, Non-U.S. Gov't Review.

67. Salvati EP. Nonoperative management of hemorrhoids: evolution of the office management of hemorrhoids. Dis Colon Rectum. 1999;42(8):989–93. Lectures.

68. Su MY, Chiu CT, Wu CS, Ho YP, Lien JM, Tung SY, et al. Endoscopic hemorrhoidal ligation of symptomatic internal hemorrhoids. Gastrointest Endosc. 2003;58(6):871–4.

69. Kanwal F, Dulai G, Jensen DM, Gralnek IM, Kovacs TO, Machicado GA, et al. Major stigmata of recent hemorrhage on rectal ulcers in patients with severe hematochezia: Endoscopic diagnosis, treatment, and outcomes. Gastrointest Endosc. 2003;57(4):462–8. Research Support, U.S. Gov't, P.H.S.

70. Robert JR, Sachar DB, Greenstein AJ. Severe gastrointestinal hemorrhage in Crohn's disease. Ann Surg. 1991;213(3):207–11.

71. Robert JH, Sachar DB, Aufses Jr AH, Greenstein AJ. Management of severe hemorrhage in ulcerative colitis. Am J Surg. 1990;159(6):550–5. Comparative Study.

72. Denton A, Forbes A, Andreyev J, Maher EJ. Non surgical interventions for late radiation proctitis in patients who have received radical radiotherapy to the pelvis. Cochrane Database Syst Rev. 2002;1:CD003455. Review.

73. Taylor JG, DiSario JA, Buchi KN. Argon laser therapy for hemorrhagic radiation proctitis: long-term results. Gastrointest Endosc. 1993;39(5):641–4. Research Support, U.S. Gov't, Non-P.H.S.

74. Silva RA, Correia AJ, Dias LM, Viana HL, Viana RL. Argon plasma coagulation therapy for hemorrhagic radiation proctosigmoiditis. Gastrointest Endosc. 1999;50(2):221–4.

75. Hui AJ, Wong RM, Ching JY, Hung LC, Chung SC, Sung JJ. Risk of colonoscopic polypectomy bleeding with anticoagulants and antiplatelet agents: analysis of 1657 cases. Gastrointest Endosc. 2004;59(1):44–8.

76. Rosen L, Bub DS, Reed 3rd JF, Nastasee SA. Hemorrhage following colonoscopic polypectomy. Dis Colon Rectum. 1993;36(12):1126–31. Review.

77. Yousfi M, Gostout CJ, Baron TH, Hernandez JL, Keate R, Fleischer DE, et al. Postpolypectomy lower gastrointestinal bleeding: potential role of aspirin. Am J Gastroenterol. 2004;99(9):1785–9. Comparative Study.

78. Rex DK, Lewis BS, Waye JD. Colonoscopy and endoscopic therapy for delayed post-polypectomy hemorrhage. Gastrointest Endosc. 1992;38(2):127–9.

79. Colon Cancer Screening (USPSTF Recommendation). US preventive services task force. J Am Geriatr Soc. 2000;48(3):333–5. Guideline Practice Guideline.

Nicole Fox

Introduction

Colonic volvulus was first recorded in the Ebers Papyrus in ancient Egypt. The authors astutely recognized that detorsion of the colon was crucial and that if the colon did not spontaneously reduce, it "rotted." Early management of colonic volvulus was nonoperative and various techniques evolved from ancient Egypt until the late nineteenth century. Hippocrates proposed the insertion of a suppository, 12 in. in length to promote detorsion. Other practitioners used air insufflation, oral ingestion of metal and lead balls as well as external manipulation in order to relieve the volvulus and concomitant bowel obstruction [1]. In 1859, Gay published his observations in an article entitled "Fatal obstruction from twisting of the meso-colon." Through his work on cadavers, he observed that insertion of a rectal tube detorsed sigmoid volvulus, which led him to propose that all patients with sigmoid volvulus have a rectal tube inserted [2]. By the late nineteenth century, nonoperative treatment was well established. Operative treatment was avoided, as surgical mortality rates were high. In 1851 Malgaigne warned "you cannot be too reserved" in operating on volvulus. Trousseau echoed this sentiment and suggested that laparotomy be reserved for cases where "there was imminent danger to life."[1]

In the twentieth century, as surgical mortality rates declined, the transition to prompt operative management of volvulus began. In 1883, Atherton published the first reported case of successful operative reduction of sigmoid volvulus in the United States. Senn recognized the high rate of recurrence after simple detorsion of the colon and advocated an operative approach that included mesenteric shortening [3]. Surgeons used a variety of operative approaches during this time period including simple detorsion, sigmoidopexy and sigmoid resection. By the end of the twentieth century, immediate surgical treatment was standard and nonoperative management was abandoned. This persisted until 1947 when Bruusgaard challenged this paradigm with the results of his success using nonoperative decompression in 91 patients with sigmoid volvulus. Reduction with a combination of proctoscopy and a rectal tube was successful in 123 attempts. Surgery was required acutely in 18 patients. Overall mortality for the 91 patients was 14.2%. These results swung the pendulum back to the middle and affirmed that in the acute phase, "treatment may be either non-operative or operative."[4]

Sigmoid Volvulus

Epidemiology

The word volvulus originates from the Latin "volvere," which means to twist around. Colonic volvulus is the cause of 5–7% of large bowel obstructions in the United States. In other regions such as India, Turkey, Russia, Iran, Norway, and Africa, however, it is the most common cause of large bowel obstruction. The most common location of volvulus in the large bowel is the sigmoid (60–80%) followed by the cecum (20–40%) [5].

Incidence, age distribution, and etiology vary by geographic region. For example, in Brazil, Chagas' disease results in megacolon. In one study of 365 patients, 30% of patients with megacolon developed sigmoid volvulus. Volvulus is the most common cause of intestinal obstruction in pregnancy. Jain and colleagues reviewed 182 cases of bowel obstruction in pregnant women in which 44% were caused by sigmoid volvulus [6]. Adhesions from prior abdominal surgery may also contribute to the development of volvulus. In their series of 59 patients with sigmoid volvulus, Ballantyne et al. found that 53% had a previous abdominal operation [5].

N. Fox, M.D., M.P.H. (✉)
Department of Trauma, Cooper Medical School of Rowan University,
Cooper University Hospital, 1 Cooper Plaza, Camden, NJ 08103, USA
e-mail: fox-nicole@cooperhealth.edu

L.J. Moore et al. (eds.), *Common Problems in Acute Care Surgery*,
DOI 10.1007/978-1-4614-6123-4_30, © Springer Science+Business Media New York 2013

In the United States, the most common patient presenting with sigmoid volvulus is chronically ill, elderly, and/or institutionalized. In a series of 99 patients with sigmoid volvulus published by Arnold et al., the average age was 66 and 13 patients were admitted from nursing homes [7]. It is proposed that patients of long-term care facilities and patients who require psychotropic medications have chronic constipation, which promotes colonic lengthening and results in a redundant sigmoid colon. A number of studies confirm the relationship between chronic constipation and sigmoid volvulus. Sinha documented that 85% of 211 patients with volvulus were chronically constipated. Of 45 cases reviewed by Hines et al., 73% of the patients reported severe, chronic constipation [8]. Regardless of the etiology, the twisting of the sigmoid colon on its mesentery results in decreased arterial inflow and venous outflow leading to intestinal ischemia. Prompt intervention is necessary to avoid progression to intestinal necrosis.

Clinical Presentation and Diagnosis

The sigmoid colon is, on average, 38 cm in length but may range from 15 to 50 cm. The arterial supply to the sigmoid originates from the inferior mesenteric artery with two to six sigmoid branches that form collaterals with the left colic artery. These arterial arcades also contribute to the marginal artery of Drummond. Venous and lymphatic drainage follows the arterial supply. In general, the sigmoid colon is mobile with a long and floppy mesentery. Two anatomic features contributing to the development of sigmoid volvulus are acquired and include a redundant sigmoid colon along with a narrow, elongated mesentery. As stated previously, altered intestinal motility from factors such as chronic constipation, diets high in fiber and vegetables and psychotropic medications is believed to promote colonic lengthening [5].

Colonic volvulus is a surgical emergency that must be recognized and treated promptly. Delayed intervention leads to significant morbidity and mortality from intestinal ischemia and bowel necrosis. Patients with sigmoid volvulus generally present with evidence of large bowel obstruction. Signs and symptoms include abdominal pain and/or distention, nausea, vomiting, constipation, and obstipation. Abdominal distention is the most significant clinical exam finding. In some cases the distention is so pronounced that it interferes with cardiac and respiratory function. Up to 60% of patients presenting with sigmoid volvulus have a history of similar episodes. In cases where volvulus has progressed to intestinal ischemia, patients may exhibit systemic manifestations including: peritonitis, fever, tachycardia, and leukocytosis.

Although the patient's history and physical exam findings may suggest a diagnosis of sigmoid volvulus, radiographic

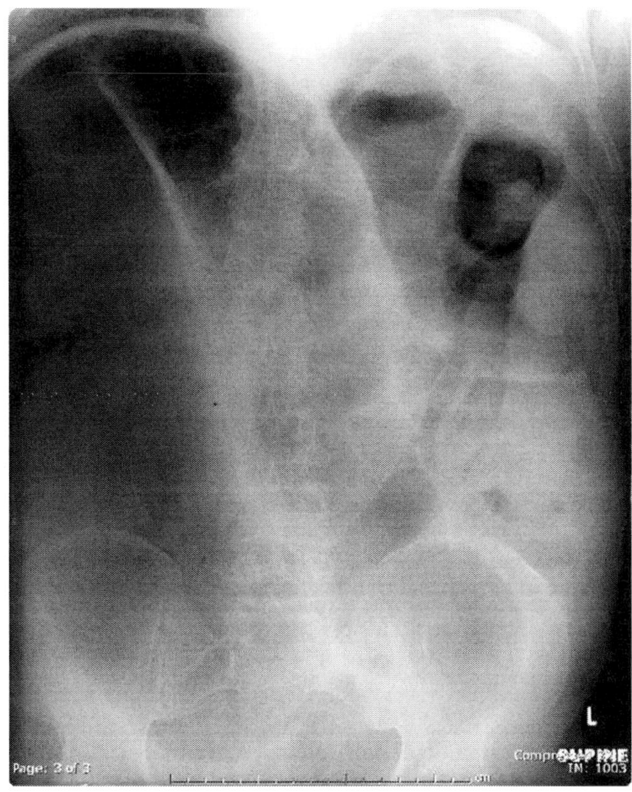

Fig. 30.1 "Bent inner tube" sign associated with sigmoid volvulus. Published with permission from William Herring, MD, FACR, learningradiology.com

imaging is used for confirmation. Plain abdominal X-rays are diagnostic in over 50% of cases and have a reported specificity of 85%. The volvulus will appear as a "bent innertube," with a markedly dilated, ahaustral colon (Fig. 30.1). This characteristic shape is also referred to as an "omega," with the convex aspect pointing toward the right upper quadrant (Fig. 30.2). The addition of a barium enema increases the diagnostic accuracy of plain X-rays to 90%. On these contrast studies the distal colonic tapering produces the classic "bird's beak" appearance. Using a contrast enema to attempt reduction of sigmoid volvulus, however, is not recommended because of the risk of colonic perforation. Computed tomography (CT) may also be used in the diagnostic process. The twisted mesentery seen on CT is referred to as a "whirl" sign, created by the rotation of afferent and efferent bowel loops around the point of obstruction. The advantage of CT scan over plain radiographs is that other sources of abdominal pathology can be identified if the diagnosis is not sigmoid volvulus.

Management

The initial management of sigmoid volvulus involves preparing the patient for intervention. Typically, patients are volume depleted and may have electrolyte abnormalities. A nasogastric tube and urinary catheter should be inserted. Broad spectrum antibiotics are recommended due to the potential for bacterial translocation through the compromised bowel wall. Depending on the severity of systemic manifestations, central venous pressure (CVP) monitoring should be considered to help guide in the resuscitation.

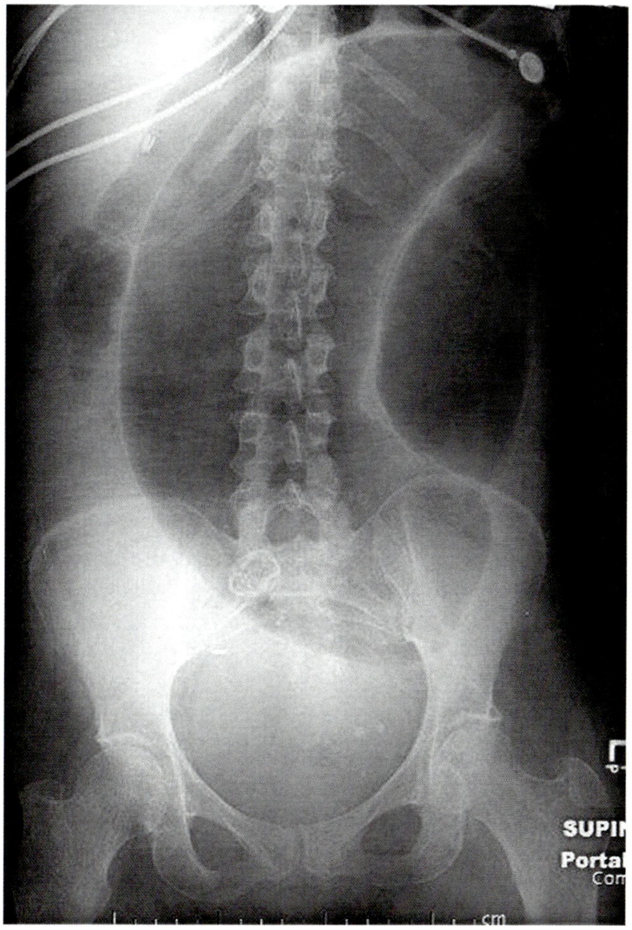

A proposed algorithm for the management of sigmoid volvulus is presented in Fig. 30.3. Since the publication of Bruusgaard's article in 1947, nonoperative decompression is considered the initial treatment of choice for patients with sigmoid volvulus. However, the first decision that must be made is whether or not the patient is a candidate for nonoperative reduction. If there is any evidence that the patient has colonic ischemia, there should be no delay in operative treatment and the patient should proceed immediately to surgery. These patients should *not* have an attempt at endoscopic reduction. Mortality rates for patients with sigmoid volvulus increase dramatically in the presence of compromised bowel. In a study published more than 100 years ago by Moynihan looking at patients with sigmoid volvulus, mortality was 80% in patients with gangrenous bowel as compared to 10.6% in patients with viable colon [9]. This has not changed dramatically. In 2000, Madiba and Thompson cited an overall 38% mortality rate in patients with gangrenous colon, which (similar to the Moynihan study) is eight times higher than the mortality rate for those with viable bowel [10].

Patients with peritonitis or any signs of bowel ischemia should proceed directly to the operating room. Likewise, patients who fail endoscopic decompression or those that have evidence of ischemia on endoscopic evaluation also

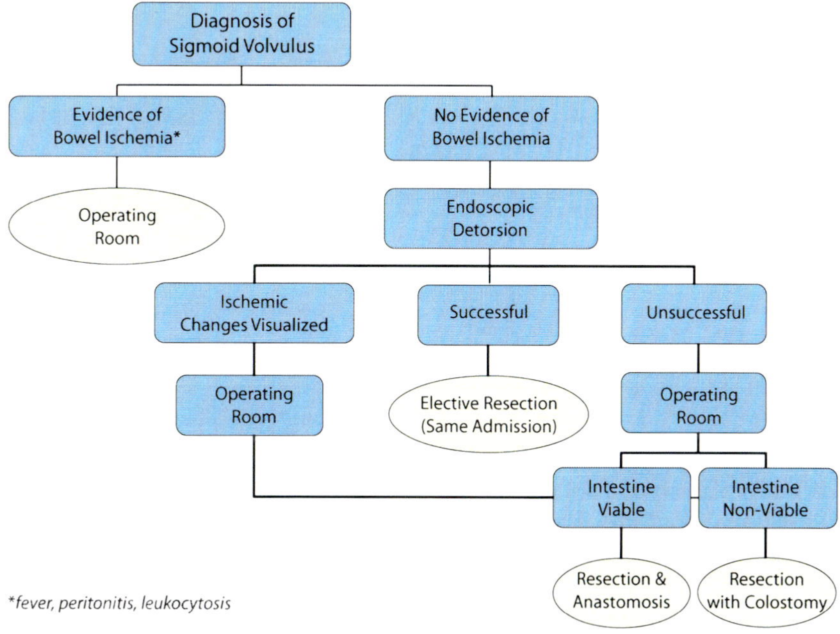

Fig. 30.2 "Omega" sign associated with sigmoid volvulus. Published with permission from William Herring, MD, FACR, learningradiology. com

Fig. 30.3 Algorithm for the management of sigmoid volvulus

require surgical resection. The type of operation in this case will depend on the viability of the colon and the patient's clinical condition. Although there are reports describing non-resectional operations for sigmoid volvulus such colopexy, mesosigmoidoplasty and laparoscopic fixation, they are not considered standard and are beyond the scope of this chapter. Therefore, only resectional options are discussed. If the colon is viable at the time of operation it is appropriate to proceed with sigmoid resection and primary anastomosis. The extent of sigmoid resection should be limited to the area of sigmoid colon that is redundant and freely mobile. If the bowel is ischemic and/or the patient is hemodynamically unstable, the operation of choice is a sigmoid resection and end colostomy (Hartmann procedure). As stated previously, if the volvulus has progressed to the point of intestinal gangrene at the time of colectomy the mortality rate is extremely high (50–80%). Cirocchi et al. reviewed 23 patients with sigmoid volvulus and separated them into two groups: patients who were completely obstructed and those with symptoms considered "sub-occlusive." The mortality rate in the obstruction group overall was 44% but increased to 57% in patients who had signs and symptoms of peritonitis and required sigmoid resection with end colostomy. In the group with sub-occlusive symptoms, mortality increased from 35 to 50% in patients with a delayed diagnosis who required sigmoid resection with end colostomy [11].

If there is no evidence of ischemia, the first step in management is endoscopic detorsion. As mentioned previously, in the Bruusgaard series, reduction was achieved 123 times with a combination of proctoscopy and rectal tube placement. A review of 19 American series involving a total of 596 patients also confirmed that endoscopic decompression is successful in the majority of cases. In these patients, nonoperative reduction was successful 417 times. Nineteen percent of cases were reduced with proctoscopy, 40% with a combination of proctoscopy and rectal tube and 0.2% with colonoscopy [1]. A more recent study, published in 2010 by Tan et al. reviewed their 9-year experience with sigmoid volvulus. Seventy-one patients were admitted 134 times for acute sigmoid volvulus. The authors were able to achieve endoscopic decompression with a success rate of 78%. They used flexible sigmoidoscopy as their modality of choice. Decompression with a rectal tube only was successful in 57.1% of cases. Their results also reinforce the benefits of endoscopic decompression as the mortality rate for emergency surgery in their series was 17.6% [12].

Endoscopic decompression may be performed with either a rigid or flexible scope. An advantage of the flexible scope is that it is longer and easier to maneuver. The rigid scope, however, allows for the placement of a rectal tube through the lumen of the scope. The patient should be positioned supine, on their left side with knees flexed towards the chest. The scope is gently inserted through the anus and advanced

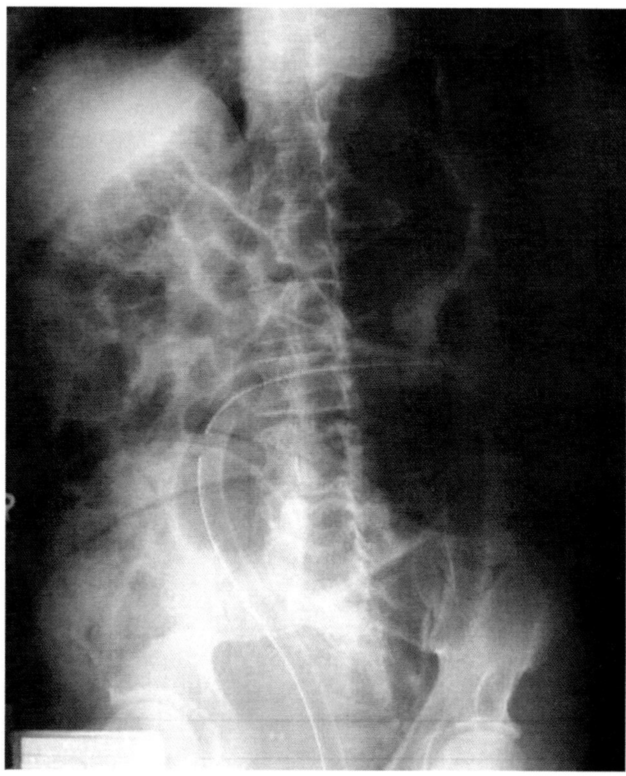

Fig. 30.4 Decompressed sigmoid colon after rectal tube placement. Published with permission from William Herring, MD, FACR, learningradiology.com

slowly to the point of obstruction. The most common location of obstruction is around 15 cm above the anal verge. It should be noted that if there is *any* evidence of intestinal ischemia or necrosis, the scope should be terminated and the patient taken immediately to the operating room. In the case of viable mucosa, gentle insufflation and advancement is employed until the loop of colon is decompressed. This is usually verified by the scope passing into a more dilated segment of colon along with a return of flatus and stool. The evacuation of flatus and stool may be immediate so the practitioner should be prepared and dressed in a gown, gloves and mask. When using the rigid scope, a rectal tube can be inserted via the lumen. If a flexible scope is used it should be gently withdrawn and a rectal tube advanced. It is appropriate to use either a red rubber catheter or Foley catheter as the rectal tube. This must be secured to the thigh or perineal region to prevent dislodgement and left in place for 48–72 h. Fig. 30.4 shows successful decompression of the colon after rectal tube placement.

Although nonoperative reduction of sigmoid volvulus spares the patient emergent surgery, it is not considered definitive treatment as patients decompressed by endoscopy are likely to recur. In a study from Northwestern, the recurrence rate after endoscopic decompression was 90% [13]. In the Tan study, the rate of recurrence after successful nonoperative reduction was

60.9%. Furthermore, a 15.4% mortality rate is associated with detorsion without resection. Brothers et al. reviewed 39 patients with colonic volvulus over a 9-year period. Twenty-nine attempts were made at reduction with either colonoscopy or sigmoidoscopy with a success rate of 55%. The recurrence rate after successful decompression, however, was 57% [14].

Endoscopy is a temporizing measure that allows the patient to be prepared for elective resection, ideally with primary anastomosis. Once detorsion is achieved, the patient can be adequately hydrated and undergo bowel preparation for surgery scheduled during the same hospital admission. Elective resection would proceed as described previously with removal of the redundant and freely mobile segment of sigmoid colon involved in the volvulus. This procedure is associated with low morbidity and mortality rates and an approximately 5% anastomotic leak rate. In a small percentage of cases, the remaining colon is massively dilated (megacolon) as a result of the distal obstruction caused by the volvulus. If megacolon is present and there is concern for the viability of the remaining colon, the surgeon should consider a total abdominal colectomy with either ileo-rectal anastomosis or end ileostomy and planned reconstruction at a second operation. This is a rare circumstance and typically not encountered at operation for sigmoid volvulus.

Summary

Sigmoid volvulus is a clinical entity that has been recognized and treated since ancient times. It is a surgical emergency that the practicing acute care surgeon must recognize and treat promptly. Diagnosis is based on physical exam findings in combination with radiographic imaging. As mentioned previously, patients with evidence of bowel ischemia must proceed directly to the operating room without delay. In the absence of signs of bowel ischemia, the initial treatment is endoscopic decompression followed by definitive operative intervention. Overall the patients who have the best outcomes after sigmoid volvulus are those that undergo successful endoscopic detorsion followed by resection and primary anastomosis of prepared bowel on the same hospital admission.

Cecal Volvulus

Epidemiology

Cecal volvulus was first described by Hildanus in the sixteenth century and later by Rokitansky in 1837. It is a surgical emergency, resulting from an axial twist of the cecum, distal ileum and proximal colon around a mesenteric pedicle. It is the second most common location for colonic volvulus

following the sigmoid and is responsible for 20–40% of all cases. The overall incidence of cecal volvulus in the general population is approximately 2.8–7.1 million people per year [5]. Unlike sigmoid volvulus in which the predisposing anatomic factors are acquired, cecal volvulus has a congenital etiology. The right colon is a midgut structure that initially leaves the abdominal cavity during fetal development and rotates counterclockwise around the superior mesenteric artery. When the midgut structures return to the abdominal cavity at 9 weeks gestation, the ascending colon assumes a fixed retroperitoneal position. Patients who present with cecal volvulus have a mobile cecum that lacks normal retroperitoneal fixation. In a review of 125 cadavers at Northwestern, 11.2% were found to have freely mobile right colons and 25.6% had enough cecal mobility to allow volvulus to occur [5].

The age, geographic distribution, and predisposing factors of patients who present with cecal volvulus are different than those with sigmoid volvulus. In 1949, Donhauser reviewed 100 patients with cecal volvulus; the mean age of presentation was 40 [16]. Rabinovici and colleagues reviewed 561 cases of cecal volvulus from 1959 to 1989. This is the largest review in the literature to date. The mean age at presentation was 53.3 years and there was a slight female predominance [15]. In the Ballantyne series of 71 patients with cecal volvulus, the mean age at presentation was 59 years and the authors also noted a female-to-male predominance (59% versus 41%) [5]. More recent literature reflects an increase in age at presentation but this may be due to the aging of the population. Cecal volvulus is more prevalent in India where it accounts for 4.3% of cases of acute obstruction. In the United States, Britain and Western Europe, cecal volvulus is the cause of 1% of acute obstructions [7].

Although a mobile cecum is the anatomic predisposing factor for volvulus, not all individuals with cecal mobility will develop volvulus. Precipitating factors for cecal volvulus include prior abdominal surgery, pregnancy, mental illness, obstructing lesions of the distal colon, and the presence of other acute medical conditions. Adhesions from prior surgery may act as a fixed point for the colonic volvulus. Rabinovici found that 39% of patients with cecal volvulus had a history of prior abdominal surgery and Ballantyne noted that 68% of their patients had a prior abdominal operation [5, 15]. During pregnancy the gravid uterus can displace a mobile cecum from its normal anatomic position. In the Rabinovici series, 10% of patients with cecal volvulus were pregnant, which is consistent with the findings of Donhauser et al. in 1949 [15, 16]. Similar to sigmoid volvulus, acute medical illnesses, including psychiatric disorders, are associated with the development of cecal volvulus. The mechanism for this is not entirely clear but is most likely related to the chronic constipation associated with these conditions. Finally, mechanical factors also play a role in cecal volvulus.

In 1969, Krippaehne found that 8 out of 22 patients with cecal volvulus had distal colonic obstruction [17]. Two patients in the Ballantyne series had distal colonic obstruction. Although patients may present without any of the risk factors outlined previously, it is crucial to obtain a thorough history on initial presentation.

Clinical Presentation and Diagnosis

The cecum is a sac-like portion of the ascending colon. It has a diameter of 7.5 cm and a length of 10 cm. The arterial supply to the cecum is derived from the ileocolic branch of the superior mesenteric artery. Although the cecum is thin walled and can tolerate distention, there is a risk of perforation and necrosis when it reaches a diameter of ≥ 12 cm. True cecal volvulus involves axial torsion, or a twist of 180–360°, along the longitudinal axis of the ascending colon. A subset of patients may present with the "loop" type of cecal volvulus. In this case, the cecum and often the terminal ileum twist *and* invert into the left upper abdominal quadrant. It is important to differentiate these from a separate entity, cecal bascule, which is often confused with cecal volvulus. Cecal bascule is an anteromedial *fold* of the cecum in relation to the ascending colon that creates a mechanical obstruction at the site of cecal flexion. It does not result from a lack of retroperitoneal fixation and ischemic changes are infrequent. It is found in 10–33% of patients who undergo surgery for cecal volvulus. A consistent operative finding in patients with cecal bascule is a constricting band across the ascending colon of unclear etiology.

Patients with cecal volvulus present with signs and symptoms of small bowel obstruction. Early diagnosis is critical as cecal volvulus creates a closed loop obstruction and 20–30% of patients with cecal volvulus will have gangrenous bowel at the time of laparotomy. The most common symptoms of cecal volvulus in the Rabinovici series (in order of frequency) were: abdominal pain, abdominal distention, constipation, nausea/vomiting and diarrhea. The most common abdominal signs in the same series (in order of frequency) were: distention, hyper-peristalsis, peritoneal signs, abdominal mass and hypoperistalsis [15]. Many patients with cecal volvulus report a history of waking from sleep with the sudden onset of pain leading some to hypothesize that the normal movements during sleep may displace a predisposed right colon to an abnormal location.

In addition to history and physical exam findings, radiographic imaging is used to diagnose cecal volvulus. Plain abdominal X-rays have a specificity of 60% and show the dilated cecum directed upwards into the left upper quadrant with a characteristic "coffee bean" appearance (Fig. 30.5). In the case of cecal bascule, abdominal X-rays show the cecum located more centrally, rather than towards the left upper

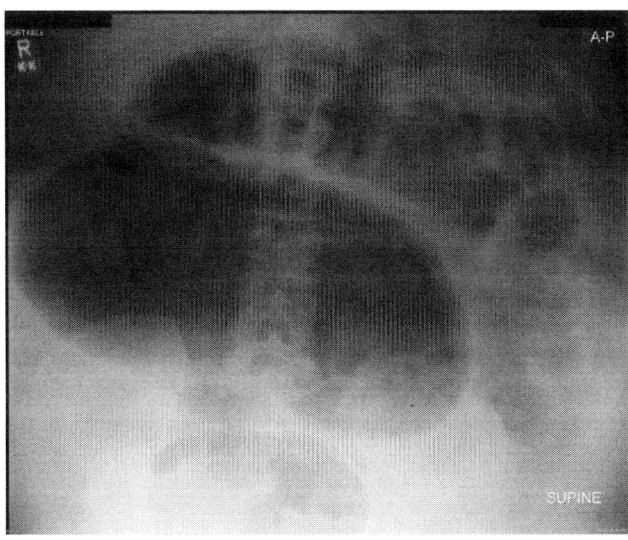

Fig. 30.5 Cecal volvulus on plain X-ray. Image courtesy of the Department of Radiology, Cooper University Hospital

quadrant. Ballantyne diagnosed 38% of patients with cecal volvulus based solely on abdominal radiographs. In the Rabinovici series, 46% of plain abdominal X-rays were concerning for cecal volvulus; 30% were misinterpreted as small bowel obstruction. Only 17% were diagnostic [15]. The addition of water-soluble contrast or barium enema may aid in diagnosis if plain films are equivocal. Rabinovici found that the addition of barium enema to plain films increased accuracy to 88% [15]. Over the past several years, CT scan has become the more common initial imaging for patients presenting with acute abdominal pain. The benefits of CT versus plain X-rays are that they are more sensitive at detecting complications of volvulus such as ischemia and perforation. The first indication of the presence of cecal volvulus visualized on CT scan is massive dilation of the cecum with displacement into the left upper quadrant, similar to what is seen on abdominal radiographs (Figs. 30.6 and 30.7). Haustral markings on the enlarged cecum indicate that it is large bowel despite its abnormal anatomic position. Two CT scan findings, typically attributed to sigmoid volvulus, which are also applied to cecal volvulus are the "bird beak" and the "whirl" sign. The bird beak is created by the tapering of both ends of the closed loop obstruction. The whirl is created by loops of collapsed large bowel along with an engorged, twisted colonic mesentery [18].

Management

Endoscopic detorsion is *only* advised for volvulus of the sigmoid colon. Although there is a reported success rate of 5–25% for endoscopic detorsion of cecal volvulus in the literature, it is not the appropriate treatment for this disease

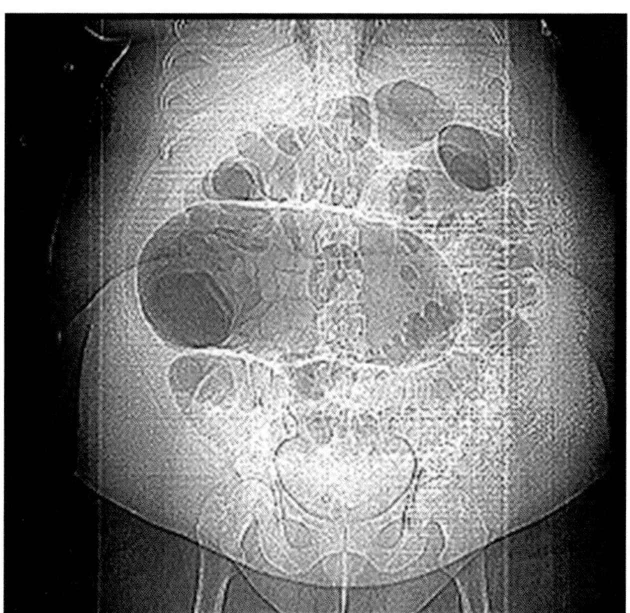

Fig. 30.6 CT scan "scout" film of patient with cecal volvulus. Image courtesy of the Department of Radiology, Cooper University Hospital

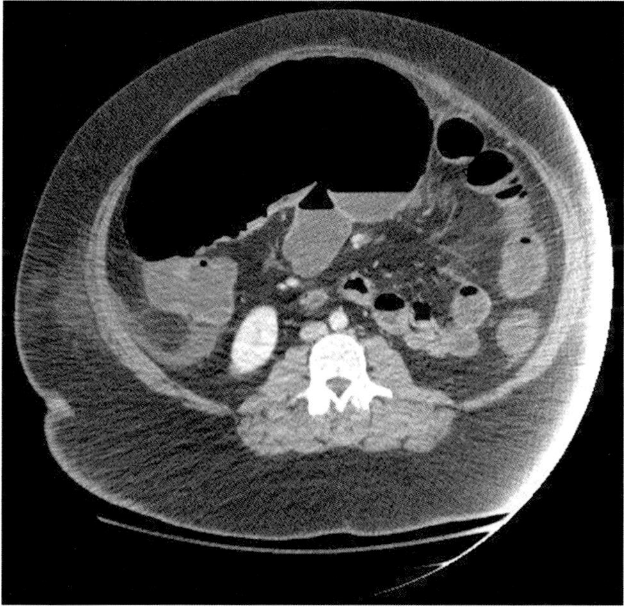

Fig. 30.7 Cecum located in *left* upper quadrant on CT scan. Image courtesy of the Department of Radiology, Cooper University Hospital

process [19]. Several reports demonstrate that while detorsion of the cecum is feasible, it is technically difficult, often unsuccessful and not considered standard of care. Once the diagnosis of cecal volvulus is made, the patient will need operative intervention. Early recognition and operative intervention are essential to avoid colonic ischemia, perforation, sepsis and death [20]. Patients with bowel obstruction from cecal volvulus must be prepared for prompt surgical management. They may be volume depleted with electrolyte abnormalities. Intravenous access must be secured to allow for fluid resuscitation and a nasogastric tube and Foley catheter inserted. As in the case of patients with sigmoid volvulus, broad spectrum antibiotics should be administered preoperatively.

A proposed algorithm for the management of cecal volvulus is presented in Fig. 30.8. Patients with any evidence of or concern for bowel ischemia are taken immediately to the operating room. For this patient population a resectional procedure, right hemicolectomy, is advised. The decision of whether or not to perform a primary anastomosis after right hemicolectomy is based upon findings at the time of operation and sound surgical judgment. If the bowel is viable and the patient is stable, it is appropriate to proceed with a right hemicolectomy and ileocolic anastomosis. If the patient is unstable and/or the bowel viability is in question, a right hemicolectomy with end ileostomy is the surgical procedure of choice. In the Ballantyne series, 27 patients had a right hemicolectomy with primary anastomosis. None had recurrence during the follow-up period which ranged from 4 months to 20 years. Of the patients that required right hemicolectomy with end ileostomy, none had subsequent gastrointestinal complications and all had bowel continuity restored [5]. In rare cases of hemodynamic instability and bowel necrosis, damage control laparotomy is an option. In this procedure, necrotic bowel is resected, bowel continuity is *not* restored at the first operation and the patient returns to the operating room in 24–48 h after resuscitation in an intensive care setting. A full discussion of damage control surgery is beyond the scope of this chapter. However, the acute care surgeon should be familiar with the principles of damage control surgery and prepared to utilize this technique if the patient's condition requires it.

In patients diagnosed with cecal volvulus where there is no concern for bowel ischemia, operative intervention must still be prompt. There are surgical options for viable colon that do not involve resection, which include detorsion, cecopexy, and cecostomy. Cecal detorsion does not address the underlying issue and is not currently recommended—it simply relieves the obstruction and is associated with high rates of recurrence (10–20%). Cecopexy involves suturing the right colon to the right paracolic gutter. One technique involves creating a flap from the parietal peritoneum and securing it anteriorly to the cecum and ascending colon. This creates a retroperitoneal "pocket," which secures the cecum in place. Cecopexy does not involve resection or anastomosis and consequently, is associated with low rates of infection. However, the placement of sutures through a thin walled and distended cecum is difficult and may result in perforation. Recurrence rates with cecopexy are also high (20–38%) and the mortality rate associated with cecopexy is approximately 9% [20].

Fig. 30.8 Algorithm for the management of cecal volvulus

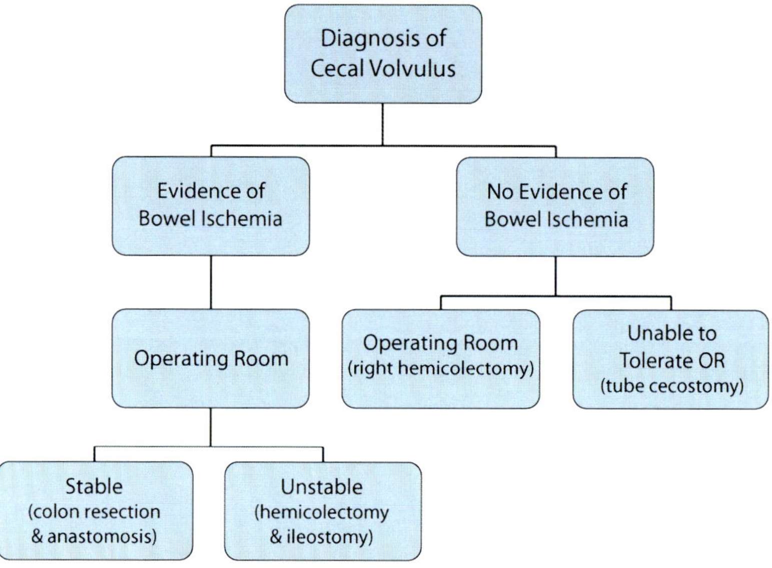

Historically, cecostomy tube placement was utilized as a non-resectional alternative for cecal volvulus. Cecostomy involves the creation of an enterotomy in the cecum to facilitate the placement of a soft rubber tube. Circumferential purse-string sutures are placed in the cecal wall prior to enterotomy. Once the catheter is placed through the enterotomy the purse string sutures are secured. For added security, the cecum may be affixed to the anterior abdominal wall. This provides bowel decompression as well as fixation. In some series, cecostomy was associated with low rates of recurrence (1–2%). In the Rabinovici series, however, cecostomy tube placement was associated with the highest rate of complications. The authors noted a 52% complication rate, 22% mortality rate and 14% recurrence rate after tube cecostomy [15]. Complications included wound infection, abdominal wall necrosis, cecal necrosis, and intra-abdominal leakage around the cecostomy tube. The authors strongly recommended in their conclusions that "cecostomy should be abandoned." Currently, cecostomy tube placement is reserved only for patients who are too unstable to undergo colonic resection because of medical comorbidities. Tube cecostomy can be performed safely under local anesthesia.

Although non-resectional procedures were described and utilized into the 1990s, Meyers et al. advocated as early as 1972 that patients with cecal volvulus undergo right colon resection whenever possible [21]. A right hemicolectomy precludes the possibility of recurrent volvulus and is currently considered the standard operative treatment for patients with cecal volvulus who have viable bowel. Although an open operation is most commonly performed, laparoscopic approaches are described. Right hemicolectomy is safe and effective and morbidity and mortality rates are low. If a cecal bascule is encountered at operation for diagnosis of cecal volvulus, there are two possible options: ileocecectomy or right hemicolectomy. If it is a true cecal bascule (limited to the cecum only with a normally fixed ascending colon), ileocecectomy is appropriate. If the ascending colon is mobile and not fixed to the retroperitoneum, a right hemicolectomy should be performed [22].

Summary

Cecal volvulus was recognized in the sixteenth century and is considered a surgical emergency. As in the case of sigmoid volvulus, delay in diagnosis and treatment is the leading cause of morbidity and mortality. Diagnosis is based on physical exam findings in conjunction with the results of radiographic imaging. Approximately 30% of patients who present with cecal volvulus will have bowel compromise at laparotomy. In comparison to sigmoid volvulus, complications from surgical treatment for cecal volvulus are much lower. Therefore, an aggressive approach to management which involves colonic resection and primary anastomosis is advocated. Although non-resectional options have been described, they are primarily of historical interest. Cecostomy tube placement is still reserved for patients with a diagnosis of cecal volvulus who are unable to tolerate operative intervention. Overall, patients who have the best outcomes after cecal volvulus are those that are diagnosed early and have immediate operative intervention.

Conclusion

Although colonic volvulus is not the most common cause of bowel obstruction in adults, it is a serious condition that the acute care surgeon may encounter in their practice. Any patient presenting with signs and symptoms of bowel obstruction must be evaluated promptly and colonic volvulus should be included on the list of differential diagnoses. The type of intervention depends on the location of the volvulus and the patient's clinical presentation. The information and algorithms provided in this chapter are intended to serve as a guide for the acute care surgeon when faced with this relatively uncommon yet life-threatening disease process.

References

1. Ballantyne G. Review of sigmoid volvulus: history and results of treatment. Dis Colon Rectum. 1981;24:630–2.
2. Gay J. Fatal obstruction from twisting of the meso-colon. Trans Pathol Soc London. 1859;10:153–4.
3. Senn N. The surgical treatment of volvulus. Med News. 1889;55:590–8.
4. Bruusgaard C. Volvulus of the sigmoid colon and its treatment. Surgery. 1947;22:466–78.
5. Ballantyne G, Brandner M, Beart R, Ilstrup D. Volvulus of the colon: incidence and mortality. Ann Surg. 1985;202:83–92.
6. Jain BL, Seth KK. Volvulus of intestine: a clinical study. Indian J Surg. 1968;30:239–46.
7. Margolin D, Whitlow C. The pathogenesis and etiology of colonic volvulus. Semin Colon Rectal Surg. 2007;18:79–86.
8. Sinha RSA. A clinical appraisal of volvulus of the pelvic colon. Br J Surg. 1980;67:433–5.
9. Moynihan BGA. Abdominal operations. Philadelphia, PA: WB Saunders Co.; 1905.
10. Madiba TE, Thomson SR. The management of sigmoid volvulus. J R Coll Surg Edinh. 2000;45:74–80.
11. Cirocchi R, Farinella E, La Mura F, et al. The sigmoid volvulus: surgical timing and mortality for different clinical types. World J Emerg Surg. 2010;5:1–5.
12. Tan K, Chong C, Sim R. Management of acute sigmoid volvulus: an institution's experience over 9 years. World J Surg. 2010;34:1943–8.
13. Hines JR, Guerkink RE, Bass RT. Recurrence and mortality rates in sigmoid volvulus. Surg Gynecol Obstet. 1967;124:567–70.
14. Brothers T, Strodel W, Eckhauser F. Endoscopy in colonic volvulus. Ann Surg. 1987;206:1–4.
15. Rabinovici R, Simansky D, Kaplan O, et al. Cecal volvulus. Dis Colon Rectum. 1990;33:765–9.
16. Donhauser JL, Atwell S. Volvulus of the cecum. Arch Surg. 1949;58:129–47.
17. Krippaehne WW, Veto RM, Jenkins CG. Volvulus of the ascending colon: a report of twenty-two cases. Am J Surg. 1967;114:323–32.
18. Moore C, Corl F, Fishman E. CT of cecal volvulus: unraveling the image. Am J Roentgenol. 2001;177:95–8.
19. Drelichman E, Nelson H. Colonic volvulus. In: Cameron J, editor. Current surgical therapy. Philadelphia, PA: Elsevier Mosby; 2004. p. 179–83.
20. Bimsotn D, Stryker S. Volvulus of the colon. In: Fazio V, editor. Current therapy in colon and rectal surgery. Philadelphia, PA: Mosby, Inc.; 2005.
21. Meyers JR, Heifetz CJ, Baue AE. Cecal volvulus: a lesion requiring resection. Arch Surg. 1972;104:594–9.
22. Martin MJ, Steele SR. Twists and turns: a practical approach to volvulus and intussusception. Scand J Surg. 2010;99:93–102.

Michelle L. Cowan and Marc Singer

Introduction

Benign anorectal emergencies are among the most commonly encountered surgical emergencies in the acute care setting. Although nearly all anorectal emergencies are benign in nature, and rarely life threatening, the severity of pain often demands the most immediate attention. This chapter reviews the acute presentations of fissure, hemorrhoids, abscess, fistula, and anorectal trauma. In order to fully appreciate the nature of these disease processes, and the most appropriate therapies, a review of basic anorectal anatomy is required.

Anatomy

The surgical anal canal measures approximately 4 centimeters (cm) in length, originating from the rectum as it passes through the levator ani muscle where the puborectalis muscle loops behind the anorectal junction (the anorectal ring), and extending distally to the anal verge. Within the anal canal, the dentate line lies 2 cm proximal to the anal verge. This is a critical surgical landmark demarcating the transition of columnar epithelium proximally and stratified squamous epithelium distally. In fact, the mucosa 1 cm proximal to the dentate line may be columnar, cuboidal, or squamous, and is therefore termed the transitional, or cloacogenic, zone. The columns of Morgagni reside in this zone. The dentate

line also serves as a point of division for the nervous system, vascular supply, and lymphatic drainage of the anal canal. Proximal to the dentate line, the anorectal mucosa is innervated by the autonomic nervous system and relatively insensate. Distal to the dentate line, the anoderm and anal mucosa is richly innervated by the somatic nervous system, which accounts for the significant pain associated with anorectal diseases. The vascular supply to the anal canal is highly collateralized and supplied by the inferior mesenteric artery (IMA) via the superior rectal (hemorrhoidal) artery, the internal iliac arteries via the middle rectal arteries, as well as the internal pudendal arteries via the inferior rectal arteries. Proximal to the dentate line, venous return is via the inferior mesenteric vein (IMV) to the portal circulation, with lymphatics draining into the inferior mesenteric and internal iliac nodes. Distal to the dentate line, venous drainage proceeds through the systemic circulation by way of the internal iliac and internal pudendal veins, with lymphatic drainage primarily to the inguinal lymph nodes.

The internal sphincter is a continuation of the circular smooth muscle of the rectum, is innervated by the autonomic system, and under involuntary control. On the contrary, the external sphincter is a continuation of the skeletal longitudinal muscle layer of the rectum and is under voluntary control. The space between the internal and external anal sphincters is termed the intersphincteric space and normally contains 6–10 anal glands, which are implicated in anal abscess and fistula formation. There is a preponderance of glands at the posterior aspect of the anal canal.

In order to communicate findings of physical examination, accurate anatomic description is required. Historically, locations related to the face of a clock have been commonly used to describe pathology around the anus. However, without knowing the patient position during the exam—i.e., prone jackknife, lateral, lithotomy—it is impossible to correlate clock location to anatomic location. Therefore, all terminology should be with reference to the patient, independent of positioning, such as anterior/posterior and right/left lateral positions.

M.L. Cowan, M.D.
Department of Surgery, University of Chicago Medical Center, Chicago, IL, USA

M. Singer, M.D., F.A.C.S., F.A.S.C.R.S. (✉)
Section of Colon and Rectal Surgery, NorthShore University HealthSystem, University of Illinois at Chicago, Evanston, IL 60612, USA
e-mail: msinger1@northshore.org; msinger123@gmail.com

L.J. Moore et al. (eds.), *Common Problems in Acute Care Surgery*,
DOI 10.1007/978-1-4614-6123-4_31, © Springer Science+Business Media New York 2013

Anal Fissure

Epidemiology/Pathophysiology

Anal fissure is one of the most common reasons for patients to present with severe anal pain. Anal fissure, also called fissure-in-ano, is a linear ulcer in the squamous epithelium of the anoderm. Fissures are typically found in the posterior midline extending from the dentate line to the anal verge. This condition affects both men and women equally and is often seen in young adults, as well as peripartum women. The process begins with a break in the anal mucosa as a result of hard stool, diarrhea, or direct trauma (anal intercourse, vaginal delivery). A majority of these epithelial disruptions heal spontaneously; however, some fissures do not heal and become chronic. Increasing evidence suggests that the acute fissure causes spasm of the internal sphincter, perhaps due to pain and inflammation. Spasm of the internal sphincter diminishes perfusion to the fissure, resulting in relative ischemia. This theory is supported by documentation that increased sphincter pressures cause ischemia, and that perfusion of the posterior midline, the most common location of fissure, suffers the most significant ischemia [1, 2]. Schouten et al. established this relationship between prolonged spasm of the internal anal sphincter, increased anal pressures, decreased blood flow to the posterior anal canal, and non-healing of the fissure [3]. For this reason, treatment modalities, both medical and surgical, are directed towards treating the hypertonicity of the internal anal sphincter, which restores perfusion, and subsequent healing of the fissure.

Clinical Manifestations

The most common symptom reported by patients with anal fissure is severe anal pain, which can be incapacitating. This pain is typically described as sharp or tearing. The pain is precipitated by the passage of stool and may last hours after a bowel movement due to internal sphincter spasm. Characteristic symptoms also include hematochezia, usually described as a few drops of bright red blood on the toilet paper, and less commonly pruritus or drainage. A history of constipation and/or diarrhea can sometimes be elicited either as a precipitating factor or a consequence due to severe pain.

Diagnosis

Although the diagnosis can often be made by the clinical history, confirmation requires physical exam. In the office or the emergency room, the ability to perform a digital rectal exam (DRE) or anoscopy is often limited secondary to pain and thus should be appropriately deferred. Gentle spreading of the buttocks, without DRE, will usually reveal the distal edge of the anal fissure. In approximately 90% of cases, the anal fissure is identified at the posterior midline, but can be seen in the anterior midline in 10–20% cases. Fissures occurring in lateral or ectopic locations, as well as multiple fissures, require a more thorough and specialized workup as this raises the suspicion of an underlying disease such inflammatory bowel disease (Crohn's disease), acquired immunodeficiency syndrome (AIDS), syphilis, tuberculosis, trauma, or systemic malignancy.

In patients with acute fissures (less than 6 weeks), the exam will often reveal a simple tear in the anoderm, whereas patients with chronic fissures demonstrate more edema and fibrosis around the fissure. Specifically, a sentinel skin tag ("sentinel pile") can be seen at the distal aspect of the fissure. This is often confused with a painful hemorrhoid by both the patient and physician. Close inspection of the base of the fissure will reveal exposed fibers of the internal sphincter. There may also be a hypertrophied anal papilla proximal to the fissure within the anal canal.

Treatment

All treatment strategies are directed at breaking the cycle of pain, sphincter spasm, ischemia, and non-healing of the fissure. The first line of treatment for most fissures is medical management, which includes stool bulking agents (fiber), stool softeners or lubricants, and increased water intake in order to reverse or prevent constipation. Patients should also be advised to take warm sitz baths three to four times daily, which relaxes the internal sphincter. Additionally, some surgeons prescribe lidocaine ointment for topical anesthesia. This may provide symptomatic relief; however, it is ineffective at relieving sphincter spasm. All patients should be reevaluated after 4–8 weeks of continuous therapy. Some patients may require oral analgesics, and should be informed regarding the constipating effects of narcotics. Acute anal fissures will often heal with resolution of symptoms during this time, and these patients should be advised to continue on a high-fiber diet to prevent recurrent constipation.

Patients with severe or persistent symptoms should be offered further therapy with topical nitrates or calcium channel blockers (CCB). Topical therapy with nitric oxide donors, such as nitroglycerin (NTG), or calcium channel blockers (CCB), such as nifedipine or diltiazem, is thought promote healing by causing muscle relaxation, with accompanying vasodilation and increased blood flow. The healing rate associated with nitrates is approximately 50–60%. A recent Cochrane review concluded that topical NTG therapy remains only marginally better than placebo for the treatment of anal fissures [4]. Once nitrate therapy has stopped, anal pressures may return to pretreatment levels, and thus, the recurrence rates after nitrate treatment when compared with operative treatment are dramatically higher [5]. Treatment with nitrate therapy can also be associated with significant headaches in 20% of patients, resulting in cessation of therapy. There is little data directly comparing CCB therapy to placebo; however, clinical trials suggest healing rates similar to nitrates, without a significant incidence of headaches [4]. In the case of both nitrate and CCB therapy, increasing dosage does not improve healing, but instead increases the dose-dependant incidence of headaches [6]. A typical dosing regimen is 0.2% NTG ointment or 0.3% nifedipine ointment applied three times daily to the anal margin for 8 weeks.

For those patients who have failed medical management, an additional treatment option is botulinum toxin injection, which inhibits the release of acetylcholine from presynaptic nerve endings, thereby promoting relaxation of the internal sphincter. Due to significant variations in dose (10–100 U), injection location (intersphincteric space versus internal or external sphincter), and number of injections, the true effectiveness of botox injections remains unclear. A recent recommendation from the American Society of Colon and Rectal Surgeons supports botox injection as a second line therapy for patients who have failed other medical therapies. Published healing rates are within the range of 60–80%, and subsequent recurrence rate of 40% [7]. The effects of botox are temporary, typically lasting 3 months, which is adequate time for the fissure to heal. This temporary effect of botox is appealing to patients, since a major side effect is incontinence to flatus and/or stool in up to 18% of patients. The effect is temporary and resolves as the effects of botox dissipate over time.

Surgical therapy remains the treatment of choice for patients with refractory anal fissures unresponsive to nonoperative therapy, or those whose symptoms are so severe that they cannot tolerate a trial of medical therapy. In the majority of cases, surgical therapy can be done on an elective basis. The "gold standard" of surgical therapy is lateral internal sphincterotomy (LIS), which has been shown to be superior to the historical method of anal dilation with regard to healing and complications rates. Indeed, anal dilation has largely been abandoned due to inefficacy and unacceptable incontinence rates. Lateral internal sphincterotomy is an operation in which a portion of the internal anal sphincter is divided. This operation yields 95% initial healing rate with only 3% recurrence [8]. The complication rates are similar between the open and closed technique and include bleeding, infection, and incontinence to flatus or stool in 10–20% of patients. Kang et al. suggested that closing the anoderm after open sphincterotomy may decrease the complication rates associated with bleeding and infection, but not incontinence [9].

Lateral sphincterotomy has historically been described at the left lateral location; however, an incision at the right lateral position avoids the left lateral hemorrhoidal plexus. There is no specific length of the sphincterotomy that can be standardized. Some authors have advocated that the sphincterotomy should extend proximally to the base of the fissure. A recent Cochrane review suggested that a longer sphincterotomy, extending to the dentate line, is associated with a lower risk of recurrence without a significant increase in incontinence [8]. If a sentinel pile is present, it should be excised in order to promote healing of the fissure.

Complications

The major complications of lateral internal sphincterotomy include bleeding, infection, and incontinence. Although the incidence of incontinence with LIS is very low, it is highly morbid. For this reason, most surgeons will begin treatment with a trial of bowel regulation and NTG or calcium channel blockers. If the patient fails, then botox or sphincterotomy is indicated.

Follow-up

Initial treatment is usually continued for 6–8 weeks with subsequent reevaluation of symptoms. Failure of therapy, and ongoing pain, will result in many patients progressing to additional therapy prior to that time. Once the fissure is successfully treated, long-term follow-up can be performed as needed. Bleeding should be further investigated in appropriate patients with colonoscopy after the fissure is healed.

Hemorrhoids

Epidemiology/Pathophysiology

Hemorrhoids are one of the most common anorectal disorders affecting more than 15 million people annually in the United States [10]. Men and women are equally affected by hemorrhoids. Symptoms usually develop in patients greater than 30 years of age, and the incidence increases further with advancing age. However, the true prevalence of hemorrhoidal disease is unknown since both patients and practitioners alike falsely attribute many, if not most, anorectal complaints to hemorrhoids, regardless of the true pathology (i.e., fissure, fistula, abscess, incontinence, etc.). In addition, the large majority patients with symptomatic hemorrhoids do not seek professional treatment, or self-medicate with over-the-counter remedies.

Although the term "hemorrhoids" typically refers to a state of symptoms, hemorrhoids are a normal part of anal anatomy and require treatment only when they acquire pathologic changes associated with symptoms. Hemorrhoids are classified into two types based on their location with respect to the dentate line: internal and external. Internal hemorrhoids consist of three, thick vascular cushions that lie in the submucosa of the transitional zone immediately proximal to the dentate line. These three fibrovascular cushions lie in the left lateral, right anterior, and right posterior positions of the anal canal. Internal hemorrhoids are thought to engorge during defecation in order to protect the anal canal from abrasions. The internal hemorrhoids also engorge during coughing, sneezing, or straining so as to complete the closure of the anal canal and maintain continence during times at highest risk for incontinence. In comparison, external hemorrhoids are also vascular cushions; however, they are located distal to the dentate line covered with squamous epithelium. Hemorrhoids become symptomatic due to factors that cause prolonged or substantially increased intra-abdominal pressure, thus increasing vascular pressures, which results in hemorrhoidal engorgement. Traditionally, these factors include chronic constipation/diarrhea, prolonged straining or attempts at defecation (i.e., reading on the toilet), low-fiber diets, obesity, increased use of laxatives/enemas, as well as pregnancy and vaginal delivery.

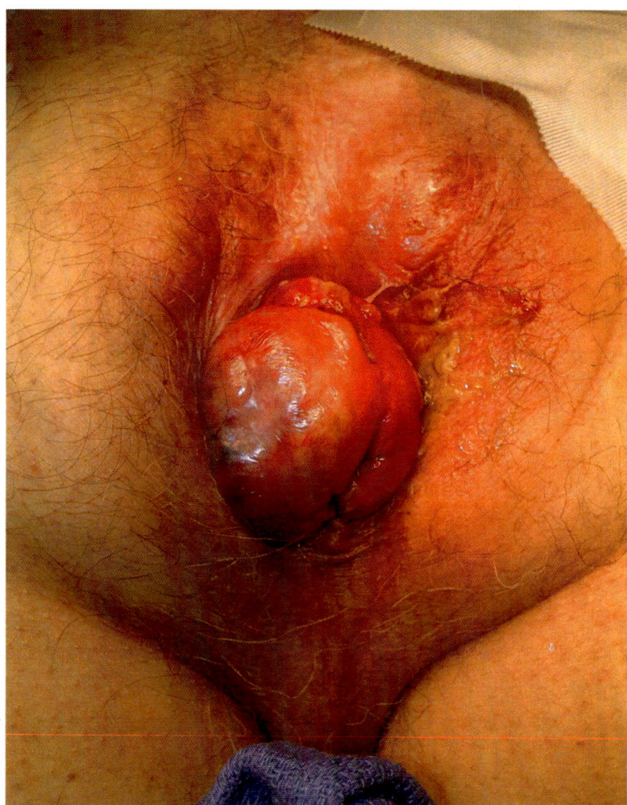

Fig. 31.1 Acute presentation of massive thrombosed external hemorrhoids. This patient was brought to the operating room for emergent hemorrhoidectomy

Clinical Presentation

The most common presentation to an acute care surgeon is likely that of symptomatic external hemorrhoids, specifically a thrombosed external hemorrhoid (an intravascular clot within a sinusoid of an external hemorrhoid). Because of their location distal to the dentate line within the richly innervated anoderm, a thrombosed external hemorrhoid can cause acute, severe pain (Fig. 31.1). The pain typically peaks within 48 h, thus prompting the patient to seek immediate medical attention. When not thrombosed, external hemorrhoids can be mistaken for simple skin tags and are commonly associated with only mild discomfort and swelling. Additionally, external hemorrhoids may cause irritation, itching, and may interfere with proper anal hygiene.

Internal hemorrhoids, on the other hand, rarely present with pain because of their location proximal to the dentate line. In the absence of an obvious thrombosed external hemorrhoid, a complaint of severe pain should alert the surgeon to search for another diagnosis. Patients with symptomatic internal hemorrhoids typically present with painless bleeding as the overlying mucosa becomes thin and friable. The bleeding associated with internal hemorrhoids typically occurs with defecation and is described by patients as bright red blood on the toilet paper. Occasionally, the blood will be

Table 31.1 Grading of internal hemorrhoids

Grade I	Prominent hemorrhoidal tissue without prolapse
Grade II	Prolapse on straining with spontaneous reduction
Grade III	Prolapse on straining requiring manual reduction
Grade IV	Prolapse is irreducible. Incarcerated and/or strangulated

noted to drip into the toilet bowl. Additionally, as a consequence of excessive straining and increased intra-abdominal pressure there is prolonged and increased engorgement of the internal hemorrhoidal plexus. Over time, the bulky hemorrhoids lose their attachment to the underlying anorectal wall, resulting in prolapse. The severity of internal hemorrhoids is graded according to severity of prolapse based on a classification system described below in Table 31.1.

Patients with prolapse may experience mucous drainage causing irritation and inflammation of the perianal skin, and some patients may report the feeling of incomplete evacuation. It is only in the rare circumstance of strangulation that a patient will experience pain associated with an internal hemorrhoid.

Diagnosis

The completion of a full history is followed by a thorough rectal exam, starting with external inspection. Inspection should make note of any evidence of perianal skin irritation caused by anal discharge, skin tags, external hemorrhoids or evidence of an alternative diagnosis such as the external opening of a perianal fistula. During inspection, the surgeon may also ask the patient to "bear down" in order to demonstrate the prolapse of internal hemorrhoids with strain. Following visual inspection is the digital rectal exam; however, hemorrhoids are not easily palpated on DRE. Therefore, the clinician should proceed to anoscopy. Although anoscopy often reduces any prolapsed internal hemorrhoids, the physician will be able to visualize the redundancy of the engorged hemorrhoidal cushions.

For patients who present with bleeding, it is necessary to recommend a full colonoscopy, once their acute issues related to hemorrhoids have resolved, to rule out a more proximal source of bleeding as well as other potential diagnoses including inflammatory bowel disease and cancer. This colonoscopy can be done as an outpatient and should be done in patients older than 40 years of age, as well as in younger patients with other risk factors, such as family history, and in whom hemorrhoids are the not the obvious source of bleeding.

Treatment

Since hemorrhoids are a physiologic part of normal anatomy, the decision to treat should be based on the frequency and severity of symptoms. For thrombosed external hemorrhoids—the most common presentation of hemorrhoidal disease to an acute care surgeon—treatment options include excision or observation. For patients that present within the first 48 h from the onset of pain, current guidelines recommend surgical excision in order to provide the patient with the most rapid relief from pain. Excision can easily be performed in the emergency room under local anesthesia, or if desired in the operating room. Excision is preferable to simple unroofing and evacuation of clot due to higher rates of recurrence and re-thrombosis with the latter. Post-procedure the wound can be left open with or without packing (based on surgeon preference), with postoperative care focused on pain control and proper hygiene. Patients should be instructed to soak in warm sitz baths after each bowel movement to aid in cleanliness. Beyond 48 h, the clot begins to reabsorb, and patients will often report improvement in pain. Subsequently, supportive treatment with sitz baths, analgesics, and prevention of constipation with fiber supplements are usually effective without the need for excision. After treatment, patients should be advised of the risk of possible recurrence: 25% after supportive nonsurgical therapy and 6.5% after excision [11].

For internal hemorrhoids, the treatment options can be classified based on the degree of symptoms and grade of hemorrhoids. For Grade I and II internal hemorrhoids associated with minor symptoms such as bleeding and do not significantly interfere with daily activities, the initial treatment should begin with conservative therapy, which includes fiber supplements and a high-fiber diet. The rationale is to produce soft, bulky stools that decrease the need for straining. Patients should also be advised to avoid prolonged straining or attempts at defecation. The addition of sitz baths may provide symptomatic relief as well as over-the-counter topical therapies; however, there are no studies that demonstrate their efficacy. In contrast, conservative therapy has not demonstrated significant efficacy in Grade III or IV hemorrhoids with significant prolapse and therefore treatment should begin with more aggressive treatment modalities discussed as follows.

For hemorrhoids that do not respond to conservative management, as well as Grade III and IV hemorrhoids with significant prolapse, the first line of therapy is rubber band ligation, with other options including sclerotherapy and infrared photocoagulation. All of these therapies are techniques of fixation. By securing the hemorrhoids to the normal anatomic location, high in the anal canal, the incidence and degree of prolapse diminishes, the venous drainage of the hemorrhoids improves, and the size of the hemorrhoids ultimately diminishes. Sclerotherapy is the oldest treatment and similar to that used for esophageal varices. It works by injecting a sclerosing agent into the submucosa, resulting in fibrosis and fixation of the hemorrhoidal cushion. Infrared photocoagulation has been well studied, and alternatively causes tissue destruction by delivery of heat via an infrared light source. However, the most commonly used treatment for severely prolapsed or refractory internal hemorrhoids is rubber band ligation. In a recent meta-analysis reviewing over 18 prospective, randomized controlled trials comparing rubber band ligation to sclerotherapy and infrared photocoagulation, rubber band ligation was more effective, with a decreased recurrence rate; albeit with a higher incidence of post-procedure pain [12].

Rubber band ligation can be performed in the office, or emergency room, using a fenestrated anoscope. A circular rubber band is then placed around the base of the internal hemorrhoid resulting in an inflammatory response, which causes fixation to the sphincter. By constricting the blood supply, the tissue and the band will typically slough within 5–10 days, and the patient should be informed that this is normal. Typically, banding all three hemorrhoidal cushions at once is avoided due to increasing patient discomfort with increased banding. However, one or two hemorrhoids can be banded simultaneously, with further ligations done at 4-week intervals. During placement, it is imperative that placement of the band is proximal, and not including, the dentate line so as to avoid pain associated with somatic nerve fibers. A band that has slipped or is placed too distally should be suspected in patients who complain of immediate, severe pain. The band should be removed and replaced correctly. Rubber band ligation is not painless and even when the band is placed properly patients will experience some mild discomfort usually secondary to sphincter spasm. Post-procedure, patients should be advised to take sitz baths to reduce their pain as well as oral analgesics as needed. They should also be advised to increase their dietary fiber or add supplements to their diet. The success rate of rubber band ligation approaches 80% [13].

Excisional hemorrhoidectomy is the gold standard and most effective therapy for symptomatic hemorrhoids, and is recommended for those patients who have failed less invasive treatment options, those who have combined symptomatic external and internal hemorrhoids, as well as those with severe symptoms including incarcerated or strangulated Grade IV internal hemorrhoids. Surgical hemorrhoidectomy is performed in the operating room as a Ferguson closed hemorrhoidectomy. This procedure involves an elliptical incision starting at the anal margin with extension to the anorectal ring, making sure to include both the internal and external hemorrhoidal plexus. Dissection is carried out in the submucosal plane taking care to avoid injury to the sphincters. The wound is completely closed using running suture. The primary complaint postoperatively is significant pain, which is treated with analgesics, sitz baths, and bulk laxatives starting on postoperative day 1.

Although excisional hemorrhoidectomy is considered the "gold standard," it is not without complications, including significant pain, urinary retention, and possible anal stenosis. As a less painful alternative to excisional hemorrhoidectomy, stapled hemorrhoidopexy, or the procedure for prolapsed hemorrhoids (PPH), was introduced [14]. In lieu of hemorrhoidal excision, this procedure makes use of a specially engineered circular stapler to divide the hemorrhoidal blood supply, excise the redundant submucosal tissue, and suspend the prolapsing internal hemorrhoids. The staple line lies entirely within the anal canal, proximal to the dentate line. This eliminates very painful external incisions. A recent Cochrane review compared PPH to conventional excisional hemorrhoidectomy, and concluded stapled hemorrhoidectomy is associated with decreased postoperative pain and hospital stay; however, it is associated with increased recurrence, increased prolapse, and an increased need for further procedures. Therefore excisional hemorrhoidectomy is still considered the "gold standard" of surgical care [15].

Complications

Complications for most procedures include bleeding, infection, urinary retention, and pain. After excision for external hemorrhoids, complications are rare but may include bleeding and perianal abscess and/or fistula [11]. After rubber band ligation, the most common complications include pain due to malpositioning of the band, as mentioned previously, as well as bleeding. For this reason, it is recommended that patients taking nonsteroidal anti-inflammatory drugs (NSAIDs) or anticoagulants stop therapy seven days prior to anticipated banding. For the rare instance when a patient presents post-banding with a triad of delayed pain, urinary retention, and fever, one must be suspicious of infection and/or perianal sepsis, which can be fatal if not immediately diagnosed and treated with antibiotics +/− drainage of associated infection/abscess. Due to this risk, albeit low, some surgeons avoid rubber band ligation in immunocompromised patients who are at increased risk of morbidity from this complication.

Complications of excisional hemorrhoidectomy include: bleeding (2–4%), urinary retention (2–32%), anal stenosis (0–6%), and infection (0–5%). Coagulopathic patients and immunocompromised patients pose a unique problem due to already high risk of bleeding and the morbidity of a potential non-healing with an open wound. Furthermore, for patients with portal hypertension, although the incidence of pathologic hemorrhoids does not increase, bleeding from hemorrhoids can be life-threatening and difficult to stop. In addition to correcting any abnormal coagulopathy, the recommended treatment is to suture ligate the bleeding hemorrhoid including the mucosa, submucosa, and underlying muscle in order to effectively stop bleeding. Excisional hemorrhoidectomy in these patients should be reserved for when suture ligation fails.

Follow-up

The follow-up for hemorrhoids is dependant on the treatment prescribed. For thrombosed external hemorrhoids that were treated with supportive management or internal hemorrhoids treated with conservative management, no follow-up is necessary unless they experience recurrent symptoms. However, patients who underwent excision for thrombosed external hemorrhoids should be reevaluated within 1–2 weeks to check for proper healing. After rubber band ligation, the patient should be seen in 4–6 weeks unless they develop signs of infection or sepsis. At this interval, further banding can be performed if necessary. After either conventional or stapled hemorrhoidectomy, the patient should be seen soon after surgery and then at 4–6 weeks to ensure proper healing. All suitable patients with bleeding should be considered for colonoscopy upon completion of treatment for hemorrhoids.

Anorectal Abscess

Epidemiology/Pathophysiology

The large majority of anorectal abscesses result from infection of the anal glands and crypts, called crypto-glandular infection, and are thought to be part of the same disease process as anorectal fistula, which is discussed later. The abscesses are the acute manifestation of disease and fistula represent the chronic stage. Anorectal abscesses can affect patients at all ages; however, they most often present during the third decade of life. They are more common in men than women and typically affect healthy individuals; however, there are some conditions that predispose patients to abscess and these include diabetes mellitus, trauma (i.e., foreign body or surgery), Crohn's disease, malignancy, radiation, human immunodeficiency virus (HIV), or other immunosuppressed states that may leave the patient susceptible to opportunistic infection.

The pathogenesis of an anorectal abscess is thought to start with infection of one of the 6–10 anal glands that lie in the intersphincteric space and normally function to secrete mucous and lubricate stools. These glands traverse the internal anal sphincter and empty into the 10–15 anal crypts, which lie circumferentially around the dentate line. Therefore, infection of the anal gland or crypt, usually by blockage, follows the path of least resistance and spreads along one of several planes in the anorectal region to form a perianal or perirectal abscess. Indeed, anorectal abscesses are classified according to location (Table 31.2), which aids in diagnosis as well as treatment and requires the surgeon to be familiar with the anatomy of anorectal spaces.

Table 31.2 Classification of anorectal abscesses.

Perianal abscess	Most common. Lies beneath the anal verge and lateral to, without traversing, the external anal sphincter
Intersphincteric abscess	Occurs between the internal and external anal sphincters, commonly posterior. Most commonly associated with fistula and likely to recur
Ischiorectal (Ischioanal) abscess	A progression of the intersphincteric abscess that traverses the external sphincter and occupies the area bounded by the levators superiorly, the transverse perineal septum inferiorly, the external sphincter and anal canal medially and the ischial tuberosity laterally. May cross the midline posteriorly to form a *horseshoe abscess*
Supralevator abscess	Occurs above the levator ani

Clinical Presentation

The presentation of an anorectal abscess may depend on its location; however, the initial presentation of most abscesses, regardless of location, is anal pain. This pain is usually described as dull or achy and is often independent of defecation. However, patients may note that the pain worsens with straining, coughing, or even walking. In rare circumstances, patients may present with fever, chills, urinary retention, and signs of sepsis suggestive of systemic illness, which should raise the suspicion of a necrotizing soft tissue infection.

Diagnosis

Diagnosis starts with a complete history and physical eliciting pertinent past medical history including comorbidities and predisposing risk factors as listed previously, as well as a focus on prior abscesses or prior anorectal surgery. Physical exam should include a thorough abdominal and rectal exam, as well as a bimanual exam in women to rule out involvement of the vaginal wall. In the case of a perianal abscess, external inspection may reveal perianal swelling with associated erythema, cellulitis, and/or fluctuance. Intersphincteric abscess are usually without external signs, yet digital rectal exam will often elicit severe tenderness. Ischiorectal abscesses have the potential to be large and DRE may elicit lateral swelling and pain, however, with less obvious external findings. Supralevator abscess are the most difficult to diagnose since they may be the result of a cephalad progression of perianal infection or a manifestation of an intra-abdominal process such as diverticulitis. Therefore, computed tomography (CT) scan may be required to confirm the diagnosis. If there is ever a doubt as to the diagnosis or location of an anorectal abscess, an exam under anesthesia should be performed to allow for confirmation of the diagnosis as well as an opportunity for treatment.

Treatment

The treatment for an anorectal abscess is incision and drainage. Perianal abscesses are often superficial and the easiest to drain, and can be performed in the emergency room under local anesthesia. An elliptical or cruciate incision should be made over the most prominent, fluctuant part of the abscess, taking careful measures to avoid injury to the sphincter muscles. The incision should also be made large enough so as to prevent premature closure of the skin before complete drainage of the abscess has occurred, and should also be made close to the anal verge in order to limit the extent of any potential fistulas that may develop in the future. The abscess cavity should then be thoroughly irrigated and loculations broken by either the surgeon's finger or a blunt hemostat. No packing is necessary if the incision is adequate; however, a superficial dressing is ideal to prevent drainage onto the patient's clothing. An ischiorectal abscess can be drained by a similar method, but may require a larger incision with a more thorough evacuation of the abscess. In the case of a horseshoe abscess that spreads posteriorly to both ischiorectal fossas, drainage often necessitates regional or general anesthesia in the operating room. At that time, an incision is made either posterior to the anus or over each ischiorectal fossa with a Penrose placed to allow for adequate drainage of the postanal space. The surgical drainage for intersphincteric abscesses is slightly more complicated in that it requires an incision in the anal mucosa overlying the abscess, followed by a partial division of the internal anal sphincter in order to access and fully clear the abscess. Again, packing is not necessary after drainage. Finally, in the case of supralevator abscesses, the treatment requires accurate diagnosis and identification of location prior to drainage. If the cause originates from cephalad spread of an ischiorectal or intersphincteric abscess then the drainage should be performed as discussed previously via the ischiorectal fossa or the rectum, respectively. For those supralevator abscesses caused by an intra-abdominal source, drainage is performed via the most direct route and often requires CT-guided drainage. Post-procedurally, patients should be given analgesia and instructed to take sitz baths three to four times a day to keep the area clean.

If a fistula is identified at the time of draining the abscess, then a seton may be placed through the fistula tract. This will keep the fistula open at both the internal and external openings, and promote drainage. Suture material or silastic vessel loops may be used as the seton. The fistula will not heal while the draining seton is in place, but it will protect the patient from recurrent abscess. Subsequently, the seton must be removed, or the fistula treated operatively in order to heal.

The success of incision and drainage for an anorectal abscess averages 50% with approximately 20–30% developing a recurrent abscess or fistula [16]. Recurrence is thought to be more common with ischiorectal fossa abscesses, potentially secondary to inadequate primary drainage; however, recurrence should also prompt the surgeon to look for a possible underlying disease such as Crohn's disease or malignancy. Historically, surgeons prescribed post-procedure antibiotics to decrease this relatively high recurrence of abscess or fistula; however, data from a recent randomized control trial demonstrate that adjuvant therapy with antibiotics does not decrease the incidence of fistula formation at 1 year [17]. Certain patient populations should, however, be given adjuvant antibiotics, and likely require hospitalization. These groups include those patients who are immunocompromised, patients with diabetes mellitus, those with prosthetic devices or valvular heart disease as well as those

patients with extensive cellulitis or a necrotizing soft tissue infection [18].

Complications

The main complication with abscesses, as previously discussed, is abscess recurrence or development of a fistula at the time of diagnosis. The risk of abscess recurrence increases significantly if there is a concurrent anal fistula. Fittingly, the role of primary fistulotomy at the time of anorectal abscess drainage has been debated as a method to reduce recurrence. While initial studies looking at the success of a combined procedure concluded no difference in the rate of abscess recurrence in those patients treated with incision and drainage alone versus the addition of a fistulotomy, a recent Cochrane review demonstrates that simultaneous fistula treatment and incision and drainage of the anorectal abscess does indeed decrease the incidence of persistent or recurrent abscess as well as the need for repeat surgical procedures [19]. A small number of patients may experience incontinence after this combined procedure; however, it is often transient. In our experience, when a fistula is discovered at the same time of abscess drainage, it is best to avoid extensive exploration of the tract due to the risk of creating false passages, and instead we place a seton to identify the tract for future definitive therapy once the inflammation surrounding the abscess has resolved. With proper drainage of the abscess, the fistula may heal on its own without the need for any further procedures.

Follow-up

After definitive incision and drainage of an anorectal abscess, complete healing takes approximately 4–8 weeks. Postoperatively, patients should be evaluated soon after surgery, within 1–2 weeks, and then again closer to 8 weeks to ensure proper healing. Afterward, patients only need to be seen on an as-needed basis based on recurrence of symptoms. Follow-up in patients with underlying Crohn's disease or those who are immunosuppressed should, however, be more aggressive with almost weekly office visits to ensure healing without signs of perianal sepsis.

Anorectal Fistula

Epidemiology/Pathophysiology

The term "fistula" is defined as an abnormal communication between two epithelial lined surfaces. In the case of anorectal fistulas, or fistula-in-ano, they are communications between an external opening at the perianal skin and an internal

Table 31.3 Classification of anorectal fistula (incidence)

Intersphincteric (70%)	Fistula tract lies within the intersphincteric space with an external opening in the perianal skin near the anal verge. Often results from a perianal abscess
Transsphincteric (23%)	Fistula tract starts in the intersphincteric space and traverses the external sphincter to the ischiorectal fossa and then perianal skin. Often results from an ischiorectal abscess
Suprasphincteric (5%)	Fistula tract starts in the intersphincteric space and tracts cephalad above the puborectalis muscle, then back downward through the ischirectal fossa to the perianal skin
Extrasphincteric (2%)	Often derived from trauma or a foreign body since the fistula tract is derived from the rectal wall (not the anus) and tracts downward through the levator into the ischiorectal fossa and perianal skin without traversing anal sphincter muscle

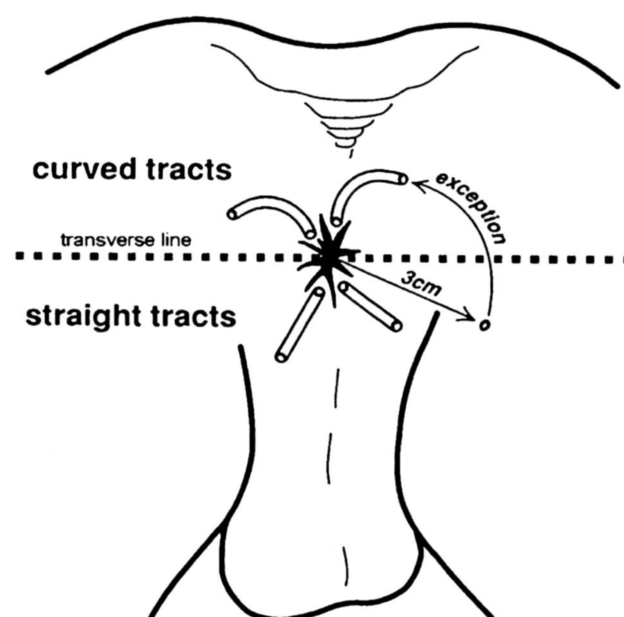

Fig. 31.2 Goodsall's rule

opening within the anal canal at the dentate line. As mentioned in the previous section, anorectal fistulas represent the chronic inflammatory process after incomplete drainage or healing of a previous acute anorectal abscess. Therefore, their incidence is analogous with abscesses and similarly, conditions such as Crohn's disease, malignancy, radiation, and trauma increase the predisposition for fistula development. Persistent infection resulting in fistula formation is usually crypto-glandular in origin and the course of the fistula can often be predicted by the location of the previous abscess such that a drained perianal abscess typically results in an intersphincteric fistula, and an ischiorectal abscess typically forms a transphincteric fistula. The tract formed by the fistula as it courses from the internal opening at the dentate line to the external perianal skin can be classified based on its location with respect to the anal sphincter and described in Table 31.3. More recently, the term "complex" fistula has been used to identify fistulas involving >30% of the anal sphincter, high fistulas or those with multiple tracts, as well as those occurring in setting of underlying disease such as local irradiation or Crohn's.

Clinical Presentation

The most common symptom of an anorectal fistula is drainage—either intermittent or constant—with a history of anorectal abscess. Additionally, patients may experience perianal itching and irritation as well as discharge. Pain is rare in the absence of a recurrent anorectal abscess and in those circumstances often manifests as cyclical pain. In patients who complain of recurrent or non-healing fistulas, one should be suspicious of an underlying disorder such as Crohn's disease or malignancy.

Diagnosis

Delineation of the fistula tract is the most important part of diagnosis and subsequent treatment. In the clinic or the emergency room, external inspection of the anus often reveals the external opening as a red cluster of granulation with or without spontaneous drainage. However, determination of the internal opening and extent of sphincter involvement typically requires an exam under anesthesia performed in the operating room. Anoscopy and the use of a probe can often track the fistula from the external opening to the internal opening using the principles of Goodsall's rule, which helps relate the position of the internal fistula opening to the external opening (Fig. 31.2). Specifically, the rule states that fistulas with an external opening anterior to an imaginary transverse anal line, tract directly to the dentate line in a short, linear fashion. On the other hand, fistulas with external openings posterior to this imaginary transverse anal line will likely tract in a curvilinear fashion to internal opening at the posterior midline. An exception to this rule is when an anterior external opening lies greater than 3 cm from the anal margin. In these cases, the fistula tracts to the posterior midline. One should be careful, however, not to make false passages with the probe. If it does not pass easily, do not force it. In cases where the internal opening still cannot be found, one can inject dilute methylene blue or hydrogen peroxide into the external opening and look for ejection of the respective fluid from the internal opening.

In the event that the internal opening still cannot be located, recent data suggests the use of magnetic resonance imaging (MRI) and/or transrectal ultrasound (TRUS) as

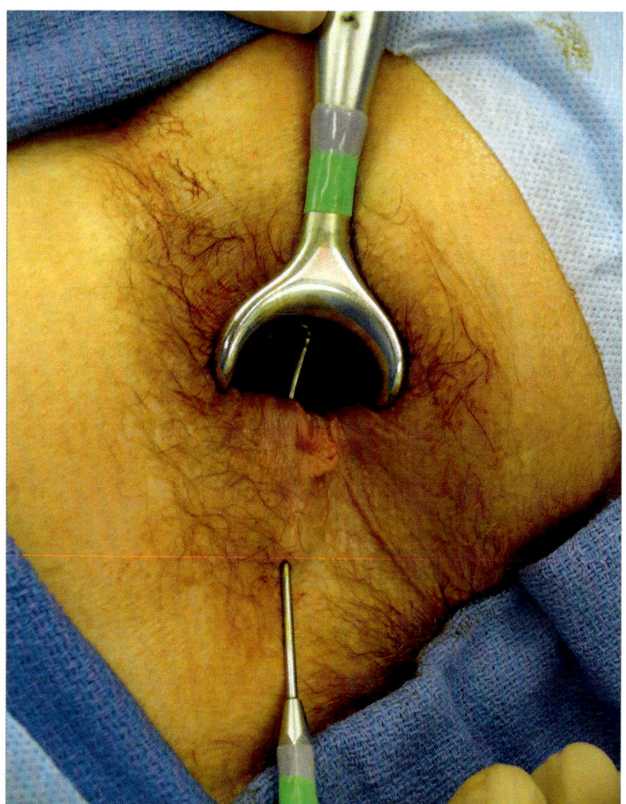

Fig. 31.3 Fistula identified by probing the tract during an examination under anesthesia

adjuncts to examination under anesthesia (EUA). The use of MRI in delineating fistulous tracts has significantly improved the accuracy of diagnosis, especially in the case of supras-phincteric and extrasphincteric fistulas, which are more difficult to fully identify, and allows the surgeon to visualize the fistula tract in relation to the surrounding anatomy as well as track progress after healing [20]. Specifically, data suggests that MRI, as well as TRUS, are more accurate in diagnosis when compared to digital exam, correctly diagnos-ing the extent of the fistula in 90%, 81%, and 61%, respec-tively [21]. As a result, surgeons are starting to use MRI preoperatively to accurately locate and evaluate the extent of fistulization in complex cases involving perianal sepsis or Crohn's disease (Fig. 31.3).

Of note, in cases of recurrent or non-healing fistula where there is a concern for Crohn's disease or malignancy, as men-tioned previously, a proctoscopy or sigmoidoscopy should be performed along with biopsies of the fistula tract to aid in diagnosis.

Treatment

Treatment of anorectal fistulas is based on the dual goals of closing the fistula and preserving continence. Choice of operation is based on the classification, location, and extent of the fistula, as well as the patient's bowel function and con-tinence. Most fistula operations can be done in the operating room on an outpatient basis using local anesthesia combined with intravenous sedation. While there is not one procedure that is ideal for all fistulas, the "gold standard" operation for anorectal fistulas is fistulotomy. Fistulotomy is typically rec-ommended for intersphincteric as well as low transphincteric fistulas involving only a small amount of sphincter muscle and is the preferred surgical option. Fistulectomy has mostly been abandoned due to the creation of a larger wound and higher rates of incontinence. Fistulotomy is performed by first placing a probe through the fistula in order to document the entire length of the track, including the internal opening. Then, using electrocautery, the tissues overlying the probe are divided all the way from the internal opening to the exter-nal opening on the perianal skin. Once unroofed, epithelial-ized tissue is removed from the fistula tract using a curette and hemostasis is obtained. Finally, marsupialization of the wound edges has been shown to accelerate wound healing as well as decrease postoperative bleeding [22, 23]. Success rates of fistulotomy approach 95%, however, not without a high incidence of postoperative incontinence reported any-where from 20 to 50%. Therefore, other treatment options have evolved in an attempt to heal anal fistulas without the associated incidence of incontinence. These other treatment options include fibrin glue, fistula plug, seton placement, as well as endorectal advancement flap.

Treatment with fibrin glue has gained increasing popu-larity due to the low risk–benefit ratio and is now recom-mended as one of the first-line treatments for anorectal fistulas [18]. The fistula should be prepared with an indwell-ing draining seton for 6 weeks prior to fibrin glue injection in order to minimize the inflammatory process within the tract. The injection procedure for fibrin glue requires one enema as a bowel preparation the morning of the procedure followed by inspection and identification of the entire fistula tract. Once identified, the tract is irrigated and gently debri-ded with a curette or cytology brush in order to remove any remaining pus or fibrotic epithielized tissue. Retained pus or gross infection may sabotage the effectiveness of the fibrin glue. Once cleared, fibrin glue is injected into the entire fistula tract. Advantages of fibrin glue treatment for anorec-tal fistulas include the elimination of incontinence as a side effect since this treatment does not require division of the anal sphincter. Additionally, the procedure is simple and can be repeated multiple times without complicating or preclud-ing future fistula operations if indicated. The success rate of fibrin glue therapy with regard to complete healing for sim-ple fistulas is 60%, with failures typically due to expulsion of the glue or persistent infection, prompting some to explore the option adding antibiotics to the sealant [24]. Furthermore, randomized controlled trials have now

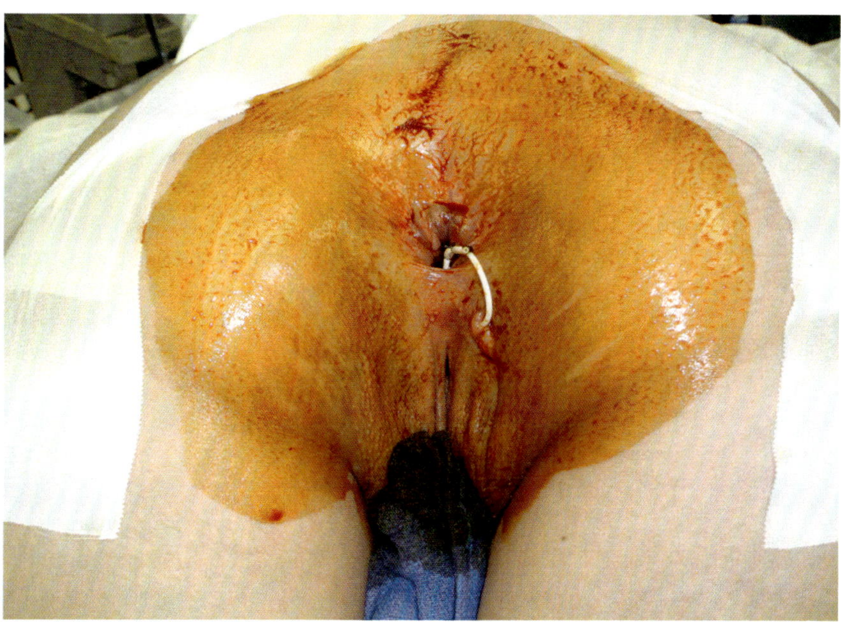

Fig. 31.4 Silastic vessel loop as draining seton

proposed fibrin glue as an option for complex fistulas and demonstrate increased success rates after fibrin glue treatment for complex, high anal fistulas when compared to conventional fistulotomy [25].

Similar to the fibrin glue, surgeons have also started using a synthetic product, the collagen plug, to treat fistulas. The collagen plug is commercially available lyophilized porcine intestinal submucosa. The fistula should be prepared with a draining seton for 6 weeks prior to plug insertion in order to minimize the inflammation within the tract. In the operating room, the plug is inserted into the fistula tract and secured with sutures at the internal opening. It does not carry any risk of incontinence because there is no disruption of the sphincter. Early fallout of the plug can be problematic, but the main drawback is the modest healing rate. Some authors have reports >80% success, but most publications suggest 20–40% rate of healing [26, 27].

For high transsphincteric and suprasphincteric fistulas that involve a greater amount of sphincter muscle, initial treatment involves placement of a seton, either cutting or loose. A cutting seton is typically a heavy suture (silk) that is tightened every 2 weeks with the theory that slow division of the external anal sphincter allows for fibrosis and scar formation, which hopefully decreases the rate of associated incontinence by decreasing the muscular defect and acute retraction of the sphincter muscle as seen with conventional fistulotomy. Alternatively, a loose, non-cutting seton can be placed to allow for drainage and mark the fistula tract for a later, staged fistulotomy after adequate control of the perianal sepsis (Fig. 31.4). In fact, a loose draining seton is now the more preferred method of treatment when compared to

cutting setons secondary to the significant pain associated with cutting setons as well as their incidence of incontinence, which approaches 2–20%, albeit less than that seen with fistulotomy.

High fistulas may also be treated with an endorectal advancement flap, which is considered to be a sphincter sparing surgical procedure. Flaps are utilized in patients in whom the risk of postoperative incontinence prevents fistulotomy, such as patients with some degree of fecal incontinence, anterior fistulas in women, patients with Crohn's disease, etc. In these patients, the risk of incontinence with fistulotomy would be unacceptably high. Creation of the flap involves elevation of a broad based, U-shaped mucosal flap starting at the internal opening of the fistula and progressing cephalad. Once elevated, the fistula tract is debrided with curettage and the internal opening sutured closed. At that time the flap is then brought down to cover this closure and sutured to the distal anal canal. Although endorectal advancement flaps are successful in approximately 60–90% of patients, it is technically demanding and takes a significant time to learn and, therefore, is not commonly performed in the acute care setting but instead performed by experienced colorectal surgeons.

In the special cases of patient's with Crohn's disease, perianal disease with fistulas can be very morbid. Often, these fistulas are multiple and disobey the rules typically applied to anorectal fistula. Contrary to the surgical options described previously, aggressive surgical intervention is discouraged in Crohn's patients with perianal fistulas with the reasoning that they typically do not heal well and even minimal division of the sphincter may result in significant incontinence or new fistulas. For these patients, any abscess should be appropriately drained and a loose seton placed in the fistula to keep the tract open for further drainage. Once complete, the primary treatment modality for these patients should be medical therapy. In a landmark randomized controlled trial published in 1999, Present et al. tested the chimeric, monoclonal, tumor necrosis factor (TNF) antagonist antibody infliximab (Remicade) against placebo for the treatment of fistula in patients with Crohn's. This trial demonstrated a significant reduction in the percentage of draining fistulas in those patients treated with infliximab versus placebo, with 40–50% complete healing at 3 months in the infliximab treated group compared to 13% in the placebo group [28]. Therefore, infliximab therapy remains the primary medical therapy offered to Crohn's patients suffering from perianal fistula.

Complications

Treatment for anal fistula requires balancing the desire to provide a cure without sacrificing continence. With the exception of fibrin glue or a collagen plug, all treatment options for anal fistula involve some degree of postoperative incontinence. Overall, sphincter cutting procedures, such as fistulotomy, offer the best chance of cure, however, with the highest rates of incontinence. Also, complex fistulas are associated with a higher risk of postoperative incontinence when compared to simple fistula. This morbidity is exacerbated if the complex fistulas are treated with sphincter cutting procedures versus sphincter sparing procedures such as fibrin glue or endorectal advancement flap, which may be less effective but have a more favorable risk–benefit ratio [29].

Follow-up

Healing after treatment for anal fistula may take 3 months and patients should be made aware of this prior to treatment. Postoperatively, patients should be given oral analgesics and advised to take sitz baths three to four times daily to keep the area clean and prevent recurrent infection. They should also maintain bulk in their diet to avoid constipation and straining. Office follow-up should be performed initially within the first 3 weeks to ensure there is not premature closure of the fistula tract, and then again closer to the 8–10 weeks period to ensure proper healing. During follow-up patients should be questioned for symptoms of incontinence, especially those with preoperative risk factors as discussed previously. For those treated with cutting setons, follow-up is more regular, usually at 2 week intervals to check progress and perform tightening of the seton itself.

Anorectal Trauma

Epidemiology/Pathophysiology

As a result of the location deep within the pelvis, anorectal trauma is less common than that of colonic trauma. Penetrating trauma accounts for approximately 95% of anorectal injuries, with a majority of these secondary to gunshot wounds as compared to stab wounds. Blunt trauma accounts for the remaining 5% of anorectal trauma injuries and is usually secondary to pelvic fracture; however, injury may also occur as a consequence of transanal impalement by a foreign object usually secondary to assault, sexual misadventure, or even body packing used by drug traffickers. Although reported in all ages, a retained foreign body is often seen in young men in the second to third decades of life. Fundamental to understanding the pathophysiology of anorectal trauma is a basic knowledge of rectal anatomy since it influences the clinical presentation and diagnosis as well as guides surgical treatment options and subsequent outcomes. Of particular importance is the distinction between intraperitoneal versus extraperitoneal rectal injuries. The anterior two-thirds of the rectum both anteriorly and laterally are covered with peritoneum, whereas the posterior-upper two-thirds and lower one-third of the rectum circumferentially are devoid of peritoneal serosa. This anatomic distinction divides the overall group of anorectal trauma injuries into a heterogenous collection of injuries, each with their own clinical picture.

Clinical Presentation

The recognition of anorectal injuries requires a high degree of suspicion, and this begins with the patient history. For penetrating trauma injuries, the history is significantly easier to ascertain as it relates to mechanism and timing of the injury. On the contrary, patients with foreign body injuries are often reluctant to fully disclose their history. Regardless of mechanism, patients often present with abdominal and/or pelvic pain. Based on the severity of the injury as well as the timing of presentation in relation to the timing of the injury, patients may also present with obstructive signs such as nausea and/or vomiting, blood per rectum, peritonitis, or in the most severe instances, shock.

Diagnosis

The same level of suspicion exercised during the patient history should be maintained during the physical exam and subsequent workup. In obvious penetrating trauma after completion the primary trauma survey, the surgeon must carefully examine the abdomen for signs of peritonitis or other abnormalities, as well as the perineum, thighs, buttocks, and external anus for any gunshot or stab wounds. Patients with extraperitoneal injuries may not develop peritonitis. Additionally, other traumatic injuries should be catalogued including pelvic fractures, ureteral injuries, and bladder injuries that are located near the rectum and may imply associated injury. For all patients with suspected anorectal trauma, regardless of cause, digital rectal exam is mandatory. This is especially important in cases of foreign body insertion since low items may be palpated on exam. Identification of gross blood by DRE implies an anorectal injury; however, a negative DRE does not rule out injury. Therefore, rigid proctoscopy should be performed in all cases of suspected anorectal injury regardless of the presence of blood on DRE. Often this exam is performed in the operating room and with the patient in lithotomy position. Proctosopy may clearly identify the injury as well as its anatomic location; however, it may not and instead be obscured by blood or stool. The presence of blood on proctoscopy is a positive indicator of anorectal injury and visualization of the injury itself is not essential. In cases of suspected perforation after penetrating trauma, imaging with plain X-ray is often performed, however, not useful since even in the absence of extra-luminal air the patient may still have an injury that needs repair, i.e., extraperitoneal injuries. However, plain X-ray is useful in cases of suspected foreign objects as they often identify the retained object(s). Additionally, the use of CT scan with rectal contrast as well as water-soluble contrast studies can be onerous and are typically only performed after completion of the aforementioned workup to aid in the diagnosis of equivocal cases in stable patients.

Treatment

The treatment of anorectal trauma has evolved from wartime surgical experience. In response to the morbidity associated with war-related colonic injuries, in 1943 the Surgeon General announced mandatory exteriorization or diverting colostomy for colonic injuries [30]. This was substantiated by Ogilvie who soon after reported on the severe complications in patients undergoing primary repair in lieu of diversion, including sepsis and death [31]. However, treatment options have changed over the last several decades from mandated diversion to more current therapies based on anatomic location, extent of injury, as well as patient stability [32].

Intraperitoneal rectal injuries should be treated as colonic injuries. As previously mentioned, in the past these injuries were treated with routine fecal diversion. However, multiple trials examining civilian injuries studies, as well as a recent Cochrane review, have established that primary repair is now the accepted standard of care for penetrating colon injuries [33, 34]. Exceptions to this rule may include patients who present in hemodynamic shock, those requiring a massive transfusion of more than 6 U of blood, those who present greater than 6 h after the injury, and those with gross fecal spillage. However, even in the presence of these risk factors, data shows that primary anastomosis with or without resection can still be performed, with surgeons often adding a diverting proximal loop ileostomy/colostomy. Furthermore, studies have also shown that the method of anastomosis, either stapled or hand-sewn, does not affect postoperative complication rates [35]. Thus, primary repair is advocated for intraperitoneal rectal injuries; however, the specific procedure performed is ultimately the surgeon's choice based on the type of injury and patient factors.

Extraperitoneal rectal injuries can be divided into two categories: high (proximal) and low (distal). High extraperitoneal injuries are often extensions of intraperitoneal wounds and can usually be easily accessed. Therefore, they are treated in a similar manner to intraperitoneal injuries. On the other hand, distal or low extraperitoneal injuries present a difficult challenge, as they are frequently difficult to access. In the instances where the injury can be seen at the time of laparotomy, a primary repair should be performed with a proximal diversion. However, more commonly, the injury is not easily exposed and in these situations the traditional treatment is proximal diversion with placement of presacral drains in order to avoid the complication of a retrorectal or presacral abscess. Presacral drainage is typically performed by creating an incision posteriorly between the anus and the coccyx in combination with the placement of drains. Recently, however, the value of presacral drainage has been challenged with some data strongly supporting drain placement quoting a significant decrease in abscess formation, whereas in contrast, there is prospective data that suggests there is no difference in outcome; however, it is difficult to distinguish those wounds that were repaired versus not repaired in the latter [36, 37]. Therefore, it is our practice to continue presacral drain placement in the case of distal rectal injuries not amenable to primary repair, with the goal of decreasing pelvic sepsis.

The management of a retained foreign body within the rectum deserves special attention, as it will likely present itself for care by an acute care surgeon. Possible approaches for removal include a transanal approach, an endoscopic approach as well as a standard laparotomy taking care regardless of approach, to make sure that the impacted foreign body is not broken, which may lead to further rectal damage [38]. Oftentimes, the removal of the foreign object requires an examination under anesthesia in the operating room in order to achieve the necessary patient relaxation. In the transanal approach, the patient is placed in lithotomy and if palpable, the object is removed using blunt surgical graspers or the

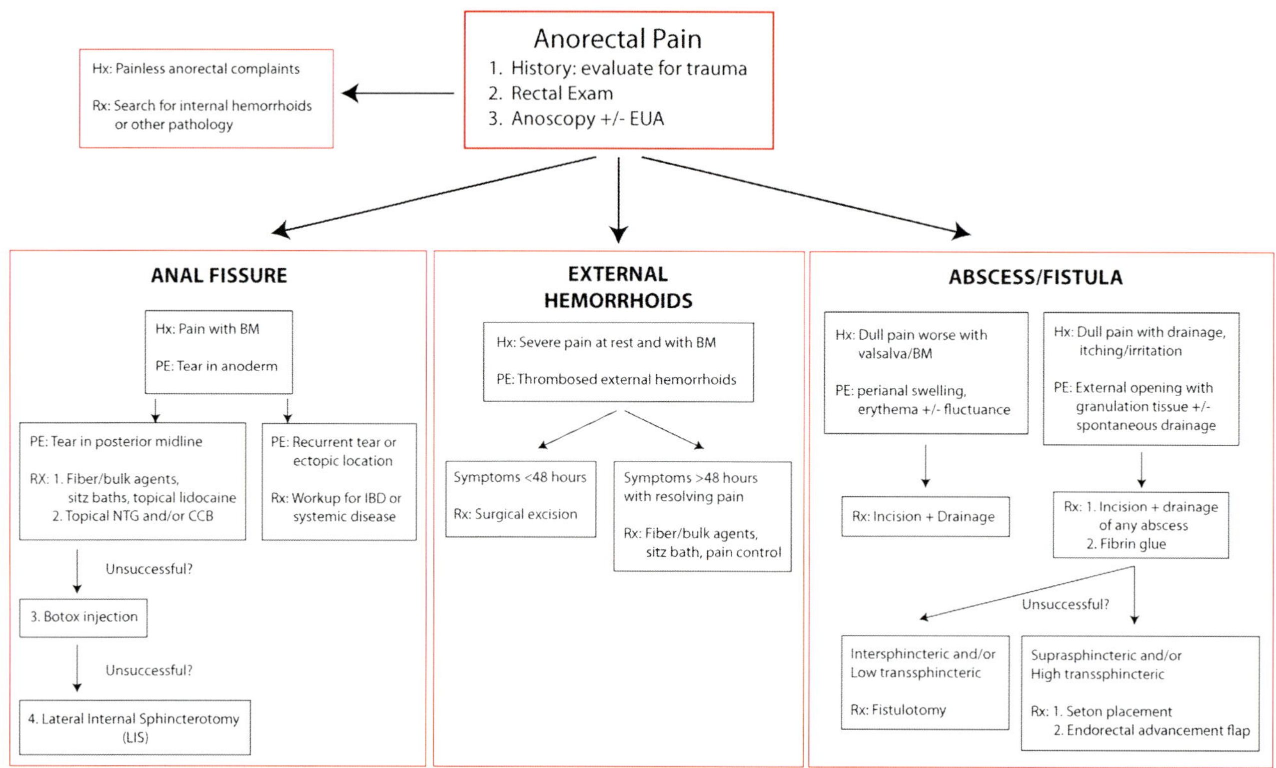

Fig. 31.5 Anorectal pain algorithm. *EUA* examination under anesthesia, *Hx* history, *PE* physical exam, *Rx* treatment, *BM* bowel movement, *NTG* nitroglycerin, *CCB* calcium channel blockers, *IBD* irritable bowel disease

surgeon's fingers. In higher objects or objects that are difficult to grab, such as jars or light bulbs, a catheter can be placed alongside the object, within the rectum, to break the vacuum seal and together with gentle valsalva the object can be dislodged. For object even more proximal within the rectum, endoscopy has proven useful for visualization and extraction. After either of these procedures, once the object is removed, proctoscopy should be performed to rule out residual objects or injuries. If neither of the aforementioned approaches is successful, then the patient should undergo standard laparotomy for object removal. Milking the object from proximally to distally with subsequent transanal extraction is the preferred method, and in the most infrequent of circumstances, colostomy with removal can be required.

Complications

The most common complication after anorectal trauma is infection; however, other complications include fistula, stricture, hernia, obstruction, urinary or fecal incontinence, as well as the need for possible colostomy closure. Infection may take on a number of different manifestations including retrorectal or presacral abscess as mentioned previously, surgical site infections, necrotizing soft tissue infection, and pelvic sepsis. In the absence of obvious wound or soft tissue infection, an abscess should be suspected in patients who postoperatively develop worsening pain, leukocytosis, or fever. A CT scan is usually sufficient for diagnosis and if an abscess is identified, drainage is imperative either through interventional radiology or if inaccessible, operative drainage.

Follow-up

Once discharged from the hospital, patients should be seen according to standard postoperative protocols. In patients who underwent proximal diversion as part of their surgical treatment, our practice is to schedule colostomy reversal no sooner than 2–3 months post-op providing that they have completely healed without active complications. Prior to colostomy reversal, we routinely obtain preoperative contrast studies to evaluate for anastomotic leak.

Conclusion

Fig. 31.5 shows an algorithm to identify the sources of anorectal pain and possible treatments.

References

1. Gibbons CP, Read NW. Anal hypertonia in fissures: cause or effect? Br J Surg. 1986;73(6):443–5.
2. Lund JN, Binch C, McGrath J, Sparrow RA, Scholefield JH. Topographical distribution of blood supply to the anal canal. Br J Surg. 1999;86(4):496–8.
3. Schouten WR, Briel JW, Auwerda JJ. Relationship between anal pressure and anodermal blood flow. The vascular pathogenesis of anal fissures. Dis Colon Rectum. 1994;37(7):664–9.
4. Nelson R. Non surgical therapy for anal fissure. Cochrane Database Syst Rev. 2006;(4):CD003431.
5. Evans J, Luck A, Hewett P. Glyceryl trinitrate vs. lateral sphincterotomy for chronic anal fissure: prospective, randomized trial. Dis Colon Rectum. 2001;44(1):93–7.
6. Bailey HR, Beck DE, Billingham RP, Binderow SR, Gottesman L, Hull TL, et al. A study to determine the nitroglycerin ointment dose and dosing interval that best promote the healing of chronic anal fissures. Dis Colon Rectum. 2002;45(9):1192–9.
7. Perry WB, Dykes SL, Buie WD, Rafferty JF. Practice parameters for the management of anal fissures (3rd revision). Dis Colon Rectum. 2010;53(8):1110–5.
8. Nelson RL. Operative procedures for fissure in ano. Cochrane Database Syst Rev. 2010;(1):CD002199.
9. Kang GS, Kim BS, Choi PS, Kang DW. Evaluation of healing and complications after lateral internal sphincterotomy for chronic anal fissure: marginal suture of incision vs. open left incision: prospective, randomized, controlled study. Dis Colon Rectum. 2008;51(3):329–33.
10. Johanson JF. Evidence based approach to the treatment of hemorrhoidal disease. Evid Based Gastroenterol. 2002;3:26–31.
11. Greenspon J, Williams SB, Young HA, Orkin BA. Thrombosed external hemorrhoids: outcome after conservative or surgical management. Dis Colon Rectum. 2004;47(9):1493–8.
12. MacRae HM, McLeod RS. Comparison of hemorrhoidal treatment modalities. A meta-analysis. Dis Colon Rectum. 1995;38(7):687–94.
13. Cataldo P, Ellis CN, Gregorcyk S, Hyman N, Buie WD, Church J, et al. Practice parameters for the management of hemorrhoids (revised). Dis Colon Rectum. 2005;48(2):189–94.
14. Longo A. Treatment of hemorrhoids disease by reduction of mucosa and hemorrhoidal prolapse with a circular suturing device: a new procedure. In: Proceedings of the sixth world congress of endoscopic surgery. Rome, Italy; 1998:777–84.
15. Jayaraman S, Colquhoun PH, Malthaner RA. Stapled versus conventional surgery for hemorrhoids. Cochrane Database Syst Rev. 2006;(4):CD005393.
16. Nelson R. Anorectal abscess fistula: what do we know? Surg Clin North Am. 2002;82(6):1139–51. v–vi.
17. Sozener U, Gedik E, Kessaf Aslar A, Ergun H, Halil Elhan A, Memikoglu O, et al. Does adjuvant antibiotic treatment after drainage of anorectal abscess prevent development of anal fistulas? A randomized, placebo-controlled, double-blind, multicenter study. Dis Colon Rectum. 2011;54(8):923–9.
18. Whiteford MH, Kilkenny 3rd J, Hyman N, Buie WD, Cohen J, Orsay C, et al. Practice parameters for the treatment of perianal abscess and fistula-in-ano (revised). Dis Colon Rectum. 2005;48(7):1337–42.
19. Malik AI, Nelson RL, Tou S. Incision and drainage of perianal abscess with or without treatment of anal fistula. Cochrane Database Syst Rev. 2010;(7):CD006827.
20. Joyce M, Veniero JC, Kiran RP. Magnetic resonance imaging in the management of anal fistula and anorectal sepsis. Clin Colon Rectal Surg. 2008;21(3):213–9. PMCID: 2780208.
21. Buchanan GN, Halligan S, Bartram CI, Williams AB, Tarroni D, Cohen CR. Clinical examination, endosonography, and MR imaging in preoperative assessment of fistula in ano: comparison with outcome-based reference standard. Radiology. 2004;233(3):674–81.
22. Ho YH, Tan M, Leong AF, Seow-Choen F. Marsupialization of fistulotomy wounds improves healing: a randomized controlled trial. Br J Surg. 1998;85(1):105–7.
23. Pescatori M, Ayabaca SM, Cafaro D, Iannello A, Magrini S. Marsupialization of fistulotomy and fistulectomy wounds improves healing and decreases bleeding: a randomized controlled trial. Colorectal Dis. 2006;8(1):11–4.
24. Singer M, Cintron J, Nelson R, Orsay C, Bastawrous A, Pearl R, et al. Treatment of fistulas-in-ano with fibrin sealant in combination with intra-adhesive antibiotics and/or surgical closure of the internal fistula opening. Dis Colon Rectum. 2005;48(4):799–808.
25. Lindsey I, Smilgin-Humphreys MM, Cunningham C, Mortensen NJ, George BD. A randomized, controlled trial of fibrin glue vs. conventional treatment for anal fistula. Dis Colon Rectum. 2002;45(12):1608–15.
26. Ky AJ, Sylla P, Steinhagen R, Steinhagen E, Khaitov S, Ly EK. Collagen fistula plug for the treatment of anal fistulas. Dis Colon Rectum. 2008;51(6):838–43.
27. Christoforidis D, Etzioni DA, Goldberg SM, Madoff RD, Mellgren A. Treatment of complex anal fistulas with the collagen fistula plug. Dis Colon Rectum. 2008;51(10):1482–7.
28. Present DH, Rutgeerts P, Targan S, Hanauer SB, Mayer L, van Hogezand RA, et al. Infliximab for the treatment of fistulas in patients with Crohn's disease. N Engl J Med. 1999;340(18):1398–405.
29. Bokhari S, Lindsey I. Incontinence following sphincter division for treatment of anal fistula. Colorectal Dis. 2010;12(7 Online): e135–9.
30. States SGotU. Care of the wounded in theaters of operation. National Archives Records Admin. and Records of US Army Surgeon General. SGO Circular Letter. Oct 1943;178.
31. Ogilvie WH. Abdominal wounds in the Western Desert. Surg Gynecol Obstet. 1944;78:225–38.
32. Weinberg JA, Fabian TC, Magnotti LJ, Minard G, Bee TK, Edwards N, et al. Penetrating rectal trauma: management by anatomic distinction improves outcome. J Trauma. 2006;60(3):508–13. Discussion 13–14.
33. Emetriades D, Murray JA, Chan L, Ordonez C, Bowley D, Nagy KK, et al. Penetrating colon injuries requiring resection: diversion or primary anastomosis? An AAST prospective multicenter study. J Trauma. 2001;50(5):765–75.
34. Nelson R, Singer, M. Primary repair for penetrating colon injuries. Cochrane Database Syst Rev. 2003;(3):CD002247.
35. Demetriades D, Murray JA, Chan LS, Ordonez C, Bowley D, Nagy KK, et al. Handsewn versus stapled anastomosis in penetrating colon injuries requiring resection: a multicenter study. J Trauma. 2002;52(1):117–21.
36. Burch JM, Feliciano DV, Mattox KL. Colostomy and drainage for civilian rectal injuries: is that all? Ann Surg. 1989;209(5):600–10. Discussion 10–1. PMCID: 1494065.
37. Gonzalez RP, Falimirski ME, Holevar MR. The role of presacral drainage in the management of penetrating rectal injuries. J Trauma. 1998;45(4):656–61.
38. Goldberg JE, Steele SR. Rectal foreign bodies. Surg Clin North Am. 2010;90(1):173–84.

Complications of Laparoendoscopic Surgery

Nicholas M. Brown, Michelle Shen, and Erik B. Wilson

Introduction

The use of advanced surgical techniques in the realm of endoscopic and laparoscopic therapy is constantly evolving and for many surgical procedures these techniques are now considered the standard of care. In the USA, an estimated 14.2 millioncolonoscopiesand9millionesophagogastroduodenoscopies (EGDs) are performed annually in the USA [1, 2]. The therapeutic applications of these procedures have also been expanded in recent years.

Laparoscopy has also been in a constant state of evolution over the last quarter century. Since Mühe performed the first laparoscopic cholecystectomy in 1985, the application of laparoscopy has expanded into all areas of surgery, including hernia, solid organ, colorectal, anti-reflux, and bariatric surgery. In fact, in the field of bariatrics an estimated 200,000 procedures are performed annually and this number is on the rise [2].

These innovations in surgical technology have offered many benefits to patients. However, with the advent of these minimally invasive techniques, we have also seen a unique set of complications that have accompanied these procedures. Patients with these complications often present to emergency rooms and it is important that these problems be recognized so that prompt intervention can ensue for optimal outcomes. The purpose of this chapter is to highlight the unique complications that occur with upper and lower endoscopy as well as those complications that occur with some of the most commonly performed laparoscopic procedures performed today. While not every surgeon may perform all these procedures described in this chapter, it is important for the acute care surgeon to be familiar with these procedures and their unique complications. This chapter describes the presentation of these complications as well as recommendations for their management.

N.M. Brown, M.D. • M. Shen, M.D. • E.B. Wilson, M.D. (✉)
Department of Surgery, University of Texas Health Science Center,
6431 Fannin Street, Suite 4.164, Houston, TX 77030, USA
e-mail: erik.b.wilson@uth.tmc.edu

Complications of Upper Endoscopy

Upper endoscopy is performed in the USA today by a variety of health care providers. Predominantly used as a diagnostic modality, the use of EGD can also be therapeutic by means of controlling upper gastrointestinal (UGI) bleeding, retrieval of foreign bodies, treatment of esophageal malignancies, dilatation and stenting of benign and malignant esophageal strictures, achalasia, and gastric outlet obstruction, and also placement of enteral access for nutrition. It is in the therapeutic application of upper endoscopy that we see the most common complications that include infection, perforation, hemorrhage, and pain.

Complications of Endoscopic Hemostasis

UGI endoscopy has been an important modality in the treatment of UGI bleed. The most commonly employed modalities for controlling upper GI bleed are endoscopic sclerotherapy, band ligation, or thermal electrocoagulation.

Bleeding from esophageal varices is a major complication of portal hypertension and can occur in up to 30% of patients with chronic liver disease and the mortality rate of an initial bleed is 30–50% [3–14]. Endoscopic techniques are the first-line therapy employed to manage acutely bleeding esophageal varices. The techniques most commonly employed are sclerotherapy and band ligation. Complications occurring after both of these procedures include ulceration, bleeding, esophageal stricture, and perforation.

The overall complication rate for sclerotherapy has been reported between 3 and 56% with a procedure related mortality rate of 0–5% [4, 14]. Sclerotherapy can cause esophageal erosions and ulceration in 70–100% (many of which are asymptomatic) and this can lead to recurrent bleeding in 2–13% of patients. Perforation can occur from direct iatrogenic injury or esophageal necrosis and may occur acutely in 2–5% of patients after undergoing sclerotherapy. Delayed perforation can also occur, but the incidence of this is unknown. Perforation is also a diagnostic dilemma as up to 50% of patients undergoing sclerotherapy can have chest pain, but this usually resolves within 24–48 h. Dissemination of the sclerosant can also cause pleural effusion, pneumonia, and bacteremia [4, 14].

Endoscopic band ligation is the preferred intervention for the treatment of esophageal varices as it has been proven to be superior with regard to control of active bleeding and has a more favorable side effect profile. Ulcer formation is seen in only 5–15% and there is a lower tendency for bleeding from these ulcers as compared to sclerotherapy [4, 5, 14]. Perforation has been reported in <1% of patients undergoing band ligation. Many of these perforations were reported with use of an overtube to facilitate passage of the endoscope, which have been eliminated with the development and common use of multifire devices.

Nonvariceal hemostasis is usually obtained endoscopically by means of injection of sclerosants and/or thermal electrocoagulation [6]. As is the case of sclerosant therapy for esophageal varices, injections of sclerosants (most commonly epinephrine) can lead to tissue necrosis and ulceration at the injection site due to vasoconstriction. Perforation after epinephrine injection has not been seen in randomized trials [12]. Thermal energy is used to obtain hemostasis in nonvariceal bleeding by means of multipolar electrocoagulation, heater probes, or laser. Bleeding is common and occurs in up to 5% of cases. Heater probes and multipolar electrocoagulation have similar rates of perforation of 0–2%.

Management of the complications associated with endoscopic management of homeostasis depends on the timing and nature of the complication. With regard to ulcer formation, proton pump inhibitors (PPIs) do not appear to prevent the formation of these ulcers, but can play a role in the healing of these ulcerations. Recurrent bleeding can be approached with repeat endoscopy regardless of the underlying etiology. In the case of bleeding from varices, repeated episodes of bleeding that cannot be controlled with repeat endoscopy should be managed with temporary balloon tamponade and transjugular intrahepatic portosystemic shunt (TIPS) or surgical shunt, but further details of this are outside the scope of this chapter. In the cases of nonvariceal UGI bleeding, repeat endoscopy is comparable with surgical intervention with regard to transfusion requirements, mortality, and duration of hospital stay. If the bleeding cannot be controlled endoscopically or if patient is persistently hemodynamically unstable, then surgery is indicated for definitive management. Patients who are poor surgical candidates can alternatively be managed with percutaneous angiography and selective embolization. Stricture can be managed with endoscopy and dilatation regardless of the underlying etiology. Often serial or repeat dilatations are needed. Management of perforation is largely dependent on timing, location, and clinical condition of the patient. In a retrospective review done by Fernandez et al. the recommendations was that if a perforation is detected at the

time of endoscopy, it should initially be treated endoscopically (by hemostasis, fibrin sealing, clip, or stent) [15]. If an injury was suspected they recommended an early esophagogram or contrasted CT scan and then treatment strategy was based on the clinical symptoms, the preexisting disorders, and the general condition of the patient. Cervical perforations of the esophagus rarely require surgical intervention other than simple drainage. The management of intrathoracic esophageal perforations is more controversial. Intramural perforations are rare, but usually can be treated conservatively. Possible endoscopic therapeutic measures after esophageal perforation are fibrin sealing, clipping, and bridging of the leakage with a stent. Perforations into the mediastinum can also be managed with aggressive conservative therapy consisting of nasogastric suction, intravenous antibiotics, and parenteral hyperalimentation. Exceptions to this are contrast leaks into the pleural or peritoneal cavity. Thoracotomy almost always is indicated if the visceral pleura is injured and a recent esophageal perforation with the corresponding clinical symptoms should be treated with immediate surgical interventions. If a perforation is not diagnosed until a few days after the injury, and if the patient is without symptoms, a watch-and-wait strategy is proposed. A study done by Merchea et al. quoted an 18% failure rate for nonoperative management and stated that nonoperative management is feasible if there is no evidence of contrast extravasation or free fluid on radiographic studies [16].

Complications of Endoscopic Foreign Body Retrieval

The majority of foreign body ingestion occurs in the pediatric population, but it is not uncommon to have adults present in the acute setting secondary to esophageal foreign body. The most common esophageal foreign body in adults is impacted meat or food bolus, but a myriad of other true foreign bodies can also be encountered in the patient population with psychiatric disorders, mental retardation, or impairment caused by alcohol or other drugs. Endoscopy is often used in the retrieval of these foreign bodies with a reported complication rate of up to 8% of cases [17, 18]. It is difficult to determine if these complications are truly due to the endoscopy or to the foreign body itself. Impaction, perforation, or obstruction most often occurs at areas of acute angulation or physiologic narrowing—most notably in upper endoscopy at the level of the cricopharyngeus muscle. Passage of foreign bodies through the esophagus predicts morbidity as most ingested foreign bodies pass through the rest of the GI tract without further complications. When dealing with esophageal foreign bodies, the primary goal is to not only remove the foreign body, put do so in a safe manner. Aspiration and mucosal injury can be reduced by use of an esophageal overtube, but overtubes have been associated with bleeding and perforation themselves and that should be considered when determining their utility. Mucosal injury can be reduced by placing a latex hood over the endoscope and when dealing with sharp or pointed object, assuring that the sharp or pointed end if trailing. With regard to impacted meat, use of meat tenderizer should be avoided due to increased risk for perforation. It is not always necessary to retrieve the foreign body, especially in the case of impacted food as the push technique, in which the impacted food is pushed past the area of obstruction, has a reported success rate up to 97% [19]. The important consideration in dealing with esophageal foreign bodies is to reinsert the endoscope after removal or clearance of the foreign body to reassess for bleeding, mucosal injuries, or underlying pathology. Most of these injuries can be treated conservatively at the time of detection by either observation alone or fibrin sealing, clipping, or stenting if the injury is more extensive. Prolonged bleeding can be treated with the same techniques as listed previously.

Complications of Treatment of Esophageal Malignancies and Stenting

Endoscopy has offered many benefits in both the treatment and palliation of esophageal malignancy. Ablative techniques such as injection of sclerosants, thermal methods (bipolar cautery, laser, argon plasma coagulation), and photodynamic therapy (PDT) are all susceptible to similar complication profiles including the minor complications of pain, edema, and strictures with major complications such as perforation or development of fistulae in up to 10% [20–24]. Unique to PDT is sun photosensitivity, and dysphagia may initially worsen after PDT. Endoscopic mucosal resection has also proven to be extremely beneficial in the treatment of early esophageal squamous-cell carcinoma or high-grade intraepithelial neoplasm with a reported overall complication rate of 20–30% with these complications being minor stenoses and bleeding [21, 22]. Esophageal stenting has been employed as a palliative measure in advanced esophageal carcinoma. These self-expanding metal stents have a post-deployment complication rates from 20 to 40% and include tumor ingrowth or overgrowth, stent migration, hemorrhage, and food impaction [23, 24]. Tumor ingrowth or overgrowth can be avoided by use of a covered stent or treated with an ablative technique or placement of an additional stent. Stent migration has been reported to occur in 2–8% of cases [23, 24]. The majority of migrated stents have an indolent course and can either be removed nonsurgically, allowed to exit the body spontaneously, or be allowed to remain in the body in an uncomplicated state. Only 2–4% of migrated stents causing bowel obstruction require surgical intervention [23, 24].

Complications of UGI Dilatation

Endoscopic dilatation is used in the treatment of benign and malignant esophageal strictures, and gastric outlet obstruction. Complication rates are largely dependent on the underlying pathology. For benign esophageal strictures, the main complications are perforation, hemorrhage, and bacteremia. The reported rate of perforation is 0.3% and this is higher when dealing with dilatation of caustic strictures [25]. The majority of perforations can be treated with conservative management. Hemorrhage can usually be managed with conventional endoscopic therapy.

Transient bacteremia has a low incidence and the rate of bacterial endocarditis or other complications can be avoided by use of the appropriate antibiotic prophylaxis [26]. With regard to malignant esophageal strictures, the rate of perforation is higher than for benign strictures with a rate up to 10% [25]. The same management principles apply as with benign dilatation complications. Dilatation of gastric outlet obstruction (GOO) has also proven to be successful with a perforation rate of 2–6.7% and most perforations occurring when attempts to dilate the gastric outlet exceed 1.5 cm diameter [25]. Again, conservative management can be employed with perforation after dilatation of GOO with surgery reserved for those who do not respond to medical management.

Complications of Percutaneous Endoscopic Gastrostomy Tube Placement

Percutaneous endoscopic gastrostomy (PEG) placement has become the modality of choice for providing enteral access for long-term nutritional support. It should be considered in patients who have a functional, non-obstructed GI tract but are unable to take adequate nutrition PO to meet metabolic needs or in those requiring gut decompression secondary to abdominal malignancies causing chronic obstruction or ileus. PEG placement is generally considered safe, but can be associated with many potential complications as well. Minor complications occur in 13–43% of patients and include skin maceration from leakage around the tube, tube occlusion, and pain that is usually self-limited [27–29]. These complications can usually be managed by local wound control and good tube maintenance. Major complications have an occurrence rate of 0.4–8.4% with a procedure related mortality rate of 1–2% [27, 28]. These major complications include wound infection, necrotizing fasciitis, aspiration, device dislodgement, colon injury, and colocutaneous fistula. Antimicrobial prophylaxis it is cost-effective and may reduce the risk of peristomal wound infection. Necrotizing fasciitis is a rare complication of PEG placement and has been linked with not making the abdominal incision large enough to allow adequate drainage. Patients with preexisting comorbidities such as malnutrition, diabetes, wound infections, and impaired immunity are at increased risk. Treatment requires wide debridement, antibiotics, and planned reoperation to assess the wound. The risk of aspiration after PEG placement is 0.3–1.0% with the majority of aspirations events occurring at a later time unrelated to the PEG procedure [27, 28]. This is largely due to the fact that many patients undergoing PEG placement have neurologic sequelae of traumatic brain injury or stroke. Despite the fact that most aspiration events occur unrelated to placement of the PEG, the endoscopist should avoid excessive sedation, thoroughly aspirate gastric content before and after the procedure and perform the procedure efficiently. Inadvertent early PEG dislodgment occurs in 1.6–4.4% of patients and is a unique challenge [27, 28]. Typically PEG tract maturation begins to occur in roughly 7–10 days but in the malnourished, diabetic, and immunocompromised patient this can take significantly longer. If the dislodgement occurs prior to 1 month since placement, repeat endoscopy should be performed to replace the tube, as the stomach may have separated from the anterior abdominal wall resulting in free perforation. If recognized early, the replacement PEG can be placed either through the same site or close to it. If recognition is delayed, the patient should be made NPO, a nasogastric tube should be placed and broad-spectrum intravenous antibiotics started. If the clinician believes that the tube has become dislodged through a mature tract, then a water-soluble contrast study should be obtained after the tube is replaced prior to reinstituting use of the tube. Surgical exploration is indicated if sign of peritonitis or sepsis are present. Colon injuries can occur during placement of a PEG tube. This can be avoided during placement by assuring adequate gastric insufflation, appropriate transillumination, and endoscopically visualized depression of the gastric wall on trans-abdominal palpation. Colonic injuries usually present with peritonitis and often require surgical intervention, but nonoperative management can be attempted in the hemodynamically stable patient without signs of abdominal sepsis.

Complications of Lower Endoscopy

Lower endoscopy serves as both a diagnostic and management tool for colonic and rectal disorders. Its diagnostic capabilities include evaluation of abnormalities, gastrointestinal bleeding, colorectal cancer screening, surveillance, examination of prior colorectal surgery, evaluation and surveillance of inflammatory bowel disease or abnormal bowel habits, and intraoperative uses including tumor or hemorrhage localization. At the same time, it is also an effective tool for managing active bleeding lesions, excision of polyps, reduction of sigmoid volvulus, removal of foreign bodies, decompression, and dilation of strictured areas. Overall complication rates for lower endoscopy falls around 0.3% [30–33].

Patients who are at higher risks for complications include those with perforated viscus, severe acute diverticulitis, or an active inflammatory process. Moderate risk factors include uncooperative patients, inadequate bowel preparation, medical comorbidities, or abdominal pathology.

Despite its numerous functional capabilities, there are many risks of complications that can occur during colonoscopies such as bleeding, perforation, and solid organ injury.

Hemorrhage

The most common complication of colonoscopy is hemorrhage, and it has an occurrence of about 0.03% [30–33]. Significant hemorrhage after a colonoscopy is defined as lower gastrointestinal bleeding requiring transfusion, hospitalization, re-intervention, or surgery. The source of bleeding may be from the biopsy site, endoscopic induced laceration to the colonic mucosa, and tearing of the mesentery or splenic capsule [30, 31]. Once the bleeding has been identified, management depends on timing and severity of the bleeding.

If bleeding is identified at the time of the colonoscopy, it can be controlled by reapplication of the snare to the pedicle with electrocautery or strangulation of the bleeding point for 5–10 min if electrocautery is deemed unsafe. Delayed hemorrhage may occur up to 29 days after the procedure, but most of these bleeds may be managed conservatively. However, if these bleeds fail conservative management, repeat endoscopy with sclerotherapy, bipolar cautery, or heater-probe application may be necessary.

Perforation

Perforations that occur during lower endoscopy often result from mechanical forces against the bowel, barotrauma, or direct insults from therapeutic procedures. Most often perforations occur within the sigmoid colon [32, 33].

Perforation should be suspected if intraperitoneal structures are visualized, or if there is inability to maintain insufflation. Early post-procedural signs include persistent abdominal pain and abdominal distension with later manifestations to include fever and leukocytosis.

If the perforation is recognized early on then surgical intervention with primary repair is sufficient. However, there remains controversy in those who are asymptomatic or minimally symptomatic with delayed presentation and pneumoperitoneum. Conservative management including bowel rest, broad-spectrum antibiotics, and serial abdominal examinations can be employed.

Solid Organ Injury

Iatrogenic splenic injury after lower endoscopy is extremely rare but a potentially fatal complication [31]. Mesocolon avulsion, serosal tear, or splenic hematoma causing extraluminal intra-abdominal bleeding is extremely rare but does occur. The most common reason for splenic rupture after colonoscopy is due to forceful stretching of the splenocolic ligament. It is often due to the aggressiveness of instrumentation at the splenic flexure and the degree of adhesions at the splenocolic ligament. However, the exact incidence of splenic injury during colonoscopy is unknown despite large reviews reported in the literature.

Patients often present with symptoms of splenic injury 24 h following a colonoscopy. Most often the chief complaint is abdominal pain that should raise a high level of suspicion and warrant a computed tomography (CT) scan of the abdomen.

Colonoscopy-induced splenic injuries often have a higher grade of injury needing earlier operative intervention. Conservative management may be used until patient's hemodynamic status deteriorates despite aggressive resuscitation. It may be feasible to perform a laparoscopic splenectomy; however, it should be based on the comfort level of the operating surgeon.

Complications of Bariatric Surgery

With the introduction of minimally invasive techniques, the field of bariatric surgery has grown exponentially over the last 15 years. More than 200,000 bariatric operations are performed per year [34–36]. The most commonly performed operations today are the laparoscopic Roux-en-Y gastric bypass (RGYB), the laparoscopic adjustable gastric band, and the laparoscopic sleeve gastrectomy. While rates of major complications from these procedures are low as a whole [37], it is not uncommon for patients having undergone these procedures to present to emergency rooms and it is important for the on-call surgeon to be able to recognize and manage the unique problems that may be encountered in these patients.

Complications of Laparoscopic Access

Trocar injuries are potentially preventable complications in laparoscopic surgery and are often the most serious. Most frequent organs injured during insertion of trocars include small bowel, iliac artery and vein, and less commonly the bladder.

Incidence of major vascular injuries from trocars and Veress needles averages around 0.1% [38–41]. Most commonly injured vessels include iliac vessels, then the aorta or IVC, and less commonly mesenteric vessels [38–41].

Early recognition is essential in management of the above states injuries. Small bowel or bladder injuries can often be repaired laparoscopically, but major vascular injuries often require conversion to an open procedure to repair.

Complications of Laparoscopic RYGB

Anastomotic Leaks

Anastomotic leak is typically an early complication of laparoscopic RYGB with an incidence of 0–5.2% [42–49]. Most patients present in the first 7–10 postoperative days with nonspecific symptoms of sepsis including tachycardia, fever, and abdominal pain. They may or may not have leukocytosis. Radiologic diagnosis is often a dilemma as these patients' body habitus often precludes obtaining a CT scan. CT also has a low sensitivity for the detection of leaks seen in one large case series as being 56% [46]. Upper GI series also has a low sensitivity (30%) as shown in this same case series and the combination of the two was shown in this series to detect leaks 70% of the time [46]. With the sensitivities of these studies being relatively poor, any patient with tachycardia and sepsis in the early post-op period should be considered for re-laparoscopy. Management of these patients is often determined by their timing of presentation. Many of these patients will already be discharged home and present to the on-call surgery team [50]. Many patients can be managed nonoperatively with retaining surgically placed drains, intravenous antibiotics, and withholding oral intake. In the unstable patient, a laparoscopic washout and drain placement can be a temporizing measure until the bariatric team is available for definitive management. In stable patients, it is sometimes possible to stent leaks endoscopically, thus avoiding high-risk surgery. Percutaneous drainage of localized, contained leaks is also possible, but these measures should both be done in coordination with the bariatric team.

Gastrointestinal Bleeding

The incidence of GI hemorrhage after laparoscopic RYGB ranges from 1.1 to 4% [51, 52]. Patients with GI hemorrhage present either early (within 48 h) or late (after 48 h). Early bleeding is usually from poor hemostasis at the time of surgery or bleeding from staple lines. There are four potential areas for staple line bleeds: the gastric pouch, the gastrojejunostomy, the jejunostomy, and the bypassed stomach. Patients usually present with hematemesis, hematochezia, and/or hypotension. The initial management of GI hemorrhage consists of fluid resuscitation and preparation for blood transfusions. Ongoing bleeding in the early group with a decline in hematocrit indicates active bleeding that will likely require intervention. Endoscopic therapy can be employed to control staple line bleeding by injection of epinephrine or thermal coagulation. Endoscopic management is usually limited to the gastric pouch and the gastrojejunostomy due to the long Roux limb length but successful endoscopic management at the jejunojejunostomy has been described. Reoperative intervention is indicated in the hemodynamically unstable patient. It consists of either laparoscopy or open surgery based on the degree of instability as laparoscopy is relatively contraindicated in the unstable patient as pneumoperitoneum can result in worsened hemodynamics. In the event that bleeding is from the bypassed stomach, a gastrotomy can be performed in the distended remnant stomach and clot evacuated. It is important to oversew the staple line in the remnant stomach and it may be necessary to place a gastrostomy tube in the remnant stomach for decompression, potential radiography, and feeding. Late bleeding, usually after the first postoperative week is commonly associated with ulceration at the anastomosis or ulceration due to nonsteroidal anti-inflammatory drugs (NSAIDs). It can also be commonly associated with gastritis, and evaluation is usually by upper endoscopy. If no bleeding is visualized on upper endoscopy it may be prudent to repeat endoscopy using a longer scope to visualize the more distal jejunojejunostomy. Treatment of late bleeding can usually be accomplished by endoscopic intervention as needed, acid reducing therapy, and identification and eradication of *Helicobacter pylori* infection.

Internal Hernias

The overall incidence of internal hernia in the laparoscopic RYGB is estimated to be between 3 and 4.5% [53–56]. Depending on the type of procedure performed, there are up to three potential hernia spaces at the mesenteric defect of the jejunojejunostomy, the Peterson defect (posterior to the Roux limb) and in the case of a retrocolic anastomosis at the transverse mesocolon. Internal hernias can result in intestinal obstruction, ischemia, or both. Presenting symptoms are usually intermittent abdominal pain and, less commonly, emesis. When bilious emesis is present, more distal obstruction should be expected. Laboratory findings are also nonspecific and only about one-quarter of patients will be present with leukocytosis. Radiologic evaluation is often unreliable with UGI (33–55% positive for obstruction) and CT (48–90% positive for obstruction) [57]. The presence of a mesenteric swirl sign is a more reliable indicator of internal hernia (sensitivity 61–83% and specificity 67–94%) [57]. With nonspecific symptoms, laboratory values and a potentially unremarkable radiologic workup, the on-call surgeon should have a low threshold for exploring patients when internal hernia is clinically suspected or patients fail to improve. Laparoscopic management of internal hernia after gastric bypass is feasible in 83–100% of patients with low conversion rates of 7–17% [55]. Resection of necrotic bowel

segments should be performed, but is rarely necessary if exploration is performed promptly and all hernias should be reduced and the mesenteric defects closed [53].

Anastomotic Stricture

Stricture can follow any anastomosis and in the case of RYGB is most common at the gastrojejunal anastomosis with a reported incidence between 3.1 and 15.7% [58–60]. The method in which the gastrojejunal anastomosis was performed is important as circular staplers seem to have higher rates of stricture than linear staplers or a hand-sewn anastomosis. Causes of stricture include subclinical leak, fibrosis secondary to ulceration, ischemia or technical error. Patients present dysphagia, nausea and or obstruction typically between 3 weeks and 3 months after surgery. Diagnosis can usually be made based on history alone. A UGI study may be helpful, but is only diagnostic. An EGD can be both diagnostic and therapeutic. Endoscopic dilatation of the stricture is the treatment of choice and is successful in 55–83% of cases after a single dilatation to 15–18 mm [58]. Serial dilatation may be required in late anastomotic strictures. Perforation is a potential complication of dilatation (2.1%) particularly if dilatation is done in the first month after surgery [58, 59]. Revisional surgery is occasionally recommended for resistant stenosis, but typically not in the acute setting.

Marginal Ulceration

Marginal ulcers occur in approximately 1–16% of patients [61–64]. They usually occur on the jejunal side of the gastrojejunal anastomosis because while acid reduction is significant following a RYGB, the jejunum does not have the defense mechanisms against acid exposure that are present in the duodenum. The etiology of ulcer formation following RYGB is likely multifactorial. Potential etiologies for this complication include gastric acid causing peptic digestion of the unprotected jejunal mucosa as discussed above, foreign body (staples or nonabsorbable suture) inflammatory reaction, exogenous substances (alcohol, tobacco, NSAIDs), and *H. pylori* infection [61–64]. The clinical presentation of marginal ulceration is that of severe pain, nausea, unheralded bleeding, or, rarely, perforation. The diagnosis can be made on clinical presentation, but upper endoscopy is usually the employed in making the diagnosis and this also allows for a tissue sample for *H. pylori* testing. Treatment is usually medical initially and includes acid suppression and eradication of *H. pylori* if present. Predisposing factors such as alcohol, tobacco and NSAIDs are also discontinued. At the time of endoscopy, when suture material of staples are observed it may be prudent to remove them endoscopically if this can be done safely. Treatment with PPIs and sucralfate often promote resolution of the ulcers. Duration of treatment is not clearly defined, but studies recommend 6 weeks to 6 months duration of treatment followed by repeat endoscopy to evaluate success of medical treatment [61–64]. Surgical treatment is reserved for marginal ulcers refractory to medical treatment or, as is more prudent for this chapter, those patients who present with acute perforation. Acute perforation occurs in approximately 1% of patients according to a large retrospective review of 3,430 patients undergoing laparoscopic RYGB [64]. Treatment options are similar to that of a perforated peptic ulcer and are based on the size of the perforation, amount of contamination and clinical condition of the patient. One surgical option is the open or laparoscopic placement of an omental patch and/or closure of the perforation. This is the most prudent procedure for the clinically unstable patient. Another option is resection of the anastomotic segment containing the ulcer along with gastric resection to reduce the pouch size (and thus the amount of acid secreted) and re-creating the gastrojejunostomy with or without a vagotomy. A gastrostomy tube may also be placed in the remnant stomach to facilitate postoperative enteral nutrition. All patients with perforation should be maintained on acid reducing therapy for a minimum of 3 months or indefinitely in those patients who refuse to make lifestyle modifications (i.e., cessation of smoking, alcohol abuse and NSAIDs).

Complications of Laparoscopic Adjustable Gastric Band

Infection

Infection can be divided into intra-abdominal and port-site infection. The laparoscopic adjustable gastric band (LAGB) is a foreign body and thus acts as a potential nidus for infection and may precipitate infection and abscess formation [50, 65–68]. In the presence of an intra-abdominal abscess, the band should be removed and the area widely drained and the stomach tested for occult leaks. Port-site infections are classified as early or late [69]. Early infections manifest with signs similar to those of cellulitis: pain, edema, and erythema. These early port-site infections can usually be treated with oral antibiotics. In the event that these infections do not clear, then IV antibiotics should be used. When the infection does not respond to antibiotics and is limited to the port, then the infection requires adjustment port removal. The wound is then allowed to heal by secondary intention while antibiotics are tailored to cultures obtained from the adjustment port. Late port-site infections are due to erosion until proven otherwise. The band should be removed, cultured and the even if there is no erosion present, the stomach and esophagus should be tested for occult leak.

Gastric Prolapse

Gastric prolapse or band slippage occurs with cephalad herniation of the body of stomach through the band (posterior slip) or caudal migration of the band (anterior slip). Historically, it has been reported to be as high as 25%, but this has decreased to less than 5% with widespread adoption of the pars flaccida technique for band placement [50, 65, 66]. Up to 20% of patients may be asymptomatic or present with dysphagia, nausea, vomiting and reflux [50, 65, 66]. Abdominal pain may be an ominous sign when dealing with gastric prolapse indicating possible gastric ischemia. Gastric prolapse is diagnosed radiographically with a UGI study. With the pars flaccida technique for band placement, the most common type of gastric prolapse after LAGB is anterior slip. Posterior slip was more common with the peri-gastric technique of band placement. Either type can lead to UGI bleeding, aspiration pneumonia, or complete obstruction of the stomach, gastric perforation, or ischemia of the prolapsed stomach. The treatment of all types of gastric prolapse is first to remove fluid from the band as this can sometimes improve the patient's condition. Gastric prolapse does require operative intervention and sometimes this needs to be done acutely in the patient with abdominal pain as this can indicate gastric ischemia. Most of the time surgery can be accomplished laparoscopically. Some surgeons remove and replace the band, others take down the plicated fundus and attempt to reposition the band. For a surgeon who is not familiar with treatment of this complication or in the presence of gastric ischemia, the most appropriate management is band removal. The band can either opened, but this is often a difficult maneuver and the simplest option is sharp transection of the band.

Gastric Pouch Dilatation

Gastric pouch dilatation is a common occurring late complication of LAGB, occurring in 5–25% of cases [50, 65–69]. It may involve the stomach, the esophagus, or both. Symptoms included dysphagia, vomiting, reflux, and heartburn. It is thought to occur secondary to overinflation of the band or overeating with resulting high pressure within the pouch. It is diagnosed by means of a UGI contrast study or by upper endoscopy. The first-line treatment and the important step to remember for the on-call surgeon who may not be familiar with troubleshooting a LAGB is band deflation with a follow-up contrast study in 4–6 weeks [50]. If the pouch size returns to normal then attempts at re-inflating the band may be done at this time. If the patient cannot tolerate band fills or if the pouch fails to return to its original size on repeat UGI then surgical revision is often required with replacement of the band at a higher position.

Band Erosion

Band erosion is an uncommon complication of LAGB with an incidence less than 1% [67, 68]. It is a slow process and rarely results in perforation and peritonitis. As stated previously, the band is exposed to gastric flora and the tubing can become infected. Many patients are asymptomatic, but some patients present with weight-gain as the band loses its restrictive effect. Some patients present with epigastric pain and gastrointestinal bleeding, but one of the most common presentations are recurrent port-site infections. Diagnosis can be made with contrast studies, endoscopy, or both. Band removal can be accomplished either laparoscopically or use of endoscopy depending on degree of erosion. Our institution is currently investigating a method of placing a stent across a partially eroded band to complete the erosion allowing later facilitation of endoscopic removal. There have been case reports of an eroded band migrating and causing small bowel obstruction, but rarely is emergent surgery necessary with this complication [68]. In some instances, band removal may be delayed for many months in the asymptomatic patient to facilitate endoscopic removal of the eroded band.

Complications of Laparoscopic Sleeve Gastrectomy

Laparoscopic sleeve gastrectomy is the newest bariatric procedure that is commonly done today. This procedure has been utilized in the past as a staged procedure for inpatients undergoing a duodenal switch procedure but has recently been utilized as a standalone procedure in bariatric surgery. Studies quote excess body weight loss at 1 year to be around 50% [70–73]. The procedure is attractive to both patients and surgeons as it does not require a gastrointestinal anastomosis or intestinal bypass and is thought to be less technically demanding than RYGB. It also eliminates the presence of a foreign body as in the LAGB. The commonly identified complications of laparoscopic sleeve gastrectomy are abscess, hemorrhage, sleeve stricture, gastric fistula, and leak. Abscess formation is an uncommon occurrence and can be managed by percutaneous drainage and antibiotics. Unlike the LAGB, the laparoscopic sleeve gastrectomy does not involve a foreign body requiring explantation in the event of intra-abdominal infection. Hemorrhage is reported in the literature as occurring in 0–15.8% of cases and usually occurs from the staple line [71]. Most bleeding is self-limited and resolves with conservative management. Bleeding causing hemodynamic instability can often be addressed endoscopically by injection of epinephrine or thermal coagulation at the staple line. Laparoscopy or open surgery to oversew the staple line is reserved for patients who are unresponsive to surgical measures and usually involves oversewing the staple line or looking for other intra-abdominal injuries (i.e., liver and splenic lacerations). Sleeve stricture is another uncommon complication, with sleeve stricture presenting in <1% of patients and usually presenting 3–4 weeks after surgery [71]. This can be managed most of the time with endoscopic dilatation. Gastric fistula is another potential complication reported in one

prospective study as being as high as 5.1% [72]. This was diagnosed in this series either by UGI contrast study or CT scan at a median time of diagnosis of 4.8 days. Patients in this series were treated with IV antibiotics, parenteral nutrition, and somatostatin analogues. This complication can be treated with conservative therapy as stated previously, along with endoscopic stent placement and/or histoacryl glue. The most dreaded complication following laparoscopic sleeve gastrectomy is gastric leak. Its incidence is reported in the literature as 0–5.5% [73]. Leaks can present with signs of sepsis including fever, tachycardia, and abdominal pain as well as leukocytosis on lab evaluation. A study done by Tan et al. defined an algorithm for management of leaks following laparoscopic sleeve gastrectomy [73]. The principle behind the treatment of these patients was control of sepsis, nutritional supplementation, and definition of anatomy of the leak for definitive therapy. Early leaks in patients with signs of sepsis with no discernible abscess were treated with either laparoscopic or open washout with drain placement, and either an omental patch or insertion of a T-tube into the defect. A feeding jejunostomy was also placed at this time. If a drainable abscess was identified on CT scan, a percutaneous drain was placed and a nasojejunal feeding tube was placed for enteral nutrition. In non-septic patients and late leaks, an NJT was placed for enteral nutrition and if there was a drainable collection it was either drained percutaneously or with surgery [73].

Complications of Laparoscopic Cholecystectomy

Bleeding can arise at many different points during a laparoscopic cholecystectomy [74]. Such instances may include trocar insertion injuring abdominal vessels that can be detected under direct visualization. Bleeding can be controlled with a figure of eight stitch placed under direct visualization with a suture passer or a straight needle. Another option may be inserting a Foley catheter into the trocar site to tamponade the bleeding for several hours.

Liver bed bleeding can also be problematic, if not controlled with electrocautery; other options include direct pressure with sponges, and packing with hemostatic agents or fibrin sealant. If bleeding continues to persist, clipping or electrocautery may be used, however, with extreme caution due to high risk of bile duct or hepatic vessel injuries. If bleeding still cannot be adequately controlled, conversion to an open approach should be done immediately.

Bile leaks after laparoscopic cholecystectomy occurs in approximately 1% of the patient population [74]. Most often, these patients have already been discharged home. Patients often present with persistent abdominal pain, distention, or leukocytosis. Diagnostic imaging includes ultrasound and if a fluid collection is visualized, a hepatobiliary iminodiacetic acid (HIDA) scan is performed to confirm presence of a bile leak.

If a bile leak is confirmed, it can be drained percutaneously in addition to cholangiography (magnetic resonance cholangiopancreatography [MRCP] or endoscopic retrograde cholangiopancreatography [ERCP]) performed to define the biliary anatomy. Most often the source of bile leak is the cystic duct. These are often managed conservatively with percutaneous drainage, endoscopic sphincterotomy with temporary stenting.

If the leak is from a major bile duct, it is advisable to place drains at the time of surgery and refer care to an experienced biliary surgeon for the definitive therapy.

Complications of Laparoscopic Hernia Repair

Laparoscopic Inguinal Hernia Repair

Laparoscopic inguinal hernia repair (LIHR) offers many advantages to traditional open hernia repair including decreased level of post-op pain, earlier return to normal activities, and the ability to visualize the contralateral side and repair both hernias at the same time [75–79]. The two widely recognized approaches to laparoscopic inguinal hernia repair are the trans-abdominal pre-peritoneal repair (TAPP) and the totally extraperitoneal repair (TEP). Postoperative complications following LIHR include seroma, chronic pain secondary to nerve entrapment and neuralgia, and there have been reports of small bowel obstruction (more common after the TAPP repair) [79]. Additional complications include bowel or bladder injury from trocar placement or intraoperative manipulations, vessel injury (mainly epigastric vessels), transection of the ductus deferens, and scrotal emphysema, but these are usually appreciated and managed at the time of surgery. Seroma formation, which occurs in approximately 3% of patients, usually has an indolent course and most resolve without need for any intervention [76, 77]. Occasionally, large and persistent scrotal seromas may require needle drainage or possible even formal exploration and treatment for hydrocele. Chronic pain and/or parasthesia secondary to nerve entrapment and neuralgia (including the genital branch of the genitofemoral nerve, the lateral femoral cutaneous nerve, and the ilioinguinal nerve) have become less common as surgical techniques have improved. In the event of pain or paresthesia secondary to nerve entrapment, conservative management is the best initial option as most of these symptoms will resolve on their own without intervention. Repeat laparoscopy is sometimes required with removal of the offending staple or suture causing the entrapment. The use of absorbable sutures and tacks is thought to make nonoperative management of these complications even more feasible. Small bowel obstruction following LIHR has been reported in the literature at 0.5% for TAPP repairs and 0.07% for TEPP

repairs [79]. These are usually secondary to peritoneal tears not repaired at the time of surgery. Small bowel obstruction in the perioperative period following LIHR is best managed with surgically as the hernia is likely at a peritoneal defect causing mechanical obstruction. This can usually be managed laparoscopically with reduction of the hernia and closure of the peritoneal defect.

Laparoscopic Ventral Hernia Repair

Laparoscopic ventral hernia repair (LVHR) has been widely adopted for repair of both ventral and incisional hernias due to its decreased rate of wound complications, visualization of the entire abdominal wall and intra-abdominal placement of mesh with generous overlap and fixation to healthy abdominal wall fascia to ensure a successful repair [80, 81]. The most common complications following LVHR are ileus, seroma, suture site pain, and missed or delayed bowel injury. Ileus can occur in patients undergoing any type of surgery, but those undergoing repairs of ventral hernias requiring extensive adhesiolysis or those with large defects are more prone to development of ileus. Most of the time, the ileus will resolve on its own with conservative management with IV fluids and possibly pro-motility agents. Persistent ileus is present in <1% of all patients undergoing LVHR [80–82]. The importance is to not mistake persistent ileus for internal herniation between the mesh and the abdominal wall. This is a rare complication, but can present as a bowel obstruction of the mesh is not properly secured or if fixation devices fail. This can be diagnosed by abdominal series and/or CT scan. Incidence of seroma increases with size of the defect repaired as fluid fills the space formerly occupied by the hernia contents—in essence, almost all ventral hernia repairs will develop some sort of seroma. Persistent seromas (lasting >4 weeks) are very common after LVHR occurring in 4–10.7% of the population [80–82]. These are usually asymptomatic and can be treated conservatively. In the event that they become symptomatic, the common presentation is pain and these seromas can be aspirated if needed, but again, most seromas resolves and the complication of draining the seroma is that introduction of the needle can lead to infection. Persistent suture site pain is present in 2–3.3% of the population and is usually due to the transfixion sutures used in the repair [80–82]. Occasionally a tacking device can also cause persistent pain by nerve entrapment. Many of these patients will present to the emergency room with complaints of pain at the incision site. Management is usually by the use of anti-inflammatory medications and the pain will usually resolve over time. Local injections are sometimes used in persistent suture site pain and, in the rare occasion, sometimes removal of the anchoring suture is needed to alleviate the pain. The most devastating complication in LVHR is delayed or missed bowel injury. Enterotomy is not an uncommon complication during LVHR occurring in up to 6% of patients undergoing LVHR [80–82]. These are usually appreciated intraoperatively and can be addressed at that time. However, when an injury is missed or delayed, patients will present the first few days after surgery with worsening abdominal pain and may begin showing signs of sepsis such as fever, hypotension, tachycardia, and oliguria. Lab results usually reveal a leukocytosis. These patients should be watched closely and stable patients should undergo radiologic evaluation with a CT scan to rule out an intra-abdominal source for their presentation. If a missed or delayed bowel injury is strongly suspected or proven by radiographic studies, then reoperation with mesh removal should be prompt as this can prove to be a fatal injury.

Complications of Anti-reflux Surgery

Although the majority of gastroesophageal reflux disease (GERD) is treated medically, anti-reflux surgery remains as appropriate and effective management for the treatment GERD refractory to medical treatment or those on lifelong acid suppression. As anti-reflux procedures have evolved, morbidity and mortality have decreased for these procedures as well, but complications do exist for this procedure and can be divided into complications occurring early and late. Early complications occur in 2–3% of patients and include severe dysphagia, gas bloating, bleeding, pneumothorax, wrap herniation, wrap ischemia, and perforation [83–85]. The most common late complication is failure of anti-reflux surgery with return of symptomatic GERD. Failure of surgery as a late complication rarely necessitates immediate operative intervention. Severe dysphagia and food impaction occurs in the postoperative patient between postoperative day 10 and usually resolves within 3 weeks. This is usually due to postoperative edema and usually will resolve on its own. Severe cases lasting longer than 6 weeks will sometimes require esophageal dilatation. If this is necessary than serial dilatations with Savary dilators is preferred over balloon dilatation as it is less likely to disrupt the wrap. Gas bloat is another complication of anti-reflux surgery that usually manifests from a wrap that is too tight or persistent edema. Commonly, this is associated with preoperative delayed gastric emptying. Workup for this is primarily a patient's history. The main complaint is postprandial abdominal pain that makes belching or vomiting difficult. Most of these symptoms will resolve without further intervention, but in some cases it is necessary to perform a gastric emptying study to determine contributing factors to the patient's symptoms. If the symptoms persist, then consideration may be given to placement of a PEG tube as a vent to control the patient's symptoms. In some patients with significant delayed gastric emptying a

pyloroplasty is needed to alleviate the gas bloat symptoms. Postoperative bleeding is unusual occurring in <1% of anti-reflux surgery patients [85]. It is commonly due to hepatic or splenic injury at the time of surgery or from the short gastric vessels. UGI bleeding from a peptic ulcer or gastritis can also occur, but is rare. Management in the stable patient is conservative with possible contrasted CT study to determine a site of bleeding if thought to be from inadvertent injury to the liver or spleen. If the patient presents with hematemesis, then an EGD should be performed to determine the etiology. The limitation of this is that the wrap itself cannot be visualized. In the case of unidentified UGI bleeding in the hemodynamically unstable patient, urgent laparoscopy or laparotomy with take down of the wrap should be performed to allow for endoscopic visualization of the remainder of the stomach. Pneumothorax is another potential complication of anti-reflux surgery secondary to entrance into the pleural cavity during trans-hiatal dissection. It is usually identified at the time of injury, but occasionally this can present in the postoperative period. Small pneumothoraces can be managed conservatively by placing patients on oxygen and serial chest X-rays to determine resolution. Larger and symptomatic pneumothoraces require tube decompression. Wrap migration has an incidence of 7–20% and accounts for up to 84% of failed laparoscopic repairs [83–85]. Acute wrap herniation occurs in 0.5–1.3% [83–85]. This is most commonly preceded by a sudden increase in intra-abdominal pressure as a result of postoperative emesis or coughing. Acute wrap herniation can present with intractable midepigastric abdominal pain, nausea, vomiting, or dysphagia, or in some instances as new onset dysphagia. Workup includes a UGI contrast study that is diagnostic. Early wrap herniation (within the first postoperative week) warrants reoperation involving reduction of the hernia and reconstruction of the esophageal hiatus. If wrap herniation is discovered past the first postoperative week then surgery should be delayed secondary to potential for dense adhesions making the repair tedious. Wrap ischemia with or without perforation is fortunately a rare complication occurring in <1% of all anti-reflux procedures [83–85]. If a leak is suspected then an early UGI contrast study can help aid in the diagnosis. Elderly vasculopathic patients are particularly prone to this complication. Urgent reoperation is indicated when this complication is suspected and can usually be managed laparoscopically. If minimal contamination is encountered then a primary repair covered by a fundoplication or omental patch is a reasonable option. A drain and gastrostomy tube should also be placed in this situation. In the event of gross contamination then drainage with diversion and a venting gastrojejunostomy may be the best option. In the event of gastric ischemia, the resection of the ischemic segment is warranted.

References

1. Seeff LC, Richards TB, Shapiro JA, Nadel MR, Manninen DL, Given LS, Dong FB, Winges LD, McKenna MT. How many endoscopies are performed for colorectal cancer screening? Results from CDC's survey of endoscopic capacity. Gastroenterology. 2004;127(6):1670–7.

2. Sonnenberg A, Amorosi SL, Lacey MJ, Lieberman DA. Patterns of endoscopy in the United States: analysis of data from the Centers for Medicare and Medicaid Services and the National Endoscopic Database. Gastrointest Endosc. 2008;67(3):489–96. Epub 2008 Jan 7.

3. Eisen GM, Baron TH, Dominitz JA, Faigel DO, Goldstein JL, Johanson JF, Mallery JS, Raddawi HM, Vargo JJ, Waring JP, Fanelli RD, Wheeler-Harbough J, American Society for Gastrointestinal Endoscopy. Complications of upper GI endoscopy. Gastrointest Endosc. 2002;55(7):784–93.

4. Svoboda P, Kantorová I, Ochmann J, Kozumplík L, Marsová J. A prospective randomized controlled trial of sclerotherapy vs. ligation in the prophylactic treatment of high-risk esophageal varices. Surg Endosc. 1999;13:580–4.

5. Tait IS, Krige JE, Terblanche J. Endoscopic band ligation of esophageal varices. Br J Surg. 1999;86(4):437–46.

6. Barkun AN, Bardou M, Kuipers EJ, Sung J, Hunt RH, Martel M, International Consensus Upper Gastrointestinal Bleeding Conference Group, et al. International consensus recommendations on the management of patients with nonvariceal upper gastrointestinal bleeding. Ann Intern Med. 2010;152:101–13.

7. Imhof M, Ohmann C, Röher HD, Glutig H, DUESUC Study Group. Endoscopic versus operative treatment in high-risk ulcer bleeding patients—results of a randomised study. Langenbecks Arch Surg. 2003;387:327–36.

8. Kim SK, Duddalwar V. Failed endoscopic therapy and the interventional radiologist: non-variceal upper gastrointestinal bleeding. Tech Gastrointest Endosc. 2005;7:148–55.

9. Lau JY, Sung JJ, Lam YH, Chan AC, Ng EK, Lee DW, et al. Endoscopic retreatment compared with surgery in patients with recurrent bleeding after initial endoscopic control of bleeding ulcers. N Engl J Med. 1999;340:751–6.

10. D'Amico M, Berzigotti A, Garcia-Pagan JC. Refractory acute variceal bleeding: what to do next? Clin Liver Dis. 2010;14(2):297–305.

11. Fleischer DE. Therapy for gastrointestinal bleeding. In: Geenen JE, Fleischer DE, Waye JD, editors. Techniques in therapeutic endoscopy. 2nd ed. New York: Gower Medical Publ. 1992;1.1–1.27.

12. Llach J, Elizalde JI, Guevara MC, Pellisé M, Castellot A, Ginès A, Soria MT, Bordas JM, Piqué JM. Endoscopic injection therapy in bleeding Mallory-Weiss syndrome: a randomized controlled trial. Gastrointest Endosc. 2001;54(6):679–81.

13. Jensen DM. Endoscopic control of nonvariceal upper gastrointestinal hemorrhage. In: Yamada T, Alpers DH, Laine L, Owyang C, Powell DW, editors. Textbook of gastroenterology. Philadelphia, PA: Lippincott Williams and Wilkins; 1999. p. 2857–79.

14. Schmitz RJ, Sharma P, Badr AS, Qamar MT, Weston AP. Incidence and management of esophageal stricture formation, ulcer bleeding, perforation, and massive hematoma formation from sclerotherapy versus band ligation. Am J Gastroenterol. 2001;96(2):437–41.

15. Fernandez FF, Richter A, Freudenberg S, Wendl K, Manegold BC. Treatment of endoscopic esophageal perforation. Surg Endosc. 1999;13(10):962–6.

16. Merchea A, Cullinane DC, Sawyer MD, Iqbal CW, Baron TH, Wigle D, Sarr MG, Zielinski MD. Esophagogastroduodenoscopy-associated gastrointestinal perforations: a single-center experience. Surgery. 2010;148(4):876–80. discussion 881–2. Epub 2010 Aug 14.

17. Wu WT, Chiu CT, Kuo CJ, Lin CJ, Chu YY, Tsou YK, Su MY. Endoscopic management of suspected esophageal foreign body in adults. Dis Esophagus. 2011;24(3):131–7.

18. Eisen GM, Baron TH, Dominitz JA, Faigel DO, Goldstein JL, Johanson JF, Mallery JS, Raddawi HM, Vargo 2nd JJ, Waring JP, Fanelli RD, Wheeler-Harbough J, American Society for Gastrointestinal Endoscopy. Guideline for the management of ingested foreign bodies. Gastrointest Endosc. 2002;55(7):802–6.

19. Vicari JJ, Johanson JF, Frakes JT. Outcomes of acute esophageal food impaction: success of the push technique. Gastrointest Endosc. 2001;53(2):178–81.

20. Freeman RK, Van Woerkom JM, Ascioti AJ. Esophageal stent placement for the treatment of iatrogenic intrathoracic esophageal perforation. Ann Thorac Surg. 2007;83(6):2003–7. discussion 2007–8.

21. Pech O, Bollschweiler E, Manner H, Leers J, Ell C, Hölscher AH. Comparison between endoscopic and surgical resection of mucosal esophageal adenocarcinoma in Barrett's esophagus at two high-volume centers. Ann Surg. 2011;254(1):67–72.

22. Pech O, May A, Gossner L, Rabenstein T, Manner H, Huijsmans J, Vieth M, Stolte M, Berres M, Ell C. Curative endoscopic therapy in patients with early esophageal squamous-cell carcinoma or high-grade intraepithelial neoplasia. Endoscopy. 2007;39(1):30–5.

23. Ko HK, Song HY, Shin JH, Lee GH, Jung HY, Park SI. Fate of migrated esophageal and gastroduodenal stents: experience in 70 patients. J Vasc Interv Radiol. 2007;18(6):725–32.

24. De Palma GD, Iovino P, Catanzano C. Distally migrated esophageal self-expanding metal stents: wait and see or remove? Gastrointest Endosc. 2001;53(1):96–8.

25. Siersema PD. Treatment options for esophageal strictures. Nat Clin Pract Gastroenterol Hepatol. 2008;5(3):142–52. Epub 2008 Feb 5.

26. Hirota WK, Petersen K, Baron TH, Goldstein JL, Jacobson BC, Leighton JA, Mallery JS, Waring JP, Fanelli RD, Wheeler-Harbough J, Faigel DO, Standards of Practice Committee of the American Society for Gastrointestinal Endoscopy. Guidelines for antibiotic prophylaxis for GI endoscopy. Gastrointest Endosc. 2003;58(4):475–82.

27. Schrag SP, Sharma R, Jaik NP, Seamon MJ, Lukaszczyk JJ, Martin ND, Hoey BA, Stawicki SP. Complications related to percutaneous endoscopic gastrostomy (PEG) tubes. A comprehensive clinical review. J Gastrointestin Liver Dis. 2007;16(4):407–18. Review.

28. Nicholson FB, Korman MG, Richardson MA. Percutaneous endoscopic gastrostomy: a review of indications, complications and outcome. J Gastroenterol Hepatol. 2000;15(1):21–5. Review.

29. ASGE Standards of Practice Committee, Jain R, Maple JT, Anderson MA, Appalaneni V, Ben-Menachem T, Decker GA, Fanelli RD, Fisher L, Fukami N, Ikenberry SO, Jue T, Khan K, Krinsky ML, Malpas P, Sharaf RN, Dominitz JA. The role of endoscopy in enteral feeding. Gastrointest Endosc. 2011;74(1):7–12.

30. Reissman P, Durst AL. Splenic hematoma: a rare complication of colonoscopy. Surg Endosc. 1998;12:154–5.

31. Pothula A, Lampert J, Mazeh H, Eisenberg D, Shen H. Splenic rupture as a complication of colonoscopy: report of a case. Surg Today. 2010;40:68–71.

32. Levin TR, Zharo W, Conell C, Seeff LC, Manninen DL, Shapiro JA, et al. Complications of colonoscopy in an integrated health care delivery system. Ann Intern Med. 2006;145(12):880–6.

33. Waye JD, Kahn O, Auerbach ME. Colonoscopy: a prospective report of complications. J Clin Gastroenterol. 1992;15:347–51.

34. Flegal KM, Carroll MD, Ogden CL, Curtin LR. Prevalence and trends in obesity among US adults, 1999–2008. JAMA. 2010;303(3):235–41.

35. Consensus Development Conference Panel. Conference NIH: gastrointestinal surgery for severe obesity. Ann Intern Med. 1991;115:956–61.

36. Steinbrook R. Surgery for severe obesity. N Engl J Med. 2004;350:1075–9.

37. Monkhouse SJ, Morgan JD, Norton SA. Complications of bariatric surgery: presentation and emergency management—a review. Ann R Coll Surg Engl. 2009;91(4):280–6. Epub 2009 Apr 2. Review.

38. Chandler JG, Corson SL, Way LW. Three spectra of laparoscopic entry access injuries. J Am Coll Surg. 2001;192(4):478–90.

39. Geers J, Holden C. Major vascular injury as a complication of laparoscopic surgery. Am Surg. 1996;62:377–9.

40. Saville LE, Woods MS. Laparoscopy and major retroperitoneal vascular injuries. Surg Endosc. 1995;9:1096–100.

41. Hashizume M, Sugimachi K. Needle and trocar injury during laparoscopic surgery in Japan. Surg Endosc. 1997;11:1198–201.

42. Suter M, Donadini A, Calmes J-M, Romy S. Improved surgical technique for laparoscopic Roux-en-Y gastric bypass reduces complications at the gastrojejunostomy. Obes Surg. 2010;20:841–5.

43. Edwards MA, Jones DB, Ellsmere J, Grinbaum R, Schneider BE. Anastomotic leak following antecolic versus retrocolic laparoscopic Roux-en-Y gastric bypass for morbid obesity. Obes Surg. 2007;17(3):292–7.

44. Gonzalez R, Haines K, Gallagher SF, Murr MM. Does experience preclude leaks in laparoscopic gastric bypass? Surg Endosc. 2006;20(11):1687–92. Epub 2006 Sep 6.

45. Gonzalez R, Sarr MG, Smith CD, Baghai M, Kendrick M, Szomstein S, Rosenthal R, Murr MM. Diagnosis and contemporary management of anastomotic leaks after gastric bypass for obesity. J Am Coll Surg. 2007;204(1):47–55. Epub 2006 Nov 17.

46. Lee S, Carmody B, Wolfe L, Demaria E, Kellum JM, Sugerman H, Maher JW. Effect of location and speed of diagnosis on anastomotic leak outcomes in 3828 gastric bypass cases. J Gastrointest Surg. 2007;11(6):708–13.

47. Madan AK, Lanier B, Tichansky DS. Laparoscopic repair of gastrointestinal leaks after laparoscopic gastric bypass. Am Surg. 2006;72(7):586–90. discussion 590–1.

48. Nguyen NT, Hinojosa M, Fayad C, Varela E, Wilson SE. Use and outcomes of laparoscopic versus open gastric bypass at academic medical centers. J Am Coll Surg. 2007;205(2):248–55. Epub 2007 Jun 27.

49. Schweitzer MA, Lidor A, Magnuson TH. A zero leak rate in 251 consecutive laparoscopic gastric bypass operations using a two-layer gastrojejunostomy technique. J Laparoendosc Adv Surg Tech A. 2006;16(2):83–7.

50. Kirshtein B, Lantsberg L, Mizrahi S, Avinoach E. Bariatric emergencies for non-bariatric surgeons: complications of laparoscopic gastric banding. Obes Surg. 2010;20(11):1468–78. Epub 2010 Jan 15.

51. Papakonstantinou A, Terzis L, Stratopoulos C, Mablekou E, Papadimitriou N, Hadjiyannakis E. Bleeding from the upper gastrointestinal tract after Mason's vertical banded gastroplasty. Obes Surg. 2000;10(6):582–4.

52. Goergen M, Arapis K, Limgba A, Schiltz M, Lens V, Azagra JS. Laparoscopic Roux-en-Y gastric bypass versus laparoscopic vertical banded gastroplasty: results of a 2-year follow-up study. Surg Endosc. 2007;21(4):659–64. Epub 2006 Dec 16.

53. de la Cruz-Muñoz N, Cabrera JC, Cuesta M, Hartnett S, Rojas R. Closure of mesenteric defect can lead to decrease in internal hernias after Roux-en-Y gastric bypass. Surg Obes Relat Dis. 2011;7(2):176–80. Epub 2010 Oct 16.

54. Ahmed AR, Rickards G, Husain S, Johnson J, Boss T, O'Malley W. Trends in internal hernia incidence after laparoscopic Roux-en-Y gastric bypass. Obes Surg. 2007;17(12):1563–6. Epub 2007 Nov 15.

55. Cho M, Pinto D, Carrodeguas L, Lascano C, Soto F, Whipple O, Simpfendorfer C, Gonzalvo JP, Zundel N, Szomstein S, Rosenthal RJ. Frequency and management of internal hernias after laparoscopic antecolic antegastric Roux-en-Y gastric bypass without division of the small bowel mesentery or closure of mesenteric defects: review of 1400 consecutive cases. Surg Obes Relat Dis. 2006;2(2):87–91. Epub 2006 Mar 3.

56. Garza Jr E, Kuhn J, Arnold D, Nicholson W, Reddy S, McCarty T. Internal hernias after laparoscopic Roux-en-Y gastric bypass. Am J Surg. 2004;188(6):796–800.

57. Lockhart ME, Tessler FN, Canon CL, Smith JK, Larrison MC, Fineberg NS, Roy BP, Clements RH. Internal hernia after gastric bypass: sensitivity and specificity of seven CT signs with surgical correlation and controls. AJR Am J Roentgenol. 2007;188(3):745–50.

58. Takata MC, Ciovica R, Cello JP, Posselt AM, Rogers SJ, Campos GM. Predictors, treatment, and outcomes of gastrojejunostomy stricture after gastric bypass for morbid obesity. Obes Surg. 2007;17(7):878–84.

59. Nguyen NT, Stevens CM, Wolfe BM. Incidence and outcome of anastomotic stricture after laparoscopic gastric bypass. J Gastrointest Surg. 2003;7(8):997–1003. discussion 1003.

60. Goitein D, Papasavas PK, Gagné D, Ahmad S, Caushaj PF. Gastrojejunal strictures following laparoscopic Roux-en-Y gastric bypass for morbid obesity. Surg Endosc. 2005;19(5):628–32. Epub 2005 Mar 11.

61. Rasmussen JJ, Fuller W, Ali MR. Marginal ulceration after laparoscopic gastric bypass: an analysis of predisposing factors in 260 patients. Surg Endosc. 2007;21(7):1090–4. Epub 2007 May 19.

62. Gumbs AA, Duffy AJ, Bell RL. Incidence and management of marginal ulceration after laparoscopic Roux-Y gastric bypass. Surg Obes Relat Dis. 2006;2(4):460–3.

63. Dallal RM, Bailey LA. Ulcer disease after gastric bypass surgery. Surg Obes Relat Dis. 2006;2(4):455–9.

64. Felix EL, Kettelle J, Mobley E, Swartz D. Perforated marginal ulcers after laparoscopic gastric bypass. Surg Endosc. 2008;22(10):2128–32. Epub 2008 Jun 14.

65. Eid I, Birch DW, Sharma AM, Sherman V, Karmali S. Complications associated with adjustable gastric banding for morbid obesity: a surgeon's guides. Can J Surg. 2011;54(1):61–6. Review.

66. Allen JW. Laparoscopic gastric band complications. Med Clin North Am. 2007;91(3):485–97. xii. Review.

67. Mozzi E, Lattuada E, Zappa MA, Granelli P, De Ruberto F, Armocida A, Roviaro G. Treatment of band erosion: feasibility and safety of endoscopic band removal. Surg Endosc. 2011;25(12):3918–22. Epub ahead of print.

68. Shah KG, Molmenti EP, Nicastro J. Gastric band erosion and intraluminal migration leading to biliary and small bowel obstruction: case report and discussion. Surg Obes Relat Dis. 2011;7(1):117–8. Epub 2010 Feb 6.

69. O'Brien PE, Dixon JB. Weight loss and early and late complications—the international experience. Am J Surg. 2002;184(6B):42S–5.

70. Shi X, Karmali S, Sharma AM, Birch DW. A review of laparoscopic sleeve gastrectomy for morbid obesity. Obes Surg. 2010;20(8):1171–7. Review.

71. Lalor PF, Tucker ON, Szomstein S, Rosenthal RJ. Complications after laparoscopic sleeve gastrectomy. Surg Obes Relat Dis. 2008;4(1):33–8. Epub 2007 Nov 5.

72. Fuks D, Verhaeghe P, Brehant O, Sabbagh C, Dumont F, Riboulot M, Delcenserie R, Regimbeau JM. Results of laparoscopic sleeve gastrectomy: a prospective study in 135 patients with morbid obesity. Surgery. 2009;145(1):106–13. Epub 2008 Sep 30.

73. Tan JT, Kariyawasam S, Wijeratne T, Chandraratna HS. Diagnosis and management of gastric leaks after laparoscopic sleeve gastrectomy for morbid obesity. Obes Surg. 2010;20(4):403–9.

74. Wherry DC, Marohn MR, Malanoski MP, et al. An external audit of laparoscopic cholecystectomy in the steady state performed in medical treatment facilities of the department of defense. Ann Surg. 1996;224(2):145–54.

75. Soper NJ, Swanstrom LL, Eubanks WS. Mastery of endoscopic and laparoscopic surgery. 3rd ed. Publisher Lippincott Williams and Wilkins, 2009

76. Pavlidis TE. Current opinion on laparoscopic repair of inguinal hernia. Surg Endosc. 2010;24(4):974–6. Epub 2009 Sep 19.

77. Ramshaw B, Shuler FW, Jones HB, Duncan TD, White J, Wilson R, Lucas GW, Mason EM. Laparoscopic inguinal hernia repair: lessons learned after 1224 consecutive cases. Surg Endosc. 2001;15(1):50–4.

78. Balakrishnan S, Singhal T, Samdani T, Hussain A, Shuaib S, Grandy-Smith S, Nicholls J, El-Hasani S. Laparoscopic inguinal hernia repair: over a thousand convincing reasons to go on. Hernia. 2008;12(5):493–8. Epub 2008 May 22.

79. McKay R. Preperitoneal herniation and bowel obstruction post laparoscopic inguinal hernia repair: case report and review of the literature. Hernia. 2008;12(5):535–7. Epub 2008 Feb 9. Review.

80. Heniford BT, Ramshaw BJ. Laparoscopic ventral hernia repair: a report of 100 consecutive cases. Surg Endosc. 2000;14(5):419–23.

81. Perrone JM, Soper NJ, Eagon JC, Klingensmith ME, Aft RL, Frisella MM, Brunt LM. Perioperative outcomes and complications of laparoscopic ventral hernia repair. Surgery. 2005;138(4):708–15. discussion 715–6.

82. Bedi AP, Bhatti T, Amin A, Zuberi J. Laparoscopic incisional and ventral hernia repair. J Minim Access Surg. 2007;3(3):83–90.

83. Morgenthal CB, Lin E, Shane MD, Hunter JG, Smith CD. Who will fail laparoscopic Nissen fundoplication? Preoperative prediction of long-term outcomes. Surg Endosc. 2007;21(11):1978–84. Epub 2007 Jul 11.

84. Smith CD, McClusky DA, Rajad MA, Lederman AB, Hunter JG. When fundoplication fails: redo? Ann Surg. 2005;241(6):861–9. discussion 869–71.

85. Singhal T, Balakrishnan S, Hussain A, Grandy-Smith S, Paix A, El-Hasani S. Management of complications after laparoscopic Nissen's fundoplication: a surgeon's perspective. Ann Surg Innov Res. 2009;3:1.

Robert G. Martindale, Clifford W. Deveney, Sara Bubenik, and Svetang Desai

Introduction

There has been a virtual explosion in the number of bariatric procedures done in the USA and globally in the past 5 years. It is anticipated that more than 200,000 bariatric procedures will be done in the USA in 2012. Bariatric procedures carried out today are generally safe, in most cases effective, and commonly cost-effective in the total health care cost of this population [1]. This chapter reviews the short- and long-term complications of bariatric procedure.

Bariatric operations are designed to reduce excess weight by either reducing the amount of food one consumes (restrictive) or by causing malabsorption and/or maldigestion of an ingested meal. Numerous variations on this theme of procedures have been attempted with variable success [2]. Presently, there are two widely accepted procedures that are purely restrictive: laparoscopic adjustable gastric band (LAGB) and sleeve gastrectomy (SG). There are three widely utilized bariatric procedures which are a combination of restrictive and malabsorptive. Roux-en-Y gastric bypass (RYGBP) is primarily restrictive but does have a malabsorptive component from the bypassed stomach, duodenum, and proximal jejunum. Biliopancreatic diversion with duodenal switch (BPD-DS) is primarily malabsorptive, but has a restrictive component because a sleeve gastrectomy is performed as part of this procedure. Biliopancreatic diversion (BPD) as described by Scopanaro is a purely malabsorptive procedure. Because of the relatively high frequency of metabolic complications (e.g.,

malnutrition, osteoporosis) following procedures that rely on malabsorption primarily (BPD, BPD-DS), these procedures are less often performed in the USA. Descriptions of these procedures can be found in several articles [1, 2].

The complications following bariatric surgery can be loosely divided into metabolic, nutritional, infectious, and anatomic. The complications can also be divided into acute perioperative complications and long-term complications (Table 33.1). While nearly all patients develop some metabolic or nutritional compromise in the months to years following bariatric surgery, the infectious and anatomic complications occur in a small percentage [3–5].

Anatomic Complications Following Bariatric Surgery

When discussing anatomic complications, it is worthwhile to separate those problems directly related to surgery (e.g., anastomotic leakage, pneumonias, pulmonary embolus, etc.) versus those that occur as a result of the anatomy of the operation (i.e., internal hernias, diarrhea, hypoglycemia, etc.).

Overall, the surgical mortality and morbidity from bariatric procedures is very low when procedures can be performed laparoscopically, except under extenuating circumstances (e.g., extensive intra-abdominal adhesions, extremely high body mass index). Factors associated with increased mortality and morbidity were nicely described by Wolfe et al. [1, 6].

Obviously, the technically easier operations have lower complication rates than the most complex operations. That is to say that complication rates for LAGB (technically the easiest operation) report fewer complications than for BPD-DS with GS and RYGBP having complication rates between these two extremes. In a study involving outcomes of 4,776 patients undergoing bariatric surgery from ten centers, the 30-day mortality was 0.3% with 4.3% of patients having at least one adverse outcome [1]. These numbers are quite low and are very acceptable when one examines risks versus gains from the surgery.

R.G. Martindale, M.D., Ph.D. (✉)
C.W. Deveney, M.D. • S. Bubenik, M.D.
Division of General Surgery, Department of Surgery,
Oregon Health and Science University,
3181 SW Sam Jackson Park Road, L223A, Portland,
OR 97239, USA
e-mail: martindr@ohsu.edu

S. Desai, M.D.
Division of Gastroenterology, Duke University
Medical Center, Durham, NC, USA

L.J. Moore et al. (eds.), *Common Problems in Acute Care Surgery*,
DOI 10.1007/978-1-4614-6123-4_33, © Springer Science+Business Media New York 2013

Table 33.1 Complications of bariatric surgery

Complications of bariatric surgery	
Short-term (first 30–90 days)	Long-term
Nausea/vomiting	Fistulae • Gastro-gastric, gastro-cutaneous, etc.
Dehydration	Diarrhea • Maldigestion, malabsorption, bacterial overgrowth
Fatigue	Dumping
Anastomotic stricture	Reactive hypoglycemia
Leaks/sepsis	Failure to maintain weight loss
GI bleed • Marginal/anastomotic ulcerations • Staple line hemorrhage	Vitamin and mineral deficiency
Venous thromboembolic disease/DVT	Bowel obstruction • Adhesions, internal hernias
Wound complications	Ventral hernia
Band slippage	Anastomotic stricture Anastomotic ulcerations Gallstones Gastric band erosion Gastric band slippage Band infections

Immediate Perioperative Complications

Although immediate postoperative complication rates in bariatric surgery are relatively low, they are potentially lethal. In the morbidly obese person, symptoms of a complication may be subtle and extremely difficult to diagnose often yielding a delay in treatment. The physician caring for these patients should be aware of the potential complications and their presentation, however subtle they may be. Recent litigation would indicate that even surgeons who do not perform bariatric surgery are required to understand and be aware of the complications of bariatric surgery if they see surgical consults involving bariatric patients in the emergent setting [7, 8].

For any operation involving suture or staple lines (i.e., RYGBP, BPD, SG), one worries about leakage from a suture line. Leak from a suture line can produce a collection of findings that are associated with sepsis. Mental changes (agitation, disorientation), sustained tachycardia ($p > 120$/min), fever, and renal failure are all manifestations of a suture line leak. These symptoms often occur without overt signs of peritonitis secondary to the difficulty of the abdominal exam in the morbidly obese [9]. The patient often presents with only one or two of these manifestations, so the physician must have a high index of suspicion. When recognized early and treated promptly, the patient usually survives with little morbidity. If diagnosis is delayed until the patient becomes overtly septic (i.e., hypotensive, in respiratory and renal failure), the

prognosis is much worse, and in some instances will lead to death. If one suspects a suture line leak and the patient is stable, the leak can be confirmed or excluded by computed tomography (CT) scan with oral contrast. Anastomotic breaches may also be investigated with an endoscopic approach. If the leak is noted at the time of endoscopy, there have been numerous reports of covered metal stents across the leak with initiation of oral nutrition leading to closure of the leak [10–12]. This study has been shown to be effective in up to 81% of patients (17 of 21) [13]. Recent studies have shown leaks with fistualization can also be treated endoscopically [14].

If the surgeon is relatively sure that a leak is present and the patient is unstable, the patient should be taken to the operating room for exploratory laparoscopy or laparotomy. Commonly, intraoperative endoscopy is helpful in finding the location of small areas of leak from the staple lines. Operative treatment of the leak consists of irrigation, reinforcement of the suture line, and wide drainage [9, 15, 16]. With this treatment, the leak often stops or an enterocutaneous fistula occurs along the drain tract. If the fistula is resulting from a small leak, it will commonly close with conservative management. With larger leaks, a secondary surgery will be required for closure several months later. Attempting to do major reconstructive surgery in the face of a leak and infection is fraught with complications and results in anastomotic failure commonly [9]. While surgery with drainage is the mainstay of therapy, their stable patients can be managed non-operatively as long as adequate drainage can be assured.

Fortunately, leakage from a suture or staple line occurs in less than 2% of patients undergoing a primary bariatric procedure. Again, the patient's obesity and recent surgery makes the abdominal exam much less reliable in diagnosing postoperative leaks. Therefore, the surgeon or emergency department physician must have a high level of suspicion and rely on evaluating multiple criteria (e.g., pulse rate, respiratory status, temperature, white blood cell count, etc.), which could help determine evidence of leak.

Other acute complications in bariatric surgery populations that occur in the immediate postoperative period are similar to those non-obese patients undergoing abdominal major surgery with the exception of wound infection, which occurs in 20–30% of obese patients undergoing an open (non-laparoscopic) bariatric procedure [17]. Wound infections should be treated as any other post-op wound infections with the caveat that the risk of deep fluid/purulent collections that are inadequately drained are more common than in the lower body mass index (BMI) patient [18]. Bariatric surgeons are concerned about the potential for post-op thrombophlebitis and pulmonary embolus in these patients; and prophylactic low molecular weight heparin, as well as anti-embolus stockings, is recommended in the postoperative period. The reported incidence of clinical pulmonary embolus is low (0.3–0.6%) and compares with the incidence in non-obese patients [19]. Pulmonary embolus often presents as persistent O_2 desaturation as measured by pulse oximeter or arterial blood gas. When suspected, pulmonary embolus (PE) should be excluded with a pulmonary angio CT scan, and if PE is present, the patient should be fully anticoagulated for 6 weeks.

Most bariatric patients are thoroughly assessed for coronary artery and pulmonary disease preoperatively; and consequently, the incidence of postoperative respiratory failure, heart failure, or pneumonia is extremely low [20].

Lap bands have the potential to develop a unique set of postoperative complications, including band slippage, unrecognized perforation of the esophagus, infection, and erosion into the stomach. Bands can "slip" in the acute setting following surgery or long after the initial procedure. The slippage occurs when the band "slips" more distal along the greater or lesser curvature and the distal stomach herniates through the band. This complication is usually manifested by the inability to tolerate anything by mouth and rather severe abdominal pain [21]. The diagnosis is made by a contrast swallow. Water soluble contrast is suggested as the first attempt; and if no leaks are present, barium can be used to better define the anatomy [22]. A slipped band should be acutely repositioned surgically; this can usually be done laparoscopically. If adequately skilled bariatric surgical support is unavailable to reposition the band should be removed. This procedure can be usually be done by freeing up the band cautiously with cautery then when adequately exposed just cut the band and remove. If concern for gastric injury exists, the band removal can be combined with endoscopy to evaluate for small leaks. Allowing the slipped portion of the stomach to remain for prolonged periods will often result in ischemia and full thickness necrosis of the herniated segment of stomach [23]. (See "Band Slippage" in next section.)

Long-Term Complications

Long-term complications in bariatric patients fall into three groups: post-op adhesions, metabolic complications, and complications which are procedure specific.

As with any intra-abdominal surgery, postoperative adhesions causing bowel obstruction are a risk when bariatric procedures are performed. Most bariatric procedures are now performed laparoscopically, and there are minimal adhesions following laparoscopic procedures.

Postoperative incisional hernias are very common (up to 30%) following open bariatric procedures [24, 25]. Trocar site hernias following laparoscopic bariatric procedures are reported to occur between 0 and 5.2% of the time [26, 27].

Patient risk factors for trocar site hernias are older age and higher body mass index. Technical risk factors for trocar site hernias are related to the design and size of trocars [26].

Internal Hernia

Both biliopancreatic diversion with or without duodenal switch and gastric bypass are procedures that employ Roux-en-Y reconstruction; and with this reconstruction, the patients can develop internal hernias. Three types of internal hernias make up the majority of these herniations following bariatric procedures. These include (1) hernia through the transverse mesocolon into the lesser sac, (2) internal rotation of the biliary limb under the Roux-en-Y limb (often called Petersen Hernia), and (3) herniation through the divided leaves of the mesentery where the jejunojejunostomy was performed [4, 28]. The usual presentation for internal hernias is quite variable. The presentation can be from subtle vague intermittent cramping epigastric pain to severe unrelenting constant abdominal pain making this diagnosis very difficult. It may present as closed loop bowel obstruction with ischemia or necrosis of the loop [29]. One must remember also that with the Roux-en-Y reconstruction, the biliary limb can become obstructed without having the alimentary limb obstructed; and thus a standard upper gastrointestinal (GI) series with small bowel follow-through may appear normal when the biliary limb is obstructed. CT scan is the best test to diagnose obstruction of the biliary limb and internal hernia in general [29, 30]. When a patient presents with post-gastric bypass abdominal pain or has abdominal pain from biliary pancreatic diversion, a CT scan should be performed to help rule out obstruction of the biliary limb; the scan will sometimes diagnose internal hernias. If the CT is negative, laparoscopy or laparotomy may be required to rule out internal hernia.

Marginal Ulcerations

Roux-en-Y reconstruction consists of anastomosing jejunum to gastric pouch (in RYGBP) or duodenum (in BPD). This reconstruction is ulcerogenic, as the jejunum is without buffering components from pancreatic and biliary secretions, so marginal ulcers can occur after these two procedures [31, 32]. If the ulceration occurs on the jejunal side, it is most likely secondary to acid exposure and will most likely respond to treatment with H_2 receptor antagonists or proton pump inhibitors. However, if the ulcer occurs on the gastric pouch side of the anastomosis, it is most likely due to ischemia in that part of the pouch and may need resection. The majority of these patients will respond to treatment with proton pump inhibitors (PPI), which confirms that unbuffered acidity is the major cause of these lesions. The incidence of anastomotic ulcers varies from 3 to 12%. These ulcers may be under diagnosed since a substantial (>5%) number may be asymptomatic. The majority of these ulcers occur acutely, that is within 1 year from surgery [33, 34]. The development of marginal ulcers is higher in patients who had history of *H. pylori* infections even when eradication has been attempted [35]. Marginal ulcer formation is also common source of blood loss. Most bleeds can be managed conservatively with proton pump inhibitors (PPI) via IV or infusion and blood transfusion; however, if the bleeding remains persistent, endoscopic evaluation is warranted. When source of bleeding is noted, hemostasis should be achieved with the use of endoscopic clips over cautery or epinephrine injection as the clips do not produce additional tissue injury [36]. Although most marginal ulcerations heal with PPI therapy, there will be some that are recalcitrant to PPI therapy or that result in an anastomotic stricture not amenable to dilatation. These ulcers are treated with resection of the gastrojejunostomy with formation of a new gastrojejunostomy [37].

Anastomotic strictures can be secondary to technical problems constructing the anastomosis, chronic inflammation of the tissue around the anastomosis, an ulcer at the anastomosis, or ischemia. Strictures are primarily treated with PPIs and balloon dilation up to 15–18 mm. This has been shown to have a success rate of up to 93% in symptom resolution and subsequent resumption in weight loss [38]. It is often necessary to dilate multiple times, but if the stricture recurs following the third dilatation, it is usually an indication for elective resection and making a new anastomosis. Like marginal ulcers, strictures occur rather acutely following surgery, and it is unusual to see a new stricture forming after 1 year. Anastomotic strictures following bariatric surgery occur about 3% of the time, and it is often difficult to determine the exact etiology (i.e., technical versus ulcer or ischemia [39]). The symptoms produced by marginal ulcers or anastomotic strictures are chronic epigastric pain and often symptoms of gastric outlet obstruction. The diagnosis is made endoscopically, and the treatment is proton pump inhibitors at least initially [40].

Patients following Roux-en-Y gastric bypass are also known to have a higher incidence of intussusception of small intestine [41, 42]. When a patient who has had a Roux-en-Y gastric bypass presents with bowel obstruction and epigastric pain, one must consider intussusception as a possible cause. The bloody or "currant jelly" stools often seen in ileocolic intussusception is not commonly seen in intussusception following gastric bypass surgery [43].

Surgeons and emergency department (ED) physicians are often presented with a patient who has had RYGH or BPD who presents with abdominal pain or symptoms suggestive of bowel obstruction; one must consider not only adhesions as the cause, but also internal hernia and intussusception. In someone presents with epigastric pain or occult hemorrhage and possible symptoms of gastric outlet obstruction, marginal ulcer or stricture is a probable diagnosis.

Slippage of the Gastric Band

Those patients with LAB have minimal to no problems with adhesions or internal hernias since their anatomy has not been altered. Their problems are related to the band and its attachments (i.e., tubing and reservoir). These problems are principally slippage of the band, erosion of the band, infection of the port site, and malfunction of the insufflation system (leakage from the port, tubing, or the balloon on the inside of the band [44–46]).

Symptoms of slippage are often manifested by symptoms of gastric outlet obstruction; that is, early satiety, nausea, and vomiting. This slippage occurs when the posterior and greater curvature aspects of the stomach herniate through the band, placing a significantly greater amount of stomach on the proximal or cephalad side of the band. Slippage can occur acutely or gradually. The diagnosis is best made with an upper GI (UGI) series, which will demonstrate the herniated stomach with limited or no passage of contrast beyond the band [22]. A plain film of the abdomen may show the band at an inappropriate angle or tilt [22]. When this problem occurs acutely, it is an emergency and should be treated promptly because the herniated stomach may be at risk for ischemia and perforation [22]. Repositioning of the band with reduction of the hernia can often be done; however, occasionally, it is necessary to remove the band. These procedures can virtually always be performed laparoscopically unless it is associated with band erosion [22].

Band Erosion

Band erosion occurs when the band erodes through part or all of the gastric wall. This process occurs gradually and most commonly does not produce peritonitis from free leakage of gastric content into the peritoneal cavity [47]. The erosion may be asymptomatic and manifest by weight gain, as the constrictive effect of the band can be lost [47]. Another common manifestation of transmural band erosion is infection of the port site on the abdominal wall. As the contamination from gastric contents seeds the exposed gastric band, it forms a biofilm containing viable bacteria along the length of the tubing to the port [45, 48]. Upper GI hemorrhage, often acute and severe, can also occur secondary to band erosion [49, 50]. When band erosion is suspected for any of these symptoms, endoscopy should be performed, and a segment of the band will most often be seen on the luminal side of the stomach. If on plain X-ray of the abdomen the band is unusually angled, this also would suggest erosion.

CT is very helpful in making diagnoses of the more subtle band erosions. It will usually show the change in angulation and often show air outside the lumen of the stomach at the site of the band erosion [51].

In virtually all cases of transmural erosion, the band should be removed because it has the potential to produce infectious complications (i.e., infection of the extra-gastric parts of the band and local abscesses and hemorrhage) and because it usually loses its effectiveness in weight loss. Eroded bands can sometimes be removed endoscopically when the buckle has eroded into the stomach [52, 53]. They are most often removed laparoscopically and can in some cases be removed endoscopically [54]. Following removal the surgeon must insure that no unsecured or unrecognized defects in the gastric wall remain. This is done by combining endoscopy with air insufflation watching for leaks. Once removed and leaks are ruled out, the patient usually can undergo a subsequent bariatric procedure such as sleeve gastrectomy or gastric bypass.

Biliary Disease

Rapid weight loss that occurs following bariatric procedures leads to gallstone formation in up to 50% of patients [55]; however, only 10% will develop symptomatic gallstones, and these patients can be treated with cholecystectomy [56, 57]. Treatment with Ursodiol for 6 months postoperatively will lower the incidence of gallstones by as much as 50% [58]; therefore, the most common algorithm in performing bariatric surgery is to not perform cholecystectomy in the patient who is asymptomatic at the time of his or her bariatric procedure and to prophylactically treat with Ursodiol for 6 months postoperatively. However, these patients are at risk to develop cholecystitis in the future and should have cholecystectomy when and if they become symptomatic. To evaluate a symptomatic patient for the presence of stones magnetic resonance imaging in the form of magnetic resonance cholangiopancreatography (MRCP) or computed tomography is preferred to ultrasound because body fat can distort imaging leading to missed diagnosis [59, 60]. Proven gallstones via imaging should still be approached with endoscopy. Given the complex postsurgical anatomy Laparoscopic-assisted and enteroscopy with either balloon or rotational device have been used to achieve stone extraction prior to cholecystectomy [61].

Metabolic and Nutritional Complications

Restrictive and malabsorptive bariatric surgery significantly alters anatomical space and digestive physiology commonly prompting certain nutritional deficiencies and metabolic complications. Globally in bariatric surgery, the most common nutritional deficits encountered are iron, protein, calcium, vitamin B12, and vitamin D deficiencies. Complications after the restrictive/malabsorptive (RYGPB) and malabsorptive (BPD, BPD-DS) procedures contribute to the majority of observed short-term and long-term metabolic imbalances and overt deficiencies (Table 33.2). More specific nutritional complications are observed after restrictive procedures (banding); however, these deficits are much less common and usually related to changes in dietary patterns, food choices

Table 33.2 Etiology of postoperative nutritional deficiencies

Etiology of postoperative nutritional deficiencies
• Caution: estimated 15% deficient pre-op!
○ Altered dietary intake
○ Decreased intake
○ Small pouch
○ Change in food preferences
• Anatomic post-op complications of the procedure
• Malabsorption of ingested nutrients
○ Decreased intestinal absorptive surface area
○ Altered mixing and preparation
• Deficiency will depend on:
○ The procedure performed
○ The individual patient compliance
• Deficiency can develop years later
• Serum levels often not accurate measure of deficiency

and noncompliance with the post-op nutritional supplement recommendations.

At least 30% of bariatric surgery patients will develop some nutrition-related complication [62]. These complications are typically a macronutrient or micronutrient deficiency, and commonly both deficiencies develop [63, 64]. Numerous specific nutrient related complications have been widely reported, and these include anemia iron; folate; vitamins B12, A, and E, copper and zinc deficiencies; all of which can result in anemia and/or metabolic bone disease resulting from calcium and/or vitamin D deficiency. Other specifics include protein-energy malnutrition, steatorrhea, Wernicke encephalopathy (thiamine), polyneuropathy and myopathy (thiamine, copper, vitamins B12 and E), visual disturbance (vitamins A and E, thiamine), skin rash (zinc, essential fatty acids, vitamin A), and a litany of non-symptomatic or clinically silent micronutrient deficiencies. The etiology of most nutrition deficiencies following bariatric surgery is multifactorial, with contributions from reduced dietary intake, altered dietary choices, and malabsorption.

The most common trace mineral deficiency following RYGB and BPD is iron with up to one-third of patients having low ferritin stores [65, 66]. Deficiencies in B12, although less common than iron depletion, typically follow bariatric procedures as well. Two mechanisms are known to cause depleted ferritin stores and decreased B12, they include decreased intake of foods rich in these nutrients and/or anastomotic changes related to these bariatric procedures. These anastomotic changes can cause inadequate digestion of meats to release B12 and iron. If not released from the native source, B12 is not able to bind with R protein or intrinsic factor thereby decreasing net absorption. Supplementation of B12 is required following RYGB. Folic acid deficiency occurs less frequently than iron or vitamin B12 deficiency; however, one-third of patients with folic acid deficiency are also depleted in serum vitamin B12 [30]. Folate supplementation is important in all women of childbearing age, but becomes critically important in women who are post-bariatric procedures, to prevent fetal neural tube defects. Serum deficiencies are easily corrected with vitamin supplementation [67].

The frequency of thiamine deficiency is relatively rare after bariatric surgery; but when it occurs, the consequences can be serious and life threatening. Thiamine deficiency may lead to Wernicke encephalopathy, which has been described after gastric bypass surgery [68, 69]. As previously described, the reduction in dietary intake of thiamine is often the primary cause, but malabsorption and bacterial overgrowth of the small bowel also play a role. A common scenario occurs after several visits to an ED for nausea and vomiting with inadequate PO intake between visits. This is usually a result of an anastomotic stricture. The patient receives IV hydration and D5 and then develops acute Wernicke's encephalopathy. Supplementation of IV multivitamins with the hydration should correct or prevent this deficiency; however, in serious cases IM/IV thiamine is warranted.

In general, vitamin D deficiency is common in the obese population both preoperatively and postoperatively. Patients within 3–9 months after gastric bypass have an increase in bone resorption associated with a decrease in bone mass as compared to controls [30, 70]. Vitamin D and calcium are absorbed preferentially in the jejunum and ileum. Nonetheless, there have been reports of osteomalacia and secondary hyper-parathyroidism after RYGB [71]. Daily supplementation of 400 IU of vitamin D and 1,500 mg of elemental calcium is adequate to maintain sufficient levels. Deficiencies of fat-soluble vitamins A, D, and K will be deficient in two-thirds of these patients within 4 years after surgery [62].

Protein deficiencies are uncommon with RYGB and have a higher association with BPD procedures. Two retrospective studies demonstrated that decreased serum albumin was negligible in both RYGB and BPD 1–2 years after the procedure. Many of the cases are secondary to noncompliance with protein supplements or a relative meat intolerance of unknown etiology. Often following duodenal switch, patients have either decreased protein intake or suffer from protein malabsorption resulting in hypoalbuminemia, anemia, edema, weakness, and alopecia, which characterize a serious potential late complication [72].

Adhering to dietary and post bariatric surgery nutritional supplement recommendations will alleviate most, if not all, nutrient specific deficiencies. Patients should be aware that compliance with these recommendations following bariatric surgery is essential for reducing the risk of acute and chronic nutritional deficiencies.

Restrictive and malabsorptive bariatric surgery significantly alters anatomical space and digestive physiology commonly prompting certain nutritional deficiencies and metabolic complications. Globally in bariatric surgery, the most common nutritional deficits encountered are iron, protein, calcium, vitamin B12, and vitamin D. Complications after the restrictive/ malabsorptive (RYGPB) and malabsorptive (BPD, BPD-DS) procedures contribute to the majority of observed short-term and long-term metabolic imbalances and overt deficiencies. More specific nutritional complications are observed after restrictive procedures (banding); however, these deficits are much less common and usually related to changes in dietary patterns, food choices, and noncompliance with the post-op nutritional supplement recommendations.

Conclusion

Medical and surgical management of the bariatric patient presenting with post surgical complications are fortunately relatively uncommon. Now that more bariatric procedures are being done in American College of Surgeons Centers of Excellence for Bariatric Surgery fewer patients are presenting to emergency departments and hospitals without ability to have immediate bariatric surgeon call coverage. However, with more than 200,000 bariatric procedures being done in the USA in 2012, many bariatric patients will present with complications in the immediate perioperative period while many others will present months to years following bariatric surgery with a more insidious indolent presentation of serious complications. The acute care surgeon, gastroenterologist, and emergency room physician must be aware of the difficulty in early recognition, management, and potential endoscopic and surgical needs. This population by nature of their size is at especially high risk for major complications, including death, if a delay in diagnosis ensues.

References

1. Longitudinal Assessment of Bariatric Surgery (LABS) Consortium, Flum DR, Belle SH, et al. Perioperative safety in the longitudinal assessment of bariatric surgery. N Engl J Med. 2009;361(5): 445–54.
2. Deveney CW, Martindale RG. Factors in selecting the optimal bariatric procedure for a specific patient and parameters by which to measure appropriate response to surgery. Curr Gastroenterol Rep. 2010;12(4):296–303.
3. Segaran E. Provision of nutritional support to those experiencing complications following bariatric surgery. Proc Nutr Soc. 2010; 69(4):536–42.
4. Hamdan K, Somers S, Chand M. Management of late postoperative complications of bariatric surgery. Br J Surg. 2011;98(10): 1345–55.
5. Maciejewski ML, Livingston EH, Smith VA, et al. Survival among high-risk patients after bariatric surgery. JAMA. 2011;305(23): 2419–26.
6. Smith MD, Patterson E, Wahed AS, et al. Thirty-day mortality after bariatric surgery: Independently adjudicated causes of death in the longitudinal assessment of bariatric surgery. Obes Surg. 2011;21(11): 1687–92.
7. Sokol DK. How can I avoid being sued? BMJ. 2011;343:d7827.
8. Raper SE, Sarwer DB. Informed consent issues in the conduct of bariatric surgery. Surg Obes Relat Dis. 2008;4(1):60–8.

9. Gonzalez R, Sarr MG, Smith CD, et al. Diagnosis and contemporary management of anastomotic leaks after gastric bypass for obesity. J Am Coll Surg. 2007;204(1):47–55.

10. Eubanks S, Edwards CA, Fearing NM, et al. Use of endoscopic stents to treat anastomotic complications after bariatric surgery. J Am Coll Surg. 2008;206(5):935–8. Discussion 938–9.

11. Serra C, Baltasar A, Andreo L, et al. Treatment of gastric leaks with coated self-expanding stents after sleeve gastrectomy. Obes Surg. 2007;17(7):866–72.

12. Babor R, Talbot M, Tyndal A. Treatment of upper gastrointestinal leaks with a removable, covered, self-expanding metallic stent. Surg Laparosc Endosc Percutan Tech. 2009;19(1):e1–4.

13. Salinas A, Baptista A, Santiago E, Antor M, Salinas H. Self-expandable metal stents to treat gastric leaks. Surg Obes Relat Dis. 2006;2(5):570–2.

14. Bege T, Emungania O, Vitton V, et al. An endoscopic strategy for management of anastomotic complications from bariatric surgery: a prospective study. Gastrointest Endosc. 2011;73(2):238–44.

15. Ballesta C, Berindoague R, Cabrera M, Palau M, Gonzales M. Management of anastomotic leaks after laparoscopic Roux-en-Y gastric bypass. Obes Surg. 2008;18(6):623–30.

16. Gonzalez R, Nelson LG, Gallagher SF, Murr MM. Anastomotic leaks after laparoscopic gastric bypass. Obes Surg. 2004;14(10):1299–307.

17. Chopra T, Marchaim D, Lynch Y, et al. Epidemiology and outcomes associated with surgical site infection following bariatric surgery. Am J Infect Control. 2012;40:815.

18. Anaya DA, Dellinger EP. The obese surgical patient: a susceptible host for infection. Surg Infect (Larchmt). 2006;7(5):473–80.

19. Winegar DA, Sherif B, Pate V, DeMaria EJ. Venous thromboembolism after bariatric surgery performed by bariatric surgery center of excellence participants: analysis of the bariatric outcomes longitudinal database. Surg Obes Relat Dis. 2011;7(2):181–8.

20. Kuruba R, Koche LS, Murr MM. Preoperative assessment and perioperative care of patients undergoing bariatric surgery. Med Clin North Am. 2007;91(3):339–51. ix.

21. Vijgen GH, Schouten R, Pelzers L, Greve JW, van Helden SH, Bouvy ND. Revision of laparoscopic adjustable gastric banding: success or failure? Obes Surg. 2012;22(2):287–92.

22. Ponce J, Fromm R, Paynter S. Outcomes after laparoscopic adjustable gastric band repositioning for slippage or pouch dilation. Surg Obes Relat Dis. 2006;2(6):627–31.

23. Kirshtein B, Lantsberg L, Mizrahi S, Avinoach E. Bariatric emergencies for non-bariatric surgeons: complications of laparoscopic gastric banding. Obes Surg. 2010;20(11):1468–78.

24. Newcomb WL, Polhill JL, Chen AY, et al. Staged hernia repair preceded by gastric bypass for the treatment of morbidly obese patients with complex ventral hernias. Hernia. 2008;12(5):465–9.

25. Capella RF, Iannace VA, Capella JF. Reducing the incidence of incisional hernias following open gastric bypass surgery. Obes Surg. 2007;17(4):438–44.

26. Swank HA, Mulder IM, la Chapelle CF, Reitsma JB, Lange JF, Bemelman WA. Systematic review of trocar-site hernia. Br J Surg. 2012;99(3):315–23.

27. Rao RS, Gentileschi P, Kini SU. Management of ventral hernias in bariatric surgery. Surg Obes Relat Dis. 2011;7(1):110–6.

28. Quigley S, Colledge J, Mukherjee S, Patel K. Bariatric surgery: a review of normal postoperative anatomy and complications. Clin Radiol. 2011;66(10):903–14.

29. O'Rourke RW. Management strategies for internal hernia after gastric bypass. J Gastrointest Surg. 2011;15(6):1049–54.

30. Shikora SA, Kim JJ, Tarnoff ME. Nutrition and gastrointestinal complications of bariatric surgery. Nutr Clin Pract. 2007;22(1):29–40.

31. Csendes A, Torres J, Burgos AM. Late marginal ulcers after gastric bypass for morbid obesity. Clinical and endoscopic findings and response to treatment. Obes Surg. 2011;21(9):1319–22.

32. Garrido Jr AB, Rossi M, Lima Jr SE, Brenner AS, Gomes Jr CA. Early marginal ulcer following Roux-en-Y gastric bypass under proton pump inhibitor treatment: prospective multicentric study. Arq Gastroenterol. 2010;47(2):130–4.

33. Csendes A, Burgos AM, Altuve J, Bonacic S. Incidence of marginal ulcer 1 month and 1 to 2 years after gastric bypass: a prospective consecutive endoscopic evaluation of 442 patients with morbid obesity. Obes Surg. 2009;19(2):135–8.

34. Sapala JA, Wood MH, Sapala MA, Flake Jr TM. Marginal ulcer after gastric bypass: a prospective 3-year study of 173 patients. Obes Surg. 1998;8(5):505–16.

35. Rasmussen JJ, Fuller W, Ali MR. Marginal ulceration after laparoscopic gastric bypass: an analysis of predisposing factors in 260 patients. Surg Endosc. 2007;21(7):1090–4.

36. Tang SJ, Rivas H, Tang L, Lara LF, Sreenarasimhaiah J, Rockey DC. Endoscopic hemostasis using endoclip in early gastrointestinal hemorrhage after gastric bypass surgery. Obes Surg. 2007;17(9):1261–7.

37. Datta TS, Steele K, Schweitzer M. Laparoscopic revision of gastrojejunostomy revision with truncal vagotomy for persistent marginal ulcer after Roux-en-Y gastric bypass. Surg Obes Relat Dis. 2010;6(5):561–2.

38. Peifer KJ, Shiels AJ, Azar R, Rivera RE, Eagon JC, Jonnalagadda S. Successful endoscopic management of gastrojejunal anastomotic strictures after Roux-en-Y gastric bypass. Gastrointest Endosc. 2007;66(2):248–52.

39. Schwartz ML, Drew RL, Roiger RW, Ketover SR, Chazin-Caldie M. Stenosis of the gastroenterostomy after laparoscopic gastric bypass. Obes Surg. 2004;14(4):484–91.

40. Lee JK, Van Dam J, Morton JM, Curet M, Banerjee S. Endoscopy is accurate, safe, and effective in the assessment and management of complications following gastric bypass surgery. Am J Gastroenterol. 2009;104(3):575–82. Quiz 583.

41. Howard DD, DeShazo ME, Richards WO, Rodning CB. Retrograde jejunojejunal intussusception status following Roux-en-Y gastrojejunostomy. Int Surg. 2010;95(2):177–82.

42. McAllister MS, Donoway T, Lucktong TA. Synchronous intussusceptions following Roux-en-Y gastric bypass: case report and review of the literature. Obes Surg. 2009;19(12):1719–23.

43. Shaw D, Huddleston S, Beilman G. Anterograde intussusception following laparoscopic Roux-en-Y gastric bypass: a case report and review of the literature. Obes Surg. 2010;20(8):1191–4.

44. Spivak H, Abdelmelek MF, Beltran OR, Ng AW, Kitahama S. Long-term outcomes of laparoscopic adjustable gastric banding and laparoscopic Roux-en-Y gastric bypass in the United States. Surg Endosc. 2012;26(7):1909–19.

45. Tog CH, Halliday J, Khor Y, Yong T, Wilkinson S. Evolving pattern of laparoscopic gastric band access port complications. Obes Surg. 2012;22(6):863–5.

46. Himpens J, Cadiere GB, Bazi M, Vouche M, Cadiere B, Dapri G. Long-term outcomes of laparoscopic adjustable gastric banding. Arch Surg. 2011;146(7):802–7.

47. Hainaux B, Agneessens E, Rubesova E, et al. Intragastric band erosion after laparoscopic adjustable gastric banding for morbid obesity: imaging characteristics of an underreported complication. AJR Am J Roentgenol. 2005;184(1):109–12.

48. Facek M, Receveur I, Darbar A, Richardson A, Leibman S, Smith G. Prosthesis related sepsis following laparoscopic adjustable gastric banding. ANZ J Surg. 2010;80(7–8):506–9.

49. Rao AD, Ramalingam G. Exsanguinating hemorrhage following gastric erosion after laparoscopic adjustable gastric banding. Obes Surg. 2006;16(12):1675–8.

50. Iqbal M, Manjunath S, Seenath M, Khan A. Massive upper gastrointestinal hemorrhage: an unusual presentation after laparoscopic adjustable gastric banding due to erosion into the celiac axis. Obes Surg. 2008;18(6):759–60.

51. Freeman L, Brown WA, Korin A, Pilgrim CH, Smith A, Nottle P. An approach to the assessment and management of the laparoscopic adjustable gastric band patient in the emergency department. Emerg Med Australas. 2011;23(2):186–94.

52. Abu-Abeid S, Szold A. Laparoscopic management of lap-band erosion. Obes Surg. 2001;11(1):87–9.

53. Egberts K, Brown WA, O'Brien PE. Systematic review of erosion after laparoscopic adjustable gastric banding. Obes Surg. 2011;21(8):1272–9.

54. Mozzi E, Lattuada E, Zappa MA, et al. Treatment of band erosion: feasibility and safety of endoscopic band removal. Surg Endosc. 2011;25(12):3918–22.

55. Iglezias Brandao de Oliveira C, Adami Chaim E, da Silva BB. Impact of rapid weight reduction on risk of cholelithiasis after bariatric surgery. Obes Surg. 2003;13(4):625–8.

56. Caruana JA, McCabe MN, Smith AD, Camara DS, Mercer MA, Gillespie JA. Incidence of symptomatic gallstones after gastric bypass: is prophylactic treatment really necessary? Surg Obes Relat Dis. 2005;1(6):564–7. Discussion 567–8.

57. Swartz DE, Felix EL. Elective cholecystectomy after Roux-en-Y gastric bypass: why should asymptomatic gallstones be treated differently in morbidly obese patients? Surg Obes Relat Dis. 2005;1(6):555–60.

58. Sugerman HJ, Brewer WH, Shiffman ML, et al. A multicenter, placebo-controlled, randomized, double-blind, prospective trial of prophylactic Ursodiol for the prevention of gallstone formation following gastric-bypass-induced rapid weight loss. Am J Surg. 1995;169(1):91–6. Discussion 96–7.

59. Keith JN. Endoscopic management of common bariatric surgical complications. Gastrointest Endosc Clin N Am. 2011;21(2):275–85.

60. Fiegler W, Felix R, Langer M, Schultz E. Fat as a factor affecting resolution in diagnostic ultrasound: possibilities for improving picture quality. Eur J Radiol. 1985;5(4):304–9.

61. Attasaranya S, Cheon YK, Vittal H, et al. Large-diameter biliary orifice balloon dilation to aid in endoscopic bile duct stone removal: a multicenter series. Gastrointest Endosc. 2008;67(7):1046–52.

62. McClave SA, Kushner R, Van Way 3rd CW, et al. Nutrition therapy of the severely obese, critically ill patient: summation of conclusions and recommendations. JPEN J Parenter Enteral Nutr. 2011;35(5 Suppl):88S–96.

63. Schweiger C, Weiss R, Berry E, Keidar A. Nutritional deficiencies in bariatric surgery candidates. Obes Surg. 2010;20(2):193–7.

64. Fujioka K. Follow-up of nutritional and metabolic problems after bariatric surgery. Diabetes Care. 2005;28(2):481–4.

65. Shankar P, Boylan M, Sriram K. Micronutrient deficiencies after bariatric surgery. Nutrition. 2010;26(11–12):1031–7.

66. Mason ME, Jalagani H, Vinik AI. Metabolic complications of bariatric surgery: diagnosis and management issues. Gastroenterol Clin North Am. 2005;34(1):25–33.

67. Moliterno JA, DiLuna ML, Sood S, Roberts KE, Duncan CC. Gastric bypass: a risk factor for neural tube defects? Case report. J Neurosurg Pediatr. 2008;1(5):406–9.

68. Aasheim ET. Wernicke encephalopathy after bariatric surgery: a systematic review. Ann Surg. 2008;248(5):714–20.

69. Loh Y, Watson WD, Verma A, Chang ST, Stocker DJ, Labutta RJ. Acute wernicke's encephalopathy following bariatric surgery: clinical course and MRI correlation. Obes Surg. 2004;14(1):129–32.

70. Bacci V, Silecchia G. Vitamin D status and supplementation in morbid obesity before and after bariatric surgery. Expert Rev Gastroenterol Hepatol. 2010;4(6):781–94.

71. De Prisco C, Levine SN. Metabolic bone disease after gastric bypass surgery for obesity. Am J Med Sci. 2005;329(2):57–61.

72. Ziegler O, Sirveaux MA, Brunaud L, Reibel N, Quilliot D. Medical follow up after bariatric surgery: nutritional and drug issues. General recommendations for the prevention and treatment of nutritional deficiencies. Diabetes Metab. 2009;35(6 Pt 2):544–57.

Joseph F. Sucher and Michael Klebuc

Epidemiology

Abdominal wall hernia repair is one the most common groups of major operations in acute care surgery, with more than a million hernia repairs performed annually in the United States alone [1]. The latest understanding of hernia epidemiology in the United States comes from studies performed in 1996 by the National Center for Health Statistics [2]. Abdominal wall hernias can be classified broadly into two groups: ventral hernias (including flank and lumbar) and groin hernias. The most common abdominal hernia operation performed is groin herniorrhaphy, totaling more than 75% of the abdominal wall hernia repairs. Ventral hernia repairs comprise the remaining 25% [1].

Ventral Hernia Epidemiology

Ventral hernias (including flank and lumbar) have two etiologies—primary and acquired (traumatic or incisional)—and can be further subclassified by their respective locations. In 2009, Muysoms et al. proposed an anatomic classification scheme, based primarily on location relative to the midline (Figs. 34.1 and 34.2) [3]. Additionally, there are specific ventral hernias classified by their eponyms, i.e., Spigelian ("lateral hernia" at or below the linea arcuata, bound medi-

ally by the rectus and laterally at the linea semilunaris), Grynfelt's (superior lumbar triangle), and Petit's (inferior lumbar triangle). Some eponyms describe a structure that is contained in the hernia, irrespective of location, i.e., Richter's (hernia strangulating single wall of intestine), Littre's (Meckel's diverticulum in hernia sac), and Maydl's (incarceration of two adjacent loops of intestine). Women appear to be nearly twice as likely to develop incisional hernias as men (65% to 35%) but are only slightly more at risk for primary ventral hernias (57% to 43%) (Tables 34.1 and 34.2) [2]. Incisional hernia repair is the most common ventral hernia operation, owing to the more than 2 million laparotomies performed each year in the United States with a complication rate of hernia formation of 2–23% [4, 5]. Repair of such hernias has a dismal 31–63% failure rate following open primary suture repair, and 12–24% failure following open mesh repair. [4, 6–10] There are numerous risk factors for ventral incisional hernia including surgical technique, morbid obesity, smoking, chronic obstructive pulmonary disease, postoperative wound complications (such as infection or seroma), renal failure, chronic corticosteroid use, malignancy, male gender, and prostatism. [4] Postoperative wound infection and aneurysmal disease are independent risk factors in the development of incisional hernia [4]. Studies looking at time to incisional hernia formation reveal that half are detected within the first year, and over 90% by the third year, with a 2% per year failure rate thereafter [4]. Surgical technique is the most controllable of all the variables, and the two most recent meta-analyses [11, 12] reveal that incisional hernia formation risk is lowered by (1) mass closure, (2) simple running technique, (3) the use of nonabsorbable monofilament suture, and (4) suture-to-wound length ration of 4:1 first documented by Jenkins [13]. More recent work regarding defects in collagen metabolism, the ratio of Type I to Type III procollagen, cathepsin G, tropoelastin, and matrix metalloproteinase (MMP) activity may help to shed light into individual risk of incisional and primary hernia formation in the future.

J.F. Sucher, M.D., F.A.C.S. (✉)
Department of Surgery, The Methodist Hospital,
Weill Cornell Medical College, 6550 Fannin Street,
Smith Tower 1661, Houston, TX 77030, USA
e-mail: jfsucher@tmhs.org

M. Klebuc, M.D.
Department of Plastic and Reconstructive Surgery,
The Methodist Hospital, Weill Medical College,
Cornell University, Houston, TX, USA

L.J. Moore et al. (eds.), *Common Problems in Acute Care Surgery*,
DOI 10.1007/978-1-4614-6123-4_34, © Springer Science+Business Media New York 2013

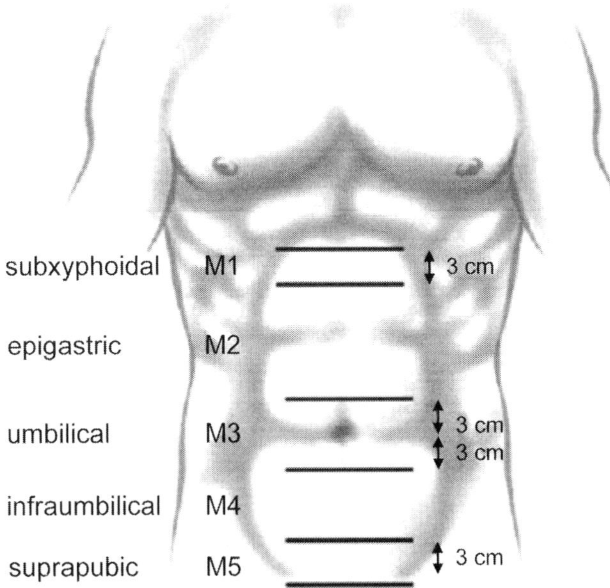

Fig. 34.1 Classification of ventral hernias between the two lateral margins of rectus muscles. Five zones are defined. (Reprinted with permission from Muysoms FE, Miserez M, Berrevoet F et al. Classification of primary and incisional abdominal wall hernias. Hernia. 2009;13(4): 407–414)

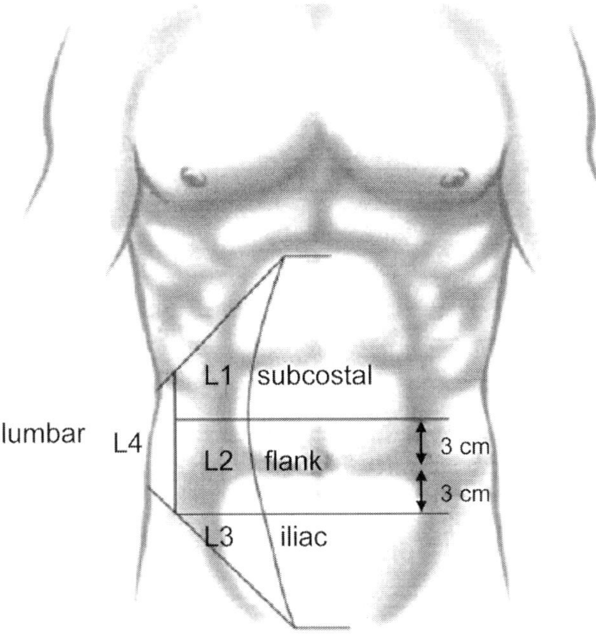

Fig. 34.2 For lateral hernias, 4 zones lateral to the rectus sheath are defined. (Reprinted with permission from Muysoms FE, Miserez M, Berrevoet F, et al. Classification of primary and incisional abdominal wall hernias. Hernia. 2009;13:407–414)

Groin Hernia Epidemiology

Groin hernias are divided into inguinal and femoral types. Inguinal hernias are subdivided into direct and indirect based on the relation of herniation to that of the epigastric vessels.

Table 34.1 Abdominal wall hernia operations in the USA during 1996

Type of hernia	Number of outpatient procedures	Number of inpatient procedures	Total number of procedures
Inguinal hernia			
Unilateral repair	458,000	62,000	520,000
Bilateral repair	73,000 (76,000[a])	15,000 (30,000[a])	176,000[a]
Total repairs	604,000[a]	92,000[a]	696,000[a]
Femoral hernia	19,000	6,000	25,000
Umbilical hernia	120,000	46,000	166,000
Incisional hernia	40,000	57,000	97,000
Other abdominal wall hernias (epigastric, Spigelian)	45,000	31,000	76,000

The numbers do not include US Veterans' Administration and other federal facilities, so to compensate, the number of groin hernia repairs should be increased by an estimated 5%. Adapted from [2]
[a]The number of bilateral repairs has been doubled to account for the total number of individual bilateral inguinal hernia repairs

Table 34.2 The age and gender of herniorrhaphy patients in the United States during 1996

Type of hernia	Gender (%)		Age (%)			
	Male	Female	<15 years	15–44 years	45–64 years	>65 years
Inguinal hernia	90	10	18	29	23	30
Femoral hernia	30	70	<1	19	29	48
Umbilical hernia	57	33	13	33	36	17
Incisional hernia	35	65	<1	25	35	39
Other abdominal wall hernias (epigastric, Spigelian, etc.)	43	57	1	32	40	25

The numbers do not include US Veterans' Administration and other federal facilities, so the actual number of groin hernia repairs is likely to be higher among males. Adapted from [2]

Indirect hernias are lateral to the epigastric vessels and are generally related to a congenital weakness via a patent processus vaginalis. Direct hernias are medial to the epigastric vessels and bound by Hesselbach's triangle, whose lateral border is the epigastric artery, the medial border is the lateral aspect of the rectus muscle, and the inferior border is the inguinal ligament. A Pantaloon hernia is an inguinal hernia with its sac extending through both the direct and indirect spaces. Numerous eponyms for femoral hernias exist based on anatomic location, such as Cooper's (a hernia with extension into the femoral space and a second sac anterior to the femoral vessels), Hesselbach's (hernia medial to the femoral vessels), Velpeau's (hernia anterior to the femoral vessels), Serafini's (hernia posterior to the femoral vessels), Laugier's (hernia through the lacunar ligament), and Cloquet's (hernia through the pectineal fascia). There are also eponyms based on what is contained in the hernia sac, i.e., Amyand's (appendicitis in inguinal hernia sac), De Garengeot's (appendicitis in femoral hernia sac), and Busse's (testicle in hernia sac). The term "sliding hernia" when referring to a groin hernia is one in which a wall of hernia sac is composed of an organ, such

Table 34.3 Comparison of groin hernia classifications schemes

Traditional updated	Gilbert	Nyhus	Schumpelick
Indirect			
1. Small	1. Snug	I. Indirect, small normal internal ring, sac in canal	L1 < 1.5 cm
2. Medium	2. Moderately dilated ring	II. Indirect, medium enlarged internal ring, sac not in scrotum	L2 1.5–3 cm
3. Large	3. Greater than 2 finger-breadths	III. B. Combined–indirect large, encroaching into direct floor	L3 > 3 cm
Direct			
4. Small	4. Diverticular	III. A. Direct–Floor only. No more than one finger-breadth	M1 < 1.5 cm
5. Medium	–	III. A.	M2 1.5–3 cm
6. Large	5. Entire floor	–	M3 > 3 cm
Combined			
7. Pantaloon	6. Combined	III. B.	Mc
Femoral			
8. Femoral	7. Femoral	III. C. Femoral	F
0. Other	–	–	–
Recurrent	–	IV. Recurrent A. Direct B. Indirect C. Femoral D. Combinations of A-B-C	–

Adapted from [15, 16]

as the bladder or colon. Finally, Gilmore's groin, AKA sportsman's hernia, is understood to be groin pain associated with dilated external ring and/or tears in the musculature or tendonous insertions in the area of the inguinal canal. Approximately 96% of groin hernias are inguinal and 4% are femoral. The overall lifetime risk of developing an inguinal hernia is 27% for men and 3% for women [14]. There is a 9:1 male-to-female predominance for inguinal hernias and a 7:3 female-to-male predominance for femoral hernias [2]. Groin hernia classification is important for purposes of literature review and comparison of techniques. As with most classification systems, numerous have been developed. However, the traditional classification of indirect, direct, and femoral remains the most consistent over time. In such, the most commonly used classification systems utilize these basic anatomic descriptors as seen in Table 34.3 [15, 16]. In 2002, the "Updated Traditional Classification" was proposed at a consensus conference and serves as the current method most commonly agreed upon today [16].

Clinical Presentation, Diagnosis, and Therapeutic Options

The acute care surgeon will encounter all types of abdominal wall hernias. Fortunately, there is little dilemma in the diagnosis of most abdominal wall hernias. As with any problem in surgery, careful history and physical examination will provide most all of what is needed to make the diagnosis. However, the diagnoses of some hernias, such as sportsman's, Spigelian, femoral, and lumbar hernias can be challenging. The "sportsman's hernia" incidence remains unclear, and its diagnosis relies almost completely on history and symptoms

alone. Spigelian hernias only constitute 0.12% of all hernias [17], femoral hernias make up 2–8%[18] of all groin hernias, and lumbar hernias are so rare that it is likely most general surgeons will only have the opportunity to repair one in his/her lifetime [19]. Therefore, for these latter three hernias, the surgeon needs to have a high index of suspicion and employ judicious utilization of abdominal-pelvic computed tomography (CT) scanning to make a definitive diagnosis.

More often, the acute care surgeon will be faced with the emergent presentation of hernias with associated incarceration, obstruction, strangulation, and/or contamination, along with complex giant ventral hernias related to catastrophic loss of abdominal wall integrity. As such, this chapter will focus on the diagnosis and management of these two issues. Of note, although an important tool, even in the emergency setting, laparoscopic repair is not discussed in this chapter. One of the pitfalls we have encountered in this age of hernia repair is that many surgeons entering practice have performed very few "tissue-only repairs" (repairs without some type of mesh). This is especially salient when faced with the need to perform groin herniorrhaphy in a contaminated field.

Groin Hernias

The focus of groin hernia repair in this chapter has been limited to emergent tissue-only repair in a contaminated environment. In situations, where the surgeon encounters obstructed, strangulated bowel or perforated bowel, mesh placement is generally unfavorable. In these instances, the fundamentals of tissue-only repair remain immutable and the tenets of identifying bowel viability and control of contamination with bowel resection remain paramount.

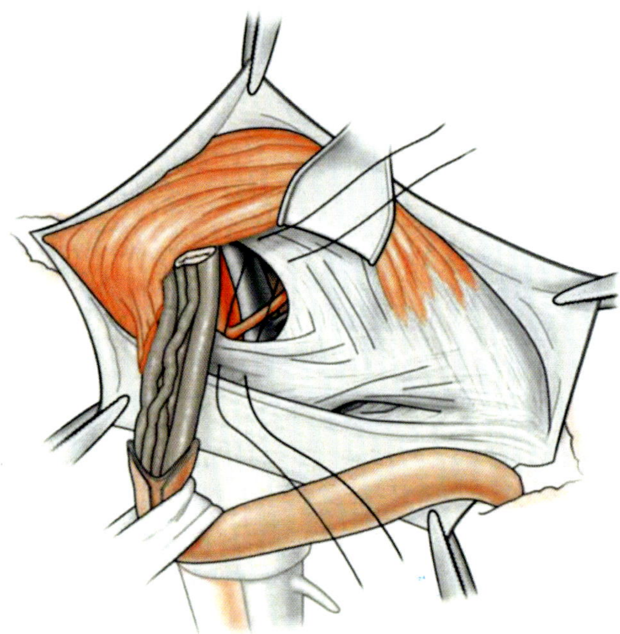

Fig. 34.3 Marcy repair. (Reprinted with permission from Fitzgibbons RJ, Richards AT, Quinn TH. "Open Hernia Repair" in: ACS Surgery: Principles and Practice 2004. Wilmore DW et al. (eds) 603–624. WebMD Professional Publishing, 2004. In: ACS Surgery Online. Ed: Ashley SA. Decker Intellectual Properties (2012). http://www.acs-surgery.com)

This is not to say that laparoscopic repair or mesh repair is absolutely contraindicated in emergency groin surgery; rather we have chosen to establish an updated reference of open tissue-only repairs for surgeons whose training may have focused on tension-free and laparoscopic mesh repairs. More than 70 tissue-only repairs have been described [20], with a handful remaining especially important for the acute care surgeon. Four tissue-only repairs provide an excellent foundation for groin hernia surgery in settings where the implantation of mesh is at high risk for infection. These are reviewed as follows.

Indirect and Direct Inguinal Hernia Tissue-Only Repairs

The Marcy repair is optimal for the small indirect hernias that are more often encountered in children and young adults. After dissecting the hernia sac free, the cord structures are retracted laterally and the hernia sac is ligated high. Subsequent approximation of the transverse aponeurotic arch to the iliopubic tract with one or two monofilament sutures (Fig. 34.3), returns the deep inguinal ring to its normal size, completing the repair.

The Bassini technique is a three-layer repair that can be employed for any indirect, direct, or pantaloon groin hernias. The external abdominal oblique aponeurosis is divided along its fibers and the cord is identified and encircled. The cremasteric fibers are incised longitudinally. The medial flap is avascular and resected entirely, the lateral flap contains the genitofemoral nerve and spermatic vessels that can be divided and ligated. The indirect hernia sac (if present) can be ligated high or reduced. The surgeon then divides the transversalis fascia from the deep ring to the pubic tubercle and actualizes the preperitoneal space allowing for repair of the "triple layer" (transversalis fascia, transversus abdominis, and internal oblique muscle) (Fig. 34.4a). Nonabsorbable suture is used in an interrupted fashion to approximate the "triple layer" supero-medially to Poupart's ligament infero-laterally. This begins at the pubic tubercle medially and ends with the recreation of a normal sized deep inguinal ring (Fig. 34.4b). If necessary, a relaxing incision can be performed medially to the internal abdominal oblique aponeurosis to reduce the tension prior to the repair.

The Shouldice repair [21] for indirect, direct, or pantaloon hernias incorporates the same initial steps as the Bassini repair. Following the opening of the transversalis fascia, a relaxing incision is created over the medial internal abdominal oblique aponeurosis. The repair uses two running nonabsorbable monofilament sutures (originally a 32- or 34-gauge steel wire), with the first starting at the pubic tubercle, approximating the iliopubic tract laterally to the undersurface of the transverse aponeurotic arch (transversalis fascia, transverses abdominis and internal abdominal oblique) (Fig. 34.5a). This moves supero-laterally to the deep ring, picking up the lateral stump of the cremasteric muscle to form the new deep ring, and returning back along the medial edge of the transverses and internal oblique to Poupart's ligament, ending at the pubic tubercle and tied to itself (Fig. 34.5b). The second running suture begins at the internal ring grabbing the internal oblique and transversus muscles laterally and brings them to the external oblique aponeurosis just superficial to Poupart's ligament. The direction is reversed and runs just superficial to itself, ending at the internal ring. Thus 4 suture lines are created in this repair.

Finally, the McVay repair is best suited for reconstruction of a femoral hernia with high risk for postoperative infection. Like Bassini and Shouldice, the initial steps of the dissection remain the same. After opening of the transversalis fascia and creating a relaxing incision medially, the repair is begun at the pubic tubercle with interrupted nonabsorbable monofilament suture. The transverse aponeurotic arch (lateral) is affixed to the deep and medial Cooper's ligament (instead of the inguinal ligament as performed in the Bassini repair). This proceeds supero-laterally up to the medial and anterior femoral sheath, with a "transition stitch" into the inguinal ligament (Fig. 34.6). From here, the repair proceeds laterally as in the Bassini repair. Affixing the aponeurotic arch to Cooper's ligament accomplishes the task of narrowing the femoral canal. Additionally, the complete repair fixes the deep ring, the myopectineal orifice and Hesselbach's triangle. Thus, it addresses all areas of potential herniation.

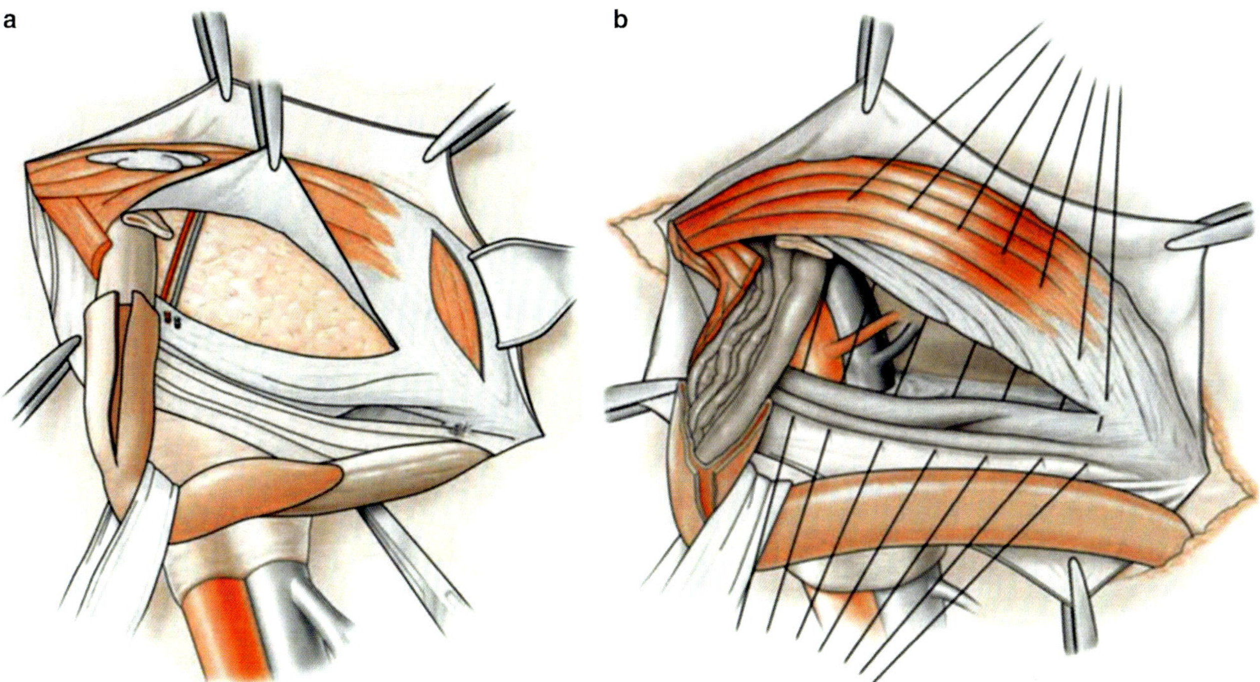

Fig. 34.4 (**a, b**) Bassini repair. (Reprinted with permission from Bergman S, Feldman L, "Inguinal Hernia Repair" in: ACS Surgery: Principles and Practice, 6th Edition, Wilmore DW et al. (eds) BC Decker Inc, 2009. In: ACS Surgery Online. Ed: Ashley SA. Decker Intellectual Properties (2012). http://www.acssurgery.com)

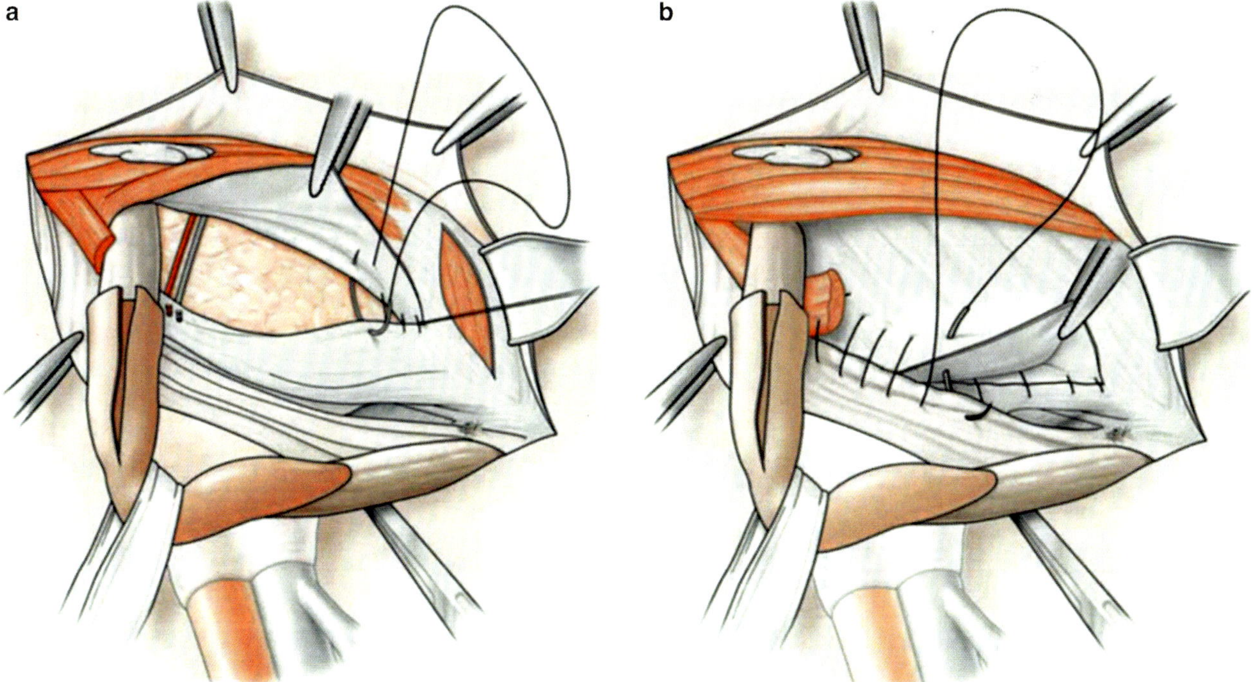

Fig. 34.5 (**a, b**) Shouldice repair. (Reprinted with permission from Bergman S, Feldman L, "Inguinal Hernia Repair" in: ACS Surgery: Principles and Practice, 6th Edition, Wilmore DW, et al. (eds), BC Decker Inc, 2009. In: ACS Surgery Online. Ed: Ashley SA. Decker Intellectual Properties (2012). http://www.acssurgery.com)

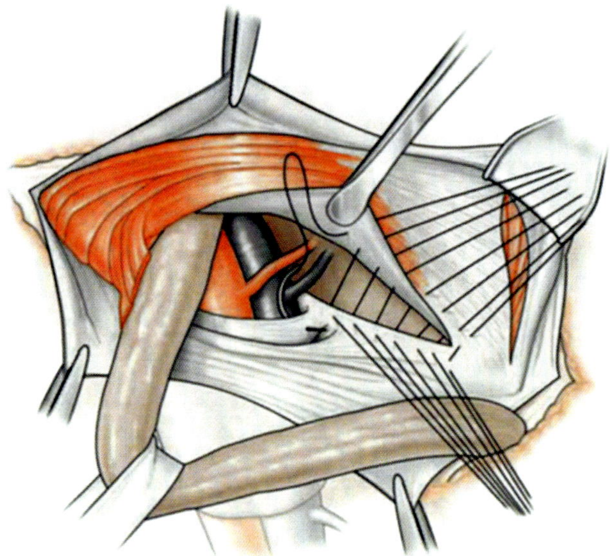

Fig. 34.6 McVay repair. (Reprinted with permission from Bergman S, Feldman L, "Inguinal Hernia Repair" in: ACS Surgery: Principles and Practice, 6th Edition, Wilmore DW et al. (eds) BC Decker Inc, 2009. In: ACS Surgery Online. Ed: Ashley SA. Decker Intellectual Properties (2012). http://www.acssurgery.com)

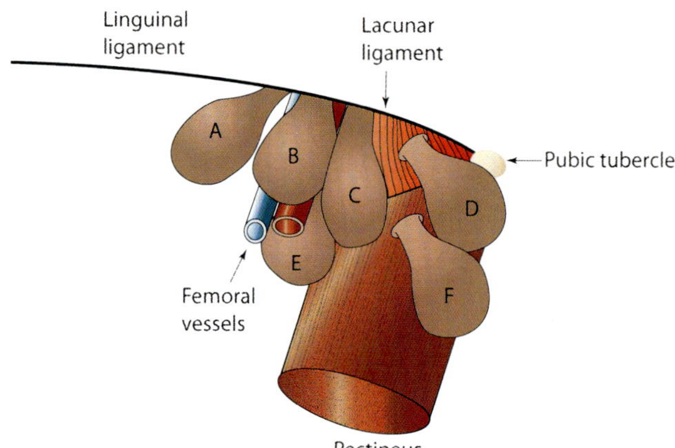

Fig. 34.7 Variable locations of femoral hernias. (**a**) Hesselbach's hernia. (**b**) Velpeau's hernia (prevascular). (**c**) Femoral hernia. (**d**) Laugier's hernia. (**e**) Serafini's hernia (retrovascular). (**f**) Cloquet's hernia. (Adapted from [22])

Femoral Hernia Tissue-Only Repairs

Due to its low incidence and complexity, emergency femoral hernia repair remains a vexing problem in acute care surgery. They are the most common incarcerated groin hernia, and due to its higher incidence of bowel strangulation it carries a mortality of up to 14% [18]. Additionally, due to its multiple configurations (Fig. 34.7) [22], diagnosing its presence, choosing an optimal approach, and constructing an appropriate repair can be challenging. While the McVay repair is the mainstay for the inguinal approach to repair femoral along with any associated indirect or direct hernias, it is not a panacea. The acute care surgeon often faces tightly incarcerated, strangulated, or even grossly contaminated femoral hernias. The approach will be predicated on numerous factors, including size of hernia, the state of its contents, the ability to reduce the hernia and whether the diagnosis of femoral hernia was made preoperatively (versus misidentifying the hernia as inguinal preoperatively). Generally speaking, an inguinal incision 1 cm above the medial half of the inguinal ligament, will allow access to visualize the femoral hernia both above and below the inguinal canal [18]. In simple, non-contaminated cases with easy reduction of the bowel and sac, a repair can be accomplished by approximating the lacunar ligament to the pectineal ligament, thus closing the femoral space. In complex cases, when contents cannot be reduced but are viable, division of the lacunar ligament, from below the inguinal ligament, generally grants enough room to achieve reduction. The surgeon should ovoid dividing the inguinal ligament, as restoration of this structure is challenging at best.

In cases where the contents are nonviable, the surgeon can proceed with two different approaches via the same incision. First, for large hernia defects, a trans-inguinal approach can be easily achieved. The transversalis fascia is opened and the neck of the strangulated bowel can isolated at its healthy point. Here the bowel is divided and a primary anastomosis can be performed. The necrotic bowel can be delivered distally from under the inguinal ligament and a McVay repair can be performed. Second, for smaller hernia defects, a preperitoneal approach can be achieved by developing a plane over the external oblique and then entering into the rectus sheath at the linea semilunaris. The rectus is retracted medially and the transversus is incised. The preperitoneal space can be developed toward the inguinal ligament. Here the neck of the hernia sac can be encountered. Again, the peritoneum can be opened and the bowel resected as above. After performing the primary anastomosis, the peritoneum is closed and a mesh-free repair can be achieved by approximating Cooper's ligament to the iliopubic tract (Fig. 34.8) [23].

Complex Ventral Hernias in Acute Care Surgery

Complex ventral hernias constitute large (>10 cm diameter or 100 cm^2) abdominal wall defects with a range of associate problems such as loss of abdominal domain, skin and soft tissue integrity deficiencies, enteric fistulas, and/or acute peritonitis with gross contamination. For 25 years, we contributed to the increase in complex abdominal wall problems through a practice of massive crystalloid resuscitation, thus promoting abdominal compartment syndrome with subsequent problems in the management of the open abdomen leading to fistulas and giant abdominal wall defects [24]. With the improving understanding of shock resuscitation, we might expect to see a decrease in the incidence of abdominal compartment syndrome and the need for the

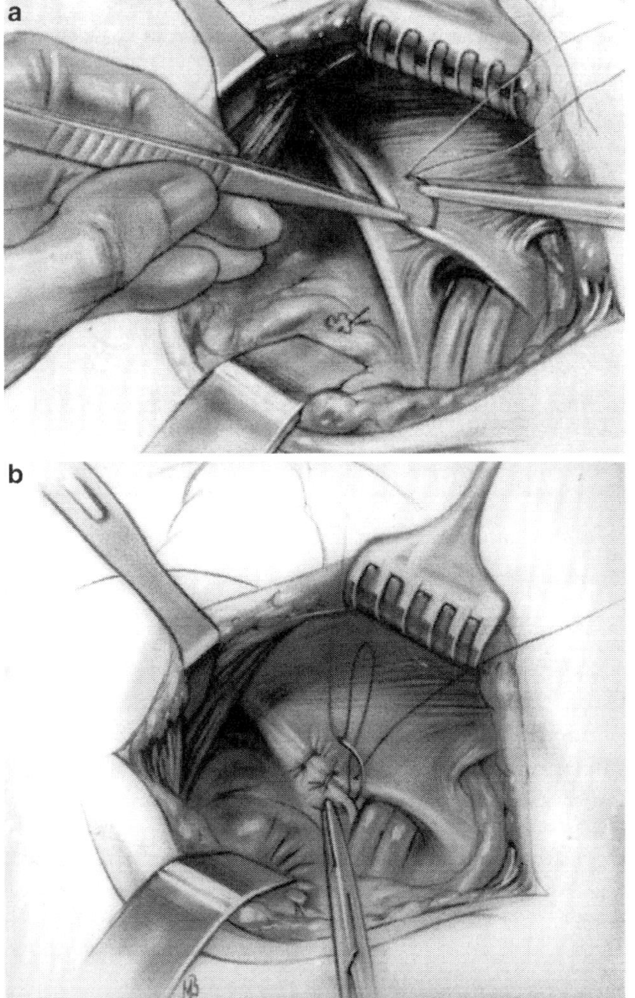

Fig. 34.8 Posterior preperitoneal approach to femoral hernia repair (Reprinted with permission from Nyhus LM. The posterior (preperitoneal) approach and iliopubic tract repair of inguinal and femoral hernias—an update. Hernia. 2003;7(2):63–67)

Table 34.4 Recommendations of the Ventral Hernia Working Group (VHWG) for the technique of repair of incisional ventral hernias

Recommendation	Strength of recommendation	Level of evidence	Evidence source (first author)
1. Reinforcement recommended for repair of all incisional ventral hernias	1	A/B	Burger [26] Espinosa-de-los-Monteros [27] Luijendijk [10]
2. Centralize and reapproximate rectus muscles when feasible under physiologic tension	1	C	de Vries Reilingh [28] Espinosa-de-los-Monteros [27] Kolker [29] VHWG opinion
3. Reduce bioburden prior to repair	1	B	Mangram [30] VHWG opinion
4. Placement of repair material: Underlay is the recommended technique for the placement of appropriate repair material for open and laparoscopic repairs; overlay placement of repair material should only be considered when complete fascia-to-fascia repair has been achieved	2	B	Awad [31] Espinosa-de-los-Monteros [27] Korenkov [32] VHWG opinion
5. In the setting of gross, uncontrolled contamination, it is appropriate to consider delayed repair	1	C	VHWG opinion

Adapted from [25]

management of the open abdomen. However, on the flip side, patients may be more likely to survive from abdominal catastrophes due to improvements in surgical critical care, management of septic shock, and advancements in the care of complex enterocutaneous and "entero-atmospheric" fistulas. Three management strategies have evolved to address the repair of these complex problems. As it pertains to large defects (>10 cm), the first option is primary closure with bridging mesh. The second option is transfer of autologous tissue by rotational or free flap transfer with or without mesh reinforcement. Finally, the third option is components separation with or without mesh reinforcement.

The overarching theme for the approach to the management of ventral hernias is to restore abdominal wall integrity and dynamic function in a tension-free manner [4]. Five recommendations from the Ventral Hernia Working Group (VHWG) provide the evidence-based foundation for this goal (Table 34.4) [10, 25–32]. To accomplish this "meticulous attention to technique, timing, utilization of new technology, and tension-free repair in a clean, well-vascularized wound continue to be the cornerstones of the ideal repair" [33]. Therefore, performing a primary repair with bridging mesh is suboptimal, as restoration of dynamic function is not achieved. Reconstruction with rotational or free flaps is not desirable as they demand reduction of function and distortion of the donor site with poor functional results at the recipient site [34]. With this in mind, the utilization of components separation techniques (Fig. 34.9) pioneered by Donald H. Young in 1961 [35] and popularized by Oscar M Ramirez et al. in 1990 [36] has accelerated significantly in the past decade. Since 1990 there have been many modifications of the Ramirez components separation technique. In 1994 Fabian et al. [37] reported their modification with a more recent long-term follow-up report by DiCocco et al. that stated that their modification (Fig. 34.10) "…allows for more extensive mobilization and local advancement of autologous tissue,

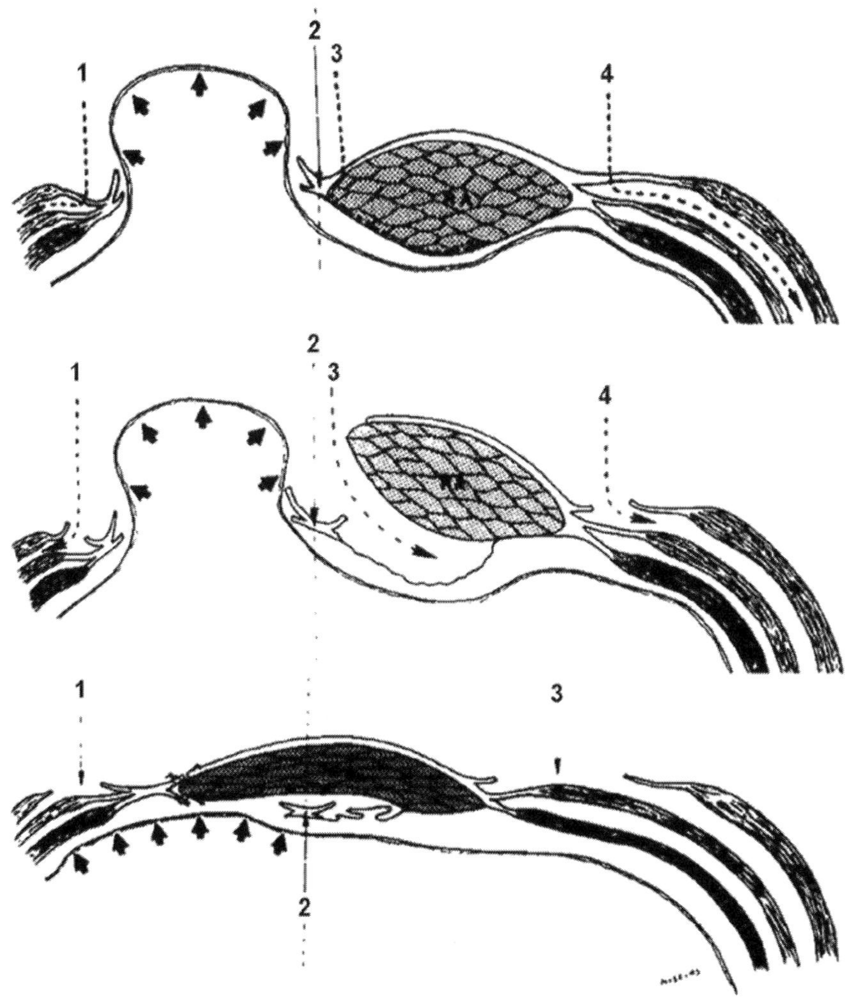

Fig. 34.9 Cross-sectional diagram of components separation. (Reprinted with permission from Ramirez OM, Ruas E, Dellon AL. "Components separation" method for closure of abdominal-wall defects: An anatomic and clinical study. Plast Reconstr Surg. 1990;86:519)

essentially doubling the mobilization compared with the original description" [38]. In the report by DiCocco, a variety of techniques were employed, including standard components separation (SCS) alone, modified components separation (MCS) alone, or SCS or MCS with prosthetic mesh implantation. They had a follow-up of 14.6 years (mean 5.3 years) of 114 patients with a 14% overall recurrence, but only a 5% recurrence when the MCS technique was employed without any prosthetic implantation. Interestingly, they had a fourfold increase in recurrence when a prosthetic mesh was used. This observation is disputed in other studies, which show that the addition of mesh reduces recurrence rates [27–29, 39–41].

There are no data to support or refute utilization of the components separation technique to achieve definitive abdominal closure in the face of acute illness associated with massive trauma or surgical sepsis. However, given recurrence and wound complication rates of 4–53% and 8–84%, respectively [25, 28, 33, 42, 43] for this technique, one should give strong consideration to winning the immediate battle and coming back later for the definitive closure procedure.

A staged approach to the management of these complex problems has become accepted and may be necessary to reduce the risk catastrophic failures in order to increase overall long-term success [37, 42, 44–46]. In general, when faced with a patient who presents with multiple comorbidities in a high inflammatory state during the acute phase of trauma or sepsis, the surgeon should consider limiting the extent of the index abdominal closure to restoration of integrity only. Then, if necessary, the second stage can focus on restoration of both integrity and function, and can be delayed until such time as the patient recovers fully from their initial insult. The following three general scenarios utilizing components separation for repair of complex ventral hernias form the foundation of techniques that should be in the armamentarium of the acute care surgeon.

Scenario 1. Large Complex Ventral Hernia with Enterocutaneous Fistula

Enterocutaneous fistula(s) in the presence of a large ventral hernia can be safely managed as a single stage procedure [45, 47, 48]. Preoperative planning and preparation begin

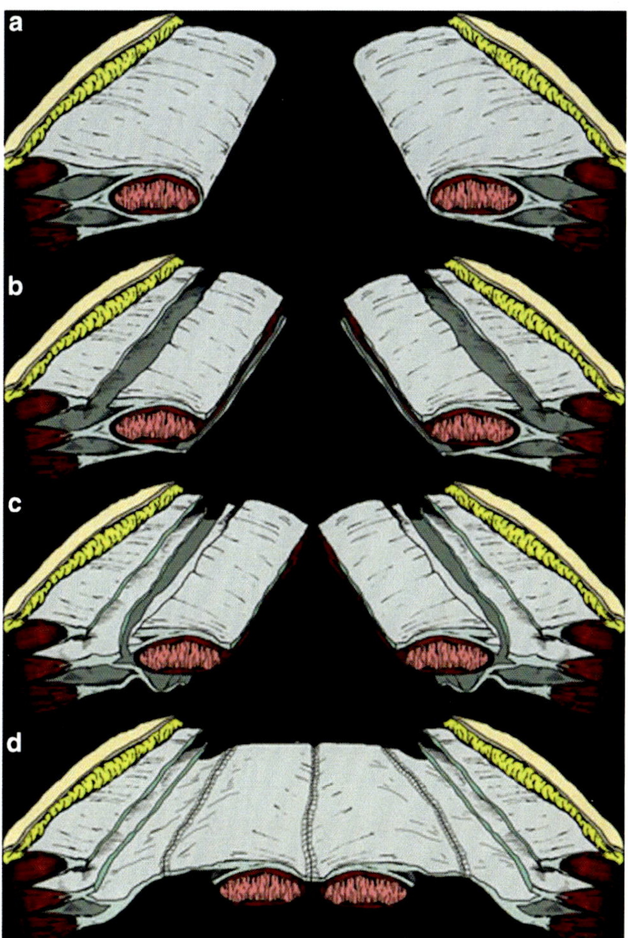

Fig. 34.10 Modified components separation technique for abdominal wall reconstruction. (**a**) Normal anatomy above the arcuate line. (**b**) The posterior rectus sheath is mobilized from the rectus muscle, and the external oblique fascia is divided. (**c**) The internal oblique component of the anterior rectus sheath is divided down to the arcuate line. (**d**) Completed repair, suturing the medial border of the posterior sheath to the lateral border of the anterior sheath, with approximation of the medial portion of the anterior sheath in the midline. Illustration by Steven P Goldberg. (Reprinted with permission from DiCocco JM, Magnotti LJ, Emmett KP, et al. Long-term follow-up of abdominal wall reconstruction after planned ventral hernia: a 15-year experience. J Am Coll Surg. 2010;210(5):686–695, 695–698)

with local management of the fistula with special focus on protecting the skin from further damage and allowing for complete healing of the surrounding tissues. Attention must be paid to optimal nutritional support along with fluid and electrolyte control. For those patients who require total parenteral nutrition, optimizing wound care for rapid healing is critical, as these patients are at high risk for catheter related bacteremia and sepsis. The more complex "entero-atmospheric" fistulas will require massive time resources, attention to detail, extreme patience, and ingenuity (Fig. 34.11a–e). However, when taken care of well, the results can be truly amazing (Fig. 34.11f).

Once the wound is optimized (Fig. 34.12a), definitive repair is undertaken. We advocate utilizing the technique of components separation [36, 49] with an underlay of a biologic mesh implant. Although there is convincing evidence that the use of synthetic mesh with components release (tension-free repair) is superior to that of components release only [40, 50], there is no definitive evidence to support or refute the use of biologic mesh in conjunction with components release. The current literature has not provided significant controlled studies or even a large case series that standardize the patient characteristics, technique, or biologic product used. Therefore, given the high-risk of wound complications with components separation technique and the potential for catastrophic consequences of synthetic mesh infection, our opinion is that the use of biologic reinforcement in conjunction with components separation for contaminated cases is safe and efficacious.

The initial step is to isolate the enterocutaneous fistula and ensure bowel integrity along its entire length (Fig. 34.12b). A partial enterectomy with primary anastomosis is performed, removing the damage portion of bowel in its entirety. The components separation (Fig. 34.12c, d) is performed as described by Ramirez et al. [51] with or without mesh reinforcement. As mentioned, we recommend the placement of biologic mesh in an underlay fashion in cases where there is any tension bringing the midline together, or when unable to completely close the hernia defect. Figure 34.13a–c show the outcome after a single stage procedure.

Scenario 2. Large Complex Ventral Hernia with Loss of Abdominal Domain

Loss of abdominal domain is the inability to restore the abdominal viscera to the confines of the abdominal cavity without an undue increase in intra-abdominal hypertension, potentially resulting in impaired pulmonary, cardiac, and/or renal function (abdominal compartment syndrome). To avoid this, preoperative planning and proper patient selection are paramount. Figure 34.14 shows a patient whose ventral hernia has been left unattended for more than 25 years, resulting in liver and almost all of the intestinal tract herniated outside the true abdominal cavity, thus resulting in complete loss of abdominal domain. Although radical techniques, such as intestinal resection for reducing abdominal visceral contents, have been performed successfully [52], this patient was unsuitable for abdominal wall reconstruction, not withstanding advanced age (>80 years) and multiple comorbidities. However, this is an extreme case. Most giant abdominal wall defects are able to be reconstructed with proper attention paid to the preoperative patient risk assessment along with focused assessment of the abdominal wall anatomy as it relates to its structural (musculofascial units) and coverage (skin and soft tissue) components (Fig. 34.15). In fact, performing components separation for abdominal reconstruction

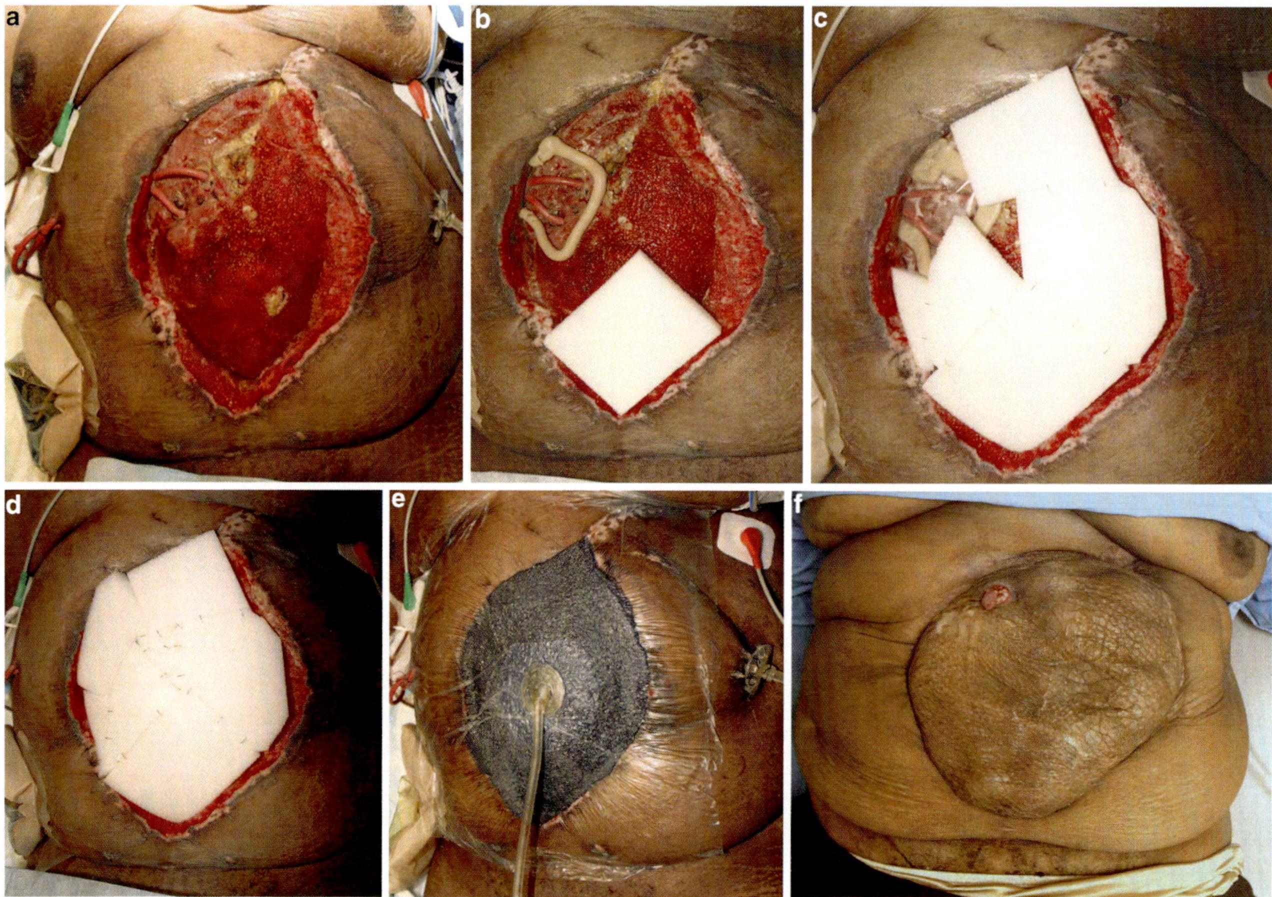

Fig. 34.11 (**a**) Patient with open "frozen" central abdomen and two entero-atmospheric fistulae. Two red rubber catheters have been tunneled laterally and enter directly into the fistulae to divert enteric contents away from the open wound. (**b**) Stoma paste is placed around the fistulae providing a barrier between the enteric leak and the rest of the open wound. A clear plastic sheet is placed over this area, providing an anterior barrier. White dense foam sponge (VersaFoam—KCI, Kansas City, MO) is placed directly over the granulating bowel. (**c**) White dense foam sponge (VersaFoam) covers all of the granulating bowel. (**d**) White dense foam sponge (VersaFoam) covers the entire granulating bowel. (**e**) Black foam (GranuFoam—KCI, Kansas City, MO) is placed over this and a sterile sticky plastic barrier is applied and a hole is cut in the plastic barrier for the KCI TrackPad with suction tubing to cover. Suction at 125 mmHg can be applied. This system is changed at least every 3 days, or as needed. (**f**) Post split thickness skin graft. Duodenal fistula remains in right upper abdomen

may reduce the risk of intra-abdominal hypertension [53]. The patient in Fig. 34.16a, b is a good example of how giant abdominal wall defects can be closed with use of tissue expansion techniques in conjunction with components separation. This patient has a 21×20 cm ventral hernia defect with associated muscle, skin, and soft tissue loss. The skin and soft tissue assessment reveals that there is not enough to provide coverage to the midline. However, there is enough local tissue for expansion, which was achieved by endoscopic placement of subcutaneous tissue expanders (Fig. 34.17a, b). Serial expansion was performed over a 6-week period of time, gaining a significant increase in skin volume (Fig. 34.18). An additional benefit of local tissue expansion is the incitement of neovascularization during capsule formation around the expanders. This well vascularized tissue capsule can be seen at time of removal of the expanders (Fig. 34.19). The patient underwent components separation with an underlay of a bridging biologic mesh and primary soft tissue closure. The patient has had no hernia recurrence in a 4-year postoperative follow-up visit (Fig. 34.20 shows 4 weeks postoperative).

Scenario 3. Large Complex Ventral Hernia with Peritonitis

Not uncommonly, the acute care surgeon will be faced with a patient who presents with peritonitis in the face of a chronic giant ventral hernia (Fig. 34.21a, b). The algorithm for the management with this presentation becomes more focused on resolving the peritonitis and achieving abdominal wound coverage more so than repairing the structural integrity by closure of the hernia defect (Fig. 34.15). As noted previously, the postoperative wound complications alone in an elective

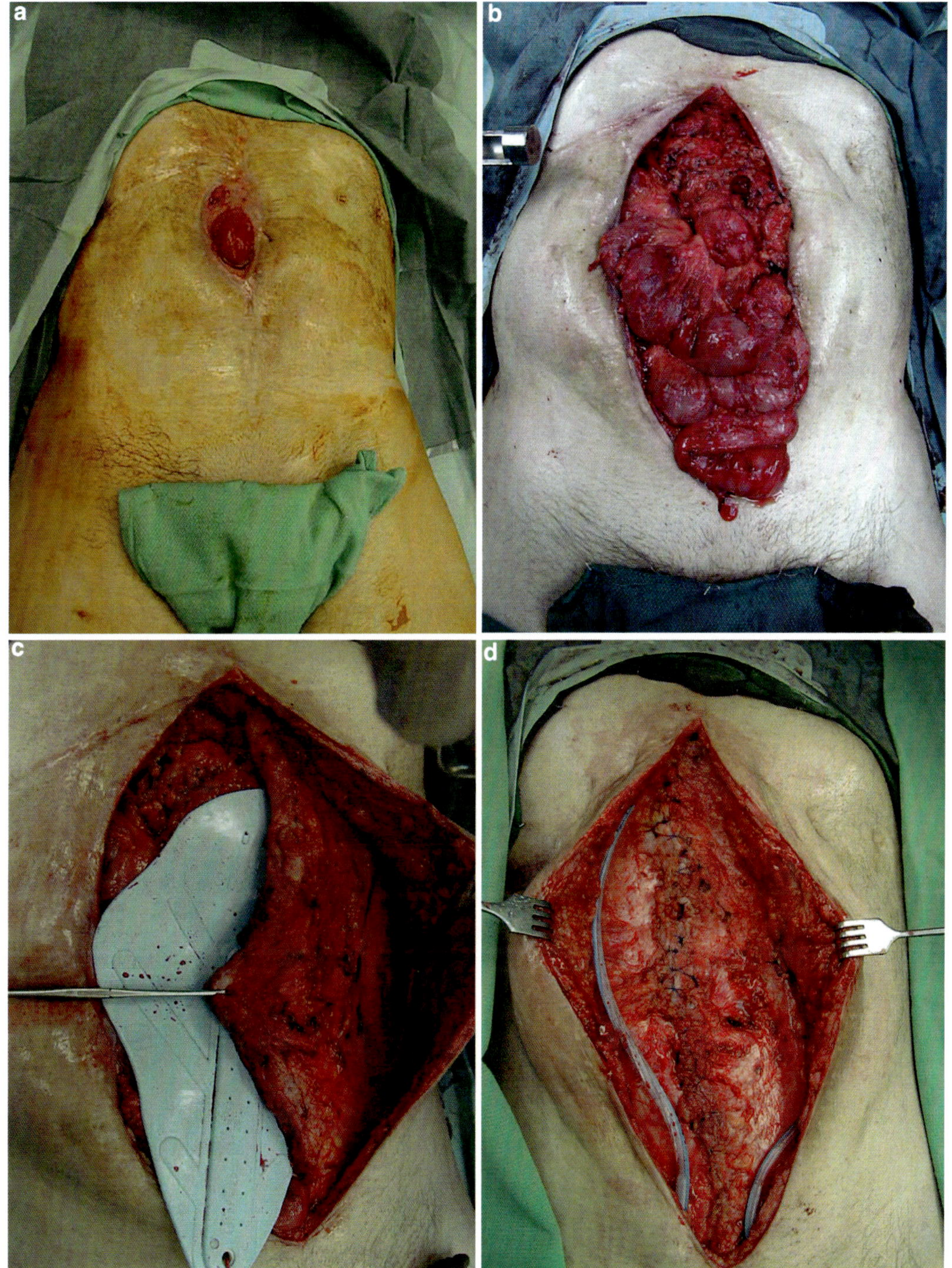

Fig. 34.12 (**a**) Large enterocutaneous fistula with associated giant hernia. (**b**) Isolation of EC fistula prior to complete resection of the damage bowel. (**c**) Components separation. (**d**) Midline fascial closure

setting should caution the surgeon on engaging in attempting to reconstruct the musculofascial defect by employment of components separation in this emergent setting. The patient in Fig. 34.21a, b presented with an acute abdomen, giant ventral hernia, morbid obesity, and loss of skin abdominal skin integrity. An emergent laparotomy revealed perforated appendicitis with gross peritonitis (Fig. 34.22). An appen-

dectomy was performed, the gross peritonitis was cleared, and the unviable skin was excised. We elected to close the giant central defect (150 cm^2) without components separation by placement of a large biologic implant in an underlay fashion (Fig. 34.23). The skin was closed over 4 large subcutaneous drains. The patient had an uneventful recovery with good results in a 6-week postoperative visit (Fig. 34.24a, b).

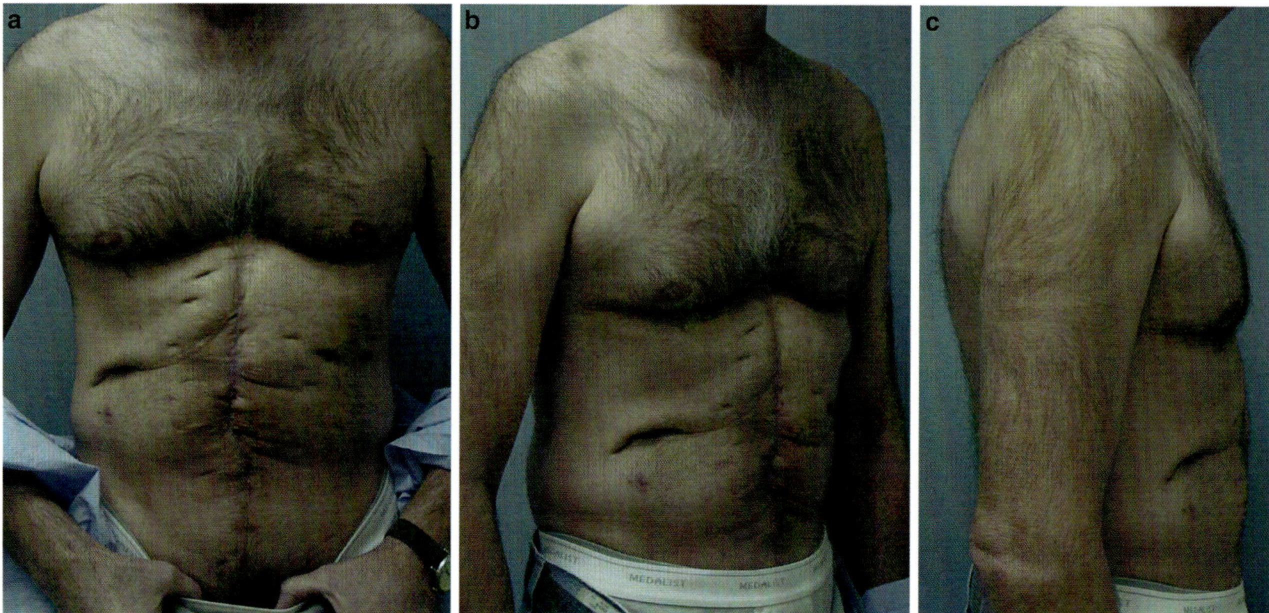

Fig. 34.13 (**a, b, c**) Post-op outcome

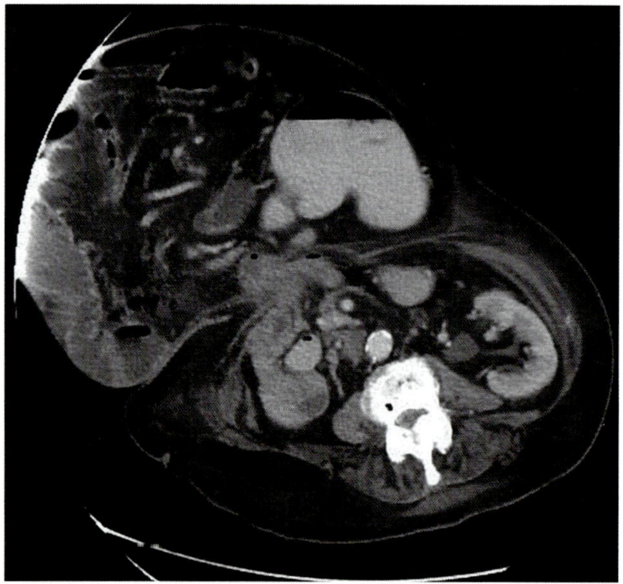

Fig. 34.14 Patient with history of more than 10 previous abdominal operations and >25 year history of ventral hernia. CT shows massive loss of abdominal domain

Although bridging fascial defects with biologic mesh implants is known to have recurrence rates of 21–50% [54], we advocate its employment for two reasons (instances). First, standard practice of simply closing the skin or bridging the defect with absorbable mesh such as Polyglactin 910 has a 100% recurrence rate, whereas bridging with a biologic implant has a potential for a long lasting repair. Caution is warranted because, as noted previously, there is a high incidence of recurrent herniation when bridging with biologic implants. However, new products and careful, long-term, prospective studies remain to be published. Second, the current biologic products hold up well to infected environments with a 3% fistula rate, as compared to Polyglactin 910 fistula rate of 9–12% during management of open abdomens [37, 54, 55].

Complications/Outcomes

Open Emergency Groin Hernia Repair

Emergency groin hernia surgery carries an increased morbidity and mortality as compared to elective surgery. Patients that present emergently do so in a delayed fashion, tend to be older (>60 years old), have a threefold higher incidence of femoral hernias, and an increased risk of bowel obstruction or strangulation, thus leading to a six- to ninefold increase in mortality [56–59]. The mortality increases 20-fold if bowel resection is required, which occurs in 4.5–19% of emergency cases [58, 60]. Other common acute morbidities include bleeding, cardiac and pulmonary complications, along with wound and urinary tract infections with an overall 30-day complication rate of 12–31%. Recurrence after groin hernia operation is 2.3–20% for inguinal repairs and 11.8–75% for femoral repairs, depending on presentation, anatomy, and

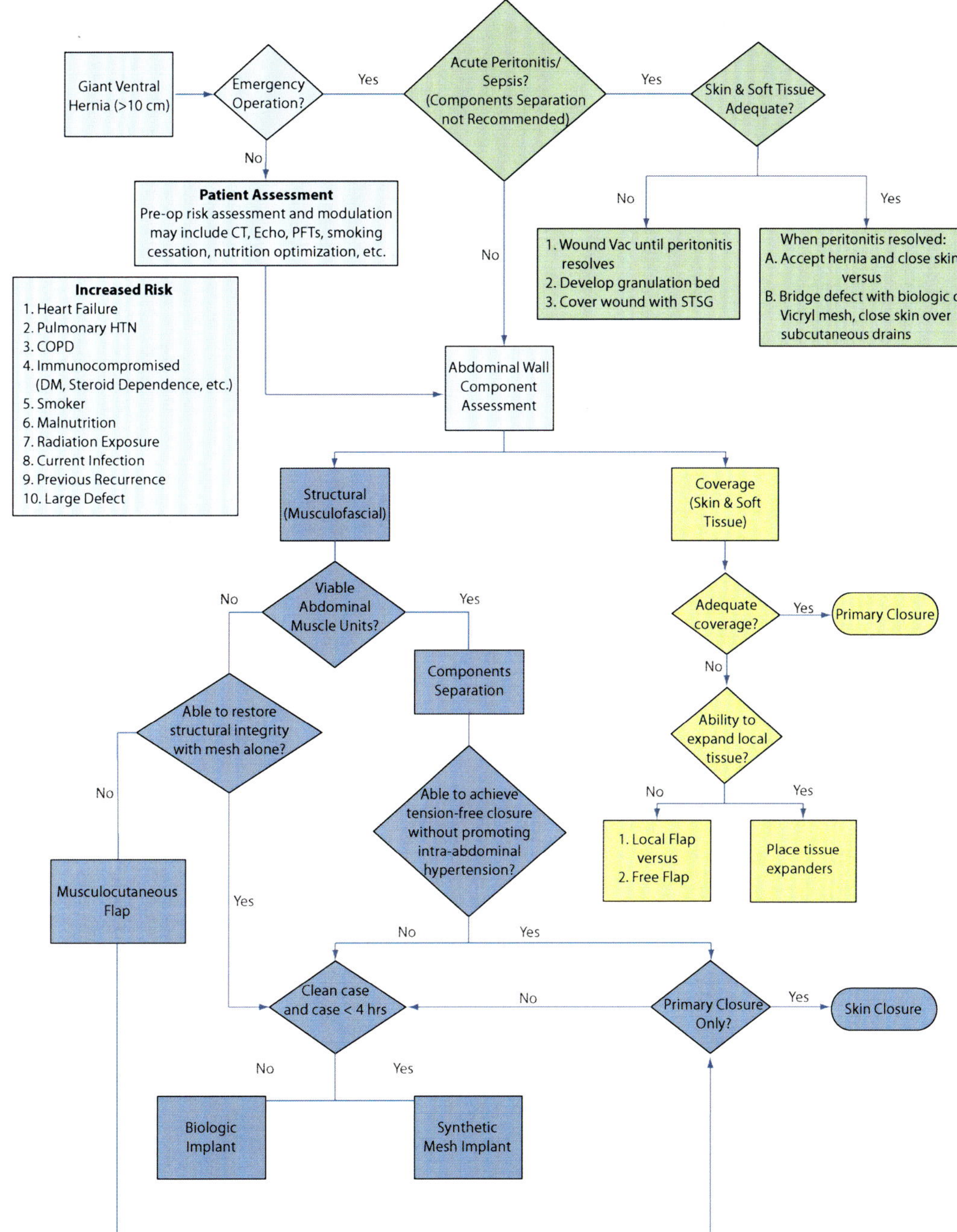

Fig. 34.15 Algorithm for repair of giant abdominal wall defects

surgeon experience [56, 58, 61]. Early postoperative pain is common, with an incidence of 15–20% due to neuropraxias and hypesthesias. However, chronic pain is generally seen in only 5% of patients [61]. Other less common, but significant complications are ischemic orchitis, testicular atrophy, disruption of the vas deferens or lymphatics, and osteitis pubis. Risk mitigation for these complications occurs by attention to careful surgical technique with avoidance of aggressive dissection of the spermatic cord and avoidance of suture fixation to the pubic tubercle.

Open Complex Ventral Hernia Repair

The repair of giant complex ventral hernias has an overall morbidity of 24–53% and mortality less than 2% [27, 38, 39,

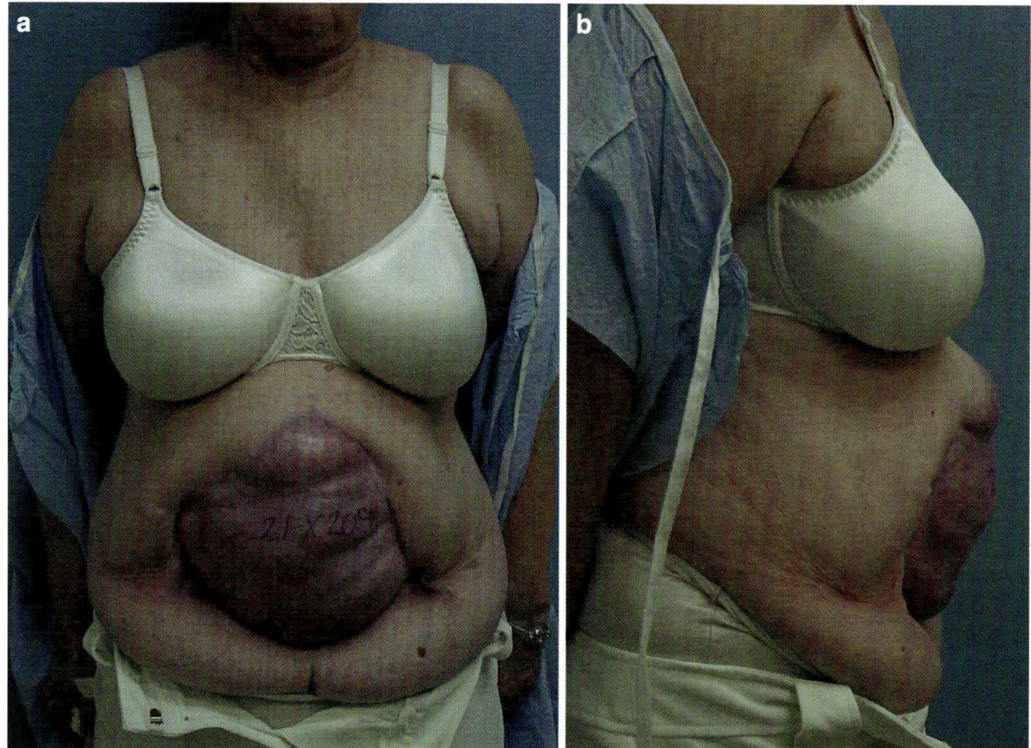

Fig. 34.16 (**a, b**) Stage I. Anatomical assessment of abdominal wall components

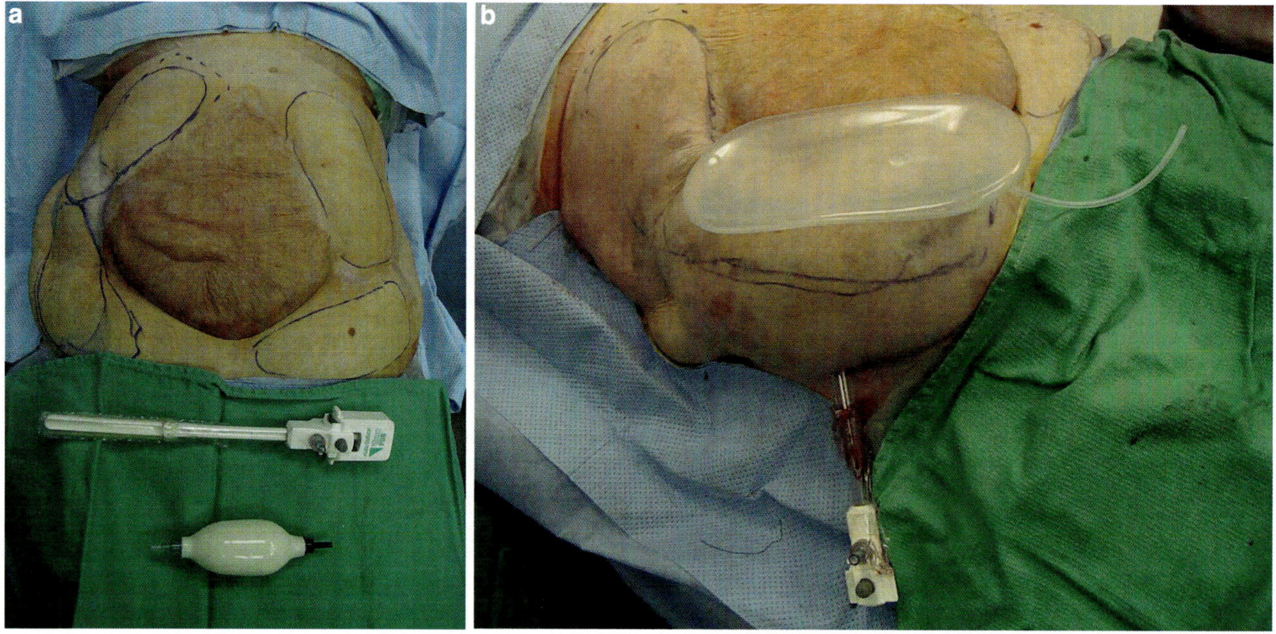

Fig. 34.17 (**a, b**) Stage II endoscopic expansion of skin and soft tissues

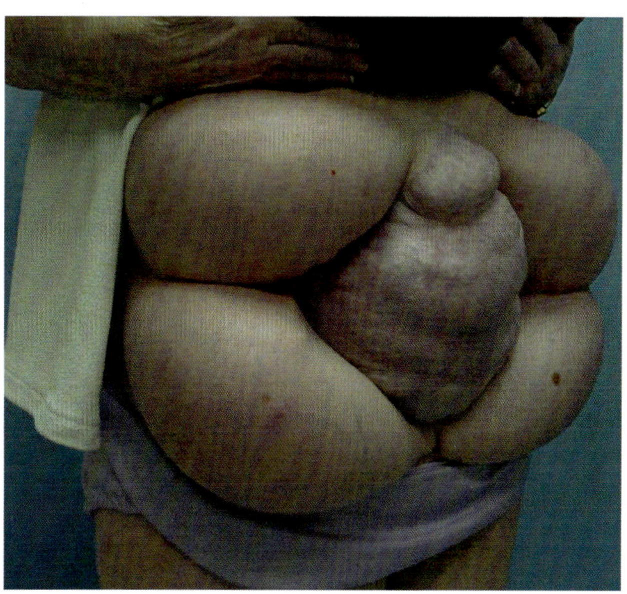

Fig. 34.18 Stage III serial balloon expansion of skin and soft tissues

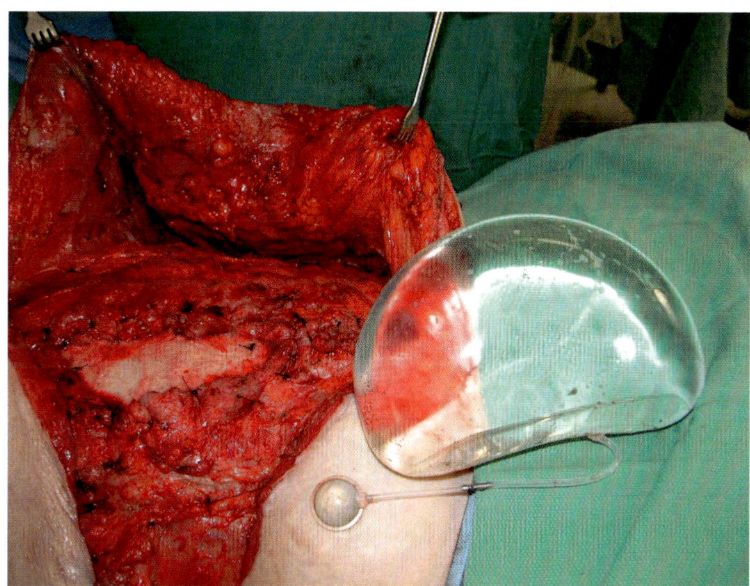

Fig. 34.19 Stage IV removal of balloon expanders, components separation, and placement of bridging underlay of biologic implant

55, 62–71]. Proper patient selection through appropriate preoperative evaluation and optimization is necessary to maintain the current low mortality rate. However, the morbidity remains significant and long-term outcomes of repairs utilizing the components separation technique remain unclear due to the retrospective nature of the studies along with a heterogeneous patient mix and lack of standardization of techniques. While the follow-up period for most is 2 years or less, there are two recent publications with mean periods of 5 years and large numbers of patients (114 and 545) [38, 71]. Table 34.5 summarizes the current literature and shows that the recurrence rate is 5–32% after repair of complex ventral hernias with components separation technique with or without mesh prosthesis.

Wound complications are the most vexing issues related to components separation. The original Ramirez technique requires dissecting from the midline laterally, raising large soft-tissue flaps to reach the external abdominal oblique fascia.

Fig. 34.20 Four weeks post-op

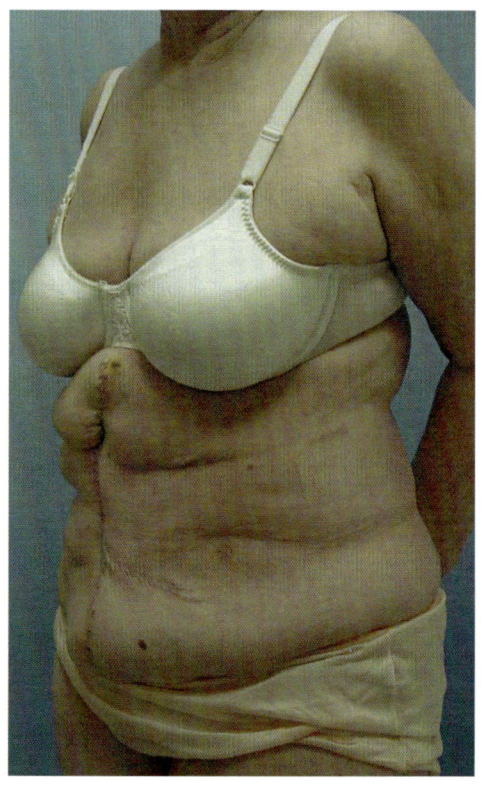

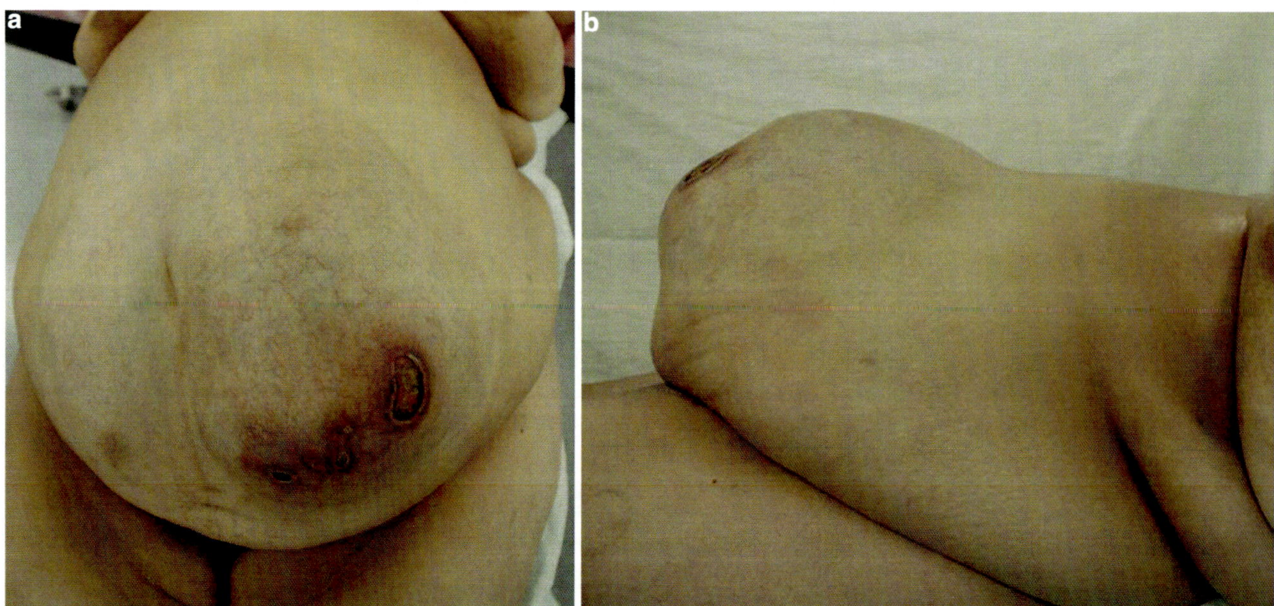

Fig. 34.21 (**a, b**) Giant hernia with peritonitis and loss of skin integrity

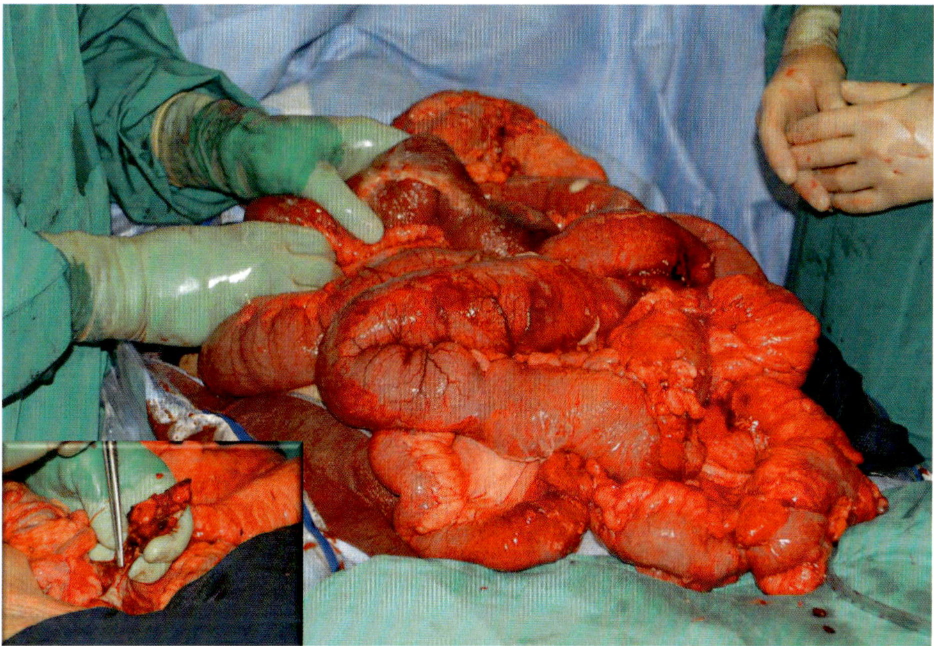

Fig. 34.22 Gross peritonitis with dilated and inflamed small intestine due to perforated appendicitis (Inset)

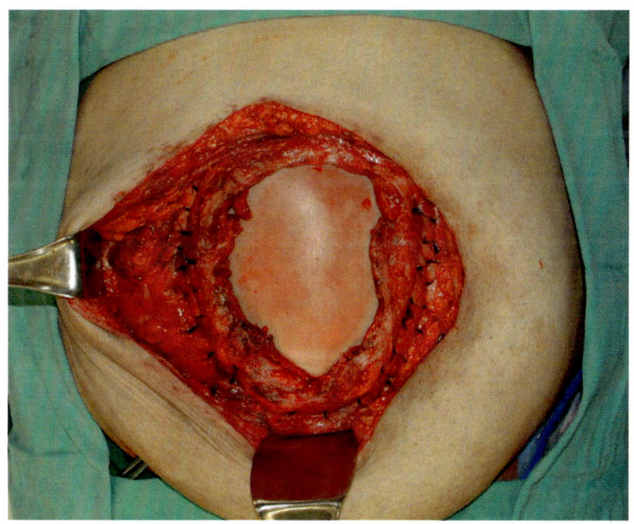

Fig. 34.23 Biologic implantation as underlay, bridging hernia defect

Doing so often requires interruption of the perforators supplying blood to the soft tissue of the anterior abdominal wall via the deep epigastric arcade. This leaves the blood supply coming from the superficial epigastric and circumflex iliac arteries as well as the intercostals, resulting in a risk of ischemia to the midline closure [64]. Additionally, the dissection leaves a large subcutaneous space, increasing the risk of seroma or hematoma formation with a concomitant rise in the risk for surgical site infections. More recently, minimally invasive approaches for components separation have been popularized to reduce the risk of tissue ischemia and seroma/hematoma formation [64, 72–78]. Endoscopically assisted components separation appears to have similar results for achieving midline fascial closure with comparable hernia recurrence rates but with significantly reduced wound complications (0–33%).

Conclusion

Finally, as it relates to reduction of hernia recurrence, the type of mesh reinforcement or whether to use mesh at all is difficult to understand based on the current studies. As noted previously in this chapter, DiCocco's review of their 15-year experience with 152 patients showed that "the highest recurrence rates occurred in patients with prosthetic-assisted repairs" [38]. There was a 5–8% recurrence rate for patients undergoing components release only versus 20–44% recurrence rate if mesh was used. However, this may be explained by placing more prosthetics in patients with higher risk for re-herniation, potentially due larger defect size, and increased midline closure tension. In a review of 200 consecutive patients, Ko et al. [40] observed a higher re-herniation rate when acellular cadaveric dermis was used as an underlay versus soft polypropylene mesh (33% vs. 0%). However,

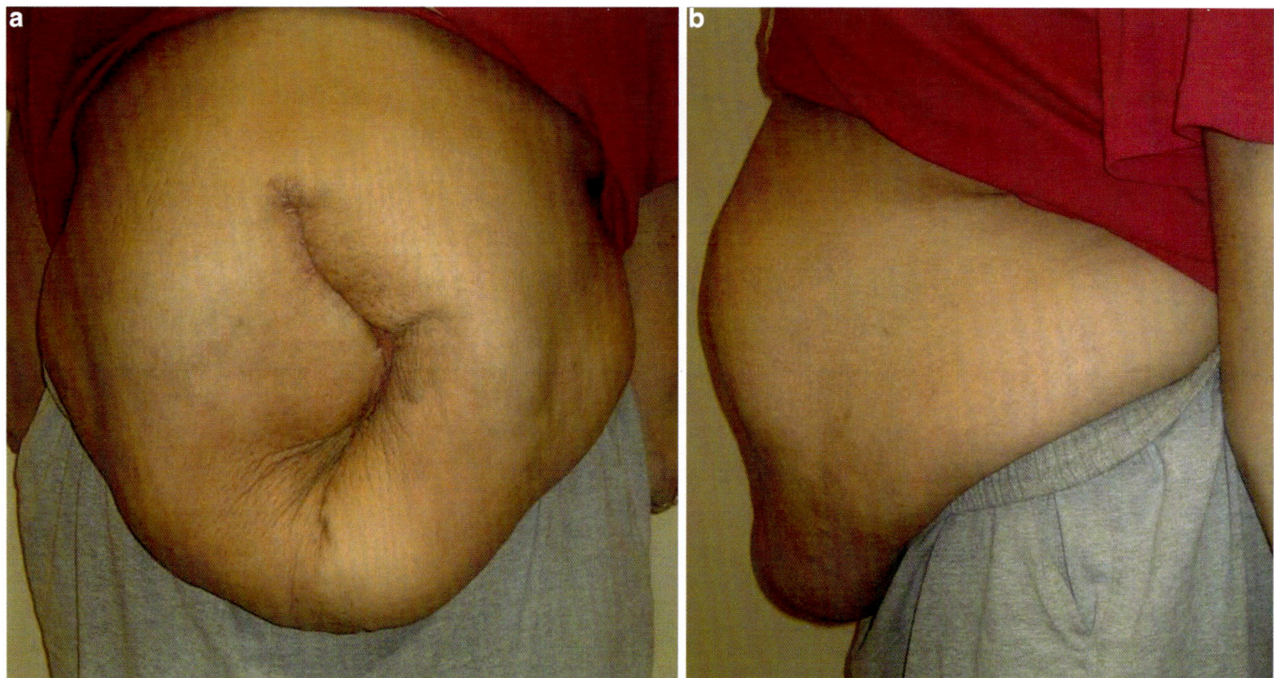

Fig. 34.24 (**a**, **b**) Six weeks post-op

Table 34.5 Publications with 30 or more patients, utilizing various methods of components separation (CS) with or without mesh prostheses (synthetic or biologic)

First author	Year	No.	Wound complications[a] no. (%)	Other major complications[b] no. (%)	Overall morbidity no. (%)	Mortality no. (%)	Recurrence no. (%)	Mean follow-up (range) months
DiBello	1996	35	5 (14)	0	5 (14)	0	3 (9)	22 (1–43)
Girotto	1999	37	14 (38)	5 (14)	19 (51)	0	2 (5)	21 (6–57)
Lowe[c]	2000	37	31(84)	19 (51)	?	0	4 (13)	12 (?)
Girotto	2003	96[d]	25 (26)	?	?	?	21 (22)	26 (6–96)
de Vries Reilingh	2003	43	14(33)	2 (5)	17 (40)	1 (2)	12 (32)[e]	15.6 (12–30)
Jernigan	2003	73	?	?	?	0	4 (5)	24 (2–60)
Gonzalez	2005	42	14 (33)	0	14 (33)	0	3 (7)	16 (?)
Espinoza-de-los-Monteros	2007	39	(26)	0	13 (34)		2 (5)	15 (?)
Moore	2008	90	23 (26)	8 (9)	31 (34)	1 (1)	5 (6)	50 (1–132)
Ko[f]	2009	200	?	?	86 (43)	?	43 (22)	10 (0–74)
Sailes	2010	545	41 (8)	?	?	?	100 (18)	66 (?)
DiCocco[g]	2010	114	?	?	?	?	16 (14)	63.6 (9–175)
Hultman[h]	2011	136	?	?	?	?	26 (19)	? (?-120)
Yegiyants	2011	34	11 (32)	9 (26)	18 (53)	0	2 (6)	47 (4–92)
Giurgius[i]	2011	35	12 (34)	2 (6)	14 (40)	0	1	8 (1–21)

[a]Wound Complications—infection, hematoma, seroma, ischemia, dehiscence

[b]Other Major Complications—UTIs, bacteremia, acute kidney injury, fistulas, mesh erosion, cardiopulmonary complications, chronic pain

[c]Mixed Open ($n = 30$) and Endoscopic ($n = 7$) Components Release

[d]This is one arm of a three arm retrospective study. These patients underwent CS and mesh placement

[e]38 patients available for follow-up

[f]Most patients (158) were treated with CS only (without prosthetic reinforcement). Study separated complications by "major" (24%) and "minor" (19%)

[g]11% did not undergo CS

[h]Paper focuses on recurrent hernia of 26 patients out of the original 136

[i]Comparison of Open ($n = 14$) to Endoscopic ($n = 21$) CS. Endoscopic had 20% wound complications compared to the Open group with 57% wound complications

there were few patients ($n = 18$) in the study, which was not powered to make any conclusions on this observation. Ultimately, most would support the use of synthetic mesh in clean cases and reserve the use of biologic mesh for those cases where there is contamination.

References

1. Rutkow IM. Demographic and socioeconomic aspects of hernia repair in the United States in 2003. Surg Clin North Am. 2003;83(5):1045–51. v–vi.
2. Rutkow IM. Epidemiologic, economic, and sociologic aspects of hernia surgery in the United States in the 1990s. Surg Clin North Am. 1998;78(6):941–51. v–vi.
3. Muysoms FE, Miserez M, Berrevoet F, et al. Classification of primary and incisional abdominal wall hernias. Hernia. 2009;13(4):407–14.
4. Shell 4 DH, de la Torre J, Andrades P, Vasconez LO. Open repair of ventral incisional hernias. Surg Clin North Am. 2008;88(1):61–83. viii.
5. den Hartog D, Dur AHM, Tuinebreijer WE, Kreis RW. Open surgical procedures for incisional hernias. Cochrane Database Syst Rev. 2008;(3):CD006438.
6. Cassar K, Munro A. Surgical treatment of incisional hernia. Br J Surg. 2002;89(5):534–45.
7. Heniford BT, Park A, Ramshaw BJ, Voeller G. Laparoscopic repair of ventral hernias: nine years' experience with 850 consecutive hernias. Ann Surg. 2003;238(3):391–9. discussion 399–400.
8. Ramshaw BJ, Esartia P, Schwab J, et al. Comparison of laparoscopic and open ventral herniorrhaphy. Am Surg. 1999;65(9):827–31.
9. Flum DR, Horvath K, Koepsell T. Have outcomes of incisional hernia repair improved with time? Ann Surg. 2003;237(1):129–35.
10. Luijendijk RW, Hop WC, van den Tol MP, et al. A comparison of suture repair with mesh repair for incisional hernia. N Engl J Med. 2000;343(6):392–8.
11. Hodgson NC, Malthaner RA, Ostbye T. The search for an ideal method of abdominal fascial closure: a meta-analysis. Ann Surg. 2000;231(3):436–42.
12. Ceydeli A, Rucinski J, Wise L. Finding the best abdominal closure: an evidence-based review of the literature. Curr Surg. 2005;62(2):220–5.
13. Jenkins TP. The burst abdominal wound: a mechanical approach. Br J Surg. 1976;63(11):873–6.
14. Primatesta P, Goldacre MJ. Inguinal hernia repair: incidence of elective and emergency surgery, readmission and mortality. Int J Epidemiol. 1996;25(4):835–9.
15. Zollinger Jr RM. Classification systems for groin hernias. Surg Clin North Am. 2003;83(5):1053–63.
16. Zollinger Jr RM. An updated traditional classification of inguinal hernias. Hernia. 2004;8(4):318–22.
17. Mittal T, Kumar V, Khullar R, et al. Diagnosis and management of Spigelian hernia: a review of literature and our experience. J Minim Access Surg. 2008;4(4):95–8.
18. Sorelli PG, El-Masry NS, Garrett WV. Open femoral hernia repair: one skin incision for all. World J Emerg Surg. 2009;4:44.
19. Stamatiou D, Skandalakis JE, Skandalakis LJ, Mirilas P. Lumbar hernia: surgical anatomy, embryology, and technique of repair. Am Surg. 2009;75(3):202–7.
20. Amid PK. Groin hernia repair: open techniques. World J Surg. 2005;29(8).1046–51.
21. Bendavid R. The Shouldice technique: a canon in hernia repair. Can J Surg. 1997;40(3):199–205, 207.
22. Papanikitas J, Sutcliffe RP, Rohatgi A, Atkinson S. Bilateral retrovascular femoral hernia. Ann R Coll Surg Engl. 2008;90(5):423–4.
23. Nyhus LM. The posterior (preperitoneal) approach and iliopubic tract repair of inguinal and femoral hernias—an update. Hernia. 2003;7(2):63–7.
24. Moore FA. The use of lactated Ringer s in shock resuscitation: the good, the bad and the ugly. J Trauma: Inj Infect Crit Care. 2011;70:S15–6.
25. Breuing K, Butler CE, Ferzoco S, et al. Incisional ventral hernias: review of the literature and recommendations regarding the grading and technique of repair. Surgery. 2010;148(3):544–58.
26. Burger JWA, Luijendijk RW, Hop WCJ, et al. Long-term follow-up of a randomized controlled trial of suture versus mesh repair of incisional hernia. Ann Surg. 2004;240(4):578–83. discussion 583–585.
27. Espinosa-de-los-Monteros A, de la Torre JI, Marrero I, et al. Utilization of human cadaveric acellular dermis for abdominal hernia reconstruction. Ann Plast Surg. 2007;58(3):264–7.
28. de Vries Reilingh TS, Van Goor H, Charbon JA, et al. Repair of giant midline abdominal wall hernias: components separation technique versus prosthetic repair: interim analysis of a randomized controlled trial. World J Surg. 2007;31(4):756–63.
29. Kolker AR, Brown DJ, Redstone JS, Scarpinato VM, Wallack MK. Multilayer reconstruction of abdominal wall defects with acellular dermal allograft (AlloDerm) and component separation. Ann Plast Surg. 2005;55(1):36–41. discussion 41–42.
30. Mangram AJ, Horan TC, Pearson ML, Silver LC, Jarvis WR. Guideline for prevention of surgical site infection 1999. Hospital Infection Control Practices Advisory Committee. Infect Control Hosp Epidemiol. 1999;20(4):250–78. quiz 279–280.
31. Awad ZT, Puri V, LeBlanc K, et al. Mechanisms of ventral hernia recurrence after mesh repair and a new proposed classification. J Am Coll Surg. 2005;201(1):132–40.
32. Korenkov M, Paul A, Sauerland S, et al. Classification and surgical treatment of incisional hernia. Results of an experts' meeting. Langenbecks Arch Surg. 2001;386(1):65–73.
33. Ghazi B, Deigni O, Yezhelyev M, Losken A. Current options in the management of complex abdominal wall defects. Ann Plast Surg. 2011;66(5):488–92.
34. Maas SM, van Engeland M, Leeksma NG, Bleichrodt RP. A modification of the "components separation" technique for closure of abdominal wall defects in the presence of an enterostomy. J Am Coll Surg. 1999;189(1):138–40.
35. Young D. Repair of epigastric incisional hernia. Br J Surg. 1961;48:514–6.
36. Ramirez OM, Ruas E, Dellon AL. "Components separation" method for closure of abdominal-wall defects: an anatomic and clinical study. Plast Reconstr Surg. 1990;86(3):519–26.
37. Fabian TC, Croce MA, Pritchard FE, et al. Planned ventral hernia. Staged management for acute abdominal wall defects. Ann Surg. 1994;219(6):643–50. discussion 651–653.
38. DiCocco JM, Magnotti LJ, Emmett KP, et al. Long-term follow-up of abdominal wall reconstruction after planned ventral hernia: a 15-year experience. J Am Coll Surg. 2010;210(5):686–95. 695–698.
39. DiBello Jr JN, Moore Jr JH. Sliding myofascial flap of the rectus abdominus muscles for the closure of recurrent ventral hernias. Plast Reconstr Surg. 1996;98(3):464–9.
40. Ko JH, Wang EC, Salvay DM, Paul BC, Dumanian GA. Abdominal wall reconstruction: lessons learned from 200 "components separation" procedures. Arch Surg. 2009;144(11):1047–55.
41. Mathes SJ, Steinwald PM, Foster RD, Hoffman WY, Anthony JP. Complex abdominal wall reconstruction: a comparison of flap and mesh closure. Ann Surg. 2000;232(4):586–96.
42. Hultman CS, Pratt B, Cairns BA, et al. Multidisciplinary approach to abdominal wall reconstruction after decompressive laparotomy for abdominal compartment syndrome. Ann Plast Surg. 2005;54(3):269.

43. de Vries Reilingh TS, van Goor H, Rosman C, et al. "Components separation technique" for the repair of large abdominal wall hernias. J Am Coll Surg. 2003;196(1):32–7.

44. Perathoner A, Margreiter R, Kafka-Ritsch R. Surgical treatment of the open abdomen in patients with abdominal sepsis using the vacuum assisted closure system. World J Surg. 2009;33(6):1332–3. author reply 1334.

45. van Geffen HJAA, Simmermacher RKJ, van Vroonhoven TJMV, van der Werken C. Surgical treatment of large contaminated abdominal wall defects. J Am Coll Surg. 2005;201(2):206–12.

46. Leppäniemi A, Tukiainen E. Planned hernia repair and late abdominal wall reconstruction. World J Surg. 2011. Available at: http://www.ncbi.nlm.nih.gov/pubmed/21713574. Accessed 2 Nov 2011.

47. Wind J, van Koperen PJ, Slors JFM, Bemelman WA. Single-stage closure of enterocutaneous fistula and stomas in the presence of large abdominal wall defects using the components separation technique. Am J Surg. 2009;197(1):24–9.

48. Alaedeen DI, Lipman J, Medalie D, Rosen MJ. The single-staged approach to the surgical management of abdominal wall hernias in contaminated fields. Hernia. 2007;11(1):41–5.

49. Shestak KC, Edington HJ, Johnson RR. The separation of anatomic components technique for the reconstruction of massive midline abdominal wall defects: anatomy, surgical technique, applications, and limitations revisited. Plast Reconstr Surg. 2000;105(2):731–8. quiz 739.

50. Mathes SJ, Steinwald PM, Foster RD, Hoffman WY, Anthony JP. Complex abdominal wall reconstruction: a comparison of flap and mesh closure. Ann Surg. 2000;232(4):586–96.

51. Ramirez OM, Ruas E, Dellon AL. "Components separation" method for closure of abdominal-wall defects: an anatomic and clinical study. Plast Reconstr Surg. 1990;86(3):519–26.

52. Buck 2nd DW, Steinberg JP, Fryer J, Dumanian GA. Operative management of massive hernias with associated distended bowel. Am J Surg. 2010;200(2):258–64.

53. Agnew SP, Small Jr W, Wang E, et al. Prospective measurements of intra-abdominal volume and pulmonary function after repair of massive ventral hernias with the components separation technique. Ann Surg. 2010;251(5):981–8.

54. Maurice SM, Skeete DA. Use of human acellular dermal matrix for abdominal wall reconstructions. Am J Surg. 2009;197(1):35–42.

55. Jernigan TW, Fabian TC, Croce MA, et al. Staged management of giant abdominal wall defects: acute and long-term results. Ann Surg. 2003;238(3):349–55. discussion 355–7.

56. Malek S, Torella F, Edwards PR. Emergency repair of groin herniae: outcome and implications for elective surgery waiting times. Int J Clin Pract. 2004;58(2):207–9.

57. Nilsson H, Stylianidis G, Haapamäki M, Nilsson E, Nordin P. Mortality after groin hernia surgery. Ann Surg. 2007;245(4):656–60.

58. Tiernan JP, Katsarelis H, Garner JP, Skinner PP. Excellent outcomes after emergency groin hernia repair. Hernia. 2010;14(5):485–8.

59. Oishi SN, Page CP, Schwesinger WH. Complicated presentations of groin hernias. Am J Surg. 1991;162(6):568–70. discussion 571.

60. Suppiah A, Gatt M, Barandiaran J, Heng MS, Perry EP. Outcomes of emergency and elective femoral hernia surgery in four district general hospitals: a 4-year study. Hernia. 2007;11(6):509–12.

61. Bendavid R. Complications of groin hernia surgery. Surg Clin North Am. 1998;78(6):1089–103.

62. Moore M, Bax T, MacFarlane M, McNevin MS. Outcomes of the fascial component separation technique with synthetic mesh reinforcement for repair of complex ventral incisional hernias in the morbidly obese. Am J Surg. 2008;195(5):575–9. discussion 579.

63. Girotto JA, Ko MJ, Redett R, et al. Closure of chronic abdominal wall defects: a long-term evaluation of the components separation method. Ann Plast Surg. 1999;42(4):385–94. discussion 394–395.

64. Lowe JB, Garza JR, Bowman JL, Rohrich RJ, Strodel WE. Endoscopically assisted "components separation" for closure of abdominal wall defects. Plast Reconstr Surg. 2000;105(2):720–9. quiz 730.

65. Girotto JA, Chiaramonte M, Menon NG, et al. Recalcitrant abdominal wall hernias: long-term superiority of autologous tissue repair. Plast Reconstr Surg. 2003;112(1):106–14.

66. de Vries Reilingh TS, van Goor H, Rosman C, et al. "Components separation technique" for the repair of large abdominal wall hernias. J Am Coll Surg. 2003;196(1):32–7.

67. Gonzalez R, Rehnke RD, Ramaswamy A, et al. Components separation technique and laparoscopic approach: a review of two evolving strategies for ventral hernia repair. Am Surg. 2005;71(7):598–605.

68. Ko JH, Salvay DM, Paul BC, Wang EC, Dumanian GA. Soft polypropylene mesh, but not cadaveric dermis, significantly improves outcomes in midline hernia repairs using the components separation technique. Plast Reconstr Surg. 2009;124(3):836–47.

69. Hultman CS, Tong WMY, Kittinger BJ, et al. Management of recurrent hernia after components separation: 10-year experience with abdominal wall reconstruction at an academic medical center. Ann Plast Surg. 2011;66(5):504–7.

70. Yegiyants S, Tam M, Lee DJ, Abbas MA. Outcome of components separation for contaminated complex abdominal wall defects. Hernia. 2011. Available at: http://www.ncbi.nlm.nih.gov/pubmed/21786148. Accessed 2 Nov 2011.

71. Sailes FC, Walls J, Guelig D, et al. Synthetic and biological mesh in component separation: a 10-year single institution review. Ann Plast Surg. 2010;64(5):696–8.

72. Maas SM, van Engeland M, Leeksma NG, Bleichrodt RP. A modification of the "components separation" technique for closure of abdominal wall defects in the presence of an enterostomy. J Am Coll Surg. 1999;189(1):138–40.

73. Maas SM, de Vries RS, van Goor H, de Jong D, Bleichrodt RP. Endoscopically assisted "components separation technique" for the repair of complicated ventral hernias. J Am Coll Surg. 2002;194(3):388–90.

74. Milburn ML, Shah PK, Friedman EB, et al. Laparoscopically assisted components separation technique for ventral incisional hernia repair. Hernia. 2007;11(2):157–61.

75. Harth KC, Rosen MJ. Endoscopic versus open component separation in complex abdominal wall reconstruction. Am J Surg. 2010;199(3):342–6. discussion 346–347.

76. Parra MW, Rodas EB. Minimally invasive components separation—an updated method for closure of abdominal wall defects. J Laparoendosc Adv Surg Tech A. 2011;21(7):621–3.

77. Rosen MJ, Jin J, McGee MF, et al. Laparoscopic component separation in the single-stage treatment of infected abdominal wall prosthetic removal. Hernia. 2007;11(5):435–40.

78. Giurgius M, Bendure L, Davenport DL, Roth JS. The endoscopic component separation technique for hernia repair results in reduced morbidity compared to the open component separation technique. Hernia. 2011. Available at: http://www.ncbi.nlm.nih.gov/pubmed/21833851. Accessed 22 Nov 2011.

John A. Harvin and Rondel P. Albarado

Introduction

Temporary closure of the abdomen following a laparotomy for trauma or emergency surgery (open abdomen) is an invaluable tool that improves patient outcomes. It allows the surgeon to control bleeding or sepsis with as little physiologic stress to the patient as possible. Ongoing resuscitation in the intensive care unit (ICU) in the patient with an open abdomen followed by the definitive procedure can, in select patients, improve outcomes. Unfortunately, the open abdomen also has many potential, associated complications. This chapter discusses the history of the open abdomen, indications for temporary closure of the abdomen, the evolution of the care of the laparotomy wound, abdominal closure techniques following the open abdomen, and complications of the open abdomen.

The History of the Open Abdomen

Sir William H. Ogilvie first described temporarily closing the abdomen of a patient during World War II. He used a piece of canvas or cotton cloth to bridge the defect in the abdominal wall. He postulated that the device prevented retraction of the gap, kept the intestines from protruding through the defect, and allowed the abdominal wall to be used for breathing [1].

J.A. Harvin, M.D.
Department of Surgery, University of Texas Health Science Center at Houston, Houston, TX, USA

R.P. Albarado, M.D. (✉)
Division of Acute Care Surgery, The University of Texas Medical School at Houston, 6431 Fannin Street, MSB 4.284, Houston, TX 77030, USA
e-mail: rondel.albarado@uth.tmc.edu

In actuality, the modern history of temporary abdominal closure evolved simultaneously with the management of hepatic trauma by packing. The first surgeon to describe hepatic packing was James Hogarth Pringle in his seminal paper in which he also described mass occlusion of the portal triad as a method to hepatic hemorrhage control. In this manuscript, he advocated en masse ligation of hepatic tissue as the preferred method of controlling hemorrhage, but acknowledged that hepatic packing is sometimes the only alternative [2]. Hepatic packing fell out of favor during the middle of the twentieth century [3]. Not until the 1970s did it return as an acceptable method for the management of hepatic trauma [4–6]. In 1975, Stone et al. documented the rapid and effective control of hepatic venous bleeding via autogenous omental packing [4]. This was followed in 1980 by a larger series with almost uniform success in patients with non-penetrating injury [5]. Feliciano and colleagues further identified hepatic packing to be a "life saving maneuver in highly selected patients in whom coagulopathies, hypothermia, and acidosis make further surgical efforts likely to increase hemorrhage" [6].

Around the time of the reemergence of hepatic packing, reports of abbreviated laparotomy and temporary abdominal closure were also being published. Stone et al. discussed the "protocol for abdominal tamponade" and resultant "initial abortion of laparotomy" [7]. By doing so, they documented a decreased need for blood product transfusion and increased survival in patients packed who were coagulopathic [7]. The term "Damage Control" was first coined by Rotondo and colleagues [8]. They defined it as the "initial control of hemorrhage and contamination followed by intraperitoneal packing and rapid closure" [8]. This allowed for aggressive resuscitation in the ICU and the definitive procedure to follow. The authors documented that in patients with major vascular injury and two or more visceral injuries, damage control resulted in improved survival. Importantly, a damage control laparotomy did not improve survival in the entire cohort.

Table 35.1 Indications for temporary abdominal closure in trauma and emergency surgery

Moore [9]
- Medical bleeding due to coagulopathy
- Inaccessible major venous injury
- Need for a time-consuming procedure in an under-resuscitated patient
- Need for control of extra-abdominal, life-threatening injury
- Inability to close laparotomy incision
- Desire to reassess abdominal contents

EAST [10]
- Abdominal compartment syndrome
- Intra-abdominal packing after severe abdominal trauma
- Severe intra-abdominal sepsis
- Inability to close the abdomen

EAST—Eastern Association for the Surgery of Trauma

Indications for Temporary Closure of the Abdomen

As experience with temporary abdominal closure increased, a consensus on indications emerged. These indications were best summarized by Dr. Gene Moore during his Thomas G. Orr Memorial Lecture at the 1996 Southwestern Surgical Congress [9] and by the Eastern Association for the Surgery of Trauma (EAST) in 2009 [10]. These indications are listed in Table 35.1.

Many researchers have attempted to find objective data as an indication for an abbreviated laparotomy [11–13]; however, these data are highly heterogeneous and the indications in Table 35.1 appear to be the most consistently agreed upon.

Laparotomy Management

The ideal temporary abdominal closure device should be universally available, be easy to apply, control fluid losses, leave the skin and fascia intact, not react to viscera, and be easy to change [14]. The first generation of temporary abdominal closures included towel clips to the skin and the use of synthetic materials to bridge the abdominal defect. Towel clips were certainly quick and easy to apply, but did not prevent abdominal compartment syndrome or fascial retraction, and interfered with postoperative radiologic evaluation of the abdomen. The use of a sterile crystalloid bag (i.e., a Bogota bag), synthetic mesh, or Velcro (i.e., the Wittmann Patch®, NovoMedicus, Nokomis, FL) were and are commonly used. These devices help to prevent abdominal compartment syndrome, but do not allow for the control of fluid loss and nor do they prevent fascial retraction.

Second-generation temporary abdominal closure devices focus on all of the above with a primary focus on fluid control. The vacuum pack was one such device that covered the viscera with a plastic drape followed by a surgical towel. Sump drains were then placed over the towel and the laparostomy wound covered with an adhesive drape [15]. Certainly, this device controlled the fluid losses better than first generation devices, but it did not prevent loss of abdominal wall domain. The most commonly employed devices now are negative pressure wound therapy devices (i.e., the Wound V.A.C.®, KCI, San Antonio, TX; and the Renasys™, Smith & Nephew, London, United Kingdom). These devices use negative pressure to both control fluid loss and to prevent retraction of the abdominal wall. Unfortunately, no device currently available meets all of the ideal criteria for a temporary abdominal closure device.

Abdominal Closure Techniques Following the Open Abdomen

The right time to start thinking about closing an open abdomen is precisely when it is decided to leave an abdomen open. A step-wise, multifaceted approach to abdominal closure provides the surgeon with the best chance to close the abdomen as quickly as possible.

First, the decision to leave an abdomen open should be made with great caution. In Rotondo et al.'s paper coining the phrase "damage control," only the most severely injured patients benefited from an open abdomen, not all patients. In fact, there is evidence that on-demand laparotomy is as safe as planned relaparotomy, while saving health care dollars and operations [16]. By properly selecting those patients who require a damage control operation, morbidity, survival, and costs can be reduced [17, 18].

Second, the resuscitation strategy used for trauma and emergency surgery patients greatly affects the ability to close an open abdomen. One of the major factors in failure to close an open abdomen is intestinal edema. Permissive hypotension, early blood and plasma resuscitation, and limited crystalloid administration can prevent or minimize intestinal edema. Plasma has been shown to prevent and partially reverse the endothelial dysfunction that leads to capillary permeability and interstitial edema [18, 19]. Excessive crystalloid administration leads directly to intestinal edema and has in fact been found to be an iatrogenic cause of abdominal compartment syndrome [20–29].

Third, proper selection of a temporary abdominal closure device can assist in preventing loss of abdominal wall domain. Negative pressure wound therapy appears to help prevent fascial retraction and is associated with increased likelihood of early fascial closure [25]. Additionally, there are many institution-specific pathways for abdominal closure that focus on constant tension on the fascia and repetitive, partial fascial closure.

Reported useful adjuncts for facilitating early fascial closure include the use of hypertonic saline to decrease bowel edema and third spacing, and early enteric feeding to decrease bowel distension [21, 22]. In addition, the early short-term use of neuromuscular blocking agents has been associated with more rapid and frequent primary fascia approximation in patients managed with damage control laparotomy [23].

When primary fascia approximation is not feasible, the skin may be closed directly over the granulation tissue covering the bowel. If skin approximation is not possible, a split thickness skin graft may be fixed over the granulation bed. Delayed abdominal wall reconstruction is then considered after 6 months. The early reconstruction utilizing bridging techniques and biologics has been associated with recurrence rates up to 80% and can potentially increase complications like small bowel fistula [26, 28]. The delayed abdominal wall reconstruction can be accomplished with a sandwich technique of mesh reinforcement in conjunction with the separation of components to restore a functional abdominal wall with acceptably low hernia recurrence rates [27]. In large defects not amenable to separation of components, bridging with nonabsorbable mesh is appropriate at this time. In select patients, early definitive fascia approximation can be obtained with separation of components in lieu of skin closure or split thickness skin graft during initial hospitalization. Endoscopic component separation techniques offer a minimally invasive alternative to open techniques, thus reducing the complications associated with large skin flaps communicating directly with contaminated spaces [29].

Complications of the Open Abdomen

Although the use of damage control can be a life-saving maneuver in select patients, a surgeon should be well versed in the complications associated with the open abdomen.

Nutrition and Fluid Loss

The open abdomen is a source of large amounts of fluid and protein loss in the critically ill patient [30]. Though the nitrogen and protein content of the abdominal fluid is similar to that of extremity wound exudates, the sheer volume lost through an open abdomen can lead to significant protein deficit if not appropriately accounted for in nutritional supplementation. The open abdomen has been associated with up to 25 g/day protein loss [31].

Incisional Hernia

The rate of incisional hernia formation following an open abdomen can be as high as 30%. Patients discharged from the hospital with an open abdomen have a significantly lower quality of life than societal norms. In this group of patients, a successful abdominal wall reconstruction does not restore the patient's quality of life to that of societal norms, nor does it significantly improve the quality of life compared to those who underwent unsuccessful abdominal wall reconstruction [32].

Fistulae

An open abdomen is associated with higher rates of enterocutaneous and enteroatmospheric fistulae than a closed abdomen [33]. In fact, abdominal closure at the first take back is associated with a significantly lower rate of fistula formation [34]. The routine use of negative pressure wound therapy is associated with lower fistula rates than other mixed modalities including placement of absorbable mesh [28]. As to be expected, the formation of an enteric fistula is associated with longer intensive care and hospital lengths of stay and a higher economic burden, not to mention the nutritional deficiencies and fluid losses that can occur [35].

Infection, Sepsis, Organ Failure

Patients with an open abdomen who are closed at the first take back have significantly fewer abdominal infections, intestinal dysfunction, wound complications, pulmonary complications and failure, and renal failure [34].

Conclusion

In conclusion, damage control laparotomy is a method by which a surgeon can improve survival in select trauma and emergency general surgery patients. Although temporary abdominal closure can improve survival in these critically ill patients, an open abdomen also serves as the cause of multiple morbidities. The decision to leave an abdomen open should be done so with much caution and be followed immediately by the implementation of a comprehensive plan to close the abdominal wall as soon as possible.

References

1. Ogilvie WH. The late complications of abdominal war-wounds. Lancet. 1940;2:253–6.
2. Pringle JH. Notes on the arrest of hepatic hemorrhage due to trauma. Ann Surg. 1908;48(4):541–9.
3. Walt AJ. The surgical management of hepatic trauma and its complications. Ann R Coll Surg Engl. 1969;45(6):319–39.
4. Stone HH, Lamb JM. Use of pedicled omentum as an autogenous pack for control of hemorrhage in major injuries to the liver. Surg Gynecol Obstet. 1975;141:92–4.

5. Fabian TC, Stone HH. Arrest of severe liver hemorrhage by an omental pack. South Med J. 1980;73(11):1487–90.

6. Feliciano DV, Mattox KL, Jordan GL. Intra-abdominal packing for control of hepatic hemorrhage: a reappraisal. J Trauma. 1981;21(4):285–90.

7. Stone HH, Strom PR, Mullins RJ. Management of the major coagulopathy with onset during laparotomy. Ann Surg. 1983;197(5):532–5.

8. Rotondo MF, Schwab CW, McGonigal MD, et al. 'Damage control': an approach for improved survival in exsanguinating penetrating abdominal injury. J Trauma. 1993;35(3):375–82.

9. Moore EE. Staged laparotomy for the hypothermia, acidosis, and coagulopathy syndrome. Am J Surg. 1996;172(5):405–10.

10. Diaz Jr JJ, Cullinane DC, Dutton WD, Jeomre R, Bagdonas R, Bilaniuk JW, et al. The management of the open abdomen in trauma and emergency general surgery: part 1-damage control. J Trauma. 2010;68(6):1425–38.

11. Asensio JA, McDuffie L, Petrone P, et al. Reliable variables in the exsanguinated patient which indicate damage control and predict outcome. Am J Surg. 2001;182:743–51.

12. Burch JM, Ortiz VB, Richardson RJ, Martin RR, Mattox KL, Jordan GL. Abbreviated laparotomy and planned reoperation for critically injured patients. Ann Surg. 1992;215(5):476–83.

13. Morris JA, Eddy VA, Blinman TA, Rutherford EJ, Sharpe KW. Staged celiotomy for trauma. Ann Surg. 1993;217(5):576–84.

14. De Waele JJ, Leppaniemi AK. Temporary abdominal closure techniques. Am Surg. 2011;S48(77):S46–50.

15. Smith LA, Barker DE, Chase CW, Somberg LB, Brock WB, Burns RP. Vacuum pack techinque of temporary abdominal closure. Am Surg. 1997;63(12):1102–7.

16. Van Ruler O, Mahler CW, Boer KR, Reuland EA, Gooszen HG, Oprneer BC, et al. Comparison of on-demand vs planned relaparotomy strategy in patients with severe peritonitis: a randomized trial. JAMA. 2007;298(8):865–72.

17. Higa G, Friese R, O'Keefe T, Wynne J, Bowlby P, Ziemba M, et al. Damage control laparotomy: a vital tool once overused. J Trauma. 2010;69(1):53–9.

18. Pati S, Matijevic N, Doursout MF, Ko T, Cao Y, Deng X, et al. Protective effects of fresh frozen plasma on vascualar endothelial permeability, coagulation, and resuscitation after hemorrhagic shock are time dependent and diminish between days 0 and 5 after thaw. J Trauma. 2010;69(S1):S55–63.

19. Kozar RA, Peng Z, Zhang R, Holcomb JB, Pati S, Ko TC, Paredes A. Plasma restoration of endothelial glycocalyx in rodent model of hemorrhagic shock. Anesth Analg. 2011;112(6):1289–95.

20. Balogh Z, McKinley BA, Cocanour CS, Kozar RA, Valdivia A, Sailors RM, Moore FA. Supranormal resuscation causes more cases of abdominal compartment syndrome. Arch Surg. 2003;138(6):637–42.

21. Oda J, Ueyama M, Yamashita K, et al. Hypertonic lactated saline resuscitation reduces the risk of abdominal compartment syndrome in severely burned patients. J Trauma. 2006;60:64–71.

22. Collier B, Guillamondegui O, Cotton B, et al. Feeding the open abdomen. J Parenter Enteral Nutr. 2007;31:410–5.

23. Abouassaly CT, Dutton WD, Zaydfudim V, et al. Postoperative neuromuscular blocker is associated with higher primary fascial closure rates damage control laparotomy. J Trauma. 2010;69(3):557–61.

24. Martin MJ, Hatch Q, Cotton BA, Holcomb J. The Use of temporary abdominal closure in low-risk trauma patients: helpful or harmful? J Trauma. 2012;72(3):601–8.

25. Hatch QM, Osterhout LM, Ashraf A, et al. Current use of damage-control laparotomy, closure rates, and predictors of early fascial closure at the first take-back. J Trauma. 2011;70(6):1429–36.

26. Blatnik J, Jin J, Rosen M. Abdominal hernia repair with bridging acellular dermal matrix—an expensive hernia sac. Am J Surg. 2008;196(1):47–50.

27. Satterwhite TS, Miri S, Chung C, et al. Outcomes of complex abdominal herniorrhaphy: experience with 106 cases. Ann Plast Surg. 2012;68:382–8.

28. Becker HP, Willms A, Schwab R. Small bowel fistulas and the open abdomen. Scand J Surg. 2007;96:263–71.

29. Rosen MJ, Jin J, McGee MF, et al. Laparoscopic component separation in the single-stage treatment of infected abdominal wall prosthetic removal. Hernia. 2007;11:435–40.

30. Cheatham ML, Safcsak K, Brzezinski SJ, Lube MW. Nitrogen balance, protein loss, and the open abdomen. Crit Care Med. 2007;35(1):127–31.

31. Hourigan LA, Linfoot JA, Chung KK, Dubick MA, Rivera RL, Jones JA, et al. Loss of protein, immunoglobulins, and electrolytes in exudates from negative pressure wound therapy. Nutr Clin Pract. 2010;25(5):510–6.

32. Zarzaur BL, DiCocco JM, Shahan CP, Emmett K, Magnotti LJ, Croce MA, Hathaway DK, Fabian TC. Quality of life after abdominal wall reconstruction following open abdomen. J Trauma. 2011;70(2):285–91.

33. Fischer PE, Fabian TC, Magnotti LJ, Schroeppel TJ, Bee TK, Maish GO, Savage SA, Laing AE, Barker AB, Croce MA. A ten-year review of enterocutaneous fistulas after laparotomy for trauma. J Trauma. 2009;67(5):924–8.

34. Hatch QM, Osterhout LM, Podbielski J, Kozar RA, Wade CE, Holcomb JB, Cotton BA. Impact of closure at the first take back: complication burden and potential overutilization of damage control laparotomy. J Trauma. 2011;71(6):1503–11.

35. Teixeira PG, Inaba K, Dubose J, Salim A, Brown C, Rhee P, Browder T, Demetriades D. Enterocutaneous fistula complicating trauma laparotomy: a major resource burden. Am Surg. 2009;75(1):30–2.

Zsolt J. Balogh and Osamu Yoshino

Introduction

Abdominal compartment syndrome (ACS) is a life-threatening condition associated with organ dysfunction/failure due to increased intra-abdominal pressure (IAP). Based on consensus, ACS is defined as IAP > 20 mmHg and vital organ dysfunction related to it. Increased IAP without organ dysfunction is considered intra-abdominal hypertension (IAH) and graded (I: 12–15 mmHg, II: 16–20 mmHg, III: 21–25 mmHg, IV: >25 mmHg) [1, 2]. The physiological compromise from increased IAP was first described in the nineteenth century in the clinical setting, and then during the early twentieth century in the laboratory setting [3, 4]. The avoidance of increased IAP, and its resultant catastrophic respiratory and renal function consequences, was first advocated by pediatric surgeons using silos to close large omphaloceles [5]. The term ACS was coined by Fietsam et al. who described the syndrome as a complication of the management of ruptured abdominal aortic aneurisms [6]. Damage control surgery made it possible to salvage patients from previously irreversible traumatic shock and resuscitate them to reach the intensive care unit (ICU) in critical condition [7, 8]. Among these severe shock/trauma patients, ACS was a frequent cause of death, unplanned returns to the operating room, and prolonged ICU stays [9, 10]. Based on the trauma experience, acute care surgeons have applied the principles of prevention, recognition, and management to acute general surgical patients. In the same time, most surgical and nonsurgical specialties have reported on ACS from their experience.

Z.J. Balogh, M.D., Ph.D., F.R.A.C.S., FAOrthA, F.A.C.S. (✉)
O. Yoshino, M.D., Ph.D
Division of Surgery, Department of Traumatology, John Hunter Hospital and University of Newcastle, Lookout Road, Newcastle, NSW 2305, Australia
e-mail: zsolt.balogh@hnehealth.nsw.gov.au

Pathophysiology

The pathophysiological effects of increased pressure in a closed body compartment are well described in other body regions (e.g., tension pneumothorax, pericardial tamponade, increased intracranial pressure, extremity compartment syndrome, etc.) and are taught in the basic medical curriculum. The abdominal cavity is a "neglected" compartment [11]. The volume of the abdominal cavity is limited by its least tensile component—the fascia. Increased pressure can be due to an increase in the volume of the abdominal contents or to a decrease in the volume of the "container." After IAP increases to greater than 20 mmHg, the abdominal cavity is on the steep portion of its pressure–volume curve, and as a result, small increases in content volume or decreases in cavity volume can result in dramatic increases in IAP. This is when close monitoring of IAP (preferably continuously) and organ function is essential for timely intervention.

Response of Individual Organ Systems

Cerebral perfusion is compromised due to the increased IAP forcing the diaphragm cephalad, thus decreasing the size of the thoracic cavity, and ultimately causing intrathoracic pressures to increase. High intrathoracic pressures increases jugular venous pressures and impede venous return from the brain. This may increase intracranial pressure, and consequently decrease cerebral blood flow [12–14]. The effect of IAH on intracranial pressure is especially relevant in severe blunt trauma secondary to the frequent coexistence of head and abdominal injuries.

Increased IAP impedes venous return to the heart causing sequestration of blood in the lower extremities, while increased intrathoracic pressures increase central venous pressure and pulmonary capillary wedge pressure, but does not increase the right or left ventricular end-diastolic volumes. In other words, when intrathoracic pressure is increased, central venous and pulmonary capillary wedge pressures are not reliable indices for assessing the adequacy of preload. Simultaneously, left ventricular afterload increases owing to increased systemic vascular resistance. Increased intrathoracic pressure can increase right ventricular afterload, potentially leading to right ventricular failure and dilation, with consequent leftward displacement of the ventricular septum and impairment of left ventricular filling. Cardiac failure with elevated pulmonary capillary wedge pressure, increased systemic vascular resistance, and decreased cardiac index is a typical finding in profound IAH and defines ACS [15–19]. The cardiac index usually does not respond to fluid challenges, which can be detrimental if the underlying cause (ACS) is not treated. The cardiac index's response to decompression is predictive of outcome; patients who survive have a significantly greater increase in cardiac index after decompression than do those who subsequently die [10].

Increased IAP forces the diaphragm into the thoracic cavity. As such, thoracic compliance decreases and increased airway pressure is required for mechanical ventilation. In the setting of massive resuscitation, these changes can be misinterpreted as being caused by acute lung injury. Historically, ACS was diagnosed by the presence of a firm abdomen in the setting of oliguria and increased airway pressures [18–20]. Although airway pressure promptly decreases in response to abdominal decompression, this finding does not differentiate survivors from non-survivors. The peak airway pressure is an important parameter to monitor during attempted primary fascial closure after laparotomy when ACS is a possible complication.

Oliguria or anuria despite aggressive fluid resuscitation is a typical sign of ACS. Mechanisms responsible for decreased renal function include direct compression of the renal parenchyma, decreased perfusion of the kidneys due to decreased cardiac index, and increased water and sodium retention due to activation of the renin–angiotensin system [21–23]. The usual threshold for defining acute oliguria, urinary output less than 0.5 mL/kg/h, should be used cautiously and considered in the context of the magnitude of the resuscitation. Among patients who require massive resuscitation, the index of suspicion for ACS should be high when the urinary output is less than 1 mL/kg/h [10].

Increased IAP impairs splanchnic perfusion by decreasing the cardiac index and increasing splanchnic vascular resistance. When severe, tissue ischemia can result. Intestinal perfusion can be assessed objectively using gastric tonometry. Decreased gastric intramural pH (pHi), increased gastric regional partial pressure of carbon dioxide (PCO_2), and a wide gap between gastric regional PCO_2 and end-tidal PCO_2 are all indicators of impaired abdominal visceral perfusion [24, 25]. Combined with urinary bladder pressure measurements, the newer semi-continuous tonometers are an excellent adjunct for the early identification of impending ACS. Moreover, the physiologic response to decompression can be evaluated by assessing changes in pHi and related parameters using gastric tonometry [26, 27].

Increased IAP increases femoral venous pressure, increases peripheral vascular resistance, and reduces femoral artery blood flow by as much as 65%.

Laboratory studies have shown that decompression of ACS causes circulating neutrophils to increase CD11b adhesion receptor expression. Decompression of ACS is also associated with the release of cytokines into the portal circulation and increased lung permeability, similar in degree to that seen after hemorrhagic shock and resuscitation [28]. Moreover, when ACS decompression is appropriately sequenced with hemorrhagic shock, it can serve as a "second hit" (i.e., ACS decompression 8 h after hemorrhagic shock causes more intense acute lung injury than does ACS decompression 2 or 18 h after shock) [29, 30].

Classification

The simple clinically relevant classification would start with the determination of the acuity (acute versus chronic) of the increased IAP. In trauma and acute care surgery, the clinically relevant problem is the acutely elevated IAP and the resultant IAH/ACS. The acute care surgeon has to be aware of the chronic conditions (such as morbid obesity) that could result in pathologically elevated baseline IAP measurements. The acute IAH/ACS can be further classified based on etiology: post-injury, acute surgical, post-burn, medical sepsis, etc. From a practical management perspective, ACS can be classified as primary (the pathology is from the abdomino-pelvic region) or secondary ACS (pathology/injury outside of the abdomen). Recurrent ACS is defined as pathological elevations in IAP and subsequent organ dysfunction that develop in the open abdomen following prophylactic or therapeutic decompression [1, 2, 10].

Epidemiology

The accurate epidemiology of IAH and ACS is difficult to determine, and depends on the patient population, institutional resuscitation strategy, and frequency of IAP monitoring. During the late 1990s, the incidence was up to 15% among severely injured patients requiring shock resuscitation in busy shock trauma ICUs [31]. Primary and secondary ACS were equally frequent with up to a 50% incidence of multiple organ failure (MOF) and mortality [10]. Following the identification of independent predictors, liberal preventive open abdomen strategies, and the evolution of resuscitation, the incidence of ACS exponentially decreased. Recent prospective cohorts identified that post-injury ACS has become rare, and the still prevalent IAH in trauma the population is not associated with worse outcomes [32]. The incidence of IAH among general surgical patients undergoing laparotomy is 33–81%, depending on the definition (20 or 18 mmHg) [23]. In a study of medical patients, Malbrain et al. reported that the incidence of IAH was only 18%, despite using a liberal cutoff value (12 mmHg) [33].

Population at Risk

In trauma and acute surgical practices, most patients who require ICU admission are at risk of IAH/ACS [34]. In general terms, any pathology increasing the size of the abdominal contents (intestinal obstruction, edema, abdominal packs) or decreasing/limiting the volume of the cavity (circumferential burns, pressure dressings, positive pressure ventilation) will increase the IAP, thus placing the patient at risk for ACS. Whole-body ischemia–reperfusion injury due to traumatic, hemorrhagic, or septic shock and the consequent resuscitation are consistently described risk factors for both primary and secondary ACS. Certain clinical patterns such as major pelvic fractures with hemorrhage and massive resuscitation, severe acute pancreatitis, injuries requiring abdominal packing during damage control surgery, and exsanguinating torso trauma patients requiring aortic cross clamping are alarming with almost certain development of IAH and a high risk for ACS [35–41].

Monitoring

The clinical examination is inaccurate in determining the magnitude of the IAP [42, 43]. The monitoring of IAP has been described with many techniques through several routes. The general premise requires a noninvasive, accurate, reproducible tool without using an additional tube/catheter system. Many techniques (intra-gastric, trans-rectal, and direct intra-peritoneal) have been shown to be safe and feasible in both the laboratory and clinical settings, but none have been widely used in clinical practice [44–46]. The most widely utilized method is the intra-vesicular measurement (the urinary bladder pressure) in the ICU environment. There are sophisticated proprietary devices available but the technique can be easily performed with a clamped Foley catheter and a zeroed pressure transducer connected to the bedside monitor. Previously recommended large volume (50 mL and more) normal saline instillation before measurement has been scientifically refuted. In fact, only minimal fluid content provides a continuous column for accurate pressure measurements. The frequency of monitoring is institution dependent and varies based on the clinical scenario from hourly to once a nursing shift. It is sensible to measure IAP in all high-risk patients on ICU admission and in the case of IAH,

monitor it regularly (every 2–4 h) according to the disease acuity. If the initial IAP is normal, it is probably safe to monitor IAP again in case of impending organ dysfunction or abdominal distension. The continuous intra-vesicular pressure measurement technique has been well validated. This method utilizes a standard three-way urinary catheter, where the irrigation port is used for continuous monitoring [47]. This method is valuable for the highest risk shock resuscitation patients and potentially can guide intraoperative closure likewise. Based on retrospective studies, the abdominal perfusion pressure (APP) (APP=mean arterial pressure minus IAP) has been advocated as a superior measurement value with a cut-off of 60 mmHg, differentiating poor from favorable outcomes [48]. Unfortunately, APP has not been found to be very useful in posttraumatic cases, where the IAH is frequently a temporary (first 24 h) problem [32].

Prevention

Prospective data suggest that the mortality rate for ACS, even with early decompression and resuscitation, is very high [10]. In addition, early favorable physiologic responses to decompression do not necessarily correlate with improved outcomes. Accordingly, the prevention of ACS is paramount. The avoidance of fascial closure following high-risk laparotomies reduces the incidence of MOF and mortality [49]. In the operating room, monitoring for increases in peak airway pressures during the attempted fascial closure is valuable in the absence of IAP measurements. In the ICU, all patients with severe shock and subsequent resuscitation (whole-body ischemia–reperfusion injury), regardless of the cause (burn, trauma, sepsis, or hypovolemia), benefit from IAP monitoring [41, 50, 51].

ACS is strongly associated with the magnitude and quality of resuscitation. Uncontrolled, goal-oriented resuscitation of trauma victims is harmful [41]. To eliminate uncontrolled resuscitation, treatment of the underlying cause of shock is crucial. Timely hemorrhage control and the elimination of septic foci should occur early. There is increasing evidence that Ringer's lactate solution is pro-inflammatory, and its use may serve as an independent predictor of post-injury ACS [52]. During burn and trauma resuscitation, crystalloid limits should be implemented, and after reaching them, alternative resuscitation fluids should be used. The best resuscitation fluid during impending ACS has yet to be determined.

In post-injury primary ACS, correction of the bloody vicious cycle of coagulopathy, acidosis, and hypothermia should be an early goal. Abbreviated laparotomies save lives, but the often required tight abdominal packing increases the risk of ACS. The use of topical hemorrhage control techniques (i.e., fibrin sealants) offers a workable solution [53]. When abnormalities in respiratory and renal function are identified, ACS should be included in the differential diagnosis.

Treatment

The support of early organ dysfunction by traditional ICU interventions is often necessary in patients with impending ACS; however, these may aggravate the underlying pathophysiology (aggressive ventilator strategies with high peak end-expiratory pressures, fluid boluses to overcome suspected pre-renal failure) [54, 55]. Patients with similar demographic characteristics, injuries, and shock severity without impending ACS respond very well to preload-directed resuscitation (appropriate increase in cardiac index). However, patients with impending ACS do not respond with an increase in cardiac index, despite vigorous crystalloid infusion. Vigorous attempts to increase preload (especially with crystalloid infusions) in patients with IAH may have a detrimental effect on outcome (futile crystalloid cycle) [56].

Theoretically, other nonsurgical interventions may be beneficial in cases of IAH/ACS, but their efficacy is unproven. These methods are nonspecific and are in general, are part of the non-evidence based attempts to overcome pseudo-obstruction/paralytic ileus. Alternative resuscitation fluids have been utilized in post-burn IAH/ACS in the laboratory setting [57]. Continuous external application of negative abdominal pressure with a suction device has shown some promise in morbidly obese patients with cerebral symptoms secondary to chronic ACS [58].

If IAH or ACS is caused by acute or chronic fluid collections, symptoms can be relieved by percutaneous drainage [59]. Case reports describe the successful drainage of abdominal fluid in burn patients with secondary ACS and the drainage of blood in nonoperatively managed liver injuries [60]. The major limitation of the technique is that it is applicable only when a significant amount of fluid is causing the increased IAP. This technique will not work and might be dangerous when extensive bowel edema or a retroperitoneal hematoma is the dominant contributing factor.

Surgical decompression remains the primary recommended intervention in acute surgical cases. Decompression is achieved by opening the midline fascia (avascular plane) along its full length. Virtually all reports describe appropriate physiologic responses to decompression, but this does not necessarily translate into better outcomes [10]. The best predictors of survival are post-decompression improvement in cardiac index and urine output. The decision to undertake surgical decompression is a difficult one, because it results in a chronically open abdomen that is associated with numerous hazards. Several case series have shown that early decompression is associated with better outcomes. However,

in those studies, "late" decompression was often carried out days after the initial signs of ACS. If decompression is carried out within 12 h of hospital admission, timing has no significant effect on outcome [38, 40]. Patients with ACS are in critical condition and require mechanical ventilation and other forms of organ support. Any unnecessary intra-hospital transportation of these patients can be detrimental. Thus, if no other intra-abdominal surgical intervention is needed, decompression can be performed at the bedside in the ICU. More recently, alternatives of midline laparotomy (transverse laparotomy and linea alba fasciotomy) were described. These approaches were popularized in cases of severe acute pancreatitis, where transverse laparotomy can be the surgical access of choice. The (subcutaneous) linea alba fasciotomy can prevent peritoneal contamination in selected pancreatitis cases, where laparotomy is not required just the reduction of the IAP [61, 62].

Conclusion

Post-injury and post-burn ACS is well characterized and has been eliminated in many centers [63, 64]. Active surveillance is essential to keep this lethal complication low [32]. ACS can occur in a wide range of critically ill acute surgical patients. This population requires better characterization based on etiology and the acuity of the various conditions in order to develop efficient preventive and therapeutic strategies similar to post-injury ACS. The significance of long standing acute IAH in general surgical patients is associated with worse outcomes, but the cause and effect relationship has not yet been proven. Primary ACS remains apparent after major abdominal catastrophes and in critical damage control laparotomy patients, but with a controlled low incidence. The occurrence of secondary ACS in burn, medical, and trauma ICUs should serve as a negative performance indicator as it is often the result of over-resuscitation, late hemorrhage, and/or poor septic focus control.

References

1. Malbrain ML, Cheatham ML, Kirkpatrick A, et al. Results from the international conference of experts on intra-abdominal hypertension and abdominal compartment syndrome. I. Definitions. Intensive Care Med. 2006;32:1722–32.
2. Cheatham ML, Malbrain MLNG, Kirkpatrick A, Sugrue M, Parr M, De Waele J, Balogh Z, Leppäniemi A, Olvera C, Ivatury R, D'Amours S, Wendon J, Hillman K, Wilmer A. Results from the conference of experts on intra-abdominal hypertension and abdominal compartment syndrome. Part II: recommendations. Intensive Care Med. 2007;33:951–62.
3. Wendt E. Ueber den Einfluss des intraabdominalen Druckes auf die Absonderungsgeschwindigkeit des Harnes. Arch Physiol Heilkunde. 1867;8:527–75.

4. Emerson H. Intra-abdominal pressures. Arch Intern Med. 1911;7:754–84.

5. Gross R. A new method for surgical treatment of large omphalocoeles. Surgery. 1948;24:277–92.

6. Fietsam Jr R, Villalba M, Glover JL, et al. Intra-abdominal compartment syndrome as a complication of ruptured abdominal aortic aneurysm repair. Am Surg. 1989;55:396–402.

7. Rotondo MF, Schwab CW, McGonigal MD, et al. "Damage control": an approach for improved survival in exsanguinating penetrating abdominal injury. J Trauma. 1993;35:375–82.

8. Morris Jr JA, Eddy VA, Blinman TA, et al. The staged celiotomy for trauma: issues in unpacking and reconstruction. Ann Surg. 1993;217:576–84.

9. Ivatury RR, Diebel L, Porter JM, Simon RJ. Intra-abdominal hypertension and the abdominal compartment syndrome. Surg Clin North Am. 1997;77:783–800.

10. Balogh Z, McKinley BA, Holcomb JB, et al. Both primary and secondary abdominal compartment syndrome can be predicted early and are harbingers of multiple organ failure. J Trauma. 2003;54:848–61.

11. Balogh ZJ, Leppaniemi A. The neglected (abdominal) compartment: what is new at the beginning of the 21st century? World J Surg. 2009;33(6):1109.

12. Bloomfield GL, Ridings PC, Blocher CR, et al. A proposed relationship between increased intraabdominal, intrathoracic and intracranial pressure. Crit Care Med. 1997;25:496–503.

13. Josephs L, McDonald J, Birkett D, et al. Diagnostic laparoscopy increases intracranial pressure. J Trauma. 1994;36:815–9.

14. Bloomfield GL, Ridings PC, Blocher CR, et al. Effects of increased intraabdominal pressure upon intracranial and cerebral perfusion pressure before and after volume expansion. J Trauma. 1996;40:936–40.

15. Richardson JD, Trinkle JK. Hemodynamic and respiratory alterations with increased intra-abdominal pressure. J Surg Res. 1976;20:401–4.

16. Kasthan J, Green JF, Parsons EQ, et al. Hemodynamic effects of increased abdominal pressure. J Surg Res. 1981;30:249–55.

17. Robotham JL, Wise RA, Bomberger-Barnea B. Effects of changes in abdominal pressure on left ventricular performance and regional blood flow. Crit Care Med. 1985;12:803–8.

18. Ridings PC, Blocher CR, Sugerman HJ. Cardiopulmonary effects of raised intra-abdominal pressure before and after intravascular volume expansion. J Trauma. 1995;39:1071–5.

19. Cullen DJ, Coyle JP, Teplick R, Long MC. Cardiovascular, pulmonary and renal effects of massively increased intra-abdominal pressure in critically ill patients. Crit Care Med. 1989;17:118–21.

20. Obeid F, Saba A, Fath J, et al. Increases in intra-abdominal pressure affect pulmonary compliance. Arch Surg. 1995;130:544–7.

21. Richards WO, Scovill W, Shin B, et al. Acute renal failure associated with increased intra-abdominal pressure. Ann Surg. 1983;197:183–7.

22. Harmann PK, Kron IL, McLachlan HD, et al. Elevated intra-abdominal pressure and renal function. Ann Surg. 1982;196:594–7.

23. Sugrue M, Buist MD, Hourihan F, et al. Prospective study of intraabdominal hypertension and renal function after laparotomy. Br J Surg. 1995;82:235–8.

24. Diebel LN, Dulchavsky SA, Wilson RF. Effects of increased intraabdominal pressure on mesenteric arterial and intestinal mucosal blood flow. J Trauma. 1992;33:45–9.

25. Rasmussen IB, Berggren U, Arvidsson D, et al. Effects of pneumoperitoneum on splanchnic hemodynamics: an experimental study in pigs. Eur J Surg. 1995;161:819–24.

26. Sugrue M, Jones F, Lee A, et al. Intraabdominal pressure and gastric intramucosal pH: is there an association? World J Surg. 1996;20:988–91.

27. Ivatury RR, Porter JM, Simon RJ, et al. Intra-abdominal hypertension after life-threatening penetrating abdominal trauma: prophylaxis, incidence, and clinical relevance of gastric mucosal pH and abdominal compartment syndrome. J Trauma. 1998;44:1016–23.

28. Oda J, Ivatury RR, Blocher CR, et al. Amplified cytokine response and lung injury by sequential hemorrhagic shock and abdominal compartment syndrome in a laboratory model of ischemia-reperfusion. J Trauma. 2002;52:625–31.

29. Rezende-Neto J, Moore EE, Melo de Andrade MV, et al. Systemic inflammatory response secondary to abdominal compartment syndrome: stage for multiple organ failure. J Trauma. 2001;53:1121–8.

30. Rezende-Neto JB, Moore EE, Masuno T, et al. The abdominal compartment syndrome as a second insult during systemic neutrophil priming provokes multiple organ injury. Shock. 2003;20:303–8.

31. Balogh Z, McKinley BA, Cox Jr CS, et al. Abdominal compartment syndrome: the cause or effect of postinjury multiple organ failure. Shock. 2003;20:483–92.

32. Balogh ZJ, Martin A, van Wessem KP, et al. Postinjury abdominal compartment syndrome: the mission completed? Arch Surg. 2011;146:938–43.

33. Malbrain ML. Abdominal pressure in the critically ill: measurement and clinical relevance. Intensive Care Med. 1999;25:1453–8.

34. Balogh ZJ, Leppäniemi A. Patient populations at risk for intra-abdominal hypertension and abdominal compartment syndrome. Am Surg. 2011;77:S12–6.

35. Meldrum DR, Moore FA, Moore EE, et al. Cardiopulmonary hazards of perihepatic packing for major liver injuries. Am J Surg. 1995;170:537–42.

36. Chen RJ, Fang JF, Chen MF. Intra-abdominal pressure monitoring as a guideline in the nonoperative management of blunt hepatic trauma. J Trauma. 2001;51:44–50.

37. Kopelman T, Harris C, Miller R, Arrillaga A. Abdominal compartment syndrome in patients with isolated extraperitoneal injuries. J Trauma. 2000;49:744–9.

38. Balogh Z, McKinley BA, Cocanour CS, et al. Secondary abdominal compartment syndrome: an elusive complication of traumatic shock resuscitation. Am J Surg. 2002;184:538–43.

39. Ivy ME, Atweh NA, Palmer J, et al. Intra-abdominal hypertension and abdominal compartment syndrome in burn patients. J Trauma. 2000;49:387–91.

40. Biffl WL, Moore EE, Burch JM, et al. Secondary abdominal compartment syndrome is a highly lethal event. Am J Surg. 2001;182:645–8.

41. Balogh Z, McKinley BA, Cocanour CS, et al. Supra-normal trauma resuscitation causes more cases of abdominal compartment syndrome. Arch Surg. 2003;138:637–43.

42. Kirkpatrick AW, Brenneman FD, McLean RF, et al. Is clinical examination an accurate indicator of raised intra-abdominal pressure in critically injured patients? Can J Surg. 2000;43:207–11.

43. Sugrue M, Bauman A, Jones F, et al. Clinical examination is an inaccurate predictor of intraabdominal pressure. World J Surg. 2002;26:1428–31.

44. Lacey SR, Bruce J, Brooks SP, et al. The relative merits of various methods of indirect measurement of intraabdominal pressure as a guide to closure of abdominal wall defects. J Pediatr Surg. 1987;22:1207–11.

45. Iberti TJ, Lieber CE, Benjamin E. Determination of intra-abdominal pressure using a transurethral bladder catheter: clinical validation of the technique. Anesthesiology. 1989;70:40–5.

46. Kron IL, Harman PK, Nolan SP. The measurement of intra-abdominal pressure as a criterion for exploration. Ann Surg. 1984;199:28–30.

47. Balogh Z, Jones F, D'Amours S, et al. Continuous intra-abdominal pressure measurement technique. Am J Surg. 2004;188:679–84.

48. Cheatham ML, White MW, Sagraves SG, et al. Abdominal perfusion pressure: a superior parameter in the assessment of intra-abdominal hypertension. J Trauma. 2000;49:621–6.

49. Offner PJ, de Souza AL, Moore EE, et al. Avoidance of abdominal compartment syndrome in damage-control laparotomy after trauma. Arch Surg. 2001;136:676–81.

50. Gecelter G, Fahoum B, Gardezi S, Schein M. Abdominal compartment syndrome in severe acute pancreatitis: an indication for a decompressing laparotomy? Dig Surg. 2002;19:402–4.
51. Ivy ME, Possenti PP, Kepros J, et al. Abdominal compartment syndrome in patients with burns. J Burn Care Rehabil. 1999;20:351–3.
52. Rhee P, Wang D, Paul R, et al. Human neutrophil activation and increased adhesion by various resuscitation fluids. Crit Care Med. 2000;38:74–8.
53. Holcomb JB, Pusateri AE, Harris RA, et al. Dry fibrin sealant dressings reduce blood loss, resuscitation volume, and improve survival in hypothermic coagulopathic swine with grade V liver injuries. J Trauma. 1999;47:233–40.
54. Sugrue M, D'Amours S. The problems with positive end expiratory pressure (PEEP) in association with abdominal compartment syndrome (ACS). J Trauma. 2001;51:419–20.
55. Burch JM, Moore EE, Moore FA, Franciose R. The abdominal compartment syndrome. Surg Clin North Am. 1996;76:833–42.
56. Balogh Z, McKinley BA, Kozar RA, et al. Patients with impending abdominal compartment syndrome do not respond to early volume loading. Am J Surg. 2003;182:602–7.
57. Oda J, Ueyama M, Yamashita K, Inoue T, Noborio M, Ode Y, Aoki Y, Sugimoto H. Hypertonic lactated saline resuscitation reduces the risk of abdominal compartment syndrome in severely burned patients. J Trauma. 2006;60(1):64–71.
58. Sugerman HJ, Felton III WL, Sismanis A, et al. Continuous negative abdominal pressure device to treat pseudotumor cerebri. Int J Obes Relat Metab Disord. 2001;25:486–90.
59. Yang EY, Marder SR, Hastings G, Knudson MM. The abdominal compartment syndrome complicating nonoperative management of major blunt liver injuries: recognition and treatment using multimodality therapy. J Trauma. 2002;52:982–6.
60. Corcos AC, Sherman HF. Percutaneous treatment of secondary abdominal compartment syndrome. J Trauma. 2001;51:1062–4.
61. Leppäniemi A, Mentula P, Hienonen P, Kemppainen E. Transverse laparostomy is feasible and effective in the treatment of abdominal compartment syndrome in severe acute pancreatitis. World J Emerg Surg. 2008;30:6.
62. Leppäniemi A. Surgical management of abdominal compartment syndrome; indications and techniques. Scand J Trauma Resusc Emerg Med. 2009;14:17.
63. Cotton BA, Au BK, Nunez TC, et al. Predefined massive transfusion protocols are associated with a reduction in organ failure and postinjury complications. J Trauma. 2009;66:41–8. Discussion 48–9.
64. Duchesne JC, Kimonis K, Marr AB, et al. Damage control resuscitation in combination with damage control laparotomy: a survival advantage. J Trauma. 2010;69:46–52.

Lillian S. Kao

Introduction

Necrotizing soft tissue infections (NSTIs) are a group of rare but fulminant type of complicated skin and soft tissue infection. The US Food and Drug Administration (FDA) differentiates complicated from uncomplicated skin and soft tissue infections based on several criteria including the need for surgical intervention [1]. These infections are typically characterized by advancing tissue necrosis and are known colloquially as being caused by "flesh-eating bacteria." Other terms that are used to describe NSTIs include: gas gangrene, streptococcal gangrene, gangrenous cellulitis, necrotizing cellulitis/erysipelas, bacterial synergistic gangrene, Meleney ulcer/gangrene, and Clostridial myonecrosis. NSTIs of the perineum are referred to as Fournier's gangrene. NSTIs have been described as early as 500 BCE by Hippocrates as a complication of erysipelas [2]. Later described as "hospital gangrene" by British naval surgeons in the eighteenth and nineteenth centuries, NSTIs were first reported in the United States by army surgeon Dr. Joseph Jones during the Civil War. Although NSTI is often used synonymously to mean necrotizing fasciitis (which was coined by Dr. Wilson in 1952), NSTIs have now come to represent a spectrum of diseases that range from necrotizing cellulitis to myonecrosis (Fig. 37.1).

Epidemiology

Incidence

The incidence of NSTIs in the United States has been estimated from large administrative databases and has been

L.S. Kao, M.D., M.S. (✉)
Department of Surgery, University of Texas Health Science Center, 5656 Kelley Street, Suite 30S 62008, Houston, TX 77026, USA
e-mail: lillian.s.kao@uth.tmc.edu

noted to have increased since the 1980s [3, 4]. Whether the increase represents a true rise in the number of infections or simply better identification and reporting of NSTIs is unclear. An analysis of medical claims data from 1997 to 2002 reported the incidence rate of NSTIs, or the probability of developing the disease over a specific period of time, as 0.04 per 1,000 person-years [5]. A review of more than 28 million patients in the Nationwide Inpatient Sample (NIS) database in the years 2001 and 2004 identified a total of 10,940 or 0.04% of hospitalized patients as having an NSTI [6]. Although rare, it is estimated that clinicians, whether surgeons or primary care physicians or specialists, will encounter at least one NSTI patient in their lifetime [7].

Classification

There are several methods for describing NSTIs, although there is no standard classification system. NSTIs can be described by their depth of invasion (Fig. 37.1); necrotizing fasciitis is characterized by pathological findings at the level of the subcutaneous fat (i.e., thrombosed vessels) and deep fascia (i.e., necrosis). NSTIs can also be classified by their anatomic location (i.e., Fournier's gangrene for NSTIs of the perineum). Another method for describing NSTIs is based on their microbiology: Type I, II, or III. Type I NSTIs are the most common type, accounting for 55–75% of infections. They are polymicrobial and include organisms such as gram-positive cocci (i.e., *Staphylococcus aureus*), gram-negative bacilli (i.e., *Escherichia coli*), and anaerobes (i.e., *Clostridium* and *Bacteroides* species). They have been associated with multiple predisposing factors including surgical procedures, diabetes, and peripheral vascular disease. Type II NSTIs are caused by Group A beta hemolytic *Streptococci* with or without *S. aureus*. These infections are less common than Type I infections and can occur in young, healthy individuals. Type III NSTIs have been attributed to *Vibrio* species by some authors and to *Clostridium* species by other authors [8].

L.J. Moore et al. (eds.), *Common Problems in Acute Care Surgery*,
DOI 10.1007/978-1-4614-6123-4_37, © Springer Science+Business Media New York 2013

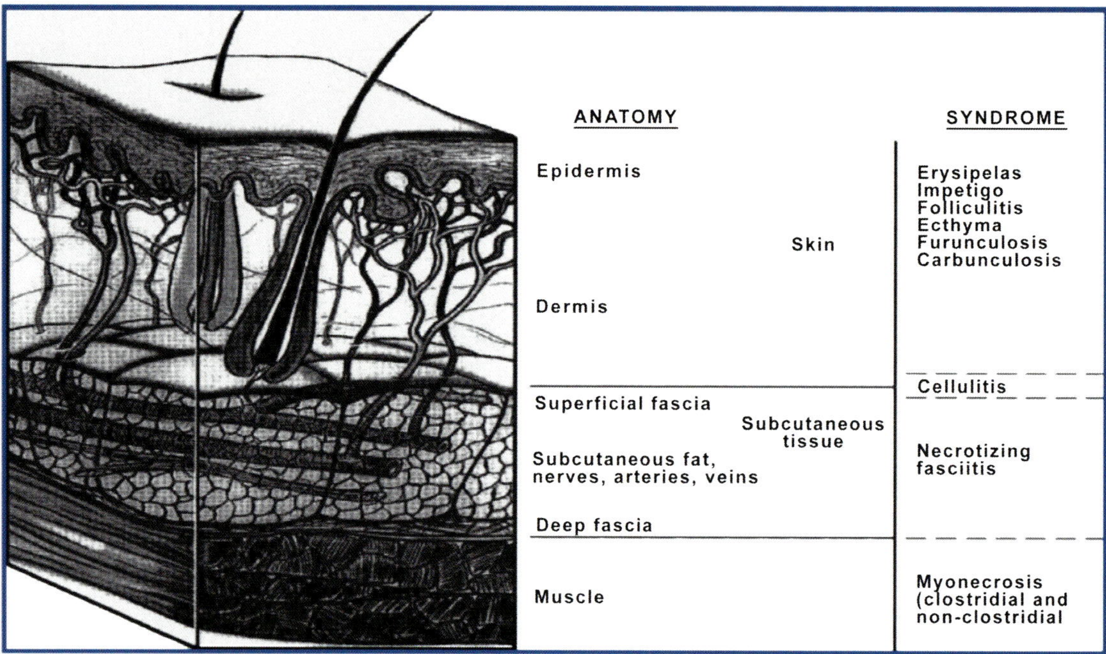

Fig. 37.1 Anatomy of skin and soft tissue and infectious processes associated with each layer

An alternative classification system was proposed by Bakleh et al. based on histopathologic findings [9]. They proposed three stages based on combinations of inflammatory response and gram-stain results. Grades of the inflammatory response were characterized by the degree of neutrophilic infiltration and presence of necrosis or microabscesses. The histopathologic stages correlated with mortality, although only unadjusted analyses were performed due to small sample size.

Risk Factors

Although there are multiple risk factors for NSTIs that include medical comorbidities and other factors, NSTIs often develop in young, healthy hosts. Comorbidities include diabetes mellitus, peripheral vascular disease, obesity, chronic renal failure, cirrhosis, heart disease, acquired immunodeficiency syndrome (AIDS), and immunosuppression. Injection drug use and alcoholism are associated with NSTIs as well. Infections may develop as a result of insect bites, abscesses, recent trauma, or surgery [3, 10].

Microbiology

As previously described, NSTIs may be polymicrobial or monomicrobial depending upon the patient's comorbidities, risk factors, and clinical setting. One study of patients from the late 1980s and early 1990s found an average of 4.4 organisms per infection [11]. Cultures may identify gram-positive and gram-negative bacteria, aerobic and anaerobic bacteria, and fungi. Historically, monomicrobial NSTIs were attributed to *Group A Streptococcus* (GAS), *Clostridium* species, and *Vibrio* species, but as described as follows, any number of microorganisms may cause monomicrobial NSTIs.

The two most common gram-positive cocci isolated from patients with NSTIs are *Staphylococci* and *Streptococci* [1, 11]. *S. aureus* is the most common pathogen present in serious soft tissue infections in North America, Latin America, and Europe [12]. Over time, its virulence and resistance has changed; there has been a concomitant decrease in infections caused by methicillin-sensitive *Staphylococcus aureus* (MSSA) and an increase in infections caused by methicillin-resistant *Staphylococcus aureus* (MRSA) [13]. Furthermore, there has been an increase in the prevalence of community acquired MRSA (CA-MRSA), which was first described in the 1990s [14]. Initially CA-MRSA infections were primarily present only in specific sub-populations such as prisoners or sports participants, but now CA-MRSA is on its way to becoming the predominant strain of MRSA in hospitals [15]. Similarly, CA-MRSA was not previously common in patients with NSTIs [16]. In 2005, Miller et al. described 14 patients with NSTIs and positive cultures for CA-MRSA, 12 of who had monomicrobial infections [16]. These patients had risk factors that included medical comorbidities such as diabetes and hepatitis, history of injection drug use, homelessness, and prior MRSA infection. All of the infections were due to the USA300 clone and had similar genotypes including the presence of the Panton–Valentine leukocidin (pvl) gene, which encodes an exotoxin that causes leukocyte destruction. Several series of patients have reported high rates of MRSA NSTIs, although genotyping was not performed in all of the series [17–20]. In one case series, MRSA was the most frequent cause of monomicrobial NSTIs [18]. There is a suggestion that mortality may not be as high in patients with CA-MRSA, but because of its increasing prevalence, empiric coverage should be started in patients with suspected NSTIs [16–20].

Streptococcus pyogenes is a type of Group A beta-hemolytic *Streptococcus* (GAS) that can cause a spectrum of diseases from bacterial pharyngitis to necrotizing fasciitis and myositis to toxic shock syndrome. In a European population-based study, the crude rate of *S. pyogenes* infection was 2.79 per 100,000 population [21]. Eight percent (308 patients) of all of the cases were diagnosed with necrotizing fasciitis, of which 50% were associated with toxic shock syndrome (TSS). Streptococcal TSS has been reported to be an independent predictor of mortality [22]. Risk factors for GAS infections include comorbidities such as liver disease or underlying malignancy and behaviors such as injection drug use, but these infections can also occur in healthy immunocompetent patients as well [23]. GAS NSTIs have a predisposition for the lower extremities and tend to spread rapidly. These organisms have a number of factors that contribute to their virulence including M protein, which facilitates attachment to the host cells and prevents bacterial phagocytosis, enzymes that facilitate the spread of infection and that prevent the migration of neutrophils to the site of infection, and superantigens that stimulate a pro-inflammatory response [8].

Gram-negative rods have been associated with NSTIs including *Klebsiella* species, *Enterobacter* species, *Pseudomonas* and *Aeromonas*, *Vibrio* species, *Acinetobacter* species, *Eikenella corrodens*, and *Citrobacter frundii* [1, 11]. Liver disease is a risk factor for NSTIs due to gram-negative rods, particularly *Vibrio*, *Klebsiella*, and *Aeromonas* [24]. Furthermore, these gram-negative rod NSTIs appear to have a higher prevalence in Asian countries [24]. *Vibrio* infections occur in immunocompromised hosts such as those with cirrhosis, diabetes mellitus, adrenal insufficiency, and chronic renal insufficiency; they are associated with contact with seawater or ingestion of raw seafood [24–28]. These infections may have an atypical presentation; increased level of suspicion should occur in these patients, particularly when hemorrhagic bullae are present given an increased associated mortality [25, 26]. *Klebsiella* NSTIs are more common in Asia, but has been reported to have been acquired nosocomially in a patient with underlying malignancy in the Western hemisphere [29].

Clostridum is a genus of gram-positive bacteria that are obligate anaerobes. Multiple species including *Clostridium perfringens* have been identified in NSTIs [1]. Clostridial infections may cluster in areas with heavy injection drug use.

For example, King County, Washington, has a high prevalence of drug users who inject heroin. In a review of 10 years' of autopsies of patients who died due to NSTIs, clostridial infections were identified as being significantly associated with injection drug use of black tar heroin [30, 31]. Different species were noted including *Clostridium sordellii*. A retrospective review of patients treated in Seattle, Washington, similarly identified an association between clostridial infections and injection drug use. Furthermore, clostridial infections were significantly associated with an increase in mortality and limb loss [30]. NSTIs caused by *Clostridium septicum* are often associated with an underlying colonic malignancy [32, 33].

Fungi (i.e., *Candida* species) may also be found in both polymicrobial and monomicrobial NSTIs. There have been case reports of monomicrobial NSTIs due to *Aspergillus* [34, 35]. Zygomycotic NSTIs from *Apophysomyces* have been reported in trauma patients and in immunocompetent hosts [36–38]. Cryptococcocal NSTIs have also been reported, largely in immunocompromised patients [39, 40].

Pathophysiology

Spread of pathogens that cause NSTIs occurs through the production of a variety of endotoxins and exotoxins, many of which have already been mentioned. Toxins may cause tissue destruction, ischemia, and necrosis; endothelial damage, which results in increased tissue edema and impaired capillary blood flow; increased escape from host defenses such as phagocytosis and neutrophil infiltration at the site of infection; and activation of the coagulation cascade, which may cause vascular thrombosis and worsened tissue ischemia [3].

Clinical Presentation

NSTIs can be difficult to distinguish from other non-necrotizing infections. Early manifestations may include swelling, erythema, and warmth, which are nonspecific findings that are also present in patients with cellulitis (Fig. 37.2). Pain out of proportion to physical exam may be present. By the time NSTIs become clinically apparent and patients manifest "hard signs," the associated morbidity and mortality are increased because of the delay in diagnosis [41–43]. Hard signs include late skin manifestations such as bullae, crepitus, or skin necrosis (Figs. 37.3 and 37.4). Wang et al. performed an observational study of patients and developed a staging system based on the time course of symptoms and signs (Table 37.1) [44]; such hard signs are classified as Stage III or late findings. Furthermore, NSTI patients may

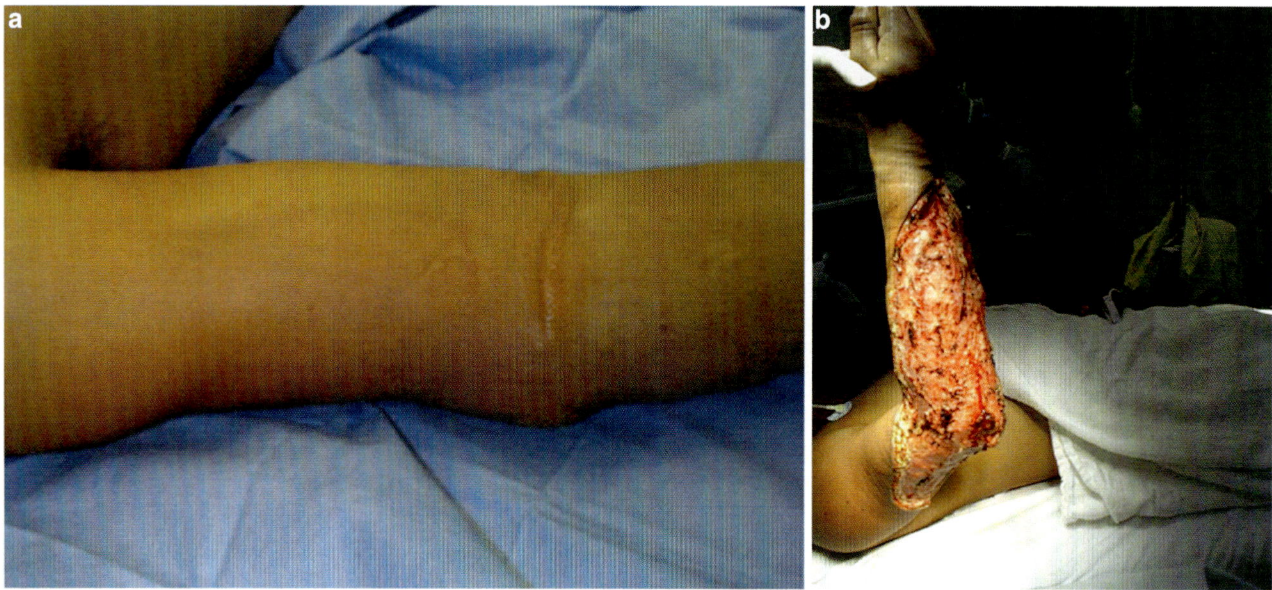

Fig. 37.2 (**a**) This patient has minimal skin manifestations of NSTI other than erythema and swelling, characteristic of Stage I or early NSTI as proposed by Wang et al. [44] (**b**) The same patient after debridement of necrotic infected tissue

Fig. 37.3 This patient has multiple blisters filled with serous fluid, characteristic of Stage II

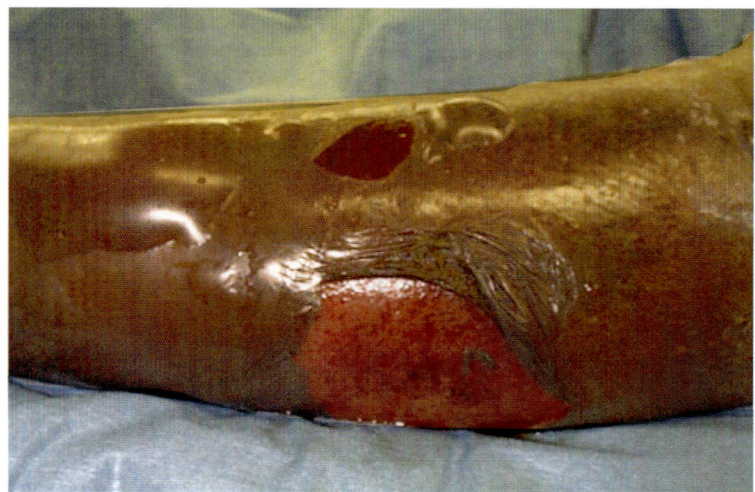

Fig. 37.4 This patient had skin necrosis and crepitus characteristic of Stage III. (Reprinted with permission from Wang YS, Wong CH, Tay YK. Staging of necrotizing fasciitis based on the evolving cutaneous features. Int J Dermatol. Oct 2007;46(10):1036–1041.)

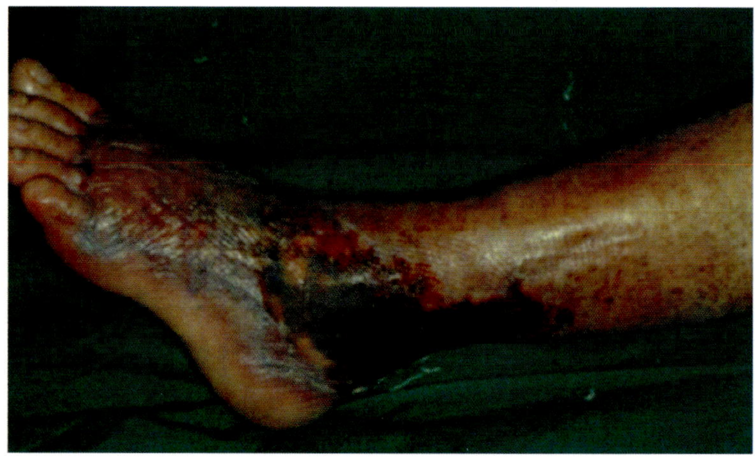

Table 37.1 Stages of evolving necrotizing soft tissue infection based on cutaneous changes [44]

Stage	Time course	Symptoms and signs
Stage I	Early	Tenderness to palpation (extending beyond the apparent area of skin involvement)
		Erythema
		Swelling
		Warmth
Stage II	Intermediate	Blister or bullae formation (serous fluid)
Stage III	Late	Crepitus
		Skin anesthesia
		Skin necrosis with dusky discoloration

Table 37.2 Laboratory Risk Indicator for Necrotizing Fasciitis (LRINEC) score; [48] a cutoff 6 points had a 92% positive predictive value and a 96% negative predictive value

Variable, units	Score
C-reactive protein, mg/dL	
<150	0
≥150	4
Total white cell count, per mm³	
<15	0
15–25	1
>25	2
Hemoglobin, g/dL	
>13.5	0
11–13.5	1
<11	2
Sodium, mmol/L	
≥135	0
<135	2
Creatinine, μmol/L	
≤141	0
>141	2
Glucose, mmol/L	
≤10	0
>10	1

present with hemodynamic instability and organ failure; the number of dysfunctional organ systems at admission is predictive of mortality [45].

Diagnosis

Multiple studies have demonstrated an association between a delay in diagnosis and worsened outcome from NSTIs [41–43]. The diagnosis may be obvious in the setting of the hard signs described above such as hemodynamic instability and late skin manifestations [46]. However, these findings are only present in a small percentage of NSTI patients; in a matched case-control series, necrotic skin and hypotension each occurred in only 5% of patients and no patients had crepitance [47]. Furthermore, as described previously, by the time bullae, crepitus, or skin necrosis are apparent on physical examination, the NSTI has already progressed to an intermediate or late stage [44].

Compounding the difficulties in diagnosis are the similarities in presentation between early stage NSTIs and cellulitis such as fever, pain, swelling, tenderness, erythema, and warmth [47]. In a matched case-control study, Wall et al. compared physical examination findings, laboratory values, and radiologic findings in patients with necrotizing fasciitis to those with a non-necrotizing soft tissue infection. They found that the parameters with the highest sensitivity for necrotizing fasciitis were white blood cell count greater than 14×10^9/L, sodium less than 135 mmol/L, and blood urea nitrogen greater than 15 mg/dL [47]. The parameters with the highest specificity (100% for all) were tense edema, bullae, sodium less than 135 mmol/L, and chloride less than 95 mmol/L [47]. Based on these findings, Wall et al. developed a simple model to assist in diagnosing NSTIs. A corrected serum sodium (for glucose) of less than 135 mmol/L or a white blood cell count of greater than 14.3×10^9/L had a 90% sensitivity and a 76% specificity for necrotizing fasciitis [46]. This model correctly classified 18/19 (95%) of patients who had no "hard signs" [46].

Another commonly used model for diagnosing an NSTI is the Laboratory Risk Indicator for NECrotizing fasciitis (LRINEC) score [48]. Six laboratory parameters are included in the score and are weighted from 1 to 4 points for a total possible score of 13 (Table 37.2). The probability of necrotizing infections was less than 50% with a cutoff score of less than or equal to 5, but increased to greater than 75% with a cutoff score of greater than or equal to 8 [48]. A cutoff score of 6 had a positive predictive value (PPV) of 92% and a negative predictive value (NPV) of 96% in the original validation dataset [48]. The LRINEC score has not been validated across other patient populations and settings [49, 50], although one study suggested that it may function as both a diagnostic and prognostic tool [51]. Thus, the LRINEC score may be useful in select patient populations in increasing the suspicion for a necrotizing infection, but further studies are required. As with all diagnostic tools, the predictive values are dependent on the incidence of the disease in the population, and the utility of a test in changing management depends on the level of suspicion for the disease (or the pretest probability).

Radiographic imaging may be helpful. In the case-control study by Wall et al., 39% of patients with necrotizing fasciitis had gas on plain film versus 5% of patients with a non-necrotizing infection [47]. However, gas on X-ray only had a sensitivity of 39%. Ultrasonography has been used in a few case reports and case series as an aid in the diagnosis of NSTIs [52–54]. Ultrasound can be performed rapidly at the bedside unlike other imaging modalities such as computed tomography (CT) scans and magnetic resonance imaging (MRI). Findings of increased echogenicity of the subcutaneous tissue may be seen in NSTIs but can also be present in cellulitis. Fluid greater than 4 mm in thickness or tracking along the deep fascia may be more suggestive of an NSTI [54]. Currently, however, there is insufficient evidence to recommend routine use of ultrasound in the diagnosis of NSTIs.

Traditionally, although CT and MRI have been reported to be useful adjuncts in the diagnosis of NSTIs, there has been a hesitation to recommend their routine use due to potential delays in obtaining the studies. However, as technology continues to evolve, these studies may become more useful. Findings on CT scans consistent with NSTIs have included subcutaneous air, fascial edema and thickening, non-enhancement of necrotic tissues, gas across tissue planes, or fluid collections [55–57]. In a study of 67 patients without indication for immediate surgical exploration for NSTI, CT scans had 100% sensitivity and 81% specificity for diagnosing NSTIs [57]. Three out of eight patients with a false-positive CT scan had fluid collections identified that ultimately were diagnosed as abscesses associated with pyomyositis [57]. Another study by McGillicuddy et al. reported that 305/715 (43%) of NSTI patients diagnosed over a 10-year period at a single center underwent CT scan. They developed a scoring system of five CT findings to aid in the diagnosis of NSTIs (Table 37.3). A score of greater than 6 had 86% sensitivity, 92% specificity, 64% PPV, and 86% NPV [58]. Further prospective validation studies are planned.

MRI has been used to diagnose NSTIs, but like CT has a high sensitivity but a low specificity [3]. Findings on T2-weighted images have included: gas or low signal intensity in the deep fascia, [59, 60] abnormal deep fascial thickening with or without contrast enhancement [59, 61, 62], peripheral high signal intensity in muscles [59, 63], extensive involvement of the deep fascia [59], and involvement of three or more compartments in one extremity [59]. Concerns about availability, potential delay in diagnosis and subsequent intervention, and lack of well-defined criteria for distinguishing NSTIs from non-necrotizing infections still limit the widespread use of MRIs in establishing the diagnosis.

Fluid and tissue sampling have also been suggested for diagnosing NSTIs. A 22-gauge needle with a 10-mL syringe has been used to aspirate fluid in the setting of soft tissue infections [64]. In a study of 50 patients in whom aspiration biopsy was performed, cultures were positive in 81% of patients not on antimicrobial therapy, but the percentage dropped to 30% in patients receiving antimicrobial treatment. Growth of an organism on aspirate was not specific as the cultures were taken from patients with cellulitis, ulcers,

Table 37.3 Computed tomography (CT) NSTI Scoring System: [58] a score of >6 points had an 86% sensitivity and a 92% specificity for the diagnosis of NSTI

Variable	Points
Fascial air	5
Muscle/fascial edema	4
Fluid tracking	3
Lymphadenopathy	2
Subcutaneous edema	1

Table 37.4 Histologic criteria for the diagnosis of necrotizing fasciitis [65]

Necrosis of superficial fascia
Polymorphonuclear infiltration of the deep dermis and fascia
Fibrinous thrombi of vessels passing through the fascia
Angiitis with fibrinoid necrosis of vessel walls
Presence of microorganisms within the destroyed tissue on Gram stain
No muscle involvement

chronic osteomyelitis, and infected surgical wounds. Furthermore, although the organisms on aspirate were similar to those in surgical specimens among patients who were subsequently debrided, there was often a delay to growth of an organism in the aspiration fluid (up to 72 h) [64]. There is inadequate evidence to recommend the routine use of aspiration biopsy to diagnose NSTIs.

Ultimately, the diagnosis of a NSTI is confirmed by surgical exploration, either at the bedside (if the patient is clinically unstable) or in the operating room. Typical gross findings include loss of tissue resistance to blunt dissection, thrombosis of subcutaneous vessels, presence of foul-smelling and/or dishwater fluid, and grayish appearance of fascia with or without obvious tissue necrosis. These findings are sufficient to confirm the diagnosis, but if the surgeon is still uncertain, frozen-section biopsy can be performed. Frozen-section biopsy for rapid and early diagnosis of necrotizing fasciitis was advocated by Stamenkovic and Lew in 1984 [65]. They recommended obtaining at least a $10 \times 7 \times 7$ mm incisional biopsy of soft tissue under local anesthetic. Their criteria for the histologic diagnosis are listed in Table 37.4. In their small case series, which included eight subsequently confirmed cases of necrotizing fasciitis, the histology revealed intact superficial epidermis and dermis and a combination of edema, vasculitis and thrombosis, neutrophilic infiltration, and microorganisms in the deeper layers including deep dermis, subcutaneous fat, and fascia [65]. Histologic samples from patients who did not undergo frozen section biopsy demonstrated further extension of the necrosis representative of progressive disease. Use of frozen section biopsy, however, is limited by the availability of a pathologist to read the samples, and necrotizing infections are usually associated with obvious findings such as those described previously.

Management

The mainstay of treatment for NSTIs is administration of broad spectrum antibiotics and prompt and aggressive surgical debridement of infected tissues (Fig. 37.5). Randomized trials of adjunctive treatments are lacking, and synthesis of observational studies is hampered by: (1) a lack of standardized terminology and (2) heterogeneity in patient populations, bacteriology, and management strategies.

Surgical Management

Recognizing the lack of randomized trials to guide management, the Surgical Infection Society (SIS) Guidelines for the Treatment of Complicated Skin and Soft Tissue Infections strongly recommend timely and adequate surgical debridement to improve outcome [1]. General caveats for operative debridement include complete resection of necrotic tissues and drainage of fluid collections. Non-viability of tissues is often marked by easy separation from surrounding structures, thrombosis of blood vessels and lack of arterial bleeding, and lack of muscle contraction. Tissue should be cultured to guide postoperative antibiotic management.

Source control may require aggressive surgical management. Ten to 25% of patients required amputations in several cases series [18, 30, 41, 66], and approximately a quarter of patients with extremity involvement required amputation in two series [18, 30]. Guillotine or through-joint amputations can be done expeditiously at the initial operation if the patient is hemodynamically unstable and/or the level of involvement is not clearly defined. Anaya et al. identified heart disease, shock defined as a systolic blood pressure less than 90 mmHg at hospital admission, and *Clostridial* infection as independent predictors of limb loss [30].

SIS guidelines recommend frequent reevaluation or return to the operating room within 24 h of the initial debridement to determine the adequacy of source control and to verify the lack of progression [1]. Repeat operative exploration is continued until source control has been achieved and no more tissue requires debridement. In a population-based analysis of more than 10,000 NSTI patients, the mean number of surgical procedures was 4.6 ± 3.1 for patients treated at burn centers and 4.3 ± 3.3 for patients treated at non-burn centers [6]. Management of the open wounds has traditionally been to employ wet-to-dry dressings, but there have been increasing reports of negative pressure wound therapy usage [67]. Ultimately, large wounds that do not heal by secondary intent may require coverage with split thickness skin grafts or musculocutaneous flaps.

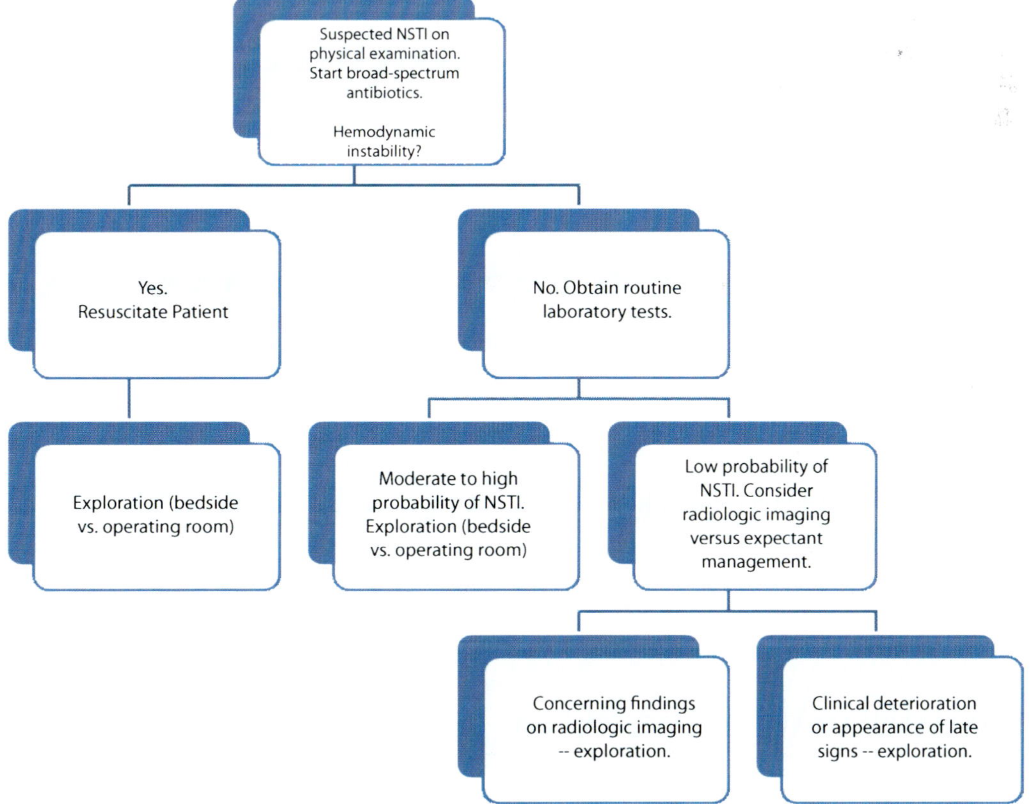

Fig. 37.5 Algorithm for management of a patient with a suspected NSTI

Table 37.5 Accepted antibiotic regimens for NSTIs (from Howell and Rosengart) [8]

Monotherapy agents	Imipenem-cilastin
	Meropenem
	Ertapenem
	Piperacillin-tazobactam
	Tigecycline
Multidrug regimens	Penicillin or cephalosporin PLUS aminoglycoside or fluoroquinolone PLUS clindamycin or metronidazole
	Add vancomycin, linezolid, or daptomycin for MRSA if indicated
	Add protein synthesis inhibitor (clindamycin or linezolid) in severe or rapidly progressive infections

Antibiotic Therapy

Early, empiric, broad-spectrum antibiotics are strongly recommended for the treatment of NSTIs. Antibiotic coverage should include activity against aerobic and anaerobic gram-positive and gram-negative organisms. The SIS Guidelines recommend several effective single-agent regimens including carbapenems (i.e., imipenem/cilastin, meropenem, ertapenem), other beta-lactam antibiotics (i.e., piperacillin/tazobactam and ticarcillin/clavulanate), and glycylcyclines that are similar to tetracyclines (i.e., tigecycline) [1]. However, antibiotic combinations with the same coverage can also be used. For severe, rapidly progressive infections, combination antibiotic therapy that includes a protein synthesis-inhibiting agent such as clindamycin, erythromycin, or linezolid should be used [1]. Further antibiotic therapy should be tailored based on the level of suspicion for specific organisms. For example, if MRSA is suspected, antibiotics with anti-MRSA activity should be considered such as vancomycin, linezolid, quinipristin/dalfopristin, daptomycin, and tigecycline [1, 68]. If Group A streptococcal infections are suspected, penicillin is the drug of choice with or without a protein synthesis-inhibitory agent [1]. If clostridial infections are suspected, a protein synthesis inhibitor is again recommended to prevent production of exotoxins that contribute to the organism's rapid spread. If *Vibrio* infections are suspected, tetracyclines (i.e., doxycycline), quinolones (i.e., ciprofloxacin), and third-generation cephalosporins or carbapenems can be used. In severe cases with rapidly progressive infections, combination therapy with cell-wall-active agents and a tetracycline should be used. Table 37.5 lists several acceptable antibiotic regimens. There are no evidence-based guidelines regarding the length of antibiotic therapy—whether a set duration should be predetermined or whether clinical criteria should be used such as 3 days after the resolution of signs of systemic toxicity and local infection have resolved [68, 69].

Supportive Care

While the mainstays of therapy are rapid and aggressive surgical debridement and antibiotic therapy, supportive care is important as well given that these patients are at high risk of death. Perioperative resuscitation of patients with septic shock and severe sepsis should be performed using evidence-based guidelines [70]. Postoperative care should include supplemental nutrition, preferentially enteral, given the increase in predicted energy requirements of NSTI patients [68].

Adjunctive Therapies

There are a number of adjunctive therapies that have been suggested but there is a paucity of high quality evidence to support their use. Hyperbaric oxygen has been proposed to have a biologic rationale for improved outcome—the resultant increased partial pressure of oxygen in infected tissues [71] may improve polymorphonuclear leukocyte function and improve wound healing. Retrospective studies have conflicting results as to whether or not hyperbaric oxygen confers a mortality benefit in NSTI patients [72–74]. These uncontrolled studies may have an inherent selection bias in that hemodynamically stable patients may be more likely to be able to be safely transported to the hyperbaric chamber and therefore have improved outcomes. Furthermore, it is unknown whether there is a potential harm in transporting these patients or whether use of hyperbaric oxygen may delay definitive surgical therapy. The SIS guidelines conclude that there is insufficient evidence to make a recommendation regarding hyperbaric oxygen for treating NSTIs [1].

Intravenous immunoglobulin (IVIG) has been suggested in patients with severe Group A streptococcal or staphylococcal infections or TSS. The proposed mechanisms of action include binding of bacterial toxins and inhibition of binding of bacterial superantigens to T-cell receptors with resultant down-regulation of the inflammatory response. Despite the biological plausibility, data are limited to case reports and expert opinion. The only randomized trial of IVIG in streptococcal toxic shock syndrome was terminated early due to slow recruitment and was underpowered to identify either a mortality benefit or harms from adverse effects [75]. The SIS guidelines gave only a weak recommendation based on low or very low quality evidence for the use of IVIG in patients with TSS due to staphylococcal or streptococcal NSTIs [1].

Plasmapheresis has also been suggested as an adjunctive therapy for NSTI patients, but evidence specific to this patient population is limited to a single case report [76]. Plasmapheresis has been studied in the treatment of septic shock and severe sepsis. The biological rationale is that separation of the cellular and plasma components of circulating blood allows circulating inflammatory mediators or toxins to be removed. One small single-center trial of plasmapheresis in severe sepsis and septic shock demonstrated a reduction in 28-day all-cause mortality [77], but confirmatory multicenter effectiveness trials are lacking. The SIS guidelines determined that there was insufficient evidence to make a recommendation regarding plasmapheresis or other extracorporeal treatments for NSTIs [1].

Prior to the recent withdrawal of drotrecogin alfa (activated) or recombinant human activated protein C from the market, its use in NSTI patients was suggested in case reports [78, 79]. Although initial randomized trials suggested a mortality benefit to drotrecogin alfa in patients with severe sepsis, only a small number of enrolled patients had NSTIs. Moreover, despite this initial evidence, a recent unpublished trial demonstrating no mortality benefit resulted in withdrawal of the drug from the market. This example demonstrates the caution that should be employed in using therapies with unproven benefit, even in diseases with a high risk of mortality.

Potential Complications

Mortality

The acute mortality of NSTIs had been reported to be unchanging for many decades, ranging from 25 to 35% [3]. A review of 27 case series of NSTIs published between 1980 and 1998 reported mortality rates of 6–73%, with an overall mortality rate of 32% for 862 patients [80]. Since then, several case series have reported lower mortality rates between 10 and 20% [6, 18, 25, 80, 81]. Mortality in an analysis of more than 10,000 hospitalized patients with NSTIs was 10.9% [6]. This apparent recent reduction in mortality may be due to a true improvement in the diagnosis and management of NSTIs or to changing patient populations, inconsistency in the definition of NSTIs, or differences in the virulence of bacterial strains causing NSTIs.

There are multiple predictors of mortality reported in the literature including advanced age, presence of comorbidities, and severity of disease on admission (i.e., presence of shock and/or organ failure) [30, 42, 66]. Furthermore, delay in intervention has also been associated with increased mortality [41, 42, 66]. Other authors have proposed weighted scoring systems for predicting mortality. As previously mentioned, the LRINEC score greater than 6 has been associated with increased mortality [51]. Anaya et al. developed a scoring system that assigned points based on six variables: heart rate >110 beats per minute, temperature <36 °F, creatinine >1.5 mg/dL, age >50 years, white blood cell count greater than 40,000/mm^3, and hematocrit greater than 50% [81]. This model was 87% accurate in predicting mortality in

a validation set derived from two different patient populations but needs to be validated in larger multicenter studies.

Morbidity

There is a paucity of studies evaluating morbidity among NSTI survivors. Amputations are common amongst patients with extremity involvement. Two series reported that approximately a quarter of patients with extremity involvement require an amputation [18, 30]. Anaya et al. identified ischemic heart disease, shock defined as a systolic blood pressure less than 90 mmHg, and clostridial infection as independent predictors of amputation [30]. Pham et al. evaluated the functional impairment of NSTI survivors at a large tertiary referral center treated between 2002 and 2006 with up to 1-month post-discharge follow-up [82]. Thirty percent of patients had mild to severe physical limitation at hospital discharge. On univariate analysis, worsened functional status was associated with extremity involvement, a higher Acute Physiology and Chronic Health Evaluation (APACHE) II score, longer intensive care stay, and delay in consult for therapy. On multivariate analysis, extremity involvement, independent of amputation status, was associated with a higher functional limitation class [30]. Given the short follow-up period of this study, further study is required to determine the longer-term functional limitations of surviving NSTIs.

Follow-up

In addition to an acute mortality risk, NSTI patients have an increased risk of long-term mortality and morbidity. Light et al. performed a study of 345 NSTI survivors followed for 15 years; the estimated median age of death was significantly younger than that for population-based controls [83]. In particular, there was a significantly increased risk of subsequent death due to infectious causes in NSTI survivors (14% versus 2.9%) [83]. The authors recommended the following: counseling patients regarding the increased mortality risk; broadening indications for immunizations; and pursuing aggressive modification of other risk factors for death such as obesity, diabetes, smoking, and atherosclerotic disease [83]. They also identified a need for further research into the genetic and social determinants of this excess mortality risk.

Conclusion

NSTIs are associated with significant morbidity and mortality. Despite advances in critical care, the mainstays of therapy have remained largely unchanged over the last several decades: prompt recognition, early and aggressive debridement, and broad spectrum antibiotics. Diagnosis remains challenging given the lack of specificity of many of the early signs and symptoms, but advances in imaging may prove to be helpful. Further studies are required to identify adjunctive therapies and to determine their benefit in treating NSTIs.

References

1. May AK, Stafford RE, Bulger EM, et al. Treatment of complicated skin and soft tissue infections. Surg Infect (Larchmt). 2009;10(5):467–99.
2. Descamps V, Aitken J, Lee MG. Hippocrates on necrotising fasciitis. Lancet. 1994;344(8921):556.
3. Sarani B, Strong M, Pascual J, Schwab CW. Necrotizing fasciitis: current concepts and review of the literature. J Am Coll Surg. 2009;208(2):279–88.
4. Salcido RS. Necrotizing fasciitis: reviewing the causes and treatment strategies. Adv Skin Wound Care. 2007;20(5):288–93. quiz 294–85.
5. Ellis Simonsen SM, van Orman ER, Hatch BE, et al. Cellulitis incidence in a defined population. Epidemiol Infect. 2006;134(2):293–9.
6. Endorf FW, Klein MB, Mack CD, Jurkovich GJ, Rivara FP. Necrotizing soft-tissue infections: differences in patients treated at burn centers and non-burn centers. J Burn Care Res. 2008;29(6):933–8.
7. Anaya DA, Dellinger EP. Necrotizing soft-tissue infection: diagnosis and management. Clin Infect Dis. 2007;44(5):705–10.
8. Howell GM, Rosengart MR. Necrotizing soft tissue infections. Surg Infect (Larchmt). 2011;12(3):185–90.
9. Bakleh M, Wold LE, Mandrekar JN, Harmsen WS, Dimashkieh HH, Baddour LM. Correlation of histopathologic findings with clinical outcome in necrotizing fasciitis. Clin Infect Dis. 2005;40(3):410–4.
10. Endorf FW, Supple KG, Gamelli RL. The evolving characteristics and care of necrotizing soft-tissue infections. Burns. 2005;31(3):269–73.
11. Elliott D, Kufera JA, Myers RA. The microbiology of necrotizing soft tissue infections. Am J Surg. 2000;179(5):361–6.
12. Moet GJ, Jones RN, Biedenbach DJ, Stilwell MG, Fritsche TR. Contemporary causes of skin and soft tissue infections in North America, Latin America, and Europe: report from the SENTRY Antimicrobial Surveillance Program (1998–2004). Diagn Microbiol Infect Dis. 2007;57(1):7–13.
13. Fry DE, Barie PS. The changing face of Staphylococcus aureus: a continuing surgical challenge. Surg Infect (Larchmt). 2011;12(3):191–203.
14. Zetola N, Francis JS, Nuermberger EL, Bishai WR. Community-acquired methicillin-resistant Staphylococcus aureus: an emerging threat. Lancet Infect Dis. 2005;5(5):275–86.
15. Cooke FJ, Brown NM. Community-associated methicillin-resistant Staphylococcus aureus infections. Br Med Bull. 2010;94:215–27.
16. Miller LG, Perdreau-Remington F, Rieg G, et al. Necrotizing fasciitis caused by community-associated methicillin-resistant Staphylococcus aureus in Los Angeles. N Engl J Med. 2005;352(14):1445–53.
17. Fagan SP, Berger DH, Rahwan K, Awad SS. Spider bites presenting with methicillin-resistant Staphylococcus aureus soft tissue infection require early aggressive treatment. Surg Infect (Larchmt). 2003;4(4):311–5.
18. Kao LS, Lew DF, Arab SN, et al. Local variations in the epidemiology, microbiology, and outcome of necrotizing soft-tissue infections: a multicenter study. Am J Surg. 2011;202(2):139–45.
19. Lee TC, Carrick MM, Scott BG, Hodges JC, Pham HQ. Incidence and clinical characteristics of methicillin-resistant Staphylococcus aureus necrotizing fasciitis in a large urban hospital. Am J Surg. 2007;194(6):809–12. discussion 812–803.
20. Lee YT, Lin JC, Wang NC, Peng MY, Chang FY. Necrotizing fasciitis in a medical center in northern Taiwan: emergence of methicillin-resistant Staphylococcus aureus in the community. J Microbiol Immunol Infect. 2007;40(4):335–41.
21. Lamagni TL, Darenberg J, Luca-Harari B, et al. Epidemiology of severe Streptococcus pyogenes disease in Europe. J Clin Microbiol. 2008;46(7):2359–67.
22. Golger A, Ching S, Goldsmith CH, Pennie RA, Bain JR. Mortality in patients with necrotizing fasciitis. Plast Reconstr Surg. 2007;119(6):1803–7.
23. Garcia-Casares E, Mateo Soria L, Garcia-Melchor E, et al. Necrotizing fasciitis and myositis caused by streptococcal flesh-eating bacteria. J Clin Rheumatol. 2010;16(8):382–4.
24. Lee CC, Chi CH, Lee NY, et al. Necrotizing fasciitis in patients with liver cirrhosis: predominance of monomicrobial Gram-negative bacillary infections. Diagn Microbiol Infect Dis. 2008;62(2):219–25.
25. Hsiao CT, Weng HH, Yuan YD, Chen CT, Chen IC. Predictors of mortality in patients with necrotizing fasciitis. Am J Emerg Med. 2008;26(2):170–5.
26. Kuo YL, Shieh SJ, Chiu HY, Lee JW. Necrotizing fasciitis caused by Vibrio vulnificus: epidemiology, clinical findings, treatment and prevention. Eur J Clin Microbiol Infect Dis. 2007;26(11):785–92.
27. Tsai YH, Hsu RW, Huang KC, et al. Systemic Vibrio infection presenting as necrotizing fasciitis and sepsis. A series of thirteen cases. J Bone Joint Surg Am. 2004;86-A(11):2497–502.
28. Tsai YH, Huang TJ, Hsu RW, et al. Necrotizing soft-tissue infections and primary sepsis caused by Vibrio vulnificus and Vibrio cholerae non-O1. J Trauma. 2009;66(3):899–905.
29. Kelesidis T, Tsiodras S. Postirradiation Klebsiella pneumoniae-associated necrotizing fasciitis in the western hemisphere: a rare but life-threatening clinical entity. Am J Med Sci. 2009;338(3):217–24.
30. Anaya DA, McMahon K, Nathens AB, Sullivan SR, Foy H, Bulger E. Predictors of mortality and limb loss in necrotizing soft tissue infections. Arch Surg. 2005;140(2):151–7. discussion 158.
31. Dunbar NM, Harruff RC. Necrotizing fasciitis: manifestations, microbiology and connection with black tar heroin. J Forensic Sci. 2007;52(4):920–3.
32. Mao E, Clements A, Feller E. Clostridium septicum sepsis and colon carcinoma: report of 4 cases. Case Report Med. 2011;2011:248453.
33. Schade VL, Roukis TS, Haque M. Clostridium septicum necrotizing fasciitis of the forefoot secondary to adenocarcinoma of the colon: case report and review of the literature. J Foot Ankle Surg. 2010;49(2):159. e151–8.
34. Johnson MA, Lyle G, Hanly M, Yeh KA. Aspergillus: a rare primary organism in soft-tissue infections. Am Surg. 1998;64(2):122–6.
35. Singh G, Ray P, Sinha SK, Adhikary S, Khanna SK. Bacteriology of necrotizing infections of soft tissues. Aust N Z J Surg. 1996;66(11):747–50.
36. Snell BJ, Tavakoli K. Necrotizing fasciitis caused by Apophysomyces elegans complicating soft-tissue and pelvic injuries in a tsunami survivor from Thailand. Plast Reconstr Surg. 2007;119(1):448–9.
37. Andresen D, Donaldson A, Choo L, et al. Multifocal cutaneous mucormycosis complicating polymicrobial wound infections in a tsunami survivor from Sri Lanka. Lancet. 2005;365(9462):876–8.
38. Kordy FN, Al-Mohsen IZ, Hashem F, Almodovar E, Al Hajjar S, Walsh TJ. Successful treatment of a child with posttraumatic necrotizing fasciitis caused by Apophysomyces elegans: case report and review of literature. Pediatr Infect Dis J. 2004;23(9):877–9.
39. Begon E, Bachmeyer C, Thibault M, et al. Necrotizing fasciitis due to Cryptococcus neoformans in a diabetic patient with chronic renal insufficiency. Clin Exp Dermatol. 2009;34(8):935–6.

40. Baer S, Baddley JW, Gnann JW, Pappas PG. Cryptococcal disease presenting as necrotizing cellulitis in transplant recipients. Transpl Infect Dis. 2009;11(4):353–8.

41. McHenry CR, Piotrowski JJ, Petrinic D, Malangoni MA. Determinants of mortality for necrotizing soft-tissue infections. Ann Surg. 1995;221(5):558–63. discussion 563–555.

42. Malangoni MA. Necrotizing soft tissue infections: are we making any progress? Surg Infect (Larchmt). 2001;2(2):145–50. discussion 150–42.

43. Wong CH, Wang YS. The diagnosis of necrotizing fasciitis. Curr Opin Infect Dis. 2005;18(2):101–6.

44. Wang YS, Wong CH, Tay YK. Staging of necrotizing fasciitis based on the evolving cutaneous features. Int J Dermatol. 2007;46(10):1036–41.

45. Elliott DC, Kufera JA, Myers RA. Necrotizing soft tissue infections. Risk factors for mortality and strategies for management. Ann Surg. 1996;224(5):672–83.

46. Wall DB, Klein SR, Black S, de Virgilio C. A simple model to help distinguish necrotizing fasciitis from nonnecrotizing soft tissue infection. J Am Coll Surg. 2000;191(3):227–31.

47. Wall DB, de Virgilio C, Black S, Klein SR. Objective criteria may assist in distinguishing necrotizing fasciitis from nonnecrotizing soft tissue infection. Am J Surg. 2000;179(1):17–21.

48. Wong CH, Khin LW, Heng KS, Tan KC, Low CO. The LRINEC (Laboratory Risk Indicator for Necrotizing Fasciitis) score: a tool for distinguishing necrotizing fasciitis from other soft tissue infections. Crit Care Med. 2004;32(7):1535–41.

49. Tsai YH, Hsu RW, Huang KC, Huang TJ. Laboratory indicators for early detection and surgical treatment of vibrio necrotizing fasciitis. Clin Orthop Relat Res. 2010;468(8):2230–7.

50. Holland MJ. Application of the laboratory risk indicator in necrotising fasciitis (LRINEC) score to patients in a tropical tertiary referral centre. Anaesth Intensive Care. 2009;37(4):588–92.

51. Su YC, Chen HW, Hong YC, Chen CT, Hsiao CT, Chen IC. Laboratory risk indicator for necrotizing fasciitis score and the outcomes. ANZ J Surg. 2008;78(11):968–72.

52. Hosek WT, Laeger TC. Early diagnosis of necrotizing fasciitis with soft tissue ultrasound. Acad Emerg Med. 2009;16(10):1033.

53. Yen ZS, Wang HP, Ma HM, Chen SC, Chen WJ. Ultrasonographic screening of clinically-suspected necrotizing fasciitis. Acad Emerg Med. 2002;9(12):1448–51.

54. Wronski M, Slodkowski M, Cebulski W, Karkocha D, Krasnodebski IW. Necrotizing fasciitis: early sonographic diagnosis. J Clin Ultrasound. 2011;39(4):236–9.

55. Becker M, Zbaren P, Hermans R, et al. Necrotizing fasciitis of the head and neck: role of CT in diagnosis and management. Radiology. 1997;202(2):471–6.

56. Wysoki MG, Santora TA, Shah RM, Friedman AC. Necrotizing fasciitis: CT characteristics. Radiology. 1997;203(3):859–63.

57. Zacharias N, Velmahos GC, Salama A, et al. Diagnosis of necrotizing soft tissue infections by computed tomography. Arch Surg. 2010;145(5):452–5.

58. McGillicuddy EA, Lischuk AW, Schuster KM, et al. Development of a computed tomography-based scoring system for necrotizing soft-tissue infections. J Trauma. 2011;70(4):894–9.

59. Kim KT, Kim YJ, Won Lee J, Park SW, Lim MK, Suh CH. Can necrotizing infectious fasciitis be differentiated from nonnecrotizing infectious fasciitis with MR imaging? Radiology. 2011;259(3):816–24.

60. Yu JS, Habib P. MR imaging of urgent inflammatory and infectious conditions affecting the soft tissues of the musculoskeletal system. Emerg Radiol. 2009;16(4):267–76.

61. Arslan A, Pierre-Jerome C, Borthne A. Necrotizing fasciitis: unreliable MRI findings in the preoperative diagnosis. Eur J Radiol. 2000;36(3):139–43.

62. Loh NN, Ch'en IY, Cheung LP, Li KC. Deep fascial hyperintensity in soft-tissue abnormalities as revealed by T2-weighted MR imaging. AJR Am J Roentgenol. 1997;168(5):1301–4.

63. Seok JH, Jee WH, Chun KA, et al. Necrotizing fasciitis versus pyomyositis: discrimination with using MR imaging. Korean J Radiol. 2009;10(2):121–8.

64. Lee PC, Turnidge J, McDonald PJ. Fine-needle aspiration biopsy in diagnosis of soft tissue infections. J Clin Microbiol. 1985;22(1):80–3.

65. Stamenkovic I, Lew PD. Early recognition of potentially fatal necrotizing fasciitis. The use of frozen-section biopsy. N Engl J Med. 1984;310(26):1689–93.

66. Wong CH, Chang HC, Pasupathy S, Khin LW, Tan JL, Low CO. Necrotizing fasciitis: clinical presentation, microbiology, and determinants of mortality. J Bone Joint Surg Am. 2003;85-A(8):1454–60.

67. Baharestani MM. Negative pressure wound therapy in the adjunctive management of necrotizing fascitis: examining clinical outcomes. Ostomy Wound Manage. 2008;54(4):44–50.

68. Endorf FW, Cancio LC, Klein MB. Necrotizing soft-tissue infections: clinical guidelines. J Burn Care Res. 2009;30(5):769–75.

69. DiNubile MJ, Lipsky BA. Complicated infections of skin and skin structures: when the infection is more than skin deep. J Antimicrob Chemother. 2004;53 Suppl 2:37–50.

70. Dellinger RP, Levy MM, Carlet JM, et al. Surviving Sepsis Campaign: international guidelines for management of severe sepsis and septic shock: 2008. Crit Care Med. 2008;36(1):296–327.

71. Korhonen K, Kuttila K, Niinikoski J. Tissue gas tensions in patients with necrotising fasciitis and healthy controls during treatment with hyperbaric oxygen: a clinical study. Eur J Surg. 2000;166(7):530–4.

72. Escobar SJ, Slade Jr JB, Hunt TK, Cianci P. Adjuvant hyperbaric oxygen therapy (HBO2) for treatment of necrotizing fasciitis reduces mortality and amputation rate. Undersea Hyperb Med. 2005;32(6):437–43.

73. Riseman JA, Zamboni WA, Curtis A, Graham DR, Konrad HR, Ross DS. Hyperbaric oxygen therapy for necrotizing fasciitis reduces mortality and the need for debridements. Surgery. 1990;108(5):847–50.

74. Shupak A, Shoshani O, Goldenberg I, Barzilai A, Moskuna R, Bursztein S. Necrotizing fasciitis: an indication for hyperbaric oxygenation therapy? Surgery. 1995;118(5):873–8.

75. Darenberg J, Ihendyane N, Sjolin J, et al. Intravenous immunoglobulin G therapy in streptococcal toxic shock syndrome: a European randomized, double-blind, placebo-controlled trial. Clin Infect Dis. 2003;37(3):333–40.

76. Simmonds M. Necrotising fasciitis and group A streptococcus toxic shock-like syndrome in pregnancy: treatment with plasmapheresis and immunoglobulin. Int J Obstet Anesth. 1999;8(2):125–30.

77. Busund R, Koukline V, Utrobin U, Nedashkovsky E. Plasmapheresis in severe sepsis and septic shock: a prospective, randomised, controlled trial. Intensive Care Med. 2002;28(10):1434–9.

78. Purnell D, Hazlett T, Alexander SL. A new weapon against severe sepsis related to necrotizing fasciitis. Dimens Crit Care Nurs. 2004;23(1):18–23.

79. Bland CM, Frizzi JD, Reyes A. Use of drotrecogin alfa in necrotizing fasciitis: a case report and pharmacologic review. J Intensive Care Med. 2008;23(5):342–6.

80. Gunter OL, Guillamondegui OD, May AK, Diaz JJ. Outcome of necrotizing skin and soft tissue infections. Surg Infect (Larchmt). 2008;9(4):443–50.

81. Anaya DA, Bulger EM, Kwon YS, Kao LS, Evans H, Nathens AB. Predicting death in necrotizing soft tissue infections: a clinical score. Surg Infect (Larchmt). 2009;10(6):517–22.

82. Pham TN, Moore ML, Costa BA, Cuschieri J, Klein MB. Assessment of functional limitation after necrotizing soft tissue infection. J Burn Care Res. 2009;30(2):301–6.

83. Light TD, Choi KC, Thomsen TA, et al. Long-term outcomes of patients with necrotizing fasciitis. J Burn Care Res. 2010;31(1):93–9.

Roman Kosir and Andrej Cretnik

Introduction

An extremity compartment syndrome develops when the tissue pressure within a limited space of the body reaches the point where the circulation, nerve function, and muscle function of that space are compromised. For this to occur, the compartment must have a relatively fixed space (i.e., enveloped by fascia) preventing inner tissue expansion and there needs to be a source of increased tissue pressure, either externally or internally.

The German surgeon Richard Von Volkmann first described the late sequelae of extremity compartment syndrome in 1881—termed Volkmann's ischemic contracture [1]. Later, in 1912 Wilson described exertional compartment syndrome and in 1956, Mayor reported on chronic compartment syndrome. Since then, there have been numerous cases of extremity compartment syndrome reported in the literature. It has been identified in a wide variety of clinical situations including tetanus, meningococcemia, malignant hyperthermia, frostbite, horseback riding, and childbirth [2–6]. Typically, it occurs following traumatic events, most commonly those involving orthopedic fractures or vascular trauma with subsequent ischemia reperfusion injuries. Recent literature documents an increased incidence of secondary extremity compartment syndrome in 2% of severely injured patients [7–9]. This typically occurs following massive resuscitation in patients with otherwise uninjured extremities. The incidence of extremity compartment syndrome varies depending on the patient population studied and its etiology. In a subset of patients with leg pain, 14% were noted to have anterior compartment syndrome of the lower leg according to Qvarfordt et al. [10]. In those with lower extremity fractures, it was seen in 1–9% of patients [11].

The most commonly affected body region is the lower extremity, specifically the four compartments of the lower leg (anterior, peroneal (lateral), superficial posterior, and deep posterior). This is followed in incidence by the volar and dorsal compartments of the forearm. Other potential compartments include the deltoid and biceps compartment of the arm, the interosseus compartment of the hand, the gluteal compartment of the buttock, the quadriceps compartment of the leg, and the interosseus, medial, central, and lateral compartments of the foot [12–15].

The etiology of extremity compartment syndrome varies and can be divided into three major categories: decreased compartmental volume, increased compartmental content, and externally applied pressure. Common causes seen in acute care surgery are presented in Table 38.1 [16]. Of these categories, increased compartmental content is the most prominent. Pathophysiologically, increasing the volume in a space limited by noncompliant fascia results in an exponential rise in the intracompartmental pressure. This is fairly straightforward when it comes to bleeding into a compartment. However, post-ischemic swelling or reperfusion-injury is more complex, as it produces a "double ischemic insult." The initial ischemic insult leads to dysfunction of the tissues, including the nerves, muscles, and microvasculature Increased vascular permeability following this initial ischemic insult leads to post-ischemic swelling, and thus ultimately increased compartmental volume and compartment syndrome, which causes additional injury to the neuromuscular component of the compartment. Secondary to this, the physical examination in patients with a reperfusion injury may be unreliable [16].

Clinical Presentation

In awake, alert patients, most extremity compartment syndromes can be diagnosed by clinical examination alone. The common clinical signs include the five Ps: pain, pulselessness, pallor, paresthesias, and paralysis. Additional Ps to

R. Kosir, M.D. (✉) • A. Cretnik, M.D., Ph.D.
Trauma Department, University Clinical Center Maribor,
Ljubljanska 5, Maribor, 2000, Slovenia
e-mail: roman.kosir@siol.com; andrej.cretnik@guest.arnes.si

L.J. Moore et al. (eds.), *Common Problems in Acute Care Surgery*,
DOI 10.1007/978-1-4614-6123-4_38, © Springer Science+Business Media New York 2013

Table 38.1 The most common causes of increased compartment pressures in acute care surgery

Decreased compartmental volume	• Excessive traction with fracture immobilization • Closure of fascial defects following trauma
Increased compartmental content	• Intracompartmental bleeding secondary to fractures, vascular injury, or bleeding disorders • Increased capillary filtration following reperfusion after ischemia, embolectomy, soft tissue trauma, burns, or fracture fixation
Externally applied pressure	• Tight immobilization of fractures • Lying on limb

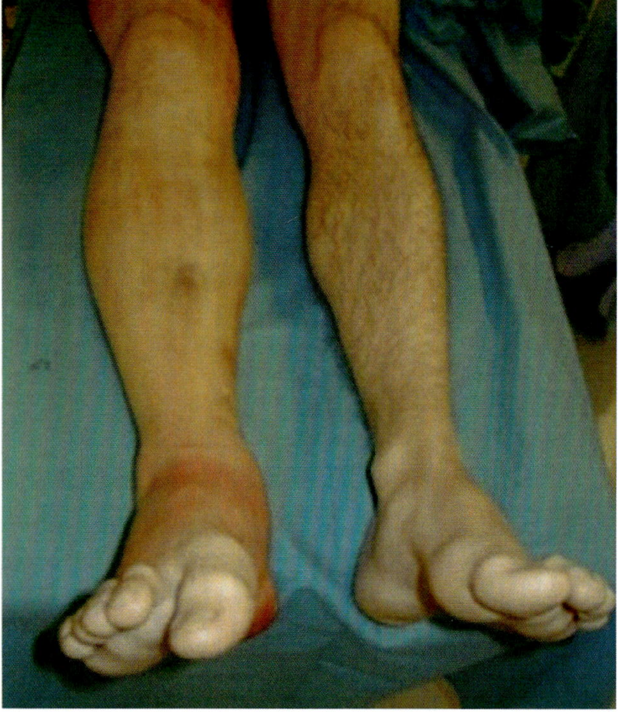

Fig. 38.1 A case of right lower extremity compartment syndrome secondary to an isolated tibial fracture. Pain, swelling, and the inability of dorsal flexion of the toe was noted on examination

consider include pressure (swelling and tenseness of the compartment), and poikilothermy (Fig. 38.1). Other signs to look for are skin edema, blisters, swelling, and subcutaneous blood suffusions (Fig. 38.2).

To make a diagnosis, a physician must first have an evidence of increased intracompartmental pressure. If so, the signs do not occur simultaneously, but they develop with time. One of the first signs is a swollen or tight compartment in combination with severe pain that is out of proportion of what it is expected to be and which is not relieved by regular analgesia. Other signs are late presentation and often, when this is present, an irreversible damage to soft tissues has occurred. There are numerous other pathophysiological events that can cause a similar clinical picture. In fact, a large meta-analysis of studies comparing clinical signs with development of acute lower extremity compartment syndrome showed sensitivity of 13–19%, specificity of 97%, positive predictive value of 11–15%, and negative predictive value of 98% [17]. Thus, the absence of this sign does rule out compartment syndrome, but the presence rarely confirms the correct diagnosis.

Nevertheless, clinical observation of the suspected compartment is what is recommended, since the hourly progress of the symptoms is what should be noted first before making a definitive diagnosis and starting definitive treatment. A useful tool for observation could be a simple sheet with notes about date, time, location, pain level, motor, and sensory testing. To do this, one must know the anatomical position of various compartments and their vascular and nerve content. Figure 38.3 shows an example of a screening form of the most commonly observed acute lower extremity compartment [18].

Diagnosis

To make a diagnosis of compartment syndrome we must have evidence of increased tissue pressure, inadequate tissue perfusion, and loss of tissue function. When all the three factors are present, the diagnosis may be made with assurance; when one or more of these factors are absent, the diagnosis is less secure. Evidence of increased tissue pressure may include complaints of tightness or pressure in the involved area. By palpation, the physician may perceive the tenseness of the compartmental envelope [19].

Evidence of inadequate perfusion of local tissue pressure may include the symptom of pain that is out of proportion to what would be anticipated from the clinical situation. Patients requiring increasing analgesic medication in a properly immobilized leg should raise suspicion. Pain on passive stretching of the intracompartmental muscles is another useful indication of increased pressure, especially if muscles have not been injured. Reduced peripheral pulses are very late signs of compartment syndrome; in fact, studies have shown normal pulses with Doppler signals in otherwise severely elevated intracompartmental pressures. Arterial flow is rarely compromised in elevated tissue compartment pressures. On the other hand, diminished pulses could be a result of other causes (e.g., vascular lesions) and in combination with reperfusion injury could also lead to development of compartment syndrome [19].

Evidence of abnormal tissue function includes weakness of the intracompartmental muscles and nerves, including sensory branches that cross-involve compartments and their lesion produces hypoesthesia. Both nerve and muscle function may be altered by direct injury; therefore, evidence of progressive loss of function over time may be a better sign [19].

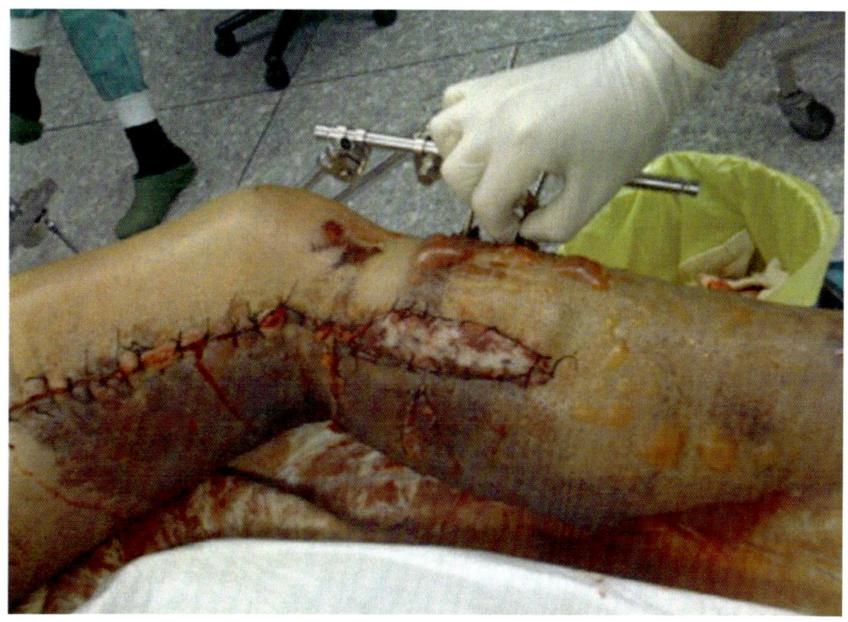

Fig. 38.2 A case of left lower left extremity compartment syndrome following a popliteal artery injury and subsequent revascularization in combination with a proximal tibial fracture externally fixed. Several hours following this management, there are obvious signs of compartment syndrome to include swelling, skin discoloration and blistering, and functional loss

To summarize, in awake and cooperative patients who can be reexamined frequently, the diagnosis of compartment syndrome is associated with the following findings:

1. Pain that is out of proportion to what is anticipated from the clinical situation
2. Weakness of the muscles in the compartment
3. Pain on passive stretching of the muscles in the compartment
4. Hypoesthesia in the distribution of the nerves coursing through the compartment
5. Tenseness of the compartmental envelope

Since clinical signs are progressing and because they do not appear all at once, the clinical decision-making results in a conundrum [12, 20–22]. Especially in critically ill patients who are unable to cooperate because of head trauma, sedation, or even neuromuscular blocking drugs, the diagnosis cannot be made based on clinical examination alone [18].

Although the clinical examination should be a cornerstone of the diagnosis of compartment syndrome, it has disadvantages of being subjective and requires patient cooperation [12, 17, 23]. Therefore, tissue pressure measurement should be performed to add vital information for establishing the diagnosis and starting immediate treatment. The normal interstitial tissue pressure in the compartment is around 5 mmHg. Capillary blood flow becomes compromised at 20 mmHg, pain develops at pressures between 20 and 30 mmHg. A tissue pressure of more than 45 mmHg has been reported to be usually associated with compartment syndrome, and a pressure of more than 60 mmHg can confirm diagnosis [24–26]. But, the tolerance of tissue for increased pressure may be reduced by other factors, such as arterial occlusion, limb elevation, and shock [25, 27]; with these conditions compartment syndrome may occur at significantly lower interstitial pressures. According to arteriovenous gradient theory, the local blood flow (LBF) depends on the pressure gradient between arteries (P_a) and veins (P_v) and local vascular resistance to flow (R). This condition describes the formula [28]:

$$LBF = (P_a - P_v) / R$$

Local blood flow should be maintained to deliver enough oxygen to the tissues. According to this relationship, it is not the interstitial pressure that increases resistance, the only factor that reduces blood flow. The arterial pressure is also important, whereas venous pressure is somehow related to interstitial pressure. Increasing interstitial pressure also increases venous pressure, and furthermore decreases blood flow.

Because tolerance of tissues to increased intracompartmental pressure varies among different individuals and there are more factors that influence local blood flow, only one isolated measurement of interstitial pressure could not be enough to diagnose this condition. For example, higher compartment pressures may be necessary before injury occurs to peripheral nerves in patients with systemic hypertension [25], while compartment syndrome may develop at lower pressures in those with hypotension and/or peripheral vascular disease [29, 30]. It has been proposed that the difference between diastolic pressure and intracompartmental pressure is a better marker for compartment syndrome. A δP is calculated as follows:

$$\delta P = DBP \, (\text{diastolic blood pressure})$$
$$- IP \, (\text{interstitial pressure})$$

Fig. 38.3 Acute lower extremity compartment syndrome screening tool [18]

Acute Lower Extremity Compartment Syndrome
Screening Form

Start Date: ___/___/____

Start Time: ___________

CLINICAL DIAGNOSES

Increased tissue pressure / swelling	YES / NO

Pain — *Assess according to scale from 1 to 10*

Calf Pain - Calf pain at rest
PPSF - Pain with passive stretch, foot in plantarflexion
PPSE - Pain with passive stretch, foot in extension/dorsiflexion

Vascular Exam		Pulse	Scale
DPA – Dorsal Pedal Artery		Palpable	4
		Diminished	3
PTA – Posterior Tibial Artery		Non-palpable, Doppler positive	2
		Non-palpable, Doppler negative	1

Neurologic Exam - Motor	Strength	Scale
DPN - Deep Peroneal Nerve	Movement against gravity with full resistance	6
DPN-M Foot dorsiflexion	Movement against gravity with some resistance	5
	Movement against gravity only	4
TN - Tibial Nerve	Movement with gravity eliminated	3
TN-M Foot plantar flexion	Visible/palpable muscle contraction	2
	Without movement, no contraction	1

Neurologic Exam - Sensory	Touch Sensation	Scale
DPN Deep Peroneal Nerve		
DPN-S 1st to 2nd toe web space	Normal	3
TN Tibial Nerve	Diminished	2
TN-S Sole	Absent	1

If unable to assess – write N/A

Left \ Right	Initial exam	Exam 4h	Exam 8h	Exam 12h	Exam 16h	Exam 20h	Exam 24h	Exam 28h	Exam 32h	Exam 36h	Exam 40h	Exam 44h	Exam 48h
Date													
Time													
Swelling													
Calf Pain													
PPSF													
PPSE													
DPA													
PTA													
DPN-M													
DPN-S													
TN-M													
TN-S													

YOUR Hospital Name

Your Department Name

Acute Lower Extremity Compartment Syndrome Screening

Patient Sticker

It is suggested to be more than 30–35 mmHg, but a specific threshold does not exist [31–34].

There are numerous methods of tissue pressure measurements [35–38]. The most commonly used are commercial handheld pressure monitors (e.g., Stryker™ device, Stryker, Kalamazoo, Michigan), a simple needle manometer system, and the wick or slit catheter technique. The question is accuracy, since there are reports that the arterial line manometer is the most accurate device [39]. The arterial line manometer device has another advantage of being able to monitor pressure continuously. Whichever method is used to measure compartment pressures, accuracy depends upon proper calibration of the measuring device and placement of the needle of pressure sensor in the level of the injured compartment. The principle of tissue pressure measurement in the case of acute lower extremity compartment syndrome is shown in Fig. 38.4.

Use of near-infrared spectroscopy for detection of low tissue oxygenation and therefore development of compartment syndrome is controversial. It has been reported as a useful noninvasive tool in diagnosing compartment syndrome after surgical revascularization of lower limb ischemia, whereas other studies did not prove its use due to severe edema of the soft tissues and inability to measure StO_2 inside the muscle compartment [21, 33, 40–42].

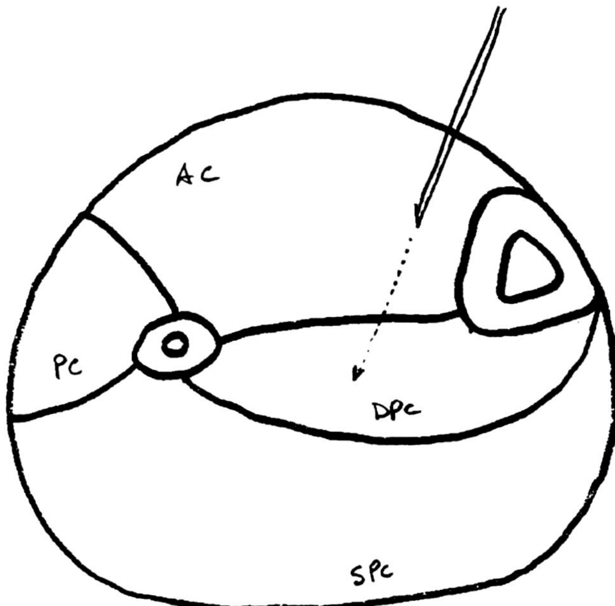

Fig. 38.4 An anatomical cross section of the lower leg and the location for needle placement in the anterior compartment (then proceeding into the deep posterior compartment) for pressure measurements. *AC* anterior compartment, *PC* peroneal (lateral) compartment, *DPC* deep posterior compartment, *SPC* superficial posterior compartment

In establishing a diagnosis of compartment syndrome we have to rule out other causes of pain-producing symptoms or we have to confirm a cause of elevated intracompartmental pressure. Especially with trauma, consider obtaining workup for rhabdomyolysis (creatinine phosphokinase (CPK), renal functions, urinalysis, and urine myoglobin). Extremity X-ray or CT scan can confirm the presence of fracture. MRI or ultrasonography can show muscle tears. Doppler ultrasonography or arteriography can detect vascular abnormality.

Management

The objective of treatment of a compartmental syndrome is to minimize deficits in muscular and neurological function by promptly restoring local blood flow. Certain nonoperative measures may be effective, such as eliminating external pressure and maintaining local arterial pressure. When there is external pressure that causes compartment syndrome, such as tight casts, it is essential to release the envelope immediately (remove and exchange for noncircular splint) when there is only one symptom or sign present. Usually this is pain and is most often observed in patients with fracture splints several hours after treatment. Restoration of normal limb perfusion has priority over closed fracture treatment and this is postponed until the perfusion returns to normal. Before using operative methods for reducing tissue pressure, we have to consider improvement of local blood flow if it has

been reduced by shock, peripheral vascular disease, or elevation of the limb above the heart. All causes of systemic hypotension should be treated. Limb elevation should be avoided, because it lowers local arterial pressure and does not help to reduce swelling [43, 44]. Use of vasodilatating drugs or sympathetic blockade appears to be ineffective, because in this condition local maximal vasodilatation is already present. The use of phosphodiesterase inhibitor in experimental animals caused modulation of compartmental pressures. In a large study of trauma patients with isolated arterial injury, early anticoagulation with heparin has been found to reduce the incidence of compartment syndrome without significant bleeding as a consequence [45, 46].

The primary goal of treating compartment syndrome is to decrease intracompartmental pressures. Surgical decompression of all limiting envelopes is the gold standard of treatment indicated in the presence of a characteristic clinical picture of compartmental syndrome in a cooperative patient. When clinical exam is unreliable or difficult to obtain we have to consider pressure measurement, where either pressure should not exceed 45 mmHg or rather deltaP should not be below 30 mmHg.

The standard way of treatment is long skin incision and fasciotomy of all involved compartments and debridement of obvious nonviable tissue. Procedure should be performed without a tourniquet to avoid prolonging of ischemia and to permit the surgeon to assess degree of viability and restoration of blood flow. The skin is incised through the entire length of the involved compartment. There is obvious muscle bulging observed in a true compartment syndrome. Only obvious necrotic muscle should be removed, because tissue may have potential for reperfusion and recovery. The sign of contractility with electro stimulation should not be used initially. After fascial release we should anticipate post-ischemic swelling, and therefore, the skin should be left open and the wound temporarily closed with a patch of compliant artificial temporary skin closures. If release of the compartment is not complete, "rebound" compartment syndrome may occur.

After surgical decompression and temporary skin closure, sterile dressings are applied and the extremity is usually splinted in a functional position. In presence of fractures we have to consider fixation with external fixators, rarely with plates or intramedullary nails. This stabilization is performed immediately after fascial decompression and greatly facilitates later care of the wound, limb, and fracture. Passive stretching exercises are instituted to maintain range of joint motion. Skin closure may usually be accomplished 3–5 days after surgical decompression, usually by mesh-graft, rarely by direct suturing (Fig. 38.5). At that time, additional debridement of nonviable tissue can be performed. Fascial closure is not recommended, because this requires closure under tension and can lead to development of the compartment syndrome again. Muscle hernia is left behind and should be

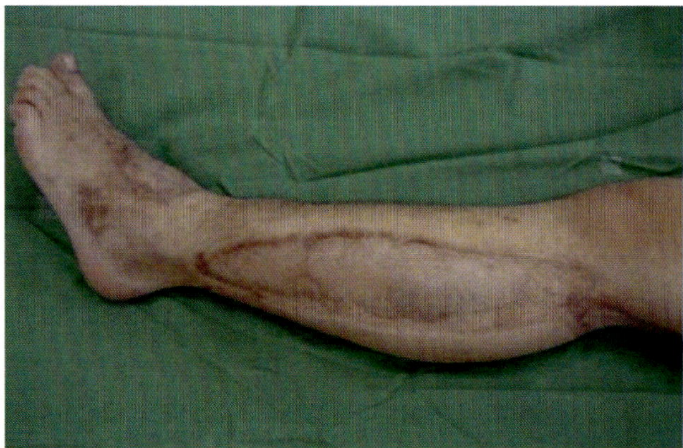

Fig. 38.5 Cosmetic result of a lower extremity compartment syndrome following split thickness skin grafting

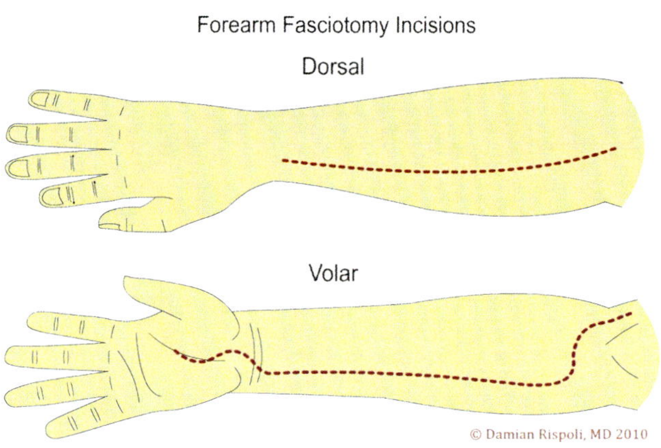

Fig. 38.6 Fasciotomy of the forearm—dorsal and volar aspects. Reprinted by permission of Data Trace Internet Publishing, LLC. *Wheeless Textbook of Orthopaedics*, Copyright 2011

large enough not to cause additional late problems. When optimal cosmetic result is desired, one may progressively approximate the wound edges over 7–14 days with sutures to achieve direct skin closure.

Negative pressure wound care closure devices can be useful in the management of fasciotomy wounds. Negative pressure decreases wound edema, facilitates approximation of the skin edges, enhances local blood flow, promotes granulation tissue, and decreases bacterial colonization. There are no prospective randomized trials comparing standard sterile dressings compared to negative pressure treatment. But in retrospective analyses, negative pressure led to a significantly higher rate of complete skin closure and decreased time to skin closure [47, 48]. Hyperbaric oxygen as an adjunct to management following fasciotomy is reported in some case reports and animal studies, but there is lack of evidence to show an advantage compared to current practices [49–53].

Fasciotomy Techniques

The fasciotomy technique depends on the underlying condition or mechanism that caused compartment syndrome. The length of the lower extremity skin incisions have been debated for a long time. Minimal skin incisions with more extensive fascial incisions could place patient at risk for recurrent compartment syndrome [54–56]. The degree of muscle swelling after reperfusion cannot be predicted. Peak edema occurs several hours later after surgery.

Fasciotomies of the Upper Extremities

The upper extremity is anatomically divided into the brachium, antebrachium, and hand. Each of these anatomical segments has a different number of compartments with various muscle functions. The techniques for release of these compartments have to be discussed separately.

Fasciotomy of the Arm

The arm has two compartments: anterior, which includes the biceps and brachioradialis muscles, and posterior with the triceps muscle. Fasciotomy technique includes lateral skin incision from deltoid insertion to lateral epicondyle. Care must be taken to avoid damage to larger cutaneous nerves. At fascial level, intermuscular septum between anterior and posterior compartment is identified and fascia overlying each compartment is released with longitudinal incisions. The radial nerve should be protected as it passes through the intermuscular septum prom posterior compartment to the anterior compartment just below the fascia.

Fasciotomy of the Forearm

The antebrachium has three muscular compartments: mobile wad proximally, volar compartment, and dorsal compartment. Fasciotomy technique consists of a longitudinal centrally placed incision over the extensor compartment and a curvilinear incision on the flexor aspect beginning at the antecubital fossa (Fig. 38.6). A palmar incision is made between the thenar and hypothenar muscles in the palm, where the carpal tunnel can be released if needed. The incision is extended transversely across the wrist flexion crease to the ulnar side of the wrist, then arched across the volar forearm back to the ulnar side at the elbow. At the elbow, the incision is curved just radial to the medial epicondyle across the elbow flexion crease and the deep fascia is released. At the antecubital fossa, the fibrous band overlying the brachial artery and median nerve is carefully released. This incision allows for soft tissue coverage of the underlying neurovascular structures at the wrist and elbow and prevents soft tissue contractures from developing at flexion creases.

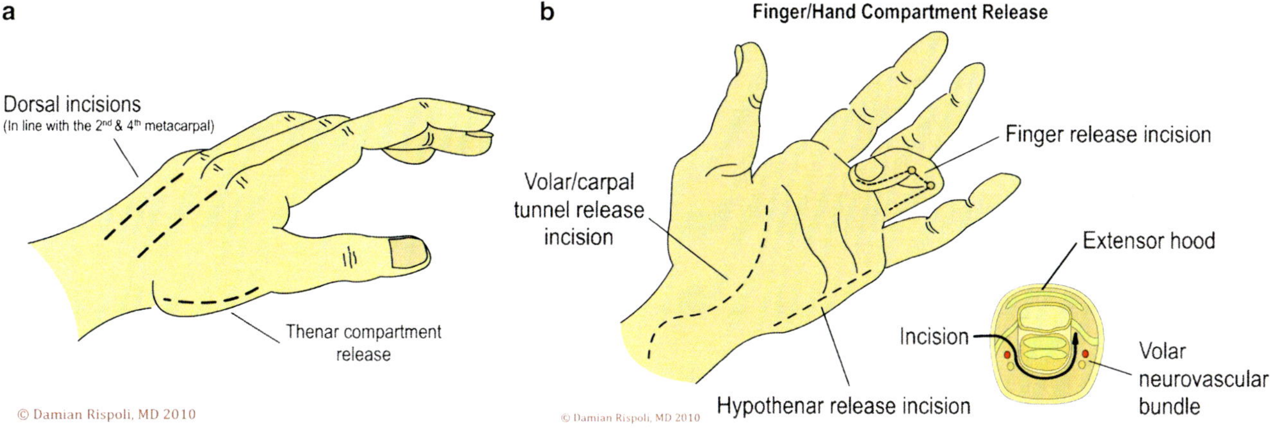

Fig. 38.7 Fasciotomy of the hand—(**a**) dorsal and (**b**) volar aspects. Reprinted by permission of Data Trace Internet Publishing, LLC. *Wheeless Textbook of Orthopaedics*, Copyright 2011

Fig. 38.8 Fasciotomy of the leg. Reprinted by permission of Data Trace Internet Publishing, LLC. *Wheeless Textbook of Orthopaedics*, Copyright 2011

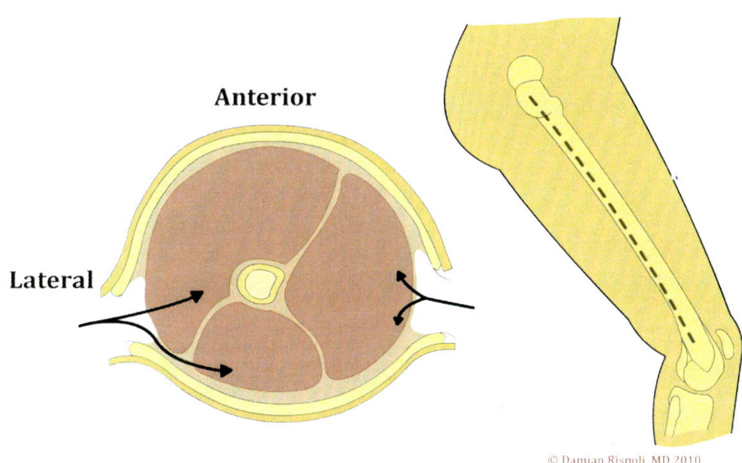

A second straight dorsal incision can be made to release the mobile wad if necessary.

Fasciotomy of the Hand

The hand has a unique anatomy with ten separate fascial compartments: four dorsal and three volar interossei, thenar muscles, hypothenar muscles, and adductor pollicis. The fasciotomy technique consists of four incisions (Fig. 38.7). One incision on the radial side of the thumb metacarpal releases the thenar compartment. A dorsal incision over the index finger metacarpal is used to release the first and second dorsal interossei and to reach the ulnar-to-index finger metacarpal and to release the volar interossei and adductor pollicis. A dorsal incision over the ring finger metacarpal is used to release the third and fourth dorsal interossei and to reach down along the radial aspect of the ring finger and small finger metatarsal to release the volar interossei. An incision placed at the ulnar aspect of the small finger is used to release the hypothenar muscles.

Fasciotomies of the Lower Extremities

The lower extremity is anatomically divided into three parts: thigh, lower leg, and foot. As in the upper extremity, each anatomical segment has a different number of compartments with various muscle functions. Techniques for release of these compartments are discussed separately as well.

Fasciotomy of the Thigh

The thigh has three compartments: anterior (quadriceps), medial (adductors), and posterior (hamstrings) (Fig. 38.8). Because of its large volume compartment and also the blending of the fascial compartments with the hip (which may allow extravasation of blood outside the compartments), compartment syndrome in the thigh is less likely to occur, but can be seen especially in patients with high-energy femoral fractures or hip fractures. The fasciotomy technique consists of a lateral incision made from the greater trochanter to the lateral condyle of the femur. The iliotibial band is incised and the vastus lateralis reflected off the intermuscular septum bluntly, releasing the anterior compartment. The intermuscular septum is then incised over the length of the incision, releasing the posterior compartment. This release should not be done closely to the femur because of a series of perforating vessels passing through the septum from posterior to anterior near the bone. The medial compartment is released through a separate *anteromedial incision*.

Fasciotomy of the Lower Leg

Lower extremity compartment syndrome is the most common due to the unique anatomy of the lower leg's compartments. Most of the studies have been done in this part of the body and most of the current knowledge about epidemiology and treatment are based on lower extremity compartment syndrome studies. The lower leg has four compartments: peroneal (lateral) (peroneus brevis and longus), anterior (extensor hallucis longus, extensor digitorum longus, tibialis anterior, and peroneus tertius), superficial posterior (gastrocnemius and soleus), and deep posterior (flexor hallucis longus, flexor digitorum longus, and tibialis posterior). The anterior compartment is the most commonly involved, followed by the deep posterior compartment. In case of compartment syndrome of any of the compartments, release of all four is recommended.

There are two operating techniques for release of all four compartments in the lower leg: the one incision technique and the two-incision technique. There is no strong evidence showing which technique has an advantage over the other. It seems that due to its simplicity, the two-incision technique is more often used. In case of tibial fractures, any exposure of the fracture is not recommended; therefore, use of the one-incision technique may have some advantage. Single-incision technique also causes only one surgical wound and less related complications were described in one study [57].

Fasciotomy of the Lower Leg: Single-Incision Technique

Single-incision technique is technically more difficult; its disadvantage is that it is difficult to visualize the deep posterior compartment, and therefore, there is increased risk of injury to the peroneal artery and nerve. This technique starts with a skin incision 1–2 cm anterior to the fibula and parallel to it, just inferior from the fibular head to 3–4 cm proximal of the lateral malleolus. An anterior flap enables exposure of the anterior and peroneal (lateral) compartments. Longitudinal incisions are made in the fascia and care must be taken to avoid damage to the common, superficial, and deep peroneal nerves at the fibular head. A lateral flap is exposed more posteriorly to visualize the superficial posterior compartment. The gastrocnemius should be identified and the fascia is incised longitudinally. The deep posterior compartment is identified later after exposure of the posterior side of the fibula with dissection of the soleus muscle. Fasciotomy of

deep posterior compartment is performed right at the medial border of fibula. Here, peroneal vessels should be retracted and protected posteriorly to avoid injury.

Fasciotomy of the Lower Leg: Two-Incision Technique

This technique uses medial and lateral longitudinal incisions that should be long enough to completely release all four compartments. In adults, the incisions can be up to 30 cm long. The lateral incision starts about 5 cm lateral to the anterior border of the tibia. The underlying fascia of the anterior and peroneal (lateral) compartments are identified and released. The intermuscular septum should be identified to ensure that both compartments are released. Care must be taken not to damage the common peroneal nerve proximally, as it passes around the fibular head; therefore, skin incisions should not reach to the fibular head level. Distally, it ends about 5 cm above the lateral malleolus. The medial incision of the two-incision technique starts 2 cm medial to the tibial margin. It is used to release both posterior compartments. Sometimes, the length of incision is shorter than the lateral—this depends on the degree of intracompartmental pressures. Care must be taken to avoid saphenous nerve and vein damage and these structures should be identified before fasciotomy of the compartments. The superficial posterior compartment is decompressed by incising the gastrocnemius fascia in a longitudinal direction from proximal to distal. The posterior compartment is decompressed by dividing the attachments of the soleus muscle to the tibia.

Fasciotomy of the Foot

Acute compartment syndrome of the foot most commonly occurs due to crush injury, and it is not very common that fasciotomy is needed. There are five compartments in the foot: intraosseous, lateral, central, medial, and calcaneal. Foot fasciotomy can be performed through either a dorsal, lateral, or medial approach. Each of the compartments should generally be released; some debate exists if the superficial compartment should be included. A dorsal approach is most commonly used and requires less dissection than the other two approaches. It starts with dual dorsal longitudinal incisions over the medial side of the second metatarsal bone and the lateral side of the fourth metatarsal bone. Each of the four intraosseous compartments is released first between metatarsal bones. The medial compartment may be released by accessing medial to the second metatarsal and lateral compartment by accessing lateral to the fourth metatarsal bone. The calcaneal compartment lies underneath the second interosseus space and can be released through medial incision. The superficial compartment is accessed through the calcaneal compartment by blunt dissection of the adductor hallucis muscle. Sometimes release of this compartment is not required, since it predominantly contains tendons of finger flexors and it is not a "true" muscular compartment.

Potential Complications

Delay of treatment of compartment syndrome can lead to irreversible complications and left untreated can lead to death. Complications may occur also as a sequel of surgical procedures performed and wound management. Late sequel of compartment syndrome includes persistent hypoesthesia, dysesthesia, persistent motor weakness, infection, myoglobinuric renal failure, contractures, amputation, and death. The initial management should be focused not only to preserve tissue viability in the compartment but also to initial management of systemic complications of reperfusion injury, which requires restoration of intravascular volume, prevention of hyperkalemia, and treatment of metabolic acidosis and myoglobinuria, which may lead to acute kidney injury.

Technical complications of fasciotomy are preventable by considering the anatomy of the important structures. Persistent or recurrent compartment syndrome can occur if fascial incisions are not adequate to permit complete decompression of the compartment or if selective fasciotomy has been performed [54].

Persistent neurologic deficits following fasciotomy are common. Nerve injury can occur due to an initial traumatic event or due to prolonged ischemia or as a consequence of fasciotomy dissection and tissue debridement. The most common neuropathic syndrome is altered sensation at the margins of the incision, and chronic pain syndromes are described [58]. Impaired neurologic function after lower extremity fasciotomy is described in 7–36% of injured limbs [59–61].

Wound complications after fasciotomy may occur immediately or be delayed for months to years. Early wound complications occur in up to 40% of patients following lower extremity fasciotomy [59, 62, 63]. Risk factors are related to the presence of vascular injury and lower extremity site and premature or delayed closure of the wound [63]. Wound infection occurs in 4–7% of extremity fasciotomies [59, 62]. Prophylactic antibiotics should be given at the time of fasciotomy and discontinued after 24 h. Repeated debridement of devitalized tissue may protect from severe wound infections and sepsis. Late wound complications are reported in 4–38% of limbs [58, 59, 62, 63]. Delayed wound complications are tethered scars and tendons, muscle hernias, and poor healing and ulceration especially in patients with underlying vascular diseases. Venous insufficiency can predispose patient to chronic venous disease after fasciotomy.

Acute extremity compartment syndrome is associated with significant risk for limb loss [64]. Major amputation will require 5–21% of limbs treated with fasciotomy [59, 60, 62, 63, 65]. Combined orthopedic and vascular injury, other severe injuries, and systemic factors may contribute to the need for amputation in severely injured patients. The highest amputation rate occurs in patients with severe vascular injuries with occlusion [59]. Amputation of the upper extremity following fasciotomy is rare.

The most severe cases of compartment syndrome left untreated may cause death. Reported mortality ranges from 11 to 25% and depends on epidemiology of compartment syndrome [54, 60, 62, 65]. Mortality is most often due to massive trauma, severe hypovolemic shock, and multisystem organ failure, and cannot be attributed only to the need for fasciotomy. Especially in severely injured patients with massive shock resuscitation, the mortality after fasciotomy in one study reached 67% [18].

Conclusion

The patient who undergoes fasciotomy requires a physical therapy program to regain function. Postoperative care and rehabilitation is just as important as the procedure itself. During the immediate postoperative period, weight bearing is limited, and assistive devices (e.g., crutches) are needed. Within a few days, and with adequate pain control, the use of crutches can be discontinued. The rehabilitation program then involves range of motion (ROM) and flexibility exercises involving the muscles of the affected compartment. Adjacent joints need to be exercised to maintain their normal ROM.

Once the patient is able to ambulate with a normalized gait pattern, a program of graduated resistive exercises (depending on the person's regular activities or work) is initiated. In the case of athletes, sports-specific exercises are started with the intention of returning to a regular athletic schedule. Cross training is also beneficial for these athletes. Activities such as swimming, pedal exercises, water jogging, or running help athletes to regain muscle strength and flexibility without loading the affected compartment.

With surgical intervention for decompression, occupational therapy consultation should be considered early in the postoperative period for assessment of appropriate treatment and of the patient's deficits with regard to activities of daily living (ADL), as well as for instruction in the use of any necessary assisted devices.

References

1. Volkmann R. Die ischaemischen muskellahmungen und kontrakturen. Zentralbl Chir. 1881;51:801–3.
2. Davies MS, Nadel S, Habibi P, et al. The orthopedic management of peripheral ischemia in meningococcal septicemia in children. J Bone Joint Surg Br. 2001;82:383–6.
3. Jyothi NK, Cox C. Compartment syndrome following postpartum hemorrhage. BJOG. 2000;107:430–2.
4. Loren GJ, Mohler LR, Pedowitz RA. Bilateral compartment syndrome of the leg complicating tetanus infection. Orthopedics. 2001;24:997–9.

5. Nicholson P, Devitt A, Stevens M, et al. Acute exertional peroneal compartmental syndrome following prolonged horse riding. Injury. 1998;29:643–4.

6. Johnson IA, Andrzejowski JC, Currie JS. Lower limb compartment syndrome resulting from malignant hyperthermia. Anaesth Intensive Care. 1999;27:292–4.

7. Cara JA, Narvaez A, Bertrand ML, et al. Acute traumatic compartment syndrome in the leg. Int Orthop. 1999;23:61–2.

8. Tremblay LN, Feliciano DV, Rozycki GS. Secondary extremity compartment syndrome. J Trauma. 2002;53:833–7.

9. Williams P, Shenilikar A, Roberts RC, et al. Acute non-traumatic compartment syndrome related to soft tissue injury. Injury. 1996;27:507–8.

10. Qvarfordt P, Christenson JT, Eklöf B, Ohlin P. Intramuscular pressure after revascularization of the popliteal artery in severe ischaemia. Br J Surg. 1983;70:539.

11. McQueen MM, Gaston P, Court-Brown CM. Acute compartment syndrome. Who is at risk? J Bone Joint Surg Br. 2000;82:200.

12. Elliott KG, Johnstone AJ. Diagnosing acute compartment syndrome. J Bone Joint Surg Br. 2003;85:625.

13. Köstler W, Strohm PC, Südkamp NP. Acute compartment syndrome of the limb. Injury. 2005;36:992.

14. Patel RV, Haddad FS. Compartment syndromes. Br J Hosp Med (Lond). 2005;66:583.

15. DeLee JC, Stiehl JB. Open tibia fracture with compartment syndrome. Clin Orthop Relat Res. 1981;160:175–84.

16. Matsen FA. Etiologies of compartmental Syndrome. In: Matsen FA, editor. Compartmental syndromes. New York: Grune & Stratton; 1980. p. 69–71.

17. Ulmer T. The clinical diagnosis of compartment syndrome of the lower leg: are clinical findings predictive of disorder? J Orthop Trauma. 2002;16:572–7.

18. Kosir R, Morre FA, Selby LH. Acute lower extremity compartment syndrome (ALECS) screening protocol in critically ill trauma patients. J Trauma. 2007;63:268–75.

19. Matsen FA. Diagnosis of compartmental syndrome. In: Matsen FA, editor. Compartmental syndromes. New York: Grune & Stratton; 1980. p. 85–100.

20. Fuller DA, Barrett M, Marburger RK, Hirsch R. Carpal canal pressures after volar plating of distal radius fractures. J Hand Surg Br. 2006;31:236.

21. Shadgan B, Menon M, O'Brien PJ, Reid WD. Diagnostic techniques in acute compartment syndrome of the leg. J Orthop Trauma. 2008;22:581.

22. Myers RA. Hyperbaric oxygen therapy for trauma: crush injury, compartment syndrome, and other acute traumatic peripheral ischemias. Int Anesthesiol Clin. 2000;38:139.

23. Olson SA, Glasgow RR. Acute compartment syndrome in lower extremity musculoskeletal trauma. J Am Acad Orthop Surg. 2005;13:436.

24. Mubarak SJ, Owen CA. Double-incision fasciotomy of the leg for decompression in compartment syndromes. J Bone Joint Surg Am. 1977;59:184.

25. Newton EJ, Love J. Acute complications of extremity trauma. Emerg Med Clin North Am. 2007;25:751.

26. Matsen III FA, Krugmire Jr RB. Compartmental syndromes. Surg Gynecol Obstet. 1978;147:943.

27. Zweifach SS, Hargens AR, Evans KL, et al. Skeletal muscle necrosis in pressurized compartments associated with hemorrhagic hypotension. J Trauma. 1980;20:941.

28. Matsen FA. Pathophysiology of increased tissue pressure. In: Matsen FA, editor. Compartmental syndromes. New York: Grune & Stratton; 1980. p. 36.

29. Szabo RM, Gelberman RH, Williamson RV, Hargens AR. Effects of increased systemic blood pressure on the tissue fluid pressure threshold of peripheral nerve. J Orthop Res. 1983;1:172.

30. Zweifach SS, Hargens AR, Evans KL, et al. Skeletal muscle necrosis in pressurized compartments associated with hemorrhagic hypotension. J Trauma. 1980;20:941.

31. McQueen MM, Court-Brown CM. Compartment monitoring in tibial fractures. The pressure threshold for decompression. J Bone Joint Surg Br. 1996;78:99–104.

32. Owings JT, Kennedy JP, Blaisdell FW. Injuries to the extremities. In: Wilmore DW, Cheung LY, Harken AH, Holcroft JW, Meakins JL, Soper NJ, editors. ACS surgery: principles and practice. New York: WebMD Corporation; 2002. p. 474–6.

33. Gentilello LM, Sanzone A, Wang L, et al. Near infrared spectroscopy versus compartment pressure for the diagnosis of lower extremity compartmental syndrome using electromyography determined measurements of neuromuscular function. J Trauma. 2001;51:1–8.

34. White TO, Howell GED, Will EM, Court-Brown CM, McQueen MM. Elevated intramuscular compartment pressures do not influence outcome after tibial fracture. J Trauma. 2003;55:1133–8.

35. Whitesides TE, Haney TC, Morimoto K, Harada H. Tissue pressure measurements as a determinant for the need of fasciotomy. Clin Orthop Relat Res. 1975;113:43–51.

36. Mubarak SJ, Owen CA, Hargens AR, et al. Acute compartment syndromes: diagnosis and treatment with the aid of the wick catheter. J Bone Joint Surg Am. 1978;60:1091.

37. Rorabeck CH, Castle GS, Hardie R, Logan J. Compartmental pressure measurements: an experimental investigation using the slit catheter. J Trauma. 1981;21:446.

38. Willy C, Gerngross H, Sterk J. Measurement of intracompartmental pressure with use of a new electronic transducer-tipped catheter system. J Bone Joint Surg Am. 1999;81:158.

39. Uliasz A, Ishida JT, Fleming JK, Yamamoto LG. Comparing the methods of measuring compartment pressures in acute compartment syndrome. Am J Emerg Med. 2003;21:143.

40. Heppenstall RB, Sapega AA, Izant T, et al. Compartment syndrome: a quantitative study of high-energy phosphorus compounds using 31P magnetic resonance spectroscopy. J Trauma. 1989;29:1113–9.

41. Arbabi S, Brundage SI, Gentilello LM. Near-infrared spectroscopy: a potential method for continuous, transcutaneous monitoring for compartmental syndrome in critically injured patients. J Trauma. 1999;47:829–33.

42. Giannotti G, Cohn SM, Brown M, Varela JE, McKenney MG, Wiseberg JA. Utility of near-infrared spectroscopy in the diagnosis of lower extremity compartment syndrome. J Trauma. 2000;48:396–401.

43. Matsen FA. Treatment of compartmental syndromes. In: Matsen FA, editor. Compartmental syndromes. New York: Grune & Stratton; 1980. p. 101–15.

44. Styf J, Wiger P. Abnormally increased intramuscular pressure in human legs: comparison of two experimental models. J Trauma. 1998;45:133.

45. Hakaim AG, Cunningham L, White JL, Hoover K. Selective type III phosphodiesterase inhibition prevents elevated compartment pressure after ischemia/reperfusion injury. J Trauma. 1999;46:869–72.

46. Guerrero A, Gibson K, Kralovich KA, et al. Limb loss following lower extremity arterial trauma: what can be done proactively. Injury. 2002;33:765–9.

47. Zannis J, Angobaldo J, Marks M, et al. Comparison of fasciotomy wound closures using traditional dressing changes and the vacuum-assisted closure device. Ann Plast Surg. 2009;62:407.

48. Yang CC, Chang DS, Webb LX. Vacuum-assisted closure for fasciotomy wounds following compartment syndrome of the leg. J Surg Orthop Adv. 2006;15:19.

49. Wattel F, Mathieu D, Nevière R, Bocquillon N. Acute peripheral ischaemia and compartment syndromes: a role for hyperbaric oxygenation. Anaesthesia. 1998;53 Suppl 2:63.

50. Strauss MB, Hargens AR, Gershuni DH, et al. Delayed use of hyperbaric oxygen for treatment of a model anterior compartment syndrome. J Orthop Res. 1986;4:108.
51. Tibbles PM, Edelsberg JS. Hyperbaric-oxygen therapy. N Engl J Med. 1996;334:1642.
52. Weiland DE. Fasciotomy closure using simultaneous vacuum-assisted closure and hyperbaric oxygen. Am Surg. 2007;73:261.
53. Abdullah MS, Al-Waili NS, Butler G, Baban NK. Hyperbaric oxygen as an adjunctive therapy for bilateral compartment syndrome, rhabdomyolysis and acute renal failure after heroin intake. Arch Med Res. 2006;37:559.
54. Jensen SL, Sandermann J. Compartment syndrome and fasciotomy in vascular surgery. A review of 57 cases. Eur J Vasc Endovasc Surg. 1997;13:48.
55. Sheridan GW, Matsen III FA. Fasciotomy in the treatment of the acute compartment syndrome. J Bone Joint Surg Am. 1976;58:112.
56. Cohen MS, Garfin SR, Hargens AR, et al. Acute compartment syndrome. Effect of dermotomy on fascial decompression in the leg. J Bone Joint Surg Br. 1991;73:287.
57. Cooper GG. A method of single-incision, four compartment fasciotomy of the leg. Eur J Vasc Surg. 1992;6:659.
58. Fitzgerald AM, Gaston P, Wilson Y, et al. Long-term sequelae of fasciotomy wounds. Br J Plast Surg. 2000;53:690.
59. Rush DS, Frame SB, Bell RM, et al. Does open fasciotomy contribute to morbidity and mortality after acute lower extremity ischemia and revascularization. J Vasc Surg. 1989;10:343–50.
60. Heemskerk J, Kitslaar P. Acute compartment syndrome of the lower leg: retrospective study on prevalence, technique, and outcome of fasciotomies. World J Surg. 2003;27:744.
61. Lagerstrom CF, Reed II RL, Rowlands BJ, Fischer RP. Early fasciotomy for acute clinically evident posttraumatic compartment syndrome. Am J Surg. 1989;158:36.
62. Johnson SB, Weaver FA, Yellin AE, et al. Clinical results of decompressive dermotomy-fasciotomy. Am J Surg. 1992;164:286.
63. Velmahos GC, Theodorou D, Demetriades D, et al. Complications and nonclosure rates of fasciotomy for trauma and related risk factors. World J Surg. 1997;21:247.
64. Ojike NI, Roberts CS, Giannoudis PV. Compartment syndrome of the thigh: a systematic review. Injury. 2010;41:133.
65. Ritenour AE, Dorlac WC, Fang R, et al. Complications after fasciotomy revision and delayed compartment release in combat patients. J Trauma. 2008;64:S153.

Part III

Ethics, Legal, and Administrative Considerations

Bridget N. Fahy

Introduction

Palliative care is based upon the Latin word *palliare*, to cloak. Based upon this Latin root, it follows that palliative care is care focused on providing cover or protection to patients. In its purest sense, palliative care is intended to shield or protect patients from suffering.

According to the current World Health Organization (WHO) [1], palliative care is "an approach that improves the quality of life of patients and their families facing the problem associated with life-threatening illness, through the prevention and relief of suffering by means of early identification and impeccable assessment and treatment of pain and other problems, physical, psychosocial, and spiritual." Furthermore, the following are considered essential elements of palliative care services:

- Provides relief from pain and other distressing symptoms.
- Will enhance quality of life and may also positively influence the course of illness.
- Is applicable early in the course of illness, in conjunction with other therapies that are intended to prolong life.
- Includes those investigations needed to better understand and manage distressing clinical complications.
- Integrates the psychological and spiritual aspects of patient care.
- Offers a support system to help patients live as actively as possible until death.
- Affirms life and regards dying as a normal process.
- Intends neither to hasten nor to postpone death.
- Offers a support system to help the family cope during the patient's illness and in their own bereavement.
- Uses a team approach to address the needs of patients and their families, including bereavement counseling, if indicated.

B.N. Fahy, M.D., F.A.C.S. (✉)
Department of Surgery, The Methodist Hospital, Weill Cornell Medical College, 6550 Fannin Street, SM 1661, Houston, TX 77030, USA
e-mail: bnfahy@tmhs.org

Based upon this definition and the associated key elements, palliative care is ideally suited to the care of the acute care surgical patient given its focus on pain and other distressing symptoms, its holistic approach to the patient and their family, the emphasis on a team approach to both the patient and his/her family, and its applicability in conjunction with other therapies intended to prolong life. Notably absent from the World Health Organization definition provided above is a proscription about who can provide palliative care or what specific interventions or treatments may considered palliative. The definition leaves open a role for *all* healthcare providers to utilize any and all tools available that will meet the needs of their patients and families as they face serious, life-threatening, and/or debilitating illness.

An important corollary to the essential components of palliative care is an understanding of what palliative care is not. Perhaps most importantly, palliative care is not synonymous with hospice care. Hospice is a program of services designed to provide care to patients and families in which a patient's life expectancy is 6 months or less. In contrast, palliative care is appropriate for patients with potentially curable diseases or conditions for which a complete recovery may be expected. Given this distinction, palliative care is sometimes referred to as supportive care in order to avoid confusion with patients considered to have terminal conditions. According to the "modern" conception of palliative care, palliative care can be provided in conjunction with curative treatment and at any point during a disease: from diagnosis through end-of-life care (Fig. 39.1).

Surgeon's Role in Palliative Care

Prior to the start of the hospice movement in the 1960s with the pioneering work of Dame Cicely Saunders, surgeons have long played a central role in the care of the seriously ill. This is no better illustrated than the work of surgeons who provided burn care during World War II. Burn care begins with pain control and progresses through the acute phase of

L.J. Moore et al. (eds.), *Common Problems in Acute Care Surgery*,
DOI 10.1007/978-1-4614-6123-4_39, © Springer Science+Business Media New York 2013

Fig. 39.1 Palliative care model. Adapted from United States Department of Health and Human Services

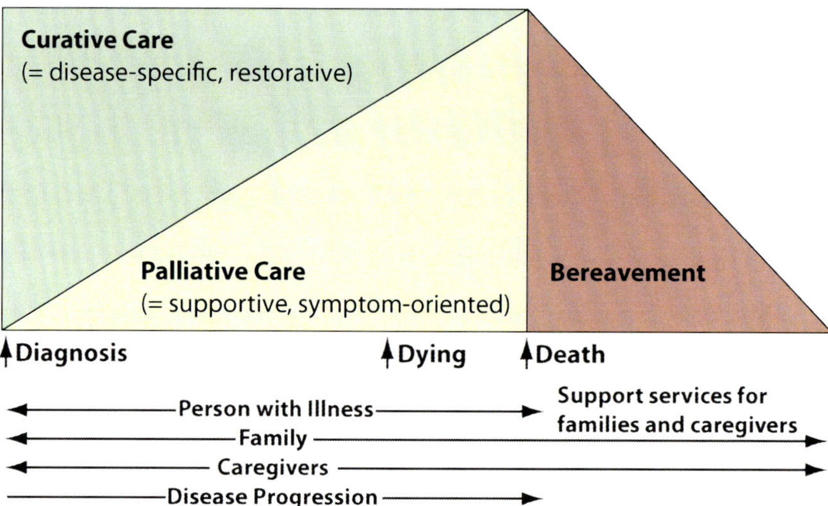

wound healing into an ongoing process of interdisciplinary care designed to restore function and quality of life. Furthermore, many operations currently or previously used to effect a surgical "cure" were originally introduced to alleviate symptoms. Perhaps the best example of such a procedure is the radical mastectomy, first used in 1881 by William S. Halstead to treat pain from locally advanced and ulcerated breast cancers and later accepted as standard curative treatment for breast cancer.

The circumstances which have led surgeons to play a central role in palliative care were aptly described by Dunn and Milch [2] as follows: "The widening spectrum of disease and life expectancy encountered in palliative care led to the inevitable arrival of the concept at the doorstep of many specialties, including surgery. With their significant presence in the setting of advanced and incurable illness, surgeons could not indefinitely avoid the social, psychological, and spiritual challenges encountered there."

The routine incorporation of palliative care into the daily practice of acute care surgery falls under von Gunten's definition of primary palliative care [3]. Primary palliative care refers to the basic skills and competencies required of all healthcare providers to relieve pain and other distressing symptoms. The application of basic palliative care principles to surgery is a fundamental component of good surgical clinical care. Surgeons can and should be expected to relieve suffering and maintain quality of life for all of their patients, not just those at the end of their life. Consequently, surgeons must be able to provide palliative treatment in conjunction with curative treatment and furthermore, must possess the skills to transition from curative to purely palliative as dictated by both the patient's disease as well as their goals.

Unlike few other medical specialties, surgeons are frequently at the forefront of providing pain and symptom control for their patients. Furthermore, surgeons from all specialties are routinely called upon to provide palliation.

The central role of surgeons as "palliativists" is perhaps illustrated best through the work of the acute care surgeon charged with "manning" the front lines against acute surgical disease. In this way, palliative surgery, and by extension palliative surgeons, are not restricted by surgical subspecialty or procedure but by the intent of the surgical intervention offered—that is, to relieve pain or other distressing symptoms.

Despite the introduction of the term "palliative care" by Balfour Mount, a Canadian urologist, in 1975, it was not until 1998 that the Board of Regents of the American College of Surgeons approved the "Principles Guiding Care at the End of Life [4] and identified key palliative care concepts for surgeons." Of the ten principles outlined, those most germane to the current discussion include the following:

- Be sensitive to and respectful of the patient's and family's wishes.
- Ensure alleviation of pain and management of other physical symptoms.
- Recognize, assess, and address psychological, social, and spiritual problems.
- Provide access to therapies that may realistically be expected to improve the patient's quality of life.
- Provide access to appropriate palliative care and hospice care.
- Recognize the physician's responsibility to forego treatments that are futile.

Notable among these principles is the focus on provision of care consistent with patient and family wishes, interventions designed to improve quality of life, and an appreciation of all symptoms—physical, emotional, psychosocial.

In 2003, the American College of Surgeons published the core competencies for surgical palliative care [5]. Structured according to the Accreditation Council for Graduate Medical Education six core competencies, the Surgeons Palliative Care Workgroup of the American College of Surgeons established core competencies in two basic elements of palliative care—pain management and communication skills—to be essential for all surgeons. Additionally, for surgeons who care for dying patients more frequently, additional skills in end-of-life care were felt to be important. While a complete review of the surgical palliative care core competencies is beyond the scope of this chapter, the competencies, as delineated by the Workgroup are fundamental to the complete care of the surgical patient, regardless of diagnosis or specialty of the surgeon providing care.

Application of Palliative Care to the Acute Care Surgery Patient

Recognizing the Acute Care Surgical Patient in Need of Palliative Care

Given that palliative care is appropriate for any patient facing a serious or life-threatening illness, many patients presenting with acute surgical illness will benefit from palliative care. Furthermore, virtually all patients with acute surgical disease are symptomatic. Symptoms commonly seen in the acute care surgical patient include: right upper quadrant pain from acute cholecystitis, right lower quadrant abdominal pain from appendicitis, left lower quadrant pain from diverticulitis, nausea and vomiting due to a small bowel obstruction, anorectal pain caused by a perirectal abscess. While many of these diseases will not be life-threatening or produce long-term debility, a significant percentage of patients with these common acute surgical problems are at risk for disease and/or treatment-related morbidity and mortality which may result in long-lasting symptoms or debility. A recent study by Moore et al. [6] found that emergency colon operations were associated with a 28% mortality rate even in the hands of experienced acute care surgeons. Ingraham et al. [7] examined the morbidity and mortality associated with emergency appendectomy, cholecystectomy, or colon resection in the National Surgical Quality Improvement Program database and reported a 15% complication rate across these three procedures. The morbidity rate was highest for colorectal resection (47%), followed by cholecystectomy (9%) and appendectomy (6%).

The first challenge facing the acute care surgeon is the identification of a patient who will benefit from a palliative procedure. In other words, "what are the characteristics of a prospective palliative care patient?" An acute care surgical patient appropriate for palliative care will typically meet the following criteria:

1. Serious or life-threatening condition.
2. Disease potentially responsive to surgical intervention.
3. Patient's premorbid health conditions do not preclude surgical intervention.

Taken together, these criteria reflect the basic tenets of surgical decision-making. As Winchester noted [8], "It is judgment that matters in this profession. Otherwise the surgeon is no more than a man (or woman) with a knife, and a license to mutilate."

While it may be argued that any surgical disease, no matter how limited or seemingly uncomplicated, may become serious or life-threatening under certain circumstances (e.g., incarcerated ventral hernia in a patient 3 months following an acute myocardial infarction). The more obvious cases involve either patients with common surgical problems in the setting of advanced underlying disease such as cancer or end stage organ dysfunction or advanced surgical disease in an otherwise healthy patient. In the case of the former, it is imperative that the acute care surgeon consider the status of the underlying disease and its associated prognosis before considering the disease-related complications or procedure-specific risks. To illustrate this point, consider the following case of Ms. O.

Ms. O is a 57-year-old woman with Stage IIIC ovarian cancer whose disease has progressed on second-line chemotherapy. She presents to the emergency department with severe anorectal pain. On physical examination, you determine that she has a perirectal abscess.

A surgical palliative care approach to Ms. O will include the following steps:

1. Global assessment of Ms. O's health, including a discussion with her oncologist regarding the status of her cancer, additional treatment options, and previous conversations regarding her prognosis.
2. Discussion with Ms. O regarding the anticipated outcomes following the proposed surgical procedure. The specific outcomes to be discussed include the likelihood that the proposed procedure will alleviate her symptom (anorectal pain), perioperative risks of the procedure considering her premorbid and treatment-related risk factors (i.e., neutropenia, thrombocytopenia, etc.), and impact of the procedure on future treatment options (i.e., potential delay in additional cancer treatment).
3. Articulation of alternate nonoperative treatment options and how this may interfere or promote her goals of treatment.

Prognostication for the Acute Care Surgical Patient

A second criterion of an acute care surgical patient appropriate for a palliative surgical approach is the presence of disease potentially responsive to surgical therapy. This criterion highlights the importance of accurate prognostication in the acute care surgical patient. Although prognostication has traditionally been listed as the third of the three great clinical skills-behind diagnosis and treatment, it may be considered second behind diagnosis when caring for the acute care surgical patient in need of palliative care. Prognosis is generally used to describe the prediction of any health outcome. When performed accurately, prognostication allows patients and their families to participate in their healthcare decision-making in a way that ensures their autonomy through a process of informed consent.

Although issues related to informed consent are addressed elsewhere in this book, it is instructive to briefly consider the informed consent process here since informed consent is a direct extension of accurate prognostication. As Robert Veatch [9] notes in his remarks regarding informed consent: "Telling the patient everything about a procedure is an impossible task. All that is being called for is adequate information." The standards used to determine adequate information include the professional standard, the reasonable person standard, and the subjective standard. According to the subjective standard, the surgeon gives the patient the information he or she would personally find meaningful. The information shared should fit with the life plan and interests of the individual patient. In the setting of palliative acute care surgery, it is the subjective standard that seems most relevant when considering prognostication and informed consent given the emphasis placed on providing treatments that may realistically be expected to improve the patient's quality of life and reflect sensitivity to, and respect for, the patient's and family's wishes.

Unlike prognostication in other medical specialties, surgical palliative care is unique in that surgeons are called upon to incorporate knowledge of the surgical disease, any relevant underlying diseases (e.g., end stage organ dysfunction), as well as the anticipated surgical outcome, when providing prognostic information to a patient and their family. Various factors have been used to formulate estimates of prognosis: clinician estimate of survival, performance status scales (e.g., Karnofsky performance status), biological parameters (e.g., preoperative albumin levels, Acute Physiology and Chronic Health Evaluation II score). The Palliative Prognostic (PaP) Score [10] was created by a group of Italian investigators who combined laboratory values, symptoms, clinician estimates, and performance status into a survival prognostication tool that can be readily calculable at the bedside. In their study of 451 terminally ill cancer patients, the PaP score was able to subdivide patients into three distinct risk groups with median survival of 14, 32, and 76 days in three groups.

The Palliative Performance Scale (PPS) is another validated prognostic tool used to estimate the survival of patients with life-threatening illness [11, 12]. The PPS provides a functional assessment of ambulation, activity level, evidence of disease, self-care, oral intake, and level of consciousness. The scale consists of 11 categories yielding a score from 0% (death) to 100% (ambulatory and healthy). A PPS score of 50% is associated with a patient who is non-ambulatory (mainly sits or lies), requires a significant amount of assistance, and has normal to reduced oral intake. At a score of 50%, extensive disease is evident, and the estimated life expectancy ranges from 2 to 4 weeks. The PPS was recently used to assess survival in an inpatient population at a university teaching [13]. A total of 310 adult inpatients with advanced cancer (60%) and other advanced (life-limiting) diseases were included in the study cohort. Three distinct survival groups were identified based upon PPS: 10–20, 30–40, and ≥50. The median survival for patients with PPS 10–20 was approximately 10 days, while that for 30–40 was approximately 40 days, and for patients with PPS of ≥50 it was not reached by 150 days. A 10% decrement in PPS was associated with a 1.65-fold increased risk of death [13].

Formulating a prognosis in other serious diseases such as congestive heart failure, chronic obstructive pulmonary disease, and various forms of dementia can be more difficult than it is in the case of malignancy due to the difference in disease trajectories. Despite these challenges, guidelines do exist to assist in determining the prognosis of patients with non-cancer diagnoses [14]. A thorough review of the guidelines for each disease is beyond the scope of this chapter, but they are nicely summarized in a review article by Lynn [15].

Communication with the Acute Care Surgical Patient

The other group of acute care surgical patients who may benefit from a surgical palliative care approach is those with advanced surgical disease but are otherwise without significant comorbidities or serious underlying disease. The case of Mr. A illustrates the vital role of communication in the setting of acute surgical disease.

Mr. A is a healthy 73-year-old man recently diagnosed with atrial fibrillation during an annual physical examination. He was started on digoxin and is heart rate is well controlled. He presents to the emergency department with acute onset of abdominal pain which woke him from sleep. His workup in the emergency department shows that he is in atrial fibrillation with a heart rate of 125 and a blood pressure of 102/58. When you examine his abdomen, you do not hear any bowel sounds, he is soft, non-tender, and non-distended. He complains of severe abdominal pain out of proportion to his physical examination. You diagnose him with mesenteric ischemia and take him to the operating room for urgent exploration. At laparotomy, his entire small bowel is ischemic but not necrotic and he has an embolus in his superior mesenteric artery for which you perform an embolectomy. You transfer him to the surgical intensive care unit intubated with a temporary abdominal closure and plan to examine his bowel again in 24 h.

A surgical palliative care approach to Mr. A will include the following steps:

1. Discussion of the intraoperative findings with Mr. A's family, including the possible outcomes from re-exploration: complete necrosis of his small intestine representing a non-survivable injury, large amount of nonviable bowel requiring a massive small bowel resection and short-gut, or little to no bowel ischemia with the prospect of full recovery.
2. Determine if Mr. A has completed an advance directive and/or a medical power of attorney to assist with medical decision-making.
3. Make referrals to a hospital social worker and/or chaplain as needed to provide support to Mr. A's family.
4. Arrange for a family meeting to follow Mr. A's re-exploration to update his family and begin planning for his next phase of care.

The case of Mr. A emphasizes the importance of prompt, clear, and direct communication. As noted above, the American College of Surgeons has identified communication one of the two basic elements of palliative care in which all surgeons must be competent. Essential components of communication in the acute care surgery setting include willingness on the part of the surgeon to disclose prognosis truthfully, an appreciation that communication with patients and/or their families is a process and not a singular event, and the skills to effectively communicate with all members of the care team. Despite the well-intentioned efforts of some surgeons to avoid giving bad news out of fear of robbing hope, there is little evidence to support this position. In his book entitled *The Dying Patient*, Simpson asserts that "Hope is based on knowledge, not ignorance" [16]. It is more likely that misguided avoidance of difficult information, or worse, blatant dishonesty about prognosis, may add to a patient or family's distress, cause them to seek treatment which they might not otherwise pursue, and rob them of precious time better spent engaged in activities that promote peace and dignity. A recent study by Wilkinson et al. [17] studied patient preferences for information and for participation in decision-making among 152 consecutive acute medical inpatients. They found that 61% of patients favored a passive approach to decision-making (physician makes the final decision). In contrast, 66% of patients sought "very extensive" or "a lot" of information about their condition. Importantly, there was no relationship between patient preferences for involvement in decision-making and for information about their medical condition. A study by Mazur and Hickam [18] of 467 veterans studied the level of involvement the patients wanted in decision-making related to invasive medical interventions. The vast majority of patients (93%) preferred that their physician disclose risk information to them and two-thirds of patients preferred shared decision-making compared to only 21% who preferred physician-based decision-making.

Taken together, these studies confirm that patients want to participate in their healthcare decisions and desire the necessary information needed to make these decisions.

Family meetings are a crucial tool for effective communication in palliative care. Optimal palliative decision-making is facilitated through effective interactions among the patient, family members, and the surgeon through a dynamic relationship described as the "palliative triangle" [19]. The "palliative triangle" is a model designed to aid in complex surgical decision-making when palliative surgical procedures are being considered. The three arms of the triangle include the patient, family and surgeon and the goals that each member of the triangle brings when palliative surgical procedures are considered. The patient's concerns, values, and emotional support are considered against existing medical and surgical alternatives. The process of aligning the concerns and interests of the three parties involved can moderate against the unrealistic expectations that each party may bring to the decision-making process. A study by Miner et al. [20] utilized the "palliative triangle" technique in 227 patients with incurable metastatic or advanced cancer considered for a palliative procedure. A palliative procedure was performed in 47% of patients, while 53% were not selected for a palliative operation. The indications for the palliative procedures included gastrointestinal obstruction in 36%, local control of tumor-related symptoms (e.g., bleeding, pain, or malodor, 25.5%), jaundice in 10%, and other symptoms in 28%. Patient-reported symptom improvement or resolution was noted following 91% of procedures. Patients who experienced symptom relief did so within 30 days of the operation. It is noteworthy that prior to the palliative procedures being performed, one or two meetings between the patient, family, and surgeons occurred before a final treatment decision was reached [20]. While there may be cases in which time for such meetings are not possible, this opportunity does exist for a significant proportion of acute care surgical patients. In the end, the highly satisfactory results published by Miner et al. [20] reflect the essential combination of appropriate patient selection, excellent surgical technique, and effective communication among the arms of the "palliative triangle." As Buckman noted, "Communication is often the most important component of palliative care, and effective symptom control is virtually impossible without effective communication" [21].

Outcomes of Palliative Procedures

Definition of Palliative Procedure

Once the surgeon has identified the acute care surgical patient in need of palliative care, the next steps, as noted above, are prognostication and communication of anticipated outcomes to patients and their families. Even after the surgeon has gathered the necessary information to discuss prognosis for a given disease process and has communicated this information effectively, she/he is faced with a formidable challenge, namely, the actual provision of a palliative procedure.

Agreement about what constitutes a palliative procedure has been the matter of debate in the existing surgical literature. First and foremost, palliative surgery care begins with a symptomatic patient. To paraphrase Blake Cady: It is impossible to palliate the asymptomatic patient [22]. The precise definition of palliative surgery is less clear, as illustrated by a study by McCahill et al. [23]. In this study, 419 members of the Society of Surgical Oncology were surveyed and asked to select the single best way they classified a procedure as palliative. They found that 41% of surgeons defined a procedure as palliative based upon the preoperative intent of the procedure, 27% defined the procedure based upon the postoperative evaluation. Surgeons in this group waited for the results of the operation to determine whether it was palliative or curative. One-third of surgeons based their definition of a palliative procedure based upon the patient's prognosis [23]. If a palliative operation is defined by its outcome and not by its intention, the possibility to effectively inform and prognosticate is severely hampered. In their article on the ethics of palliative surgery in patients with advanced cancer, Hofmann et al. [24] define palliative surgery in this select group of patients as "any invasive procedure in which the main intention is to mitigate physical symptoms in patients with non-curable disease without causing premature death." Regardless of the underlying disease process, most surgeons agree that the goals of a palliative operation include symptom relief, pain relief, and maintaining patient independence and function [23]. The logical extension of any definition of palliative operation that focuses on relief of symptoms and/ or improvement in quality of life is that no specific surgical intervention is automatically included or excluded as potentially palliative.

Morbidity and Mortality of Palliative Procedures

Regardless of the specific procedure performed or underlying disease process, the literature is clear regarding the high morbidity and mortality rates associated with palliative procedures. Mesa and Tefferi [25] reported a 30.5% morbidity and 9% operative mortality rate following splenectomy for symptom palliation from myelofibrosis with myeloid metaplasia. McCahill et al. [26] reported a 41% complication rate among their palliative-intent procedure in patients with advanced malignancy. Similar to the findings of the City of Hope group, the Memorial Sloan-Kettering Cancer Center group [27] reported that 40% of patients developed some postoperative complication and 11% of patients died within

30 days following their palliative procedure. Badgwell et al. [28] and the group from the M. D. Anderson Cancer Center reviewed the records of 442 patients with advanced or incurable cancer for whom a surgical oncology consultation for palliation was requested. A total of 119 (27%) of patients underwent a palliative surgical procedure. Sixty-seven complications occurred in 48 patients for an overall morbidity rate of 40%. The most common complications were respiratory distress or failure in 12%, wound infection/non-healing wounds in 11%, with approximately 5% of patients suffering from postoperative bowel obstructions, ileus, or bacteremia/ line sepsis. The overall mortality rate was 7%. The median survival for all patients, nonoperative patients, and patients who underwent a palliative procedure was 2.9, 2.1, and 6.9 months, respectively [28]. Compared to these older studies, there appears to be some improvement in the postoperative morbidity and mortality following palliative procedures as recently reported by Miner et al. [20]. In their study of 129 patients who underwent a palliative procedure for incurable malignancy, 20% sustained a postoperative complication and the 30-day postoperative mortality rate was 4%.

Palliative Outcomes Following Palliative Procedures

In addition to counseling patients and their families about the high morbidity and mortality associated with palliative procedures, surgeons are challenged with providing information about the anticipated success of the proposed procedure in alleviating the patient's symptom(s). The paucity of literature regarding palliative outcomes following palliative procedures was first described by Miner et al. [29]. The authors reviewed 348 studies published between 1990 and 1996 that studied outcomes following surgical procedures for cancer palliation. They found that the majority of these studies were retrospective in nature with the balance of the reports divided between review articles, prospective studies and case reports. More than two-thirds of the studies reviewed reported physiologic response, survival, and morbidity and mortality data while only 17% of the studied reported any quality of life outcomes and only 26% reported the effect of the procedure on pain control. Furthermore, less than half of the studies that considered quality of life outcomes used a validated instrument [29].

Since this study by Miner et al. [29] was published, a handful of studies have specifically examined the outcomes of palliative procedures and the majority of these studies have focused on oncology patients. Among the earliest studies to prospectively examine the outcome following palliative surgical procedures was published by McCahill and the group from the City of Hope Cancer Center in 2003 [26]. They studied 59 patients who underwent major operations for advanced malignancy; 22 operations were performed for palliation and 37 were performed with curative intent. A total of 33 patients (20 in palliative group, 13 in the curative group) were symptomatic from their tumors preoperatively. Symptom resolution was seen in 26/33 patients (79%). A large study was published in 2004 by the group at the Memorial Sloan-Kettering Cancer Center [27] in which they examined the outcomes following over 1,000 palliative procedures performed in 823 patients with advanced cancer. The indications for the procedure were gastrointestinal obstruction in 34%, neurologic symptoms in 23%, pain in 12%, and dyspnea in 9%. Eighty percent of patients experienced an improvement in their symptoms and almost half remained symptom free for a median of 135 days. Most recently, Miner et al. [20] studied the outcomes following 129 palliative procedures and found that patient-reported symptom improvement or resolution occurred following 91% of procedures. Those patients who experienced symptoms relief did so within 30 days of the operation.

On balance, the surgical literature is severely limited regarding palliative outcomes (e.g., symptom resolution) following palliative procedures. As noted by Smith and McCahill [30], "… there are educational and research opportunities among surgeons in better defining factors associated with successful surgical palliation." Although they were referring specifically to surgical palliation of advanced malignancies, their statement is equally applicable to the acute care surgical patient without malignancy.

Patient Selection for Palliative Procedures

Given the high morbidity and mortality rates associated with palliative procedures-regardless of procedure or underlying disease process-it seems that patient selection may be the single more important factor in successful surgical palliation [19]. As Smith and McCahill [30] recently noted, "The decision to pursue a major surgical intervention becomes more controversial when it is likely to be noncurative and instead has symptom relief as its major objective." The accuracy of surgeons' preoperative predictions following major surgery for advanced malignancy was recently studied by Smith and McCahill [30]. The authors correlated surgeons' preoperative estimation of each patient's life expectancy and likelihood of symptom palliation following surgery with patient self-reports of symptom palliation following surgery. They found that surgeons' preoperative estimates of patient survival agreed with survival outcomes. However, surgeons' preoperative estimates of the success of symptom improvement following surgery did not correlate in general with patients' self-assessments; surgeons underestimated their success in symptom resolution. This tendency to underestimate the success of symptom resolution may result in patients

with advanced malignancies not receiving palliative procedures.

If surgeons' predictions of symptom relief following palliative procedures cannot accurately identify those patients most likely to benefit, what other criteria are available? McCahill et al. [26] attempted to quantitate the effectiveness of palliative surgery in symptomatic patients with advanced malignancies through a Palliative Surgery Outcome Score (PSOS). The PSOS incorporates elements of treatment success (e.g., symptom relief) and treatment failure (e.g., symptom recurrence and surgical complications) and their associated hospital days. The PSOS indicates the percentage of postoperative days for which a patient was not hospitalized, free of the symptom that the operation was intended to treat, and free of major surgical complication in the 6 months after surgery. A PSOS of 70 was defined as good-excellent surgical palliation as it represented a patient who lived at least 70% of the study period outside of the hospital, free of the symptom addressed by the procedure and without major surgical morbidity. This result was achieved in 64% of patients. Given that only 36% of patients who lived <6 months achieved a PSOS of 70, the authors emphasized the significant impact of limited longevity on successful surgical palliation and stressed the importance of identifying clinical factors known to correlate with survival. In their study, preoperative serum albumin and weight loss were important predictors of survival. Similarly, the group from the Memorial Sloan-Kettering Cancer Center [27] found that poor palliative outcomes were associated with patients who had poor performance status, poor nutrition, weight loss, and no previous cancer therapy. Furthermore, a major postoperative complication reduced the probability of symptom improvement to 17%. A recent examination of the National Surgical Quality Improvement Program database for outcomes following operations for disseminated cancer identified the following independent risk factors for postoperative morbidity and mortality: increasing age, impaired functional status, weight loss >10%, dyspnea, ascites, chronic steroid use, active sepsis, elevated creatinine, hypoalbuminemia, decreased serum hematocrit, acuity of the surgical procedure, impaired respiratory function, and abnormal white blood cell count [31].

Future Directions for Palliative Care in the Acute Care Surgical Patient

Expanding the Role of Surgeons as Primary Providers of Palliative Care

Although palliative surgical care has been most consistently applied to the field of oncology, it is increasingly being applied to patients with disease processes other than oncology.

Furthermore, while physicians from nonsurgical specialties have traditionally dominated the ranks of palliative care providers, this too, is changing. Surgeons can point to Balfour Mount, Geoff Dunn, Karen Brasel, Anne Mosenthal, and others as early pioneers in palliative surgical care. Furthermore, beginning in 2008, the American Board of Surgery (along with nine other medical specialty boards) began offering a subspecialty certificate in Hospice and Palliative Medicine. As of December 2011, the American Board of Surgery has certified 26 diplomates in Hospice and Palliative Medicine. This number is expected to continue to rise as several surgeons prepare to enter the board certification process in Hospice and Palliative Medicine through the Experiential and Practice Pathways. Current surgical leaders in palliative care can be found in every surgical specialty, including acute care and surgical intensivists.

Education in Surgical Palliative Care

Despite the American College of Surgeon's publication of core competencies in palliative care in 2003 [5] few surgeons receive the education and training needed to satisfy these competencies. The lack of formal instruction in palliative care among surgical oncologists was reported by McCahill et al. in 2002 [23]. They queried 419 members of the Society of Surgical Oncology about prior education or training they had received in palliative surgery. They found that the respondents had received a mean of 5 h of palliative care education during medical school and a mean of 9.8 h of education during residency and/or fellowship. One third of respondents had received no training in residency or fellowship. Galante et al. [32] surveyed 70 surgeons from a variety of subspecialties who practiced in both academic and community settings about their palliative care education experience. The median number of hours of palliative care education during residency was zero; approximately 85% of those surveyed received no palliative care education during residency or fellowship. These studies highlight the significant need for palliative care education for surgeons at all levels of training and in all subspecialties. Given the unique perspective surgeons bring to the specialty of palliative medicine (in contrast to our non-procedural colleagues), it is imperative that education about surgical palliative care be provided by surgeons in conjunction with the other interdisciplinary palliative care team members.

Need for Surgical Palliative Care Research

The studies cited above on the morbidity and mortality of palliative-intent procedures and the paucity of research available regarding palliative outcomes following these procedures clearly demonstrates an urgent need for research specifically focused on surgical palliative care. Some of the specific areas of surgical palliative care that warrant further study include the following:

Surgical Decision-Making

Surgeons must learn how to ask "should this operation be performed for this patient at this time?" before "can this operation be done?" Establishing basic guidelines for elements to be considered prior to undertaking a palliative procedure should be a priority. Much like the computer-aided decision support models currently available to address other clinical scenarios like abdominal sepsis [33] decision support based upon evidence (when available) should also be a goal for palliative surgical decision-making. In contrast to decision support in other situations, however, patient (and family) preferences and goals of care must play a central role as defined by the "palliative triangle" [19].

Intimately related to the process of surgical decision-making is the role of prognostication. Prognostication is based upon a surgeon's ability to incorporate his/her knowledge of the natural history of disease with and without treatment and expected outcomes of a procedure to arrive at an overall prognosis. Several clinical prognostic scales and indices exist (e.g., Palliative Prognostic Score [10], Palliative Performance Scale [12], Palliative Prognostic Index [34], and Good/Bad/Uncertain [35]), although, to date, none of these scales have been specifically validated in a surgical population and most have been applied primarily or exclusively to oncology patients.

Patient and Family Decision-Making

Understanding patient and family preferences for treatment, specifically as they relate to accepting or rejecting surgical intervention as a means of palliation, is an essential area in need of research. A recent study by Kwok et al. [36] retrospectively examined inpatient surgical procedures in the year before death for Medicare beneficiaries aged ≥65 years and found that 32% (575,596) underwent a surgical procedure in the last year of their life, 18% had a surgical procedure in the last month of life, and 8% had a surgical procedure in the last week of their life. The high volume of surgical procedures performed in this one cohort raises significant questions about the utility and benefit of these procedures meeting the goals of these patients and their families given their short life expectancy. An important corollary to this study would be an examination of patient and family satisfaction with the decision to proceed with surgical intervention and factors associated with their satisfaction or dissatisfaction.

Symptom Management

On a daily basis, surgeons are faced with determining whether surgical intervention is an appropriate or optimal means of relieving patient symptoms. With rare exception (e.g., malignant gastric outlet obstruction [37]), surgeons have little evidence-based guidelines upon which to make their recommendations. For common clinical scenarios (e.g., malignant bowel obstruction), prospective randomized clinical trials are needed to effectively guide surgical decision-making about the optimal method of palliation. Furthermore, such trials must also include relevant palliation-specific outcomes such as efficacy of symptom relief, duration of symptom relief, and need for re-intervention.

Conclusion

Palliative care provides a multidisciplinary approach to patients and families facing life-threatening illness that seeks to relieve suffering in both physical and nonphysical domains. Importantly, palliative care can be initiated early in the course of disease (e.g., at the time of diagnosis) and may be provided in conjunction with therapies intended to prolong life. Palliative care principles form the basis of good surgical care and surgeons can and should be expected to possess the skills needed to provide palliative care in conjunction with/as part of their routine surgical care. The American College of Surgeons has established core competencies for surgical palliative care. Two basic elements of palliative care—pain management and communication skills—are considered core competencies for all surgeons.

The application of palliative care to the acute care surgical patient reveals a significant need in this vulnerable population. Specific needs in this setting include a prompt recognition of the acute care patient in need of surgical palliation, an accurate assessment of the patient's prognosis, and an honest and accurate discussion of prognosis with patients and their families. Essential components of the communication with the acute care surgical patient in need of palliation include a discussion of the anticipated palliation-specific outcomes following the proposed surgical intervention and a candid discussion of the significant morbidity and mortality associated with palliative procedures.

Although some progress has been made toward integrating palliative care principles into surgical practice, substantial challenges remain. These challenges, in turn, represent important opportunities for research. A few key areas prime for investigation include validation of existing palliative care prognostic scales in surgical populations, examination of patient and family decision-making for or against surgical intervention for palliation and satisfaction with these decisions, and prospective randomized trials designed to determine the optimal method of palliation for common clinical scenarios facing the acute care surgeon (e.g., malignant bowel obstruction).

References

1. World Health Organization. WHO definition of palliative care. 2012 [cited 28 Feb 2012]. Available from http://www.who.int/cancer/palliative/definition/en/
2. Dunn GP, Milch RA. Introduction and historical background of palliative care: where does the surgeon fit in? J Am Coll Surg. 2001;193(3):325–8.
3. von Gunten CF. Secondary and tertiary palliative care in US hospitals. JAMA. 2002;287(7):875–81.
4. Statement on principles guiding care at the end of life. American College of Surgeons' Committee on Ethics. Bull Am Coll Surg. 1998;83(4):46.
5. Surgeons Palliative Care Workgroup. Office of Promoting Excellence in End-of-Life Care: Surgeon's Palliative Care Workgroup report from the field. J Am Coll Surg. 2003;197(4):661–86.
6. Moore LJ, Turner KL, Jones SL, Fahy BN, Moore FA. Availability of acute care surgeons improves outcomes in patients requiring emergent colon surgery. Am J Surg. 2011;202(6):837–42.
7. Ingraham AM, Cohen ME, Bilimoria KY, Raval MV, Ko CY, Nathens AB, et al. Comparison of 30-day outcomes after emergency general surgery procedures: potential for targeted improvement. Surgery. 2011;148(2):217–38.
8. Winchester S. A Man with a knife. New York: GP Putnam's and Sons; 2003.
9. Veatch RM. The basics of bioethics. 2nd ed. Upper Saddle River, NJ: Pearson Education, Inc.; 2003.
10. Maltoni M, Nanni O, Pirovano M, Scarpi E, Indelli M, Martini C, et al. Successful validation of the palliative prognostic score in terminally ill cancer patients. Italian Multicenter Study Group on Palliative Care. J Pain Symptom Manage. 1999;17(4):240–7.
11. Anderson F, Downing GM, Hill J, Casorso L, Lerch N. Palliative performance scale (PPS): a new tool. J Palliat Care. 1996;12(1):5–11.
12. Morita T, Tsunoda J, Inoue S, Chihara S. Validity of the palliative performance scale from a survival perspective. J Pain Symptom Manage. 1999;18(1):2–3.
13. Olajide O, Hanson L, Usher BM, Qaqish BF, Schwartz R, Bernard S. Validation of the palliative performance scale in the acute tertiary care hospital setting. J Palliat Med. 2007;10(1):111–7.
14. Stuart B. The NHO Medical Guidelines for Non-Cancer Disease and local medical review policy: hospice access for patients with diseases other than cancer. Hosp J. 1999;14(3–4):139–54.
15. Lynn J. Perspectives on care at the close of life. Serving patients who may die soon and their families: the role of hospice and other services. JAMA. 2001;285(7):925–32.
16. Simpson M. Therapeutic uses of truth. In: Wilkes E, editor. The dying patient. Lancaster: MYP Press; 1982.
17. Wilkinson C, Khanji M, Cotter PE, Dunne O, O'Keeffe ST. Preferences of acutely ill patients for participation in medical decision-making. Qual Saf Health Care. 2008;17(2):97–100.
18. Mazur DJ, Hickam DH. Patients' preferences for risk disclosure and role in decision making for invasive medical procedures. J Gen Intern Med. 1997;12(2):114–7.
19. Thomay AA, Jaques DP, Miner TJ. Surgical palliation: getting back to our roots. Surg Clin North Am. 2009;89(1):27–41. vii–viii.
20. Miner TJ, Cohen J, Charpentier K, McPhillips J, Marvell L, Cioffi WG. The palliative triangle: improved patient selection and outcomes associated with palliative operations. Arch Surg. 2011;146(5):517–22.
21. Buckman R. Communication skills in palliative care: a practical guide. Neurol Clin. 2001;19(4):989–1004.
22. Cady B, Easson A, Aboulafia AJ, Ferson PF. Part 1: Surgical palliation of advanced illness—what's new, what's helpful. J Am Coll Surg. 2005;200(1):115–27.

23. McCahill LE, Krouse R, Chu D, Juarez G, Uman GC, Ferrell B, et al. Indications and use of palliative surgery-results of Society of Surgical Oncology survey. Ann Surg Oncol. 2002;9(1):104–12.

24. Hofmann B, Haheim LL, Soreide JA. Ethics of palliative surgery in patients with cancer. Br J Surg. 2005;92(7):802–9.

25. Mesa RA, Tefferi A. Palliative splenectomy in myelofibrosis with myeloid metaplasia. Leuk Lymphoma. 2001;42(5):901–11.

26. McCahill LE, Smith DD, Borneman T, Juarez G, Cullinane C, Chu DZ, et al. A prospective evaluation of palliative outcomes for surgery of advanced malignancies. Ann Surg Oncol. 2003;10(6):654–63.

27. Miner TJ, Brennan MF, Jaques DP. A prospective, symptom related, outcomes analysis of 1022 palliative procedures for advanced cancer. Ann Surg. 2004;240(4):719–26. discussion 26–7.

28. Badgwell BD, Smith K, Liu P, Bruera E, Curley SA, Cormier JN. Indicators of surgery and survival in oncology inpatients requiring surgical evaluation for palliation. Support Care Cancer. 2009;17(6):727–34.

29. Miner TJ, Jaques DP, Tavaf-Motamen H, Shriver CD. Decision making on surgical palliation based on patient outcome data. Am J Surg. 1999;177(2):150–4.

30. Smith DD, McCahill LE. Predicting life expectancy and symptom relief following surgery for advanced malignancy. Ann Surg Oncol. 2008;15(12):3335–41.

31. Tseng WH, Yang X, Wang H, Martinez SR, Chen SL, Meyers FJ, et al. Nomogram to predict risk of 30-day morbidity and mortality for patients with disseminated malignancy undergoing surgical intervention. Ann Surg. 2011;254(2):333–8.

32. Galante JM, Bowles TL, Khatri VP, Schneider PD, Goodnight Jr JE, Bold RJ. Experience and attitudes of surgeons toward palliation in cancer. Arch Surg. 2005;140(9):873–8. discussion 8–80.

33. Moore LJ, Turner KL, Todd SR, McKinley B, Moore FA. Computerized clinical decision support improves mortality in intra abdominal surgical sepsis. Am J Surg. 2010;200(6):839–43. discussion 43–4.

34. Morita T, Tsunoda J, Inoue S, Chihara S. The Palliative Prognostic Index: a scoring system for survival prediction of terminally ill cancer patients. Support Care Cancer. 1999;7(3):128–33.

35. Sloan JA, Loprinzi CL, Laurine JA, Novotny PJ, Vargas-Chanes D, Krook JE, et al. A simple stratification factor prognostic for survival in advanced cancer: the good/bad/uncertain index. J Clin Oncol. 2001;19(15):3539–46.

36. Kwok AC, Semel ME, Lipsitz SR, Bader AM, Barnato AE, Gawande AA, et al. The intensity and variation of surgical care at the end of life: a retrospective cohort study. Lancet. 2011;378(9800):1408–13.

37. Jeurnink SM, Steyerberg EW, van Hooft JE, van Eijck CH, Schwartz MP, Vleggaar FP, et al. Surgical gastrojejunostomy or endoscopic stent placement for the palliation of malignant gastric outlet obstruction (SUSTENT study): a multicenter randomized trial. Gastrointest Endosc. 2010;71(3):490–9.

Common Ethical Problems in Acute Care Surgery

Jeffrey P. Spike

Introduction

Ethics is to some degree a human rather than a natural phenomenon (or a blend of the two). So at the very least we need to recognize there will be some variation between countries, and to a lesser degree there will even be some variation between different states in the USA and even between hospitals. Nevertheless, the variation is small enough, at least within the USA that the following can be taken as guidance for ethical deliberation in any acute care surgery department in the USA.

Surgical ethics has become recognized as an important and importantly different field from medical ethics [1, 2]. Any practicing surgeon who last had ethics in medical school most likely would benefit from some continuing medical education (CME) credits specifically concerned with surgical ethics [3].

Similarly, within surgical ethics, some issues stand out as of particular importance to acute surgery. This chapter will first give a brief summary of the received view of bioethics, the standard that is taught in most medical schools in the USA and Canada. Then it will outline some of the core issues in surgical ethics in general, and acute care surgery in particular.

Biomedical Ethics: The Current Paradigm

The model of ethics in healthcare used most often is called the four principles. This was first proposed in 1977 in *The Principles of Biomedical Ethics*, by Tom Beauchamp and James Childress [4]. The four principles are autonomy, beneficence, non-maleficence, and justice.

J.P. Spike, Ph.D. (✉)
McGovern Center for Humanities and Ethics, University of Texas
Health Science Center, 6531 Fannin Street, JJL Suite 410,
Houston, TX 77030, USA
e-mail: jeffrey.p.spike@uth.tmc.edu

The principles have been widely adopted in hundreds of articles and textbooks, not just in medicine, but also in nursing, dentistry, and other fields. They have great utility, especially for the purpose of helping an interprofessional team reach a consensus. Various authors have proposed various additional principles, such as confidentiality. But to start with the four original principles is the single best way to make sure one is starting with a common and widely agreed upon set of grounding assumptions.

Another strength the principles approach offers is it represents the traditional values of medicine, or what some call Hippocratic ethics, in two of the principles (beneficence and non-maleficence), while the other two principles (autonomy and justice) represent more modern ethical values that give us freedom to question certain traditional beliefs.

The principles have also been simplified into a formula known as the four boxes, which does not differ in substance. While the four principles are more of an explanatory model, the four boxes seems closer to a description of how to operationalize the four principles.

Here is a brief summary of the four principles:

Autonomy

The surgeon ought to provide all the information patients with decision-making capacity need in order to make an informed decision. The patient is the ultimate decision-maker because what counts is as much a value judgment as a clinical judgment. (The four boxes uses the term "patient preferences.") Informed consent might be seen as the legal counterpart to the ethical principle of autonomy.

Beneficence

The surgeon ought to do whatever is determined to be in the patient's best interest, balancing benefits and burdens. This is a very high standard. It is also altruistic, as it rules out letting

L.J. Moore et al. (eds.), *Common Problems in Acute Care Surgery*,
DOI 10.1007/978-1-4614-6123-4_40, © Springer Science+Business Media New York 2013

one's own self-interest (e.g., ownership of a lab or imaging equipment) or third-party interests (e.g., an insurance company) interfere with what is best for the patient. It identifies the surgeon as a fiduciary, meaning that the surgeon is exclusively devoted to the patient's interest. (The four boxes simply calls this "best interest.")

Non-maleficence, or "At Least, Do No Harm"

The surgeon must include preventing or relieving pain and other symptoms in the equation. This is a conservative or precautionary principle to avoid heroic interventions that may make things worse; it may counsel that hospice or palliative care is the best of the available choices. (The four boxes calls this "quality of life.") Confidentiality might be seen as a legal consequence of the ethical principle of non-maleficence, though the ethical principle includes much more.

Justice

Justice is the most complex and least intuitive of the four principles. It can be seen as both a positive duty requiring that we give vulnerable people (the uninsured, the homeless, as well as the mentally ill, handicapped, or drug addicted) the same care as powerful people and as a negative duty requiring that we are careful stewards of resources, so there is enough to take care of everyone. (The four boxes calls this "contextual features," a not very descriptive catch-all term for economic factors, religious factors, etc.)

It is interesting that most ethicists would hold that a society owes every member a reasonable standard of care, regardless of income or job status. Thus, of all the fields of medicine, probably emergency medicine has the best claim to the mantle of ethical practice, thanks to EMTALA (Emergency Medicine Treatment and Active Labor Act 1986). Acute care and trauma surgery, because of its close link to the patients who are admitted through the emergency room (ER), thus would have the claim to the mantle of ethical practice within surgical specialties and subspecialties.

For an interdisciplinary team, the members might try to keep the overall balance by each advocating for one of the principles. Perhaps the surgeon would represent beneficence (the best interest of the patient from a surgical point of view), the nurse might see being a patient advocate as requiring more attention to avoiding interventions with high-risk or low-probability of success in the name of 'do no harm' (nursing ethics is often called an ethics of caring), and justice might be the domain of the social worker (who often weigh financial issues as well as family dynamics and cultural context). Decisions should involve the entire team plus the patient (autonomy).

Even with that interdisciplinary team model, it is important that everyone on the team be aware of the importance of all four principles, and that no case is "just" an autonomy case, or "just" a non-maleficence case. The only way to do a good job understanding a case is to carefully consider how each of the four principles applies. Each principle is considered to be relevant to every case *prima facie* (when you begin the analysis). Equally importantly, they are four independent principles, meaning they can conflict with each other. Thus, they are better thought of as helping you understand why a case is complex than as a way to simplify a case.

Lastly: Here is a humorous mnemonic that may help you to remember the names of the four principles: "*A*nywhere *B*ut *N*ew *J*ersey" (*A*utonomy, *B*eneficence, *N*on-maleficence, and *J*ustice).

Surgical Ethics in General and Acute Care Surgery

Following are a sample of the primary issues in general surgery and acute care surgery. Surgical ethics includes (at least) the following 12 unique issues that are rarely covered in medical ethics:

1. When (if ever) should a patient be do not resuscitate (DNR) during surgery? It can be appropriate, especially in cases of palliative surgery.
2. When (if ever) can a surgeon refuse to take a patient who might benefit from a procedure because of the risk? (Who should decide which patient is a "surgical candidate"?) This should be the result of careful weighing of the benefits and risks of surgery to the patient. Sometimes very high risk surgery is still the best option for the patient.
3. What is the ideal relationship of the surgeon to the anesthesiologist?—their relationship—having two attending physicians simultaneously responsible for one patient—has no parallel in medicine. It might often be best for the patient to discuss a planned surgery with both, and have them share responsibility for the case, rather than have one see herself as the "captain of the ship." This might help assure that the best anesthesia method for the patient and his or her recovery from surgery is chosen, rather than what the surgeon prefers.
4. What are the demarcations of role between the anesthesiologist and the surgeon? This is a unique relationship in the medical world, and there is no a priori reason that one should have greater authority than the other. For example, in some countries, it is the anesthesiologist who is most often seen as "the captain of the ship" during a surgery, and the surgeon is more the technician. At the very least, there is a movement towards having both required to see the patient before surgery, and even to have two separate consent processes.

5. Should informed consent include a description of morbidities that are not fully understood but are statistically significant, such as "pumphead" for patients who will require cardiopulmonary bypass? How much can be presumed by a "general surgical consent" and how much should be broken down into details? It is best to err on the side of sharing information, as you can never know in advance just what will be important information to the patient. But you can also try to judge in advance whether the patient is someone who likes as much information as possible, or finds it overwhelming, confusing, or frightening, and would prefer you keep it to a minimum and give them a recommendation.

6. Should informed consent include a description of your connections to companies such as medical instruments, implantable devices, biomaterials, prostheses, or other devices that you use in your surgery—investments, consulting, board membership, stock and futures ownership, paid speaker, bonus for enrolling patients into a study, etc.? There is no doubt that disclosure is the expectation now, and can be conveyed both in person (verbally) and in writing (on consent forms, advertising, brochures, etc.) because they are all potential conflicts of interest that can bias your decisions and recommendations.

7. When (if ever) does the surgeon's responsibility for a patient's best interest end? In contrast to medicine, some surgeons maintain the tradition that when one takes a patient, one has so great a responsibility for their interests that one may have some say in their future medical decisions in order to achieve the best possible outcome, and patients cannot change their mind in midcourse. However, one cannot impose this on patients—better to explain your expectations in advance. And for that to be fair, then the patient should know details such as what outcomes might occur (infections at graft sites, difficulty being weaned, physical therapy) that you consider them to be agreeing to before going into surgery.

8. How to handle errors: Yours, colleagues', and surgeons' you have never met. Here both issues of honesty (truth-telling, veracity) and professionalism come into play, and have to face the powerful forces of denial, defense mechanisms, and fear of legal retribution. If you did it, you can explain it, tell how it was repaired, and apologize. If you know someone else did it, it is better for them to tell the patient. But if the responsible person does not, then you should start a review process so the correct person of authority (rather than you) tells them to talk to the patient. This is part of the quality assurance or improvement at most hospitals now, to prevent recurrences. Studies indicate this is also the best way to prevent lawsuits, while trying to dodge responsibility is the best way to invite them (and increase the size of settlements).

9. What surgery should you do, and what should you refer out? It is always tempting to try to stretch your abilities, take on new challenges. But at the same time, experience always leads to better outcomes. So when you are a novice, you are imposing greater risks on the patient than if you referred them to a more experienced surgeon. Patients have a right to know that. And professionalism means honesty about your skill level, willingness to refer, and encouraging any patient to get a second opinion from an independent surgeon if they would benefit from it or they indicate an interest in it. Similarly, you should be willing to give honest second opinions when requested, and not see loyalty to the other surgeon as a limiting factor on being honest. General surgeons may be the best source of information for patients who want to know whether the benefits of a new, innovative procedure are being exaggerated (and its risks minimized).

While these nine issues are important in all surgical ethics, they are probably more important in elective surgery than acute care surgery. This rest of chapter will focus on three issues that are, in contrast, probably more important to discuss with regard to acute care surgery:

1. What is allowable (and what is not) in the surgical theater to maintain a sense of *esprit* or teamwork—for example, is it ever acceptable to make fun of a patient's *habitus* while they are under anesthesia?

2. What is your relationship to the police, and how does it affect your relationship to your patient?

3. Can one ever have true informed consent in acute care surgery, when most patients understand so little to begin with? In cases where time is limited and decisions are urgent, is any patient really emotionally capable of participating in informed consent? Can we assume all patients want to live, and would accept our recommendations, and spare them the fear that might be caused by informed (or misinformed) consent? How much can be presumed by a "general surgical consent"? Is there such a thing as "implied consent"? Can it ever be true consent?

Esprit, Tradition, or Unprofessional Behavior?

Surgeries are different from most medical encounters in the way there is a team that works in very close quarters, and must be well coordinated. The best teams tend to be ones that work together often, and get to know each well. Such intimacy can bring out the best in people, or the worst. At a psychological level it is, one might surmise, rather like a family gathering.

There are some practices that help surgeons maintain their calm and their focus, such as playing music, which are perfectly acceptable. But there ought to be limits, based on what is acceptable interpersonal and professional behavior.

Thus, for example, some popular songs have such vulgar lyrics that they might offend some members of the team. In that case, the surgeon ought to respect that person's feelings and not play such music.

Respect for the patient is equally important. Another unique aspect of surgery compared to medicine is that the patient is unconscious during much of the time one spends together. However, even if a patient is unconscious, there is no justification for making any sort of insulting comments. Such behavior may have once been more common, but fortunately it has become rare.

Referring to the size or shape of a person's body, or any part of a person's body, are never important to maintain a surgeon's calm or focus. These are nothing more than entertainments, and even to find them entertaining is itself an indication of poor character. An attending surgeon ought to think of being a role model at all times, whether it is to a medical student or resident or fellow, or simply as a role model of the profession to members of other professions represented in the room.

What is more, there are interesting philosophical arguments that one can harm a person without the person even knowing of it—because harms are not limited to physical injuries, but also include libel and harms to the self-esteem or reputation of a person. A person's reputation can even be harmed after they are dead. If a patient heard, from any source, that insulting things were said, they would have reason to complain to a medical board, and it could be categorized as unprofessional conduct. One occurrence might be ignored, but repeated offenses might not.

Although these are becoming rare occurrences, there continue to be reports of such behaviors. So it would be best for all surgeons to address them with the team up front, and also have all members of the department or practice agree to the same standards. One would never want all the staff to be saying, behind one's back, that they hate to work with you and would rather be on any other service.

At its extreme, this becomes the question of the disruptive physician [5–8]. It will still happen in some places that a surgeon is overheard to swear at unconscious patients, or worse—swear at nurses during a surgery. That is never acceptable. And there should be immediate reporting and sanctions against any surgeon who throws any object in the surgical theater. This behavior poses an immediate danger.

If these issues occur more in acute care surgery, it might be because of the lack of a prior relationship to the patient; empathy may benefit from a degree of familiarity to better understand another person, and a sense of mutual respect may also be nurtured in the process.

If the question is not "what must I do?" but rather "what is best?" the answer becomes clear. Act such that it would not matter if the patient was aware of everything being said. That would be the highest possible standard of behavior.

And, in the long run, it would also lead to the best *esprit de corps*, or teamwork, and hence to the best outcomes as well.

This advice can be supported by all four principles. Autonomy, sometimes called respect for persons, can be taken to require that we treat all persons with dignity and respect. Beneficence would support the practices that lead to the best overall outcomes. Non-maleficence could argue that a patient might be harmed by libelous comments, either by the rare event of unexpected levels of consciousness and memories of surgery, or by somehow hearing about what was said. And justice could hold that we ought to treat poor people as well as we treat rich people, uninsured as well as the insured, the homely as well as the beautiful, the infamous as well as the famous, and the overweight as well as the well-built.

Police and Criminal Investigations

Much of acute care surgery starts with an admission from the ER. Emergency room physicians are accustomed to the presence of police. But that does not mean they should see themselves as an arm of the law. In fact, anything that appears to be a friendly overture from the police must be taken with a grain of salt. They could be "grooming" the physician, hoping to ride the rush of excitement in an "adrenaline junkie" to get them to do things that are, in fact, professional boundary violations.

Surgeons, like physicians, are there to help patients. It is the job of the law to make their case, and decide issues of guilt and punishment. But for surgeons to get involved in judging guilt and innocence risks losing the trust patients have in doctors. It could lead to people delaying going to the hospital, a potentially lethal mistake for many situations where there is a "golden hour" for successful intervention. The best reminder for surgeons would be that a primary professional value (or virtue) in surgical providers is to be non-judgmental—quite the opposite of the police. (Remember too that the legal system rests its claim to fairness on an adversarial system in which the accused has his own lawyer and a right to a trial of his peers). A good example of maintaining a nonjudgmental attitude in the most intense situations is the obligation for military doctors to take care of enemy combatants without bias (something they do with pride).

In general, no test should be done without the consent of the patient. If the police want something done, it should only be done with a search warrant or a court authorization. Your discussions with the patient should focus on the medical situation, not what led up to it. (This is analogous to the Miranda warning: they have the right to an attorney, and to refuse to talk until they have legal representation.) If they do tell you something material to an investigation, it should still be protected by patient confidentiality and the Health Insurance Portability and Accountability Act (HIPAA) privacy rule. And unless it is clinically relevant, there would be no reason to put it in the chart.

For surgeons this should come up less often than with ER physicians. Objects removed from bodies that might be used as evidence should be properly saved; however, notes pertaining to them should be carefully worded so as not to presume any knowledge of their provenance (e.g., speculating on whether the patient was the perpetrator or the victim).

It is also important to always be up to date with state laws requiring reporting of certain things. Physical abuse of children is required in every state, usually to Child Protective Services. Gunshot wounds and knife wounds are usually reportable to the police, as is spousal abuse (but there is variation, in some states it is not required but left to the discretion of the physician). The same with clear threats of violence to an identifiable person; it is always allowed to be reported to the police (so confidentiality can be violated without consequences to you), but in some states it is required and in others it is permissible.

In each of these rules one can see how the principles apply: autonomy would suggest doing what the patient with capacity wishes, beneficence would support helping the patient even if you find some of his or her actions reprehensible, non-maleficence would support not making his or her situation worse merely because they came to a hospital for help, and justice would suggest remaining free of bias, especially against people who may have been born with every conceivable disadvantage in life.

What is Informed Consent?

While there were important precedents that led up to it, the term "informed consent" was first used in a court case in 1957 called *Salgo v. Stanford* (a case involving a cardiovascular surgeon), which asserted that this is a necessary part of medical practice, and one cannot do any procedure without first getting the approval of the patient.

The concept really originated in a 1914 court case called *Schloendorff v. New York Hospital* (also a case involving a surgeon), which stated that "Every human being of adult years and sound mind has a right to determine what shall be done with his own body; and a surgeon who performs an operation without his patient's consent commits an assault for which he is liable in damages. This is true except in cases of emergency where the patient is unconscious and where it is necessary to operate before consent can be obtained" [9]. The latter sentence is particularly helpful for those who work in acute care settings. Over 90% of patients in acute care are not unconscious or otherwise incapacitated. Thus, the mere fact of being in an acute setting like an emergency department

(ED) does not rule out the possibility of consent. The setting does not matter; informed consent is necessary in any setting unless there is imminent risk to the patient of death or serious injury and the patient is incapacitated. (Imminent is usually defined as meaning within minutes or hours, not days.)

After Nazi doctors were found guilty of crimes against humanity, the Nuremberg court wrote up guidelines for human subject research that began "the voluntary consent of the subject is absolutely essential," which solidified international recognition of consent, even though it already had clear legal roots in the USA for 30 years. Thus, the 1957 *Salgo* decision [10] can be seen as an assertion that the same rules apply to the doctor–patient relationship as to the research subject–doctor relationship, and to US doctors as well as to German doctors.

A pair of other decisions in 1960 made clear (in case there was any doubt) that a surgeon is liable for failing to properly get the consent of the patient, even if one does the medically indicated procedure, and has a good outcome. Part of the surgeon's job, one can conclude, is to talk to the patient, explain your recommendations, answer questions, and get their understanding and agreement to your plan.

And even that is too one-sided, for one does not always fail in the job if one does not get consent. It might be that the patient refuses your recommendation. As long as it is the result of the educational process, that too can be considered a successful consent process. It may be that a patient does not want to take the same risks that other patients would accept. A good consent process accepts such variation as a normal result of different people having different goals of treatment, and different goals in life. There is no reason to expect extremely religious people to always agree with totally secular people about anything else, so why should they agree about medical treatments, for example? And certainly it must be rational for 45-year-olds to have different goals in life than 80-year-olds.

Is Informed Consent Possible in Acute Care?

Some surgeons have expressed skepticism that informed consent is really possible. The reasoning is that patients are not well enough informed to understand the medical information, and cannot be adequately educated in the brief time allowed. (Perhaps it is added it would take a patient 4 years of medical school to do it.) Other surgeons put a similar skeptical view in slightly kinder terms, saying that patients are often too frightened to make a good decision. In the latter version it is also said that modern medical ethics has made autonomy into the dominant principle, and encourages surgeons to just drop decisions into patients' laps with a nonchalant attitude, as if any decision is equally acceptable.

These are important concerns. Patients certainly do understand less than their surgeons, and one of the toughest skills for many surgeons is how to communicate clearly without bias to patients of very different educational levels. But surgeons have learned many other difficult skills, and if this is posed as another competency they must master, all surgeons would. So it is important for department and hospital policies to be clear about the importance of communication to achieve required ethical and legal responsibilities.

As to autonomy, the original theory does not place any one principle above the others. It is totally acceptable to say that beneficence means one must make recommendations, and not just lay out all of the options, especially for patients who are having difficulty making a choice for any reason. And non-maleficence could be taken to imply that one should not easily let a patient refuse an intervention with great likelihood of benefit. Nonchalance is an inappropriate attitude in such circumstances. If there is time, perhaps calling an ethics consultation could help in these cases. But an angry response, "washing your hands of it," would not be appropriate.

(This reminds me of one of my favorite anecdotes. I was once in the room with a pre-op patient who was about to back out of a hernia repair. He had done the same thing once before. The surgeon came in the room, but stood by the door impatiently, very unhappy about the whole situation. He did ask the patient if he had any questions, from the doorway, and the patient asked "What will happen if I don't get the surgery?" The surgeon looked annoyed, and said in an aggrieved tone of voice "Strangulation!" Then he opened the door and left the room. As I looked at the patient's face, he looked startled. I am convinced he thought the surgeon was suggesting he just might come back and strangle him if he did not have the surgery!)

Who Can Give Informed Consent?

Informed consent should always be given by the patient if at all possible. To have such "decision-making capacity" requires they be able to understand information about what is wrong, what options are available to correct it, the likelihood of a desired outcome, and the side-effects they are likely to experience, that they are free from coercion (from both family members and aggressive or paternalistic surgeons), and possess sufficient clarity of mind to make a decision based on their own values. If you are uncertain, the best test of the last of those requirements is to ask if this decision is consistent with past decisions of the patient.

If the patient is incapable of consent (incapacitated), then one must find a surrogate. State laws vary in small degrees, but generally share a similar order of people who can serve as surrogate if the patient lacks capacity. First is not any "next of kin" but a person who was named by the patient. This is in many states called the "health care proxy," but the legal term for it is "durable power of attorney for health care." This person can make the same decisions the patient could make if the patient had capacity, but only for as long as the patient lacks capacity.

The next person on the list is the spouse, if there is one. Next is usually an adult child, or all of the adult children, or a majority of the adult children. There is considerable variation in state law on this point, but in practice one usually tries to talk to all of the adult children who are available and get a consensus.

Ethically, the most important thing to remember is that you are asking each person to decide according to what the patient would most likely want in these circumstances, not what the surrogate wants, and their authority is based on the assumption that they know the patient well enough to represent the patient. In all states, a surrogate on the list can defer to someone else on the list if they are not comfortable in the role of surrogate (for example, a spouse who is separated but not divorced).

In the acute care setting though, an important ethical issue is not which surrogate should make the decision, but why one has turned to surrogates when the patient is available. It seems that talking to patients can be uncomfortable to some surgeons, and it can be very tempting to ask the family for consent even when the patient is capable of being involved in the consent process. This is not ethically justified and can lead to ethical and legal dilemmas down the road (first, as a violation of confidentiality, as well as if the family consents to something the patient did not want).

Elements of Informed Consent

If time is limited, but the patient is awake and aware, at least tell him what is wrong, what you recommend, give an explanation of what to expect, get their agreement to the procedure, and document the discussion afterwards. These are the most basic elements of informed consent.

The purpose of informed consent is to help the patient make a decision that will be best for him, not just medically, but for his life overall. Hence, full and fair disclosure is best. The question then is how much information must be included to be full and fair?

First and foremost, in an ideal setting (for example, with all elective surgery) one must tell the patient about all of the reasonable options. Thus, for example, if there are radiological or pharmacological alternatives to surgery, those should be presented. One should also include the option of choosing not to treat the condition at all (which sometimes is a good choice, justified by "at least, do no harm"). Refusing treatment is always one of the options for patients with capacity, as the side-effects of surgery may not be worth it.

With each of the reasonable options you should give patients your best estimate of the likely risks and benefits. This should include not just during the intraoperative period, but also post-op; e.g., normal expected rehabilitation time and site. Even if telling more will not change the decision, the information could still be helpful to the patient to plan their life better (e.g., to visit a loved one before having surgery or starting chemo).

There are also some religious beliefs such as Jehovah's Witnesses and Christian Science that influence medical decisions. If an adult patient refuses transfusions, you should not deceive them. You can tell them the chance they will die as a result, you can be careful to discuss this alone with them so they do not feel pressured by a spouse or other member of the church, or you can recommend a "bloodless surgery" center.

There is then, a curious, subtle, and important asymmetry at work in this entire section: patients cannot make you do something that is not indicated, but they can stop you from doing something that is. That is referred to as the right to refuse treatment, something well supported in legal opinions.

Six Pearls About Informed Consent

1. Consent that is not fully informed is not informed consent.
2. Consent is a process, not a piece of paper.
3. "Consenting a patient" is impossible, a contradiction in terms—it is the patient that does the consenting, not the surgeon.
4. The purpose of informed consent is to protect the patient, not the surgeon.
5. If 100% of your patients agree with you, you may be giving biased information; in other words, sometimes a refusal can be a sign of success.
6. If you let others get your consents, they may not be as thorough as they should be. Delegation is dangerous, unless you are certain they can do it as well or better than you can. To do it well requires both knowledge and skill, which in turn require training.

Final Observations: Culture and Consent

The USA is one of the most diverse countries in the world. In general, this is a wonderful fact. But it can lead to some difficulties with informed consent. Here, then, are four further pearls:

7. If a patient does not speak English, communication can be more time consuming. But ethically the same requirements hold. One should use trained interpreters whenever possible, and phone translators and/or TTY as a fallback option. Family members are not a good option unless there is no other choice (e.g., a very rare language) because of the violation of confidentiality that will inevitably result, as well as the lack of sophisticated understanding that is likely.

8. Each patient comes from a different culture, and one must be sensitive to the variations in assumptions. It is up to the patient to decide which cultural norms to live by. The only way to discover this is by talking to the patient, not the patient's parents or the patient's adult children. There can be very large differences in cultural norms between first- and second-generation Americans.

9. All doctors come from a culture too. So every doctor–patient interaction can be thought of as trans-cultural. You might be from another country than the USA, so American patients might be a little foreign to you. But even if you are from the USA, your 10 years or so of training (including some premed years, med school, residency, and fellowships) can be thought of as entering "the culture of surgery," something you must be able to translate or interpret every time you talk to a patient.

10. Patients who do not want to know anything about their own treatment are rare. But they do exist, and have the right to defer all the information and decision-making to someone else. It is then incumbent on them to identify a person, using the same criteria as any patient choosing a proxy or durable power of attorney for health care. In those cases, you may help the patient by reminding them they do not need to choose their spouse if this would be a difficult responsibility for them; they can choose whomever they think is best suited to know their wishes and best able to carry them out.

References

1. Laurence C McCullough, James W Jones, Baruch A Brody, ed., Surgical ethics. Oxford, 1998: Oxford University Press; Chapters 5–7 are concerned with acute care surgical patients.
2. Jones JW, McCullough LB, Richman BW. The ethics of surgical practice: cases, dilemmas, and resolutions. New York: Oxford University Press; 2008.
3. The American College of Surgeons makes one available to members. "Ethical issues in clinical surgery," Mary H McGrath, Donald A Risucci, and Abraham Schwab. ACS, 2007. CME credit offered with their DVD "Professionalism in Surgery," 2008 available from their website.
4. Beauchamp T, Childress J. Principles of biomedical ethics. 6th ed. Oxford: Oxford University Press; 2008.
5. Spike JP. Anesthesiological ethics: commentary on an ethical case involving the interaction of surgery and anesthesia. J Clin Ethics. 2012;23(1):68–70.
6. Jones JW, McCullough LB, Richman BW. Case 56. Ethics of unprofessional behavior that disrupts. (Reprinted from J Vasc Surg. 2007;45:433–435).
7. Rosenstein AH, O'Daniel M. Disruptive behavior and clinical outcomes: perceptions of nurses and physicians. Am J Nurs. 2005;105:54–64. quiz 64–65.
8. Rosenstein AH, O'Daniel M. Impact and implications of disruptive behavior in the perioperative arena. J Am Coll Surg. 2006;203:96–105.
9. Schloendorff v. Society of New York Hospital. 211: New York Court of Appeals; 1914.
10. Salgo v. Leland Stanford, 154 Cal.App.2d 560 [Civ. No. 17045. First Dist., Div. One. Oct. 22, 1957].

Advanced Directives

Gary T. Marshall

Introduction

Acute care surgeons are working with patients at the end of their lives with increasing frequency. The elderly have been the most rapidly enlarging segment of the population over the last century due to the combined effects of the "baby boom" (the population growth during the two decades after World War II) and the increase in average life expectancy. This trend shows no signs of abating, and with the blessing of increased life span has come the burden of chronic disease and disability [1]. According to Medicare data, nearly one-third of Americans underwent surgery during the last year of their life. Further, 18% underwent procedures in the last month of life, and 8% during the last week of life [2]. Clearly it is important for the acute care surgeon to understand the issues surrounding end-of-life care. These include advanced directives and "Do-Not Resuscitate" (DNR) orders, especially in the operating room. In addition, we must have the skills needed to discuss end of life care with patients and their families with honesty and compassion, including withdrawal of non-beneficial therapies and transition to comfort measures.

This chapter reviews the history of advance directives, the DNR order, and the current form these now take. Application of these orders in the operating room and the intensive care unit setting is discussed. Attention is then directed to working with surrogate decision makers, as the naming of a surrogate decision maker for health care is common in advance directives.

G.T. Marshall, M.D. (✉)
Department of Surgery, University of Pittsburgh
Medical Center, Presbyterian University Hospital,
200 Lothrop Street, F1266.2, Pittsburgh, PA 15213, USA
e-mail: marshallgt@upmc.edu

History

In 1976 the first hospital policies on DNR orders were developed and published in the literature [3–5]. Initially these measures evoked strong controversy and emotion, and through time evolved and became accepted by both the medical and lay community. The introduction of the DNR order marked the first time orders directed that a treatment not be given. Cardiopulmonary resuscitation (CPR) is the only treatment administered in a hospital without an order, and that requires a special order not to be administered. The presence or absence of the DNR order now determines how death will ensue in the hospital setting.

Examination of the history of CPR and the DNR order is necessary to understand how medicine has arrived at this point. CPR by closed chest massage was developed in the early 1960s for patients experiencing arrest secondary to anesthesia. For this use it proved to be a simple and highly successful procedure, resulting in hospital discharge rates of 70% [6]. Following publication of initial experiences, resuscitation by closed chest massage was expanded to include nearly all hospitalized patients. With this broader application new problems developed. CPR was capable of initially returning circulation, but the process of dying was merely being prolonged. Within a decade, reports were published citing the suffering many terminally ill patients were subjected to by multiple rounds of resuscitation [7].

Studies of medical patients, in contrast with surgical patients, showed stark contrast to the initial experience. In these patients receiving CPR following cardiac arrest, successful return of circulation occurred in 41% of patients, and only 18% were discharged from the hospital [8]. Further retrospective studies in the elderly reported even more dismal outcomes. In a group of older patients only 6.5% of survived to discharge after in-hospital arrest and CPR. Further, less than half of these patients were discharged to home. For out of hospital arrest, CPR proved even less effective, resulting

L.J. Moore et al. (eds.), *Common Problems in Acute Care Surgery*,
DOI 10.1007/978-1-4614-6123-4_41, © Springer Science+Business Media New York 2013

in a survival of only 0.8% of patients [9]. These data suggested that survival ranged from 1 to 70% after CPR, and that quality of life varied significantly amongst the survivors. Carefully chosen patients in select environments fared the best, with out of hospital arrests in the elderly showing minimal benefit [10].

The growing body of evidence showing poor response to resuscitative efforts led to the next trend in hospitals: the "slow code." Also dubbed the "chemical code" and "show code" among other euphemisms, this involved the delivery of less than full attempts at resuscitation. At other times staff members would simply refuse to call a "code blue" in those situations for which they believed CPR would have no benefit. Inconsistent and institution-specific methods became common, including verbal orders passed from provider to provider, and initials or markers on charts indicating that resuscitation should not be undertaken. As a result, growing controversy over the practice developed. This centered on issues of inadequate advanced decision making, lack of informed consent, poor documentation of procedures, and lack of accountability for the events as they transpired [11].

It was out of this confusion and inconsistency that medical societies began to develop guidelines. In an effort to standardize care the American Medical Association recommended that any decision to forego resuscitation attempts should be clearly documented and communicated. The statement went on to make clear that CPR was meant for the treatment and prevention of sudden, unanticipated deaths, not for those patients expiring due to terminal and irreversible illness [12]. It was following this that explicit DNR policies developed with the goal of promoting patient autonomy by allowing self-determination. Open discussion of the options for resuscitation could now occur with patients and their families prior to the event, and the results of these discussions communicated directly and openly between the staff [11].

During this same time period the medical ethics community took interest. At the heart of the matter has always been the principle of autonomy, and assuring that the patient's wishes are placed ahead of the physician's wishes. In 1983 the President's Commission for the Study of Ethical Problems in Medicine published an influential report challenging many of the predominant beliefs of the time. This report concluded that CPR and resuscitation would be the appropriate and desired response for all arrests. This was in contrast to the multiple prior publications stating that CPR should have limited application due to poor success in terminal and irreversible conditions. With this CPR became the default standard of care, and all patients were presumed to have consented implicitly [13]. Several conclusions reached in this report deserve discussion, as they have shaped the current practice surrounding DNR orders. First, they concluded that life-sustaining therapy could be foregone by competent patients. In addition, the patient could make this decision in advance, and specify by means of an advance directive to be applied should he or she lose the capacity to make decisions. A substituted judgment standard was also proposed, allowing the patient's family to forego resuscitation for incompetent individuals when no advance directive was in place, provided they deemed the patient would choose against resuscitation for themselves. Again, these recommendations were based on the assumption that CPR is the favored option in all cases, and in order to override this implied consent there must be explicit documentation and direction that the decision is in accord with the patient's wishes. Notably omitted from the consensus statement were guidelines regarding futility of resuscitation, where the physician unilaterally determines that CPR is not indicated. This was out of concern that specific standards could not be developed due to the uncertainty of outcome for any specific patient and clinical circumstance [14].

State statutes regarding DNR orders were first enacted in New York in 1988. Under these laws, every patient was presumed to have given informed consent for CPR. For competent patients, a physician could enter a DNR order only after obtaining the patient's express consent to do so. Surrogates could consent to the DNR order on behalf of patients who had become incapacitated provided that the patient was terminally ill, in an irreversible coma, or if CPR was deemed medically futile. Providers were legally protected for following these orders to withhold care, and also for providing CPR in good faith when the provider was unaware of the DNR order. Since the New York action, nearly all states have followed in the development of statutes allowing for living wills, and most have enacted laws regarding the use of proxy or surrogate judgment [11].

In 1991, the Patient Self-Determination Act (PSDA) was passed. This came about for numerous reasons, most notably the perception that ethical standards in end-of life care were needed. This was based on evidence that age, sex, diagnosis, physician specialty, medical institution, and even hospital unit were all associated with variability in patterns of prescribing DNR [15]. The PSDA required that any health care institution receiving federal funding of any type must inform their patients about their rights in medical decision making, including the right to refuse CPR and other life sustaining care [16].

Current Advanced Directives

Current advanced directives serve to direct care in the event that the patient is incapable of making his or her own decisions. The documentation and communication of these wishes has evolved over time. Initially, the three letters "DNR" were simply entered in the chart. This lacked the ability to communicate exactly which procedures were to be withheld. In addition, many times the care team confused DNR to signify that other procedures and treatments be withheld [17]. In response, procedure-specific forms were developed in hospitals. These went on to specify exactly what interventions should or should not be performed. These lists have served to increase clarity by giving very specific direction to caregivers. This type of order is best suited for the patient on the hospital ward, where a large number of caregivers may be involved and communication may be difficult due to interruptions in the continuity of care [18]. These lists have grown to include chest compression, cardioversion, vasopressor medications, dialysis, blood and blood products, intubation, enteral nutrition, antibiotics, and others. These changes within the hospital have led to changes in the advanced directives patients develop on their own and present as they seek care. Advance directives documents usually specify which treatments the patient desires and consents to and name a surrogate decision maker. As mentioned, the directive documents take on numerous forms, and may range from very broad to highly specific, and may even dictate that all measures be taken in the event of cardiac arrest.

When overly broad in nature, definitive guidance is rarely provided, and when too specific, the actual clinical circumstances may not be addressed [19]. Adding to the confusion in many directives, patient preferences are stated with regard to a particular outcome when it is certain to occur, but fail to address situations in which the functional outcome is uncertain. Despite these drawbacks, advance directives provide benefits. They can alleviate the burden of decision making for the family, and they can lay the groundwork for end-of-life discussions between the physician and family [20].

DNR Orders in the Operating Room

There are numerous barriers to the implementation and honoring of DNR orders in the operating room (OR). These include anesthesia, the OR environment and culture, physician attitudes, and legal concerns. The first area in which conflicts arise lies in the very nature of anesthesia and surgery. Endotracheal intubation is required in nearly all major cases, yet this may be excluded in some highly specific advance directives. Outside of the OR, vasopressor administration may be considered a heroic measure; however, it is commonplace in the operative environment. It may seem logical to draw the line at CPR or electrical countershock when limiting care, but in the OR all events are witnessed, and may carry a better prognosis than events occurring outside the OR [13]. It is easy to see how the line might be blurred in determining where routine anesthesia care ends and resuscitation begins, especially for a readily reversible condition.

Another barrier arises from the physician's own interest in providing resuscitation. Any death in the OR is generally viewed as a bad outcome, and the culture tends to assume human error to be at play. In addition, physicians and anesthesiologist bear a strong and dedicated sense of responsibility for their patients and what transpires in the operating room. When iatrogenic complications arise due to anesthesia and surgery the physicians feel the natural response is to take all measures necessary to reverse the situation [21]. Another physician factor contributing to the problem may be the physician's lack of understanding of the patients desire to forego life sustaining therapies in the OR and perioperative period [22]. The lack of understanding arises due the differing values upon which the patient and physician base their decision. The physician gives priority to the imminent death, while on the other hand, the patient is basing decisions on their functional status and longer range outcomes [23].

Finally, legal considerations may impede a physician from honoring a patient's advanced directives to withhold resuscitation [24]. Physicians are frequently concerned with potential liability, especially when death is iatrogenic or in the operative setting. Concerns may arise over whether the family shares the patient's wishes to withhold treatment, or if they have changed their minds. These fears persist despite the fact that few cases have arisen or been successful as a result of a physician honoring an advanced directive. Conversely, there have been successful legal cases in which hospitals and physicians were deemed liable for damages resulting from resuscitation against the wishes of the patient and family [25]. Case law is difficult to interpret. Cases are frequently highly specific, making generalization to broader practice difficult. In addition, case law is applicable only in the jurisdiction in which the case was decided. The best recommendations for minimizing legal issues are development of an institutional policy taking local precedent and culture into consideration, and of course careful and thorough documentation of the patient's condition, prognosis, wishes, and all conversations that occur between physicians and patients or their surrogate decision makers.

The application of DNR orders and advanced directives in the operating room was initially met with significant resistance, the causes of which have been previously discussed [26]. Prior to the 1990s, policies to work with these patients were rare, and the usual practice was to suspend the DNR order in the OR and the immediate postoperative period. These policies drew criticism for forcing patients to give up their autonomy in order to qualify for surgery [27, 28]. This led to the policy of "required reconsideration," meaning that the patient or surrogate, surgeon and anesthesiologist must discuss and review the advanced directive together. This was formalized by the American Society of Anesthesiologists (ASA) in 1993. Following this discussion, the DNR order could be formally rescinded with the patient's informed consent; it could be left in place, specifying the patient's goals of care; or it could be left in place with a detailed list of exactly what procedures the patient would allow [13]. The American

College of Surgeons (ACS) echoed the views of the ASA. In their statement, they also stated that the automatic reversal of DNR status in the OR removed the patient from appropriate participation in the decision process, and that inappropriate management in the perioperative setting might result [18]. The criticism and the resulting publication of societal guidelines and hospital policies did have an effect on OR practice. A 1991 study found that 50% of hospitals had a policy regarding DNR orders in the OR, and 81% of these policies required suspension of the DNR order in the OR. A follow-up study revealed that 71% of institutions had implemented policy, and that only 26% required suspension of the DNR order in the OR. Although improvement in compliance with standard guidelines for the American Society of Anesthesiologists (ASA) was noted, several of the programs questioned had developed guidelines mandating revocation of the DNR order after adoption of the ASA guidelines [18].

As many as 15% of patients with DNR orders will undergo surgery, either related to their preexisting illness or for treatment of unrelated conditions [29]. The procedures offered may prolong life, ease suffering, or improve quality of life. Many of these procedures fall within the scope of acute care surgery, and examples may include the repair of pathologic fractures, tracheostomy and feeding tube placement, treatment of bowel obstruction, vascular access, and a wide variety of others [13, 30]. A study of patients with DNR orders in place showed that the presence of the order did not affect the likelihood that patients being considered for surgery would undergo the procedure considered. In only 18% of the patients was the DNR order reversed. Half of the patients undergoing surgery with a DNR order in place were discharged from the hospital, and 44% were alive two months following hospital discharge [30].

It is clear that institutions, anesthesiologist and surgeons will encounter patients with advance directives, and be called upon to deliver appropriate care to palliate patient suffering and facilitate end-of-life care. In order to deliver this care and respect both the patient's autonomy and the providers themselves, institutions must develop clear guidelines for patients with advanced directives. Several guidelines and recommendations have been suggested for the development of policy regarding DNR orders in the OR. These policies should address the barriers encountered in providing adequate end-of-life care, and should adopt an institutional policy establishing the patient's right to forego treatment according to their own health care wishes. Recommended standards for hospital policy are as follows:

1. The policy should be written. This will add legitimacy to the policy, and facility uniformity of application.
2. Policies should be developed at the institution level, not the level of individual departments. All groups within the hospital should be involved in the design and implementation of the policy.
3. The policy should have flexibility to allow the tailoring of DNR orders to fit each patient individual. The patient should be able to revoke DNR orders if they wish, or provide procedure specific advance directives based on their own health care values.
4. Policies should be very clear. Providers should be made aware of the available options for limiting care and a detailed description of the mechanism to carry these options out should be included. At a minimum, the policy of reevaluation of the DNR order in the perioperative period should be mandated.

In the implementation of these policies, other areas for possible inclusion are the response to iatrogenic arrest in the operative and perioperative period and the role of the OR personnel in caring for these patients should arrest occur. The role of surrogate decision makers in the process may also be delineated [25, 31].

A Practical Approach to Working with Patients

When a patient presents for surgery with a DNR order in place, the physician must not only consider the risks and benefits of the specific procedure, but also must take the time to learn the values and goals of treatment for the patient. The key to resolving the complexities surrounding perioperative resuscitation is communication. When discussions occur, the provider may learn the patient's rationale for the DNR order. Frequently the patient is far more concerned with the quality of life after CPR, not before. When the surgeon understands the goals and fears of the patient a contingency plan can be developed and implemented. Looking into these concerns may show that the patient is afraid of a long stay in the intensive care unit (ICU), or in losing independence and not wanting to spend the remainder of their life in a nursing home. By learning these fears, the surgeon and care team may adjust therapy to address these concerns. Surrogate decision makers and the anesthesiologist should be included in these discussions [10]. The addition of the surrogate will assist in ensuring that patient's wishes are respected, as it is not infrequent that the surrogate and the patient may not share the same decision making [32]. During these discussions three options are available: rescinding the DNR order, providing limited resuscitation with a procedure-directed DNR order, and providing resuscitation with a goal-directed order.

The first option is to rescind the DNR order and provide full resuscitation regardless of clinical circumstances. This avoids the question of determining what exactly constitutes resuscitation, which may prove difficult during anesthesia. In addition, it frees the treating team to act in the event of an easily reversible or iatrogenic arrest, such as an arrhythmia on induction of anesthesia. Chances for an acceptable quality of life are better during these witnessed arrests [33], and care may be withdrawn later if the outcome is unfavorable. Despite all of the concern for ethics, this is a viable and appropriate course of action so long as the patient is involved in the decision.

A procedure-directed DNR order may be developed by the patient and surgeon. In this type of order patients may specify which procedures and interventions they will consent for and those they refuse. This is appealing to some patients, as they prefer the control of being able to dictate exactly what procedures will, and more importantly, will not be performed. This imitates the type of orders most commonly employed on hospital wards. The patient may be presented with a list of possible interventions. Frequently included items are intubation, postoperative ventilation, CPR, defibrillation, vasoactive drugs, and placement of invasive monitoring devices. When adapting these lists and preparing for the OR environment, interventions deemed mandatory for anesthesia are discussed with the patient, as they may not be refused [18]. These procedure-specific orders are clear and easily understood, but they do not allow for the all clinical circumstances that may arise, or those that may be difficult to document and define preoperatively [34].

The final approach to DNR orders in the OR is to take a goal-directed approach. In this approach the physician is left to determine which specific procedures should be performed if cardiac arrest or instability occurs. In order to supplant his own judgment for that of the patient, the surgeon must know the patient's concerns regarding resuscitation and outcome. Are they worried about pain, neurologic damage, loss of independence, or the need for further surgery and procedures? By knowing these values, the physician is able to respond appropriately. For example, if a patient sustains an arrhythmia on induction that requires brief support with CPR, it could be administered, as outcome is likely to conform to the patient's wishes. Conversely, if the patient experiences a massive intraoperative myocardial infarction and arrest, CPR could be withheld, also supporting the patient's values. This approach to DNR is perhaps the most in line with preserving patient autonomy and allowing values held by the patient to be considered. The translation from theory to practice is not quite as easy. First, the surgeon and patient must understand each other, and this requires time that is not always present in emergency situations. In addition, the person responding to the arrest situation should be the same as the person who had the discussion with the patient. Clearly this is not the case for patients on hospital wards, but the OR, better than other places, provides for this continuity in care. When the continuity of care cannot be preserved, or when the trust required between patient and surgeon is not present, it is best to rely on a procedure-directed approach. When the goal-directed approach is taken, documentation in the medical record is essential. This will usually take the form of a descriptive narrative, detailing the conversations that have occurred, and the preferences the patient has expressed for goals of care [18, 34].

Discussing End-of-Life Care with Patients

In preparing for these conversations it is important to understand those factors that are considered inportant by patients, family members, and how these may differ from those of the physician. As patients consider various therapies they typically take three things into consideration: the treatment burden, the treatment outcome, and the likelihood of outcomes. When outcome is likely to be favorable, patients are typically willing to tolerate a greater treatment burden, however, this willingness diminishes as outcomes show only marginal benefit. Patients cite quality-of-life outcomes such as prolongation of inevitable death, dependence on machinery, functional dependence, and excessive fatigue and pain as important factors in their decisions. Other nonmedical concerns, such as becoming a burden on the family or society, influence these decisions as well [35]. Preparation for death, both by the family and the patient, is valued and important to the family and patient, however, physicians tend to place less emphasis on this aspect of end-of-life care. Patients also appreciate being told the expected course of their disease, the symptoms they will experience, the time course, and what can be done for them. Additionally, a sense of life completion is desired by patients, and adequate, timely communication and preparation may allow this to mature [36, 37]. Achieving the last of these goals may be very difficult for the acute care surgeon. Our practice, by its nature, frequently encounters patients in an situation that is a clear departure from their usual state of health. While those patients receiving palliative care are aware that they are terminally ill, the patient suffering an acute catastrophic event has not had the luxury of time for prepartation. Understanding the value of these aspects of the end of life will help to guide conversations and treatment planning. Specific concerns can be determined and addressed. Communication should begin early with patients once the treatment team realizes death is imminent. Despite nearly a majority of physicians realizing that death is imminent in the inpatient setting, only a small percentage will comminicate this with the patient. As the patients approach death their level of consciousness varies, and delay in communication until death is a certainty denies the family and patient adequate time to prepare [38].

During end-of-life discussions the patient or their surrogates may respond by stating that they want the physician to do "everything." This is often difficult for the physician, who frequently takes this request at face value. This may result in launching into a course of action that is burdensome to the patient and family, and unlikely to result in a positive outcome. Rather, the physician should look further into what is motivating the request. First, the clinician must discover exactly what "do everything" means to the patient. Frequently, the patient only wishes to undergo all treatments that offer a reasonable chance of benefit with a tolerable amount of treatment burden. The patient may have unspoken concerns underlying the request. Frequently patients remain fearful and anxious. They may have an incomplete understanding of their condition, or simply desire reassurance that all reasonable options have been pursued. Spiritual and family concerns may also play a role. Taking time to understand the hopes, fears, and goals of the patient will allow the concerns to be addressed and a reasonable treatment plan developed. A general framework for these discussions first involves development of a philosophy of treatment, determining whether the goals are for full and aggressive intervention, or more for treatment likely to provide benefit with tolerable burden, or to limit therapy to comfort measures. The physician should recommend a plan in support of the philosophy developed. At this time recommendations setting limits on CPR can be given. Often, treatments can be continued, but DNR orders placed if the outcome is likely to be unsatisfactory. This is an emotional decision, and physicians must attend to the emotional responses and seek to resolve any disagreements. When accord cannot be reached, and the family or patient insists on full resuscitation, the physician should adopt a harm reduction strategy and coninue to use good clinical judgement. CPR can be initiated, but discontinued after one cycle if it fails. Different than a "show code," this is a full attempt at resuscition, but clinical judgement allows the code to be terminated. The family can be assured that "everything was done," while avoiding the ordeal of a futile code for both the patient and the medical staff [39]. In applying this strategy to the surgical patient, especially when preparing for a high risk emergency operation, the surgeon will often know the patient will likely not survive to hospital discharge. This is an excellent time to discuss with the patient or family exactly what doing everything will involve, and what the outcome is likely to be. If multiple operations, feeding tubes, tracheostomy, and discharge to a nursing facility or long-term care facility are the most likely outcomes this needs to be discussed. Many times, once the family or patient knows surgery will involve a long ICU stay and ventilator dependence is the most likeley outcome, they will choose to forego treatment. This often avoids the difficult and futile operation followed by withdrawal of support in the immediate postoperative period. Foregoing surgery might allow the patient and family time together and avoid suffering. As always, providers must assure all involved that not having surgery does not mean no treatement. Treating pain and anxiety become the focus of care.

Advance Directives in the ICU

Communication

The treatment of many acute surgical patients frequently transitions to the ICU, and it is here that questions and decisions regarding advance directives play an increasing role. Surgical technique has improved to the point where nearly all patients can survive the initial operation. Unfortunately, many remain critically ill or fail to respond to surgery as hoped. In light of this, communication with patients takes on greater value, but also becomes more challenging. Patients and their families often insist on prognostic information, both in terms of lenth of life in terminal illness and in likelihood of death and other possible outcomes. This is a constant challenge to physicians. Multiple studies have demonstrated that physicians across all specialties tend to be overly optimistic. The accuracy does not increase with greater patient contact [40]. It has been found that although they consistently overestimate survival, physician predictions do correlate, showing that physicians are able to discriminate between those closer and further from death. Accurate predictions, both long and short term, are needed to allow patients to achieve a "good death" [41].

Clear communication is difficult to achieve, especially in acute situations. Studies have documented that physicians and patients or their caregivers frequently disagree on whether conversation included discussion of the possibity that the patient may die, or on the anticipated life expectancy. These finding likely result from both physician and patient factors. Physicians tend to be uncomfortable with prognostication, and may withhold information, or avoid the discussion. Patients and their caregivers may be unprepared to discuss issues around death, or may simply not understand the information presented [42]. To avoid misunderstanding physicians must be very clear, avoiding euphamisms and highly technical terms. Do not avoid the words death and dying. The information should be presented during multiple encounters and repeated as needed to assure that message is delivered and received. It has been shown that allowing more time for family conferences, held in a proactive manner, and allowing the family members adequate time to talk may lessen the burden of bereavement [43].

The Family Meeting

As fewer than 5% of ICU patients are lucid enough to take part in treatment planning, clinicians must rely on decisions made by family members and other surrogates. The first step in preparing for family discussion is to identify the surrogate. Most states in the United States have a legal order of priorty.

First, any court-appointed guardian is given priority, followed by any named durable power of attorney for health care, and then to family members. Usually the order is spouse, then parents, adult children, and finally siblings. In practice, the decision is usually made by all of those with close ties to the patient, and develops over several meetings. Clinicians should aim for consensus, as this can usally be reached [44].

The family meeting begins with adequate preparation. First, all data must be reviewed. This should include medical history, treatments, responses, and disease course. When subspecialists are involved, their input should be sought after, and elements of prognosis incorporated into the planning. If any prior discussions regarding end-of-life care have taken place, or if directives were made prior to admission, these should be reviewed. Before beginning any meeting the message should be developed. Once prepared the meeting should be arranged with the family, spiritual leaders if needed, and the medical care team. While it is good to include many voices, care must be taken to not overwhelm the family. Having nurses and social workers present may help, as they are often better known to the family and provide familiar and reassuring faces. The meeting goals and leader should be decided in advance, and possible sources of conflict should be identified and a response developed. Finally, a quiet place should be used, unless the patient is able to participate and the surrogate desires this [45, 46].

Once gathered, the meeting is usually begun with introductions of all involved. Assure the family that these meetings are a routine part of all patient care. Next, an attempt should be made to explore the family's understanding of the patient's illness and prognosis. Following this a clear statement of prognosis should be given. This usually follows a medical review of what has happened and where things stand now. Clinicians must take care not to give too much medical information, and make certain the message is not misleading. If death is imminent this needs to be said, explicitly. Uncertainty should be acknowledged, but the message must not be diluted. Once complete, remain silent. Allow the family to grieve, ask questions, and express themselves [47]. This last component is perhaps the most difficult for physicians. Most discussions with families involve the physician speaking nearly 70% of the time. They frequently miss opportunities to learn about the patient, their values, and concerns. Increasing the amount of time spent listening while the family is given time to speak has been shown to increase family satisfaction [48].

Conflict may arise during family discussions and communication may break down. The leader must recognize when confilict occurs and work to meet the needs of the family. The first source of conflict is usually lack of information. This may be the result of inacurate understanding of prognosis, inconsistent information given by various providers, confusing information, excessive information from outside sources, genuine uncertainty regarding prognosis and outcome, and finally language and cultural barriers. Confusion over the goals of care may manifest in unclear and contradictory orders such as performing CPR, but not intubating a patient. The priorities placed on the treatment of the disease and the treatment of discomfort may differ. Situations in which an acute condition, such as urosepsis, occurs in a terminal cancer patient may also confuse the goals of care. Emotions such as guilt, anger, fear, and grief lead to conflict as well. The dynamics between the team and the family and the dynamics within the family itself may be problematic. The family may have internal conflict of decisions, be dysfunctional, or simply lack the ability to make decisions. The family may also be placed in the center of disagreements between the various consulting teams. Finally, there may be a real diffence in the values held by the clinician and the family. Clearly, conflict may arise anywhere and at any time. It is important to understand these sources of conflict, identify the problem, address the cause, and continue to bring the goals of the clinician and the family into alignment [49]. Developing trust with the patient and family is essential for the delivery of quality end-of-life care. This is challenging in the short amount of time during an acute illness and hospitalization. Suggestions for the development of a trusting rapport with patient and family include encouraging them to talk and allowing them to tell you about themselves, their values, and their understanding of their disease. Take the time to recognize the patient's concerns, while being sure not to insult or contradict other health care providers. All errors that are made should be acknowledged, avoiding excuses. Throughout the discourse it is important to remain humble and demonstrate respect for the patient, the family, and their wishes. Finally, attempts to force a decision are discouraged. If a decision cannot be reached, allow the family to discuss amongst themselves, process what they have heard, and simply plan for the next meeting [50].

During these meetings strong emotions are provoked, and the physician must be prepared to deal with them appropriately. Empathy from physicians helps family members and is found to be strongly supportive and is associated with family satisfaction. When strong emotions are observed, first acknowledge the emotion. Once this is done the emotion should be ligitimized as appropriate and normal given the circumstances. Move on to explore more about the emotion and what specifically is causing it. Expressions of empathy are important, but should only be made if legitimate. Finally the conversation can be turned to exploring particular strengths and possible coping strategies [51].

During the course of meetings and discussions it is important that the clinician make recommendations. There is a tendency for physicians to present a laundry list of options and possible outcomes as if all were equal. Family members want to know what the doctor thinks is best [46]. It is especially important when the decision is to withhold or withdraw life support. The family member should not be left feeling as if they had "pulled the plug," especially when it is unlikely that any further treatment would have been of benefit [44]. As families are asked to make decisions regarding the termination of life support, clinicians may ease this decision. It is important to bring the patient's desires into the discussion, and reinforce that the surrogate is not being asked what he or she wants, but rather what the patient would want if they could speak for themselves. These decisions should not be forced upon a family, especially before they have had time to prepare. This may set up an antagonistic relationship and erode trust. It is important not to argue over facts, repeating them over and over. One of the most common fears held by family members is that withdrawal of support will be withdrawal of care. It cannot be emphasized strongly enough that the patient will continue to receive the full attention of the treatment team. The goals of care will simple be comfort-oriented, and this will be the utmost priority [52]. When discussing advanced cardiac life support (ACLS) it should not be broken down into component parts, but rather treated as a package. This may avoid incongruent orders, such as the "chemical code only." Finally, at the end of any meeting the decisions and agreements reached should be repeated, questions answered, and further meetings planned. If the decision has been made to withdraw support then the family should be educated about the process, allowed to gather all loved ones, and offered additional support if desired [44].

Time-Limited Trials

A time-limited trial of therapy may be appropriate in setting the course of medical treatment to be pursued. Time-limited trials are agreements made between the patient, surrogates, and physician to use treatments for a set amount of time and then to assess the patient's response. This allows the patient to both avoid giving up all treatment options and avoid the burden of ongoing treatment should it prove unsuccessful. If improvement is noted, then disease-directed therapy may be continued. If the course deteriorates, support may be withdrawn and comfort-oriented measures initiated. In considering a time-limited trial, the conversation begins as usual by reviewing the patient's condition and prognosis, and follows with a discussion of treatment goals. A course of care is then determined and objective measures of improvement or deterioration defined as well as the time frame to be considered. Potential actions are then proposed at the end of the trial. These plans are not meant to be binding, but to allow for adaptation as the clinical picture changes. Communication amongst all caregivers is important, and continuity needed to carry these plans out. The time used may allow the family and patient to come to terms with the situation at hand, and to be assured that all reasonable efforts have been made [53].

Emergent and acute surgical procedures fit well into time-limited trials with patients. Decisions may be made to go ahead with high risk procedures, but to agree that should operative findings be so catastophic that an acceptable quality of life not be possible the operative efforts will be terminated. At other times, the patient and family may agree to proceed with surgery, but then withdraw support if the ICU course becomes prolonged, multiple orgen system failure worsens, or ventilator weaning becomes unlikely. Key markers of failure such as unplanned return trips to the OR, need for tracheostomy of feeding tube, or institution of dialyis should be defined. These are concrete events and help to make the situation clear. In addition, many patients will have discussed these specific treatments and expressed their wishes regarding them. These trials allow for the operation to procede when a poor outcome is likely but unclear, with a clear plan to change stararegy if efforts prove unsuccessful.

Futility of Care

Cases will arise in which the physician and the family cannot come to an agreement, and the physician may feel that all further treatment is futile. At the root of this problem may be diffences in core values, and the family may be willing to accept a burdensome treatment that the physician would not want for themselves. The physician should question and determine whether the surrogate is employing substituted judgement, and speaking for the patient's best interest and wishes, or inserting their own wishes and values. In most circumstances agreement can be achieved between the doctor and the surrogate with time [54]. When they cannot resolve the conflict, the physician should avoid acting unilaterally to limit care. There is a risk of legal action, and although rarely successful, lawsuits are expensive [55]. The legal system has failed to provide clear guidelines regarding this issue, but other options are available. Ethics committees provide an outside source of action. Most committees act in an advisory capacity, but may make decisions in some states. Texas allows ethics committees to withdraw treatment deemed futile after 10 days if no other facility or provider will assume care. Experience with this extra-judicial process has proven successful in resolving these conflicts [56]. Most institutions have policies in place in accordance with local legal statutes, and although frustrating, the physician should remember time is an ally in these situations, and outside assistance is available. Until resolution can be achieved, treatment should continue.

Conclusion

Results of Advance Directives

The results of advanced directives have been debated, and at times some have declared them to have been a failure [57]. This is not the universal belief, and they have had an impact. One recent review suggested that nearly two-thirds of patients that required decision making at the end of life had living wills in place. All but a small percentage of these expressed wishes for limited or comfort care, and in the vast majority of these cases these wishes were honored. When a surrogate was named the patients were less likely to die in a hospital and to receive all care possible [58]. The quality of end-of-life medical care has been improved with advance directives. Patients with advance directives are less likely to die in the hospital. They have less frequent feeding tube placement, and avoid mechanical ventilation. Despite this, patients still have concerns for unmet pain needs and emotional support for both the patient and family. Room for improvement still exists [59].

End-of-life converstions can benefit both the patient and their caregivers. When these conversations take place there has been no observed increase in depression or worry. Similar to the results of advanced dirctives, less use of aggressive care follows, with reduced ICU admission, and reduced use of mechanical ventialtion and resuscitation. When these aggessive measures are used the quality of death is perceived as worse overall. In addition, the family members of those involved with aggressive treatments have a significantly higher risk for major depressive disorder. Hospice referral, especially when early, results in better quality of death for the patient and better caregiver quality of life in follow-up after the loss of a loved one [60].

Overall medical expenses in the last year of life continue to remain high nationally, and this trend has been consistent over the last decade despite changes in the delivery of medical care [61]. There has been some improvement when end-of-life conversations occur. Having these conversations has been associated both with significantly lower health care costs at the end of life, and a higher quality of death [62]. In the intensive care unit setting the incorporation of a communication team to work with families of patients with imminent death has been shown to significantly reduce the length of stay in the ICU and the hospital, and to significantly reduce the costs of treatment [63].

References

1. Trends in aging—United States and worldwide. MMWR Morb Mortal Wkly Rep. 2003;52(6):101–4, 6.
2. Kwok AC, Semel ME, Lipsitz SR, Bader AM, Barnato AE, Gawande AA, et al. The intensity and variation of surgical care at the end of life: a retrospective cohort study. Lancet. 2011; 378(9800):1408–13.
3. Optimum care for hopelessly ill patients. A report of the Clinical Care Committee of the Massachusetts General Hospital. N Engl J Med. 1976;295(7):362–4.
4. Fried C. Editorial: terminating life support: out of the closet. N Engl J Med. 1976;295(7):390–1.
5. Rabkin MT, Gillerman G, Rice NR. Orders not to resuscitate. N Engl J Med. 1976;295(7):364–6.
6. Kouwenhoven WB, Jude JR, Knickerbocker GG. Closed-chest cardiac massage. JAMA. 1960;173:1064–7.
7. Symmers Sr WS. Not allowed to die. Br Med J. 1968;1(5589):442.
8. Rozenbaum EA, Shenkman L. Predicting outcome of inhospital cardiopulmonary resuscitation. Crit Care Med. 1988;16(6):583–6.
9. Murphy DJ, Murray AM, Robinson BE, Campion EW. Outcomes of cardiopulmonary resuscitation in the elderly. Ann Intern Med. 1989;111(3):199–205.
10. Caruso LJ, Gabrielli A, Layon AJ. Perioperative do not resuscitate orders: caring for the dying in the operating room and intensive care unit. J Clin Anesth. 2002;14(6):401–4.
11. Burns JP, Edwards J, Johnson J, Cassem NH, Truog RD. Do-not-resuscitate order after 25 years. Crit Care Med. 2003;31(5):1543–50.
12. Standards for cardiopulmonary resuscitation (CPR) and emergency cardiac care (ECC). V. Medicolegal considerations and recommendations. JAMA. 1974;227(7):Suppl:864–8.
13. Ewanchuk M, Brindley PG. Perioperative do-not-resuscitate orders–doing "nothing" when "something" can be done. Crit Care. 2006;10(4):219.
14. President's Commission for the Study of Ethical Problems in M, Biomedical R. Deciding to forego life-sustaining treatment. Report No: Pr408:ET3L/62/2. [Book Chapter].
15. Morrell ED, Brown BP, Qi R, Drabiak K, Helft PR. The do-not-resuscitate order: associations with advance directives, physician specialty and documentation of discussion 15 years after the Patient Self-Determination Act. J Med Ethics. 2008;34(9):642–7.
16. United States. Social Security Administration. Office of Legislation and Congressional Affairs. Omnibus Budget Reconciliation Act of 1990 : H.R. 5835, Public Law 101–508, 101st Congress : reports, bills, debates, and act. Washington, D.C.: Dept. of Health and Human Services, Social Security Administration, Office of the Deputy Commissioner for Policy and External Affairs, Office of Legislation and Congressional Affairs; 1990.
17. La Puma J, Silverstein MD, Stocking CB, Roland D, Siegler M. Life-sustaining treatment. A prospective study of patients with DNR orders in a teaching hospital. Arch Intern Med. 1988;148(10):2193–8.
18. Truog RD, Waisel DB, Burns JP. DNR in the OR: a goal-directed approach. Anesthesiology. 1999;90(1):289–95.
19. Lo B, Steinbrook R. Resuscitating advance directives. Arch Intern Med. 2004;164(14):1501–6.
20. White DB, Curtis JR. Care near the end-of-life in critically ill patients: a North American perspective. Curr Opin Crit Care. 2005;11(6):610–5.
21. Walker RM. DNR in the OR. Resuscitation as an operative risk. JAMA. 1991;266(17):2407–12.
22. Wenger NS, Phillips RS, Teno JM, Oye RK, Dawson NV, Liu H, et al. Physician understanding of patient resuscitation preferences: insights and clinical implications. J Am Geriatr Soc. 2000;48(5 Suppl):S44–51.
23. Eliasson AH, Parker JM, Shorr AF, Babb KA, Harris R, Aaronson BA, et al. Impediments to writing do-not-resuscitate orders. Arch Intern Med. 1999;159(18):2213–8.
24. Meisel A, Snyder L, Quill T. Seven legal barriers to end-of-life care: myths, realities, and grains of truth. JAMA. 2000;284(19):2495–501.
25. Waisel DB, Burns JP, Johnson JA, Hardart GE, Truog RD. Guidelines for perioperative do-not-resuscitate policies. J Clin Anesth. 2002;14(6):467–73.

26. Truog RD, Waisel DB. Do-not-resuscitate orders: from the ward to the operating room; from procedures to goals. Int Anesthesiol Clin. 2001;39(3):53–65.

27. Truog RD. "Do-not-resuscitate" orders during anesthesia and surgery. Anesthesiology. 1991;74(3):606–8.

28. Cohen CB, Cohen PJ. Do-not-resuscitate orders in the operating room. N Engl J Med. 1991;325(26):1879–82.

29. Margolis JO, McGrath BJ, Kussin PS, Schwinn DA. Do not resuscitate (DNR) orders during surgery: ethical foundations for institutional policies in the United States. Anesth Analg. 1995;80(4):806–9.

30. Wenger NS, Greengold NL, Oye RK, Kussin P, Phillips RS, Desbiens NA, et al. Patients with DNR orders in the operating room: surgery, resuscitation, and outcomes. SUPPORT Investigators. Study to Understand Prognoses and Preferences for Outcomes and Risks of Treatments. J Clin Ethics. 1997;8(3):250–7.

31. Waisel D, Jackson S, Fine P. Should do-not-resuscitate orders be suspended for surgical cases? Curr Opin Anaesthesiol. 2003;16(2):209–13.

32. Coppolino M, Ackerson L. Do surrogate decision makers provide accurate consent for intensive care research? Chest. 2001;119(2):603–12.

33. Taffet GE, Teasdale TA, Luchi RJ. In-hospital cardiopulmonary resuscitation. JAMA. 1988;260(14):2069–72.

34. Waisel DB. Perioperative do-not-resuscitate orders. Curr Opin Anaesthesiol. 2000;13(2):191–4.

35. Fried TR, Bradley EH. What matters to seriously ill older persons making end-of-life treatment decisions?: A qualitative study. J Palliat Med. 2003;6(2):237–44.

36. Steinhauser KE, Christakis NA, Clipp EC, McNeilly M, Grambow S, Parker J, et al. Preparing for the end of life: preferences of patients, families, physicians, and other care providers. J Pain Symptom Manage. 2001;22(3):727–37.

37. Steinhauser KE, Christakis NA, Clipp EC, McNeilly M, McIntyre L, Tulsky JA. Factors considered important at the end of life by patients, family, physicians, and other care providers. JAMA. 2000;284(19):2476–82.

38. Sullivan AM, Lakoma MD, Matsuyama RK, Rosenblatt L, Arnold RM, Block SD. Diagnosing and discussing imminent death in the hospital: a secondary analysis of physician interviews. J Palliat Med. 2007;10(4):882–93.

39. Quill TE, Arnold R, Back AL. Discussing treatment preferences with patients who want "everything". Ann Intern Med. 2009;151(5):345–9.

40. Christakis NA, Lamont EB. Extent and determinants of error in doctors' prognoses in terminally ill patients: prospective cohort study. BMJ. 2000;320(7233):469–72.

41. Glare P, Virik K, Jones M, Hudson M, Eychmuller S, Simes J, et al. A systematic review of physicians' survival predictions in terminally ill cancer patients. BMJ. 2003;327(7408):195–8.

42. Fried TR, Bradley EH, O'Leary J. Prognosis communication in serious illness: perceptions of older patients, caregivers, and clinicians. J Am Geriatr Soc. 2003;51(10):1398–403.

43. Lautrette A, Darmon M, Megarbane B, Joly LM, Chevret S, Adrie C, et al. A communication strategy and brochure for relatives of patients dying in the ICU. N Engl J Med. 2007;356(5):469–78.

44. Curtis JR. Communicating about end-of-life care with patients and families in the intensive care unit. Crit Care Clin. 2004;20(3):363–80. viii.

45. Weissman DE, Quill TE, Arnold RM. Preparing for the family meeting #222. J Palliat Med. 2010;13(2):203–4.

46. Curtis JR, Patrick DL, Shannon SE, Treece PD, Engelberg RA, Rubenfeld GD. The family conference as a focus to improve communication about end-of-life care in the intensive care unit: opportunities for improvement. Crit Care Med. 2001;29(2 Suppl):N26–33.

47. Weissman DE, Quill TE, Arnold RM. The family meeting: starting the conversation #223. J Palliat Med. 2010;13(2):204–5.

48. McDonagh JR, Elliott TB, Engelberg RA, Treece PD, Shannon SE, Rubenfeld GD, et al. Family satisfaction with family conferences about end-of-life care in the intensive care unit: increased proportion of family speech is associated with increased satisfaction. Crit Care Med. 2004;32(7):1484–8.

49. Weissman DE, Quill TE, Arnold RM. The family meeting: causes of conflict #225. J Palliat Med. 2010;13(3):328–9.

50. Tulsky JA. Beyond advance directives: importance of communication skills at the end of life. JAMA. 2005;294(3):359–65.

51. Weissman DE, Quill TE, Arnold RM. Responding to emotion in family meetings #224. J Palliat Med. 2010;13(3):327–8.

52. Weissman DE, Quill TE, Arnold RM. Helping surrogates make decisions #226. J Palliat Med. 2010;13(4):461–2.

53. Quill TE, Holloway R. Time-limited trials near the end of life. JAMA. 2011;306(13):1483–4.

54. Smedira NG, Evans BH, Grais LS, Cohen NH, Lo B, Cooke M, et al. Withholding and withdrawal of life support from the critically ill. N Engl J Med. 1990;322(5):309–15.

55. Asch DA, Hansen-Flaschen J, Lanken PN. Decisions to limit or continue life-sustaining treatment by critical care physicians in the United States: conflicts between physicians' practices and patients' wishes. Am J Respir Crit Care Med. 1995;151(2 Pt 1):288–92.

56. Fine RL, Mayo TW. Resolution of futility by due process: early experience with the Texas Advance Directives Act. Ann Intern Med. 2003;138(9):743–6.

57. Fagerlin A, Schneider CE. Enough. The failure of the living will. Hastings Cent Rep. 2004;34(2):30–42.

58. Silveira MJ, Kim SY, Langa KM. Advance directives and outcomes of surrogate decision making before death. N Engl J Med. 2010;362(13):1211–8.

59. Teno JM, Gruneir A, Schwartz Z, Nanda A, Wetle T. Association between advance directives and quality of end-of-life care: a national study. J Am Geriatr Soc. 2007;55(2):189–94.

60. Wright AA, Zhang B, Ray A, Mack JW, Trice E, Balboni T, et al. Associations between end-of-life discussions, patient mental health, medical care near death, and caregiver bereavement adjustment. JAMA. 2008;300(14):1665–73.

61. Riley GF, Lubitz JD. Long-term trends in Medicare payments in the last year of life. Health Serv Res. 2010;45(2):565–76.

62. Zhang B, Wright AA, Huskamp HA, Nilsson ME, Maciejewski ML, Earle CC, et al. Health care costs in the last week of life: associations with end-of-life conversations. Arch Intern Med. 2009;169(5):480–8.

63. Ahrens T, Yancey V, Kollef M. Improving family communications at the end of life: implications for length of stay in the intensive care unit and resource use. Am J Crit Care. 2003;12(4):317–23. discussion 24.

James J. McCarthy

Introduction

The United States Congress passed Emergency Medical Treatment and Active Labor Act (EMTALA) in 1985. By doing so, it defined for the first time a standard of medical care and legislated how hospitals and physicians were required to practice medicine. With the passage of EMTALA, Congress effectively defined hospital emergency departments as a community resource and essentially created a federal right to emergency care [1].

> "People have access to health care in America. They can just go to the emergency room."
>
> President George W. Bush [2]

This chapter briefly describes the history of the EMTALA legislation, its change over time, its current state, and implications to physicians and hospitals providing emergency care. The subject of EMTALA could easily fill an entire book; therefore, this chapter specifically focuses on the responsibilities of the on-call physician and their obligations under EMTALA.

History

Initial Law and Intent

After being stabbed in the head, Eugene Barnes was rushed to Brookside Hospital in San Pablo, California, on January 28, 1985. The emergency physician and staff promptly

attended to him, and, as part of his evaluation, a computed tomography (CT) scan of the brain was performed, which revealed a neurosurgical emergency requiring immediate intervention. The emergency physician caring for Mr. Barnes contacted the on-call neurosurgeon who refused to come in; a second neurosurgeon (also on staff at Brookside Hospital) was contacted. He also refused to come in, as he was not on call. Over the next several hours, attempts were made to transfer the patient to two other facilities, which both refused, until finally San Francisco General Hospital agreed to accept the patient only if the emergency physician accompanied him in transport. Mr. Barnes was taken immediately for emergency surgery but, unfortunately as a result of his injuries, died 3 days later [3]. The details surrounding his death attracted national media attention [4] and, as expected, generated a public outcry. With increased scrutiny over the next several months, public outrage began to grow as multiple other stories with similar themes came to light [5].

The addition of the "active labor" language in the EMTALA statute was largely driven by the case of Sharon Ford in November of 1985. Ms. Ford, in active labor, presented to Brookside's emergency department where, prior to any medical evaluation, it was determined that she was a member of a Medicaid health maintenance organization (HMO). As a result, she was not seen or evaluated but rather referred to Samuel Merritt Hospital in Oakland (the regional HMO contract hospital). Upon her arrival to the labor and delivery suite at Samuel Merrit, her registration information could not be located in the computerized records of those covered by the HMO—this was later determined to be due to a delay in the State of California updating its records. As a result, despite the fact that she was noted to be in "active labor," she was transferred to Highland General Hospital—the local county facility where shortly after her arrival her baby was delivered stillborn [1].

These horrific stories in the lay press coincided with increasing reports of "patient dumping" in the medical literature [6, 7]. With mounting public frustration, a legislative response was perhaps inevitable.

J.J. McCarthy, M.D. (✉)
Medical Director of Emergency Medical Services,
Texas Medical Center, Memorial Herman Hospital,
University of Texas Medical School, 6411 Fannin, Suite H175.1,
Houston, TX 77030, USA
e-mail: james.j.mccarthy@uth.tmc.edu

L.J. Moore et al. (eds.), *Common Problems in Acute Care Surgery*,
DOI 10.1007/978-1-4614-6123-4_42, © Springer Science+Business Media New York 2013

These series of events at Brookside hospital and in Northern California caught the attention of local Congressman Fortney Stark who championed the initial legislative effort behind EMTALA. The initial proposed legislation was focused on "patient dumping" and had extremely harsh proposed penalties, with physicians found to have violated a patient's EMTALA rights being subject to felony charges. The proposed penalties for physician in violation were up to 5 years in jail and up to $250,000 in fines per occurrence. After measured discourse, this language and respective penalties were softened considerably during the legislative process [8].

In response to growing public pressure and media attention, Congress passed the Emergency Medical Treatment and Active Labor Act (EMTALA) as part of the Consolidated Omnibus Budget Reconciliation Act (COBRA). It was signed into law by President Ronald Reagan on April 7, 1986 [9]. Interestingly and perhaps troublingly, EMTALA was passed with very little time for public comment and with no formal hearings in either the US House or the Senate [10]. Regardless of the process, effective August 1, 1986, any person presenting to an emergency room, in a hospital that participated in Medicare, had a right to emergency medical care.

The initial intent of EMTALA was clearly to prevent "patient dumping" by creating antidiscrimination legislation to protect those without insurance who could not afford emergency care services [11]. This new legislation required that all patients be evaluated and that those with an emergency medical condition (EMC) be "stabilized" prior to transfer or discharge. There was no requirement for hospitals to accept transfers. Perhaps in some part due to the very compressed legislative process, there was no consideration in the EMTALA regulations as to hospital capabilities or requirements for on-call coverage. This oversight resulted in continued medical disasters as hospitals could simply not have "call coverage" and tertiary-care hospitals (with on-call physicians) could still refuse to accept patients from hospitals lacking subspecialty coverage.

The US Congress corrected this oversight in 1989 with an amendment to EMTALA, which required hospitals to have physicians on call to stabilize emergency cases and to require "higher-level of care facilities" to accept patients in transfer when they had the ability to care for the patient [12].

The result of the 1989 revision left hospitals and physicians with several clear responsibilities under the law.

Hospitals Obligations

1. Provide an appropriate medical screening exam (MSE) to determine if an EMC exists.
2. If an EMC is determined to exist, hospitals have a duty to either provide stabilizing medical treatment or, if they lack the capability to stabilize, transfer the patient to an appropriate facility.
3. Hospitals with specialized capabilities must accept patients requiring specialized care if they have the capacity to treat them [13].

"On-Call" Physicians Obligations

1. Respond to the emergency department to help stabilize a patient with an identified or suspected EMC.
2. Accept appropriate transfers when transfers are requested by other facilities that are unable to address a patient's EMC.

The initial legislation also defined the penalties for hospitals and physicians. Though toned down significantly from Congressman Starks' initial proposal, the penalties still carried considerable weight.

Hospital Penalties

1. Fines between $25,000 and $50,000 ($25,000 for hospitals with fewer than 100 beds) per violation.
2. Termination of its Medicare provider agreement.

Physician Penalties

1. Fines up to $50,000 per incident.
2. Excluded from Medicare and Medicaid programs.

In addition, patients who suffered personal injury from a violation could sue the hospital and physician in civil court. Receiving facilities that suffered a financial loss as a result of a transferring facility failing its EMTALA obligation could also now pursue damages.

Changes Over Time

As one can imagine, the passage of EMTALA created significant new "stresses" on the medical establishment. Numerous questions regarding the language and the enforcement of the legislation arose from hospital and physician groups. In response to these questions and concerns EMTALA, has grown significantly in scope and enforcement with multiple revisions and "clarifying statements" over the 25 years since its inception. This next section covers the major changes to the statute, the rationales behind them, and their impact to hospitals and physicians.

In response to growing questions regarding enforcement, the HCFA (Health Care Financing Administration), now known and Centers for Medicare & Medicaid Services (CMS), convened an "Anti Dumping Task Force" to review the interpretation and enforcement of EMTALA. This task force had broad representation from physician and hospital groups as well as from the insurance industry and general community. The final recommendations from the task force were presented to HCFA in January of 1997, and HCFA incorporated their recommendations into their "interpretive guidelines," which went into effect on July 14, 1998 [14]. The guidelines resulted in a more consistent enforcement of the regulations allowing hospitals and physicians to better understand their requirements and improve their efforts to comply with the regulations.

Several items of particular note from the 1998 guidelines included:

1. The MSE was clarified to be a process, not an outcome or a correct medical diagnosis. This clarification meant that failing to correctly diagnosis could not be interpreted as failing to perform an appropriate MSE.
2. Distinct responsibilities for on-call physicians were clarified.
3. Stabilization was divided into "stable for discharge" and "stable for transfer" recognizing that "stable for transfer" may not in fact be "stabilized" [15].

In 2003, after multiple updates, clarifications, legal case and "interpretive guidelines," CMS issued "The Final Rule" on September 9, 2003, which became effective on November 10, 2003. The intent of this "Final Rule" was to "clarif(y) policies relating to the responsibilities of Medicare-participating hospitals in treating individuals with emergency medical conditions who present to a hospital under the provisions of the Emergency Medical Treatment and Labor Act (EMTALA)."[16] This update's focus was centered chiefly around: seeking prior authorization from insurers, emergency patients presenting to "off-campus" outpatient clinics that do not routinely provide emergency care, "dedicated emergency departments," allowing exception to EMTALA for nonemergency cases cared for in the emergency department, hospital-owned ambulances, and the applicability of EMTALA to inpatients and physician responsibilities related to being "on call" [17].

The final rule added much needed clarity but was by no means the last adjustment. In 2005, Congress created the EMTALA Technical Advisory Group (TAG). This group's recommendations were incorporated into the CMS State operations Manual on May 29, 2009.

The new revisions address and define the following:

1. Nonphysician providers and their role in "on-call" coverage,
2. Telemedicine,
3. Newborn protection under EMTALA,
4. "Parking" of patients presenting by ambulance,
5. "False labor,"
6. Specialty Hospital Transfers,
7. Community call for on-call specialists,
8. Inpatient transfers of unstable patients, and
9. On-call coverage rules and obligations [18].

Current EMTALA Regulations

The "Final Rule" and the TAG update of 2008 largely define the current state of EMTALA. The following section discusses EMTALA in its current form and the implications to physicians and hospitals. With all of the revisions and updates, fundamental responsibilities for hospitals and physicians under EMTALA can be broken down into 3 distinct groups:

1. Requirement for a medical screening exam.
2. Stabilizations for patients with an EMC.
3. Transfer requirements—for patients with an EMC not able to be stabilized and the treating facility.
4. Requirements for a call schedule and on-call physicians.

For the purposes of simplification, we focus the following discussion around these four categories.

General Principles

EMTALA applies to any individual who presents to a hospital emergency department requesting emergency care. Citizenship or insurance status has no bearing on an individual's rights under EMTALA.

Medical Screening Exam

EMTALA mandates that hospitals provide every patient who presents seeking medical care a "medical screening examination" (MSE) to determine if they have an EMC or are in "active labor." The medical screening exam is a process rather than a discrete event. Importantly, it is not triage and must be clearly separate from the triage process. The MSE is not a discrete event but rather includes available history and physical and any required testing to determine if an EMC is present. Significantly, being incorrect in the determination of whether or not a patient has an EMC is not a violation of EMTALA. The law requires that the process be done consistently but does not cover medical judgment. If a patient presents with chest pain and the physician performing the MSE determines that the pain is not cardiac in nature, and that no EMC exists and discharges the patient who 2 h later dies of an acute myocardial infarction, the physician and facility would have no exposure under EMTALA.

Hospitals must provide an MSE and stabilizing treatment for any EMC regardless of a patient's ability to pay for the services. It is imperative that the MSE or treatment of the

EMC cannot in any way be delayed to obtain financial information.

The "final rule" further defined different scenarios in which a patient may present to a hospital and provided clarifying language as to the different responsibilities of each party.

Dedicated Emergency Departments

This definition applies to all licensed emergency departments or departments that advertise "emergency service" and includes freestanding emergency departments. For specialized facilities that have separate labor and delivery units, emergency psychiatric units, or pediatric emergency departments, this definition also applies to them.

When a patient presents to a "dedicated emergency department" the hospital must: [19]

1. Provide an appropriate medical screening exam to determine if an EMC exists; and
2. If an EMC exists, the hospital must provide stabilizing treatment and/or transfer for stabilizing treatment if the hospital lacks the capacity to treat the condition.
3. Hospitals must not delay the medical screening exam, stabilizing treatment, or transfer to obtain financial information from the patient.

When a Patient Presents to Another Location on a Hospital Property (That Has a Dedicated Emergency Department)

In this instance, the EMTALA obligation as defined previously is invoked. The fact that the patient walked in the wrong door does not relieve the facility of its obligation. Over the last 10 years, there has been significant change in what constitutes hospital property and when the EMTALA obligation starts. The current regulations are as follows: If a patient presents requesting medical attention at a facility that has an emergency department, the facility has an obligation as soon as the patient is on their property. Hospital property is now defined as the entire property including all parking lots, sidewalks, and buildings. It does not apply to nonhospital buildings on the campus like doctor's offices or restaurants [20]. This supersedes the old "250-yard" rule. However, for very large hospital campuses, the 250-yard language still is in place for the range of how far on hospital property the "EMTALA" obligation extends from the main building(s).

Requirements for Call Coverage and On-Call Physicians

The final rule attempts to clarify hospital responsibilities regarding call coverage to allow "local flexibility." Hospitals are now required to maintain an on-call list of physicians to meet the needs of the hospital's patients who present with EMCs. Hospitals are also required to have written policies to handle situations where the on-call physician is unavailable. This requirement also applies to situations when a given specialist may be on call simultaneously at multiple facilities or currently operating on an elective case when an emergency presents and thus be unavailable. Both of these situations are allowable under the current regulations with some restrictions. While these activities are permitted, hospitals must still ensure that services are available to meet the needs of patients with EMCs. Hospitals must have a predefined procedure for dealing with these conflicts [21]. This may include, but is not limited to, a backup call system or transfer in more extreme cases.

In contrast to previous guidance regarding the rule of three, CMS does not specify how often physicians must be on call or have any formal requirements for a facility to provide on-call coverage for services that is performed in an elective manner. This is a clear distinction from the previous guidance that if hospitals provide a service to the public they must provide that service to patients in the emergency department [22]. It is important to note that this is not an open door to eliminate call coverage to emergency department patients. CMS has clearly stated that they will continue to monitor and take appropriate actions if the availability of call coverage, in their interpretation, is inappropriately low after considering all relevant factors including but not limited to the following:

1. The number of physicians on staff.
2. The number of physicians in the particular specialty.
3. The other demands of the physicians.
4. The frequency in which a hospital's patients require the services of on-call physicians.
5. Provisions the hospital has made for when on-call physicians are unavailable [23].

So while there is no formal guidance, CMS, in the case of a complaint/investigation, will determine retrospectively if the hospital's on-call coverage "best meets the hospital's patients" [24].

Responsibilities of the On-Call Physician

The on-call physician must respond to the emergency department when requested by the emergency physician to either: help determine if an emergency condition exists or to help stabilize a patient with an EMC. The determination of whether a physician must respond to the emergency department or if phone consultation is sufficient is solely the discretion of the emergency physician. On-call physicians are not required under EMTALA to respond in situations where patients request a "specialist" when the physician has the ability to perform any required stabilizing treatment and would routinely do so. In cases of disagreement, however, CMS has stated clearly "any disagreement between the two (physicians) regarding the need for an on-call physician to come to the hospital and examine the individual must be resolved by deferring to the medical judgment of the emergency physician who has personally examined the individual" [25].

Physician extenders and mid level providers (MLP) can be utilized to improve access to specialized care, however, the decision on whether an MLP or the physician responds must be made by the on-call physician and not the MLP [26]. Once a patient has had their EMC stabilized and they are suitable for discharge, the on-call physician's obligation under EMTALA ends. Under EMTALA, there is no requirement for the on-call physician to provide follow-up care—though hospital bylaws and state regulations may make this requirement.

Transfer Patients

EMTALA only covers emergent transfers of patients with an EMC. Stable or lateral transfers are not covered by the statute. Hospitals and physicians who have the ability and capacity to treat patients with an EMC must accept appropriate patients in transfer from facilities without the ability to treat the EMC. It is necessary to point out that hospital capacity is not necessarily determined by a specific number of beds or resources. It is determined by behavior and operations. CMS clarified its position in 2001, "whatever a hospital customarily does to accommodate patients in excess of its occupancy limits" [27]. This is an important relaxation for the previous standard of "if they've ever done it before." One important example would be the case of a critically ill patient with a surgical emergency in the emergency department requiring an operative procedure and then admission to a surgical intensive care unit (ICU). In the case where ICU beds are frequently not available and these patients are routinely taken from the emergency department to the operating room and then held for extended lengths of time (hours to days) in the recovery room waiting for ICU opening or overflowed to a nonsurgical ICU, the same standard must be applied to transfer patients.

The question of who determines if an EMC exists and if the facility requesting the transfer can "handle" the EMC is again deferred to the treating physician who is "face-to-face" with the patient. This can be extremely frustrating to on-call physicians at referral facilities, but the language is quite clear. The physician taking care of the patient makes the call.

For the purposes of accepting transfers, there is no EMTALA requirement that the on-call specialist physician personally accepts the patient—this can be delegated. It is required that a physician sign off on all transfers if a nonphysician accepts them. This process must, however, be clearly outlined in hospital bylaws.

Importantly, in the situation where a physician refuses to accept an appropriate transfer the hospital is responsible for the physician's decision to "deny" a transfer if CMS should find the denial inappropriate, because for the purposes of transfers they are in this case acting as the hospital's agent.

The only acceptable reason to refuse to accept a patient in transfer is because the requested receiving facility lacks the capability or capacity to treat the patient. Reasons of insurance status, medical instability, and hospital affiliation are all unacceptable reasons for declining to accept a transfer. The transferring facility can choose to contact any facility they wish to request a transfer. They are not obligated to honor referral patterns, hospital affiliations, or transfer agreements. One exception would be in the case where a long distance transfer has been requested—if there are closer facilities that are available to accept the patient and the extended transport time would clearly lead to deterioration in condition, the facility could refuse as inappropriate. However, if the closer facilities are not available, then the transport distance alone cannot be used as a reason to decline transport.

The transferred patient remains the responsibility of the transferring facility until they are physically present at the accepting facility [28]. As such, the sending facility is responsible for determining the method of transportation and which service will provide the transportation. Receiving facilities cannot use mode of transportation or transportation service as a criteria for accepting or refusing the transfer.

When does EMTALA end? EMTALA obligation ends when a "qualified medical person" has made the determination that:
1. There is no EMC, or
2. An EMC exists and requires transfer to an appropriate facility, or
3. An EMC exists and the patient is admitted for further treatment and stabilization.

EMTALA does not, in its current form, apply to hospital inpatients.

EMTALA Violations

EMTALA has several "teeth" in its provision. The largest and biggest stick is clearly the ability to exclude hospitals and physicians from participation in Medicare. Individual fines of up to $50,000 per violation can be assessed to facilities and physicians. Importantly, these are administrative penalties and typically not covered by malpractice premiums. In addition, the law allows those who have been harmed, as a result of a physician or facility failing to meet their EMTALA obligation, to seek damages in civil court. These courts have ruled that only hospitals and not physicians are subject to these damages—however, a hospital that is sued as a result of a physician's behavior can seek damage from the physician [29].

Common Questions/Case Scenarios

Can patients be transferred if they have not been medically stabilized?

Yes. The inability to stabilize a patient may be the reason the patient required transfer in the first place. Unstable patients can be transferred in two instances: (1) when the treating facility lacks the ability/capacity to stabilize the patient and the benefits of transfer outweigh the risks of transfer, or (2) if the patient or their representative insists on transfer to another facility after being informed of the risks of transfer and the hospital's obligation under EMTALA.

If a patient in an emergency department with an abscess requests that a surgeon be called instead of the emergency physician performing the procedure, does the on-call surgeon have an EMTALA obligation to respond?

If the abscess is such that the emergency physician would routinely manage it without requiring consultation with a surgeon then there is no EMTALA obligation for the on-call physician. However, recognizing that physician experience, training, and ability varies, there is no "community standard" for what a given provider should be able to perform. So if the emergency physician requests consultation because they "lack the expertise" to handle the EMC, then an EMTALA obligation does exist even if 9 out of 10 emergency physicians would have performed the procedure without consultation.

If a request to transfer a patient with an surgical abdominal emergency comes at 6 p.m. on Friday evening from a Hospital that reports they have no surgeon on call, even though abdominal surgical procedures are routinely performed at the Hospital, does the receiving facility have an EMTALA obligation to accept the patient?

Yes. The requesting facility may, in fact, have a very legitimate reason for not having coverage at that time. However, even if they do not, and while it is possible that the sending facility may in fact be violating its EMTALA obligation, this does not excuse the receiving facility from theirs.

If a patient is seen in the emergency department and diagnosed with diverticulitis, and after telephone consultation the emergency physician and on-call surgeon agree that the patient is stable and decide on a treatment course of oral antibiotics with outpatient follow-up, does the surgeon have an EMTALA obligation to see the patient in follow-up at his/her office?

No. The EMTALA obligation ended when it was determined that the patient was stable for discharge and physician's offices are not covered under EMTALA.

What if the patient's condition deteriorates and they re-present 20 h later septic with an acute abdomen? Would the physicians and hospital be subject to an EMTALA violation for failing to provide stabilizing medical treatment during the first visit?

No. The fact that after an MSE the physicians determined that the patient was safe/stable for discharge ended their EMTALA obligation. Being incorrect in their assessment does not in and of itself imply an EMTALA obligation. One important cautionary point is that there must not be anything in the treatment plan that implies that the care was in some way determined by the patient's financial status or ability to pay for services.

If an emergency physician requests an on-call physician to evaluate a patient in the emergency department, when does the physician need to see the patient?

The on-call physician must respond in a "reasonable" amount of time. The guidelines state that the expected response time in minutes should be stated in the hospital policies [30]. Additionally, if the on-call physician fails to respond in a reasonable amount of time, the emergency physician is obligated to transfer the patient and must write on the transfer form the names and addresses of any on-call physician who failed to provide stabilizing services.

If a patient with EMC is admitted to hospital and the hospital later determines that it lacks the capacity to treat the patient and requests transfer for a "higher level of care," does the receiving facility has an EMTALA obligation to accept the patient?

This is a very delicate area with court decisions favoring both sides. Most currently consider that the EMTALA obligation for an individual patient ends with admission to a hospital. Previous interpretations have suggested that while the initial hospital may no longer have an obligation, the "higher level of care" facility *does* have an obligation. In 2008, CMS proposed [31] that even though EMTALA obligations cease upon admission for the first hospital, EMTALA obligations would nevertheless continue for a receiving hospital with specialized capabilities. After the public comment period, they retreated from this stance stating that a hospital with specialized capabilities is not required under EMTALA to accept the transfer of a hospital inpatient [32].

Do state laws regarding tort reform affect EMTALA penalties or obligations?

No. EMTALA preempts any state law that directly conflicts with its requirements. State laws could affect civil penalties as a result of CMS actions related to EMTALA violations.

Legal Examples

Inspector General v. St. Anthony Hospital

A 65-year-old male was critically injured in a motor vehicle collision and taken to a small rural hospital. The emergency physician on duty, Dr. Spengler recognized the critical nature of the patient's injuries and initiated a ground transfer to University Hospital. Prior to the transfer, Dr. Spengler noted significant deterioration and believed that the patient had an aortic injury. He arranged for aeromedical transport and recontacted University Hospital which informed him that all ORs were busy and they lacked the capacity to handle this case. Dr. Spengler then contacted Dr. Lucas (a vascular surgeon) at St. Anthony Hospital. Dr. Lucas refused to accept the patient who was ultimately transferred to Presbyterian Hospital where an angiogram revealed an aortic injury. The patient expired 3 days later. The Office of Inspector General (OIG), noting that St. Anthony Hospital, even though not a trauma center, had specialized surgical capabilities and had the capability and capacity to treat the injuries, imposed a $50,000 fine [33]. Notable in this case was the affirmation that higher level of care does not require the receiving facility to be a teaching or research facility but simply to have the capacity to treat the patient. Dr. Lucas was not fined because there is no obligation to the on-call physician to accept the patient; the risk is born completely by the hospital.

Millard v. Corrado

Dr. Corrado was providing call coverage at Audrain Medical Center. Dr. Corrado decided to attend a conference 30 miles away without notifying the hospital. During his period of unavailability, a trauma patient presented with an EMC and, because of Dr. Corrado's unavailability, required transfer to another facility. The Missouri Court of Appeals determined that the physician on call had the obligation to respond in a reasonable amount of time or to notify the hospital in light of the anticipated unavailability [34].

Conclusion

The EMTALA requirements have evolved significantly since its creation in 1985. It is critical that all providers participating in the care of emergency patients understand the current updates and their obligations when providing call coverage. The final rule, while providing significant clarification to many issues, has opened the door to allowing "gaps" in call coverage at many facilities. This change has resulted in significant increased pressure in referral centers as smaller community facilities "opt out" of providing subspecialty emergency coverage. Further updates are of course likely. In 2011 and again in 2012, CMS sought public comments on whether it should reexamine the provision that states that EMTALA obligation does not apply to hospital inpatients. Relaxation of this rule might at first seem intuitive, but from a patient-centric point of view it could easily result in massive patient "dumping" from community facilities to tertiary care facilities for every complication. We do not yet have the results of this comment period—regardless of the results we can expect further revisions and those participating in emergency care will need to keep abreast of these changes.

References

1. Bitterman RA. Providing Emergency Care under Federal Law: EMTALA, AM. College of Emergence Physicians (2000), p. xiii
2. President George W. Bush, July 10, 2007, Cleveland, OH
3. Equal Access to Health Care: Patient Dumping: Subcommittee on Homan Resources and Intergovernmental Relations to the House Comm. On Governmental Operations, H.R. REP. No. 531, 100th Cong., 2d Sess., at 6–7 (1988)
4. Dan Rather, *CBS Evening News*, Tuesday, 2/5/1985
5. Private Hospitals' Dumping of Patients, NY Times Oct 28, 1985 at A19.
6. Schiff RL, Ansell DA, Schlosser JE, et al. Transfers to a public hospital, a prospective study of 467 patients. NEJM. 1986;314:552–7.
7. McCormick B. CO public hospital dumps patients. Hospitals 1986;60(23):76
8. US House of Representatives. H.R. Rep No 241, 99th Cong, 1st Sess 5 (1985)
9. The Consolidated Omnibus Budget Reconciliation Act of 1985, Pub. L. No. 99-272 9121, 100 Stat. 82 (1986).
10. US House of Representatives. H.R. Rep No. 241, 99th Cong., 2d Sess., pt. 3, at 6,7 (1986) U.S.C.C.A.N. 726, 728.
11. Moy MM. The EMTALA Answer Book 2012 addition Wolters Kluwer Law and Business (2012).
12. US Congress. 42 USC 1395dd(g). Congressional amendments in 1989. Pub L No 101–239, Title VI, Sections 6003(g)(3)(D)(XIV), 6211(a)-(h), 103 Stat 2154, 2245 (enacted December 19,1989, effective on July 1, 1990) (codified in 42 USCA Section 1395dd (West Supp 1991).
13. US Congress. 42 USC 1395dd(a), 42 USC 1395dd(b), 42 USC 1395dd(g) Congressional amendments in 1989. Pub L No 101–239, Title VI, Sections 6003(g)(3)(D)(XIV), 6211(a)–(h), 103 Stat 2154, 2245 (enacted December 19,1989, effective on July 1, 1990) (codified in 42 USCA Section 1395dd (West Supp 1991).
14. Baker CH, Goldsmith TM. From triage to transfer: HCFA's update on EMTALA. Health Law Digest. 1998;26:3–14.
15. Health Care Financing Administration, State Operating Manual, App. V (Rev. 2, May 1998).
16. Department of Health and Human Services Centers for Medicare & Medicaid Services 42 CFR Parts 413, 482, and 489
17. Federal Register, Vol. 68, No. 174, Tuesday, September 9, 2003, p. 53250
18. Department of Health and Human Services Centers for Medicare and Medicaid Services 42 CFR Part 489.24
19. Department of Health and Human Services Centers for Medicare and Medicaid Services 42 CFR Part 489.24(d)(3)

20. Department of Health and Human Services Centers for Medicare and Medicaid Services 42 CFR Part 489.24(b)

21. HHS/CMS Program Memorandum S&C-02-35, Simultaneously On-Call (June 13, 2002). Letter from Steven A. Pelovitz, Director, CMS Survey and Certification Group

22. Bitterman RA. HCFA's New Guidelines for Enforcement of EMTALA. Emerg Department Legal Lett. 1998;9(12):113–20.

23. Interpretive Guidelines, Department of Health and Human Services Centers for Medicare and Medicaid Services 42 CFR Parts 489.24(j) (1), at 21

24. Bitterman RA. Supplement to Providing Emergency Care under Federal Law: EMTALA (April 2004)

25. Federal Register. Vol. 68, No. 174, Tuesday, September 9, 2003, p. 53255

26. HCFA Interpretive Guidelines, 42 USC 1395dd(h)

27. Federal Register. Vol. 68, No. 174, Tuesday, September 9, 2003, p. 53,244

28. HCFA Interpretive Guidelines § V-32, 42 USC 1395dd(b)(2)(D);

29. Bitterman RA. Providing Emergency Care Under Federal Law: EMTALA, AM. College of Emergence Physicians (2000), p. 184

30. U.S. Department HHS, CMS, State Operations Manual, App. V, Emergency Medical Treatment and Labor Act (EMTALA) Interpretive Guidelines, Part II, Tag A-2404/C-2404 (revised 5/29/2009)

31. CMS 2008 IPPS Proposed Rule (73 Federal Register 23669–23671)

32. 73 Federal Register 48661, Vol. 61, No. 180/Monday, 16 Sept 1996

33. St. Anthony Hospital v. U.S. Department HHS, 309 F.3d 680, 713 (10th Cir. 2002)

34. Millard v. Corrado, 14 S.W.3d 42 (Mo. App. Ct. 1999)

Index

Printed by Publishers' Graphics LLC
JCIMO130819.15.13.16